Improve International

SURGICAL NURSING

Improve
Veterinary Education

First published 2023

Published by
Improve International Ltd.
Alexandra House, Whittingham Drive
Wroughton, Swindon,
Wiltshire SN4 0QJ
United Kingdom

Tel: +44 (0) 1 793 759 159
https://improveinternational.com/uk/

Important note
Medicine is an ever-changing science, so the contents of this publication, especially recommendations concerning diagnostic and therapeutic procedures, can only give an account of the knowledge at the time of publication. While utmost care has been taken to ensure that all specifications regarding drug selection and dosage and treatment options are accurate, readers are urged to review the product information sheet and any relevant material supplied by the manufacturer, and, in case of doubt, to consult a specialist. From both an editorial and public interest perspective, the publisher welcomes notification of possible inconsistencies. The ultimate responsibility for any diagnostic or therapeutic application lies with the reader.

A Catalogue record for this book is available from the British Library

ISBN: 978-1-913352-18-9

Copywriter: Dr. Pippa Elliott
Illustrator: Elaine Leggett
Photos by the authors unless otherwise indicated.
AdobeStock pictures: Chapter 2, Figure 7; Chapter 5, Figure 103 B; Chapter 7, Figures 39, 42 and 55.

Authors

Darren Barnes

MA VetMB CertSAS DipECVS MRCVS
Darren graduated from Cambridge University in 2006, spending a one-year rotating small animal internship at the Animal Health Trust, Newmarket thereafter. He then spent five years in general practice in Bishops Stortford whilst studying for the RCVS Certificate in Small Animal Surgery under the supervision and guidance of Dick White. He returned to Cambridge University as a Staff Surgeon for one year before completing a three-year Surgery Residency training at Dick White referrals. He was awarded the Diploma in Small Animal Surgery by the European College of Veterinary Surgeons in February 2017 and continues to work as a Specialist in Small Animal Surgery at Dick White Referrals.

Claire L. Dorey-Phillips

BSc (Hons) ISFM DipFN RVN
Claire graduated from the University of Bristol in 2005 with a BSc (Hons) in Veterinary Nursing and Practice Administration. Following graduation, Claire joined a multidisciplinary referral hospital where she went onto lead various departments including surgery and medicine before becoming a head nurse and, finally, clinical nursing training manager. During this time Claire's passion for feline medicine and surgery grew and in 2015 Claire left to take up the role of a Lead Nurse primarily in Feline Medicine and to help set up another multidisciplinary hospital in Hampshire, where she was instrumental in obtaining gold Cat-Friendly Clinic status as well as obtaining her diploma in feline nursing. Claire's main interests are feline medicine/ surgery, and emergency and critical care.

Barbara Gomes

IMVM MVMV CertAVP(DI) DipECVDI MRCVS
Barbara graduated with an integrated Master's in Veterinary Medicine from the Technical University of Lisbon, Portugal in 2009. After graduation, she worked for a year in a small animal practice in Portugal. In 2011 Barbara moved to the United Kingdom to undertake a one-year rotating internship at a referral practice in Swindon followed by three years working in general practice. In 2015, she began a four-year senior clinical training scholarship in Diagnostic Imaging at the University of Glasgow's Small Animal Hospital. During her residency, Barbara obtained the RCVS Certificate in Advanced Veterinary Practice in Diagnostic Imaging in 2017 and a Master's degree investigating canine oesophageal disease in 2019. After completing the residency Barbara moved to the northeast of England to work in a multidisciplinary small animal referral practice and gained a Diploma in Small Animal Diagnostic Imaging in February 2020. In June 2020, Barbara decided to moved back to Scotland to work for a small animal multidisciplinary referral hospital in Livingston.

Nicola Grint

BVSc PhD CertVA DVA DiplECVAA MRCVS
Nicki graduated from Bristol Vet School in 2000, and stayed on to undertake an internship and then residency in veterinary anaesthesia. In 2005, she moved to Liverpool Vet School to undertake a three-year lectureship post, becoming head of division in 2007. After leaving Liverpool, Nicki locumed at the Animal Health Trust, the Royal Veterinary College, and Ross University School of Veterinary Medicine. She completed her PhD in analgesia at Bristol University and holds the RCVS Certificate and Diploma in Veterinary Anaesthesia, and is also a European Diplomate in Veterinary Anaesthesia and Analgesia. She ran the anaesthesia service at Cave Veterinary Specialists for eight years and is now an independent anaesthesia consultant.

Alison Mann

BSc (hons) Dip HE CVN Dip AVN (small animal) RVN
Alison graduated from Writtle College in 2005 with a BSc (hons) in Equine Science and qualified as a small animal VN in 2009 whilst working in mixed practice in Bristol. In 2010 she moved to Langford Vets to work as a surgical nurse. During this time she has achieved the Dip AVN (small animal). For a few years she worked as a clinical teaching nurse for the University of Bristol, teaching practicals and lectures to undergraduate VNs in the Veterinary Nursing and Bioveterinary degree course. She moved back into clinical nursing in 2018, returning to the theatre team, becoming Head Theatre Nurse in 2019. In 2021 Alison started working for Linnaeus group as a Professional Development Manager which is part of the groups central Veterinary Nursing support.

Contents

Preparation for Surgery

Darren Barnes

Orthopaedic Procedures

Alison Mann

Surgical Sampling, Surgical Complications, and Wound Management

Darren Barnes

Principles: the Clinic

Claire L. Dorey-Phillips

Chapter Summary:

- **The role of the surgical veterinary nurse/technician in practice.**
- **Types of hospital acquired infections and how they are acquired.**
- **Control and prevention of hospital acquired infections.**
- **Infection surveillance.**
- **Barrier nursing.**
- **Antibiotics and resistance.**
- **Cleaning and disinfection of the clinic, surgical equipment, and surgical personnel.**
- **Good surgical practice.**
- **Health and safety at work and in the operating theatre.**

Introduction to the Role of the Surgical Nurse/Technician

Surgery nurses and technicians play an essential part in patient care, both directly and indirectly, and are **integral to the success of the surgical team.** Expert patient care is required throughout the perioperative period, with patient outcome influenced by the nurse's knowledge, skills, and experience.

The **perioperative period** is divided into the following:
- **preoperative:** patient preparation;
- **operative:** assistance in theatre and with anaesthesia monitoring and maintenance; and
- **postoperative:** patient recovery and discharge.

Hospital Acquired Infections (HAI)

What is a Hospital Acquired Infection?

Hospital acquired infections (HAI), or nosocomial infections, are newly acquired infections contracted within the hospital environment. These infections were not present or incubating in the patient prior to hospital admission.

Hospital adquired infections **usually develop symptoms two days or more after admission,** within three days following discharge, or one month after a surgical procedure. Clinical staff can also acquire a HAI from work-related pathogens within the clinical environment. Nosocomial infections are significant because they:
- increase morbidity
- increase mortality
- increase hospitalisation time
- increase costs to the client
- are a risk to staff
- are a risk to other patients
- are difficult to treat.

Complications arising from hospital acquired infections are particularly **significant in critically ill, immunocompromised patients** (e.g. those receiving high-dose steroids, immunosuppressive agents, or chemotherapy) or other at-risk patients such as extremely young/old patients, or unvaccinated patients.

These infections are challenging to treat, particularly in the face of multi-drug resistance; and increase the duration of the hospital stay and in turn the cost of treatment. **Typical multi resistant infections seen in practice are MRSA** (methicillin-resistant *Staphylococcus aureus*) and **MRSP** (methicillin-resistant *Staphylococcus pseudintermedius*).

Types of Infectious Agents

Infection is colonisation of an individual (host) **by a foreign organism** (infectious agent). When an infectious agent is harmful to the host it is termed a pathogen.

Infections can be caused by a variety of pathogenic microorganisms:
- viruses
- prions
- fungi
- protozoa
- parasites
    - endoparasites
    - ectoparasites
- bacteria.

Transmission can take place between animals, humans, humans and animals and via fomites (inanimate objects) or vectors (e.g. flies, fleas).

Viruses

A virus is an extremely small and simple structure which is incapable of replicating outside a cell. Viruses vary in stability with a minority not able to survive within the environment. Once infection is established the virus is protected within the host's cells from the host's immune system.

Parvovirus

Canine parvovirus initially attacks the lymph nodes of the throat, before invading lymphocytes for 1–2 days and replicating. Within the lymphocytes, the virus is able to travel through the bloodstream to target the bone marrow and small intestine (and in very young dogs, the heart). The affected lymphocytes ultimately die, causing neutropoenia, in turn increasing the host's susceptibility to infection.

In the bone marrow, **the virus causes leukopenia,** weakening the host's immune system, and facilitates viral invasion of the GI tract. In the GI tract, the virus destroys the intestinal epithelium and **compromises the intestine's barrier abilities.** This causes severe diarrhoea, nausea, vomiting, hypovolaemic shock secondary to severe fluid loss, and sepsis secondary to translocation of intestinal bacteria into the bloodstream.

In cats the equivalent infection is feline panleukopenia (feline infectious enteritis).

Canine Adenovirus-1 (Distemper)

Canine adenovirus-1 (CAV-1) attacks the respiratory, gastrointestinal, and nervous systems. Dogs are usually infected following inhalation of aerosolized virus, or via fomites. Clinical signs initially include a purulent ocular discharge, which progresses to pyrexia, nasal discharge, lethargy, coughing, vomiting, and hyporexia. When the CNS is affected, circling, head tilt, muscle twitches, salivation, chewing actions, seizures, and paralysis may result. Distemper is also nicknamed hard pad disease as the footpads thicken and harden as a result of infection.

Feline Herpesvirus-1 and Calicivirus (Cat Flu)

Cat flu is caused by two viruses: **feline herpesvirus-1 (FHV-1) and feline calicivirus (FCV).** Both viruses are spread either by direct contact, inhalation of respiratory secretions, or via fomites.

Both viruses cause **upper respiratory tract infection,** with signs such as sneezing, nasal discharge, ocular discharge, conjunctivitis, lingual ulceration, pyrexia, lethargy, and anorexia.

FCV also causes chronic gingivitis/stomatitis, joint inflammation, and in very rare cases, systemic FCV infection (vsFCV) associated with particularly virulent strains of FCV (as the virus mutates readily during viral replication, different strains are common, and these strains have different pathogenicity).

FHV also causes keratitis, corneal inflammation and ulceration. FHV associated corneal ulcers are often small and branching in nature. **Dermatitis** is occasionally associated with FHV, skin inflammation, and ulceration, particularly around the nose, mouth and forelimbs.

3

Parasites

Parasites are **eukaryotic organisms** and are characterised as ectoparasitic or endoparasitic.

- **Eukaryotic:** organisms whose cells contain a nucleus and organelles, which are enclosed by a plasma membrane.

Ectoparasites

These include fleas, ticks, lice and mites. Many of these parasites also often act as biological vectors, indirectly spreading disease as part of their life cycle:

- *Ctenocephalides spp.* transmit the tapeworm *Diplydium caninum*;
- *Ctenocephalides felis* transmits *Mycoplasma haemofelis*, causing feline infectious anaemia; and
- *Ixodes spp.* transmit *Borrelia burgdorferi*, causing Lyme disease.

Endoparasites

Endoparasites cause varying host effects, depending on the species and health status of the host, (e.g. a heavy roundworm burden in a young puppy has far more disastrous effects than the same roundworm burden in an adult dog). Some endoparasites are zoonotic:

- *Toxocara canis* larvae can migrate and are typically reported in the human eye.
- The tapeworm *Echinococcus granulosus* can cause hydatid cysts to form in human hepatic or pulmonary tissue.

Protozoa

Protozoa are single-celled organisms which can be free-living or parasitic. Parasitic protozoa cause varying disease levels depending on the species and some are also zoonotic. Common protozoal infections include:

- **Giardia and coccidia:** cause gastrointestinal disease with signs such as vomiting and diarrhoea.
- **Toxoplasma:** causes pyrexia, anorexia, pneumonia, neurological signs, hepatitis and ocular signs such as uveitis.
- **Neospora:** causes muscle atrophy, dysphagia, megaoesophagus, limb paralysis and muscle contracture.

Fungi

Fungi are parasitic organisms which reproduce through fungal spores. They are broadly classified into **yeasts and moulds.** Some species of fungi are zoonotic. Common fungal infections encountered in practice are:

- **Malassezia:** a yeast found on the skin and in the ears of dogs, causing dermatitis.
- ***Microsporum canis, Trichophyton verrucosum, T. equinum,* and *T. mentagrophytes*** (**Ringworm**): zoonotic dermatophytes (type of mould) causing hair loss, crusty skin, and erythema.
- **Aspergillus:** a mould which grows in the sinuses of dogs, causing nasal turbinate bone destruction, fungal plaque formation, sneezing and nasal discharge.
- **Cryptococcus:** a yeast which grows in the nose of (mostly) cats, causing naso-facial bone deformity and swelling, rhinitis and nasal discharge. Systemic and CNS forms are also rarely reported.

Prions

Prions (proteinaceous infectious particles) are non-living, misfolded infectious proteins which have the ability to transmit their shape onto variants of the same protein, which then mutate into stable structures.

They are smaller than a virus and unique as **they do not contain nucleic acid** (DNA and RNA) unlike other pathogens. Although they do not contain nucleic acid, prions have the ability to reproduce by changing their folded form.

Prions cause brain tissue damage and consequently cell death to the surrounding brain tissue, causing fatal and transmissible neurodegenerative disease in both humans and animals. An example is Creutzfeldt-Jakob disease (CJD a.k.a. mad cow disease). Diseases involving prions can be acquired, genetic, or sporadic. It is believed that prions spread between animals via body fluids either directly or indirectly.

Bacteria

Bacteria are:

- microscopic, single-celled organisms
- do not have a nucleus
- classified as prokaryotes
- thrive in diverse environments
- have a cell wall
- vary in length and shape
- replicate at body temperature
- able to replicate outside of cells
- classified based on their shape
- Gram +ve or -ve
- anaerobic or aerobic.

Bacterial cells have a **protective outer cell wall,** which provides structural support and an inner cell membrane (plasma membrane). However, certain bacteria, such as mycoplasmas, do not have a cell wall. Some bacteria may even have a third, outermost protective layer called the capsule, which is a sticky protective layer used for attachment.

The outer surface of a bacterium is often covered by **whip-like projections:** flagella (long) or pilli (short). These projections help bacteria to move around and attach to a host. (See Figure 1).

Bacteria Structure

Capsule

The capsule is made up of complex carbohydrates (polysaccharides) and has several functions, the most important being to **prevent the bacterium from drying out.** The capsule's other important function is to prevent the bacterium from being engulfed by other larger microorganisms via phagocytosis.

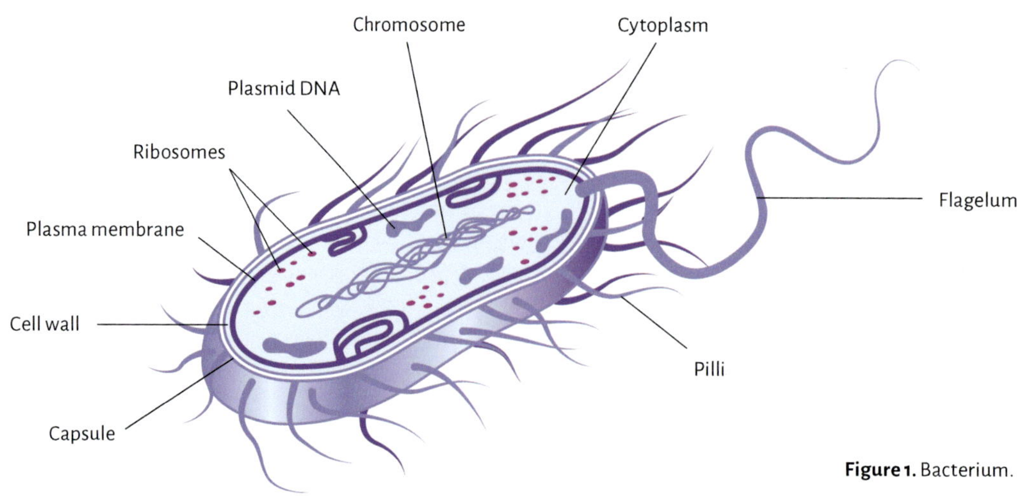

Figure 1. Bacterium.

Cell Wall

The rigid cell wall surrounds the cytoplasmic membrane, which **protects it from the environment and gives the cell shape.** It is responsible for keeping the cell from erupting when there are large differences in osmotic pressure between the cytoplasm and the environment.

The cell wall is made up of peptidoglycan, a protein-sugar (polysaccharide) molecule and provides support to appendages such as the pilli and flagella. The composition of the cell wall varies between different species of bacteria such as is seen in Gram +ve and Gram -ve bacteria.

Plasma Membrane

The cytoplasmic membrane consists of a layer of phospholipids and proteins which **regulate the flow of materials in and out of the bacterium cell.**

Ribosomes

Ribosomes consist of small and large ribosomal units, which **aid in the synthesis of proteins which are required by all living cells.** The small ribosomal units translate the genetic code from RNA and the large ribosomal units form the amino acid polypeptide chains.

Plasmid DNA

A plasmid is a molecule of extrachromosomal DNA within a cell. It is physically separated from chromosomal DNA and can replicate independently. Plasmids are mainly found as small circular double stranded DNA molecules. **They contain genes which aid in the survival of the bacterium such as conferring the selection of antibiotic resistance.**

Chromosome

A chromosome is a long piece of DNA that **contains all or part of the genetic material** of that organism.

Cytoplasm

The cytoplasm is a gel-like matrix which is composed of water, enzymes, nutrients, waste products and gases and contains cell organelles.

Flagellum

Flagella enable the bacterium to move. Not all bacteria cells have flagella. The flagella can be found at either or both ends of a bacterium, or all over its surface. The flagella beat with a propeller like motion to help the bacterium move toward nutrients, away from toxic chemicals, or, in the case of photosynthetic bacterium, towards light.

Pilli

Pilli are small hair like projections that aid the bacterium in **attaching to other cells** and surfaces.

Bacteria are **classified by** the nature of their:

- shape
- cell wall structure
- genetic makeup.

There are **three common shapes of bacteria** (Figure 2). These are:

- **Bacilli:** rod-shaped, include pathogens such as salmonella.
- **Cocci:** spherical, include pathogens such as streptococcus.
- **Spirochetes:** spiral-shaped, include pathogens such as leptospira.

These bacteria may be present alone, in chains (e.g. streptococcus), or bunches (e.g. staphylococcus).

It is important to note bacteria may **present as single cell organisms or form together in shapes** such as chains (streptococci), or as bunches to form different shapes such as squares (tetrad), and triangles (staphylococci).

Identifying Structural Differences of Bacterium

In 1882 (published 1884) a Danish bacteriologist, Hans Christian Jachim Gram (1853–1938), developed one of the most important staining techniques in modern microbiology, which is known as the Gram staining method.

Gram stain detects structural differences between different bacteria (Figure 3). Bacteria can therefore be classified as either:

- **Gram-positive bacteria** which are surrounded by a thicker peptidoglycan layer which takes up and retains the crystal violet stain after the decolourisation part of the staining process, and a lower phospholipid membrane layer. They therefore **appear purple coloured microscopically.**
- **Gram-negative bacteria** which contain a thinner peptidoglycan layer which lies between an inner and outer lipid membrane. Gram-negative bacteria cannot retain the crystal violet stain as the alcohol used in the decolourisation step of the process damages the thinner peptidoglycan layer allowing the inner and outer cell membrane to take up the counterstain (Safranin or Fuchsine) and **appear pink in colour.**

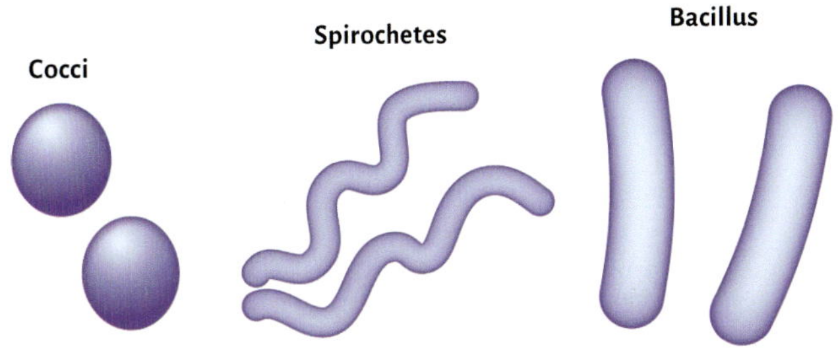

Figure 2. Bacterial shapes.

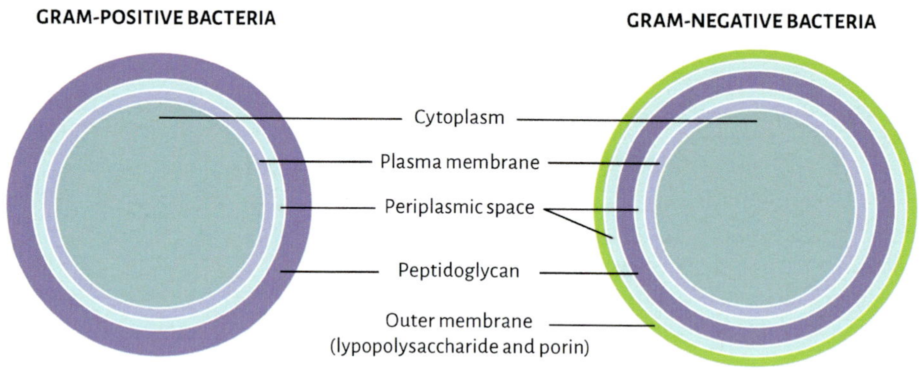

Figure 3. Gram stain.

Types of Bacteria

It is important to remember that not all types of bacteria are pathogenic. Bacteria can be classed as:

Commensal

Commensal bacteria live in or on the animal but **do not harm the host.** They use food supplied by the internal or external environment of the host. **Commensalism is a relationship between species in which one benefits, and the other is unaffected.**

In some cases, commensal bacteria (e.g. MRSA and *E. Coli*) can become pathogenic when they escape their original niche.

Facultative

Bacteria which can live under aerobic, anoxic, or anaerobic conditions.

Symbiotic or Mutualistic

Provide a benefit to the animal and themselves. For example, *Prevotella spp.* are found in cow rumens and help to digest ingested vegetation.

Obligate

These either require oxygen (obligate aerobe) or must be in an environment where oxygen is not present (obligate anaerobe) to survive.

Mycoplasma

Mycoplasma are the simplest forms of bacteria and lack a cell wall around their cell membranes which makes them naturally resistant to antibiotics that target cell wall synthesis. Mycoplasma are smaller than other bacteria with a cell wall and can be parasitic or saprotrophic. (See Figure 4).

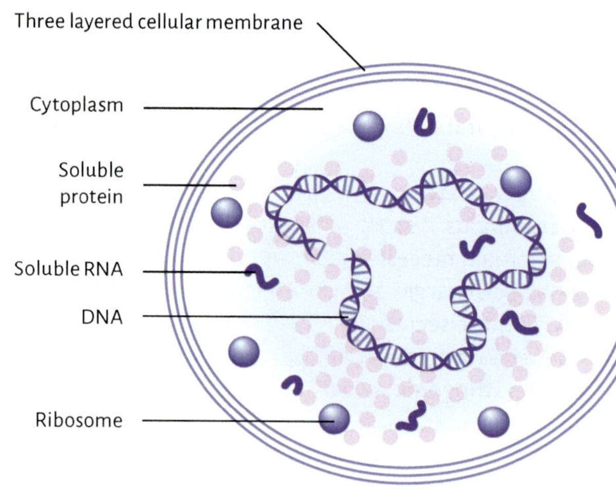

Figure 4. Mycoplasma. They have no cell wall, but a three layered cellular membrane.

Mycoplasma can be anaerobic, and the lack of cell wall means they can change their shape, making them **pleomorphic.**

Other characteristics include:

- cannot be classified as rods, cocci or spirochetes;
- fastidious growth requirements and characterized by fried-egg or mulberry-shaped colonies on agar;
- lack a nucleus and other membrane bound organelles hence **the genetic material is termed naked** as it is a single DNA duplex;
- divided into **haemotropic and non-haemotropic types,** on the basis of their ability to infect erythrocytes;
- several species are **pathogenic in humans and animals,** including *M. pneumoniae* and *Mycoplasma felis* (Greene and Chalker, 2012) and are associated with lower respiratory disease (*M. cynos, M. felis*), joint disease (*M. felis,*

Mycoplasma gatae, *Mycoplasma spumans* and *Mycoplasma edwardii*), and meningoencephalitis (*M. felis and M. canis*);
- require a rich environment for nourishment, which they find on mucosal membranes of the respiratory and urogenital tracts of animals;
- some mycoplasmas are ureaplasmas; with an **affinity for the genitourinary tract** as they require urea to grow and can subsequently cause urinary tract infections; and
- **mycoplasma infections can be found in healthy animals,** so interpretation of diagnostic findings must be in conjunction with the clinical signs observed.

Transmission Methods and Infection

Postoperative patients are amongst those at highest risk of acquiring a nosocomial infection. The latter not only increases morbidity and mortality but poses an infection risk to other patients and places a financial and emotional burden on the client. Therefore, it is the responsibility of veterinary personnel to prevent the spread of these infections and to do this requires an understanding of the transmission methods.

Infectious agents are transmitted by many methods, including in ceruminous discharge, saliva, vomit, respiratory secretions, skin/hair, faeces, blood, ocular and nasal discharge, milk, vaginal discharge, semen, and venereal contact. The pathogens in these secretions are spread via direct or indirect contact depending on the agent.

- **Direct pathogenic spread requires physical contact between two animals,** such as when sleeping, playing, grooming, fighting, or mating. Generally, the pathogens spread via this method need to live on the host to survive; they are therefore fragile and can be destroyed easily.
- **Indirect pathogenic transmission is where there is no direct physical contact between the infected and host animal.** The infected animal contaminates the environment with body fluids (urine, faeces, vomit, saliva, airborne droplets of respiratory secretions) which are then picked up by the new host. This may happen directly (e.g. by inhaling air containing respiratory secretions from a sneezing cat) or via a vector or fomite. Pathogens which spread by this method must be able to survive in the environment for long periods of time, depending on their species, and hence are difficult to destroy.
  - **Fomite:** a contaminated inanimate (non-living) object such as a food bowl, bed, or litter tray, which acts as a source of transmission of infection.
  - **Vector:** an animate (living) object which carries the pathogen/s. These can be classified as biological or mechanical vectors:
    - **Biological vector:** acts as the intermediate host in the pathogen's life cycle and is required for the pathogen's development (e.g. fleas/ticks).
    - **Mechanical vector:** plays no role in the pathogen's development, and only transports it from one animal to another. These vectors may be affected by the pathogen (paratenic host) or may remain healthy (transport host). For example, flies.

Some pathogens are transmitted by carriers. These animals secrete the pathogen (normally in intervals) and pose a risk to animals in contact with them. Carriers are classified either as convalescent or healthy carriers.

- **Convalescent carriers** are animals who have recovered from the disease but secrete the pathogen. This is particularly common during times of stress or immunosuppression, e.g. steroid use in a cat affected previously with flu due to Herpes virus which can recrudesce (reappear) at times of stress.
- **Healthy carriers** are animals who have never shown signs of the disease or are immune to it. These carriers are a particular risk to other animals, as there is no history of disease, and it is impossible to tell that they are a carrier without screening tests being performed.

7

Contracting a Pathogen

Once the pathogen enters the susceptible host, it commonly travels to the lymph nodes local to the entry site, to establish itself. Once the pathogen has replicated sufficiently, it travels throughout the body, generally via blood or lymphatic fluid, until the target area is reached. Here the pathogen exerts its effect on the desired site of action, and clinical signs develop. **This period between pathogen entry into the host, and the appearance of clinical signs, is known as the incubation period.** (See Figure 5).

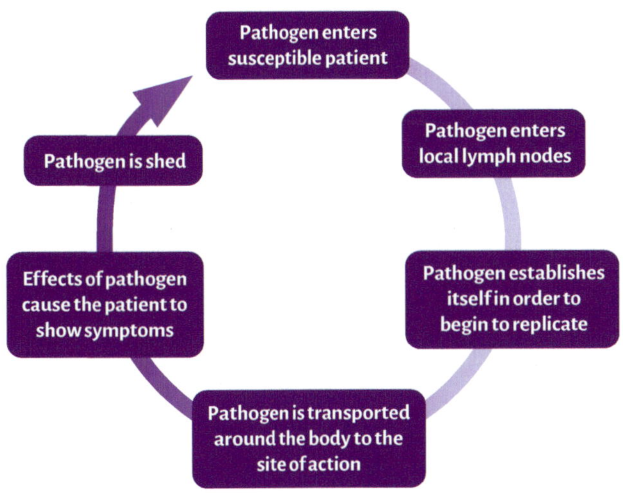

Figure 5. Stages of a generic pathogen life cycle.

The Control of Hospital Acquired Infections

There are a variety of methods by which hospital acquired infections are initially introduced to the veterinary hospital. These include:

- patients
- staff
- visitors (e.g. pharmaceutical representatives etc.)
- clients
- fomites or live vectors (e.g. faeces).

HAI's commonly present as:

1. **Urinary catheter associated infections.**
2. **Infections associated with intravenous and or arterial vascular catheters, thoracic drains, epidural catheters.**
3. **Diarrhoea.**
4. **Pneumonia.**
5. **Surgical site infections (SSI's).**

Presentations and Management

Urinary Tract Infections

The most common hospital acquired infections are urinary tract infections (Reid K. Nalamura et al., 2012) of which the **majority are associated with urinary catheterisation.** This is a result of infection ascending into the bladder from, or passing along, the urinary catheter itself.

Urinary catheters should always be placed aseptically, using sterile gloves and a sterile barrier drape.

To eliminate external contaminants, **the fur around the prepuce or vulva** should be clipped and cleaned using an appropriate antiseptic solution such as chlorhexidine or povidone iodine solution. The prepuce or vulva should also be cleaned by flushing with very dilute 0.005% chlorhexidine or 0.1% povidone-iodine solution before catheterisation is performed.

Chlorhexidine is beneficial as part of a comprehensive protocol for urinary catheters. A reduction in urinary tract infections during prolonged use of urinary catheters has been shown when using a 0.005% chlorhexidine for bladder irrigation (Lim, K. S. et al., 2008)

The type of urinary catheter is also important, for example, is the urinary catheter going to be for temporary or long-term use? Rigid catheters can cause increased irritation and discomfort when left in situ. Therefore, a softer and more flexible urinary catheter should be used to prevent trauma to the bladder and urethra.

Following placement of an indwelling urinary catheter it is important to use a closed collection system. The latter also requires aseptic management for the duration of the time the catheter is in situ. This is to prevent pathogenic organisms from ascending via the lumen of the urinary catheter and causing a urinary tract infection.

Indwelling urinary catheters should be in place for the minimum time necessary, subject to the patient's disease status and reason for catheterisation; prolonged catheterisation is a risk factor for development of urinary tract infections.

When a urinary tract infection is suspected, collect a urine sample and remove the indwelling urinary catheter aseptically to send for culture. If an infection is confirmed, only then administer the appropriate antibiotic. Maintaining a urinary catheter during treatment of an infection may aid in selection for bacterial resistance.

Urinary Catheter Management

When managing and maintaining an indwelling urinary catheter the following steps should be taken:

- Clean gloves must be worn to handle the catheter and closed collection system.
- Clean the vulva/prepuce, collection system line, and exposed urinary catheter with an appropriate diluted antiseptic solution every 4–6 hours.
- Do not disconnect the closed collection system from the urinary catheter if at all possible and store it within a protective transparent bag, stored either within a tray or up off the floor away from any sources of contaminants.

Intravenous Catheter (IV) Site Infections

Intravenous catheter related infections are associated with significant mortality and morbidity (B Salzman et al., 1995). This is due to bacteria directly entering the circulatory system and thus increasing the risk of sepsis and other complications. Intravenous catheter related infections are mainly **caused by their placement and management when in situ.**

Contamination of IV catheters occurs from extraluminal, intraluminal, or other sources. (See Figure 6).

- **Extraluminal contamination** comes from the patient's own skin microbial flora, or the skin flora of the person placing the intravenous catheter.

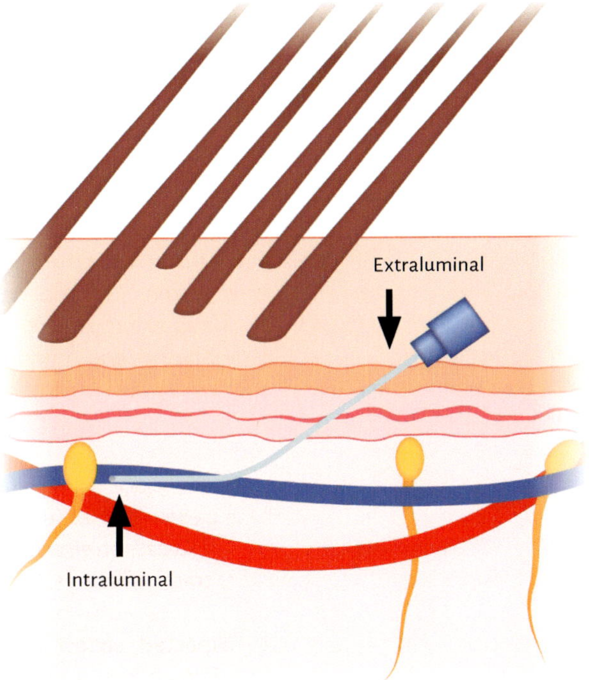

Figure 6. IV catheter in situ.

- **Intraluminal contamination** includes catheter tip contamination and the skin flora of the person placing the IV catheter.

Intravenous contamination from other sources includes **contaminated infuscate** (i.e. medications or fluids that are intravenously administered via the IV catheter) or the use of a T-connector rather than a 'Y' connector. (Jones et al., 2009).

Phlebitis

Phlebitis is the inflammation of a vein and is associated with pain, erythema, oedema, hardening and/or a palpable thread. There are various factors that can influence the development of phlebitis, such as inadequate technique when inserting the catheter, the patient's clinical situation, the characteristics of the vein, drug incompatibility, tonus and pH of the medicine or solution, ineffective filtration, catheter diameter, size, length, and material as well as prolonged use (White et al., 2001).

Diarrhoea

Diarrhoea in a hospitalised patient may arise from many different infectious causes which include bacterial infections such as *Campylobacter spp.*, viral infections (parvovirus) and protozoal infections as in the case of *Tritrichomonas foetus, Isospora spp.*, and *Giardia spp.*

There are three types of phlebitis:

- **Mechanical**
  This is the result of friction from the movement of a foreign object (cannula) within a vein causing subsequent venous inflammation.
- **Chemical**
  Results from a drug or fluid being infused through the canula and irritating the vein, resulting in venous inflammation.
- **Infective**
  - This arises from a pathogen entering a vein from a cannula, which results in venous inflammation. Before placing, handling, or administering medications hands must be washed or disinfected with an alcohol solution.
  - **Bandages should be changed, and the IV catheter site checked for signs of infection and any notable signs of phlebitis at least twice a day.** A phlebitis scoring system should be used to measure the grade and severity. Any incidence greater than two should be reported to the veterinary surgeon.
  - **The catheter should be flushed with 0.9% saline.** The IV catheter should be removed aseptically if there is any evidence of suspected phlebitis and the suspected catheter tip cultured.
  - Unnecessary disconnection of the fluid line and catheter should be avoided, and **all ports and connections cleaned with isopropyl alcohol** before syringe, needle, or fluid line connection.

The hospital setting can facilitate the spread of the infectious agents in diarrhoea. This is particularly evident in high traffic/populated areas (i.e. kennels/wards).

The spread of infection can be prevented by good hand hygiene and the use of PPE (personal protective equipment) during and between patient interaction. Cross contamination is minimised by designated exercise areas for inpatients, strict hospital cleaning and practice policies on management of inpatients which are fed a raw diet.

Pneumonia

True hospital acquired pneumonia is classically seen in patients that have been placed on mechanical ventilation. However, **pneumonia that develops** (with no prior clinical signs) **after admission over a 48 hour period** is categorized as hospital acquired pneumonia. Another type of hospital acquired pneumonia seen in veterinary practice is **aspiration pneumonia.**

The following conditions and procedures can lead to a higher risk of the patient developing aspiration pneumonia:

- laryngeal disease
- oesophageal disease
- recent anaesthesia
- sedation
- neurological diseases
- syringe feeding
- nasopharyngeal enteral feeding
- pharyngostomy tube feeding.

Surgical Site Infections

Surgical site infection (SSI) is defined as an infection occurring at the surgical site within 30 days, or one year if implants remain in situ. SSI is an important factor of morbidity and mortality in postoperative patients. Recognizing the risk factors and making a concerted effort to monitor patients for postoperative infection has a positive effect on the patient's outcome, clients, and practice.

Surgical site infections can be divided into three groups:

- **Superficial:** occur within 30 days and affect only the skin and subcutaneous tissues of the incision.
- **Deep:** occur within 30 days if no implant or one year of the procedure if an implant was used and includes deep soft tissues of the incision such as muscle and fascia tissue.
- **Organ/space:** includes any part of the body other than the incision through the skin, subcutaneous tissue, fascia, and muscle at the incision site, that is manipulated during surgery, such as osteomyelitis (bone infection) following orthopaedic surgery or septic peritonitis following celiotomy (abdominal surgery).

All surgical wounds are contaminated with bacteria, however not all will become infected. **For infection to occur a grave level of contamination is required, which is approximately 10^5 organisms per gram of tissue or ml of fluid.**

Nevertheless, this figure oversimplifies the situation as there are many variable factors involved which determine whether a level of contamination within a wound results in infection.

Bacterial contamination during a surgical procedure can originate from:

- flora found on/within the patient itself. This type of bacteria is known as endogenous bacteria;
- the environment;
- temporary skin contaminants also known as exogenous bacteria;
- the surgical team; and
- the surgical equipment/implants.

Factors that determine the risk of infection developing include the **host's resistance,** the **contaminant organisms' characteristics,** and **the interaction between the host and micro-organism** (i.e. the local wound environment). (See Figure 7).

Therefore, it is important that essential and effective aseptic and operative techniques are performed to reduce the level of tissue contamination.

Surgical Site Contamination

Most bacterial contamination occurs at the time of surgery. Consequently, **the peri- and intraoperative phases of patient management are regarded as mainstays of aseptic technique.**

The main sources of contamination in surgery are:

- theatre environment
- surgical team
- surgical equipment
- the patient.

Prevention of SSIs involves maintaining surgical asepsis, administering prophylactic antibiotics (when appropriate), identifying and managing at-risk patients, and appropriate postoperative wound care.

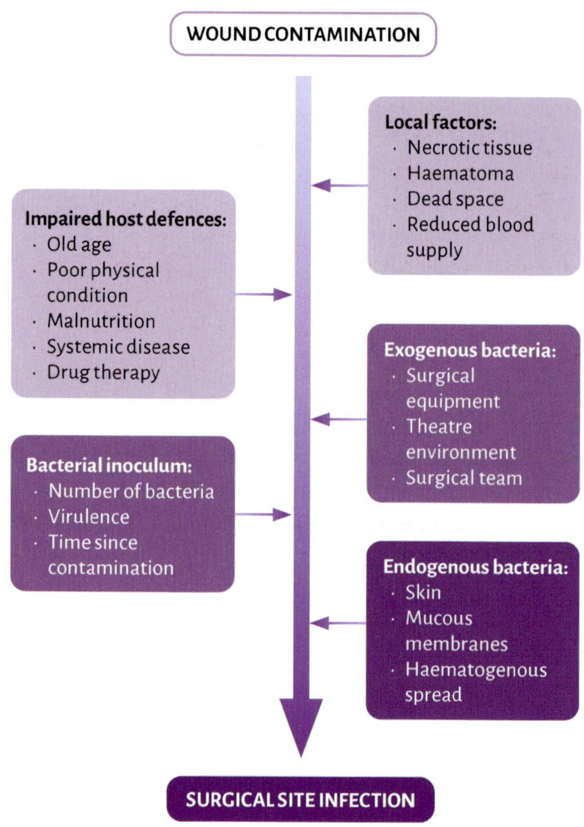

Figure 7. Factors resulting in surgical site infection.

The use of prophylactic antibiotics is not recommended in clean, uncomplicated surgeries where no implants are used, and surgical duration is less than 90 minutes.

Patients at increased risk of SSIs include hypothermic patients, patients with poor nutritional status, patients with postsurgical pain, and patients with comorbidities. Hypothermia increases risk of infection development, as the loss of thermoregulatory abilities adversely affects the immune system and reduces the body's ability to eliminate bacteria.

Animals receiving effective pain relief will heal, eat, allow effective nursing care, have effective immune function, and be discharged from hospital more rapidly, reducing risk of infection.

Postoperative wound infection is a common and potentially serious complication of surgery. The effects range from minor, quickly resolved, self-limiting infections; to serious life-threatening illnesses which can be difficult and expensive to manage. Such situations are crucial for the patient and strain relationships between surgeon and client to the limit. **Approximately 5% of small animals that undergo surgery** develop infection despite the measures taken to minimise contamination and use of antibiotics (Myhew P., 2012).

Increasingly sophisticated anaesthetic protocols and surgical expertise has resulted in larger numbers of more complex procedures being performed on patients with a significantly reduced ability to combat postoperative infection. This, along with the increased prevalence of resistance among populations of microorganisms, has placed even greater emphasis on the design of and adherence to strict surgical asepsis protocols. The principle of asepsis is the freedom of the surgical wound from microorganisms. The principle of asepsis is the adoption of surgical procedures which, while it may be impossible to eliminate all microorganisms from the site, enable the host's immunity to prevent infection from occurring.

Classification of Surgical Wounds

Surgical wounds can be classified according to the level of bacterial contamination present at the time of the procedure. To assess the risk of surgical wound infection, **a full evaluation of each patient's suitability for surgery should be carried out.** This guides the preoperative preparation, the anaesthetic risks and protocol, the surgical procedure used, and influences the postoperative care of the patient. Important considerations include the patient's physical condition, the presence of concurrent disease, and the presence of remote sites of infection. The classification of surgical wounds can be used as a starting point when considering the prophylactic antimicrobial protocol and deciding on the postoperative antimicrobial therapy. (Table 1).

Table 1. Summary of surgical would classification and characteristics of each type. (Adapted from Chris Shales, 2012).

Surgical wound classification/Type of surgical procedure	Description
Clean	· Non-traumatic elective procedure. · No entry into gastrointestinal, respiratory, urogenital tract. · No break in aseptic technique.
Clean-contaminated	· Entry into a hollow viscus with no significant spillage and no presence of infection. · A clean procedure with a minor break in aseptic technique.
Contaminated	· Fresh traumatic wound (<6–8 hours old). · Spillage from a contaminated viscus during surgery. · Entry into a hollow viscus in the presence of infection. · Clean surgery with a major break in aseptic technique.
Dirty	· Infected surgical site. · Purulent discharge encountered. · Open/traumatic wound >6–8 hours old.

Control of Hospital Acquired Infections and Preventing Pathogenic Spread

Preventing a hospital acquired infection is always preferable to treating them. Strategies for preventing the spread of disease include considering factors such as the patient, clinic/hospital environment, and staff members. Surveillance, auditing, and monitoring of infection control protocols/principles is also required, to review and reflect on infection control protocols, and implement any necessary changes.

Infection control principles begin with the front-of-house staff; when they take a call to book an appointment, the clinical signs described **over the phone should be used to triage the patient's biosecurity status.** A sneezing cat? A dog with a non-healing wound? A patient with a known infection booking a repeat consultation?

Consider infection control factors when advising the client when to arrive, which entrance/exit to use, and where to wait so as to minimize the spread of disease. If possible (contingent with the urgency of the appointment) see patients with a suspected infection at the end of consulting and possibly even ask owners to wait in the car rather than the clinic. A separate entrance/exit may also be used in cases of severely contagious disease.

Upon arrival, **infectious patients should be seen in a designated consulting room which is closed following the consultation,** until it has been fully cleaned and disinfected.

Assign each patient a biosecurity status during the consultation, prior to admission. This classification is based on the individual patient's condition (disease, immune status, vaccination status, age) plus their clinical signs and any differential or confirmed diagnoses. **Clearly mark the biosecurity status on the patient's hospital sheet** and/or kennel/ops board, to use as a visual reminder when planning procedures, treatments, or nursing care.

Biosecurity Classification Systems

There are three main classification methods which are used:
- the traffic light system
- the numerical system
- a combination of the above.

Traffic Light System

Green patients are normal patients showing no signs of contagious disease; they may be nursed within the standard ward.

Amber patients are patients with a disease unlikely to spread in hospital, such as diseases spread via direct contact (FIV through fighting etc.) and surgical site infections with sensitive bacterial isolates. These patients may be barrier nursed within the normal ward.

Red patients are patients with severely contagious or significant diseases requiring strict isolation and barrier nursing, such as multi-drug resistant infections, parvovirus, distemper, cat flu and mycobacterial infections.

This system, though very visual (a green, amber or red card is placed on the kennel door, for easy identification of these patients) and effective, does not consider patients requiring reverse barrier nursing or those staff members that are colour blind.

The Numerical System

Numerical (Table 2) and traffic light systems used together give a more perceptive biosecurity status to a patient.

Table 2. Biosecurity numerical system.

Case number	Description	Example
1	Immunocompromised patients	Those receiving chemotherapeutic drugs or high-dose immunosuppressive agents such as prednisolone/ciclosporin/ azathioprine, or unvaccinated puppies/kittens. These patients should be reverse barrier nursed within the ward, to protect them from indirect contact with other patients/pathogens.
2	"Normal" patients with no signs of contagious disease	Healthy patients in for neutering, patients with non-contagious disease processes such as CKD, orthopaedic patients etc. These patients do not require any specific infection-control related concerns (aside from the usual practice protocols).
3	Patients with mildly or moderate contagious disease	Cats and feline immunodeficiency virus or feline infectious peritonitis which typically do not require isolation, due to the nature by which the disease is spread. These patients can be strictly barrier nursed within the normal ward; they should be segregated from other cats as much as possible (e.g. use an end kennel), the barrier area marked with signs or tiger tape, and a separate supply of PPE and consumables used as well as a separate waste bag for these patients.
4	Patients with (or suspected to have) highly contagious disease	Parvovirus, distemper, kennel cough, multi-drug resistant infections, cat "flu". These patients must be isolated, and barrier nursed in an isolation unit, unless the severity of their clinical conditions means they need intensive care. In cases where ICU nursing is required (e.g. parvovirus puppies) a "makeshift isolation" should be prepared outside of the normal wards, in an area where the patient can easily observed.

Barrier Nursing

Barrier nursing is a set of environmental considerations and guidelines, used to prevent cross-contamination of infectious diseases.

Barrier nursing is achieved via **protective clothing and equipment** and using a suitable specific area to carry out barrier nursing such as **an isolation area.** The personal protective equipment (PPE)/personal protective clothing (PPC) required for individual patients varies depending on the specific infectious pathogen, transmission method, and zoonotic risk. Full PPE consists of a disposable long sleeve waterproof gown, gloves, mask, shoe covers as well as eye protection.

Reverse barrier nursing uses the same protection methods but is used to protect vulnerable patients from contracting an infectious disease. For example, patients that are unvaccinated or immunocompromised.

Infection Surveillance

Surveillance is the monitoring of clinical practices, environment, and patients.

Surveillance is classified as either **active, passive, or environmental.** Active surveillance is further subdivided into clinical, or laboratory diagnosed-based surveillance.

The purpose of surveillance is to highlight areas that are working well and identify those areas where adaptations or improvement are required.

Passive Surveillance

In veterinary practice, passive surveillance is the most common surveillance method. **Passive surveillance uses data retrospectively collected** from clinical records, or laboratory results (e.g. bacteriology results from the patient for treatment purposes which are not collected specifically for infection surveillance).

Passive surveillance is cheap and easy to perform, however as pathogens are not detected at the time of infection it is not as effective as other surveillance methods. Passive surveillance is therefore **an ineffective method for preventing hospital acquired infections** (a.k.a. nosocomial infections).

Collected data (via passive surveillance) is used to determine endemic rates of disease and susceptibility, trends, and patterns of antimicrobial agents as well as disease pattern changes. (e.g. postsurgical wound auditing).

Active Surveillance

Active surveillance is the specific gathering of data for infection control purposes, involving prospective steps to identify patients that have or may develop a hospital acquired infection. For example, the routine culturing of intravenous catheters following removal.

Generally, active surveillance is not required in most veterinary practices, unless they have an ongoing infectious disease outbreak, or they are a large practice with increased threats to infection control.

Active surveillance is more time consuming and expensive compared to passive surveillance and is based on either clinical or laboratory diagnosis.

In veterinary practice, clinical diagnosis surveillance is more commonly used. It involves creating categories based on clinical signs from HAIs. Patients which fall into these categories are then more closely monitored and further active surveillance carried out (e.g. laboratory sample collection).

Environmental Surveillance

A common source of infectious agents that give rise to hospital acquired infections is the environment itself, through contamination. Environmental bacterial cultures can help to minimise contamination and evaluate the practices' disinfection protocols.

In order for environmental surveillance to be effective, it must be **repeated regularly,** to determine the clinic's baseline bacterial number (as bacteria are present on all surfaces). Environmental cultures have an associated cost. Therefore, the frequency and interval of their use should be considered appropriate to the incidence of infection within the practice.

Investigation

If there is an **occurrence or a suspected HAI within the hospital, it is essential to identify the source quickly** and eliminate it to prevent further infection and spread. During investigation and initial treatment, **place the patient into isolation and implement rigorous barrier nursing.**

Clinical audits are an ideal method to assess the effectiveness of infection control protocols, staff compliance with protocols, and identify areas for potential improvement. They also encourage reflective practice, something all registered veterinary nurses should do. Auditing is a way of reviewing what it is being done, assessing how it can be improved, and determining what changes to make in order to do so. In addition, proof of clinical governance (specifically, surgical site infection monitoring) is a requirement for the RCVS Practice Standards Scheme.

Clinical Audits

- Assessment of infection control protocols.
- Maintain staff compliance.
- Identify areas where improvement is required.
- Reflective.
- Part of clinical governance (RCVS Practice Standard Scheme).

Investigation

- Prevention of further infection and spread.
- Source of infection is quickly identified.
- Elimination of that source.
- Isolate infection – barrier nursing.
- Treatment.

To reduce the risk of HAIs, the hospital's general cleanliness and hygiene should be maintained, using appropriate disinfectants and dilutions for each area of the hospital (depending on the risk each area poses). HAI prevention considerations for staff include wearing appropriate PPE, uniform considerations, performing effective hand hygiene, as well as the hospital layout and decoration materials/design.

Where specific risks for HAI development are present, **practice protocols should be developed.** Such situations include patients with indwelling devices such as IV catheters or urinary catheters, and patients undergoing or recovering from surgery.

Antibiotics and Resistance

There are several ways that antimicrobials damage and kill bacteria (Figure 8):

- affect protein synthesis
- affect DNA
- affect the cell wall.

Antimicrobials are used to treat bacterial disease, but resistance to them has been observed and continues to grow. However, **it is not solely the use of antimicrobials to treat bacterial disease that is the cause antimicrobial resistance.**

Bacteria have developed various mechanisms to counteract the action of antibacterial agents. Some bacteria can naturally resist certain kinds of antibiotic due to their structural or functional characteristics; while other bacteria inherit resistance, through genetic mutation within the bacterial genome or genetic transfer. In 2011 resistance genes to tetracycline were discovered in DNA from 30 000-year-old bacteria. Bacteria may therefore have the ability to modify and or replace the drug target within their cell wall and or neutralise a specific antimicrobial. (See Figure 9).

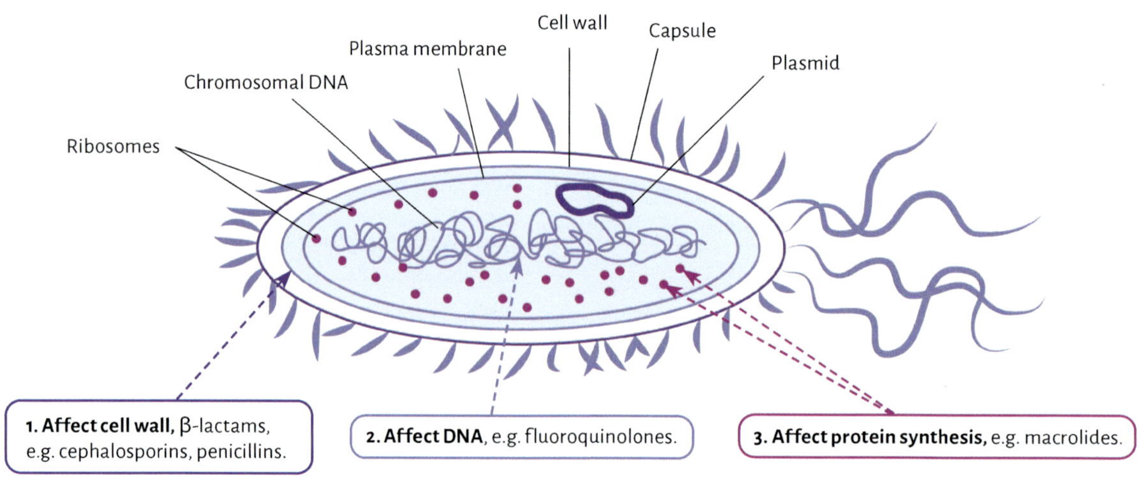

Figure 8. Ways in which antimicrobial destroy bacteria.

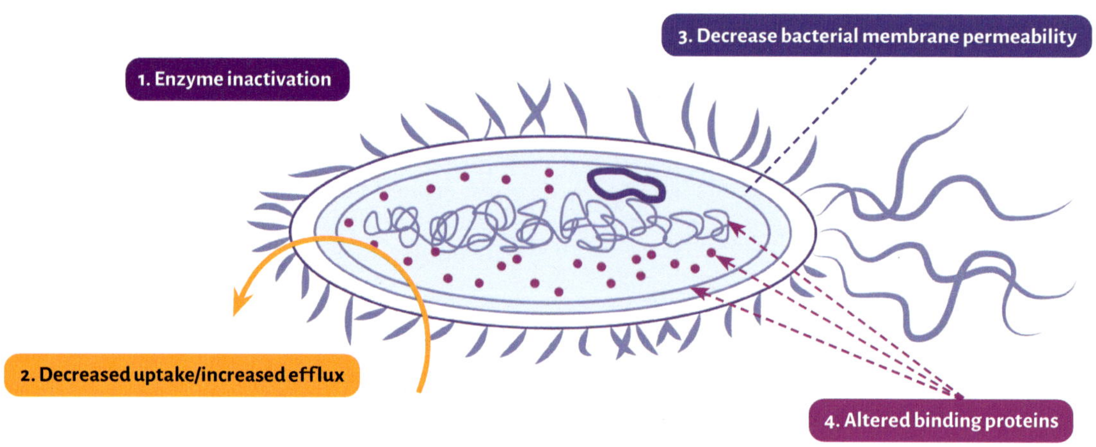

Figure 9. Ways antimicrobial resistance is conferred amongst bacteria.

Multiresistance to an antimicrobial occurs when:

- Different genes confer resistance to antibacterial agents of different classes, known as **co-selection.**
- When a single gene confers resistance to ≥2 antibacterial agents, known as **cross-selection.**

There are several ways that genes confer resistance:

- **produce enzymes** which inactivate the antimicrobial;
- develop a **membrane pump** that prevents adequate accumulation of the antibacterial agent inside the bacterial cell. This is achieved by removing the antimicrobial drug from the bacterial cell;
- **decrease bacterial membrane permeability; and**
- **mutation of the target site** on the cell wall. Therefore, altering binding proteins which in turn reduces or inhibits the affinity of the antimicrobial agent for that particular bacterium.

It is important to remember **antibacterials do not induce resistance.** Resistance to antimicrobial agents is caused by spontaneous genetic mutations that alter the structure of the cell, target molecule or the metabolism of the antibacterial agent. Mutations occur at a relatively low frequency (1 mutation per 107–109 cells).

Exposing a bacterial population to an antimicrobial applies a selection pressure for those with resistance genes to survive and proliferate.

Selection of resistance within a bacterial population is promoted by:

- **Exposure to a lower than recommended concentration of the antimicrobial (i.e. too low a dose).**
- **Exposure to the antimicrobial for insufficient time (i.e. too short a course).**

Genetic material can be dispersed by both cell division (passing genes to the next generation of bacteria) and genetic exchange (between bacteria of the same generation) resulting in bacteria spreading genetic material more efficiently and quickly than animals.

Resistance Genes

Inherent resistance is the bacterial organism's natural ability to resist the activity of a particular antimicrobial agent via its structural or functional characteristics.

Natural resistance may be due to:

- lack of affinity of a particular antimicrobial;
- alterations in the cell wall resulting in the inability to penetrate the cell wall by a particular antimicrobial agent;
- the natural production of enzymes which inactivate a particular antimicrobial agent; or
- extrusion of an antimicrobial by chromosomally encoded active exporters.

Examples of inherent resistance include:

- **Mycoplasma organisms** have inherent resistance to β-lactam antimicrobials (e.g. cephalosporins). The target site of action for β-lactam antimicrobials is the cell wall. As *Mycoplasma spp.* do not have a cell wall, they are therefore naturally resistant to β-lactam antibiotics (e.g. cephalosporins, penicillin derivatives, carbacephems).
- **Anaerobic organisms have inherent resistance to aminoglycosides** (e.g. neomicin, gentamicin) as aminoglycoside antimicrobials require oxygen dependent carriers to enter the cell wall. As anaerobic bacteria are in the presence of little to no oxygen, there is insufficient uptake of these antimicrobials.
- **β-lactamase producing organisms** (e.g. *Klebsiella*) **have inherent resistance to ampicillin.** Some bacteria naturally produce enzymes (β-lactamase) that damage antimicrobials with a β-lactam ring in their structure before the antimicrobial reaches their target, which are the penicillin binding proteins located on the bacterial cell wall.

Acquiring Resistance Genes

Resistance genes are passed on the next generation during cell division and also by genetic transfer.

Plasmids are small pieces of circular DNA carried by many bacteria (containing the resistant genes) and are transferred between the same and/or different species of bacteria. They may be transferred from a non-pathogenic form of bacteria to a pathogenic form.

Resistance genes are transferred to other bacterial organisms in three ways:

1. **Transformation.** The process by which a resistance gene is directly incorporated into the bacterial genome. Transmission between species is possible.
2. **Transduction.** Remote transfer of genes via a bacteriophage (bacterial virus).
3. **Conjugation.** Direct contact between two bacteria, with the transfer of a gene within a bacterial plasmid.

The effects of increasing antibacterial resistance are:
- limited choice of treatment leading to increased treatment costs;
- the more resistance genes there are, the greater the proportion of bacteria with resistance to antibacterials;
- treatment failures and an increased incidence of severe infection; and
- a decrease in the effectiveness of empirical treatment results and an increased need for culture and sensitivity testing in order to select the most appropriate antibacterial agent.

Antimicrobial Sensitivity Testing (AST)

Antibiotic sensitivity testing (AST) specifies antibiotic dosage and formulates a profile for empirical therapy for the proper management of an individual's health against bacterial infections. (See Figure 10).

Antibiotic sensitivity tests are used to determine which specific antimicrobial a particular bacterium is more sensitive to. AST is usually performed following or in conjunction to a Gram stain and culture.

The disk-diffusion method, also known as the Kirby-Bauer test, is the most common antibiotic sensitivity test in determining what antimicrobial to use when treating a particular pathogenic bacterium.

The test relies on evidence of a reduction of bacterial growth, which is measured under standard laboratory conditions and can be performed in practice.

The Kirby Bauer sensitivity test is performed by using cellulose (paper) discs, impregnated with a particular antimicrobial agent at the expected antimicrobial concentration at a single dose. These discs are placed onto a bacterial lawn and incubated for 24–48 hours.

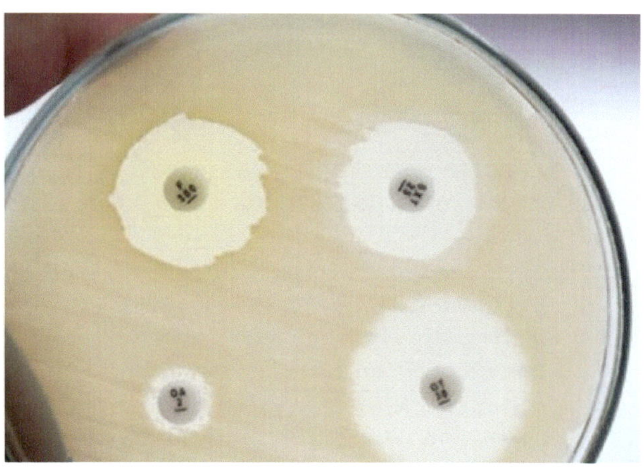

Figure 10. Antimicrobial sensitivity testing.

The test is semi quantitative, as it depends on the area around the disc which has inhibited bacterial growth. The bacterium is classified as being sensitive or resistant to the particular antimicrobial.

Resistant Organisms

Methicillin-resistant *Staphylococci*

One of the earliest penicillin drugs was methicillin and resistance to it was used as a marker for the widespread **resistance to β-lactam due to the presence of the mecA gene.**

The **mecA gene** programs an alternative penicillin binding protein on the bacterium's cell wall, which does not bind to antibacterial agents containing a β-lactam ring in their makeup and hence **inhibits their antimicrobial action.** The mecA gene is transported on the staphylococcal genome which is known as the **SCC (staphylococcal chromosomal cassette)**.

There are several types of SCC which vary in length, structure and the number of genes they contain. Therefore, methicillin resistant staphylococci that have different types of SCC can carry the gene required to program resistance to other antibacterial drugs.

Staphylococci

Coagulase is a protein enzyme produced by a number of microorganisms which allows the conversion of fibrinogen to fibrin. *Staphylococci spp.* (species) are divided into two different types:
1. **Coagulase-positive (CPS).** *S. aureus and S. intermedius.*
2. **Coagulase-negative (CNS).** *S. epidermis, S. saprophyicus, S. haemolyticus.*

Coagulase is used within a laboratory setting to distinguish between different types of staphylococcus species.

Coagulase-positive *Staphylococci spp.* are regarded as potentially pathogenic. This is because coagulase is used by the CPS to coat their surface with fibrin (forming a fibrin clot) in contact with blood. This fibrin clot protects the bacterium from phagocytosis and protects it from the hosts natural defence mechanisms.

CPS are therefore usually isolated from staphylococci associated infections. Whereas CNS are known as non-pathogenic as they are rarely the cause of an infection.

Methicillin resistance has been found in both CNS and CPS species and it is thought there is a possibility that CNS can play a role in transferring resistance genes to the pathogenic CPS organisms.

Most infections in both human and veterinary medicine are secondary, and **most humans and animals do carry commensal CPS with a low risk of pathogenic effect.**

Methicillin-resistant *Staphylococcus Aureus* (MRSA) and Methicillin-resistant *Staphylococcus Pseudintermedius* (MRSP)

It is estimated that around 30% of humans have methicillin sensitive *Staphylococcus aureus* (MSSA) within their nasal passages but only 1–3% actually carry MRSA and are asymptomatic. It is important to note that around 15% of health care workers are asymptomatic carriers of MRSA.

MRSA is the most common species of infection in both human and veterinary medicine and for this reason is the most well documented species of methicillin-resistant staphylococcus.

Research has indicated that 7–13% of veterinary personnel were colonised with MRSA and carry specific isolates of MRSA associated with their type of veterinary work (i.e. small animal, farm animal or equine). This suggests veterinary personnel are a high risk for transporting MRSA, indicating spread is associated with exposure to animal and veterinary premises.

Studies also show that >1% of healthy dogs and cats are colonised with MRSA, suggesting they are not the natural hosts and **acquire MRSA via reverse zoonosis** (transfer from humans).

MRSP (Methicillin-resistant *Staphylococcus pseudintermedius*) is more commonly associated with animals and has been isolated in 95% of canine pyoderma and studies indicate it is also the most common organism isolated from other infections in canine and feline species.

The prevalence of MRSP is however higher in the United States (70%) than continental Europe (30%) and the UK (1%).

The reason that MRSP is a concern is because the isolates in both the US and Northern Europe are the same clone, which shows this clone of MRSP has quickly spread worldwide. This MRSP clone is also highly antimicrobial resistant and therefore difficult to manage as it is resistant to five classes of antimicrobial drugs. These include penicillins, cephalosporins, fluoroquinolones, aminoglycosides, sulphonamides, macrolides tetracyclines, and fusidic acid.

Antibiotic Resistant Infections

Diagnosing Antibiotic Resistant Infections

It is the responsibility of the veterinary profession to reduce the incidence of MRSA and MRSP infections in animals. Measures which can be taken include:

- high standards of clinical practice;
- high levels of clinical hygiene;
- effective infectious disease control procedures; and
- the responsible use of antibiotics.

As discussed earlier the choice of appropriate antibiotic agent used for each infection is chosen based on culture and sensitivity results. These include the use of topical antimicrobial agents in the case of dermatological disease or wounds.

Diagnosis of MRSA and MRSP infections in particular should be suspected in cases where:

- the patient is from known **MRSA/MRSP positive households;**
- in patients with a **non-healing wound;**
- in patients with a **history of antibiotic sensitivity** where the bacteria involved is identified to be a *Staphylococcus spp.*;
- **in nosocomial** or secondary infections particularly in high-risk patients (i.e. immunocompromised); and
- in patients with **sepsis** or other invasive infections.

It is vital to **take swabs and/or tissue samples as quickly as possible** in all suspected cases and ideally send them to a laboratory with the expertise to identify MRSA/MRSP and determine their antimicrobial sensitivity.

It is equally important that samples are clearly marked as suspected MRSA/MRSP, including samples from cadavers taken at post-mortem, and specimens appropriately packaged and sealed. Sample sites include:

- surgical sites, implants and or drains;
- skin lesions and wounds;
- insertion sites of intravenous catheters;
- urine, particularly when there is or has been an indwelling urinary catheter in place and/or a urinary tract infection is present;
- faeces if diarrhoea is present;
- bronchiolar alveolar lavage fluid if there is a respiratory tract infection.

Managing Patients with an Antimicrobial Resistant Infection

In the case of methicillin-resistant *Staphylococcus aureus* (MRSA), recommended agents for treatment include tetracyclines or aminoglycosides, but the choice of agent should depend on culture and sensitivity testing results as some isolates will show more widespread antimicrobial resistance than others. However, when the veterinary surgeon decides on the treatment protocol the culture and sensitivity results, patient factors (oral vs topical), client factors (e.g. financial restrictions) and any drug interactions or potential adverse effects must be taken into account.

Patients with multi-antibiotic-resistant infections or infections such as MRSA are classified as **a biosecurity level 4 (Red classification), requiring strict isolation and barrier nursing,** depending on the type of infection, method of spread and the ability to contain that infection (e.g. resistant urinary tract infections can potentially be barrier nursed within the normal ward if a urinary catheter is present, whereas a patient with a discharging wound should be isolated).

Discharging wounds should remain covered at all times, **and all wounds should be covered with an appropriate dressing.** The movement of these patients around the hospital should be minimised, and any procedures scheduled for the end of the day. Following their discharge from hospital, the environment should be thoroughly cleaned, and disinfected, and environmental cultures collected before the kennel/isolation unit is used again.

To prevent resistant infections, antimicrobial agents should be used responsibly.

This can be achieved by:

- **Preventing the need for their use:** through regular health checks and the use of topical treatment where appropriate.
- **Using appropriately:** e.g. not in cases of viral infection, and only in ill or at-risk animals at the correct dose at the correct frequency and for an appropriate duration of treatment, ensuring clients administer the antimicrobial correctly and complete the course.
- Choosing the **appropriate agent for the pathogen:** based on practice protocols, likely pathogens, and susceptibility testing.
- **Monitoring sensitivity:** based on culture and sensitivity results.
- **Minimising use:** using only when they are strictly necessary, and when there is evidence to show use will reduce morbidity and mortality.

The Use of Antimicrobials

Antimicrobial use increases the risk of selection for resistant bacteria and thus the risk of bacterial resistance. The latter is a real concern in both human and veterinary medicine, due to over-prescribing and/or the improper use of antimicrobials in the face of every evolving pathogen. This has severe consequence for veterinary patients, livestock and food-production animals, and public health. Antimicrobial resistance is a significant contributor to morbidity and mortality, as well as increasing the duration of hospitalisation and treatment, which in turn increases treatment costs.

It is the role of the nurse or veterinary technician to educate clients. When discussing antibiotic medications with clients, ensure the client is fully aware of the dosing instructions, and that they must **complete the course even if their animal seems to be back to normal.**

Several resources are available to utilise in practice to assist with **antimicrobial stewardship,** including client resources:

- BVA "How to use antibiotics responsibly" handout: https://www.bva.co.uk/uploadedFiles/Content/News,_campaigns_and_policies/Policies/Me dicines/Antibiotic%20resistance%20client%20leaflet.pdf
- BVA "Are you antibiotic aware?" client poster: https://www.bva.co.uk/uploadedFiles/Content/News,_campaigns_and_policies/Policies/Me dicines/BVA-Antibiotic-poster.pdf
- BVA 7-Point Practice Plan: https://www.bva.co.uk/uploadedFiles/Content/News,_campaigns_and_policies/Policies/Me dicines/20170928%20BVA%20Antimicrob%20poster%202017%20v1%20WEB.pdf
- BSAVA Companion Special Issue: https://www.bsavalibrary.com/docserver/fulltext/companion/2018/11/20412495.1118.8.pd f?expires=1546772848&id=id&accname=guest&checksum=201695D3773FA5D7DA5FAE7F03D0D486

Each practice should develop guidelines on the responsible use of antibiotics; these depends on the types of patients, health conditions commonly treated, specific pathogens involved, and the antimicrobial the pathogens are likely to be sensitive to. The guidelines should include:

- when antimicrobials should/ should not be prescribed
- when to undertake culture and sensitivity
- protocols for the administration of antibiotics in surgical cases.

Some antibiotics should be **used judiciously,** never as first-line agents, and only where culture and sensitivity results indicate other agents will not work. These antibiotics include fluoroquinolones (such as enrofloxacin, marbofloxacin and pradofloxacin), and third and fourth generation cephalosporins (such as cefovecin).

Antimicrobials are divided into first, second, and third choice agents.

- **First choice agents.** These are **broad-spectrum antibiotics** that cover most commonly present infections. They are appropriate for initial treatment, not necessarily based on culture and sensitivity, or may be prescribed whilst waiting for culture and sensitivity results to be returned (typically 3–5 days).
- **Second choice agents.** These are prescribed based on **culture and sensitivity results** where no first-choice treatment is available.
- **Third-choice agents.** Reserved for serious or **life-threatening infections only,** based on culture and sensitivity results and where no first or second-choice agents are available.

It is to be noted that the use of some agents is **not advised in veterinary practice.** This is because they are the last-choice agents for resistant human infections. **Such agents include imipenem and vancomycin.**

The Clinical Environment

The design, construction and layout of the hospital facilities, as well as room protocols, affect how readily the principles of infection control can be applied. The following basic design elements may not be possible due to lack of space or finance; however, the **basic principles apply to the smallest of practices.**

Basic Principles

Asepsis

Asepsis is the absence of pathogenic microbes on living tissue and is not synonymous with sterilisation (only inanimate objects can be completely sterile).

All surgical incisions are contaminated with bacteria, however elective surgical procedures should be of a standard which does not result in clinical infection and or disease. A surgical incision is therefore described as being aseptic.

Most bacterial contamination occurs at the time of surgery. Consequently, **the mainstays of aseptic technique are management of the peri- and intraoperative phases** of patient care. Whereby, an aseptic technique is defined as the principles employed to prevent cross contamination during a surgical procedure and therefore minimise contamination of a surgical wound.

The main sources of contamination in surgery are:
- theatre environment
- surgical equipment
- surgical team
- the patient.

The Hospital Environment

Areas within the clinic/hospital include:
- reception and waiting areas
- consultation rooms
- pharmacy/dispensary
- canine ward
- feline ward
- isolation ward
- utility/washing area/patient food preparation
- high dependency/intensive care ward
- staff areas (i.e. staff room/kitchen +/- on call rooms, offices)
- surgical areas (preparation rooms, induction, theatres and recovery).

Prevention of the spread of disease is paramount and should be kept in mind when designing the above areas and layout of the practice/hospital environment. This section focuses on the clinical areas, but reviewing all other areas regarding their layout, design, and the materials used is also recommended.

Wards

All wards should be easy to clean, with minimal furniture where dust could build up, as well as closed storage cupboards, washable walls, and floors with coving (to avoid build-up of dirt in cracks and crevices).

Wards should be separated into species such as canine, feline and +/-exotic small animal wards (the latter being subdivided into small mammals, raptors, and reptiles).

Kennels should be made of an **impervious and strong material,** such as stainless steel (canine kennels) or polypropylene/waterproof construction board (WCB) for cat kennels. Walk-in kennels should be lined from floor to ceiling with uPVC and all kennels ideally be fitted with glass doors for easy cleaning. Kennels should also not be placed directly facing each other.

All ward areas should be well ventilated to reduce the transmission of airborne infection.

Isolation

The isolation ward must be kept separate from all other hospitalisation areas and have its own supply of:

- water and hand washing facilities
- bedding
- personal protective equipment
- food and water bowls
- litter trays
- other consumables.

It should have its own **dedicated entrance and exit** away from the main hospital entry/exit point to allow animals to be transported to isolation without travelling through other wards/clinical areas.

It is important that the isolation ward has its **own area for canine inpatient walking,** which is away from public, staff, or other patient walking areas. This area should ideally be cordoned off and attached to the isolation area, as well as being clearly marked.

The isolation ward should have **separate heating and ventilation facilities** to the main hospital; to prevent airborne contamination and be effectively heated and cooled, to maintain patient comfort and normothermia.

Within the isolation ward should be an area for examination, treatment, and minor procedures (e.g. blood sample collection, IV catheter placement) in isolated patients. It should also have its own sink(s). Separate washing (including the use of soluble laundry bags to segregate infectious bedding) and waste disposal facilities, and the area should be easy to clean and disinfect. **Soluble laundry bags** can be used to segregate infectious washing and prevent contamination; these plastic bags dissolve in the washing machine, keeping infectious bedding contained until clean. Washing should be performed at ≥60 °C, with the addition of disinfectant at the appropriate dilution.

A separate supply of equipment, consumables, and utensils must be available, which are stored in closed cupboards, to minimise equipment on surfaces and therefore facilitate efficient cleaning/disinfection. Equipment within the isolation area should be **of single use if possible,** or if not, used only for that patient during their stay, and thoroughly disinfected before being used again.

Bedding should be colour-coded (isolation bedding separate from main ward bedding) and washed separately. In addition to separate utensils for the isolation area, the type of items used should be considered. For example, plastic food/water bowls become scratched, which can increase contamination and prevent effective disinfection. Metal bowls are effectively disinfected and autoclavable, but may be disliked by some patients, especially cats. Ceramic bowls are easy to clean and well tolerated, but if they chip or crack, they can increase contamination and become challenging to disinfect, so should be disposed of.

Waste disposal requirements differ for infectious patients. **Infectious waste must be incinerated,** unlike non-hazardous, offensive waste which can be treated before disposal in landfill. Guidance from your waste management company should be followed and appropriate bags and containers used for infectious waste: typically, orange bags, or orange-topped plastic bins. Colour coding differs depending on area and country.

Separate cleaning and disinfection equipment should also be used in barrier nursing areas, again, **colour-coded** to prevent accidental use in the main ward.

If the clinic does not have an isolation facility, then a clearly marked barrier nursing area should be setup. Marking an area on the floor with tiger tape works well, and acts as an effective visual reminder for staff.

A footbath should be placed at the entrance to the isolation/ barrier nursing area, it should contain appropriately diluted disinfectant and used any time the area is entered/exited. The **disinfectant must be changed regularly** (at least daily), to prevent organic matter reducing the efficacy of the disinfectant.

Surgical Areas

In modern veterinary practices the operating facilities vary from a single room to large multiple-theatre surgical suites. The following basic design elements may not be possible due to lack of space or finance; however, the basic principles apply to even the smallest of practices.

Surgical areas should be located where there is low traffic flow, so as to reduce contamination levels from personnel and other patients. To minimise traffic, there should be **one entrance,** and if a second entrance is required due to fire regulations, the exit should be clearly marked as for emergency use only and this precedence not abused by personnel.

Surgical Facilities

Surgical facilities should be divided into **clean and contaminated areas.**

1. **Clean areas** include:
   - operating theatres
   - scrub areas
   - instrument sterilisation
   - sterile stores
2. **Contaminated (dirty)** areas include:
   - patient preparation areas
   - changing areas
   - radiography
   - induction
   - recovery.

Both areas should be separated by a **clear divide via closed doors** to ensure and minimise the risk of contamination entering the clean area.

All surgical personnel should wear surgical attire when entering a clean area. The clean area should ideally be entered via the changing area, located between the clean and contaminated areas. If this is not possible, when in contaminated areas surgical attire should be covered with a clean coat. **Surgical footwear specifically for clean areas** should be worn.

Thought should be given to the access to radiography and the ease with which pre- and postoperative radiographs can be taken. Foot traffic should be reduced to surgical staff only and all areas easy to clean.

It should be ensured that the **operating theatre is in an end room,** with minimal furniture/fittings to avoid build-up of dust and facilitate regular thorough cleaning and disinfection. Ventilation and heating must not cause air flow which could contaminate the surgical field (i.e. fan heaters).

The preparation area should be located near theatre, and used for all anaesthetic inductions, clipping surgical sites, and initial skin disinfection. Likewise, the scrub area should be near the operating theatre but not within it, separated by swing doors for ease of surgeon movement whilst reducing contamination.

Sterile equipment should be kept in closed cupboards that are accessible from the operating theatre, but not kept within the theatre itself. Double-sided cabinets work well, which are stocked from the outside with instruments accessible from inside theatre during procedures.

Induction and Preparation Area

The induction and patient preparation room is considered part of the **contaminated area.** Depending on the number of practice staff, it should be a separate room for a quiet patient anaesthetic induction.

Separate rooms should be designated for feline and canine patient induction in order to reduce patient stress and anxiety and reduce environmental noise. Once the patients are under anaesthesia, they can be transferred to the larger preparation room.

In the preparation room, the ideal workflow involves carrying out **clean procedures first and dirty procedures last.** The room should be well equipped with appropriate materials and equipment for patient preparation and inducing/maintaining anaesthesia. It is important the **room is well lit,** with moveable spotlights an advantage for close patient examination. Tables can be fixed or mobile, with **adjustable height** for personal health and safety.

For dirty procedures, especially when copious cleaning or lavage is required, then fixed sinks or scrub tables are advantageous. When moving patients through to theatre, a height-adjustable trolley is required, with a separate trolley available in the clean area; this avoids trolley wheels transferring dust, dirt, and hair into the surgical area. If it is not possible to use a separate clean trolley, then the use of sticky floor mats helps reduce the transfer of dust and dirt.

The transition from contaminated to clean areas should be clearly marked; this can be achieved by different floor colours or floor lines.

Changing Areas, Nurses' Station, and Sterile Stores

Ideally, the **changing area(s)** should be located next to the clean area, thus allowing staff to change into surgical attire before entering the clean area. If this is not possible, scrubs should be covered with a clean (ideally disposable) coat and personnel should wear outside surgical shoes when not in clean areas. Ideally, changing areas should contain personal cleaning (i.e. showers) and convenience facilities to reduce the level of contamination into and from dirty procedures.

A **nurses' station** allows for a point of contact between the clean area and elsewhere in the practice/hospital. This facilitates the performance of administrative tasks whilst minimizing traffic in and out of the clean area of the surgical facility. Equipment should include a computer and telephone, and storage for theatre equipment manuals and surgical supplier contracts.

Storage space for sterile surgical instruments and consumables is essential. This includes providing adequate shelving for a logical arrangement of sterile kits and equipment, to facilitate finding items and stock taking. It is best to store sterile instruments and kits in closed cabinets, to extend their period of sterility. **Glass shelves and doors** allow for easy cleaning and equipment identification. Theatre pass-through cabinets, situated between the sterile corridor and theatre, allow for easy access to instruments whilst reducing traffic in and out of the operating room.

Surgical Preparation Area

Scrubbing produces water droplets which are a potential source of contamination. To prevent this, **the scrub area should be close to (but separate from) the operating area and sterile stores.** The surgical preparation area should contain a **stainless-steel sink** with taps operated by foot, knee, elbow, or infrared to allow an aseptic scrubbing technique. This is ideally positioned at **waist height** to minimize splashing. Also, beside the sink should be a supply of sterile scrub brushes and infrared or elbow operated soap dispenser. The floor around the scrub sink should be made of **non-slip anti-microbial material** in order to maximise personnel health and safety.

An area within the surgical preparation area should be set aside for aseptic gowning and gloving, which includes a clean surface away from the surgical sink. Note that with the use of timed alcohol-based hand preparation scrubbing techniques surgical sinks for surgical hand preparation are becoming outdated.

Recovery Area

All theatre and or procedure suites require a **patient recovery area,** located next to the clean area, where patients can be carefully monitored until fully recovered from anaesthesia prior to transfer to the main ward.

Each patient should have an individual heated cage, with those patients requiring intensive care transferred directly to the **intensive care unit (ICU).** Incubators are advantageous for smaller patients during recovery, as they allow ease of patient monitoring alongside control of the temperature and oxygen levels.

To reduce postoperative hypothermia the **recovery area should be warmer** than other areas of the surgical facility, at around 22–24 °C. Warming cabinets, which contain warm fluids and blankets, or patient warming blankets with an electric heating element or hot air pump, are useful to aid in patient warming.

The recovery area should be equipped with a **well-stocked crash cart and oxygen supply,** to deal with postoperative emergencies. Moreover, this area requires a higher number of nurse personnel to patients, to allow for more intensive postoperative/procedure nursing.

Operating Theatre Design

The operating theatre must be large enough to accommodate staff and the necessary surgical/ anaesthetic equipment without compromising asepsis.

Theatre Suites

Operating rooms should be:

- simple design
- avoid clutter
- avoid ledges and other areas that trap dust
- easy to clean.

The surfaces of **walls, floors and ceilings should be a non-porous, easily cleanable material** and able to withstand regular wet cleaning with harsh chemicals. Ideally walls should be covered with **PVC sheeting** as it produces the smoothest, knock resistant surface and with welded joins that are easily and effectively cleaned.

Coverings should be used where the floor meets the walls and the **floor edges curved** to prevent debris lodging in corners and for ease of cleaning. **Theatre doors should swing open both ways** to allow scrubbed personnel to move through without breaking aseptic technique, and the doors be wide enough for easy access with large patients.

Ideally there should be **no outside windows.** Any windows that are present, should be sealed to prevent opening and hence avoid contamination from the outside.

There should be **no sinks/taps within the operating theatre** itself to prevent water droplets from contaminating the sterile field. Similarly, operating theatres should not contain any drains or gullies in the floor as these acts as a source of contamination and a reservoir for bacteria.

Operating theatres should have a good supply of **grounded power outlets,** either wall or pendular mounted to ensure safety of personnel. Ideally, theatres should have piped anaesthetic gases, compressed surgical air and suction, and a scavenging system as this reduces the amount of equipment in theatre and the traffic in and out to change cylinders.

An **anaesthetic trolley is preferable** to a wall mountable anaesthetic unit. The former allows more flexibility for certain procedures, whereby the anaesthetist is moved from the head of the patient to allow the surgeon more access to the surgical site. However, a disadvantage is trolleys take up room, which makes them inappropriate in smaller theatres.

All operating and procedure rooms should contain a working wall mounted clock, flush to the wall to prevent a dust trap. Facilities to view radiographs (either digital or conventional) should also be available.

Ventilation

Within an operating theatre, one of the **aims of ventilation is to reduce airborne contamination.** This is because the air becomes laden with skin squames and respiratory droplets form theatre personnel; exchanging that contaminated air for fresh, clean air reduces the risk of particulates entering the surgical site.

All moving matter generates particles. In the operating theatre environment potential particulate sources include the movement of theatre staff, electric motors (on surgical equipment), and airflow through supply ducts. From the later the particles can include metal oxides from the duct itself or mould/spores growing within it.

There are two types of ventilation systems used in operating theatres:

1. Laminar Flow Ventilation

Laminar flow ventilation (Figure 11) creates a dust-free, abacterial air environment. Air from the room passes through a **HEPA (high-efficiency particulate air) filter** and is fed into the working chamber by a **unidirectional** vertical descending flow. This type of ventilation is expensive and contrary to previous opinion, a recent study in the Lancet (2017) concluded there was no advantage in the incidence of SSI when laminar flow ventilation was used over conventional air flow ventilation.

2. Conventional Ventilation

Operating theatres should be fitted with a **positive ventilation system (PPV)** which produces 20 air changes per hour, as each air change reduces airborne contamination by approximately 37%. The ventilation system should also use a **HEPA filter,** located close to the air supply outlet to reduce/prevent gross contaminants such as dust and insects from entering the operating theatre.

PPV systems prevent contaminated air from entering the operating theatre by producing a pressure gradient between the clean and contaminated areas of the theatre. Therefore, air which is of higher pressure in the operating theatre forces air towards the contaminated areas, which is of a lower pressure. (See Figure 12).

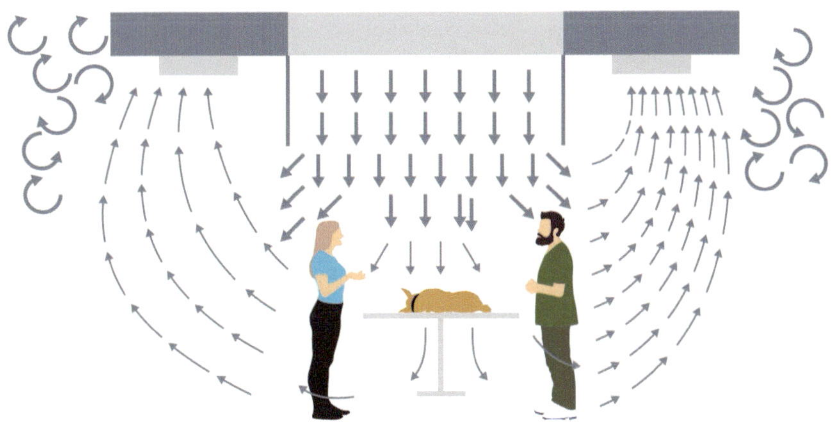

Figure 11. Laminar air flow.

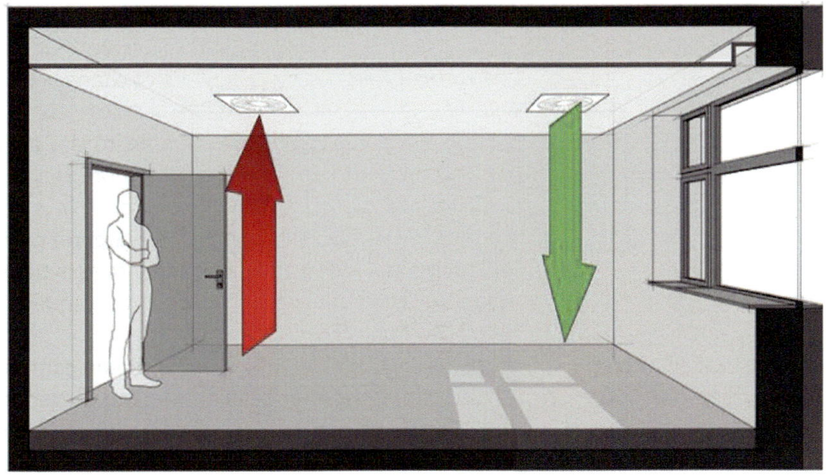

Figure 12. Conventional air ventilation.

Lighting

Good lighting is an essential part of any operating theatre, to ensure visibility of the surgical site whilst creating minimal glare and eye strain for the surgeon. **Fluorescent lights** are suitable for background lighting, accompanied by **two sets of theatre lights** directed at different angles to ensure maximum illumination of the surgical site. These lights are used for long periods of time and so should be designed to avoid emitting excessive heat which could cause tissue desiccation.

There are several different types of lamps used within operating-light fixtures:

- **Gas-filled incandescent bulbs**
  - tungsten
  - quartz gas filled incandescent lamps
  - xenon halogens
- **Light emitting diodes** (LEDs) – non-incandescent lamp.

Currently, **LEDs are the main bulbs used in surgical lights.** This is because they use less energy and produce a crisper, cooler illumination, which is uniform and reduces glare related eye strain. They can also maintain an optimal colour temperature which is important as it influences the colour and rendition of body tissue and fluids.

The **colour rendering index (CRI)** is a percentage scale that indicates how accurate a particular light source is at reproducing colours of objects faithfully in comparison with an ideal or natural light. The higher the CRI, the better the colour representation ability is. Light sources with a CRI of 85% to 90% are considered good at colour rendering. Note that **regular lighting can distort the colour and appearance of objects,** something which should be avoided during a surgical procedure.

Some operating lights have a red balance control which allows the surgical team to differentiate between tissues of similar colour (i.e. red tissue). This is achieved by adjusting the temperature of the light colour without affecting the intensity of the light.

The surgical light quality is a function of the amount of useful light within the surgical cavity; this is the balance between the amount of light and the ability to manage shadows, of which there are two types:

a. Cast shadows:
- interfere with visibility
- influenced by the surface of the light source, how light is guided towards the operating field, where it's most needed, and the number of light sources

b. Contour shadows:
- help to gauge depth and volume.

In summary, effective lighting minimizes cast shadows while enhancing contour. This is achieved with **several individual light beams,** which increases shadow dilution and improves surgeon visibility.

Some ceiling-mounted surgical lights are configured with multiple arms which can support additional surgical light heads, high-definition monitors, and high-definition video cameras. High-definition monitors provide a variety of options to connect a HD monitor to a video source or video switch.

There are two types of surgical lights, floor-standing, and ceiling mounted. Ideally, the operating theatre should be fitted with ceiling mounted as they avoid clutter in the operating room and are more easily positioned via their hinged arms. All surgical lights should be capable of being focused and equipped with removable sterile handles to allow the surgeon to adjust their position during surgical procedures.

Heating and Humidity

The ambient temperature of the operating theatre should be 20–21 °C, to provide a comfortable working environment for surgical staff whilst minimising hypothermia for the patient.

Temperatures of ≥24 °C may be more appropriate for patients prone to hypothermia, such as paediatric patients. Operating theatres should be heated via warm air through the PPV ventilation system, if this is not possible then care should be taken that other systems do not attract dust and dirt on their surfaces (e.g. radiators). Fan heaters should be avoided as they cause dust and air movement.

A **humidity regulator** ensures the humidity of the operating theatre remains between 40–60% to maximise personnel comfort and prevent environmental multiplication of bacteria.

Theatre Equipment

The amount of furniture within the operating theatre should be minimised, and it should be constructed of stainless steel and glass or an easily cleanable material that does not harbour bacteria. Ideally the operating theatre should contain:

Height Adjustable Operating Table

A **tilting table** is advantageous for certain procedures. Patient warming devices are helpful and the table should have anchor points for patient ties.

Positioning Aids

A variety of aids should be available to position patients for specific procedures. These include:

Cradles/Troughs

Troughs are an excellent way of keeping patients in dorsal recumbency, however they may limit abdominal surgery and reduce access to the thorax for thoracic surgery.

Sandbags

Clean sandbags are versatile for keeping the patient in dorsal recumbency, particularly during thoracic surgery. They may also be used as supports e.g. for the head and neck.

Vacuum Bags/Foam Cushions

Positioning aids such as foam cushions and vacuum bean bags also prevent patient injury such as neuropathies from poor support or poor cushioning.

Wipe clean bean bags conform to the patient when air is removed and maintain the position of the patient. However, these can puncture easily, and the air valve can be accidently knocked and opened during surgery, and/or limit patient repositioning during the procedure.

Ties

Ties help secure the patient in position and prevent movement with tilting/moving of the table, however these require careful use to prevent neuropathies and circulation issues.

Extension Arms

For orthopaedic procedures some veterinary surgeons find extension arms preferable to support the patient's limbs, especially if they do not have a scrubbed assistant.

Extension arms are beneficial during surgery on larger patients as they support/prevent forelimbs/hindlimbs from hanging off the surgery table, which may compromise blood flow to these limbs.

To prevent cross-contamination positioning aids should be impermeable, easily cleanable, and designated to theatre and thus kept separate from other poisoning aids in other parts of the practice/hospital.

Basic/Advanced Anaesthetic Monitoring Equipment

This depends on the type of procedure planned for the particular operating theatre, but includes capnography, echocardiography (ECG) and pulse oximetry. Other anaesthetic equipment includes fluid/drug administration devices such as fluid pumps and syringe drivers.

Stainless Steel Instrument Trolleys

There are many different types of instrument trolleys on the market. The type of trolley used depends on the procedure, must be easily cleanable, and specific to the operating room. i.e. not removed from the operating suite. More than one trolley may be needed in the operating room.

Patient-warming Facilities

Many types of patients warming devices are available, such as a circulating warm-water bed, circulating warm-air blanket (i .e . Bair hugger™), or a semi-conductive polymeric fabric that delivers safe and effective heat to the patient (i.e. Hot dog™). **Care should be taken when using electric heat pads as there is a higher risk of causing thermal burns to the immobile patient.**

Patient warming devices help reduce patient hypothermia during anaesthesia and there may be need for more than one type depending on the patient and procedure being performed.

Patients undergoing body cavity surgery (thoracic or abdominal) are often warmed with lavage solution at the end of the procedure, and a fluid warming cabinet is a practical way to store preheated sterile fluid bags/bottles for this purpose.

Surgical Suction

It is essential surgical suction is available with its many applications: removing effusions, lavage, clearing the surgical field of blood, and clearing fluid/secretions from the oral/respiratory tract. A variety of different end piece attachments for the suction are useful for the evacuation of different regions.

Diathermy

Diathermy, also called electro- diathermy, electrocautery, or vascular coagulation; is used to either **cut or destroy tissue or to coagulate vessels of less than 1.5–2 mm in diameter.**

Diathermy uses a high frequency (approximately 0.5–3 MHz) of radio-wave electrical current which alternates in polarity. The radio frequencies generated by the diathermy unit heat the tissue to create intracellular oscillation of cellular molecules.

The high frequencies used do not interfere with the lower electrical currents generated via cardiac and skeletal muscles of the patient, therefore the natural electrical physiology of the patient is unaffected by its use.

Different temperatures result in either cutting or coagulation of the tissue.

Coagulation

- Occurs when the cells dehydrate, at temperatures of between 60–99 °C.
- Consists of short surges of radio-frequency electrical current at a low power which produces enough heat to dry out the tissues (**desiccation**) slowly and hence does not produce any electrical sparks. Thus, leading to coagulation.
- When higher voltage of electrical current is used, **fulguration** (destruction) of tissues occurs as the higher power creates sparks which cause the intermittent heating of tissues so that the cells dry out faster, rather than burst due to steam.

Cutting

- Takes place when tissue vaporises, and occurs at temperatures of approximately 100 °C.
- Consists of a continuous waveform at a low voltage, but a higher current than that used for coagulation. This

- creates a high density of current in a focal area of tissue for a short time. The intense localised heat causes the cells to explode and vaporise and produces a clean cut of the tissue.
- Please note there is also a mixed (or blend) mode. This is a combination of both coagulation and cutting, which is used when haemostasis is required as the tissues are cut.

There are two types of diathermy, both of which require the electrical circuit to be complete.

1. Monopolar

The electrical current oscillates between the surgeon's electrode and the grounding/earthing plate, via the patient's body. The grounding/earthing plate is positioned underneath the patient to complete the circuit and ideally positioned as close to the surgical site as possible ensuring good contact with the patient.

It is essential there is **good contact between the patient and the ground plate** when monopolar diathermy is in use. A decreased surface area of patient contact can result in the patient acquiring **electrical burns.** For this reason, the earthing plate should not be positioned over a bony prominence, metal prosthesis, distal to a tourniquet, over scar tissue, on hairy surfaces, or on pressure points and **kept as dry as possible.** (See further information later in the chapter).

2. Bipolar

In bipolar diathermy the **current is passed between electrodes** which are located on the handpiece itself and used in tandem. Hence, limiting the need for a dispersive electrode and earthing plate. This is advantageous in microsurgery and in the few veterinary patients with pacemakers. Traditional bipolar cautery can be used for coagulation but not for making surgical incisions. (See further information later in the chapter).

Cleaning and Disinfection

An effective cleaning and disinfection protocol is vital for the management of pathogenic microorganisms which could cause nosocomial infections. This requires a knowledge of:

- disinfectant chemicals
- effective cleaning procedures (in both clinical and surgical areas)
- instrument reprocessing
- processes for removing microorganisms
- an understanding of biofilms.

It is important to distinguish between the **terms sterilisation, disinfection, asepsis, antisepsis, and cleaning,** which are fundamental in the surgical setting.

Therefore, the following definitions apply:

Sepsis: presence of pathogens and their toxic products in the tissues of a patient.

Asepsis: absence of pathogenic microbes in living tissues.

Antiseptic: agent that either kills pathogenic microorganisms or inhibits their growth, whilst the two remain in contact. Term reserved for agents that are applied to the body.

Disinfectant: germicidal or biocide chemical substance which kills microorganisms on inanimate objects outright. These chemicals are usually too caustic to be used on living tissue without causing cellular damage but are used to clean surfaces.

High-level disinfectant: a disinfectant that has the capacity to achieve sterilization if an increased exposure time is used.

Disinfection: removal of microorganisms but not necessarily their spores.

Sterilisation: complete elimination of microbial viability, including both vegetative forms of bacteria and spores. This may be achieved by either physical or chemical means.

Aseptic technique: is a set of specific practices and procedures performed to make equipment and areas free from all microorganisms and to maintain that sterility. (i.e. for a surgical procedure).

Biofilms

Biofilms are defined as: **communities of microorganisms attached to a surface, or one another, and encased within a matrix of extracellular polymeric substance which provides them with protection, and resistance to disinfectants and antimicrobials.**

The largest component of a biofilm is the **extracellular polymeric substance,** and this accounts for 80% of the biomatrix volume. The biological environment is generally composed of polysaccharides, proteins, glycolipids, blood products, cellular debris, extracellular enzymes, metal ions, and extracellular DNA; this physical and chemical configuration determines the characteristics and properties of the biofilm.

It was thought that bacteria exist in a planktonic state as individual organisms. However, it has been shown that bacteria accumulate on a wide range of surfaces in **inactive communities.**

Research has shown (National Institute of Health, 2002) that **biofilms are responsible for over 80% of microbial infections**

in patients. This is because they grow on biological tissue (e.g. tooth plaque) and on implanted medical devices such as orthopaedic implants and catheters. **Biofilms thrive upon moist or wet surfaces** and all the above surfaces are "periodically or continuously suffused with water". However, multiple environmental conditions determine the extent to which a biofilm grows. These factors also determine whether the biofilm is made of only a few layers of cells or significantly more.

A biofilm can survive in environments for millions of years, as there is fossil evidence of biofilms that date back 3.25 billion years.

The proximity of the different species of microorganisms enables:

- substrate exchange
- distribution of metabolic products
- removal of toxic end products
- protection from antimicrobials
- protection from shear forces
- protection from the host's immune system.

For this reason, biofilm formation is a great cause of concern **because bacteria within a biofilm are more resistant to antimicrobials and disinfectants** used to control them.

There are **four main stages of biofilm formation** (Figure 13):

1. initial reversible attachment to a surface
2. irreversible attachment to a surface (formation of a monolayer and matrix production)
3. irreversible attachment to a surface (formation of the multilayer "microcolony")
4. maturation dispersion.

Disinfection

Disinfection is the killing of all pathogens (except bacterial spores) that may result in infection on an inanimate object/surface (non-living) and is generally achieved chemically.

Antisepsis is the process of removal of pathogenic organisms from animate objects (living), such as the skin and mucous membranes but with some resident flora remaining.

Both processes may not eliminate all microorganisms because some viruses and bacterial spores are not inactivated by disinfection alone. Thus, bacterial numbers are reduced to a level that can be controlled by the patient's immune system should there be a break in the patient's normal protective barrier (i-e. skin).

Disinfectants and Antiseptics

Both antiseptics and disinfectants are nonselective, anti-infective agents, which are **topically applied to surfaces.** Their activity ranges from reducing the number of microorganisms to safe levels, to destroying all microorganisms on the surface to which they are applied. Generally, antiseptics are applied to tissues to reduce or prevent microbial infection.

Many different disinfectant agents are available, with different indications for different products. The properties of the ideal disinfectant include:

- broad-spectrum activity
- fast acting

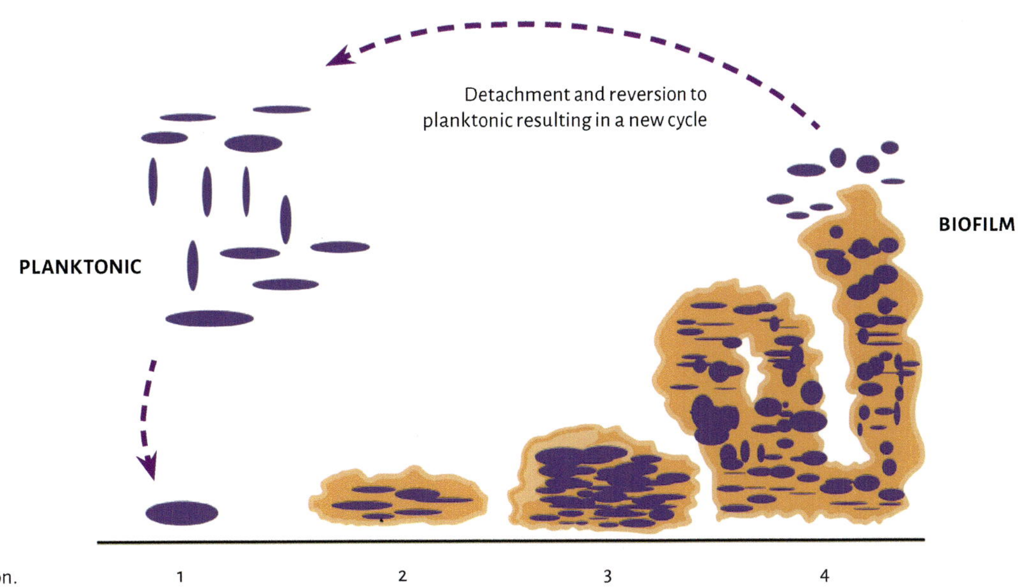

Figure 13. Biofilm formation.

- not affected by environmental factors
- nontoxic
- environmentally friendly
- wide surface compatibility
- odourless
- soluble and stable in nature
- easy to use
- environmentally friendly
- economical.

Areas to consider when selecting a disinfectant include:
- the potential pathogens against which it is effective
- the range of activity
- contact time
- cost of the product
- compatibility with other chemicals
- toxicity to staff or animals.

Examining the health and safety information, and manufacturer's product data sheets helps when selecting an appropriate product for a particular clinic. There are several chemical disinfectant groups.

Disinfectant Groups

1. Alcohols (e.g. Surgical Spirit™)

For alcohols to be effective at destroying microorganisms they must be able to pass through cell membranes. Therefore, **alcohols are most effective when diluted in distilled water.**

A mixture of 70% ethanol and 30% distilled water or isopropanol alcohol is effective against a broad spectrum of bacteria; however, higher concentrations are often needed to disinfect wet surfaces.

Alcohols are flammable and not effective on areas which have been soiled with organic matter.

2. Quaternary Ammonium Compounds (Quats)

- inexpensive
- fast acting
- broad-spectrum
- quats can be formulated with a variety of detergents to provide both cleaning and disinfecting ability
- combined with alcohol are effective against non-enveloped virus
- are positively charged (cation) surface active agents
- bactericidal and virucidal (mainly enveloped viruses)
- destroy cell membranes.

3. Chlorine Compounds (halogen-based biocides, e.g. Falcon™/ Swift™/bleach)

These are comprised of an aqueous solution of chlorine, hypochlorite, or hypochlorous acid (e.g. household bleach) and are **effective against bacteria and viruses** (including resistant) at concentrations of <1 ppm. They are also fast acting, inexpensive, irritant, corrosive, and cause discoloration of surfaces.

Because of their oxidizing power, they **lose potency quickly** and should be made fresh and used within the same day as preparation. They can also produce chlorine gas (toxic) when mixed with acid solutions.

4. Aldehydes (e.g. Anigene HLD4V™)

Formaldehyde and glutaraldehyde (mainly used):
- wide range of microbiocidal activity
- sporicidal
- fungicidal
- partly inactivated by organic matter
- a slight residual activity
- can cause health issues (e.g. asthma associated with glutaraldehyde)
- some bacterial resistance (i.e. glutaraldehyde)
- biocidal action is through alkylation of carboxyl, hydroxyl and sulfhydryl groups on proteins
- formaldehyde has an irritating odour and is carcinogenic.

5. Iodophors (halogen-based biocides, e.g. Betadine™)

- both an antiseptic and disinfectant
- a combination of iodine and a solubilizing agent
- needs to be made up in cold water to prevent breakdown of the disinfectant
- stains surfaces
- penetrates the cell walls and membranes of microorganisms and interferes with DNA synthesis.

6. Phenolic Compounds (e.g. Jayes Fluid™)

- carbonic acid derivatives (Phenol)
- act through membrane damage
- effective against enveloped viruses, rickettsiae, fungi, vegetative bacteria and pathogenic bacteria including mycobacterium
- more active in the presence of organic material
- toxic and corrosive
- may damage surfaces
- may have disposal restrictions
- used in both antiseptics and disinfectants
- acts by denaturing and coagulating proteins
- are protoplasmic toxic.

7. Oxidising Agents

Act by oxidising the cell membrane, resulting in the loss of cell structure, cell lysis and death. Examples include ozone, hydrogen peroxide and potassium permanganate:
- highly effective when combined with other chemicals
- used as antiseptics and as disinfectants.

8. Accelerated Hydrogen Peroxide (e.g. Oxivir®)

- broad spectrum
- fast acting
- sustainable
- safe
- contains surfactants
- patented synergistic blend of safe chemicals, which when combined at low levels dramatically increase the germicidal potency of hydrogen peroxide.

Disinfectant Use

Treatment of inert surfaces and heat labile materials can be accomplished using disinfectants, provided the following factors are considered:

- type and level of microbial contamination
- concentration of active ingredient
- duration of contact between disinfectant and item to be disinfected
- pH
- temperature
- humidity
- presence of organic matter or soil load.

> **Common pitfalls of disinfection include:**
>
> - **Eyeballing dilutions instead of measuring them:** the manufacturer's instructions should always be followed, and dilutions measured out. If a solution is too weak, the efficacy may be inadequate. If it is too strong, the product is wasted.
> - **Not reaching the required contact time:** the surface should be kept wet with disinfectant for the full contact time, as advised by the manufacturer. Wiping the area immediately after cleaning with a dry cloth reduces contact times and should be avoided.
> - **Not knowing the shelf-life of the agent:** it is important to always check how long, once diluted, the solution is effective for, and change diluted solutions at the recommended interval.
> - **Topping up bottles of solution** instead of replacing them and mixing old and new solutions can lead to an over-diluted or inactivated mixture, which will not work effectively .
> - **Mixing chemicals:** this carries a potentially dangerous risk of chemical interactions, plus the risk of one chemical inactivating the other.

Disinfectants are used alone or in combination (e.g. hydrogen peroxide and peracetic acid). Commercial formulations based on these chemicals are considered the unique product.

No one product is suitable for use in all practices and across all situations, and the decision of which product/s to use is influenced by the practice environment, the caseload, and the surfaces and equipment requiring disinfection. Typically, these agents may be used at a lower concentration in low-risk areas, and a **higher concentration in high-risk areas;** it is vitally **important to check the dilution rates** advised by the manufacturer and ensure appropriate dilutions are used in each area, based on a risk assessment.

Once an appropriate agent has been selected, it is important to **ensure it is used correctly.**

Cleaning

High and Low-risk Areas

To prevent nosocomial infections, it is important all staff understand the **cleaning protocols and processes involved within each clinical area,** and **who is responsible** for cleaning these areas and the equipment contained therein.

When considering a cleaning and disinfection protocol for the clinic, **a risk assessment should be performed for each area.**

- **High-risk items include hand-touch areas** such as telephones, keyboards, switches, door handles, touch-operated hand disinfectant pumps, kennels and kennel equipment, spray bottles, thermometers, infusion pumps, floors, examination tables, and surgical tables.
- **Low-risk areas** include walls, blinds, windows, doors, ceilings, extractor fans, and air conditioning units.

This information should be used to develop specific cleaning and disinfection protocols for each room of the hospital. It is important to include non-clinical areas, such as offices and the staff room, in these protocols in addition to clinical areas.

Take the feline ward area in a practice for example. For each item identify whether it is of high or low risk for pathogenic transmission (Table 3).

A range of detailed clinic disinfection guidelines (for each room in the clinic) are available on the Bella Moss Foundation website: https://www.thebellamossfoundation.com/practice-guidelines.

Cleaning equipment should be colour-coded (Table 4) throughout the hospital and used only for specific areas, and isolation should have its own supply. A separate practice cleaning and disinfection protocol should exist for the isolation area, compared with the main hospitalisation areas.

Table 3. High and low risk areas within a veterinary practice.

Item	Risk	Frequency	How to clean
Bowls/ cutlery	High	After each use	Detergent then disinfectant
Leads	High	Used per patient – after discharge	Washing machine
Bedding	High	After each use	See laundry protocol
Door handle	High	Once a day or when soiled	Disinfectant, disposable cloth
Kennel	High	Twice a day or when soiled	Detergent then disinfectant
Floors	High	Between procedures/spot clean, full clean SID	Vacuum then clean mop head
Walls	Low	Spot clean, wash down SID	Vacuum, disposable cloth
Windows	Low	Clean weekly, dusty daily	Glass cleaner/ duster

Table 4. Example of colour coding system for cleaning equipment in clinical areas.

Colour of cleaning equipment	Area	Rooms
Yellow	Front-of-house	Reception, pharmacy, waiting areas and consultation rooms.
Blue	Hospitalisation	Dog and cat wards, treatment, laundry/utility and grooming/ bathing areas.
Green	Surgical non-sterile	Preparation and imaging rooms.
Orange	Surgical sterile	Scrub area, theatre and instrument processing rooms.
Red	Isolation	Isolation ward.
Purple	Chemotherapy	Chemotherapy areas: administration room and kennelling of patients receiving chemotherapy.
Black	ICU	Intensive care units and emergency rooms.

Laundry

Bedding acts as a fomite and ineffective laundering of contaminated bedding is a source of infection in veterinary practice. Ideally, laundry used for infectious cases is restricted to single-use, disposable items; however, this is not economical, and risks reduced comfort for the patient if only incontinence pads or newspaper are used. A protocol for managing bedding in the hospital should therefore be established.

All washable items should be separated into categories:

- surgical items (drapes, scrubs, gowns, hats, and shoes)
- routine non-infectious bedding
- isolation or infectious bedding
- mop heads and cleaning equipment.

Each category should be laundered separately and where possible a different washing machine and tumble dryer should be used for surgical items. Soluble laundry bags (which dissolve in the washing machine) can also be used to separate washing.

Prior to laundering contaminated bedding, any physical soiling (e.g. solid faecal matter) should be manually removed and the items presoaked in bleach solution (1-part bleach to 9 parts warm water for 15 minutes) to facilitate effective cleaning and disinfection.

Appropriate personal protective equipment should be worn whilst handling the bedding; the exact PPE items required depend on the suspected pathogen and route of transmission. Gloves should be worn as a minimum in all cases of laundry handling, with gowns, masks and eye protection required when handling infectious bedding. Hands should be washed after handling of any contaminated laundry.

Bedding should be laundered at a temperature above 71.1 °C to ensure effective disinfection. Most household/domestic machines do not reach this temperature, even on a hot wash setting, and a commercial washing machine is required.

Ideally, the washing machine cycle maintains a temperature above 65 °C for 10 minutes and above 71 °C for 3 minutes. **When laundering specific materials that require a cold wash, a disinfectant detergent solution** should be used, which is approved for cold-water use. Disinfectant should be added to infectious waste cycles.

In addition to cleaning the bedding, **the washing machine must be appropriately cleaned and maintained,** as organic material impairs cleaning and disinfection of bedding. The seals and detergent drawer should be regularly cleaned and disinfected, and a hygiene cycle run at least weekly.

Following washing, **tumble drying is an essential step** of laundry management. Dryers should be operated on the hottest possible temperature, as the heat from drying is another important method of infection control, reducing bacterial counts on the items within. Ideally, all items should be machine dried.

The exposure to UV-light in hang-dried items is beneficial for infection control, but as direct sunlight exposure to the entire item surface is required, this is often an ineffective method compared with tumble drying.

Theatre Cleaning

To ensure a **gold standard of aseptic technique, a thorough cleaning protocol should be established and closely monitored.** Before the procedure list is started each day, **all clinical surfaces should be damp dusted** (not dry dusted as this merely moves the dust) with a dilute disinfectant solution.

Operating theatres must have their own easily designated cleaning utensils which are colour coded and stored away from the theatres but within the clean area of the surgical suite/facility. Surfaces should be cleaned with paper towel or disposable cloths which are lint free and disposed of after each use. Each day the **mop heads should go through a hot wash** and be dry before storing to reduce microbial growth.

Between cases the table, equipment, and floor (if soiled) **should be thoroughly cleaned.** All surfaces should be scrubbed and cleaned with disinfectant, including all items that came in contact with the patient (e.g. BP cuffs, stethoscopes, thermometers etc.).

Decontamination must precede disinfection for the disinfectant chemicals to work effectively; this is because organic matter inhibits their action. All gross contamination should be removed with disposable cloths which are discarded after use.

A **broad-spectrum disinfectant solution should be used, at the correct dilution and contact time,** which also has detergent properties that remove organic debris and is active against a range of contaminants, including *Pseudomonas spp.*

All clinical waste bags generated by each procedure should be removed and labelled with the theatre list number, so that any issues relating to that surgery can be easily checked.

At the end of the surgery day, all equipment and furniture should be removed from theatre so as to efficiently clean and disinfect the walls, ceilings, floors, doors, and lights. All surfaces of equipment and furniture, including any joints and undersides should be cleaned and disinfected. Wheeled equipment/furniture should be wheeled through a disinfectant-soaked mat to ensure all wheeled surfaces are thoroughly disinfected. All floors should be carefully swept with a microfibre brush before being cleaned and disinfected.

Every week there should be a thorough cleaning session when all equipment is removed from the room. All walls and ceilings should be thoroughly cleaned, and floors scrubbed with a rotary cleaner. All equipment, including the operating table, should receive similar meticulous cleaning. Ventilation grills should be vacuumed to remove accumulated dust. Ideally, **an airborne disinfectant** is used after each weekly clean. These cleaning schedules should be logged as part of the clinical governance records.

Environmental Testing

Ideally, environmental microbial testing should be performed regularly, particularly if there is an increase in postoperative surgical site infections.

The appropriate number of swabs should be collected, and the interval at which this is done is determined based on the individual clinic, caseload, and incidence of infection seen, balancing the additional cost of the associated laboratory fees with the risk of infection.

Environmental swabs should be collected after the treatment of/cleaning after patients with multi-drug resistant infections. This is to ensure environmental eradication. Other key areas to consider for swab collection include the surgical suites and wards.

Hygiene auditing is easily achievable through apps such as the Bella Moss Foundation's "Practice Hygiene Self-Audit" tool. This tool allows practices to objectively assess and compare the general cleanliness of their clinic. The tool assesses each room in the hospital, and generates a score for each, highlighting specific rooms or areas to work on. Areas assessed are:

- equipment
- waste disposal
- laundry facilities
- hand hygiene
- cleaning instructions.

Instrument Reprocessing

Many surgical instruments are composed of stainless steel and subsequently contain a certain amount of chromium, which increases resistance to corrosion (as all steel corrodes under particular conditions). This layer requires maintenance to protect the instrument and ensure the longevity of instrument use.

Surgical instruments, such as scissors, must be hard enough to take and keep a cutting edge or have a certain spring in the case of artery forceps. The steel which has these characteristics contains more carbon than chromium and consequently has an increased likelihood of staining and corroding.

The exposed surfaces of stainless-steel instruments are protected by a thin layer of chromium oxide (when chromium within the steel reacts with oxygen in the air). Processes which physically or chemically remove this protective layer of chromium oxide result in staining and corrosion (rusting) of the instrument. Therefore, protecting the chromium layer is paramount in preventing instrument corrosion and consequently increasing the instrument's useful lifetime.

The chromium layer increases with age, so new instruments are at increased risk of corrosion and damage, compared to older instruments. Protection and maximisation of this layer is achieved through appropriate handling and use, cleaning, processing, and sterilisation; products such as stainless-steel conditioners can also be used as part of the instrument preparation process to maintain the condition of instruments.

All surgical instruments should be handled carefully and only used for their designed purpose. There are seven steps in instrument reprocessing:

- preparation/preprocessing
- cleaning and disinfection
- visual inspection and lubrication
- care and repair
- packaging
- sterilisation
- storage.

Regardless of the technique used, first all instruments and surgical equipment should be cleaned to remove all gross contaminants ensure the efficiency of the sterilization process itself.

Therefore, instruments and equipment must undergo the cleaning cycle detailed (Figure 14) to decrease the risk of them becoming a fomite contributing to contamination in the direct and indirect transmission process of pathogenic microorganisms.

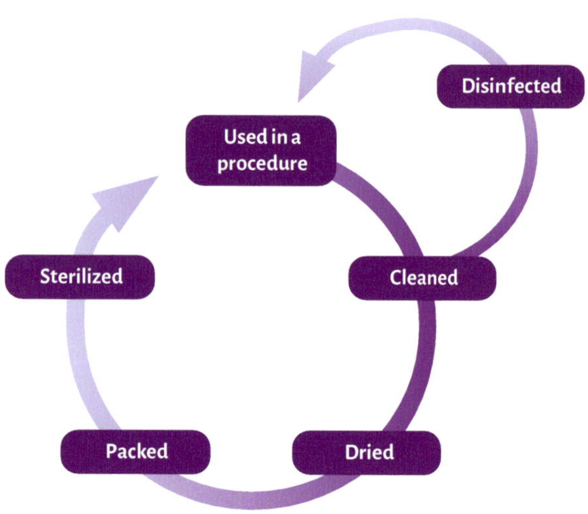

Figure 14. Instrument processing cycle.

Cleaning

Cleaning is the physical removal/reduction of surface contaminants such as dust, soil and organic matter (i.e. blood, faeces and vomit) using water and detergent and is an important prior step to disinfection. Failure to remove surface debris adequately impacts on the effectiveness of subsequent disinfection and sterilisation by creating a biofilm over the item's surface . In other words, creating a physical barrier that protects microorganisms or by inactivating the disinfectant or sterilant used.

It is imperative that instruments are cleaned as soon as possible after use, either manually and/or by an ultrasonic cleaner.

A. Precleaning

Preparation or preprocessing is the precleaning process and should take place **immediately after instruments are used** (at maximum, within 10 minutes).

After use, **instruments should be rinsed in cold water,** this prevents plasma proteins coagulating on the surface of the instrument and makes it easier to remove blood. Alternatively, before manual or mechanical cleaning, instruments can be soaked in warm water which contains an effective enzyme cleaner.

Stainless steel is not technically stainless (despite the name) and dried blood leads to staining and rusting of instruments, reducing their lifespan, and risking contamination.

All articulated instruments should be opened to allow access to box joints and ratchets.

Next, **instruments should be separated according to material** (to ensure different metals are cleaned separately), and soaked in warm water (not hot water, which causes blood and fluid to coagulate, complicating the cleaning process). Commercial pretreatment products are available containing surfactants and enzymatic agents, which can be used at this time to stop soiling from drying onto the instrument.

B. Manual Cleaning

Following soaking, instruments should be scrubbed in warm water and **an appropriate neutral pH instrument cleaning solution.** Chlorine-containing solutions such as saline or chlorhexidine, and dishwashing agents should not be used as they cause corrosion of the stainless steel as they are too alkaline and damage the instrument surface.

Soft nylon brushes are best to remove adherent materials. In some cases, such as orthopaedic instruments (i.e. burrs and drills) more aggressive cleaning is required. In this case a soft brass or stainless-steel brush can be used. Wire wool or DIY wire brushes should be avoided at all costs as this scratch and damage the surface allowing for the adherence of moisture and thus corrosion.

Instruments with a lumen (e.g. suction tips), should first be flushed with water and then cleaned with a pipe cleaner or small bottle brush. Finally, the lumen is flushed with air to remove any water droplets prior to packing.

C. Ultrasonic Cleaning

Following scrubbing, instruments should be rinsed with tap water for three minutes.

Ideally, instruments are placed into **an ultrasonic cleaner for 10 minutes at 50 °C.** This process is up to 16 times more effective than manual cleaning and uses a method known as micro-cavitation (the ultrasound causes formation of billions of tiny bubbles hitting the surface of each instrument) to effectively clean. This results in faster cleaning and removes any debris that is not reached by manual brushing alone, particularly in hard-to-reach areas.

> Note: **Ultrasonic cleaners should not be used for sharp instruments** **as this may cause them to become blunt more quickly.**

In the ultrasonic cleaner an appropriate enzymatic instrument cleaning solution should be used at the appropriate dilution, and for the correct contact time, according to the manufacturer's guidelines. The manufacturer's instructions should also be followed for ultrasonic devices to determine the optimal cycle run time.

To avoid instrument damage, heavy instruments are placed at the bottom of the cleaner with lighter more delicate instruments at the top. Instruments should be thoroughly rinsed in clean warm water and then left to air dry. They should be laid flat and fully opened to ensure effective drying.

Automatic Washers/Disinfectors (AWD)

Automatic washers come in various sizes and at a range of prices. It is recommended that **all surgical instruments (suitable to go in a washer) are indeed washed in an automated washer disinfector (AWD).** A well-designed AWD can clean surgical instruments effectively and is energy and water efficient. Automated washers for medical devices are very different to a dishwasher; programmed and validated with specialized, controlled cycles based on the medical devices being cleaned.

There are various phases of program cycles which run at different temperatures, dispensing appropriate water levels and chemicals at specific concentrations. Automatic washers are designed with special spray arms which dispense water and cleaning chemicals at the correct pressure and times to provide the required mechanical action to remove organic matter. The force of the water spray used on instruments (impingement value) is an important factor for effective cleaning and it is therefore important to check the spray nozzles for blockages as well as ensuring the spray arms are free to rotate.

For efficient and effective cleaning in an automated washer disinfector the following points should always be considered:

- instrument trays should not be overloaded;
- all hinged instruments should be open;
- trays used in the washer should be meshed and allow for water penetration;
- hollow items should be loaded upside down;
- the correct rack configuration for items in the load should be used.

D. Rinsing and Drying

Once the cleaning cycle is complete (with any of the cleaning methods mentioned), the instruments are removed from the bath and rinsed thoroughly using distilled water (not tap water) to reduce ionic charges which may cause corrosion.

If chemical disinfection is required (e.g. for items which cannot be autoclaved), they should be soaked in instrument disinfectant solution at the appropriate dilution and contact time, before rinsing with sterile water prior to use (not saline, as the chloride content can cause instrument corrosion).

Following cleaning, items should be dried thoroughly. Air drying of instruments can lead to water spotting and corrosion and is best avoided. Instead, a lint-free wipe can be used to manually dry each instrument.

E. Care/repair, Lubrication, and Inspection

Prior to packaging, individual items should be inspected visually. Paying close attention to any damage or remnants of debris/dirt. In particular:

a. the cutting edges: cutting edges should be free of damage;
b. teeth: there should be no missing teeth;
c. jaws: should meet with no twisting;
d. thumbscrews: thumbscrews should be tight; and
e. box joints: inspect for any cracks.

After the inspection, **leave any box joints and ratchets open** and mark any damaged instruments (for example, using plastic instrument tags) for disposal or repair. If repair is indicated, thoroughly decontaminate, and sterilise the items as normal prior to sending for repair.

To maintain the quality of the instrument and to facilitate the movement of the box joint, **individual instruments should be lubricated** prior to packing. This is an essential part of reprocessing and should be performed after each instrument use.

A variety of **instrument lubricants** are available, including an instrument milk in which to bathe items, lubricating sprays, and oils. When applying instrument lubricant, follow the manufacturer's guidelines, and keep sprays away from sources of oxygen.

Specialist Equipment

Some items commonly used in clinics have their own reprocessing considerations such as rigid endoscopes and powered surgical equipment.

1. Rigid Endoscopes

Rigid endoscopes do not require leak testing and their reprocessing requirements are simpler to that of flexible endoscopes. They are cleaned using an enzymatic cleaner, their working channels brushed, and manually flushed for the appropriate contact time. They should then be rinsed in distilled water and dried thoroughly, before being ethylene oxide sterilised. Some rigid scopes can be autoclaved on a lower heat cycle – check with the equipment manufacturer (it is also often written on the endoscope itself) before autoclaving the item. If neither autoclave or EtO (Ethylene oxide) sterilisation is possible, then the endoscope should be soaked in instrument disinfectant and rinsed with sterile water immediately prior to use.

2. Powered Equipment

Powered surgical equipment typically includes air or battery-powered orthopaedic equipment such as saws, drills, and burrs. Usually, these items cannot be soaked in any solutions or water; prior to cleaning, always follow the manufacturer's guidelines to prevent water-associated damage. In many cases, removal of all attachments (e.g. drill chucks) followed by thorough cleaning of the external surfaces, lubrication of moving parts, and sterilisation is recommended. Some items are autoclavable at a lower temperature, whereas others are only suitable for ethylene oxide sterilisation. In some cases, orthopaedic drills and saws are neither submersible nor autoclavable; in these cases, an autoclavable cover is used to maintain sterility through the procedure, and careful handling of the item whilst the surgeon wraps it is indicated, to prevent surgical field contamination.

Packing and Sterilization

Packing, sterilisation, and storage are important steps in the reprocessing procedure of surgical equipment. Undertaking these three steps incorrectly increases the risk of breaking aseptic technique and the risk of surgical site infections.

Packing

Once items are cleaned, dried, and inspected, those requiring sterilisation should be wrapped in packaging appropriate for the sterilisation process (Table 5).

Table 5. Method of sterilization and associated appropriate wrapping material.

Method of sterilisation	Wrapping material
EtO	Muslin cotton, paper, polypropylene fabric, polyethylene, paper/Mylar®, Tyvek®/Mylar®
Steam	Muslin cotton, paper, polypropylene fabric, polyethylene, paper/Mylar®
H_2O_2 gas plasma	Tyvek®/Mylar®, polypropylene

Instruments are either packed individually or grouped into kits for specific procedures, depending on their intended surgical use. Packing instruments enhances the ease of sterilisation and aids in the preservation of sterility.

A variety of materials are used to pack a surgical instrument. The packaging material must be a barrier to microbes to prevent contamination of instruments within the pack itself. It must also have sufficient permeability for the method of sterilisation and be non-reactive to the sterilant. Ideally, the material should durable, non-linting, and easy to handle (Table 6).

Table 6. Characteristics of wrapping materials.

Characteristic	Goal
Barrier effectiveness	Ability to prevent microbial penetration and maintain sterility of surgical pack and prevents penetration of liquids.
Penetrability (steam)	Allows steam to penetrate.
Penetrability	Allows sterilising gases or plasmas to penetrate.
Aeration	Allows aeration poststerilisation.
Ease of use	Easy to use by personnel.
Drapeability	Conforms to equipment pack contours smoothly and closely.
Flexibility	Enough sizes to accommodate any size or shaped item.
Puncture resistance	Resists punctures.
Tear strength	Resists tears.
Toxicity	Nontoxic.
Odour	No odour.
Waste disposal	Adheres to local and state solid waste disposal rules.
Linting	Minimal linting during use.
Cost	Low cost to use.
Transparency	Allows verification of pack´s internal contents before opening the pack.

There are several choices of method to maintain sterility of surgical instruments:

- rigid containers;
- peel-open pouches (e.g. self-sealed or heat-sealed plastic and paper pouches);
- roll stock or reels (i.e. paper-plastic combinations of tubing designed to allow the user to cut and seal the ends to form a pouch);
- sterilization wraps (woven and non-woven).

Originally sterilisation wraps were 140-thread count muslin cloth. These were advantageous because they were soft, reusable, inexpensive, absorbent, and have good drapability. However, the woven openings between the threads were larger than most microorganisms and thus the fabric did not provide an adequate microbial barrier. The introduction of polypropylene allowed the development of wraps that possessed strength, formed a barrier, and had repellent properties.

The most common material used for instrument kit wrapping today is **polypropylene paper** for its ability to withstand high temperatures particularly under steam sterilisation. Also popular are a combination of textiles, non-woven, laminated film pouches, and paper bags.

Plastic pouches consist of one side made from a non-permeable PVC or polyester (Mylar®) and the other side from a newer material known as Tyvek®, which is a form of polyethylene fibres which are more resistant to microbial penetration.

Table 7. Advantages and disadvantages of surgical instrument wrapping materials.

Material	Sterilisation method suitable for	Advantage	Disadvantage
Cotton muslin	Steam and EtO	· Reusable · Easily handled	· Double wrapping required · Not waterproof
Paper	Steam and EtO	· Inexpensive	· Double wrapping required · Not waterproof
Polypropylene fabric	Steam, EtO, H_2O_2	· Extremely durable · Resistant to damage	· Single-use · Double wrapping required
Pouch	Steam (only paper/Mylar®), EtO, H_2O_2, gas plasma	· Water-resistant · Single wrap · Long shelf life	· The pouch may be punctured by instruments

This makes the pouches more repellent to liquid, durable, and transparent making it easier to view the contents directly, whilst remaining permeable to gaseous sterilant.

Pouches are usually used for single instruments or small kits, with **paper drapes used to wrap larger surgical kits** for more complex surgeries.

Wrapping Technique

Wrapping is an important part of the process for instrument/equipment reprocessing. When the incorrect wrapping technique is used the instruments cannot be considered sterile and ready for use as they may be damaged during the sterilisation process. To minimise microbial contamination of the instruments inside, double sequential wrapping is sometimes used.

How the instrument and/or kit is wrapped affects whether the instrument can be opened aseptically and hence prevent contamination. Wrapping of kits/instruments should take place in a clean environment away from high traffic areas and dust (i.e. kit reprocessing room).

Individual packed items are often packed in paper and or laminated pouches which are heat sealed or have a special adhesive flap. It is imperative the correct size pouch is used so the pouch seals are not damaged during packing, which can lead to the pouch breaking during steam sterilisation. This occurs when the pouch expands under the applied pressure of autoclave sterilisation. Air should be removed before the pouch is sealed and it is important that pouches with an adhesive flap are sealed correctly via the flap perforation (50% on the laminate and 50% on the paper). If taping is used, the ends should be double folded, then taped along the bottom and at least 3 cm around the bag.

Items which have been packed should be placed in pouches so that the **handles are at the end of the pouch when opened by the surgeon,** ensuring safe and proper instrument handling.

Sharp points or edges on instruments should be protected with small sterilization covers, which are compatible with the sterilization process to avoid them from penetrating through the wrapping material and compromising sterility.

When double wrapping using pouches, it is important that two different pouch sizes are used (one smaller than the other), wrapped so the inner pouch's paper side is on the paper side of the outer. **Never fold pouches over by more than a third** as this prevents the sterilant from penetrating to the instruments.

To ensure efficient sterilisation, **instruments with hinges should be sterilized with their box lock joints fully open** and instruments that come apart should be sterilized in their dissembled state (e.g. lone star retractor).

For large items not packed in sterilisation pouches, it is imperative the packing materials are folded with small flaps, facing outward for ease of access when unpacking. This is to avoid contaminating to the inner packed layer/item.

Larger kits should be wrapped in a manner that avoids tenting and gaps. **The sequential wrap technique** uses two sheets of standard sterilisation wrap, one wrapped after the other. This procedure creates a package within a package. **The non-sequential process** uses two sheets wrapped at the same time so that the wrapping needs to be performed only once. This latter method provides multiple layers of protection for surgical instruments from contamination and saves time since wrapping is only done once.

Multiple layers are still common practice due to the rigors of handling within the clinic even though the barrier efficacy of a single sheet of wrap has improved over time. The most common method of wrapping large surgical kits is the envelope method.

The package should be taped closed with autoclave tape, and identified with pack name, initials of personnel, and date of sterilisation.

Masking tape should never be used to secure the wrapped kit, as the glue used was not designed to get wet and will therefore not hold. Additionally, surgical personnel cannot differentiate a kit that has been in an autoclave from one that has not. Instead, all kits should be sealed with sterilisation indicator tape; this has stripes which change colour to indicate adequate sterilisation processing (discussed later).

Storage of Surgical Packs

It is essential that all sterile products, whether sterilised within the clinic or purchased from an outside manufacturer, are stored in such a way that sterility is maintained until the kit, instrument, or product is used.

The sterile storage area is the area in the clinic designed or designated for the storage of medical devices/sterile equipment. The sterile storage area is the largest supply of sterile equipment, however operating theatres and procedure rooms may also have a supply of sterile equipment ready for use in certain procedures.

To ensure the sterility and function of sterile equipment, the practice should adopt standard operating procedures such that sterile supplies are maintained until use.

There are several reasons why sterile equipment may not be maintained:

A. Physical Damage to the Package

Holes and tears in packaging can be caused by:

- excessive or improper handling;
- compression of packages on storage shelves (when packages are packed too tightly);
- stacking packages and instrument sets;
- crushing packages when personnel are carrying them in their arms;
- improper packaging (e.g. sharps can penetrate the package);
- storage conditions;
- tears and holes allow airborne bacteria and dust to penetrate the package, compromising the sterility of the device within.

B. Moisture

- allows microorganisms from the air and surfaces to wick through packaging materials. Potential for condensation issues should be avoided by not placing warm packages on a cool surface;
- sterile supplies should never be stored near sources of moisture (e.g. sinks, exposed water pipes) or against an outside wall;
- excessive humidity levels in the sterile storage area or handling packages too soon after sterilisation also affects sterility;
- humidity and temperature of storage areas should be checked daily;
- sterile stores should have a low humidity of between 30–70%.

C. Soiling

- can compromise sterility;
- visibly soiled or stained packages must be considered contaminated, and the contents reprocessed or discarded;
- affected by storage or improper handling.

Therefore, **sterile items should always be protected from dust, moisture, and damage.** Ideally, they should be stored in a clean, closable glass cupboard within a low traffic area, away from moisture.

The degree of protection and the length of time the items remain sterile for (shelf life), depends on the wrapping material used (Table 8).

Sterilization

Processes of Sterilisation

Sterilisation is the process of destruction of all forms of microbial life, including bacteria, virus, fungi, algae, and protozoans.

Table 8. Material and shelf life.

Material	Shelf life
Two-layer single wrapped cotton muslin	One week
Four-layer doubled wrapped cotton muslin	Six weeks
Single-wrapped cotton muslin over a single layer of paper	Two months
Doubled-wrapped cotton muslin within a tape-sealed waterproof cover	Three months
Doubled-wrapped cotton muslin within a heat-sealed waterproof cover	Eight months
Double-wrapped polypropylene (non-woven)	Nine months
Heat-sealed plastic pouch	>12 months

Sterilization also completely eliminates dominant bacterial spores which are highly resistant to changes within the environment and able to survive within the environment for a long period of time (i.e. years). Sterilisation is an absolute phenomenon, and an item cannot be partially sterile.

There are many ways in which surgical equipment and materials can be sterilised, each with advantages and disadvantages. The decision on which method is used is based on a number of factors:

- process speed
- efficacy of process
- compatibility of instrument/material
- equipment cost
- staff safety
- training of staff
- ease of monitoring the process
- ease of use.

There are two main groups of sterilisation methods:

- **Physical:**
  - **heat**
  - **ionizing radiation**
  - **filtration**
- **Chemical sterilization:**
  - **gaseous**
  - **liquid.**

Sterilisation Using Heat

Heat destroys microbes by coagulating the proteins within their cells. Thus, microbes can be killed by either dry heat (e.g. an oven) or by moist heat (e.g. steam). Microbial death occurs more quickly and at a lower temperature with steam because moisture catalyses the chemical reactions of denaturation.

Steam Sterilising (autoclaves)

For a fixed volume sterilisation chamber, an increase in the pressure results in a temperature increase (Boyle's Law). (See Figure 15). **Steam heats and destroys microbes by a condensation process.**

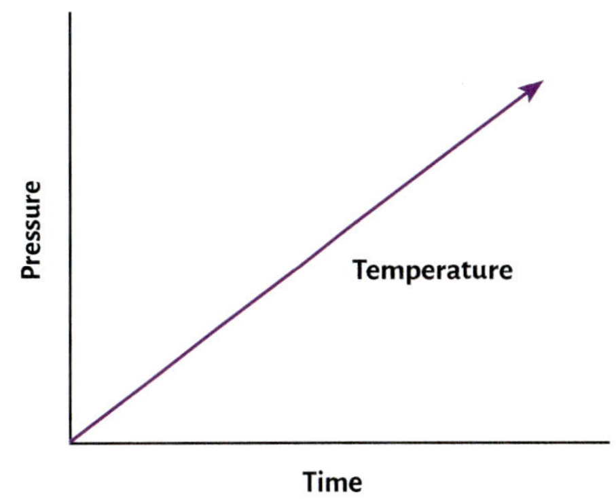

Figure 15. Influence of pressure and time on temperature.

Sterilisation with saturated steam under pressure is the most dependable and widely used method of microbial destruction.

Steam penetrates each pack and porous article, giving off heat as it condenses. It depends on direct contact and so items impenetrable by the steam are unsuitable for this method as are heat sensitive items. Surgical packs must be appropriately packed to facilitate steam penetration.

Air present in the steriliser reduces the penetration of the steam, limits condensation, and reaching the high temperatures necessary. Modern steam sterilisers differ principally in the mechanism by which air is excluded during the sterilisation procedure.

Steam sterilisers are known as autoclaves, which means self-closing and refers to the fact that the door is prevented from opening due to a high chamber pressure during the process cycle.

Moist Heat (boiling)

Boiling is not guaranteed to kill all microorganisms and their spores as, at standard atmospheric pressure, the maximum temperature attained is 100 °C. Therefore, it should not be considered as a means of sterilisation.

Dry Heat

Dry heat kills microorganisms by causing oxidative destruction of bacterial protoplasm. Equipment suitable for this method is restricted to that which is not easily damaged by the conditions. Hot air ovens have largely been superseded by autoclaves.

Autoclaves

There are two types of autoclaves:

- gravity-displacement autoclave
- pre-vacuum.

Gravity-displacement Autoclave

Gravity-displacement autoclaves (Figure 16) are also known as **downward-displacement autoclaves.** They work on the principle that steam is lighter than air. Steam enters the top of the inner chamber under pressure and displaces the heavier air downwards. A disadvantage is that air can become trapped in hollow items such as receptacles and suction tips, thus preventing exposure of sterilizing steam to their entire surface, resulting in the items not being effectively sterilised (i.e. the item is not sterile).

The displacement air is released by a thermostatic valve at the bottom of the autoclave and is released into the environment. As more steam is introduced (under pressure) to the inner chamber, more air is displaced, the pressure increases, which in turn increases the inner chamber's temperature producing condensation .

The minimum standard time and temperature for this type of autoclave is 13 minutes at 120 °C (125 °F).

Pre-vacuum

This type of autoclave is the most commonly found autoclave in UK veterinary practices. It works by actively removing the air from the inner sterilisation chamber before steam is introduced; hence, creating a vacuum. (See Figure 17).

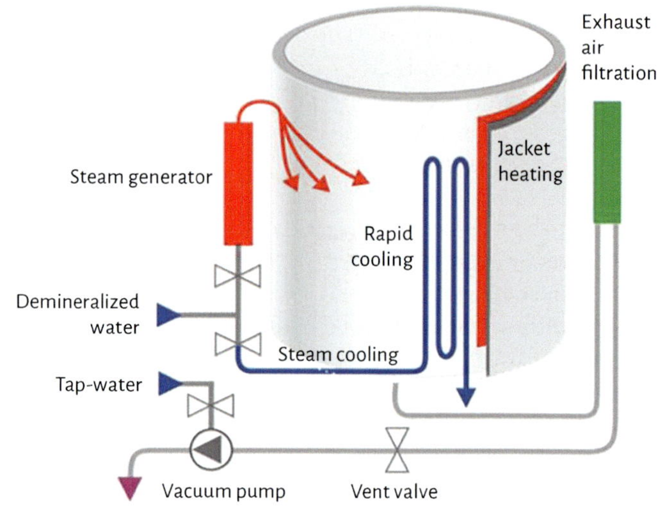

Figure 17. Vacuum autoclave.

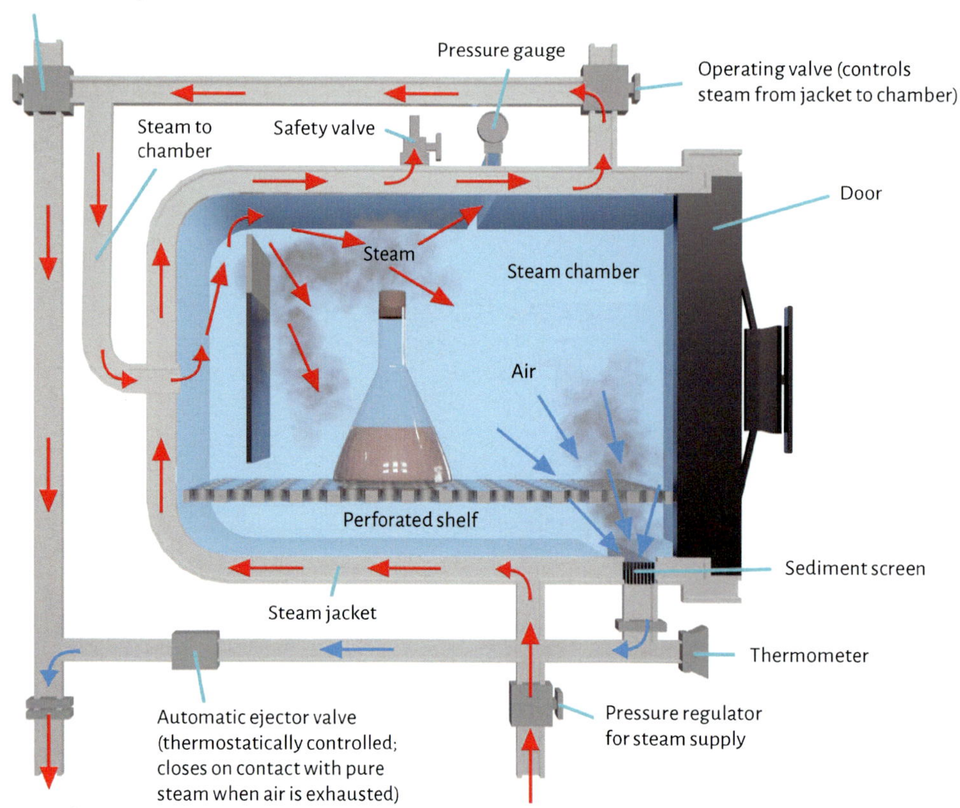

Figure 16. Gravity displacement autoclave.

By creating a vacuum prior, it reduces the time required for the steam to penetrate the inner sterilising chamber. Thus, creating a more effective and efficient process, particularly because air in hollow items is actively removed unlike in a gravity-displacement autoclave.

One of the advantages is that **instruments can be sterilised quickly in emergency situations** as they can be placed onto a perforated metal tray/container and put through the sterilisation process. The tray is then carried aseptically to the operating theatre and instruments aseptically removed from the tray by the surgeon/scrub nurse. This form of sterilisation is known as **flash sterilising.**

All items to be sterilised should be arranged so that all surfaces are directly exposed to the sterilising agent. Loading procedures must allow for free circulation of steam (or another gas sterilant) around each item. Important basic principles for loading a steriliser:

- allow for proper sterilant circulation;
- perforated trays should be placed so the tray is parallel to the shelf;
- small items should be loosely placed in wire baskets;
- peel packs should be placed on the edge in perforated or mesh bottom racks or baskets.

For effective steam sterilisation via an autoclave, a safe minimum standard is that the autoclave must reach and **maintain a temperature of 121 °C and pressure of 15 psi for a minimum of 30 minutes** to destroy the most resistant microbes. **Emergency sterilisation is carried out at 131 °C for three minutes.** The cycle times are longer to account for heat up and dry times depending on the autoclave.

γ-Irradiation

γ-irradiation is a physical means of sterilisation. The sterilisation process by irradiation does not create residues or impart radioactivity on the processed items. The process results in microbial DNA breakdown and results in inhibition of microbial reproduction.

Ionizing radiation differs from a lower energy radiation (e.g. infrared) in that the radiation has enough energy to displace the electrons within the atoms, thereby causing cellular dysfunction and death of microbial cells.

γ-irradiation sterilisation is performed by exposing the product to a radiation source, typically a **Cobalt 60 isotope, which decomposes into a Nickel 60 isotope,** firing off γ-rays in the process. These γ-rays can penetrate through the entire product, **deactivating whatever microorganisms are present.**

Because γ-rays are very penetrative the sterilisation chamber is reinforced with 2 m thick concrete. Due to its penetrative state, large quantities of items can be sterilised at the same time. γ radiation is the most effective and enables a measured dose to be administered easily. However, the process is restricted to commercial use because of its expense and hence prepackaged items (e.g. needles, syringes) are sterilised in this way. At the time of writing bone grafts and biological implants are also sterilised by γ-irradiation.

γ-sterilisation has both advantages and disadvantages which include:

- **Advantages:**
  - γ-rays have a high penetration power so multiple items can be sterilised at once
  - the method is suitable for all types of materials including dry, moist and even frozen items
  - the method is considered reliable and can be accurately controlled.
- **Disadvantages:**
  - there is some risk involved since radiation exposure may be harmful to personnel
  - it can produce undesirable changes in medicine such as colour, solubility, and texture of the product
  - it can damage the material which is being sterilised
  - it is expensive
  - a large area is required to accommodate the sterilisation chamber and its 2 m thick concrete safety jacket.

Filtration

Mechanical filtration is the technique used to sterilise liquids which cannot be sterilised by other means. This usually involves food stuffs; however, the technique is beginning to be used in the medical/biological research field, in particular for methylene blue and other liquids and emulsions. The filtration equipment is purchased as a presterile disposable unit and **filters with pore sizes of 20 nm are used to remove viruses and larger microorganisms.**

Chemical Gas Sterilisation

Chemicals used for sterilisation should not be corrosive to the items being sterilised. Items sterilised by this method are **those not suitable (too delicate) to be sterilised by heat and moisture** such as plastics, cameras, and some endoscopes and light cables.

Ethylene Oxide

Ethylene oxide (EtO) is used for items sensitive to temperatures >60 °C (e.g. optics, plastics, and electricals). It is a colourless gas which destroys microorganisms by alkylation (a chemical reaction where a hydrogen atom is replaced with a hydroxyethyl radial).

The amino acids found in proteins change their shape due to this chemical reaction and typically penetrate the cell membranes of microbes, forming a channel between the interior and exterior of the microbe cell, thereby lysing (destroying) the cells of microorganisms.

Ethylene oxide inactivates cellular DNA and prevents cell reproduction. It **destroys all known bacteria, spores, and the larger viruses,** but it is toxic, irritant to tissue and flammable (explosive at concentrations >3 %) unless mixed with carbon dioxide.

EtO diffuses quickly and is at its gas phase at a temperature of 10.5 °C and thus **an effective sterilant at room temperature at 20 °C.** It can penetrate most packaging except for nylon and polyester.

Mechanical systems (there is only one available in the UK) operate at room temperature and take 12 hours. This method is suitable for many items, but use is limited by the size of the sterilising chamber. It uses a microdose method to reduce environmental contamination/effects, and reduce the health and safety risks, whereby gas is released within a specially designed bag (containing the packaged items to be sterilised) and requires a much smaller volume of gas than historically used.

EtO is extremely toxic and can cause pulmonary oedema, respiratory mucosa, and eye irritation. Therefore, workplace exposure limits (WELs) are set, country by country. Mechanical systems use a negative pressure and vacuum system, which reduces exposure to the operator who should be adequately trained in the process.

It is important that items sterilised by EtO are surgically clean and left to air dry prior to sterilisation. EtO dissolves in water, which lowers its concentration. Items should be thoroughly dried as water droplets affect the efficiency of the process. Hot air must not be used to dry the items, as this desiccates bacterial spores and makes them resistant to the gas.

EtO should not be used to sterilise any item that has previously been sterilised by irradiation, particularly those that are made from PVC as ethylene chlorohydrin may be formed, which is a very toxic gas and is very difficult to elute.

For optimum sterilisation the temperature range is between 49–60 °C. However, in most cases, mechanical machines sterilise at room temperature which takes 12 hours (including aeration of the items) depending on items, at a concentration of 600 mg/l.

For health and safety reasons it is important items are left to air. The time that items are appropriately aerated is determined by their composition. Metals, glass, and certain plastics resist gas penetration and thus need less time for aeration whereas, rubber and some other plastics bind to the gas and require a longer time to be aerated.

EtO sterilisation time is dependent on the gas concentration, time, humidity, and the material type to be sterilised.

Gas Plasma

Hydrogen peroxide gas plasma sterilisation results in rapid inactivation of a broad spectrum of microorganisms and removal of harmful residues. It takes approximately one hour and requires no aeration. There are no reported toxic emissions or residues. Specialist equipment is required.

Chemical Liquid Sterilisation (cold sterilisation)

Cold sterilisation refers to the soaking of items in disinfectant solutions and should be considered as **high disinfection,** although some manufacturers guarantee sterilisation after 24 hours.

It is mainly used in veterinary practice for endoscopes and other items unsuitable for steam sterilisation and should not be used for items introduced beneath the surface of the body (i.e. orthopaedic implants).

Ideally the chemical used for cold sterilisation has **a high efficiency, rapid action, is nontoxic, and should be compatible with the items to be sterilised.**

Unfortunately, there is no ideal high-level disinfectant . Oxidising agents have better cidal activity than alkylating agents, which are more compatible with different materials. In veterinary practice the cold sterilant (high disinfectant) is a mix of various compounds that act synergistically to overcome the shortfalls of the more traditional chemical sterilant.

The solution must be changed regularly due to the minimum effective concentration (MEC), which is affected by dilution and contamination. Alternatively, the MEC effectiveness can be monitored by using indicator strips that are dipped into the solution to give either a negative or positive result. Some solutions such as glutaraldehyde change colour themselves to indicate the concentration has decreased below the MEC.

Most chemicals used for cold sterilisation are **irritant to the skin and mucous membranes.** Therefore, any equipment sterilised by this process should be rinsed with sterile water to remove any chemical residue before use on the patient. Appropriate PPE should be worn when using chemical sterilant.

Sterilisation Indicators

It is imperative items are sterilised effectively. The effectiveness of sterilisation depends on:

- **Human error:**
  - inadequate cleaning /drying
  - inappropriate wrapping material
  - improper loading of the sterilisation chamber.
- **Mechanical error:**
  - autoclave failure.

Sterilisation indicators confirm that sterilisation conditions have been appropriately met and mechanical failure has not occurred.

As there is a great variability in microorganisms' abilities to live in hostile environments, microorganisms are not killed instantaneously once certain conditions are met. This is because the sterilisation process is dependent on the length of time for which certain conditions are maintained.

Sterilisation indicators are classed as two types:
- chemical
- biological.

Both of which should be used in conjunction with physical monitoring (temperature, humidity and pressure), and steriliser maintenance.

Quality assurance (QA) should be set up to ensure the highest standards of surgical sterilisation are maintained. Whereby, a record is taken of multiple monitoring methods of each sterilisation load as an audit to identify a source issue if there was to be a failure in sterilisation.

Chemical Indicators

Chemical indicators are defined as the: **sterilisation process monitoring devices designed to respond with a physical or chemical change to one or more of the physical conditions within the sterilisation chamber (i.e. temperature, pressure, time).**

They identify failures in sterilisation which may occur due to human or mechanical error, and come as chemical impregnated paper strips (e.g. TST strips/ Bowie-Dick tape) or glass vials containing a liquid chemical (e.g. Browne tubes).

There are five classes of chemical indicators as defined by the Association of Advancement of Medical Instrumentation, which are based on the chemical indicator's ability to monitor one or multiple sterilisation parameters. (Table 9).

If the internal and/or external indicator suggests inadequate processing, the item should not be used as it is deemed unsterile.

It is vital to use chemical indicators correctly:

Class 1 and 2

- Place on the outside of the packed item, to indicate the item has been exposed to the sterilisation process (vacuum in the case of Bowie-Dick tape).
- Autoclave tape turns brown when the temperature reaches 120 °C.

Class 3, 4, and 5

- Place deep inside the pack/kit where there is least penetration of the sterilant (N.B. this may not be in the centre of the pack). A typical example are Brown's tubes. Brown's tubes are glass tubes filled with a chemical liquid which turns from one colour to another when exposed to a

Table 9. Chemical indicator classification.

Class	Type	Explanation
1	Process	· Most basic. · Autoclave table, indicators found on sterilisation pouches. · Used with individual items. · Distinguish between processed and non-processed.
2	Specific test	· Used for specific test procedures (Bowie-Dick tape). · Tests for air within the sterilisation chamber.
3	Single parameter	· Reacts to one of the crucial parameters (temperature/pressure).
4	Multi-parameter	· Reacts to two or more crucial parameters (e.g. time and steam pressure or time and EtO concentration.
5	Integrating indicator	· Reacts to all the crucial sterilisation parameters.

Table 10. Examples of autoclave failures.

Cause of failure	Description	Possible solution
Air leak	If air is able to leak into the autoclave chamber, the steam will be unable to penetrate the load to the point of total sterilisation.	A vacuum leak test should be run to further determine if an air leak exists or not.
Unwanted condensation	Occasionally, condensation will get trapped in the jacket of the autoclave, which can lead to cold spots at the base of the autoclave. This could also indicate a wet-steam issue.	The steam traps on the autoclave should be checked. Steam quality and wetness should be checked.
Faulty test pack	From time to time a Bowie-Dick test pack can be faulty.	The expiration date should be checked, and it should be ensured packs are being stored in the proper environment.
No warm-up cycle	A warm-up cycle allows the steriliser chamber and jacket to reach temperature.	A five-minute sterilisation cycle should be run prior to running the Bowie-Dick cycle.
Incorrect procedures	Test packs work under very specific conditions.	Test packs should be placed in an empty chamber directly over the drain on the bottom rack or shelf. They are designed for use at 270–273 °F (132–134 °C).

specific temperature (usually red to green). They come with a variety of temperature indications and methods of sterilisation which is indicated by a black spot for steam and green for hot ovens. They are reactive to heat, and therefore need to be stored in a cool, dry place.

Class 6

TST (time/steam/temperature) strips indicate the critical parameters for a sterilisation cycle. They come under class 6 and hence provide a level of validation for all three parameters. They are:

- easy to use with minimal training
- a visual reading of colour change and allow simple interpretation of results.

Bowie and Dick Test

It is also important that **an air-removal or vacuum test is performed daily** such as the Bowie-Dick test, particularly when using a prevacuum autoclave. This is to ensure efficient air removal is achieved and subsequently ensure that steam fully penetrates porous loads (i.e. cloth drapes/gowns). The Bowie-Dick test evaluates:

- **effectiveness** of the initial vacuum phase
- **steam penetration** into cavities
- **temperature and pressure** of saturated steam during the sterilisation phase.

The Bowie-Dick test should be performed after repairs and/or as part of the daily maintenance procedure (where results are recorded for clinical governance). It should also be performed if the autoclave has not been in use for long periods of time.

The Bowie-Dick test involves placing a disposable, heat sensitive, test pad that consists of several layers of paper and foam into an empty autoclave, ideally on the lowest shelf and above the chamber's drain . The sheet is impregnated with a chemical indicator which changes colour when exposed to a particular pressure of steam. The autoclave is then run for a four-minute cycle (typically known as the Bowie-Dick cycle). **This cycle should consist of 3–4 minutes prevacuum and operate at a temperature of 134 °C and at 30 psi for 3.5 minutes.**

Biological Indicators

Biological indicators are glass vials/paper strips **which contain a form of non-pathogenic, spore forming bacteria** (usually *Bacillus* or *Geobacillus spp.*) and are **more resistant to the sterilisation process than naturally occurring contaminants.**

These are subjected to the sterilisation process, the vials/ paper strips removed afterwards, and incubated for 24–48 hours. The presence of living bacteria is then checked by several methods: e.g. a colour change due to metabolism of the bacteria or fluorescence due to microbial enzymes. If there is evidence of bacterial growth, then the sterilisation process was unsuccessful.

Using biological indicators is **expensive** and is a lengthy process regarding obtaining results which can take up to seven days. For this reason, biological indicators are mainly used as part of a quality assurance (QA) regime and spore test, which should be carried out on a weekly basis, to ensure high standards of sterilisation and aseptic technique are constantly achieved.

Clinical Attire and Surgical Personnel Preparation

One of the main responsibilities of the clinical and surgical team is to prevent transmission of pathogenic microorganisms between patients and or from veterinary personnel to patients, either via nursing or the surgical procedure itself; therefore, **preventing nosocomial infections.**

Clinical Attire

Staff attire and hygiene are a major contributing factor to infection control. For example, veterinary staff were identified as high-risk individuals for the transmission of MRSA (Feilberg, 2015).

Uniforms

Uniforms can transmit pathogens from patient to patient, naturally carrying a different microbial flora within the fabric, picked up from different environments (e.g. home and work). Veterinary personnel must take care to avoid the spread of pathogens between these environments wherever possible.

Many practices do not have standard protocols regarding uniform, footwear, and personal equipment; the development of these is recommended to ensure appropriate infection control, and to standardise this amongst all members of the practice team. **Both clinical and non-clinical staff should follow these protocols.**

All staff should **wear an appropriate uniform for their role** within the clinic. This should be easy to maintain and work in. Having one clinical team follow this, whilst others wear their own clothes/shoes with a scrub top or tunic on top, defeats the point of an infection control policy. All clinical staff should **wear a full non-theatre scrub suit** or tunic/trouser uniform. Additionally, **specific workplace shoes** should form part of this uniform and should be:

- waterproof
- closed toe

- free of holes
- fully immersible in disinfectant solution.

These **shoes should be worn within work only,** and when not in use stored at work to **prevent external contamination. Uniform tops should be short sleeved** to facilitate effective hand hygiene.

As registered professionals, our uniforms should inspire public confidence. In a recent human review, healthcare professionals seen in public in their uniform (e.g. at the supermarket) was reported to lower public confidence, due to the infection control risks this poses (Loveday et al., 2007; Pratt et al., 2007; Riley, 2015).

All uniforms should be changed into, and out of, at the workplace if possible. This prevents the transfer of pathogens between the home and workplace environment, protects our patients, and protects our pets from things like flea infestations as well as bacteria and viruses.

If changing at work is not possible, a thin, long-sleeved, clean top should be worn over the uniform, which is removed on arrival at the clinic. This is then worn during the journey home and washed at the end of the day alongside the used uniform.

In the workplace, our uniforms should be visibly clean at all times: hair and scale should be removed regularly with a lint roller and soiled clothing changed as soon as possible. It is advisable to **keep a spare set of scrubs or greens in your locker** and launder the soiled set at work.

Ideally, whenever leaving the building (e.g. for lunch) uniforms should be changed, and when entering the staff kitchen or break area, protective clothing or your own clothes should be worn to prevent contamination whilst eating and drinking.

Laundry

A clean uniform should be worn every day, so the practice should issue a sufficient number of uniform sets to all staff members **(typically 3–5 sets).**

Uniforms should ideally be laundered at work to prevent transmission of pathogenic organisms outside of the clinic. **Tunics and trousers should be washed on a 60 °C wash at a cycle length ≥15 minutes** (Riley et al., 2015) and **scrub suits on a 70 °C wash at a cycle length ≥15 minutes** (Riley et al., 2015). (See Figure 18).

A recent study in 2015 (Riley et al., 2015) showed **commercial washing machines were superior** at achieving the required temperatures compared to domestic machines.

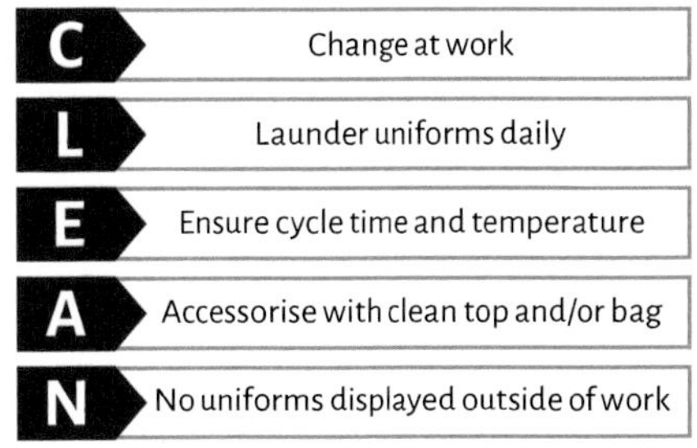

Figure 18. Acronym of uniform best practice for infection control.

After washing, **garmets should be tumble dried** to ensure sufficient reduction in bacterial load on them.

If workplace laundering is not possible, uniform sets should be transported to and from work in a protective washable bag and handled carefully at home.

Home laundering of uniforms can cause cross-contamination with household items and contamination of the washing machine itself. In addition, the consideration of economic and environmental factors often means home laundering of uniforms is often not performed at a sufficient temperature or regularly enough, causing infection control risks within the home.

There are several factors that affect how well uniforms are cleaned within the home environment:
- time between end of shift and washing
- how the uniform is transported home
- washing cycle time
- washing cycle type
- washing cycle temperature
- other items washed at the same time.

Separate bags should be used for clean and dirty items and **contaminated uniforms washed the same day** as the shift, as soon as possible after shift completion.

Disinfection of washing machines both at home (if uniformed is laundered in this way) and within the clinic should be performed. A study in 2015 showed that washing machines played an important role in bacterial transmission.

Storage in a laundry basket should be avoided as this causes cross-contamination to household clothing. **Uniforms should be washed separately to household items, at a temperature of at least 60 °C on a standard cycle** (without economical or energy-saving settings). If possible, washed uniforms should be tumble dried, as this is another important aspect of reducing bacterial contamination.

Washable items should be separated into surgical items (drapes, scrubs, gowns, hats and shoes) and in the case of surgical items, using a different washing machine and tumble dryer if possible. Soluble laundry bags (which dissolve in the washing machine) can be used to separate washing.

Personal Equipment

As well as uniform and hygiene factors, personal equipment, such as stethoscopes, scissors and equipment pouches should be used responsibly, in a way which does not risk cross contamination. Each clinical member should be responsible for ensuring their personal equipment is maintained and appropriately cleaned and disinfected after use on each patient.

Thermometers should be used with thermometer covers and equipment pouches washed at 60 °C weekly followed by tumble drying.

Other hygiene considerations for personnel infection control include:

- As well as uniforms, the appearance, and the dress code of individuals within the practice team is also an important consideration in infection control.
- Long hair should be tied back to prevent contamination of procedure sites.
- Food and drink should be avoided in all clinical areas, with food consumed in staff kitchen areas only.
- Closed-top water bottles and coffee cups should be used for cold and hot drinks.
- All PPE should be disposable and single use.
- No facial piercings and preferably only stud earrings should be worn.
- Hanging equipment such as stethoscopes around the neck should be avoided.
- Neckties and necklaces should be avoided.
- Lanyards should be worn underneath the uniform or stored in a pocket.
- Fob watches should ideally be worn on a trouser pocket or at waist height.
- A **bare below the elbow** approach should be adopted. Cuffs have been shown to harbour bacteria and cause cross contamination amongst patients and personnel.
- Mobile phone use should be avoided, or disinfection performed after each shift.
- There should be designated areas within the clinic where water bottles/drinks can be stored within reach of clinical areas, such as a shelf in a corridor next to the dog ward, or a wall-rack for bottles at the entrance to the prep room. This ensures staff wellbeing/health whilst minimising infection control concerns.

Hand Hygiene

Antiseptics

The use of antiseptics dates back to the mid-1800s. They are chemical agents which are applied to mucous membranes and the skin, which **reduce the number of microbes and hence reduce the risk of nosocomial infections.**

There are a number of different types of antiseptics, which possess specific mechanisms of action and a spectrum of microbes they target.

Antiseptics have several potential uses:

- **preventing infections on the skin,** particularly for cuts, scrapes, or minor burns;
- **dry handwashing,** between different procedures or patients;
- **cleaning the skin** before a medical procedure e.g. blood draw or surgery; and
- **cleaning/disinfecting mucous membranes,** to treat infections or before placing a urinary catheter.

The main antiseptics used in a clinical setting include:

Chlorhexidine (Hibiscrub™, Triscrub™, Bioguard™, Hydrex™)

- positively charged bisbiguanide
- binds to negatively charged bacterial cell walls resulting in disruption of cell membranes and precipitation of cellular contents
- broad spectrum (Gram +ve and -ve, fungi, enveloped viruses, mycobacteria)
- fast acting
- increased residual activity as it binds to keratin.

Povidone-iodine (Vetasept™)

- complex of povidone, hydrogen iodine and elemental iodine
- Iodination of lipids as well as the oxidization of cytoplasmic and cell membrane compounds
- broad spectrum (Gram +ve and -ve, to include spores, fungi, viruses and protozoa)
- fast acting
- reduced residual activity.

Chloroxylenol (Dettol™)

- halophenol
- disrupts microbial cell walls and inactivation of cellular enzymes
- bactericidal
- active against Gram +ve and -ve bacteria
- slow acting
- reduced residual activity.

Isopropyl Alcohol (Surgical Spirit™)

- hydrophilic alcohol
- damages cell membranes
- denatures proteins required for microbial metabolism and growth
- mixed with distilled water at a solution of 60–90 % to increase microbial activity
- fast onset
- reduced residual activity
- most effective against Gram +ve bacteria
- reduced activity against virus and fungi.

Hexachlorophene (Gamophen™, Septisol™)

- a bisphenol compound
- inhibits membrane bound electron transport disrupting cell membranes
- bacteriostatic
- active against Gram +ve cocci
- residual activity for >7 hours
- cumulative effect
- banned worldwide due to increased dermal absorption resulting in toxic effects.

Benzalkonium Chloride (Bactine™)

- a quaternary ammonium detergent
- acts by irreversibly binding to phospholipids and proteins of the membrane, disrupting the cell membrane
- effective against Gram +ve and -ve bacteria.

Triclosan (TCS)

- Used in many domestic cleaning products/toothpaste/shampoos etc as well as PDS® plus and Monocryl® plus suture materials
- polychloro phenoxy phenol
- developed in 1960's
- is a biocide at high concentrations targeting cell membranes and cytoplasm
- at low concentrations is bacteriostatic by inhibiting fatty acid synthesis
- banned in some countries due to evidence that it is associated with some cancers, hormonal imbalance, and cardiac disease in humans (still controversial)
- antibacterial and antifungal
- effective with minimal contact time
- effective against MRSA.

Hand Hygiene

Hand hygiene is considered the single most effective technique in preventing cross contamination, hospital acquired infection, and zoonotic disease transmission. It is an area which can be continually improved, especially between different groups within the practice team and during busy periods of time where hand hygiene becomes less of a priority.

It is also important to ensure hand hygiene is performed despite the use of PPE, as PPE does not replace good hand hygiene techniques.

The goal of hand hygiene is to **reduce the number of transient microbes on our hands.** These transient microbes are collected from patients, other people, handling contaminated equipment, and from the hospital environment.

In addition to this, it is important to **maintain the skin's integrity** during the decontamination process as intact skin is easier to disinfect than cracked, cut, or chapped skin. An intact skin barrier is the body's first line of defence against pathogens, and bacteria adhere more readily to inflamed or broken skin.

When to Disinfect Hands

The World Health Organisation (WHO) set guidelines for when hand hygiene needs to be performed.

These 5 Moments for Hand Hygiene can be adapted to fit veterinary patients.

Hand hygiene should be performed:

1. **Before touching a patient** or their immediate surroundings: to protect the patient against acquiring pathogens from the handler.
2. Immediately **before a procedure:** to protect the patient from harmful pathogens from entering their body during a procedure.
3. Immediately **after a procedure** or fluid exposure risk: to protect yourself and the hospital environment from pathogens.
4. **After touching a patient** or their immediate surroundings: to protect yourself and the hospital environment from pathogens.
5. After touching any **objects in the patient's surroundings,** even if they have not been touched by the patient: to protect yourself and the hospital environment from pathogens.

Additionally, the WHO recommends washing hands before or after the following:

- before, during, and after preparing food
- before eating
- after using the toilet
- after coughing, sneezing, or blowing one's nose
- after touching waste
- after touching an animal, animal feed, or animal waste
- between patients.

Hand Disinfection

The aim of hand preparation is to:

- reduce the level of resistant bacterial flora for as long as possible
- remove dirt and grease
- eliminate transient microorganisms.

The disinfectant solution used should:

- be economical
- be non-irritating to skin and other tissues
- destroy microorganisms with minimal contact time
- lather in order to remove dirt and grease
- have broad spectrum bactericidal, fungicidal, virucidal, and sporicidal activity.

Historically, the most frequently used disinfectant solutions used in practice are **chlorhexidine or iodophor based.** Recently, **alcohol-based solutions** are used (Sterillium™), which aim to help maintain skin condition and therefore the normal skin protective barrier. Chlorhexidine, however, has the highest level of residual activity because it binds to keratin. Nevertheless, the most significant factor in reducing the number of microorganisms is contact time.

All jewellery and nail varnish should be removed before hand washing. Nails should be kept short and in good condition as bacteria can be harboured under the nail, on worn or chipped nail varnish and on damaged nails.

False nails or nail extensions should not be worn by anyone directly involved in patient care, as there is evidence to show that microorganisms can be transferred from staff to patient via false nails and nail extensions.

Jewellery physically protects pathogens from antimicrobial agents during handwashing, leading to ineffective skin disinfection. In addition, rings increase the number of organisms present on the skin and can pierce gloves. A plain wedding band may be worn only if essential, with stoned or additional rings avoided. Wristwatches, bracelets, and wristbands also interfere with hand hygiene and should not be worn.

All clinical staff should adopt a bare below the elbow policy to facilitate hand hygiene and reduce contamination. It is important that all areas of the hands and forearms are disinfected. Particular attention should be paid to the nails, back of the hands, and between the fingers. Hands should be raised above the elbow so that liquid drips down the forearm to drop off the elbow. Never shake the hands as this increases environmental contamination via water droplets. Instead, **hands should be dried with a disposable paper towel.**

To aid in effective infection control, taps should be turned on and off without touching them (i.e. infrared) or via elbow control. If this is not possible, the tap should be left running during the hand washing process and then a disposable paper towel used to turn them off, which is then discarded.

Handwashing Technique

Handwashing should be performed using **antimicrobial soap and running water.** Antimicrobial soap is used to remove oily secretions, which contain microorganisms and/or organic material.

Generally, chlorhexidine or triclosan-based products are preferred, as these are effective in the presence of organic matter. Chlorhexidine is associated with skin dryness and irritation with repeated use, and so the use of a handwashing solution, rather than surgical site preparation, may be preferable. Such solutions contain emollients, which are moisturising compounds to prevent cracking, thus maintaining the barrier effect of the skin. To ensure effective handwashing and removal of microorganisms the **handwashing procedure should take 40–60 seconds.**

In order to ensure all personnel are washing their hands correctly the WHO have made hand washing posters available, to place at all hand washing facilities within the practice to remind staff of the correct hand washing techniques.

WHO hand washing guidelines: https://www.who.int/gpsc/5may/How_To_HandWash_Poster.pdf?ua=1

Hand Sanitising

Hand sanitising or hand-rubbing is generally performed using **alcohol hand rubs.** A suitable agent should be selected based on the range of pathogens it is effective against. When looking for a product to use in practice, the range of veterinary-specific pathogens as well as human ones should be taken into consideration. Note that some products use animal viruses as human virus substitutes (e.g. products listed as effective against norovirus are actually tested against feline calicivirus).

For the greatest efficacy, alcohol solutions should have an **alcohol content of above 60 %;** solutions with >70 % alcohol have been shown to kill 99.9 % of bacteria 30 seconds after application.

When hand-rubbing, ensure the hands are wet with the solution for the entire contact time of the product and the hands are allowed to air-dry thoroughly after use. The procedure should take 20–30 seconds.

Hand sanitisation is appropriate when hand washing is not possible (and there is no organic soiling), on clean hands, and between each patient, when hands are visibly soiled, alcohol products are ineffective due to organic material, and handwashing should be performed instead.

As for hand washing, it is important hand sanitisation is performed correctly for effective microbial reduction.

WHO how to hand rub poster: https://www.who.int/gpsc/5may/How_To_HandRub_Poster.pdf?ua=1

Monitoring Hand Hygiene

Approaches to monitoring hand hygiene compliance vary from simple methods (such as direct observation and product usage) to more advanced methods (such as automated electronic monitoring systems). Adopting a multimodal approach is recommended, which is complemented with staff education to increase the effectiveness of hand hygiene procedures.

Regular hand hygiene training should be performed in practice, and hand hygiene surveillance undertaken for auditing and clinical governance purposes. It is important all practice members recognise this is to continually improve clinical practices, and not to blame individual staff members.

Direct observation hand hygiene monitoring is thought to be the best type of monitoring and recommended by WHO. This is because it is the simplest and most inexpensive method for assessing staff compliance.

A trained observer is tactically positioned to accurately observe hand practice measures and should be consistent in the standardisation of their observations. Observers should document both the number of hand hygiene events as well as hand hygiene opportunities in order to calculate compliance data. Practices can also use a standardized tool to calculate hand hygiene opportunities which is provided by WHO.

However, this form of monitoring is time consuming, and only accounts for 1.2–3.5 % of all hand hygiene events within the practice. It is also influenced by the Hawthorne effect whereby staff members alter their hand hygiene behaviour when they know they are being observed.

Product usage is an indirect method for monitoring hand hygiene compliance. The consumption of paper towels, alcohol-based hand rub, and liquid soap is tracked and converted into an approximation of hand hygiene events. However, this does not ensure that hand washing/sanitisation is effective.

Electronic monitoring systems are the most effective and passive method for increasing hand hygiene compliance within a clinic; they are not time consuming or subject to human error or manipulation of the data. Electronic monitoring systems address the non-compliance of clinical staff, with hand washing and hand rubbing guidelines intended to reduce the number of nosocomial and other infections. They work by clinical staff wearing an infrared badge which senses and logs each time that a particular staff member uses the hand sanitiser or hand washing station. Again, this method does not test if the staff member is using the correct techniques and hence a training protocol should be implemented and reviewed.

Solutions are available which disclose bacteria under UV-light; to use as a training aid to improve hand hygiene techniques. Gel products are used as an alcohol hand rub and cause any areas of contamination to fluoresce; alternatively, lotions and powders are available which when applied after handwashing disclose areas to focus on in future.

Commonly missed areas during handwashing/sanitising include between the fingers, the fingertips, the thumb, and ring finger (Figure 19).

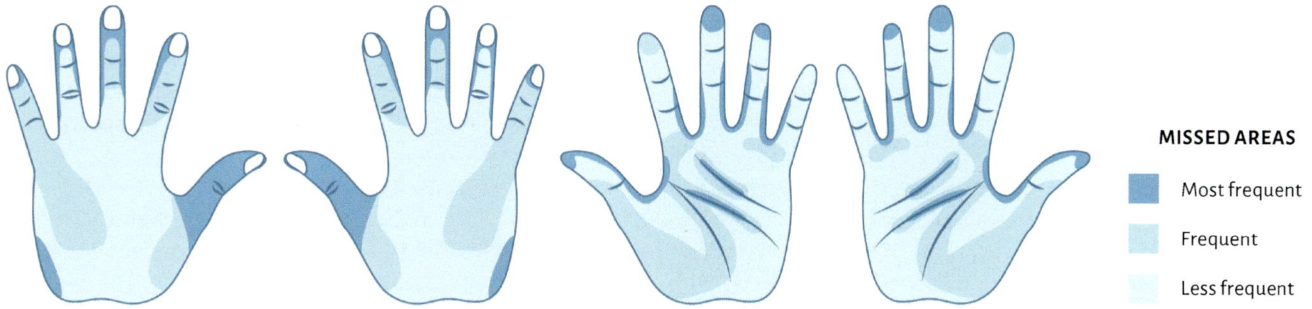

Figure 19. Commonly missed areas during hand washing. Adapted illustration from the World Health Organization 2018.

Common Pitfalls of Hand Hygiene

Common areas where hand hygiene can be improved include:
- wearing jewellery and wristwatches whilst handwashing
- not rolling up long sleeves
- applying soap before wetting the hands
- ineffective hand washing technique (e.g. not following the WHO guidelines)
- not spending sufficient time on handwashing (e.g. not achieving agent contact time)
- using alcohol gels on soiled hands, where handwashing would be indicated
- turning off taps with freshly washed hands instead of elbows, or towel
- hand operation of bin lids when disposing of hand towels.

Surgical Hand Disinfection

Similarly to hand hygiene, **the aim of surgical hand disinfection is to reduce the number of microbes that could come into contact with the patient during a surgical procedure,** particularly if there is a glove puncture, which could result in a surgical site infection (SSI).

Before starting the hand disinfection procedure, it is imperative that **all essential equipment is available and ready to use** (i.e. sterile gown, sterile hand towel, and sterile gloves).

As with hand hygiene surgical staff must adapt a **bare below the elbow approach** and remove all jewellery, such as rings and watches, as these harbour bacteria and damage surgical gloves. Similarly, nail varnish and false nails should be removed.

Commercial disposable brushes impregnated with antiseptic detergents (chlorhexidine 4% or povidone iodine) are available. They are composed of a plastic bristle brush on one side and a soft sponge on the other, also included within the pack is a disposable plastic nail pick.

Scrubbing techniques aim to:
- reduce the amount of dirt present on hands and arms;
- reduce the amount of oil present on hands and arms; and
- reduce the level of transient and endogenous bacterial flora of the surgical personnel's skin.

The antiseptic detergents/solution used must be/have:
- non-irritating to the surgeon/surgical personnel;
- fast acting;
- broad spectrum; and
- high residual activity, to prevent rapid recurrence of microbial activity under a glove.

The most commonly used surgical skin scrubbing solutions are 4% chlorhexidine, povidone iodine, and alcohol based solutions (e.g. Sterillium™).

Repeated scrubbing with a traditional scrubbing brush dries and damages the skin via removal of the surface layers, which in turn causes dermatitis and thus bacterial colonisation leading to infection. Therefore, **brushing should be limited to the tips of the fingers and nails only.**

There are various hand scrubbing techniques:

Brushless

Recent studies **discourage the use of brushes.** Mitchell et al. suggested a brushless surgical hand scrub. Research found scrubbing with a disposable sponge or combination sponge-brush reduced bacterial counts on the hands as effectively as scrubbing with a brush (Bornside, 1968 and McBride et al., 1973).

Either an anatomic timed or counted brush-stroke technique is used without the use of a brush. This technique can be used with both alcohol-based surgical hand rubs and conventional chlorhexidine.

The use of this technique using alcohol-based surgical hand rubs is dependent on the manufacturer's directions for the specific scrub solution, (e.g. Sterillium™, Vet Gel™, Hibi Liquid Hand Rub+™). Alcohol based solution is rubbed into clean dry skin for a specific time period as per manufacturer's instructions. The solution used should be proven to have a rapid and broad-spectrum antimicrobial activity.

There is evidence that alcohol-based rubs have the same immediate effect as chlorhexidine and also have a longer residual time (Verwilghen, 2011).

It is conceivable that a brush may be beneficial on visibly dirty hands before entering the operating room.

Anatomic Timed Scrub (5–6 minutes scrubbing time)

This is the most common method and involves timing the time each section of the hand/forearm is scrubbed for as recommended by the World Health Organisation. The first-hand disinfection of the day is the most meticulous and providing there is no gross contamination subsequent hand disinfection may be only three minutes in duration.

Counted Brush-stroke (5–6 minutes scrubbing time)

Instead of timing the scrub, the number of brush strokes are counted instead. Fingertips are counted as one unit and each finger and arm is considered to have four units, creating 25 anatomical regions on each hand and arm which should receive the same number of brush strokes, being between 20–30.

Note: Scrubbing longer than 10 minutes results in increased levels of positive cultures than a 5–6-minute scrub.

On completion, hands and forearms should be dried using a **four corners technique.** Whereby, one corner of the paper towel is used in turn for each hand and forearm, ensuring used parts of the towel are not touched (Figure 20).

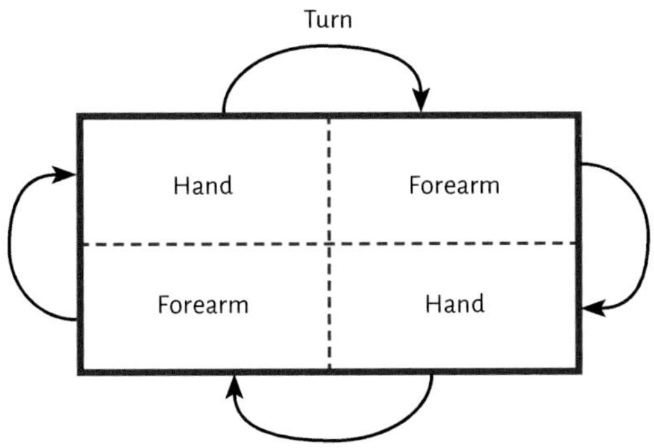

Figure 20. Technique for hand drying using a sterile towel.

Surgical Personnel Preparation

There are many methods by which the surgical team can reduce direct and indirect bacterial shedding. The most appropriate method will depend on the procedure itself. For example, scrubbed hands and sterile gloves may be adequate for a cutaneous biopsy, however for more invasive surgery full theatre attire and sterile gowns are required.

Scrub Suits

Scrub suits should be worn by all surgical personnel within the clean surgical facility; to reduce bacterial contamination from outside the clean area and instil good theatre practice.

It is imperative to wear clean suits for each theatre shift, which are changed if they become dirty. If personnel are required to leave the clean surgical suite, ideally, they should change back into other clinical, dirty area, clothes or in extreme circumstances cover their suits with a clean clinical coat. However, outside shoes should not be worn within the clean theatre suite area.

Theatre suits are made from a tight weave of the polyester/cotton-blend fabric which forms a barrier to microorganisms, and therefore proper theatre suits should be worn, with the tunic tucked into the trousers.

When scrub suits become wet the microorganism barrier is reduced. Similarly, each time the suit is laundered the material weave loosens, creating microscopic holes through which bacteria can travel, thus reducing the barrier to microorganisms. Scrub suits should be periodically sterilised and inspected for damage and signs of wear and tear.

Within the clean areas, designated footwear should be worn to prevent the transfer of hair and other particulate matter. However, this does not reduce the bacterial level on the floor, as found by Mangram et al. in 1999.

Hats

Hair and the scalp are a significant carrier of bacteria, as they act as a filter that collects microbes. Therefore, complete covering is required by scrubbed personnel, particularly as it has been shown microbial shedding from hair affects surgical wound infection rates. (McHugh et al., 2014).

Hats and/or hoods should be worn at all times within the clean area, even when a procedure is not in progress. There are many different types of surgical hats, of which it seems there is no difference in postoperative wound events and the type of hat chosen (Haskins et al., 2017). Hats come in several types, including reusable and disposable.

- **Mob cap:** a round bonnet type cap that covers the whole head.
- **Tie cap:** has a drawstring closure, which can be tightened or loosened at the back. One of the advantages of this headpiece head covering is that tightness can be controlled for a snug fit. The disadvantage of these tie-type headpieces is that it takes time to either loosen or tighten them.
- **Bouffant:** bulkier than tie caps, and they look like one type of newsboy caps. They cover a wider area, and they have enough space to keep hair in place, making them ideal for women with long hair. While bouffant caps have enough room for the head and hair, they allow little control over tightness. Hair can easily fall out, especially during activities requiring vigorous movements.
- **Disposable:** made from polypropylene fabric and elastic. They come as nurse's caps, mob cap, hoods or surgeon's tie-back style.
- **Hood:** a hood cap that covers the sides of the face, often used by surgeons who have beards, and they are particularly useful during orthopaedic joint surgeries.

Masks

There are several different types of face mask:

- fabric hygiene (non-medical)
- surgical
- PPE (FFP1, FFP2 and FFP3)
- N95 and KN95
- filtering masks.

The practice of wearing surgical masks minimises the transmission of oro- and nasopharyngeal bacteria from operating theatre staff to patients' wounds, thereby decreasing the likelihood of postoperative surgical site infections.

They have a very high exhalation filtration efficiency of around 95%. This is why they are considered a good way of limiting the spread of saliva droplets expelled when surgical personnel talk, cough, and sneeze. Some have called them **altruistic masks** because, while they effectively filter the air leaving the wearer's nose and mouth, they are not as effective at filtering the air inhaled by the wearer.

Masks should be worn at all times within the operating theatre during a procedure and worn as close to the face as possible, using the wired seam to help contour the face. Surgical masks quickly become saturated (due to respiration) which reduces the activity of the microorganism barrier.

Similarly, during exhalation microorganisms travel around the sides of the mask. The main reason for mask use is to prevent larger droplets of contamination from the mouth and nose through talking, coughing, and sneezing. They are also single use and **a new mask should be worn for each surgical procedure.**

A mask should never be allowed to dangle around the neck, put in a pocket or on a surface, and should only be handled by the ties after removal. Careful handling of a used mask by the ties prevents the spread of microorganisms throughout the surgical suite. As soon as the mask is removed it should be placed in a designated receptacle and hands washed.

Protection of the mucous membranes of the eyes, mouth, and nose from procedures that involve splashing or spraying of blood, body fluids, or bone chips is essential. Protective eyewear covering the front and side of the eyes, or full-face visors must be worn by the surgical scrub team and those performing invasive procedures. Masks are available that incorporate visors.

Gowns

Surgical gowns are a form of personal protective equipment and must be worn by all scrubbed personnel, as they provide a protective barrier to prevent fluid and microbial transmission during surgical procedures and maintain the sterile barrier between the surgical field and the surgeon's clothes and exposed arms. They provide a barrier for important areas from the shoulders to the knees and wrists.

Sterile surgical gowns and gloves should be donned from a waist height surface separate from the sterile field. Only the inner side of a sterile gown can be touched when picking it up, usually this is the neck area.

Once a sterile gown and gloves are put on, the gown's sterility is limited to the portions directly viewed by the scrubbed person. These sterile areas include:
- the front of the gown
- from the chest to the sterile field level
- the sleeves from 5 cm below the elbow to the cuff.

The neckline, shoulders, under arms, sleeve cuffs, and the back are considered unsterile. The white sleeve cuffs of the gown are made of soft, permeable material that is not waterproof. Therefore, cuffs tend to collect moisture and cannot be considered an effective bacterial barrier. Sleeve cuffs are considered unsterile when the scrubbed person's hands pass beyond the cuff. If surgical gloves do not cover the cuffs, contamination may occur from inside out or from outside in, which is especially dangerous when the surgeon's hands are deep within a body cavity.

There are two types of gowns available:

Disposable

Disposable gowns are made from non-woven cellulose or synthetic fibres closely bound together to increase the barrier effect compared to woven fabrics. They come prepacked and presterilized, with or without a reinforced paper hand towel. There are two types of disposable gowns: non-reinforced or reinforced.
- **Non-reinforced** surgical gowns are less durable and designed for surgical procedures with low to moderate fluid contact.
- **Reinforced** surgical gowns have reinforced protection in specific critical areas for more invasive and intense surgical procedures.

Some disposable gowns have an additional impervious material on the forearms and gown front to provide extra durability and increase barrier protection.

Reusable

These are made from woven cotton or a polyester/cotton-blend. Ideally, the more fibres (270 fibres per square inch) the better the barrier to microorganisms, with Gore Tex™ gowns providing the best barrier protection. However, like surgical scrubs they require regular care and inspection and do become worn and damaged reducing the effectiveness of the microbial barrier, which is also a result of repeated laundering.

Gloves

The main purpose of surgical gloves is to act as a protective barrier between the transient microflora that has not been eliminated by surgical scrubbing and the surgical site on the patient. Therefore, aiding in the prevention of SSIs and ensuring aseptic technique.

Examination gloves prevent the transmission of microorganisms between veterinary personnel and the patient or vice versa and or between patients. Additionally, they also protect veterinary personnel from harmful chemicals or pharmaceuticals (e.g. cytotoxic drugs, cleaning chemicals).

Surgical gloves are required be of a **higher quality** and are packed in pairs within a sterile packet. Surgical gloves have a **more precise range of sizing** than examination gloves (i.e. S, M and L) as it is important the glove does not impact the surgeon's or scrubbed personnel's dexterity during surgical procedures.

Surgical gloves were first used in the 1890's and are made from a variety of materials (Table 11).

Table 11. Table of glove materials.

Material	Natural/ synthetic	Pros	Cons
Latex	Natural	· Provides the best protection against viruses. · Excellent sensitivity, elasticity, and comfort. · Durable.	· Can be highly allergenic in susceptible people. · Hydrocarbon/ petroleum-based emollients must be avoided as they weaken the rubber; water-based emollients are preferred when wearing latex gloves.
Neoprene	Synthetic	· Latex-free. · High strength.	· A lower level of elasticity and comfort than latex. · More expensive than latex.
Polyisoprene	Synthetic	· Latex-free. · Similar properties to latex in terms of elasticity, comfort, and strength.	· Most expensive.
Nitrile	Synthetic	· Excellent strength and chemical protection.	· Low elasticity, comfort, and sensitivity; can be composed of a mix of nitrile and latex to improve these properties.

There are three surgical gloving techniques for putting surgical gloves on, these are:

1. **Open gloving.** This involves the hands being exposed, but only handling the inside of the glove. Thus, the chances of maintaining an aseptic technique are reduced and it is less reliable. This technique is only suitable for minor procedures when a sterile gown is not required.
2. **Closed gloving.** Hands remain inside the sleeves of the sterile gown until they are covered by the sterile gloves. Ungloved hands never touch the outside of the gown or the gloves. Hence, this technique is the most reliable way of maintaining asepsis.
3. **Assisted gloving.** This relies on the presence of an already scrubbed person who stretches open the cuff of the gloves so the wearer can plunge their hand into the glove. Because the wearers hand is exposed this means there is an increased risk of accidental contact with the outside of the glove and also pushing the cuff too far up the forearm.

It is important gloves fit snugly and hence are the correct size to ensure comfort and prevent a break in asepsis by undetected glove damage due to baggy pouches around the fingers.

Latex gloves are preferred as their elastic properties allow them to conform to the shape of the wearers hands and stretch comfortability with movement. However, latex can be difficult to put on so a lubricating agent such as powder is often used, however this is linked to surgical wound irritation. Powders may also contribute to latex allergies. Thus, powder-free gloves coated with an adherent hydrogel should be used. If required nitrile gloves may be the wearer's choice.

As gloves may become punctured during surgery, **gloves are not a substitute for a thorough skin disinfection technique.**

Double-gloving is often performed during orthopaedic procedures where sharp saws and pins /drills increase the risk of glove perforation. Although, double-gloving reduces the risk of complete perforation (via accidental means) it reduces the wearer's sensitivity and compromises surgical technique, as well as meaning the wearer is less aware when a glove becomes damaged.

In some cases, double-gloving is used during draping of the patient, whereby the outer gloves are removed to prevent accidental contamination.

To maintain asepsis, damaged gloves should be replaced immediately, which requires a non-sterile assistant to remove the glove by pulling on the glove and cuff of the gown simultaneously allowing the wearer to retract their forearm and hand back inside the gown sleeve. The wearer should then re-glove using the closed glove method.

Theatre Practice

52

The prevention of surgical site infections from the operating room is one of the main aims of the surgical team, and all activities performed by the team support this aim.

Surgical site infection rates can be improved by acting upon various factors, from the surgical environment itself to procedural aspects and staff behaviour. Operating room behaviour pertaining to asepsis and aseptic practices have the greatest direct impact upon the surgical team in helping to reduce the patient's risk of surgical site infections.

Theatre Practices

All clinical veterinary personnel have a duty to set a high standard by which to practice. These standards are taken from the focus on clinical effectiveness and evidence-based research which surgical personnel must be able to demonstrate.

Theatre practice is required to ensure good aseptic technique and reduce contamination within surgical areas. Thus guidelines/protocols should be set to which all surgical personnel entering the surgical suite are aware of and must follow. These include only entering the operating room in full theatre attire, which includes a well laundered clean two-piece scrub suit, cap, disposable mask and proper, theatre specific footwear to minimize cross infection.

The do's and don'ts in an operating room are shown in Table 12.

Patient contamination by surgical staff can be direct and indirect. The amount of air that contains bacteria is directly proportional to the movement and number of staff within the operating theatre. In order to reduce airborne bacteria within the operating **theatre the number of persons required for the procedure should be kept to a minimum** and all required consumables and equipment should be available within the operating theatre to:

1. reduce traffic in and out of theatre
2. provide an efficient theatre.

Table 12. Do's and don'ts in theatre etiquette.

Do	Don't
All personnel must wear theatre attire before entering the clean surgical areas (e.g. scrub suites and clean area footwear).	Surgical personnel should not wear jewellery.
Must wear hats and masks when within the operating theatres.	Surgical personnel should not wear nail varnish or false/long nails.
Maintain good personnel hygiene.	Non-scrubbed personnel should not pass between the surgical trolley and surgical site.
Must wash their hands on entering clean areas.	Should not enter the clean area if unwell (e.g. cold).
Access limited to a specific number of surgical staff within the operating theatre.	
Movement in theatre should be kept to a minimum, particularly on entering and exiting theatre in the middle of a procedure.	
Talking in theatre should be kept to a minimum particularly during a procedure.	
Hands must be washed between each patient.	
When non-scrubbed personnel must announce when they are moving past the surgical/scrubbed field.	
Surgical attire should be covered when leaving the surgical theatre/area.	

Thus, advance planning is essential to ensure all necessary equipment/materials are available for the procedure, including those required for possible procedure/anaesthetic risks. Additional equipment may be accessed from pass through cabinets, from within the operating theatre.

Personnel Roles and Responsibilities

To ensure safe and efficient patient care and operation of the surgical suite, the responsibilities of surgical personnel should be clearly defined. Personnel roles are defined as:

The Veterinary Surgeon (primary surgeon)

Has overall responsibility for the patient and performing the surgical procedure (which also involves directing the procedures in theatre).

Surgical Assistant

Depending on the procedure and team there may be more than one assistant, who may also be a veterinary surgeon or veterinary nurse. Their role is to assist the surgeon by passing instruments, ensuring a clean and accessible surgical field, and providing retraction if needed.

Scrub Nurse/Technician

Is in charge of the surgical trolley, ensuring all instruments are free from blood, passing instruments in the correct order for the procedure to the surgeon/assistant, ensuring all instruments and consumables are present and the swab and sharps counted prior, before closing the surgical wound, and at the end of surgery. It is particularly important the trolley is kept tidy and organised, so instruments are easily accessible.

Circulating Nurse/Technician

The circulating nurse is responsible **for the overall organisation within the particular operating theatre.** They aid in gowning and gloving the scrubbed surgical personnel, pass sterile instruments to the scrubbed personnel using aseptic technique. They record use of theatre consumables and control non-sterile equipment (e.g. diathermy/suction). They fetch items required, maintain a swab and sharp count and are responsible for completing the theatre surgical safety checklist.

Veterinary Anaesthetist

Monitors and maintains patient anaesthesia, which allows the surgeon to concentrate on the procedure. The anaesthetist and surgeon work as a team and it is important that good communication occurs as the surgery may affect patient physiology and or anaesthetic complications may occur which may affect the surgery and hence patient care.

Note: In most cases veterinary nurses monitor and maintain veterinary anaesthesia and thus do this under the direction of the veterinary surgeon. Therefore, any desired changes to anaesthesia must be made by the veterinary surgeon.

Creating Positive Surgical Outcomes

Theatre Coordination

The surgical nurse/technician plays an important role in ensuring the smooth running of the surgical procedure. This is achieved by either a designated team leader and or by an individual being given the responsibility of ensuring a particular procedure is run as smoothly and efficiently as possible.

This is achieved by:

- ensuring the correct surgical instruments and materials are **available prior to commencing the procedure.** This may be facilitated by the surgeon completing a surgical request form in advance of the procedure
- preparing the operating room
- preparing the surgical patient
- communicating with the rest of the surgical procedure team including the surgeon(s) regarding the procedure and the patient's postoperative plan
- foreseeing any potential complications which could arise and developing a plan with the surgeon to reduce and handle these complications
- ensuring a surgical safety checklist is performed
- ensuring there is an adequate number of surgical staff for the procedure and defining their roles
- ensuring that cleaning protocols are followed
- organising surgical lists.

Where there are multiple theatres, **theatres should be designated for clean or contaminated procedures** with the aim of minimising the contamination in clean theatres where clean procedures such as orthopaedics are performed involving implants. Procedures which are deemed dirty, such as debridement of a wound over six-hours old should be performed in a separate designated theatre or in the preparation room.

To maintain a gold standard of surgical asepsis, **the surgical list should be arranged relative to the highest risk of contamination from the environment.** Procedures are classified by the type of surgery (i.e. clean, clean-contaminated, contaminated and dirty) (Table 13), whereby clean procedures are started first, progressing to procedures deemed dirty, and those patients known to have a hospital acquired infection (e.g. MRSA, *Pseudomonas*) should go last. **The operating suite should be cleaned between procedures** and then again more thoroughly at the end of the surgical list.

Table 13. Procedure classification.

Procedure classification	Description
Clean	· Non-traumatic wounds. · The procedure does not enter the respiratory, gastrointestinal, or genitourinary tract.
Clean-contaminated	· The respiratory, gastrointestinal, or genitourinary tract is entered with no gross spillage. · A small break in aseptic technique.
Contaminated	· Traumatic wound <4 hours old. · A major break in aseptic technique. · Large spillage of GI contents, infected bile or urine.
Dirty	· Established bacterial tissue infection. · Traumatic wounds with gross contamination >4 hours. · Devitalized tissue. · HAI´s.

However, it is **not always possible to maintain this ideal order of procedural cleanliness, due to patient stability and urgency.** For example, a perforated gastrointestinal tract or gastric dilatation/volvulus (GDV) takes priority over an elective orthopaedic surgery. If this is the case, a thorough cleaning regime between patients is required, particularly if a positive pressure ventilation system is not used. Nevertheless, all surfaces should be cleaned between patients.

Surgical Safety Checklist

The World Health Organisation (WHO) developed and published a simple surgical safety checklist, which is a tool which brings together the whole operating team (surgeons, anaesthesia providers and nurses) to perform key safety checks during vital phases of perioperative care prior to the induction of anaesthesia, prior to skin incision, and before the team leaves the operating room.

The surgical safety checklist comprises 19 items in three parts to be completed in a total of 3 minutes at key points in surgical procedures. The items include measures such as confirming patients' names and procedures, introducing theatre staff to each other and defining their specific roles, and ensuring the appropriate use of prophylactic antibiotics to prevent surgical-site infection.

The checklist includes three moments of formalized briefings and safety checks:

- a **sign in** before induction of anaesthesia
- a **time out** before skin incision
- a **sign out** before the patient and the surgical team leaves the operating room.

Haynes et al. (2009) found that introducing the WHO surgical safety checklist into operating theatres in eight diverse hospitals was associated with marked reduction in morbidity and mortality following surgery in humans.

To apply the checklist, surgical staff must stop before the induction of anaesthesia, before skin incision, and before the patient leaves the operating theatre. In previous studies, these team practices were associated with improved safety processes and attitudes and with a marked reduction in mortality and morbidity rates.

A surgical checklist helps ensure that important safety steps are reliably followed for each and every surgical procedure to ensure a safe, positive surgical outcome. It also ensures patient and staff safety.

See https://www.who.int/patientsafety/safesurgery/checklist/en/ for further reading.

Maintaining Aseptic Technique

The main purpose of asepsis is to prevent contamination of the open surgical wound by isolating the surgical site from the surrounding non-sterile environment. The surgical team accomplishes this by creating and maintaining the sterile field and by following aseptic principles aimed at preventing microorganisms from contaminating the surgical wound.

The Association of Perioperative Registered Nurses (AORN) developed **standards and recommended practices,** which are used by the surgical team to achieve the best results from aseptic techniques.

The principles of aseptic technique play a vital role in accomplishing the goal of asepsis in the operating room environment. It is the responsibility of each surgical staff member to understand the meaning of these principles and to incorporate them into their everyday practice. **The principles of aseptic technique include the following principles.**

1. Scrubbed Personnel

The surgical team is made up of sterile and non-sterile members. Sterile members or scrubbed personnel work directly in the surgical field, while the non-sterile members work in the periphery of the sterile surgical field.

Scrubbed personnel should consider **only the front of the sterile gown from the shoulder/neckline to above the height of the operating table as sterile.** This is because the neckline, axillae and cuffs collect moisture from the wearer and thus allow bacterial strikethrough.

Scrubbed personnel should only lay out the instrument trolley in readiness prior to the first incision. In some cases, instruments and implants known not to be required until the end can remain in their sterile protective packets (i.e. skin staplers).

When sterile items are passed to the sterile field by a non-scrubbed person, they should be passed in a way that the edges of the packaging do not make contact with the sterile item.

Non-sterile personnel should not lean over the sterile field and should not pass packets over the sterile instrument trolley. It is imperative that items should not be tipped onto the surgical trolley particularly by a non-scrubbed person.

There should be minimum movement within the operating room when a surgical procedure is taking place.

2. Use of Sterile Drapes to Create a Sterile Field

Sterile surgical drapes establish an aseptic barrier minimizing the passage of microorganisms from non-sterile to sterile areas. Sterile drapes should be placed on the patient, furniture, and equipment to be included in the sterile field, leaving only the incisional site exposed. During the draping process, only scrubbed personnel should handle sterile drapes. The drapes should be held higher than the operating table with the patient draped from the prepped incisional site out to the periphery and once the sterile drape is positioned, it should not be moved or rearranged as this may drag contamination from the periphery into contact with the prepared sterile field.

After the patient and operating room tables are draped, only the top surface of the draped area is considered sterile. Towel clips should not be repositioned and once used should not be placed back in the sterile field, as they are deemed unsterile.

3. Sterility of Items

Sterile and non-sterile items/areas should not be mixed since one contaminates the other. Sterilisation provides the highest level of assurance so that all instruments, sutures, fluids, supplies, and drapes are free of microorganisms.

A sterile packet's sterility is determined by events and not by time. To ensure sterility, the packaging of all sterile items should be inspected to ensure integrity and the sterilisation process indicators, such as indicator tape and internal chemical indicators, prior to introduction into the sterile field. **If a package is compromised, it should be considered contaminated and not be used.**

Air and fluid can also contaminate a sterile package. When fluid strikethrough occurs, fluid creates a transport mechanism through which microbes can reach the sterile item.

Similarly, when a sterile package is dropped on the floor, this causes air to penetrate the sterile package, via the force. The force created when the package contacts the floor can cause the sterile barrier to be penetrated by forcing sterile air out and allowing contaminated air and particles into the package.

4. Methods to Maintain Sterility and Integrity

All sterile items should be dispensed into the sterile field by methods that preserve the integrity of the items and sterile field. The circulating nurse (non-sterile) must use good judgement when dispensing sterile items by presenting them directly to the scrubbed person or placing them securely in the sterile field. Sterile items tossed into the sterile field may displace other sterile items, penetrate the drape, or roll off the sterile field causing contamination to occur.

Sterile wrapped items which are opened by a non-sterile person, should be opened in a way that the top wrapper flap is opened away from them first, followed by the flaps on each side, with the final wrapper flap pulled towards them. The sterile item is then carefully picked up by scrubbed personnel.

This technique of opening a wrapped package ensures that the non-sterile person does not reach over the sterile item inside. Wrapper edges should be secured to prevent flipping the wrapper and contaminating the contents of the sterile package or field.

After a wrapper has been opened, the inside of the wrapper and its contents are **considered sterile with the exception of the 1-inch outer edge of the wrapper.** This one-inch outer edge of the wrapper is considered the margin of safety between sterile and non-sterile. When a package is double wrapped, only the outer package is opened, and the inner package is left for scrubbed personnel to open.

When a peel-open sterile package is opened, the non-sterile person opens the package by rolling the wrapper over their hands and presenting the inner contents of the package to the scrubbed person. **The package and its contents should be presented in such a way so as to prevent contamination of the sterile item or the scrubbed person.** When determining package content sterility, the inner edge of the heat seal is considered the line separating sterile from non-sterile.

A solution container (such as a bottle of saline) should be opened in a way so that the non-sterile person lifts the cap straight up and slowly pours the contents of the bottle into a sterile container. The sterile container is either held by the scrubbed person away from the sterile field or placed near the edge of a sterile waterproof-draped table.

It is considered that **only the top rim of the bottle top and bottle contents are sterile once the cap has been removed** from the bottle. When sterile fluids are dispensed, the entire contents of the bottle must be poured into the sterile receptacle or the fluid remaining in the bottle discarded.

5. Maintain and Constantly Monitor the Sterile Field

All surgical staff must monitor the sterile field in order to maintain its sterility. Sterility can never be absolutely guaranteed, but surgical team members should make every reasonable effort to reduce the likelihood of contamination and be vigilant to breaches in aseptic techniques and sterility. When a breach of aseptic technique occurs, team members must take immediate and appropriate action to correct the break in sterility in order to reduce further risks of contamination. This may involve discarding contaminated instruments, addition of layers of sterile drapes, and re-gloving of the surgical team, as appropriate.

The sterile field should be prepared as close as possible to the time of the procedure. The sterility of supplies can be affected by the events taking place within the operating room, and the length of time the items are exposed to the environment. Once set up, the sterile field must be monitored constantly. When the sterile field is left unattended, personnel, airborne contaminants, insects, and liquids can contaminate the sterile field. The veterinary practice should have policies and procedures in place to address these issues for the surgical team to follow (e.g. covering the sterile trolley with a disposable sterile drape during intraoperative radiographs).

6. Personnel Moving in a Manner to Maintain the Sterile Field

Scrubbed personnel should remain close to the surgical site and not wander around the room; the latter can result in contamination of the sterile field. Scrubbed personnel should move only from sterile area to sterile area. When scrubbed personnel change positions, they should maintain a safe distance from each other and always pass each other by turning back-to-back or face-to-face. This movement reduces the risk of contamination by ensuring the scrubbed persons are passing either non-sterile to non-sterile or sterile to sterile. Also, consideration should be given to the fact that the back of a sterile team member's gown does not contact the sterile field.

Scrubbed personnel should remain in the position in which they began the surgery. For example, if the surgery begins with the scrubbed person sitting and is completed with the scrubbed person standing, the portion of the gown considered sterile is uncertain.

Scrubbed personnel should always keep their arms and hands within the sterile field to avoid any accidental contact with non-sterile items or areas. Scrubbed personnel must maintain a safe distance when approaching non-sterile objects and personnel. This safe distance or margin of safety is important in identifying safe boundaries between sterile and non-sterile areas.

Non scrubbed personnel should always remain in non-sterile areas and contact only non-sterile items to prevent contamination of the sterile field. Non-sterile personnel should always face the sterile field on approach and should never walk between two sterile fields, ensuring that the sterile area is always being observed and avoiding accidental contact with the sterile field.

It is imperative that non-sterile personnel are aware of and maintain a margin of safety, which is 12 inches (30 cm) or more. When approaching sterile fields and scrubbed personnel and when opening sterile packets, they must never reach over the sterile field.

Surgical Technique

"The only weapon with which the unconscious patient can immediately retaliate upon the incompetent surgeon is haemorrhage." (William Stewart Halstead).

The technical skills of the surgeon are also important in reducing the potential for infection. By close observation of Halstead's principles of atraumatic, aseptic surgery, tissue contamination and injury are minimised. **This results in the preservation of vascularity, tissue oxygenation, and enhancement of wound healing.** The **elimination of dead space** also significantly reduces the infection rate, as well as the placement of minimum numbers of finest appropriate gauge sutures. It is important to **minimise the length of surgery,** since for every hour of surgery, the infection rate is approximately doubled. Increased duration of anaesthesia is also a significant risk factor for surgical site infection.

In the late 19th century William Stewart Halsted introduced basic principles of surgical techniques regarding tissue handling, which are still used today and aid in the prevention of SSIs. These principles are known as the Tenets of Halsted or the Halsted's principles which are:

- **Strict aseptic technique and prior to the surgical procedure.**
- **Gentle handling of tissue and preservation of blood supply.**
- **Good haemostasis (required for good visibility, limiting infection and dead space, maintaining blood volume and hence tissue perfusion).**
- **Minimum tension on tissues (when suturing).**
- **Good surgical judgement ensuring elimination of dead space and adequate removal of material.**
- **Minimisation of surgical time through knowledge of anatomy and techniques.**
- **Correct use of surgical instruments and material.**
- **Accurate tissue apposition.**

Today the following points can be added:

- **Keep tissues moist, especially abdominal, and thoracic organs.**
- **Make a skin incision large enough for the surgical procedure to be performed to prevent unnecessary tissue trauma.**
- **Take biopsies when needed, and always submit them to the laboratory for appropriate analysis.**
- **Provide adequate pain relief.**

The Surgical Assistant

The contribution of the effective surgical assistant influences a positive surgical outcome. Therefore, the **surgical assistant plays a vital role** within the surgical procedure and their role includes:

- passing surgical instruments correctly and managing the surgical trolley
- assisting the surgeon with retraction and haemostasis
- ensuring that diagnostic samples are taken and preserved appropriately
- monitoring the quantity of surgical swabs used and which are in use
- keeping instruments clean and monitoring the instrument counts at the start and after the surgical procedure prior to wound closure
- being one step ahead of the surgeon and predicting the surgeon's instrument requirements
- running continuous suture and cutting sutures. (Maintaining the tension and keeping the strand of suture out of the way of the next suture placement).

The surgical assistant may be another veterinary surgeon and/or a veterinary nurse/technician and must be well trained in aseptic techniques and have knowledge of the surgical procedure itself, the surgical plan, and the procedure steps. The assistant must have an excellent knowledge of the instruments and how they are used for each procedure.

It is imperative the operating trolley is kept organised and clean, as surgical time can be increased looking for a particular instrument. Additionally, a disorganised trolley can also lead to a break in asepsis particularly if sharps are not organised appropriately, this increases the risk of the patient developing an SSI.

During a complex procedure (i.e. total hip replacement, thoracotomy, fracture repair) it is important the surgical assistant pays attention to the surgical procedure and the instrument trolley to ensure all necessary instruments and equipment are readily available and be focused on the procedure itself.

The steps taken by the surgical assistant make the procedure more efficient and allow the surgeon to focus on the surgical field, helping to improve patient outcome and reduce morbidity.

It is important the surgeon has **excellent visualisation of the surgical site,** achieved by careful retraction of tissues. This can be either via self-retaining retractors (e.g. Gelpis, Gossets, Balfour, Wests) or via manual retractors (Langenbecks, Malleable, Hohmann, Senn), whereby the surgical assistant is essential for holding and maintaining retraction.

To prevent tissue damage the surgical assistant must have knowledge of the normal anatomy and be careful not to damage any retracted tissue or organs. They must also know which is the correct way to hold surgical instruments, as per Halsted's principles, and focus on the patient, preventing movement of the retractor which may cause unnecessary patient damage.

The surgical assistant should also have knowledge of the best practices when it comes to holding surgical instruments.

Reducing Surgical Time

Increased surgical time can increase the risk of a poor surgical outcome as the patient is at a greater risk of developing a surgical site infection.

This is because of:

- increased infection rate
- tissues drying out
- increased tissue handling
- increased environmental bacterial contamination
- prolonged anaesthetic time resulting in an increased risk of developing hypothermia, hypotension and dehydration.

Minimising surgical time can be achieved by:

- **Correct patient positioning.** It is essential that the patient is positioned correctly to enable the correct surgical approach for the particular surgical procedure, ensuring normal anatomical landmarks are visible.
- **Understanding anatomy of the surgical site area.** Knowledge of the anatomy of the surgical site is imperative to avoid damaging nerves and causing haemorrhage through damage of vessels. Additionally, time is often spent suctioning and ligating vessels and relocating retractors.
- **Correct retraction of tissues.** The correct use of self-retaining retractors and the use of a surgical assistant improves visualisation of the surgical site and reduces the surgical time as the surgeon can make timely decisions and proceed with the surgical procedure.
- **Keeping an organised surgical trolley.** An organised trolley ensures the surgeon is able to find and receive the required instrument quickly.
- **Adequate haemostasis.** Bleeding increases surgical time due to having to pause to manage the bleeding with vessel-ligation and/or cauterisation and increases surgical time due to poor visualisation of the surgical field, impairing dissection.

Health and Safety

The term health and safety is the state of being well in body and mind, and the condition of being free from danger and risks (Allen, 1991).

The surgical team's daily workload makes them susceptible to a variety of common work-related illnesses. They are exposed to a number of occupational hazards in their professional work including sharp object injuries, blood borne pathogens, latex allergy, laser plumes, hazardous chemicals, anaesthetic gases, equipment hazards, static postures, and job-related stressors.

Hazards and Risks

Health and safety in the clinical environment require the identification of hazards and risks:

- **Hazard:** anything that may cause harm (e.g. chemicals, electricity, working from ladders, an open drawer).
- **Risk:** the chance, high or low, that somebody could be harmed by these and other hazards, together with an indication of how serious the harm could be.

During a clinical procedure health and safety processes affect all those present including:

- patient
- surgeon and the surgeon's assistants
- anaesthetist
- nursing staff
- visitors to the theatre, such as students and medical representatives.

To ensure efficient and safe running of the **theatre list, a designated person** (usually the most senior) should manage it. There should be sufficient staff on duty, all with a clear understanding of their role in the team based on their skills and abilities.

All equipment should be tested before it is needed, and care taken with electrical equipment so that cables do not present a trip hazard or run across areas where there is a risk of fluids pooling. Heating should be set to a level that is safe and comfortable for patients and staff.

Every sharp object should be regarded as a potential source of injury and accepted practices in the handling of sharps adhered to, for example avoiding manual re-sheathing of needles, and disposing of sharps in containers that comply with the hazardous waste regulations act 2005.

Needles, blades, or instruments should never be passed directly from hand to hand, but via a neutral zone, for example a container. Needles and blades should be mounted using the correct instrument, never using fingers. Any sharps injury should be managed and reported.

Legislation

There are a number of pieces of UK legislation which relate to health and safety in veterinary practices. These include:

- Health and Safety at Work Act 1974 (UK).
- Management of Health and Safety at Work Regulation 1999 (UK).
- Ionising Radiation Regulations 1999 (UK).
- Control of Substances Hazardous to Health (COSHH) 2002 (UK).
- Reporting of Injuries, Diseases and Dangerous Occurrence Regulations (RIDDOR) 1995 (UK).

Legislation is dependent on country and territory area. It is therefore important all surgical staff are aware of the legislation applicable to their country/territory of employment.

Health and Safety at Work Act 1974

Health and Safety at Work Act 1974 is synonymous with workplace legislation, and the Management of Health and Safety at Work Regulations 1999 introduced more specific requirements to manage health and safety. Employers are obliged to carry out risk assessments and implement changes as necessary (Health and Safety Executive –HSE–, 2003). Equally, employees have a legal obligation to take reasonable care of their own health and safety and to follow procedures provided for their protection.

Historically, veterinary practices were not proactively inspected by the HSE as a matter of course. However, in a timely reminder of the importance of the RCVS Practice Standards Scheme to modern-day veterinary practice, the HSE has shown this is no longer the case.

All health professionals should have a clear understanding of clinical quality systems and processes for identifying and managing risk. Nurses and technicians have a duty to identify risks to patients and to work with team members to promote environments that are conducive to safe practice.

Employers should introduce new members of staff to basic health and safety laws and principles. Nurse/technician training incorporates awareness of specific legislation such as:

- Manual Handling Operations Regulations 1992 (UK).
- Reporting of Injuries, Diseases and Dangerous Occurrences Regulations 2013 (UK).
- Control of Substances Hazardous to Health 2002 (UK).

For further information on the Health and Safety at Work Act please visit the HSE website: https://www.hse.gov.uk/legislation/hswa.htm

Control of Substances Hazardous to Health (COSHH)

The COSHH Regulations require employers to control substances that are hazardous to health.

Exposure to hazardous substances is prevented or reduced by:
- finding out what the health hazards are
- keeping all control measures in good working order
- providing information, instruction and training for employees and others
- providing monitoring and health surveillance in appropriate cases
- planning for emergencies.

Hazardous substances include:
- substances used directly in work activities, e.g. cleaning agents and medicines
- substances generated during work activities, e.g. waste fumes from anaesthetic equipment
- naturally occurring substances, e.g. dust from litters
- biological agents such as bacteria and other microorganisms.

The following **steps** must be followed to comply with COSHH Regulations:
1. Assess the risks.
2. Decide what precautions are needed.
3. Prevent or adequately control exposure.
4. Ensure that control measures are used and maintained.
5. Monitor the exposure.
6. Carry out appropriate health surveillance.
7. Prepare plans and procedures to deal with accidents, incidents, and emergencies.
8. Ensure employees are properly informed, trained and supervised.

Substances classified as dangerous to health under the **Registration, Evaluation, Authorisation and Restriction of Chemicals (REACH) legislation 2007** (recognizable by their warning symbols) are:
- biological agents
- any kind of dust if concentrations in the air exceed levels specified in the COSHH regulations
- other substances that may pose a risk to health but are not covered by the Chemicals Hazard Information and Packaging for Supply Regulations (CHIP) for technical reasons, e.g. medicines.

Failure to adequately control hazards can lead to prosecution under the COSHH Regulations and civil action from injured or ill employees.

When handling chemicals, the following guidelines must be followed:
- Never eat, drink, or smoke near chemicals.
- Ensure the area is adequately ventilated.
- Read the label and data sheet before use.
- Use the PPE recommended by the manufacturer/data sheet.
- Ensure the chemical is appropriate for the intended use.
- Store chemicals in their original containers with a legible label.
- Use chemicals at the correct dilution/concentration.
- Store chemicals appropriately according to the manufacturer's instruction.
- Do not mix chemical agents.
- Wash hands after use.
- Immediately remove any spillages following the data sheet/manufacturer's recommendations, and report any necessary spillages, e.g. processing chemicals; cytotoxic spills.

RIDDOR (Reporting of Injuries, Diseases and Dangerous Occurrences Regulations) 2013. The Reporting of Injuries, Diseases and Dangerous Occurrences Regulations 2013 also known as RIDDOR, renders the responsibility of employers and the self-employed, as well as those responsible for work premises, to report directly specific situations to the health and safety executive HSE. These are:
- major or fatal accidents
- death of workers and non-workers
- fracture of the skull, spine, pelvis, or long bone of a limb;
- injury requiring amputation of a hand or foot
- loss of sight in one/both eyes
- any other accident which causes admittance to hospital as an inpatient for >24 hours
- serious burns (including scalding) which cover >10% of the body
- any crush injury to the head or thorax that results in damage to the brain and internal organs.

Occupational Diseases

- Occupational asthma: involves the employee being exposed to regular or significant amounts of a known respiratory sanitiser, e.g. airborne disinfectants.
- Cramp of the hand or forearm: which results from the person's work involving prolonged periods of repetitive movement of the fingers, hand, or arm.
- Occupational dermatitis: resulting from regular or significant exposure to a known irritant or skin disinfectant.

- Any accident or illness related to an incident at work which resulted from a >3 day absence from work:
  - slip, trip, or fall resulting in a sprain
  - post-traumatic stress
  - infected bite wound.
- Any dangerous occurrences and or near misses:
  - explosion from a gas cylinder or sterilizer
  - uncontrolled substance release (e.g. gases, vapours, or X-rays)
  - unintentional ignition or explosion
  - escape of substances which may cause inhalation-related risk, or lack of oxygen.

Health and Safety within the Operating Theatre

The characteristics of the operating theatre increase the chances of accidents occurring, from passing sharp instruments in a confined workplace which inhibit members of the surgical team being able to see what is going on. This is further complicated by the requirement of speed, fatigue, anxiety, and stress (Tietjen et al., 2003).

Sharps

In the human medical field incidents involving sharps occur mainly in theatre and are mainly due to scalpel and suture needle injuries (Tietjen et al., 2003).

Injuries involving scalpel blades occur when:
- placing and removing the scalpel blade on and from the handle
- passing the scalpel between the surgical team
- leaving the blade on the scalpel handle during the reprocessing procedure
- using fingers to spread tissues while cutting them with the scalpel
- reaching for a scalpel that is about to fall off the surgical area. i.e. not placing the scalpel back on the instrument trolley in an organised fashion
- using an overfilled sharps container.

Injuries involving suture needles occur when:
- loading the needle holder
- passing a loaded needle holder incorrectly to a surgeon/ between surgical members
- not counting suture needles after each procedure and leaving and disposing them correctly and therefore ending up in the reprocessing procedure
- not using a needle holder to suture
- using fingers to hold tissues that require suturing
- using overfilled sharps containers.

All of these incidents can be avoided by the correct use of sharp instruments, i.e. suture needles and scalpel blades. This is achieved by:
- always using forceps to hold tissue which requires suturing
- removing all sharps from the surgical site as soon as they are no longer required and organising them within a sharps area on the instrument trolley or by using sterile surgical sharps containers during surgical procedures, e.g. scalpel shields, sharps pads, sharp safety stations
- ensuring sharps containers are replaced when they become full
- using magnetic mats when and where required.

For further information on the safe handling of surgical sharps see the AfPP (The Association for Perioperative Practice) Guide to Safe Handling Procedures.

Passing Surgical Instruments Using the Hands-free Technique

Passing surgical instruments particularly those that are sharp via the hand-free technique is the safest technique (Kerrigan, 2015).

The hands-free technique consists of two methods.

Both techniques require good communication skills and cooperation of the surgical team and depend on the willingness of team members to change established routines (Ford, 2014).

- **With neutral zone.** The surgical scrub nurse/ technician places the required instrument within a receptacle such as a sterile kidney dish or commercially made hands-free device (e.g. magnetic mat or sharp passing tray) on the surgical field between them and the surgeon. This area within the sterile field is known as the **neutral zone** and the assistant/scrub nurse communicates to the surgical team that an item has been placed there. The assistant/nurse/technician ensures the receptacle is placed in such a way that the instrument's handle is pointing towards the surgeon who will pick it up. The surgeon then places the instrument back into the receptacle after use but ensures the handle is facing the scrub nurse/technician.
- **Without neutral zone.** The surgical scrub nurse/ technician places the instrument into a receptacle and directly hands the receptacle containing the instrument to the surgeon. The surgeon then picks up the instrument and places the container within the surgical field, before returning the instrument to it. The scrub nurse then retrieves the receptacle with the used instrument from the surgical field and replaces it onto the instrument trolley.

The technique was suggested by the Association of Perioperative Registered Nurses (AORN) with the idea being to lower the frequency of hand passes between the surgical team. The technique is designed to be a standardised procedure for regulating the passing of sharp items to increase the predictability amongst the surgical team who may or may not regularly work within the same team and where the wearing of facial PPE and surgical attire may distort communication (Stinger and Haines, 2006).

Items which are classed as a sharp item include:
- scalpels
- suture needles
- sharp scissors
- trocars (laparoscopy/arthroscopy)
- hypodermic needles
- and any other item that may pierce a glove.

Operating Theatre Fires and Fire Risk Assessments

Theatre fires are rare, given the fact that **the risk of a fire within an operating room is very high.** This is because for a fire to occur three important elements need to be present:
- enough oxygen in order to support combustion
- an ignition or heat source
- a fuel or combustible material.

Otherwise known as the fire triangle.

To prevent a fire from occurring a good understanding of what is known as the fire triangle is needed. A fire is the result of the combination of all these three elements. Removing one or two of the conditions helps prevent a fire.

The dynamics of an operating theatre increase the risk of these three elements being combined. These dynamics include:
- **Combustible materials** found within an operating theatre include:
  - Drapes, plastics, gauze swabs, sterile packaging, volatile anaesthetic agents, bowel gases, alcohol-based cleaning/disinfectant fluids.
- The use of high-energy heat or **ignition sources include:**
  - Diathermy, lasers.
- An **oxygen rich environment:**
  - There is an increase in the oxygen in the environment within an operating theatre compared to in a normal environment. Whereby the normal atmospheric oxygen percentage is 21%. This increase occurs from pneumatic equipment and minute oxygen leaks.
  - Additionally, if nitrous oxide is used, this can fuel a fire similarly to oxygen. The small increase in the level of oxygen within the environment supports the fire burning faster and hotter and is therefore more challenging to extinguish.

It is imperative all members of the surgical team are aware of all the dynamics that could give rise to a fire, and which are present in every surgical procedure. Precautions should be taken to ensure these dynamics do not come together, resulting in a fire.

Fire risk assessment is fundamental to the fire safety management process. A fire risk assessment should be carried out by a competent person and be in place for every building within the hospital/clinic grounds and written in accordance with the requirements of the standard Public Available Specification (PAS 79).

Fire risk assessments should **consider hazards, activities in the buildings, and the fire precautions in place.** Assessments then contain an action plan for areas identified as needing improvement that should be completed in order to maintain or reduce the risk level.

Frequency of risk assessments is determined by the hazards and activities in the building. For example, overnight accommodation or areas containing higher quantities of flammables or buildings with high occupancy levels require more frequent assessments.

Fire precautions within an operating theatre include:
- maintaining adequate ventilation under drapes
- the surgical preparation team: should pay particular attention when prepping, draping, and positioning patients undergoing head and neck procedures. Patients with their heads draped are more susceptible to fire because supplemental oxygen gathers under the drapes. Using an incise drape for surgery in this region helps prevent alcohol vapours becoming trapped and helps to ventilate oxygen (Beesley and Taylor, 2006)
- ensuring alcohol-based skin preparations have sufficient time to dry
- moistening gauze swabs in an aseptic manner so they resist ignition
- all electrical devices, e.g. diathermy and surgical lasers, must be used carefully and responsibly, at the correct setting for the intended outcome
- power cables: should be connected to the appropriate cable connections before they are switched on
- surgical machines: should be placed in standby mode or turned off when not in use
- diathermy electrodes: should be stored on a non-conductive hanger away from the patient when not in use.

All practice staff members should be **familiar with the location and operation of fire alarms and evacuation routes.** Fire procedures should be standardised across the team with fire drills held regularly. Each practice should have its own procedure if there is a fire in another part of the practice during a time when a surgical procedure is taking place and all surgical team members should be aware of this procedure.

Radiation Safety

Exposure to radiation causes intracellular water to ionise. Ionisation releases toxic products that result in the damage of cell structures such as the cell's DNA.

When a living cell meets radiation, the radiation can:

- pass through with no effect
- cause repairable cell damage
- cause non-repairable cell damage
- kill the cell.

Radiation exposure has a cumulative effect. These effects affect tissue cells in several ways. Carcinogenic effects can result in neoplasia and maybe either somatic (occur only in the lifetime of that individual) or genetic (effects are passed to future generations).

Many organ systems are sensitive to ionizing radiation; **the most sensitive systems are those that have rapidly growing and dividing cells,** such as the reproductive and the haematopoietic system.

Excessive exposure to ionising radiation can result in:

- temporary or permanent infertility
- reduced hormone production
- mutations in offspring
- reduced resistance to infection
- reduced resistance to clotting disorders
- increased incidence of squamous cell carcinoma (chronic low-level skin exposure)
- radiodermatitis (chronic low-level skin exposure).

Ionising radiation can come from any of the following sources of exposure:

- **Primary beam:** the X-ray beam prior to any interaction with the patient, grid, table, or image intensifier.
- **Scatter radiation** is defined as the X-rays degraded by collision with tissue molecules. Scatter radiation comes from the patient, floor, and sides of the table.
- **X-ray tube head:** a small amount of radiation will leak from the X-ray tube housing during an exposure. Portable X-ray equipment should therefore not be handheld.
- **Fluoroscopy:** a flow of X-rays is continuously produced, and a real-time image is viewed on a monitor. Minimizing the length of time that the fluoroscope is activated and distance from the primary beam greatly decreases the amount of exposure.

Precautions should be taken to protect clinical personnel from the damaging effects of exposure to ionising radiation, which are well understood compared with other occupational risks.

In accordance with the Ionising Radiation Regulations 1999, staff who work with ionising radiation should limit exposure to no more than is reasonably necessary and should exercise reasonable care while carrying out such work.

Lead shielding is a requirement for all staff remaining in the room while being exposed to radiation.

Lead gowns, gloves, and thyroid shields should all contain at least 0.5 mm of lead. Lead based glasses can also be worn to protect the eyes. A recent study found the use of leaded glasses alone decreased the lens dose rate by a factor of five to ten (Raymond et al., 2010). Note: The 0.5 mm of lead that is commonly used in protective apparel only decreases the primary beam exposure by 25%.

Lead gloves are used to protect the hands and forearms from scatter radiation, but they cannot protect from primary beam exposure. Lead apparel must be handled correctly to prevent damage. Lead aprons should be draped over a rounded surface without folds or wrinkles to prevent cracks in the lead or ideally hung up using an appropriate lead apron hanger facility.

Lead gloves and thyroid shields should ideally be hung on a peg mount and stored in an upright manner to prevent cracks and increase the aeration of the inner lining. If lead gloves are laid flat it is important that nothing is laid on top of them, to prevent damage.

Gloves should be radiographed every six months. Lead gowns should be screened every 12 months to check for holes and cracks in the lead.

Increasing distance from the primary beam also decreases the exposure to X-ray radiation. The law of inverse squares states that X-ray beam intensity decreases to one quarter if the distance between the X-ray source and the operator is doubled (Han, 2019).

Chemical restraint of the patient should always be used, depending on the clinical signs. If this is not possible in certain instances, personnel restraining the patient should make a point of remaining as far as possible from the X-ray source. During exposure, the person restraining the patient should lean back and look away from the beam to protect their eyes. As scatter radiation can come from any direction including from under the tabletop, placing a glove over a hand for protection does not protect from scatter radiation.

Every employee who works with ionising radiation should make full and proper use of the protective equipment provided. The number of people present in theatre should be limited to those necessary for the procedure and those present must wear lead aprons. It is advisable for pregnant personnel to avoid X-rays because radiation may cause foetal abnormalities.

In order to record the amount of radiation one receives during radiographic procedures each member of staff involved in a radiation procedure **must wear a radiation monitoring device.**

There are three types of monitoring devices:

Film Badges
This is the most widely used monitoring device. Each badge contains a small piece of film enclosed in a light proof envelope. This envelope is placed on a plastic carrier such as a ring, wristband, or clipped on to the collar.

- An MREM value correlates with the degree of blackness on the developed film.
- The amount of radiation received is proportional to the degree of blackness on the film.

> **Note: A millirem is equal to 0.001 REM. REM (Roentgen equivalent man) is the amount used to express the dose that results from exposure to ionizing radiation.**

Thermoluminescent Dosimeters (TLD)
These consist of a piece or pieces of thermoluminescent crystalline material (i.e. calcium fluoride or lithium fluoride) inside a radiolucent package. When the crystal is exposed to ionising radiation, it absorbs and traps some of the energy from the radiation in its crystal lattice. The crystal is heated resulting in the release of the trapped energy in the form of visible light. A measurement of the approximate dose of ionising radiation that the crystal was exposed to is then calculated. These monitors can only be read once.

Optically Stimulated Luminescence (OSL) Badges
Materials suitable for OSL, which are similar to those used in thermoluminescent dosimetry, i.e. crystalline solids:

- have similar principle to that of a TLD
- use aluminium oxide to absorb X-ray energy
- use laser light to stimulate trapped high energy electrons within the crystal lattice to emit visible light
- can be read several times.

An image of the filter pattern can be produced to differentiate between static (i.e. instantaneous) and dynamic (i.e. normal) exposure.

The monitoring devices are then sent to an approved laboratory to be processed every three months or less when overexposure is thought to have occurred. Personnel then receive a replacement dosimeter. The amount of radiation each badge receives is recorded under the individual's name or national security number. **To ensure correct readings,** dosimeters should be:

- worn at chest or waist level, and if a lead apron is used in an X-ray area, under the apron;
- only worn by the assigned user. Badges must not be shared;
- badges should be returned to a safe area (where there is a low radiation background area) within the practice at the end of each day and not taken out of the practice, i.e. taken home. Dosimeter monitors that are taken home are frequently lost or damaged;
- the card within the badge should not be moved except when it is changed. (i.e. in the case of TLDs);
- when cards are changed, the card number should be visible, and should be positioned the right way up in the front open window of the badge when the hinge is at the bottom (TLDs); and
- damaged holders should be replaced as soon as possible.

UK radiation employers need to consult a suitable Radiation Protection Advisor (RPA) for advice on complying with the Ionising Radiations Regulations 1999. Employers need to check that the RPA selected meets the criteria of competence in the HSE statement on radiation protection advisers and has the relevant experience to make them suitable to provide the advice needed. If an individual wishes to act as an RPA they must either:

- hold a valid certificate of competence from an organisation recognised by HSE as an Assessing Body for the certification of individual RPAs; or,
- hold a National or Scottish Vocational Qualification (N/SVQ) level 4 in Radiation Protection Practice issued within the last five years.

The hospital must appoint a Radiation Protection Supervisor (RPS) for the purpose of securing compliance with the Ionising Radiations Regulations 2017 with respect to work carried out in an area, e.g. radiography, which is subject to local rules set by the RPA.

An RPS plays a role in helping to ensure adherence to safe working practices implemented by the employer, in particular supervising safe working arrangements set out in local rules. Legal responsibility for compliance remains with the employer and cannot be delegated to the RPS.

To achieve the above an RPS is required to:

- know and understand the requirements of the regulations and local rules relevant to the type of work
- command sufficient authority from people doing the work to allow the RPS to supervise the radiation protection aspects of the work
- understand the precautions necessary to restrict exposure;
- know what to do in an emergency
- recognise the need to seek advice in certain circumstances.

An RPS is formally appointed in writing by the hospital director/practice manager and must complete an accredited and validated RPS training course.

Duties vary depending on the type and scale of work involved and the availability of additional local competent staff and support and include:

- providing support and advice to assist staff in the day-to-day control of activities using ionising radiation
- assisting in carrying out risk assessments for work involving radioactive sources and in writing local rules
- making sure staff are provided with information, instruction, and training on safe working with substances and equipment capable of emitting ionising radiation
- supervising keeping of source records for radioactive sources
- undertaking physical stock checks of radioactive sources
- setting up a regular scheme for monitoring and recording of contamination levels and/or radiation dose rates for their area of responsibility
- arranging for the immediate repair of any defective safety or warning system associated with equipment which emits ionising radiation
- coordinating the periodic testing of radiation monitoring equipment
- coordinating the periodic leak testing of sealed radioactive sources
- ensuring contingency plans exist in the event of an accident or incident, particularly if a person is accidentally exposed to ionising radiation or there is damage, theft or loss of a radioactive source.

Electrical Safety (Fixed Wiring Testing and Portable Appliance Testing)

Electrical equipment used during or in the vicinity of the treatment, monitoring or diagnosis of a patient is classed as a medical electronic device. Examples of electrical medical devices range from:

- operating tables
- infusion pumps
- hoists
- suction pumps
- scales
- diathermy
- multiparameter monitors
- syringe drivers
- clippers
- vacuums.

Before any electrical equipment is used it should be physically capable of operation, designed and constructed so that any mechanical or electrical stressors do not damage or make the equipment unsafe to use.

If electrical equipment is used in a damp environment, then battery or air powered equipment may be preferred. Alternatively, use at a lower voltage should be possible i.e. with a transformer.

Electrical equipment must be inspected each time it is to be used to ensure it is in good condition. This is to prevent any accidents and or further equipment damage from occurring.

An electrical check involves:

- **Switching off and unplugging the equipment before starting the check.**
- **Checking that the plug is not damaged and that the cable is properly secured with no internal wires visible.**
- **Checking the electrical cable is not damaged and has not been repaired with insulating tape or an unsuitable connector. Damaged cables should be replaced with a new cable by a competent person, or the equipment should be replaced.**
- **Checking that the outer cover of the equipment is not damaged in a way that will give rise to electrical or mechanical hazards.**
- **Checking for burn marks or staining that suggest the equipment is overheating.**
- **Positioning any trailing wires so that they are not a trip hazard and are less likely to be damaged.**

Portable appliance testing, also known as PAT, is the examination of electrical appliances and equipment to ensure they are safe to use. Many electrical safety defects can be found by visual examination, but some types of defects are only found by testing. It is important to understand that visual examination is an essential part of the process because some types of electrical safety defects cannot be detected by testing alone.

The UK Health and Safety Executive, along with insurance companies, expect employers to perform PAT (Portable Appliance Testing) testing to ensure compliance with certain regulations including:

- Health and Safety at Work Act of 1974.
- The Electricity at Work Regulations of 1989.
- The Provision and Use of Work Equipment Regulations of 1998.
- The Management of Health and Safety at Work Regulations of 1999.

Non-compliance with the above-mentioned regulations can result in fines of up to £5000 and/or 6 months custodial sentence.

PAT testing forms part of the RCVS practice standard scheme. Many pieces of surgical and practice electrical equipment (UK) require PAT testing and are tested to a medical standard.

It should be ensured the electrical supply is safe to use. Regular tests should be performed by a competent person, using suitable equipment and this is a good way of reducing risks. Where there is evidence that the supply may not be safe, such as damaged equipment or wiring, the supply should not be used until work has been done to correct this.

Fixed wire testing, also known as an electrical installation condition report (EICR), ensures the electrical installations or circuits within the practice/hospital conform with the latest wiring regulations, in order to comply with relevant workplace safety legislation.

Diathermy (electrosurgery)

Electrosurgical (diathermy) devices use high frequency electrical current to generate heat, which can cut and coagulate body tissue. Diathermy may be used in either monopolar or bipolar mode.

In monopolar mode the electrical current flows from the generator in the electrosurgery apparatus to an active electrode, which is the surgeon's tool. The current continues through the patient to an adhesive dispersive plate (the return electrode) placed appropriately on the patient's body so that it is earthed safely back to the electrosurgery unit, thereby preventing electrical burn. The return electrode should be placed over a vascular, muscular area to promote electrical conductivity and to dissipate heat.

In bipolar mode both active and return electrodes are combined within the same instrument. One prong of the bipolar forceps is active, and the other is the return electrode. This system is safer because the patient does not form part of the electrical circuit and therefore a dispersive plate is not required. If the patient has a pacemaker, this is the system of choice to avoid a monopolar current passing through the heart. However, the low power, low voltage waveform used with this system means it is usually incapable of cutting.

Generally, diathermy is accepted as safe, however electrosurgery-induced injuries such as surgical burns and fires can result from incorrect diathermy use.

Accidental burns are often linked to the return electrode and can arise due to one of the following mechanisms:

- at the site of the grounding electrode
- resulting from the electrode heating pooled sterilizing solutions (i.e. Surgical Spirit™)
- outside the operating field resulting from aberrant circuits generated between the active electrode and an alternate grounding source.

Diathermy can also account for surgical fires, particularly when it is used when there is pooling of flammable skin preparation fluid and during oropharyngeal/facial procedure, due to close proximity of oxygen/volatile agents within anaesthetic breathing systems.

The patient's skin should be evaluated before and after diathermy use. Correct use of equipment will ensure that skin integrity remains. The patient should not be in contact with grounded metal objects as the provision of an alternative pathway for the electrical current could result in a burn. Any metal parts of the operating table that could come into contact with the patient should therefore be padded.

Clipping may be required as fur at the dispersive site prevents complete plate contact with skin. Alternatively, ultrasound gel is usually used to ensure conductivity. The plate should not be placed over bony prominences (this can impede return current), over implanted prostheses (there is a potential for overheating), over scar tissue, or over areas distal to where adequate tissue perfusion cannot be guaranteed.

Diathermy use can also give off vapour (surgical plume) and it is suggested that this vapour may consist of toxic particles in addition to carbonised patient tissue, viral DNA tissue, bacteria, and blood particles. It is therefore recommended that filtered ventilation systems are used within the operating area.

Lasers

Laser is an acronym for Light Amplification by the Stimulated Emission of Radiation and use in the veterinary setting is expanding. Smaller reliable lasers are available for clinical use in veterinary medicine. Safety issues with the use of lasers in veterinary medicine are almost identical to those required for human surgical medicine.

A laser classification system was developed to identify the potential hazards of a laser. The manufacturer should make the laser class visible on the equipment. There may be differences in the classification of lasers between different countries and territories.

The British Standards sets out eight classes of laser products, with class 1 to 3R being used in general products such as alignment products for home improvement work.

Class 3B and 4 laser products produce higher laser emission levels and are designated in the highest hazard category. This is because radiation emitted from these devices is a hazard to unprotected eyes or skin resulting from the direct beam, its reflection and or scattering. The direct beam may also be a fire hazard if it strikes combustible materials.

A. Class 3B (e.g. lasers used for physiotherapy)
- Have an output power of ≤500 mW.
- Have sufficient power to cause ocular injury directly and indirectly.
- May produce minor skin injuries.
- Pose an ignition risk.

B. Class 4 (e.g. surgical lasers)
- Have an output power of ≤500 mW.
- No restriction on output power/emission.
- Have sufficient power to cause ocular injury directly and indirectly.
- Produce skin injuries.
- Pose an ignition risk.

Most lasers used in veterinary medicine produce an intense beam of pulsed or continuous invisible infrared light (radiation), which is used for cutting and sealing tissue.

The benefits of using laser radiation in surgery include:
- decreased bleeding as smaller blood vessels are sealed
- decreased pain in postoperative recovery
- destruction of bacteria.

It is therefore essential that all personnel involved with their use are properly educated regarding their safe use. **A brief, inadvertent exposure to high power laser radiation can cause permanent eye injury** and/or skin burns to both the patient and or personnel in the vicinity.

There are several hazards regarding the use of lasers in surgery. Examples include:
- eye damage to personnel/the patient
- skin damage to personnel/the patient
- fire, particularly if used in the same area as combustibles.

Prevention of Ocular Damage

Transmitted directly or reflected into the eye, laser light can potentially burn the retina causing a permanent blind spot. If it hits the head of the optic nerve, it may cause partial or total blindness. Since the beam is virtually non-divergent, increasing the distance from the laser confers little safety benefit.

Infrared laser light is perhaps more dangerous because it cannot be seen. The cornea, lens, and aqueous and vitreous humours are considered risk areas.

Eye protection for all personnel, including the patient, must be provided. Eyewear must be labelled with the same wavelength of laser radiation as is emitted by the laser. In addition, it must be labelled with an optical density (OD) number.

The optical density of the eyewear is unique to both the output power/energy used by the laser and the laser's wavelength. Consequently, protective eyewear must have an OD that is recommended by the laser equipment manufacturer. This is likely to be at least an OD of 5 or greater.

Eyewear must also:
- have adequate side protection: this means the eyewear must have side and top guards and fit snugly around the nose
- be regularly inspected for cracks and discoloration and replaced as required
- should not be moved between rooms, nor should they be carried in pockets between use
- be inspected regularly since small cracks, discoloration, or loose-fitting filters may permit the laser beam to reach the eye directly.

All staff, who work periodically with the laser, should have their eyes checked prior to their first occupational exposure with the laser and as further recommended by an optometrist.

Prevention of Skin Damage

If the skin is exposed to laser radiation it can cause a burning sensation and damage skin from direct and reflected laser light, which may appear as an erythematous reaction or even like severe sunburn. This can be avoided by wearing gloves and safety gowns.

Laser backstops (barriers), which protect underlying tissue, and instruments that have a non-reflective finish are used within the vicinity of a laser beam to prevent laser reflection. Windows in the laser treatment area are required to be covered with a non-flammable opaque material labelled with its optical density OD number. Window glass has an optical density of 5.0 for short wave ultraviolet and long wave infrared without being covered. All doors should be closed, and a warning entry light should also be used to avoid unprotected personnel from entering during laser operation. Skin of sedated or anaesthetised patients must also be shielded.

Laser use can also produce airborne contaminants (just like diathermy), known as surgical plume. This surgical plume may contain harmful materials such as bacteria and viruses, hazardous chemicals. Therefore, efficient ventilation systems are required.

Surgical fires can also be a result of improper laser use. Lasers should not be used in the presence of flammable anaesthetics, preparation solutions that contain alcohol, petroleum creams or flammable plastics.

Volatile liquids and gases

Theatre ventilation systems help to extract toxic gases that could lead to:

- fatigue
- nausea
- headaches.

These may play a part in a range of health problems including:
- renal problems
- hepatic problems
- neural diseases.

Any system-failure warning lights should be reported, investigated, and promptly fixed. The smoke produced when electrosurgical devices are used contains toxic substances that present biological and chemical hazards, so extraction systems should be used during procedures involving diathermy. It is advisable to avoid the use of flammable solutions with diathermy and lasers as there is the risk of ignition.

Methyl methacrylate is a volatile flammable liquid used in orthopaedic surgery to make bone cement. The vapour given off on mixing may cause irritation of the eyes and the respiratory passages or a general feeling of ill health. Anyone affected should leave the theatre immediately. Soft contact lenses should be removed when methyl methacrylate is being mixed as they are permeable to irritant vapours.

Inhalation anaesthetics may be gases or volatile liquids and require suitable equipment for storage and administration. Gas cylinders used in theatre must be clearly labelled with the name or chemical symbol of the gas on the shoulder of the cylinder and the valve. They should be stored in a cool, well-ventilated room, free from flammable materials. No lubricant of any description should be used on the cylinder valves.

Nitrous oxide, used in anaesthesia, can be dangerous to both patient and staff if used for a prolonged period in an inadequately ventilated space. Hence, its use should be regulated and used properly in closed anaesthetic breathing systems.

References

■ Ackerman, N. (2015) Antibiotic resistance in veterinary practice: a veterinary nurse's perspective. *The Veterinary Nurse.* 6 (4), 242–245.

■ Bornside, G.H., Crowder, V.H. and Cohn, I. (1968) A bacteriological evaluation of surgical scrubbing with disposable iodophor-soap impregnated polyurethane scrub sponges. *Surgery.* 64 (4), 743–751.

■ Burgess, B.A. (2019) Prevention and surveillance of surgical infections: A review. *Veterinary Surgery.* 48 (3), 284–290.

■ Dean, A. (2004) Strategies for infection control in the operating theatre. In: 2nd ed *Fundamentals of operating department practice,* Cambridge University Press, pp. 37–42.

■ Egleston, S. (2018) The forgotten complication: aspiration pneumonia in the canine patient. *The Veterinary Nurse.* 9 (3), 138–143.

■ Feilberg, E. (2015) MRSA in veterinary practice and the need for infection control link nurses. *The Veterinary Nurse.* 6 (7), 372–379.

■ Findji, L. (2014) Antibiotics in surgical patients. *Clinician's Brief. Surgery, Soft Tissue.*

■ Jones, I.D., Case, A.M., Stevens, K.B., Boag, A. and Rycroft, A.N. (2009) Factors contributing to the contamination of peripheral intravenous catheters in dogs and cats. *Veterinary Record.* 164 (20), 616–618.

■ Kümin, M. and Scarborough, M. (2017) Laminar flow ventilation during surgery. *The Lancet Infectious Diseases.* 17 (6), 581.

■ Lages, S.L.S., Ramakrishnan, M.A. and Goyal, S.M. (2008) In-vivo efficacy of hand sanitisers against feline calicivirus: a surrogate for norovirus. *Journal of Hospital Infection.* 68 (2), 159–163.

■ Lim, K.S. and Kam, P.C.A. (2008) Chlorhexidine-pharmacology and clinical applications. *Anaesthesia and intensive care.* 36 (4), 502–512.

■ Mayhew, P.D., Freeman, L., Kwan, T. and Brown, D.C. (2012) Comparison of surgical site infection rates in clean and clean-contaminated wounds in dogs and cats after minimally invasive versus open surgery: 179 cases (2007–2008). *Journal of the American Veterinary Medical Association,* 240 (2), 193–198.

■ McBride M.E., Duncan W.C., Knox J.M. (1973) An evaluation of surgical scrub brushes. *Surgery, Gynaecology & Obstetrics.* 137, 934–936.

■ McDonnell (2009) *Encyclopaedia of Microbiology* 3rd ed. Science Direct, Elsevier Inc.

■ McHugh, S.M., Corrigan, M.A., Hill, A.D.K. and Humphreys, H. (2014) Surgical attire, practices and their perception in the prevention of surgical site infection. *The Surgeon,* 12 (1), 47–52.

■ Mitchell, K.G. and Rawluk, D.J.R. (1984) Skin reactions related to surgical scrub up: Results of a Scottish survey. *British Journal of Surgery,* 71 (3), 223–224.

■ Nalamura, R.K. and Tompkins, E. (2012) Nosocomial Infections. Infectious Disease Compendium, 4(4). *Compend Contin Educ Vet,* 34 (4):E1-10; quiz E11.

■ Nelson, L.L. (2011) Surgical site infections in small animal surgery. Veterinary Clinics: *Small Animal Practice,* 41 (5), 1041–1056.

■ Nicolette, L.H. (2011) *Infection prevention and control in the perioperative setting. Alexander's Care of the Patient in Surgery, 13th ed.* St Louis, MO: Elsevier, 52.

■ O'Dwyer, L. (2017), April. Hospital-acquired infection: the cost to practice. In: *BSAVA Congress Proceedings 2017.* BSAVA Library, pp. 347–348.

■ Percival, S.L., Thomas, J.G. and Williams, D. (2010) *An introduction to the world of microbiology and biofilmology.* CRC Press: Boca Raton, pp. 1–58.

■ Salzman, M.B. and Rubin, L.G. (1995) Intravenous catheter-related infections. *Advances in pediatric infectious diseases,* 10, 337–368.

■ Sanon, M.A. and Watkins, S. (2012) Nurses' uniforms: How many bacteria do they carry after one shift? *Journal of public health and epidemiology,* 4 (10), 311.

■ Shales, C. (2012) Surgical wound infection and antimicrobial prophylaxis. In: *BSAVA Manual of Canine and Feline Surgical Principles.* BSAVA Library, pp. 220–230.

■ Spruce, L. and Braswell, M.L. (2012) Implementing AORN recommended practices for electrosurgery. *AORN journal,* 95 (3), 373–387.

■ Thornton, R.H., Dauer, L.T., Altamirano, J.P., Alvarado, K.J., Germain, J.S. and Solomon, S.B. (2010) Comparing strategies for operator eye protection in the interventional radiology suite. *Journal of Vascular and Interventional Radiology,* 21 (11), 1703–1707.

■ Weese, J.S. (2008) A review of postoperative infections in veterinary orthopaedic surgery. *Veterinary and comparative orthopaedics and traumatology,* 21 (02), 99–105.

■ White, S.A. (2001) Peripheral intravenous therapy-related phlebitis rates in an adult population. *Journal of Infusion Nursing,* 24 (1), 19–24.

■ Williams J. (2018) The why and how of antimicrobial prophylaxis, *Companion* 11, BSAVA Library, pp. 4–7.

Test

Answers on Page 70

1. FIV is transmitted via saliva through infected food bowls.

a. True.
b. False.

2. What are Protozoa?

a. A type of bacteria.
b. A single cell-organism that can be zoonotic and parasitic.
c. A type of virus.
d. A type of fungus.

3. When do hospital acquired infections occur?

a. Two days or more after hospital admission; Within three days following hospital discharge or one month after a surgical procedure.
b. The day after hospital admission; within two days following hospital discharge or two months after a surgical procedure.
c. Any time during a hospital stay.
d. Two days or more after hospital admission; within two days following hospital discharge or after a surgical procedure.

4. What type of bacteria does the following image show?

a. Gram-negative bacilli.
b. Gram-positive cocci.
c. Gram-negative cocci.
d. Gram-positive bacilli.

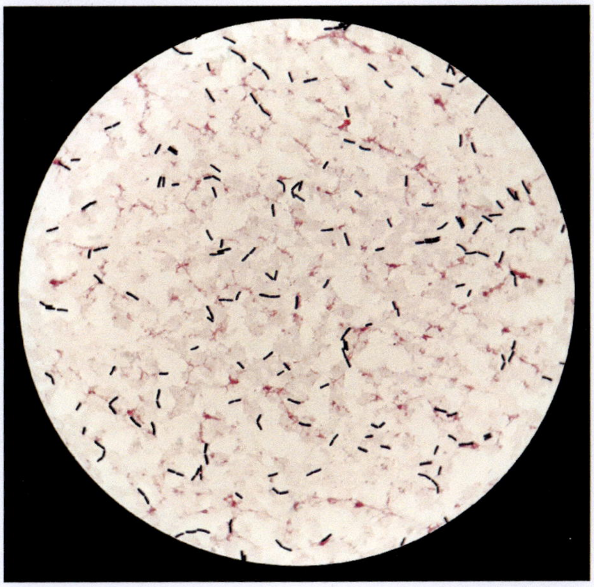

5. Which type of carrier is a higher risk to other patients?

a. Convalesce carrier.
b. Healthy carrier.

6. What does the traffic light system not consider?

a. Patients requiring reverse barrier nursing.
b. Already patient that have a contagious disease.
c. Patients which are undergoing a surgical procedure.
d. Staff that are colour blind.

7. Coagulase positive Staphylococcus are known to be pathogenic.

a. True.
b. False.

8. Chlorohexidine is an example of what type of disinfectant agent?

a. Quaternary Ammoinum Compound (Quats).
b. Phenol.
c. Aldehyde.
d. Iodophor.

9. The chromium layer of a stainless-steel surgical instrument increases with age.

a. True.
b. False.

10. Eye wear for the protection against lasers should have an optical density of:

a. 1.
b. 3.
c. 4.
d. 5 and above.

Correct Answers

1. **b.** (FIV is transmitted most effectively via direct contact through bite wounds).
2. **b**
3. **a**
4. **d**
5. **b.** Healthy carriers never shown signs of the disease, or are immune to it. These carriers are a particular risk to other animals, as there is no history of disease, it is impossible to tell that they are a carrier.
6. **a, d**
7. **a**
8. **a**
9. **a**
10. **d**

Notes

The Patient

Claire L. Dorey-Phillips

Chapter Summary:

- **Patient presurgical assessment.**
- **Patient preparation techniques and positioning required for specific surgical procedures.**
- **Nursing care plans and their use in pre-and postoperative surgical patients.**
- **The role of nutrition in the surgical patient.**
- **The importance of client communication in relation to a hospitalised patient.**

Patient Assessment

The success of a surgical procedure depends on good planning and an **awareness of potential patient risk factors.** A thorough patient preoperative assessment and selecting the optimum surgical procedure for a particular patient are imperative in order to reduce surgical risks and achieve a positive outcome.

Patient History

The aim of taking a patient history is to **obtain as much accurate information** as possible, to enable the surgeon and client to decide on the best surgical plan for the patient.

A thorough **physical examination and complete clinical history** are essential to the process. This helps evaluate the patient for underlying disease and identify other abnormalities or preexisting risk factors which may affect the surgical outcome and hence if the procedure is appropriate.

Preoperative assessment is also necessary to **select the most appropriate anaesthetic protocol** tailored to an individual patient's needs. Many anaesthetic complications result from preexisting clinical conditions, most of which are associated with abnormalities that are identifiable through a thorough clinical history and physical examination.

The clinical history should document the patient's signalment, diet, current exercise regime, how the patient copes with that level of activity, the patient's environment, past medical issues, current and recent treatment, evidence of infection and symptoms which have prompted the current clinical evaluation and possibly surgical intervention. It is vital to identify any history of seizures to avoid drugs which may precipitate seizures. Any allergies should also be clearly noted.

The consultation is the first opportunity to explore the client's expectations and aspirations, plus any financial constraints or issues which may influence the client's decision. Any reported concerns should be followed up with additional questioning to clarify the nature of the complaint. This is also the first opportunity for the client to meet the surgeon and form a judgement on their ability.

However, patients are also often presented by caretakers who may not have extensive information on the patient's background or make daily observations. The patient may live outdoors or roam free much of the time (e.g. feline patients), preventing the caretaker from making close observations.

To obtain a useful history, it **is important to phrase open questions to obtain the most accurate information possible.** Asking, "Has the patient had diarrhoea?" may prompt the client to answer "No", as they have not observed the animal to have diarrhoea. Instead, asking "Have you seen the patient's stools recently?" allows you to determine whether the client can provide an accurate description, or you may need to look to other physical signs for the information.

Patient Assessment

To reduce anaesthetic and surgical complications **a whole-body approach** should be used for the assessment. The temptation to focus on the most obvious complaint should be avoided. Developing a thorough patient assessment and physical examination is a key skill for veterinary nurses/technicians.

A good physical examination detects minor abnormalities before they become serious problems, as well as identifying major organ dysfunction without extensive and expensive diagnostic tests. This is **particularly true for geriatric, young, and neonatal patients** and those suffering major systemic disease states including major trauma. It is important to remember that old age is not a disease in itself and thus should not influence the surgical outcome.

Nevertheless, increased age does increase the risk of other diseases and concurrent organ failure (i.e. renal insufficiency and cardiac dysfunction). **Young patients are particularly prone to risk factors** such as the inability to regulate body temperature and blood glucose, thus increases in the associated anaesthetic risks.

A thorough and well-rehearsed practical and systematic evaluation (e.g. via a head to tail approach) of the patient should be carried out, which includes **all body systems.** The patient's general condition, including their body condition, demeanour, and mental status should be noted. A neurological examination and orthopaedic examination should be carried out on all traumatised patients, in addition to evaluating the respiratory, cardiovascular, urinary, and gastrointestinal systems.

Many emergency patients require stabilization and hence only a preliminary examination is possible until the patient is stabilised. Repeated reassessment is needed for trauma patients as some injuries are apparent immediately (e.g. a fractured limb) whilst others take time to develop (e.g. abdominal effusion from a ruptured abdominal organ). Additionally, patients may have also received medications (analgesia) which impact the examination findings.

When examining surgical patients, it is important to remember you are not only determining their general condition, but evaluating them for anaesthetic and surgical risk factor.

Any physical exam finding that might impact anaesthesia or surgery must be evaluated by a veterinarian before the patient is admitted for surgery so that any potential risks can be discussed with the client before the animal is admitted.

Findings that require veterinary surgeon evaluation and attention include:

- TPR values outside the normal range
- patients older than 6 years of age or younger than 12 weeks of age
- patients weighing less than 2 kg or more than 35 kg
- a history of diarrhoea or vomiting
- a history of recent trauma (past month)
- significant abnormalities on physical exam (dehydration, heart murmur, upper respiratory infection etc.).

Abnormalities or findings that might impact anaesthesia or surgery (e.g. age, physical condition, reproductive status such as oestrous or pregnancy) should be noted in the alerts area of the anaesthesia record along with notification of the anaesthesia team.

It is important to **record all results (both positive and negative) as a legal record** of a thorough examination. Colleagues use this information to evaluate and track the patient's condition, so it is crucial that examination findings are thorough and legible.

It is important to remember to sign the exam record so the next person working with the patient knows who performed this initial examination and can ask follow-up questions if necessary.

A patient examination is commonly recorded using **the SOAP method to ensure its completeness:**

- **Subjective.** The subjective evaluation of the patient; this includes information which cannot be measured in a quantifiable manner e.g. the patient's posture, demeanour and/or behaviour, assessment of pulse quality by palpation, and mucous membrane colour.
- **Objective.** Compiled from the physical exam and diagnostic test/procedures. It summarises factual information which is quantifiable and assessable in a repeatable manner with a numerical result, such as pulse rate and respiratory rate, bodyweight, blood glucose, and temperature.
- **Assessment/analysis.** This is a summary of the clinical signs and diagnosis/differential diagnoses (to assess the patient's disease process/condition), and a comparative exercise to assess patient progress in between each examination (to assess whether the patient is improving).
- **Planning.** This outlines the patient's plan and details the need for additional testing and consultation with other clinicians to address the patient's illnesses. It may also address additional steps to treat the patient and help future personnel understand what needs to be done next e.g. if the patient is beginning a new treatment protocol, or if a procedure is to be performed.

Note: **subjective and objective data are often indistinct, so it is common to combine the entries for these two sections under the heading S/O.**

Distant Assessment Process

Undertake a **brief behaviour assessment before handling or interacting with the patient.** This is to assess the patient's body language and communication methods, to detect any signs of distress, fear and or pain. Behaviours associated with stress or fear are not only detrimental to the patient but may pose a health and safety risk to clinical personnel.

These behaviours also influence the objective parameters and result in false readings.

Signs of Distress in Dogs

- changes to ear carriage and tail position e.g. ears flattened, and tail tucked between legs

- low or cowering body position
- yawning and lip-smacking
- brow furrowing
- salivation
- panting
- facial expressions
- hypervigilance
- refusing treats
- appearing sleepy (when not tired) or distracted
- involuntary urination or defecation.

Signs of Fear or Distress in Cats

- lowered body position
- flattened ears
- staring and dilated pupils
- twitching tail (agitation)
- immobility
- whiskers back
- involuntary urination or defecation.

Cats are naturally neophobic (frightened of anything new). When cats become more distressed, they make themselves smaller within a hiding position. Aggression is often a last resort when escape from the stressful situation is not possible. For further information on handling feline patients please see the AAFP-AAHA: Feline Life Stage Guidelines. "Feline handling": https://journals.sagepub.com/doi/suppl/10.1016/j.jfms.2009.12.006/suppl_file/Respect fulHandlingofcats.pdf.

The patient's disease process and or clinical signs may also change their normal behaviour and should be taken into consideration.

Before a physical assessment is performed on the patient, **the patient should be observed from a distance** to assess:

- **General appearance:** the patient should be observed from a distance and up close before any handling. Any asymmetry, differences in the size or shape of extremities, respiratory pattern, effort, and rate should be noted.
- **Respiratory assessment** (distant): initial respiratory assessment should be performed at a distance to avoid stress-induced tachypnoea. The patient's respiratory pattern, rate, and effort should be observed and monitored for increased effort and difficulty during respiration (dyspnoea). For example, is the patient showing any of the following clinical signs:
    - **increase in the expansion of the ribs** and/or abdominal muscles during respiration
    - **open mouth breathing**
    - **orthopnoea:** adopting a specific body position to aid respiration
    - **paradoxical respiration:** abnormal movement of the diaphragm during respiration. In paradoxical respiration, the chest may move inward during inspiration, and outward during expiration.

Cats in respiratory distress usually stay in sternal recumbency, with abducted elbows, an extended neck, and may or may not open mouth breathe.

If the patient has a rapid respiratory rate with deep breaths, then the patient is hyperpnoeic, whereas tachypnoea is a rapid respiratory rate with shallow breaths.

If changes in respiratory effort are seen, it should be **noted whether this occurs during inspiration, expiration, or both respiratory phases.** If tachypnoea or dyspnoea are severe or persist for prolonged periods >24–48 hours, respiratory failure can result.

Body Condition

An appropriate body condition score using standard nine-point scale (BCS = 1–9) to assess the current body fat should be used. The ideal is a patient BSC of 4–5 out of 9.

It is useful to know that in 2017, Cambridge University developed a specific BCS for pugs and other brachycephalic breeds.

Muscle condition score (MCS) is also important to determine muscle mass. Patients with acute or chronic disease have greater muscle loss than those patients that are healthy and have been deprived of food. **Muscle loss has adverse effects on wound healing and the immune system.**

A MCS should be carried out at the time of physical examination and in conjunction with the body condition score, particularly in the overweight/obese patient. The MCS is graded as:

- normal
- mild loss
- moderate loss
- severe loss.

The body condition score and muscle condition score are not directly related.

Mentation/Level of Consciousness

This is evidenced as **the patient's attentiveness and reaction to environment.**

Mental status assessment of the patient observes the way in which the patient reacts to:

- tactile, visual, and auditory stimuli
- interacts with the surroundings, owner, other animals, people, and veterinary staff.

Is the patient:

- **hyper-excitable**/over-reacting to normal stimuli
- **alert and responsive:** normal patient interaction with surroundings and people
- **depressed/dull:** reduced responsiveness to normal stimuli
- **stupor:** consciousness is reduced

– **lateral or sternal recumbency:** only responsive to strong stimuli
– **coma:** unconscious and unresponsive to any stimuli.

> **Example:** **A normal healthy patient's mentation is often bright, alert, and responsive or BAR. A healthy puppy may be described as active and playful, while a sick puppy may be moderately depressed and inactive.**

Posture, Gait, and Ambulation

The patient's gait and movement should be assessed prior to physical examination. The patient should be taken to an appropriate area to observe how they walk, and observed for abnormalities such as limping, incoordination or unsteadiness, exaggerated movements, and abnormal limb placement.

Potential gait abnormalities include ataxia, hypermetria, paresis and paralysis.

– **Ataxia is a lack of co-ordination,** which can occur in the head, trunk of the body or the limbs, or a combination of areas. Patients with a drunken appearance are typically unsteady and are classified as ataxic.
– **Hypermetria is exaggerated lifting of the limbs** when walking.
– **Paresis** may be an incomplete paralysis, or weakness, of one or more limbs, and animals with paralysis or plegia have a complete loss of motor function in one or more limbs/body parts.

Paresis and paralysis are classified as follows:

– **Paraparesis/paraplegia:** weakness/paralysis of the pelvic limbs.
– **Hemiparesis/hemiplegia:** weakness/paralysis of two limbs on the same side of the body.
– **Quadriparesis or tetraparesis:** weakness/paralysis of all four limbs.

Patients may also show other body positions, such as:

– **Kyphosis** (Figure 1): the dorsal/upward hunched curvature of the spine, often seen in patients with intervertebral disc extrusion.
– **Lordosis** (Figure 2): the ventral/downward curvature of the spine; typically seen in, in-season cats.
– **Prayer position** (Figure 3): the ventral curvature of the spine with forelimb extension, typically adopted due to abdominal pain.

Hydration Status

During the acute phase of volume depletion, physical examination findings may be the only assessment available due to the patient's ability to compensate.

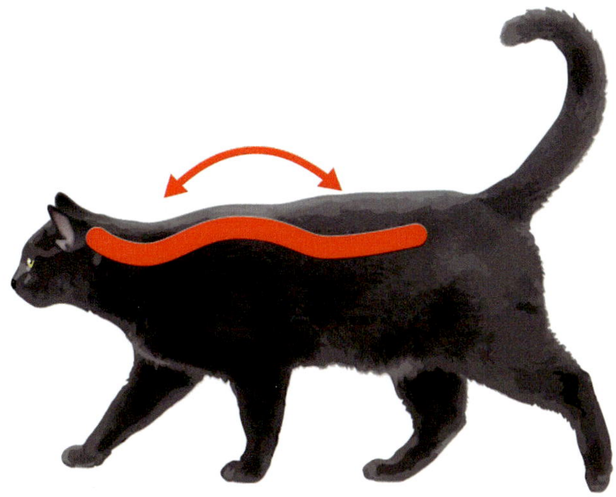

Figure 1. Kyphosis.

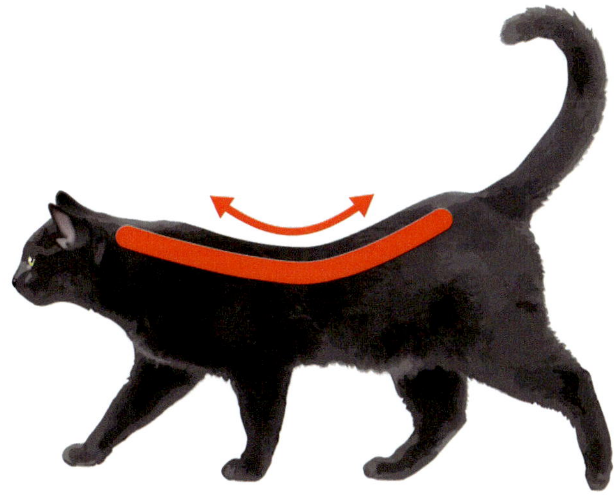

Figure 2. Lordosis.

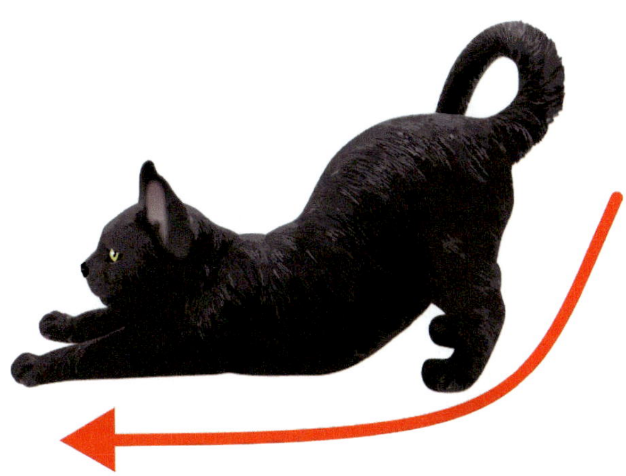

Figure 3. Prayer position.

Many physical examinations underestimate the degree of the patient's hydration status; thus, it is important to assess the patient's dehydration (if present) accordingly (Table 1). Hydration status is often expressed as percentage of body weight (0–15%) which can be subjective. **Hydration is reported as adequate, marginal, or inadequate.**

Points to remember:

- **Loss of the elasticity of the skin (skin turgor) is first sign of dehydration. The skin of the upper eyelid and the neck should be checked for tenting.**
- **Signs of dehydration are more difficult to see in some animals. Skin may tent more in emaciated animals and certain breeds (e.g. Shar-pei, Basset Hounds). Obese animals may not show skin tenting even when dehydrated.**

Table 1. Assessing dehydration.

Percentage	Hydration status	Signs
0–5%	Adequate	No abnormalities seen. Skin immediately returns to normal position after tenting. CRT normal, eyes normal, mucous membranes pink and moist.
5–8%	Marginal	Slight delay (2–4 seconds) in return of the skin to normal position, slight increase in CRT (2 sec), eyes slightly sunken in sockets, mucous membranes slightly dry or tacky.
8–10%		Obvious delay (5–10 seconds) in skin returning to normal position, increased CRT (2–2.5 sec), eyes sunken in sockets, mucous membranes dry, slightly tacky.
10–12%	Inadequate	Skin remains tented (10–30 seconds), CRT increased dramatically (3+ sec), eyes very sunken, dry mucous membranes, animal depressed, may see signals of shock (cool extremities, rapid/week pulse, tachycardia).
+12%		State of shock, death is probable.

For patients with a marginal and inadequate hydration status **a PCV should be obtained to calculate the percentage of dehydration.**

Physical Examination

The patient's vital signs should be evaluated, with the patient appropriately restrained (dependent on their behavioural assessment), in relation to their presenting complaint, history, and current health status.

Canine patients should be either restrained by their owners on a slip lead and or by another member of the clinical team. Feline patients should be restrained using cat friendly principles in line with the International Society of Feline Medicine and American Association of Feline Practitioners "Feline Friendly Handling Guidelines" by another staff member as required.

Patients suspected or confirmed to be infectious, with an open or discharging wound, or a zoonotic disease must be examined and restrained with **appropriate use of personal protective equipment (PPE).**

When performing a physical examination, it is important to adopt a logical and systematic approach, such as the **nose-to-tail approach.** However, this may not always be suited to patients that are fearful or painful.

Vital parameters, such as pulse and respiratory rate should be assessed at the start of the physical assessment or at the end depending on the individual patient. Manipulation of painful body regions should be avoided, at least until examination is otherwise complete, so as to avoid unnecessary stress for the patient.

All patients should be weighed using an appropriate animal scale. Patients weighing less than approximately 7 kg should be weighed using a small animal/paediatric scale (e.g. feline scales) to improve accuracy of measurement.

Body Temperature

The veterinary surgeon should be notified of body temperatures outside the species reference range as soon as possible. The rectal area should be examined for evidence of diarrhoea staining, parasites, and other structural abnormalities. Most animals resist having their temperature taken. The rest of the exam should be completed first, before obtaining a temperature so as to avoid agitating the animal and making the examination more difficult.

It is important to **not struggle with an aggressive patient to obtain a temperature.** If there is difficulty taking a patient's temperature, a supervising veterinarian or other clinical staff member should be consulted.

An excited/overactive patient with a temperature raised slightly above the reference range, but that has no other signs of infection/illness, may be conditionally accepted for surgery with instructions to retake the temperature after allowing them time to relax. If there is a decrease in temperature to within normal limits, then they can be cleared for surgery.

Note: Thermometer covers should be used to aid in infection control.

Head and Neck

The neck should be examined systematically from the salivary glands and mandibular lymph nodes working down towards the thorax.

Palpable superficial lymph nodes should be checked for size and shape changes, if they are attached to surrounding tissue, and pain. Several lymph nodes are easily identified in canine and feline patients while others are more difficult to locate. (Figure 4).

Lymph nodes that are normally palpable include:
- mandibular
- superficial cervical
- inguinal
- popliteal.

Lymph nodes that are not normally palpable include:
- axillary
- retropharyngeal
- deep cervical
- mesenteric and other abdominal lymph nodes
- bronchial
- sternal.

Some lymph nodes can be assessed on rectal examination: sacral, internal, and medial iliac (depending on the size of the patient).

Cardiovascular System

The patient's **cardiovascular function, peripheral perfusion, and the presence or absence of anaemia** should be checked by assessing the patient's mucus membrane colour and capillary refill time.

The heart should be auscultated in addition to the correlation of peripheral pulses with the heart rate to assess the pulse quality and **identify pulse deficits.**

Mucous Membrane Colour

Mucous membrane (MM) colour provides information about the blood flow to peripheral tissue, any abnormalities should be brought to the attention of a veterinary surgeon. See Table 2.

77

Capillary Refill Time

The capillary refill time (CRT) reflects perfusion of the peripheral tissues.

Prolonged CRT (>2 seconds) may indicate compromised circulation due to hypothermia, shock, cardiovascular disease, anaemia, or other causes and must be further evaluated by a veterinary surgeon before admitting the patient for surgery.

Pulse Rate and Quality

The external extremities should be used to evaluate the patient's pulse rate and quality (e.g. carpal or tarsal) rather than a central pulse such as a femoral pulse. Peripheral pulses

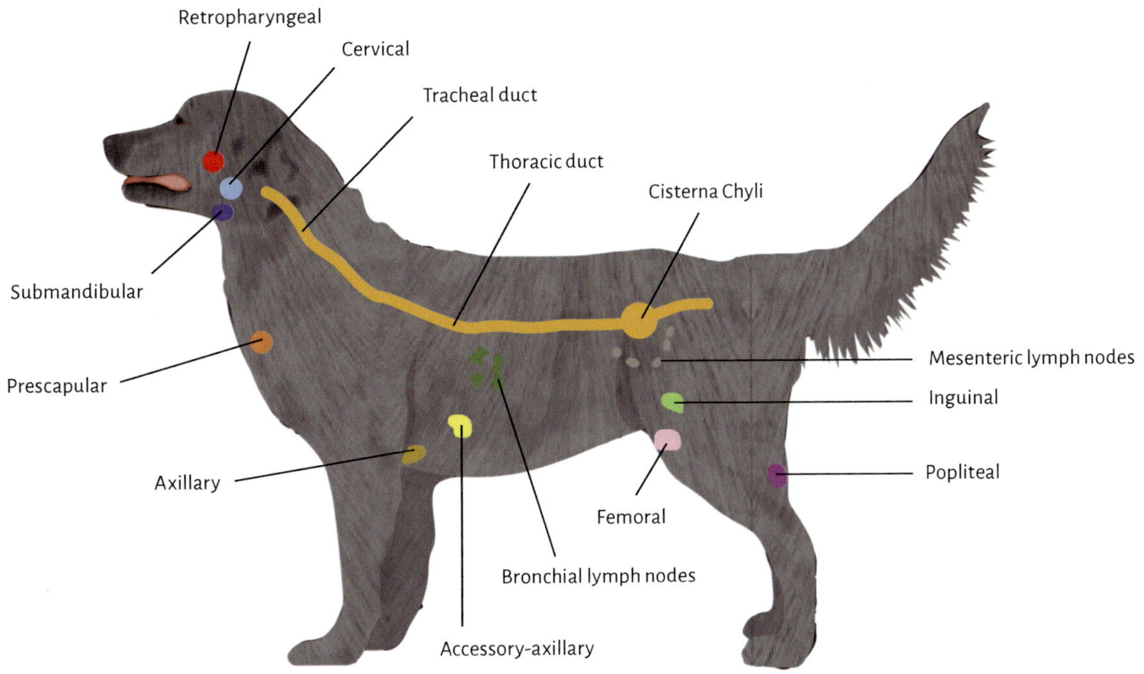

Figure 4. Lymph node locations.

provide a more accurate indication of the condition of the circulatory system, as these pulses are the first to disappear should the patient develop circulatory shock.

As well as the rate, the pulse quality and strength (e.g. strong, weak, thready, bounding) should be noted. **A normal strong pulse has a biphasic sensation on palpation.**

Evaluation of pulse deficits is performed by simultaneous cardiac auscultation, and if present, a veterinary surgeon notified immediately.

Pulse deficit = pulse rate < heart rate

Table 2. Interpretation of mucous membrane colour and possible causes.

Colour	Interpretation	Possible causes
Pink	Normal	Adequate perfusion/ oxygenation of peripheral tissues
Pale or white	Anaemia, poor perfusion, vasoconstriction	Blood loss, shock, decreased peripheral blood flow
Blue (cyanotic)	Inadequate oxygenation	Hypoxaemia
Brick red	Increased perfusion, vasodilation	Early shock, sepsis, fever, systemic inflammatory response syndrome
Yellow (icteric)	Bilirubin accumulation	Hepatic or biliary disorder and/or haemolysis
Brown	Methaemoglobinaemia	Acetaminophen toxicity in cats, intravascular haemolysis
Petechiae (red splotching)	Coagulation disorder	Platelet disorder, DIC, coagulation factor deficiencies

Cardiac Auscultation

The **heart can be assessed by palpating the area between the fourth and sixth intercostal spaces** on both sides of the thorax for the point of maximum intensity (PMI) of the heartbeat and any cardiac thrills.

Muffled heart sounds may be a result of fluid in the chest which means the heart is more distant from the bell of the stethoscope. When having difficulty hearing the heartbeat it is important not to assume it is due to lack of experience or poor technique. The veterinary surgeon should be notified.

When auscultating the patients' heart, **heart rate (HR) and rhythm (count beats for 15 seconds and multiply by 4)** should be evaluated. (Figures 5 and 6).

Normal heart sounds:

1. **Lub-Dub = should be a short time gap between heart sounds.**
2. **S1 = loud, long, low pitch (closure of AV valves). S2 = closure of the semilunar valves.**

Abnormal heart sounds:

Arrhythmia: sinus arrhythmia, atrial fibrillation, heart block, premature ventricular contractions, gallop rhythm (three or four sounds instead of two).

- **Sinus arrhythmia is the slight increase in heart rate during inspiration and decrease with expiration. This is a normal finding, particularly in healthy, fit individuals and is more common in the dog than in the cat.**

Murmurs

See Table 3: "Evaluating heart murmurs".

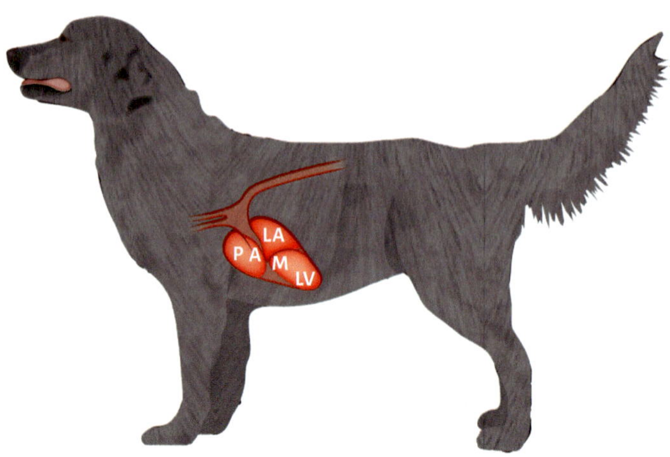

Figure 5. Left thorax landmarks for cardiac auscultation.

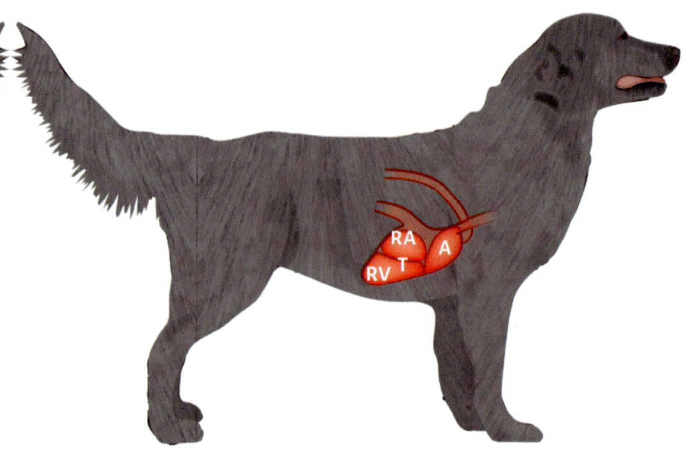

Figure 6. Right thorax landmarks for cardiac auscultation.

Table 3. Evaluating heart murmurs.

Location	Usually, the valve area over which the murmur is loudest: aortic/mitral/tricuspid/pulmonic. May also be described in relation to chest structure (e.g. sternal border).
Timing	The part of the cardiac cycle during which the murmur is heard: systole/diastole/continuous.
Duration	Refers to the duration within cardiac cycle when murmur is heard: early systole/holosystolic/diastole
Character	The quality of the murmur: · Plateau or regurgitant type (same sound for the duration of murmur). · Decrescendo, crescendo, crescendo-decrescendo or ejection type (intensity changes throughout duration of murmur). · Machinery (heard throughout systole and diastole). · Decrescendo or blowing.
Grade	Loudness. Subjective assessment, does not necessarily indicate degree of cardiac dysfunction: · 1/6: Can only be heard in quiet room after several minutes of listening. · 2/6: Can be heard immediately but is very soft. · 3/6: Low to moderate intense. · 4/6: Loud, but without a palpable thrill. · 5/6: Loud, with a palpable thrill. · 6/6: Can be heard with the stethoscope slightly off the thoracic wall.

A murmur is a repetitive series of audible vibrations during a normally silent part of the cardiac cycle. These are often heard as a soft, swooshing sound. **Murmurs are described on a basis of location, timing, duration, character, and grade.**

The heart should be auscultated in multiple locations, on both the right and left sides of the chest. A heart murmur or other abnormality may go undetected unless each valve is auscultated independently.

Locations for auscultation of specific heart valves:

- **Left 4th–6th (PMI) intercostal space just above the sternal border = mitral valve.**
- **Left 2nd–4th intercostal space above sternal border = pulmonic valve.**
- **Left 3rd–5th intercostal space at mid-thorax = aortic valve.**
- **Right 3rd–5th intercostal space at mid-thorax = tricuspid valve.**

Any doubts or concerns about an animal's cardiovascular status or the presence of a murmur or arrhythmia should be brought to the attention of a veterinary surgeon.

Respiratory Function

The patient's respiratory pattern and rate should be checked along with thoracic auscultation and percussion to evaluate the patient's ventilation capabilities. If a patient has a history of chronic respiratory disease or is showing signs of marked respiratory distress, the patient should be checked for signs of respiratory muscle fatigue and the patient's posture recorded.

Firstly, it is important to listen without a stethoscope for noisy breathing at the mouth and nares, and only then should the thorax be auscultated, in at least four areas, including right and left ventral and right and left dorsal lung fields. See Figure 7.

The following should be assessed:

– **respiratory rate** (RR): visual assessment/auscultation

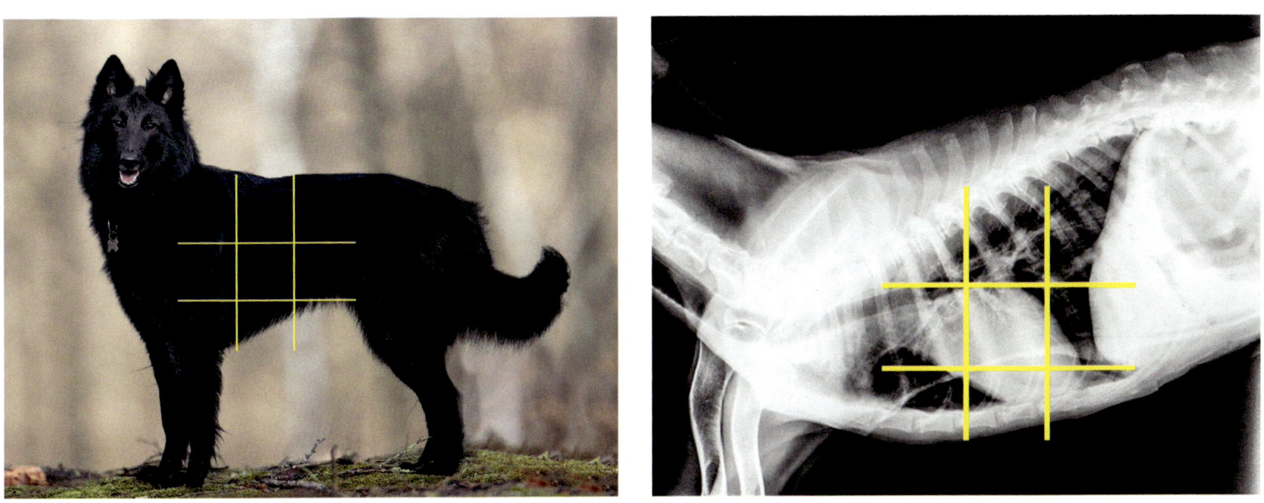

Figure 7. Locations for respiratory auscultation.

and count breaths per minute
– **depth/effort:** degree of chest movement (normal, shallow, deep) should be observed
– **character:** any sounds and/or difficulty on inspiration and/or expiration should be noted.

Normal respiratory sounds include:
– **bronchial:** an intense harsh sound heard during both inspiration and expiration
– **bronchovesicular:** a moderate sound heard at maximum inspiration and short expiration
– **vesicular**: a soft sound heard during the longer inspiratory phase.

Abnormal Lung Sounds

Changes in lung sounds may be associated with the location of respiratory system disease such as:
– loud breathing: large airway disease (nasal passages, trachea, larynx/pharynx)
– inspiratory noise or difficulty: extra thoracic airway disease (especially the larynx)
– expiratory noise or difficulty: intrathoracic tracheal disease
– rapid/shallow breathing: pleural space disease (fluid or air)
– difficulty breathing on both inspiration and expiration: lung disease
– signs of respiratory distress (dyspnoea) change as disease progresses.

See Table 4: Respiratory sounds.

Table 4. Respiratory sounds.

Respiratory sound	Location	Description
Wheezes (rhonchi)	Isolated lung fields	A continuous high or low-pitched sound heard more often on early expiration or late inspiration. Often associated with small airway disease such as feline asthma.
Rales/ crackles	Lung fields	Course to fine, discontinuous, non-musical, brief "popping" sounds heard more commonly on inspiration; may be heard when fluid is on the lungs.
Stridor	Larynx or trachea-thoracic inlet	High frequency "wheezing" sound heard during expiration.
Stertor	Larynx or trachea	Low frequency "snoring" sound heard during inspiration.
Dull	Isolated lung fields	May indicate pneumonia or consolidation.
Absence of breath sounds	Lung fields	May indicate pleural space disease (pleural effusion) or space-occupying lesions.

The first sign of respiratory compromise is usually a change in respiratory rate. This is followed by a **change in respiratory rhythm and character (depth).** Other signs include exaggerated chest or abdominal movements on inspiration, open mouth breathing and flared nostrils. In extreme cases the animal may be cyanotic. Changes in posture (e.g. standing or sitting with back arched, neck extended, and elbows out and reluctant to lie down) are a sign of very advanced respiratory disease.

It is important any abnormal lung or heart sounds or perceived abnormalities in respiratory rate or effort are assessed further by the veterinary surgeon.

Palpation of the Abdomen

The abdomen should be observed for any asymmetry or distention. Distention may arise from:
– organomegaly (e.g. hepatic)
– ascites
– intra-abdominal masses
– free gas
– gastric distention
– obesity
– pregnancy.

The entire surface of the abdomen should be assessed for surface masses, skin lesions, and hernias.

A systematic palpation of the abdomen via a cranial-caudal direction should be performed, starting gently to acclimatise the patient to the abdominal assessment. In patients with suspected abdominal pain, any painful areas should be examined last or after an appropriate analgesic. It may be that in these patients abdominal assessment is left only to the veterinary surgeon to limit the number of times the abdomen is palpated.

In both cats and dogs, the **only abdominal organs that can be palpated in their entirety are the kidneys and urinary bladder.** In canine patients only the caudal liver margins can be easily palpated in a healthy patient whereas in cases with hepatomegaly the whole liver can be easily palpated. In feline patients the liver is not generally palpable. The stomach is only usually palpable when filled with food, fluid, or distended with gas. The intestines should be evaluated for distention, masses, or foreign objects by running them through the fingers.

For **abdominal palpation of deep chested dogs, elevating their forequarters** on a chair helps displace the abdominal contents caudal to the rib cage to improve accessibility for assessment.

In cats the right kidney may be partially hidden under the caudal ribs as in both cats and dogs the right kidney is more cranial than the left. **The kidneys should be evaluated for size, shape, and symmetry.**

The bladder is more easily palpable when full. Palpation should be performed carefully, particularly after recent urinary tract surgery or in patients where pain is suspected.

Where appropriate the rectum should be examined to determine the presence of any polyps and masses associated with the rectum itself, as well as the anal sacs, and the prostate in male dogs. Mammary glands should be assessed for discharge, masses, or any abnormalities in bitches.

Pain Assessment

As part of the clinical assessment, **pain assessment is vital,** since untreated pain affects patient well-being, appetite, blood pressure and respiratory and immune function (Xu et al., 2020 and Totsch et al., 2017).

There are various types of pain which include:

- **Visceral:** originating from an organ.
- **Phantom:** the perception of pain from an area of the body which has been removed.
- **Neuropathic:** originating from injury or damage to the nerves which convey pain signals.
- **Parietal:** originating from the lining of the abdominal cavity (e.g. peritonitis).
- **Pathological/chronic pain:** pain which is still present following a painful stimulus.
- **Somatic:** originating from superficial tissues such as the skin, tissue, or muscles.
- **Referred:** caused by other pathological changes at another site within the body (e.g. intervertebral disc disease).

Patients show abdominal pain by guarding the abdomen when touched or palpated. These signs may be in conjunction with other signs such as adopting the praying position, restlessness, and the inability to settle.

Pain should be assessed with the use of a validated pain scale such as the Modified Glasgow pain scale. However, the extent to which abdominal palpation is useful depends on other factors including patient anxiety, species, obesity, and other pathological processes. (See Chapter 4: Analgesia for further information on pain).

Diagnostic Assessment

The extent of the laboratory work-up depends on the patient's physical status and the planned procedure. Laboratory work should complement clinical evaluation rather than be a substitute for a thorough examination. Results should be interpreted in light of the patient's condition.

Sample Collection

The accuracy of any laboratory analysis is determined by the quality of the sample collected. A quality blood sample should be collected via a **clean stick method** whereby "the sample was collected after a single insertion into the vessel, and there were no issues with collecting blood, such as slow draws, issues finding the vein, vein blowing, or patient movement" (Phillips, 2018).

The most commonly used sites for blood sampling are:

- dogs: cephalic vein, lateral saphenous vein, jugular vein
- cats: cephalic vein, medial saphenous vein, jugular vein
- arterial samples: dorsal pedal artery, coccygeal artery.

The patient should be appropriately restrained prior to sample collection, with the sample site prepared aseptically.

Sample collection is most commonly performed using a needle and syringe. An appropriately sized needle should be used to minimise haemolysis but maximise patient comfort. The syringe should be an appropriate size for the sample volume, whilst minimising negative pressure which can cause red blood cell lysis and venous collapse.

Recent research performed by Solbak et al. (2019) and Greenwell et al. (2014) found the use of a 25G needle did not induce any clinically significant differences in the parameters.

Venepuncture should be performed with the least tissue injury possible to minimise contamination of the needle/syringe with tissue fluid and to minimise haemolysis and clotting factor activation. The needle should be inserted at approximately a 30° angle in a smooth motion and gentle negative pressure should be applied to the syringe until the required volume of blood is aspirated. The needle should be removed from the vein and digital pressure applied at the sample site, the phlebotomist should then remove the needle and fill the required sample tubes.

Blood sampling tubes used in veterinary practice come in various sizes; smaller 0.5–1.3 ml tubes are commonly used for small animal sampling, with larger vacutainers suitable for larger sample volumes or in large animal/equine sampling. Different anticoagulants are used in these tubes depending on the intended test and are identified by colours which vary depending on country. (See Table 5).

Once the blood sample is collected, **the required blood tubes should be filled in a specific order** to maximise sample quality, avoid laboratory error, and minimise sample clotting. The order of draw dictates the order by which tubes are filled:

Table 5. Properties of different types of blood sampling tubes.

Tube colour	Anticoagulant	Purpose
Green (USA)	Sodium heparin	Plasma for biochemistry testing
Orange/light green	Lithium heparin	Plasma for biochemistry testing
Green/purple/blue	Sodium citrate	Coagulation testing
Yellow; grey (USA)	Sodium fluoride/ potassium oxalate	Blood glucose testing
White; red (USA)	Plain/no anticoagulant	Serum for biochemistry testing
Brown; yellow/gold (USA)	Gel separator and clot activator	Serum for biochemistry testing
Red/pink; purple (USA)	EDTA	Haematology testing

FILL FIRST

1. **Discard tube, if filling a coagulation tube (prior to filling citrate a small volume of blood should be discarded into a plain tube).**
2. **Blood culture bottle (for microbiology).**
3. **Sodium citrate tube (for coagulation testing).**
4. **Plain/gel (for biochemistry testing).**
5. **Heparin (for biochemistry testing).**
6. **EDTA (for haematology testing).**
7. **Fluoride/oxalate (for glucose testing).**

FILL LAST

Laboratory Data: Minimum Database

The laboratory tests which are required preoperatively are dependent on the patient, presenting condition, and proposed surgical procedure. A young patient undergoing an elective procedure (e.g. cat castration) requires less laboratory tests than a patient undergoing a complex procedure such as an adrenalectomy. Laboratory tests are also useful in establishing a baseline to assess postoperative progress.

The laboratory tests should be the minimum required for a thorough patient evaluation of the presenting condition, its systemic manifestations, and the significance of concurrent disease conditions.

In the majority of cases financial factors often determine which laboratory tests are performed and therefore priority is given to tests of paramount importance for patient evaluation.

A **minimum database** is often more than sufficient for many patients and includes:

- PCV/TP
- urea
- creatinine
- electrolytes
- urinalysis.

Geriatric patients, the critically ill and/or those that have suffered trauma, require more extensive laboratory tests such as a complete blood count (including platelet count) and serum biochemistry screen, which may or may not include coagulation assessment.

It is imperative that a full patient history is obtained, and physical examination performed to guide the veterinary surgeon when deciding which tests to perform. The veterinary nurse/technician should be able to recognise common parameters, their meaning for their patients, and their indications in patients with specific conditions.

Most veterinary hospitals/practices can perform basic laboratory tests within their clinics, and the types and complexity of in-house tests depends on the availability and the resources of each individual practice.

Biochemistry Assays

Biochemistry is the analysis of the chemical composition of a sample, where the sample is blood plasma/serum, tissue fluid, ascitic fluid, CSF, or urine. Biochemistry is an important tool to **determine how well certain organs are functioning** and can also be used to monitor response to certain treatments.

Although each individual test is not specific to one clinical condition, **the range of results across the array of tests can support a diagnosis by a process of pattern recognition.** Biochemical analysis should be accompanied by a compete blood count as evaluation of both is essential to identify many common disease patterns.

The majority of veterinary laboratories offer a basic panel of tests, which represents a minimal investigation applicable to most common circumstances.

Blood Urea Nitrogen (BUN)

A blood urea nitrogen (BUN) analysis measures the amount of nitrogen from the waste product urea. Urea is the result of the breakdown of protein by the liver and excreted via the urine. A BUN analysis evaluates the patient's kidney function, but alterations are also be associated with hydration status, hepatic disease, and gastrointestinal disease.

A significant increase in BUN is seen in patients with hypovolaemia/dehydration, due to fluid losses and in patients with gastrointestinal haemorrhage.

Patients with end-stage hepatic disease, or hepatic dysfunction such as portosystemic shunt, typically **present with low urea,** as the liver is responsible for converting ammonia into nitrogenous waste products such as urea.

Creatinine

Creatinine is the waste product which follows muscle metabolism. It is a more specific indicator of renal function than urea since it is less affected by other factors (such as diet and hydration). Creatinine is formed secondary to protein breakdown in the body and excreted by the kidneys, hence increased creatinine levels are seen in cases of renal dysfunction and reduced glomerular filtration rates. Creatinine elevations may be seen in patients with marked muscle loss or damage.

Alanine Aminotransferase (ALT) and Aspartate Aminotransferase (AST)

Alanine aminotransferase (ALT) and aspartate aminotransferase (AST) **are enzymes mainly found within the liver.** AST is also found within erythrocytes, skeletal muscle tissue, and organs such as the brain, heart, pancreas, and kidneys.

AST levels often increase after **trauma, necrosis, infection, or with hepatic neoplasia.** AST can also be found in CSF, exudates, and transudates in relation to the amount of cellular damage.

ALT and AST are used as hepatic parameters associated with hepatocellular damage. However, AST is considered "a less specific marker of hepatic injury than ALT due to its expression from other tissues" (Sharon et al., 2016). They are released due to injury to hepatic cells, (e.g. in acute hepatitis cases) and not necessarily associated with reduced hepatic function as the liver has a great reserve of functional capacity.

Alkaline Phosphatase (ALP) and γ-glutamyl Transferase (GGT)

Alkaline phosphatase (ALP) and γ-glutamyl transferase (GGT) are hepatic parameters associated with **biliary tract stasis.**

ALP plays an integral role in bone development and metabolism within the liver by dephosphorylating organic compounds. It is found within the liver on the edges of cells that join to form bile ducts and can increase when bile ducts become blocked. It can also be found in bone where it is produced by osteoblasts. Therefore, elevations in ALP are seen in cases of cholecystitis (gallbladder inflammation), hepatic neoplasia and in hepatitis. For this reason, elevations in ALP may also be seen in patients with Cushing's disease or receiving long-term steroids.

Elevations in ALP can also be seen in conditions affecting the bone, such as osteomalacia.

γ-glutamyl transferase (GGT) is found in the cell membranes of many tissues which include the kidneys, spleen, heart but predominantly bile ducts and gallbladder. Its function is to transfer amino acids across the cell membrane and to metabolise leukotrienes, the inflammatory mediator produced by leukocytes.

GGT is used in conjunction with ALP in detecting biliary tract disease whereby elevations of GGT are in fact due to biliary disease as GGT is not seen in bone diseases.

Total Bilirubin (TBIL)

Bilirubin is a compound (yellow in colour) that forms due to the catabolism of haemoglobin, where it is released into the bloodstream. Bilirubin is then transported via the bloodstream to the liver, where it is conjugated before it enters the biliary tract and small intestine for faecal and urine excretion. Increases in bilirubin levels can therefore be seen secondary to reduced liver function or liver failure, and patients may take on a jaundice appearance. Elevations can also be seen in conditions such as immune mediated haemolytic anaemia (IMHA).

Exposure to light damages the structure of bilirubin and therefore it is important to protect blood serum from illumination, particularly when analysed for total bilirubin.

Bilirubin in blood has two forms:

- **Conjugated bilirubin: water-soluble.**
- **Unconjugated bilirubin: not water-soluble.**

Total bilirubin measures both forms.

Cholesterol

Cholesterol is a type of lipid, which is an integral part of all animal cell membranes and a starting point for the body's synthesis of steroid hormones, bile acids, and vitamin D. It is mainly produced by hepatic cells.

Cholesterol levels may be increased in patients with **liver failure,** in addition to other conditions such as **canine hypothyroidism.**

Glucose

The simple sugar glucose is the most abundant monosaccharide and the most important energy source in all organisms. Glucose is stored in the liver as a polymer known as glycogen. Glucose is released in animals via glycogenolysis (breakdown of glycogen).

Hypoglycaemia is associated with sepsis, Addison's disease (Addisonian crisis), insulinoma, end-stage liver disease, and is seen frequently in paediatric patients (such as puppies with gastrointestinal signs).

Hyperglycaemia may be seen secondary to acute stress in cats (stress hyperglycaemia); which is typically transient although marked hyperglycaemia can be seen in severe cases. Additional causes of hyperglycaemia include diabetes mellitus/diabetic ketoacidosis, head trauma, and severe hypovolaemia or hypoxaemia.

Albumin

Albumin is a water-soluble globular plasma protein produced by the liver. Albumin is a transport protein which binds to various ions and molecules to transport them around the body. It **plays a key role in maintaining colloid oncotic pressure and intravascular fluid balance.** A decrease in albumin can occur due to renal or gastrointestinal disease, and inflammatory diseases, such as severe pancreatitis/systemic inflammation.

Hypoalbuminaemia is also associated with oedema, hypovolaemia, and slowed healing.

Sodium

The extracellular cation sodium has many functions, including nerve and muscle function and maintenance of normal blood pressure and body water balance. **Alterations in sodium levels are generally associated with the fluid balance,** rather than an absolute loss or gain of sodium ions, and therefore the patient's volaemic and hydration status should be evaluated when considering sodium levels.

Potassium

The intracellular cation potassium works with sodium to manage muscle and nerve function. Most of the body's potassium is sourced via the diet, and **levels depend on a variety of body processes such as renal function, blood insulin levels, cell function, and nutritional status.** When measuring blood potassium levels, it is important to consider that total potassium and serum/plasma potassium levels differ, since much of the body's potassium content is located within cells, and not within the bloodstream.

Chloride

Chloride is an extracellular anion involved in maintaining fluid balance, alongside sodium; generally, chloride levels in the body are similar to sodium levels.

Calcium

A very small amount of the body's calcium is available in the extracellular fluid, with most located within bone. Calcium within the ECF is either protein or phosphate-bound, or freely available. **Free calcium is known as ionised calcium,** and **total calcium is the sum of both the calcium bound to plasma protein (albumin) and the free calcium.** Total calcium is run on most biochemistry analysers, whereas blood gas analysers are typically required for the measurement of in-house ionised calcium. It is ionised calcium that is metabolically active.

Calcium levels are influenced by several factors including nutritional status, vitamin D levels, the presence of underlying endocrine (parathyroid gland) disease, or renal disease.

Inorganic Phosphate

Phosphate is an electrolyte that works alongside calcium to regulate many body processes. **Increases in phosphate level are seen due to renal disease, hypoparathyroidism, vitamin D toxicity, sample artefacts, and increased dietary phosphate intake.** Decreased phosphate may be due to malabsorption disorders, dietary deficiency, administration of diuretics, or from fluid shifting from the extracellular space to the intracellular space (e.g. following the release of insulin, or treatment with glucose or insulin – this is why hypophosphatemia occurs in patients with refeeding syndrome). Hypophosphataemia can cause haemolytic anaemia, therefore these patients should be monitored closely.

Total Solids (TS)

Total solids are plasma components with the most effect on the refractive index. Total solids are used to estimate the total protein (the constituents of plasma with the most effect on the refractive index). Total solids should be measured in conjunction with PCV, to obtain the most useful information.

1. A blood sample should be prepared in a microhaematocrit (capillary) tube and centrifuged for 3–5 minutes at the recommended rpm based on the centrifuge manufactures recommendations.
2. While the centrifuge is running, the refractometer should be calibrated. To do this the refractometer should be cleaned first by wiping the surface with a clean lint free tissue and distilled water prior to placing a drop of distilled water onto the reading surface and closing the lid.
3. By looking through the eyepiece it should be ensured that the line between the blue section and white section lies at 1.000 SPG (specific gravity). If it does not, then the refractometer requires calibration by using the calibration dial to bring the line to the desired 1.000 SPG position. Finally, the distilled water should be wiped off with a lint free tissue.
4. The capillary tube should be broken near the bottom of the plasma fraction/buffy coat, discarding the section that contains the packed cells.

5. Using the unbroken end of the capillary tube from the plasma containing portion, the plasma should be dabbed onto the measuring surface of the refractometer and the lid closed.
6. It is important to read from the correct scale, which is marked "Serum p; Wt; TS". If there is not enough plasma on the reading plate this appears as a blurry line between the white and blue distinctions. A first attempt at resolving this can be made by gently pressing on the lid before starting the whole process again. The reading is taken on the line that divides the blue and white portion and is multiplied by ten to get the result in g/l.

Electrolytes and Blood Gases

The main electrolytes are:
- potassium
- sodium
- calcium
- magnesium.

The concentration of electrolytes is regulated by the kidneys and various hormones. Electrolyte imbalances affect many different organs and systems including the nervous system, cardiac, and skeletal muscles and subsequently lead to mortality. Electrolytes are measured via in-house biochemistry analysers as well as point-of-care tests (POCT) such as the i-Stat (Abbot) and Epoc (Woodley). Some POCT's can also measure blood gases.

Sodium (Na)

Sodium is the major cation (positively charged ion) in extracellular fluid. Levels may be increased in patients with water deprivation and osmotic diuresis, and decreased in patients with gastrointestinal disease, Addison's disease, and congestive heart failure.

Potassium (K)

Potassium is the major cation in intracellular fluid. Levels may be increased in patients with acute kidney injury, Addison's disease, and urinary tract obstruction, and decreased in patients with anorexia, chronic kidney disease, and patients receiving diuretics.

Chloride (Cl)

Chloride is the major anion (negatively charged ion) in the extracellular fluid. Chloride and sodium levels are closely correlated.

Total Calcium (Ca)

Total calcium is the combination of ionised (freely circulating) and protein-bound calcium in the bloodstream. Only 1% of calcium is present in the bloodstream, with 99% of the total body calcium present within bone. Circulating calcium is important in maintaining neuromuscular tone, enzyme activity, coagulation, and movement of ions across cell membranes.

Ionised Calcium

Ionised calcium (Ca^{2+}) is calcium which is not attached to any proteins and therefore freely available for cellular uptake. **Ionised calcium or free calcium analysis provides a more accurate representation of the physiological calcium state** than total calcium. This is because ionised calcium stimulates or suppresses the hormones which are involved in calcium homeostasis, such as PTH, vitamin D and calcitonin. **Ideally serum should be used for analysis,** as EDTA and citrate bond with calcium and lower the ionised calcium levels. Additionally, heparin samples should not exceed 4% of total blood volume in the tube.

Serum-separator tubes or gel tubes contain calcium in the silicone gel, spuriously increasing values from the release of free ionized calcium from the gel. Also, Ca^{2+} analysis is affected by air exposure, especially if serum is mixed as this causes the pH to increase which subsequently decreases the amount of Ca^{2+}.

Magnesium

Magnesium is an intracellular cation used as a catalyst in many enzymatic reactions particularly in the sodium/potassium ATPase pump that utilizes ATP (adenosine triphosphate) and energy transfer. Approximately 1% of the body's magnesium is found within serum and exists in the body within the cells. Magnesium imbalances have a major impact on the cardiovascular and neurological systems.

Haematology

A comprehensive haematology examination includes **a quantitative and qualitative examination.**

A quantitative examination focuses on absolute cell counts and numerical data, and includes measurement of:
- **Packed cell volume (PCV):** the measurement of the proportion of blood that consists of red blood cells.
- **Haematocrit (HCT):** a measure of red blood cell percentage, calculated from the RBC level and MCV.
- **Total red blood cell (RBC) count:** the total number of red blood cells.
- **Haemoglobin (Hb) level:** the total haemoglobin level.
- **Total white blood cell (WBC) count:** the total number of white blood cells across all five white blood cell types.
- **Differential WBC counts:** total number of specific white blood cell lines including neutrophils, lymphocytes, monocytes, eosinophils, and basophils.
- **Mean corpuscular volume (MCV):** this parameter assesses the size of the red blood cells and indicates whether anaemia is normocytic or microcytic.
- **Mean corpuscular haemoglobin (MCH):** the average

mass of haemoglobin (Hb) per red blood cell (RBC) in a sample of blood.

- **Mean corpuscular haemoglobin concentration (MCHC):** assesses the haemoglobin within cells and indicates whether anaemia is normochromic or hypochromic.
- **Platelet count (PLT):** small cellular fragments which shear off large cells called megakaryocytes. Their function is to respond initially to haemorrhage by forming a primary plug, around which a blood clot is formed.
- **Mean platelet volume (MPV) level:** measures the average size of platelets.
- **Total plasma solids (TS):** measures the total dissolved solids in plasma.

A qualitative examination focuses on cellular morphology (shape, form, and structure) and is performed by examination of a blood smear.

Packed Cell Volume

Packed cell volume is expressed as a percentage and **represents the measurement of the proportion of blood made up of red blood cells,** as long as the MCV (mean corpuscular volume) is within the reference range.

A PCV is measured via a capillary tube (microhaematocrit) filled with well mixed blood and EDTA and filled to 2/3 of the tube prior to being centrifuged at 1300–2500 rpm for five minutes (higher speeds only require two minutes).

Following centrifuging erythrocytes fall to the bottom as they are the heaviest, while the white blood cells form a buffy coat on top of the erythrocytes. A layer of platelets then falls on top of the buffy coat, followed by the plasma fraction. (See Figure 8).

It is important to evaluate the plasma colour as this can indicate haemolysis, icterus and lipaemia.

The TP should be performed at the same time as the PCV for maximum information about the patient's condition. **A normal PCV is approximately 35–45%,** although sight hounds naturally have a higher PCV (up to 65% may be considered normal). (Table 6).

Table 6. Possible causes of different PCV and plasma protein levels measured using microhaematocrit.

PCV level	Plasma protein level	Description
Low	Low	Recent or ongoing haemorrhage. Plasma protein is being lost with RBC's. Mild reduction in plasma protein may be seen in cases with internal haemorrhage as plasma proteins are reabsorbed.
Low	Normal	Anaemia due to haemolysis or reduced production.
High	High	Dehydration; water loss results in both high levels of plasma proteins and RBC's.
High	Normal	Suggests absolute polycythaemia or an increase in RBC's.
Low/normal	High	Hyperglobulinaemia.

Red Blood Cells and Cell Counts

On a routine CBC the red blood cell count is the concentration of red blood cells, expressed in millions/µl of whole blood and is performed on anticoagulated whole blood. The anticoagulant of choice is EDTA, as this is superior at preserving cells, and blood smears prepared from EDTA blood also stain well.

EDTA can cause platelet clumping particularly in the feline species, and the veterinary nurse/technician should be aware of this when analysing feline haematology samples.

It is important to fill the EDTA tube precisely to the line indicated on the tube to ensure accurate results. This is because under filling the tube results in excess EDTA, which can reduce red blood cell size, resulting in a falsely low MCV.

Overfilling the EDTA tube can cause a clot to form which renders a non-diagnostic sample. In cats and small dogs, or patients where sample volumes should be minimised, 0.5 ml EDTA tubes are preferred. These allow for the collection of smaller blood volumes whilst preserving the correct anticoagulant-to-blood ratio.

As the EDTA ages the cell morphology also begins to degenerate within 12 hours of blood collection (Villers, 2016). Therefore, analysis should be performed as soon as possible after collection.

Age-related haematological changes include:

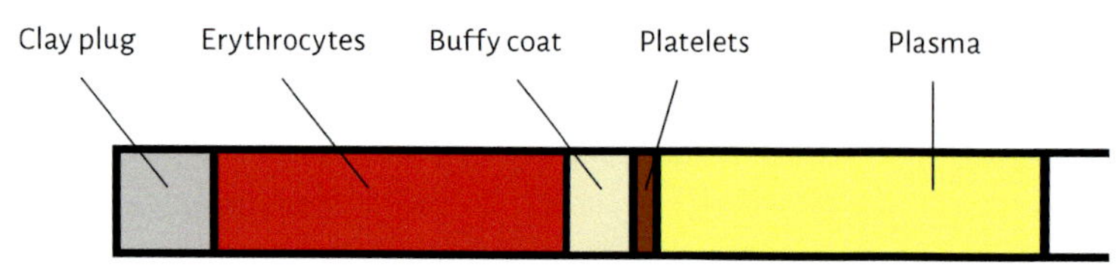

Figure 8. Cell fraction of a microhaematocrit.

- RBC crenation (misshaping)
- falsely toxic changes to white blood cells
- falsely low WBC count
- platelet clumping
- falsely low platelet count
- falsely increased MCH and MCHC
- falsely decreased RBC level and HCT
- falsely increased MCV
- falsely low platelet volume.

Blood smears should be made as soon as a blood sample (preferably via the jugular) is obtained, due to cell morphology degeneration and to ensure accurate interpretation. It is also important the sample is checked for any clots, as these cause false platelet and leukocyte counts.

Automated counts are most commonly performed using electronic impedance (Coulter principle), laser light scattering (flow cytometry) or quantitative buffy coat (QBC) analysis.

Electronic Impedance (Coulter principle) Analysers

The majority of in-house veterinary haematology automatic analysers use electronic impedance, which contain two electrodes through which electrolyte-containing conduction fluid flows. As cells move through the electrolyte-containing conduction fluid, the electrical conduction is interrupted (impeded). The duration of this impedance varies depending on the size and density (i.e. the type) of the cell, allowing analysers to differentiate between different blood cells.

These analysers require a daily background analysis, as the sample probes and reagent tubing often contain small particles which can be mistaken for cells. In addition, platelet clumping causes significantly reduced platelet counts in these analysers, and so concurrent blood film examination is often required in-house.

Flow Cytometry Analysers

Flow cytometry uses focused beams of laser light to evaluate the size and density of blood cells. As the blood passes through the laser beam, this causes light to scatter through cells in varying patterns depending on the size, volume, and density of the cell, allowing each type of white blood cell, red blood cells and platelets, to be identified. Many flow cytometry analysers use specialised stains which alter the flow of light through red blood cells, allowing the identification of reticulocytes (immature RBCs).

This type of analyser also provides additional information on the distribution of red blood cells and platelets.

Quantitative Buffy Coat (QBC) Analysers

These analysers have been replaced by electronic impedance analysers or flow cytometry analysers. They are based on the centrifugal stratification principle of blood components using a microhaematocrit tube that contains the stain acridine orange which is taken up by the cells' DNA, RNA, and lipoprotein.

After the sample has been centrifuged the cells are subjected to an ultraviolet light which causes the stained cells to emit a fluorescent light. Nucleated cells containing DNA emit a green light while white blood cells that contain lipoprotein and RNA emit a red light. The number and type of cells present are determined by the amount of red and green light produced and where the light is generated within the microhaematocrit tube (i.e. larger cells such as leukocytes will be at one end while smaller cells will fit into more space and emit more light).

However, it is assumed all cells have a normal cell volume and hence this can result in inaccurate results in certain diseases such as leukaemia where cell volumes are altered.

Different parameters are examined during haematology analysis, and the veterinary nurse/technician should be able to identify and interpret common parameters, to understand why any additional diagnostic tests are required, and how this information is used by the veterinary surgeon for the patient's treatment plan and subsequent nursing care.

RBC levels help determine whether anaemia or polycythaemia is present, and if the haematology analyser also provides a reticulocyte (immature RBC) count, it can determine whether any anaemia is regenerative or non-regenerative.

White blood cells

The WBC count and differential cell counts (individual neutrophil, leukocyte, eosinophil, monocyte, and basophil levels) are **used to determine the presence of inflammation or infection, immune system compromise, and stress responses.**

Neutrophils

This is the most common white blood cell line in both canine and feline species and is the **body's first response to injury and infection.** They also release signals (cytokines) to other white blood cells and coagulation precursors to a site of inflammation/injury.

Lymphocytes

These are the second most common white blood cell and an integral part in the immune response. Lymphocytes are subdivided as T-cells or B-cells and are both triggered by antigens found on the surface of the cell membrane of the invading cell.

T-cells control the immune response at a cellular level by helping to activate other immune cells and B-cells produce antibodies in response to antigens and are therefore part of humoral immunity as antibodies are released into the bloodstream.

An increase in lymphocytes may indicate an immune response which may be secondary to vaccination (young patients), chronic infection, or a fear flight/fight response (especially seen in cats) which is due to epinephrine being released, which in turn acutely increases the number of circulating lymphocytes.

Lymphopaenia (decreased level) is seen in stressed patients or in patients with an increase in cortisol (hyperadrenocorticism), obstruction of lymph flow (neoplasia/inflammation), in patients with decreased production (FIV, on immunosuppressive medication) or due to loss such as with chylothorax or lymphangiectasia.

Monocytes

Monocytes remove dead and damaged cells as well as microorganisms via phagocytosis. They are the largest type of white blood cell. They differentiate into macrophages and myeloid lineage dendritic cells. They interact with lymphocytes in immune reactions to produce interferon (signalling protein to other immune cells) in relation to viruses. Feline and canine monocytes differ in appearance.

Eosinophils

These white blood cells are slightly larger than neutrophils and are characterised by pink cytoplasmic granules. In the canine species these cytoplasmic granules vary in size, shape, and abundance. In particular, in Greyhound eosinophils the cytoplasmic granules do not stain and hence appear vacuolated. In cats they are found in abundance and are always a uniform rod shape (Villers, 2016).

Eosinophils are involved in parasitic defence and during hypersensitivity responses.

Basophils

These are **rare in the healthy patient** and are similar to eosinophils. They have a ribbon like nucleus and their granules are sparse in the dog and stain dark purple, whereas in cats they are abundant and stain lilac.

Platelets

Platelets are ¼ to ½ the size of erythrocytes and have no nucleus. Their cytoplasm stains pink and they also contain small granules.

Platelet levels provide information about the patient's haemostatic ability. Primary haemostasis is the formation of a platelet plug to stop haemorrhage before a blood clot forms (secondary haemostasis). Insufficient platelet levels, or platelet dysfunction, can result in spontaneous haemorrhage in severe cases.

Low automated platelet counts are a common frustration when interpreting automated results. These should always be confirmed via blood film examination.

Platelet numbers are estimated by counting the number of platelets seen per 1000 x field within the monolayer of a blood smear, once it has been established that no platelet clumps can be observed. A mean number of platelets is then calculated over five counting fields. A normal platelet count would be 10–30 platelets per 1000 x field, whereby each platelet is approximately equal to 15 x 10^9/l.

Therefore:

Number of platelets x 10^9/l = Mean number of platelets x 15

The interpretation of platelet number should be in relation to the reference range for the specific species. A low platelet count (thrombocytopaenia) is clinically more important than an increased platelet count (thrombocytosis) as the patient is at risk of haemorrhage. This is particularly important in the surgical patient.

Guidelines as to the association between platelet count and haemorrhagic risk are given in Table 7 but it is to be noted that these are based on human medicine, case reports and anecdotal data and therefore not all patients with low platelet counts will show signs of haemorrhage. (Cornell University College of Veterinary Medicine).

Table 7. Relationship between platelet count and risk of haemorrhage.

Platelet count (x 10^9/l)	Risk of haemorrhage
<10	Highest risk; at risk of spontaneous haemorrhage
10–30	Likely to be at risk of spontaneous haemorrhage
>50	At risk of trauma or surgically induced haemorrhage

Coagulation

Haemostasis

Haemostasis is characterised by **two stages (primary and secondary),** which are both triggered simultaneously.

Primary haemostasis: as the name suggests this is the first stage of haemostasis and involves **reflex constriction of the blood vessels and the formation of the platelet plug.**

Secondary haemostasis: consists of stabilisation of the platelet plug with fibrin resulting in **activation of the clotting cascade.**

Haemostasis defects are categorised as either:

- **primary haemostatic defect** caused by either quantitative or a qualitative pathology (i.e. number of platelets or defects in the vessel wall); or
- **secondary haemostatic defect** (quantitative or a qualitative).

Primary Haemostasis

- Involves interactions between the vessel wall and circulating platelets resulting in a platelet plug.
- Reflex vasoconstriction of the vessel wall aids in the reduction of bleeding. Platelets are activated and adhere to the vessel collagen at the site of damage.
- Von Willebrand's factor (vWF) is important for platelet adhesion.

Secondary Haemostasis

- Involves the formation of a fibrin mesh by coagulation factors in order to stabilise the platelet plug.
- The majority of coagulation factors are produced by the liver (except factor VIII) and are designated by Roman numerals.
- Vitamin K is required by the liver to synthesise factors II, VII, IX and X.
- Clotting factors are mainly protease enzymes, which are sequentially activated to produce a cascade phenomenon. The coagulation cascade is divided into two pathways (intrinsic and extrinsic) both leading to a common pathway.

Buccal Mucosal Bleeding Time (BMBT)

Buccal mucosal bleeding time (BMBT) is a useful and inexpensive test for the **preoperative assessment of primary haemostasis,** and thus platelet function, however **it is not disorder specific.**

A BMBT test should be carried out on surgical patients with an inherited predisposition to disorders affecting primary haemostasis such as Dobermanns (e.g. vWD) and other predisposed breeds.

1. A light gauze tie is used to hold up the upper buccal mucosa in an everted position. Care should be taken not to over tighten the tie as this restricts circulation.
2. A shallow cut should be made in the buccal mucosa via a lancet device to produce a cut of a specific length and depth, which is shallow enough to only require a platelet plug and thus primary haemostasis.
3. The time required for bleeding to stop should be counted, whilst carefully blotting away the blood without disturbing the clot.

In healthy patients the time for a clot to form is:

- restrained un-sedated/anaesthetised canine patients: 1.7–3.3 minutes
- sedated/anaesthetised canine patients: 1.7–4.2 minutes
- sedated/anaesthetised feline patients: <3.3 minutes.

Note: BMBT cannot distinguish canine patients with and without Von Willebrand factor (vWD).

Activated Partial Thromboplastin Time (APTT) and Prothrombin Time (PT)

APTT and PT are parameters used together to assess secondary haemostasis, which is a complex cascade of clotting factor activation resulting in the formation of a fibrin-based blood clot.

PT is also known as one stage prothrombin time (OSPT).

Both PT and APTT should be interpreted in conjunction with each other "because a low fibrinogen prolongs the PT (and APTT) independently of other clotting factor deficiencies (both tests rely on adequate fibrinogen to form the fibrin clot)" (Eclin path, 2020).

The clotting cascade (Figure 9) can be divided into the extrinsic, intrinsic, and common pathways.

- **APTT** evaluates the intrinsic and common coagulation pathways; and
- **PT** evaluates the extrinsic and common pathways.

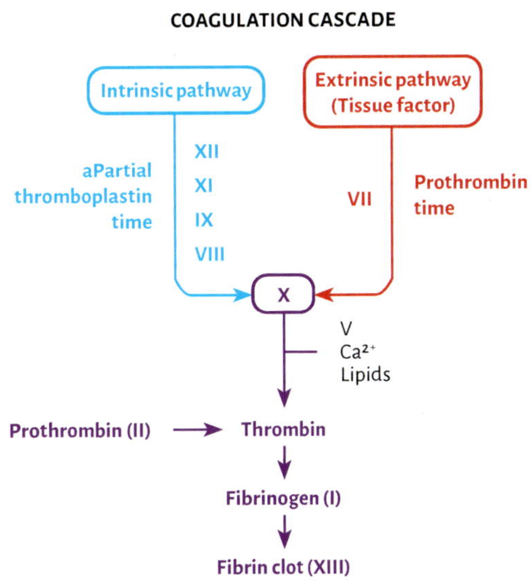

Figure 9. The clotting cascade.

There are many point-of-care tests (POCT) on the market that use either whole and or citrated blood. Each POCT has their own reference range depending on the sample used. It is essential if citrated blood is used that the **citrate tube is filled to the line** and gently mixed to ensure accurate results and manufacture guidelines are adhered to, to ensure accurate results and avoid artefacts.

If either PT or APTT is prolonged a fresh sample should be sent to an external laboratory for further evaluation which includes a thrombin clot time (TCT). **TCT evaluates the time taken for fibrinogen to be converted to fibrin.**

Urine Examination

Refrigerated urine samples should be allowed to come up to room temperature, to minimise struvite crystal artefact. Prior to any chemical analysis, the urine should be visually examined, and the colour, clarity, and odour recorded.

Colour

The urine sample should be placed in front of a plain piece of white paper in order to assess its colour effectively. The colour of urine gets its characteristic light-yellow colour from pigments called urochromes; the intensity of this yellow colour varies as the urine becomes more concentrated or diluted.

A colourless urine typically has a low specific gravity and is often seen in the polyuric/polydipsic patient, whereas **a dark yellow-to-brown urine typically has a higher specific gravity** and is seen in the oliguric patient (a patient with a urine output less than 0.5 ml/kg/hr), the dehydrated patient, and in some patients with shock, certain renal diseases, and cardiac disease.

Yellow brown to green urine contains bile pigments and forms a green foam when shaken. This can be a normal finding in dogs with very concentrated urine but is otherwise an abnormal finding.

Red or red-brown coloured urine suggests the urine sample contains erythrocytes (haematuria) or haemoglobin (haemoglobinuria). To differentiate between the two a small amount of urine should be centrifuged. If the supernatant is clear and the RBCs gravitate to the bottom of the tube, haematuria is present. If the supernatant remains red-coloured, haemoglobinuria is present.

Brown coloured urine may contain myoglobin, which indicates that the patient has muscle cell breakdown.

Certain medications can cause urine discolouration. Examples include rifampicin (an antibiotic used to treat mycobacterial infection), which turns the patient's urine (and other bodily fluids) red/orange, metronidazole (which can turn urine brown), and propofol (which can cause green discolouration).

Odour

The odour of urine is a useful indicator of infection or other specific conditions. This is because normal urine has a distinctive, **species-specific odour,** which is often stronger in intact males.

Patients with a **urinary tract infection can sometimes have a strong ammonia odour,** this is seen particularly when urease-producing bacteria (e.g. *Staphylococcus spp.*, *Proteus spp.*) are present, which cause conversion of urea to ammonia in the urine. Samples left standing at room temperature for long periods may also develop this odour, due to bacterial growth.

Ketones in urine present as a sweet or fruity smell; they are classically seen in patients with diabetic ketoacidosis, (not all personnel may be able to detect a ketone odour).

Clarity

The clarity of the urine is tested by placing the urine in front of a piece of paper with text printed on it.

In most species freshly voided urine is usually transparent. Species such as rabbits and horses can pass naturally turbid urine due to increased concentrations of calcium carbonate crystals, and mucous glands within the upper urinary tract.

Urine is classified as:
- clear
- slightly cloudy
- cloudy
- turbid (thick with suspended matter).

Cloudy samples often contain a large number of particles which when **centrifuged yield sediment for analysis.** This may be a combination of crystals, casts, epithelial cells, red and white blood cells, bacteria, and other substances; or may be seen as a result of contamination from the patient's skin/lower gastrointestinal tract, or the urine container itself. Turbid samples usually contain larger numbers of particles, which are often present in flocculent clumps large enough to see with the naked eye.

Chemical Analysis

Reagent strips are used to **test for the various chemical components of urine.** These strips contain various testing pads impregnated with reagents, which change colour when in contact with urine containing each substance. The strips are analysed manually, by visualising the colour change and comparing it to a chart or inserted into an analyser which detects the colour chart, thereby minimising subjectivity. Most commonly, a 10-test strip is used, which examines the following parameters:

- specific gravity
- pH
- glucose
- bilirubin
- ketones (acetoacetic acid)
- protein
- occult blood
- white blood cells
- nitrite
- urobilinogen.

Strips examining one or two individual parameters are also available (e.g. Keto-diastix, which evaluate just glucose and ketones). It is important to remember these **reagent strips are intended for human urine analysis** and so not all parameters are accurate in veterinary patients. Assessment of urobilinogen and nitrates is not required in veterinary patients; in addition, the leukocyte/WBC testing pad is considered unreliable, particularly in cats, and the presence of WBCs should always be confirmed via sediment examination.

When performing urine chemistry, the test strip should either be dipped in the urine and the long edge tilted against a paper towel to wick away any excess, or flooded with a pipette, ensuring that each pad is fully saturated with urine and the pads do not run into each other. **After saturation with urine, a timer should be started, and each pad should be read at the appropriate time interval.**

Specific Gravity (SG)

The specific gravity (SG) of a solution is defined as the density of a liquid, compared with the density of distilled water. SG is used to investigate the patient's hydration status and urine concentrating ability (renal function). The number and molecular weight of the components dissolved in the urine determine the urine's specific gravity.

Specific gravity is measured using a urinometer or refractometer, as this is reliable and requires only a small sample volume.

Because the specific gravity of urine is altered significantly based on the patient's food/water intake, environmental temperature, and the timing of their urination throughout the day, **an early morning, mid-stream sample is preferred** as this is when the urine is most concentrated.

Urine specific gravity is measured in a similar way to total solids ensuring that the refractometer is correctly calibrated prior to taking the measurement using the U.G scale. Because the weight is determined by the components dissolved in the urine, **SG can be measured before or after centrifugation.** Components that settle during centrifugation (e.g. crystals, cells, and casts) do not significantly alter urine SG.

The specific gravity of healthy patients is:

- **Dog: 1.025–1.030**
- **Cat: 1.030–1.035**

Based on a patient's SG, urine is categorised as isosthenuric or hyposthenuric:

1. **Isosthenuric urine** has a concentration similar to that of plasma. The urine SG is 1.008–1.015.
2. **Hyposthenuric urine** has a concentration less than that of plasma. The urine SG is <1.008.

Sediment Examination

An integral part of in-house urine analysis is the microscopic examination of the urine sample (Box 1). There are many abnormalities that may not be determined with just chemical analysis and also some of the chemical analysis results may need to be confirmed (e.g. the presence of blood and white blood cells).

Different stain pots should be used for urine and blood. Stains used to stain urine should be changed regularly so as to reduce the risk of bacterial contamination and a pipette should be used to drop the stain onto the slide rather than dipping the slide into the stain to minimise cross contamination.

A urine smear can be evaluated as an extra step to evaluate bacteria and cell morphology and is reviewed in the same way as a blood smear.

- **Epithelial cells:** occasional cells are normal, particularly in a free-catch sample. Increased epithelial cell numbers are seen with infection, irritation, or neoplasia.
- **Red blood cells:** 0–5 cells/HPF (high-power field) may be normal; increased numbers indicate haematuria or may be due to sampling method.

Box 1. Preparation of a Urine Sample for Microscopic Examination

- An Eppendorf tube should be filled with urine and labelled.
- The sample should be centrifuged at a low speed for three to six minutes depending on the centrifuged used and at the recommended speed set to the manufacture's recommendations.
- The supernatant should be poured away which leaves a small volume of urine above the sediment layer.
- The sediment should be resuspended by flicking the capped tube and gently inverting it.
- A drop of sediment solution should be transferred to a microscope slide and covered with a cover slip.
- Another slide should be prepared and preferably a drop of Sedi-Stain™ added or alternatively methylene blue stain/DiffQuick™ stain C then covered with a coverslip.
- Optionally, a urine slide smear can be prepared and left to air dry prior to staining with DiffQuick™.
- Both plain and stained slides should be evaluated so that they can be compared.
- Stained slides should be used to confirm structures seen on the plain slide and the plain slide to rule out artefacts on the stained slides that may be due to the staining process (i.e. bacteria due to contaminated stain).

- **White blood cells:** low numbers <5 cells/HPF can be normal; increased numbers indicate infection, or a sterile inflammatory process in the urinary tract. In free catch samples this may be inflammation of the urethra rather than the bladder. Figure 10 also contains epithelial cells and bacteria, indicating an infection.
- **Ammonium biurate crystals:** small, brown thorn-apple shaped crystals commonly seen in patients with liver dysfunction or portosystemic shunts.
- **Cystine crystals:** large, flat, hexagonal crystals seen in patients with renal tubular disease.
- **Normal urine is sterile:** any bacteria on a cystocentesis sample is significant, and urine collected via other methods cannot be reliably assessed due to contamination. Cocci (spherical bacteria) and/or bacilli (rod-shaped bacteria) are commonly seen; these may be alone, or in bunches or chains.
- **Casts:** cylindrical moulds of the renal tubules, made up of a matrix containing various cell types. They are associated with diseases affecting the kidneys, and several types are commonly seen, including hyaline casts, cellular casts, granular casts, and waxy casts.
- **Struvite crystals:** 6–8-sided prism-shaped crystals that form in alkaline urine.
- **Calcium oxalate crystals:** the dihydrate form are small squares containing an 'X'; these normally form in acidic urine. The monohydrate form is "picket fence"-shaped and is seen due to ethylene glycol toxicity.
- **Urate crystals:** commonly seen in Dalmatians and dogs with portosystemic shunts.

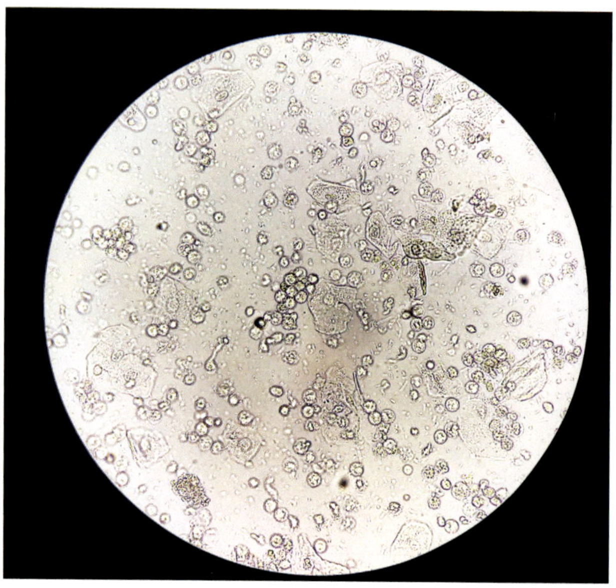

Figure 10. Moderate bacterial and white blood cells in patient with urinary tract infection.

Cytology and Histology

Histology and cytology are an integral part of analysis of the pre and postoperative patient to determine a diagnosis and treatment plan.

Histology is the study of tissues and how the cells within those tissues interact with one another, whereas **cytology is the study of cells,** harvested from tissues but no longer arranged within the tissue, which allows interpretation of the cells present but not their interaction and distribution.

Cytology

Methods of Collection

There are a number of **cytology sampling methods** available, and these include:

Fine Needle Aspirates (FNAs)

FNAs can be performed on **internal and external masses, lymph nodes, and provide fluid** or cytological information to aid diagnosis. This method is associated with less bacterial contamination but usually yields fewer cells compared to other sampling methods. FNAs can be performed under **ultrasound guidance** when sampling of deeper tissues or small target tissues is required.

Impression Smears

Impression smears can be prepared from external lesions, or from a biopsy or tissue removed at time of surgery. These generally have **fewer cells than scrapings** and may contain contamination, compared with other sampling methods. The samples collected are cleaned with saline, blotted, and placed on a clean swab or tissue. A clean glass microscope slide is then pressed against the tissue, leaving the impression of the tissue on the slide. It is advisable to **prepare several slides** so that multiple stains can be used where necessary.

Scrapings

The collection of cells via scraping yields more cells than other collection methods. Cell samples can be collected from external lesions or lesions removed via surgery. However, cells are only collected from the superficial surface and hence diagnoses may be missed.

Exfoliative Cytology

This relies on the spontaneous exfoliation of cells into fluids or onto swabs.

Fluid Cytology

Fluid cytology performed on CSF, urine, effusions, synovial fluid. These fluids are centrifuged, and the sediment used to make a smear. Alternatively, a smear can be made directly from the fluid itself.

Swab Method

Usually collected from areas where other collection methods are not feasible (e.g. reproductive tract or ear canal). A sterile cotton bud moistened in sterile 0.9% saline is used, the swab is rolled against the collection area in order to collect exfoliated cells. The swab is then gently rolled over a clean microscope slide to make a cell smear.

Preparation of Aspirated Material

Samples collected via aspiration can be prepared in four ways to produce a slide smear. These are:

- compression technique
- squash smear technique
- pull technique
- line concentration technique.

The same techniques are used for preparing blood smears; however, the spreader slide is abruptly lifted upwards after being advanced two thirds of the way. This technique is used for cystic masses and haemodiluted samples (Monti et al., 2016).

Histology

For a successful pathological evaluation, a **high quality, well-preserved sample** must be obtained. It is also important it is submitted with a thorough clinical history (a photograph of the lesion is also helpful). Tissue samples for histological analysis are collected via biopsy.

A biopsy is the surgical removal of a sample of representative tissue of the suspected lesion.

Biopsy Techniques

Punch Biopsy

This involves a biopsy punch, which come in a variety of circular circumferences. Punch biopsies are indicated for cutaneous and subcutaneous masses (skin lesions).

Punch biopsies are quick, easy, and inexpensive to obtain (Figure 11). Generally, the patient does not need to be anaesthetised. However, **the sample is limited to the circumference and depth of the punch biopsy** itself.

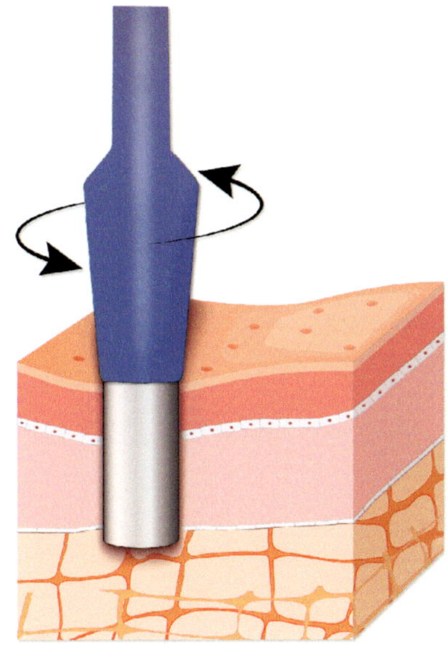

Figure 11. Punch biopsy.

Needle Core Biopsy (Tru-Cut® Biopsy)

This involves using **a large needle or special automatic Tru-Cut® biopsy needle** device to obtain a small core of tissue. A Tru-Cut® automatic needle device automatically triggers a rapid firing, side-notch, Tru-Cut®-type biopsy needle. A spring action thrusts the inner trocar forward, followed almost instantaneously by a similar forward thrust of the outer cutting cannula. The specimen is trapped in the side notch of the trocar when the cutting cannula is advanced. (Figure 12).

Tissue core biopsy has the advantage of providing the pathologist with the tissue architecture, which is essential in the diagnosis of many liver and renal diseases, and so these biopsies are usually only performed on these organs. The largest biopsy needle that can be safely used is ideal to yield more tissue, leading to a more accurate diagnosis.

Although this is a quick and easy procedure it yields a **small sample size** and is also expensive due to the instrument costs involved. Patients must be sedated or anaesthetised and not suffer from any coagulopathies. Needle core biopsies are mainly used for **ultrasound guided procedures.**

Incisional or Wedge Biopsy

This involves a small slice or wedge of tissue which is removed from a larger mass or lesion. "This technique is effective for masses in all locations and generates a larger tissue mass for the pathologist to examine. They are particularly useful for diagnosis of soft, friable, inflamed and/or necrotic tumours." (Ehrhart, 1998).

This technique is used to obtain liver samples.

Excision Biopsy

Excisional biopsies involve excision of the entire mass. The entirety of the mass (by palpation or observation) is removed including what appears to be healthy surrounding tissue. It is important to remember this technique is not curative for some lesions, such as soft tissue sarcomas and mast cell tumours, which frequently have smaller satellite lesions in the surrounding tissue.

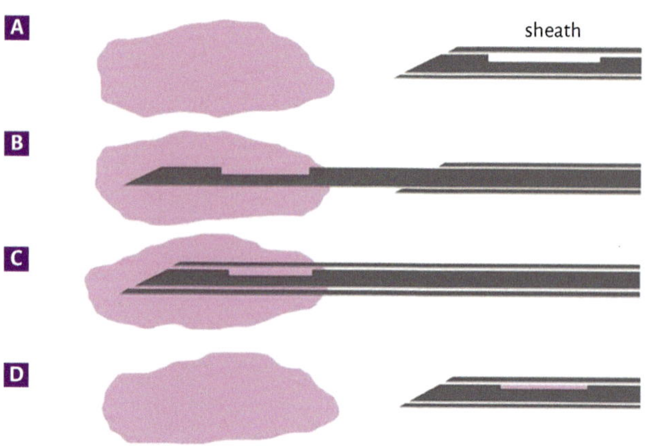

Figure 12. Automatic core or Tru-Cut® biopsies needle with coaxial needle. **A.** Needle with slot. **B.** Advancement of the needle. **C.** Slide sheath over needle to cut specimen. **D.** Tissue sample.

Tissue samples for histology should be fixed as soon as possible. The preferred **fixative is a 10% neutral buffered formalin (formal saline)** and the tissue to formal saline ratio should be 1:10. Tissues may be fixed for 24 to 48 hours depending on their thickness. Very small specimens should be placed in a tissue cassette to prevent specimen loss.

Blood Gas Analysis

Blood Oxygenation

Approximately 98% of oxygen within the vascular system is bound to haemoglobin molecules and carried to tissues within the body. Each molecule of haemoglobin is able to carry up to four molecules of oxygen. **The other 2% of oxygen within the body is dissolved in plasma.**

Both **arterial blood gas analysis and pulse oximetry** are used to evaluate the ability of the lungs to deliver oxygen to systemic arterial blood, but the information they provide is not equivalent. **Pulse oximetry measures the percentage of haemoglobin saturated with oxygen (SaO_2). Arterial blood gas analysis measures the amount of oxygen dissolved in the plasma** (expressed as the partial pressure of oxygen, or PaO_2). **The relationship between PaO_2 and SaO_2 is not linear;** the oxygen-haemoglobin dissociation curve is sigmoid in shape.

The haemoglobin dissociation curve can shift to the left or right. This depends on physiological conditions such as the patient's temperature, acid-base balance, and levels of 2,3-diphosphoglycerate in erythrocytes.

2,3-diphosphoglycerate is an anionic compound which binds to haemoglobin within the concave centre of the erythrocyte which reduces haemoglobin's affinity with oxygen, thus, becoming deoxyhaemoglobin and allowing haemoglobin to release oxygen to tissues. A decrease in 2,3-diphosphoglycerate therefore increases haemoglobin's affinity with oxygen.

If the curve (Figure 13) is shifted to the left, this indicates that the haemoglobin has a higher affinity for oxygen and thus a higher saturation for a given PaO_2. The opposite is true if the curve is shifted to the right. This means it is not possible to accurately predict the SaO_2 from the PaO_2 and vice versa.

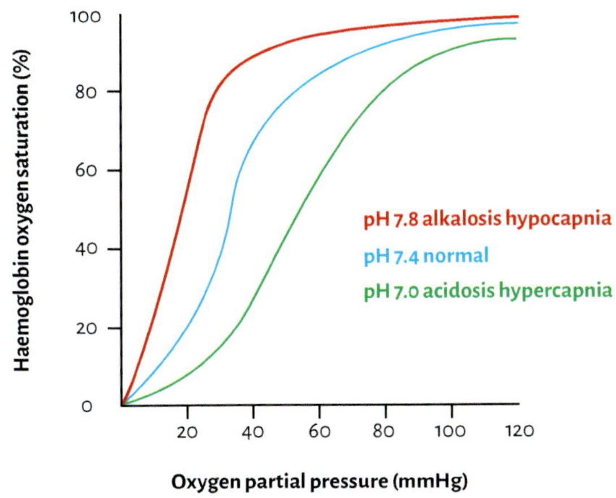

Figure 13. Haemoglobin dissociation curve.

Blood Gas Analysis

Blood gas analysis provides information on the surgical patient's pulmonary and acid-base status to enable the veterinary team to make a diagnosis and monitor patients pre-, peri- and postrespiratory surgery as well as in those with metabolic abnormalities.

A patient's acid-base status can be evaluated via either an arterial or venous sample.

However, to evaluate a patient's oxygenation status an arterial sample is required.

An arterial blood gas sample provides information on:

- **Partial pressures of oxygen (PaO_2): an accurate reflection on the ability of the lungs to transfer oxygen to the blood.**
- **Partial pressures of carbon dioxide ($PaCO_2$): indicates the effectiveness of alveolar ventilation.**
- **Blood pH: determines the acid-base status by measuring hydrogen ions (H^+).**
- **Bicarbonate concentration (HCO_3^-): serum bicarbonate levels provide information about the metabolic aspect of acid-base balance.**

The SaO_2 (pulse oximeter) measures the percentage of haemoglobin actually carrying oxygen, which is why 95–100% is normal.

Arterial Blood Sampling

An arterial blood sample is collected using either direct arterial puncture with a needle plus arterial syringe or by placing an indwelling arterial catheter.

The most common artery used for both these sampling procedures is **the dorsal metatarsal artery.** However other suitable arteries include the femoral, auricular, radial, brachial, and coccygeal arteries.

Placement of an Arterial Indwelling Catheter

Arterial indwelling catheters are placed for direct blood pressure monitoring and for repeated arterial blood sampling. As arteries are deeper and much smaller than veins, arterial catheterisation is more challenging than obtaining venous access.

Note: **Arterial blood sampling is contraindicated in patients with coagulopathies.**

The **dorsal metatarsal artery is most frequently used for catheterisation and sampling** as it is relatively superficial and located in the proximal area of the metatarsus, medial to the extensor tendon and between the second and third metatarsal bones. **A catheter size of 20–24 gauge** is used depending on patient size.

The skin over the proposed site should be clipped and prepared aseptically (but should not be scrubbed as this causes the artery to spasm). Therefore, a chlorhexidine-soaked swab should be placed over the site while the person collecting the sample carries out hand disinfection.

1. **The dorsal metatarsal pulse should be palpated** using two fingers to determine the direction of the artery.
2. While palpating the artery (between the second and third metatarsus), the catheter should be inserted through the skin, at an angle of 45–60°.
3. Once through the skin, the angle of the catheter should be reduced. Care should be taken to approach the artery at an **angle of 10–30°** to ensure the catheter is correctly aligned, which facilitates placement.
4. Because arterial walls are much thicker than venous walls, a **decisive directed motion** may be required once the tip of the inner stylet is resting just over the arterial wall.
5. Once a flashback of blood is seen in the hub of the catheter, the catheter and stylet should be advanced together for approximately 1–2 mm (to ensure the catheter itself

lies within the arterial lumen and not just the tip of the stylet) and then the needle pushed off into the artery.

6. **The catheter should be flushed with saline solution,** taped into place, and **labelled as arterial** as it should not be used for administration of fluids and medications.
7. Arterial lines should be flushed every 15 minutes or continually via a pressure bag and microtubing.

Arterial Blood Draw

1. The patient should be placed in **lateral recumbency** and the area over the collection site prepared in the same manner as for arterial catheter placement.
2. **The pulse should be palpated between the second and third metatarsal** (for the metatarsal branch of the dorsal pedal artery) with the collector's non-dominant hand.
3. With the dominant hand and via an **angle of 30°–40° the needle** is inserted slowly until there is blood-flash within the needle hub.
4. Using an arterial blood gas syringe allows the blood to automatically fill. If a non-arterial blood gas syringe is being used, the plunger can be gently pulled back.
5. Once the arterial sample has been collected the needle should be removed and the syringe capped to avoid air mixing with the sample. Direct pressure should be applied to the sample site for a minimum of 1–2 minutes, followed by a pressure bandage. The sample should be analysed promptly following sampling.

Blood gas syringes come **preloaded with dry lithium heparin anticoagulants.** The plunger stoppers have micro holes (air displacement filter) which allow air to leave the syringe as blood enters it. Thus, blood automatically fills the syringe to a set volume.

Interpretation of the arterial blood gas results are used to guide oxygen administration, fluid therapy, and requirements for blood products in combination with clinical assessment of the patient and other factors.

Diagnostic Imaging

Diagnostic imaging is an integral part of preoperative planning for surgical cases both to assess pathology that requires surgical intervention (e.g. the conformation of a fracture or the extent and invasiveness of a tumour) as well as for systemic disease and suitability for surgical intervention (e.g. the presence of pulmonary metastatic disease for a neoplastic lesion, or the presence of additional injuries following trauma).

The type of diagnostic imaging selected depends on the facilities and the veterinary expertise available to interpret the images acquired, the suspected pathological changes, the patient's clinical condition, and owner financial constraints.

Diagnostic imaging methods include:

- radiography
- ultrasonography
- computer tomography (CT)
- magnetic resonance imaging (MRI).

It is important to appreciate that **diagnostic imaging is not a priority in unstable patients,** unless essential for their stabilisation (e.g. assessment of pneumothorax on a conscious thoracic radiograph or bedside ultrasound assessment (TFAST). Unstable patients require appropriate assessment and procedures to stabilise them for further assessment, which are prioritised based on the patient's clinical status.

Radiography

The production of X-rays occurs due to the acute deceleration of fast-moving electrons when they interact with a positively charged anode, as detailed in Figure 14.

1. A current (mA) is passed through a tungsten filament which heats up the cathode. As the filament heats up the electrons within the tungsten filament become energized and are released and form an electron cloud around the filament via thermionic emission.
2. Electrons are then accelerated which gives them an increased kinetic energy. This is achieved by attracting them towards a positively charged anode, generated by the KVp (electric voltage) which forces the electrons across the tube to the positively charged anode.
3. The electrons decelerate as they hit a tungsten target on the anode. The deceleration process causes more than 99% of the energy from the electrons to be converted to heat and the remaining 1% is converted to X-rays photons. The X-ray photons are released in a beam with a range of energies (X-ray spectrum) out of the collimated window of the tube, projected towards the X-ray cassette and form the basis for X-ray image formation.

Increasing the current (mA) increases the number of electrons produced and therefore increases the amount of X-rays. Increasing the potential difference (kVp) increases the electron kinetic energy which increases X-ray energy and hence depth of tissue penetration.

There are three forms of radiography systems available on the market for veterinary use. These are:

- film-screen radiography
- digital radiography:

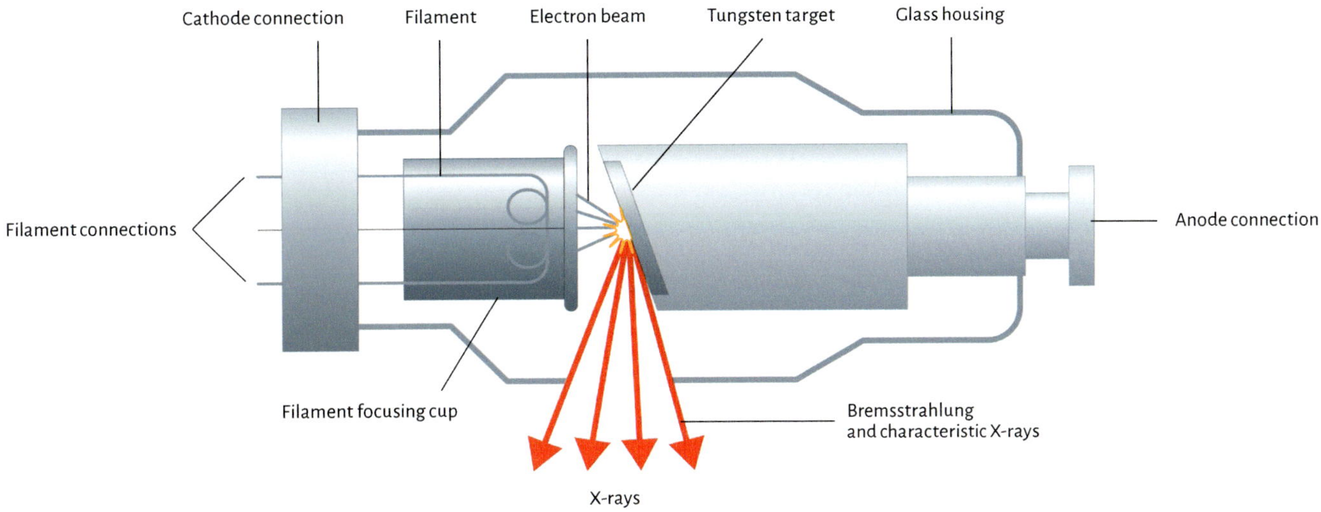

Figure 14. Production of X-rays.

- computed radiography (CR)
- direct digital radiography (DR).

Film-screen Radiography

The conventional method of producing radiographs, whereby the exposed film is processed by wet chemicals to produce an X-ray for interpretation.

Film-screen radiography requires an X-ray cassette which includes intensifying screens, radiographic film, and a chemical film processor.

Digital Radiography

Uses the same procedure to produce X-rays as film-screen radiography but the image is produced by the exposure of a capture device, which converts the image to a digital signal which is subsequently converted to a digital image. There are two types of digital radiography.

Computed Radiography (CR)

This uses a portable imaging plate containing an interior photo-stimulated luminescence screen which records the raw image created by X-rays. The plate is then manually placed into a specialised reader where the interior screen is read by a laser which converts the image to a digital image.

Direct Digital Radiography (DR)

Involves filmless X-ray capture and does not rely on a cassette to capture the image. Instead, it uses an X-ray detector plate situated on the surface of the X-ray table or mounted in the Bucky assembly which holds the X-ray cassette/plate underneath the tabletop. The digitised image is sent directly from an X-ray detector plate to the computer workstation, resulting in almost instantaneous image production.

UK health and safety regulations mandate that **personnel should not restrain patients for radiography** and so chemical restraint, sandbags, and positioning aids should be used. Local radiation safety regulations should be reviewed regularly and adhered to.

Ultrasonography

Ultrasound examination is a valuable diagnostic tool as it allows **real time, dynamic patient assessment** and is often performed with minimal restraint or without the need for sedation or anaesthesia depending on the assessment required. It is useful for evaluation of parenchymal organs within the abdomen and identifying lymph nodes for sample collection (e.g. FNAs) for cytology.

Ultrasonography allows assessment of fluid filled body cavities which on radiographs are obscured by the presence of fluid on radiographs. Thus, it is particularly useful in patients with cavity effusions, and an experienced operator can detect even small quantities of fluid between organs. Areas of interest include:

- In the abdomen:
    - between and around liver lobes
    - the bladder apex

- between the spleen and body wall.
  - In the thorax:
    - the pericardium
    - between the lung lobe fissures and the thoracic wall.

Ultrasonography uses sound waves reflected by objects of different densities within the medium it is passes through to produce an echo.

Ultrasound is particularly useful for **assessment of abdominal organ size, shape, and position,** the integrity of body cavities, and viscera such as the bladder and gallbladder as well as aiding in the assessment of congenital anatomic variations such as portosystemic shunts. Dynamic assessment is also useful for assessing vascular flow and obstruction of the urogenital and gastrointestinal tracts.

Ultrasonography can also assess the patient's cardiac function including the heart's contractility and valve function; and as such assess heart murmurs in greater depth prior to anaesthesia.

Ultrasonography is also useful to monitor for postoperative complications such as cavitary fluid accumulation with internal haemorrhage, as well as assessing the volume of urine within a patients' bladder to assess renal function, especially if there is anuria.

Computed Tomography (CT)

Computed tomography (CT) is one of the most important advancements in diagnostic imaging within veterinary medicine. It is a **computer-enhanced** X-**ray imaging procedure** that involves a narrow beam of X-rays being aimed at the patient which quickly rotate around the body to produce signals which are converted into cross-sections (or slices) of that area in the patient. The cross-sectional images are then stacked to form a 3-dimensional image of the area of interest allowing the veterinary surgeon to identify abnormalities more thoroughly than is possible with conventional radiography.

The use of **intravenous iodinated contrast media is particularly useful for vascular studies** particularly when used in conjunction with a plain study as comparing both images gives the veterinary surgeon an insight into the haemodynamic and physiological changes present, by highlighting areas of increased vascularisation. One example of the utility of CT is in patients with middle ear disease as radiographs provide limited information for surgical planning, due to the pattern of overlying structures on a radiograph.

Magnetic Resonance Imaging (MRI)

Magnetic resonance imaging (MRI) does not involve X-rays but instead uses a powerful magnet ("up to 60 000 times as strong as the magnetic field of the earth" (Lattimer, 2019)). The strength of the magnetic field is measured in Tesla (T). The magnet produces a unified magnetic field around the patient which aligns the movement of the protons within the patient's body tissues. A gradient which is composed of loops of wire or metal sheet lies just inside the bore of the MRI scanner and when an electrical current passes through it, a second magnetic field is produced which distorts (adjusts) the main magnetic field into different magnetic strengths around particular areas of interest of the patient's body (i.e. the spine). The patient is then subjected to a radiofrequency pulse (of different frequencies depending on the scan type being performed and the specific tissue of interest) which deflects the alignment of the hydrogen atoms. Once the radiofrequency is stopped the hydrogen atoms realign with the magnetic field, at a rate which is restricted by the characteristic of their individual molecules and tissue type (e.g. water, fat, bone).

These hydrogen atoms emit energy during **the realignment phase.** This energy is released as a radio wave which is detected by a coil around the area of interest. It is these radio waves which are converted to form a digital image. **Like CT these images are recorded in slices.**

The strength and duration of the frequency is evaluated to determine the chemical properties of the area of interest in a 3-dimensional plane. Unlike CT several scans are required with different magnet pulsing sequences to highlight different types of tissue in different planes.

Because MRI uses magnetic fields it is very sensitive to metals, in particular iron (found in ID chips) and cobalt, which reduce the image quality and therefore cause artefacts.

MRI is best used to image soft tissue (those tissues that are composed of H_2O) and is not reliable at imaging cortical bone and bony lesions. In veterinary practice it is mostly used to **evaluate neurological pathology of the brain and spinal cord, intervertebral discs, and meninges.** It is also particularly useful for evaluating deep blood vessels and for soft tissue structures within joints, as well as some ligaments, tendons, and muscles. **MRI needs to be performed on anaesthetised patients** due the length of time each scan takes, and the sensitivity MRI has to movement. Patients undergoing MRI must be stable, particularly as anaesthesia monitoring capability and access to the patient is reduced. Because a high-powered magnet is used, special MRI safe anaesthesia and monitoring equipment is required.

Where diagnostic imaging requires anaesthesia, it is important to consider if **both the diagnostic and surgical treatment can be performed under the same general anaesthetic.** This is advantageous for the client's finances and also to the patient if it saves unnecessary repeat anaesthesia (e.g. a paraplegic Dachshund going for MRI and then hemilaminectomy). The disadvantage of performing surgery immediately following an imaging procedure is that a vast amount of information is acquired and making rapid decisions on patient treatment may mean that diagnoses made under pressure are incomplete or incorrect which might compromise patient care. So, depending on the urgency of the surgical condition, a delay whilst waiting for a full and detailed inspection of the images acquired may benefit surgical planning and client education for the specific goals and risks of a given surgical procedure.

Patient Preparation

The patient themself is one of the major sources of contaminating microorganisms, with endogenous staphylococci and streptococci from the skin most frequently cultured from wound infections. Wounds open to the environment become contaminated with opportunistic microorganisms, which over time colonize the wound causing a wound infection. **The longer a wound is open, the higher the risk of contamination and subsequent infection.** Therefore, depending on the length of time and type of procedure, prophylactic antimicrobials are recommended. **Good aseptic technique is paramount** to ensure surgery is performed with minimal risk of microbial contamination. Antimicrobial agents alone will not eliminate negative outcomes associated with poor aseptic technique.

During a surgical procedure, the incision is exposed to:
- the environment
- the patient's own bacterial flora
- surgical personnel, instruments, and equipment.

Microorganisms and Biofilms

Reduction of the bacterial flora on the patient and the surgical team should be balanced with the potential for tissue damage caused by overzealous scrubbing, clipping and irritant chemicals.

It is important to understand there are **two types of microorganisms** originating from the patient.
- **Transient microorganisms:** these are microorganisms that do not usually colonize the skin and are acquired via contact with veterinary personnel, other veterinary patients, or the environment. They are easy to remove from the skin via physical scrubbing and eliminated by an effective antiseptic.
- **Resident or commensal microorganisms:** these are bacteria found on the patient as part of their normal flora.

Biofilms are a protective matrix which may form as the result of infection, when bacteria adhere to the patient's tissues or surgical implants such as orthopaedic plates and screws, sutures, or permanent drainage devices. **Bacteria evade the immune system within the biofilm** which is impenetrable by either antibiotics or the animal's immune system. Infection beyond the biofilm may be dampened by antibiotic therapy, but then infection recurs as further bacteria proliferate and migrate beyond the biofilm into the surrounding tissue once again.

It is imperative to **minimize the surgical incision's exposure to microorganisms.** This is achieved by:
- careful patient clipping
- meticulous skin preparation
- aseptic patient draping
- appropriate use of antibiotics depending on the expected level of surgical contamination.

Prior to premedication **the patient should be given an opportunity to void their bladder and bowel,** so as to reduce the risk of inappropriate urination and defecation during skin preparation or the surgical procedure. Clients and ward staff should be encouraged to take canine patients (in particular) for short walks (depending on the health status of the patient).

Once any patient is stable under anaesthesia, the bladder should be checked and empty via gentle expression or catheterisation if it is safe to do so. Similarly, the rectum should be manually emptied. Bladder expression/catheterisation should be avoided if there is an increased risk of causing adverse effects such as urinary tract disease. Enemas should not be used prior to patient surgery as they produce watery faeces, which increases the risk of surgical contamination.

For surgery around the rectal area (perianal surgery or total hip replacement) **the rectum should be packed with an appropriate, easily removable absorbent material, and a purse-string suture placed** around the anus if the surgical site has an increased risk of contamination during surgery via faecal material. When performing anal sacculectomy procedures, the purse-string should be placed cranial to the opening of the anal sacs, so as not to encroach on the surgical site.

A purse-string suture is a continuous stitch placed concentrically with the edges of a circular opening (e.g. anus). When placing a purse-string suture for temporary closure, care must be taken not to damage the anal sacs. Suture ends should be left long for ease of removal. (Figure 15).

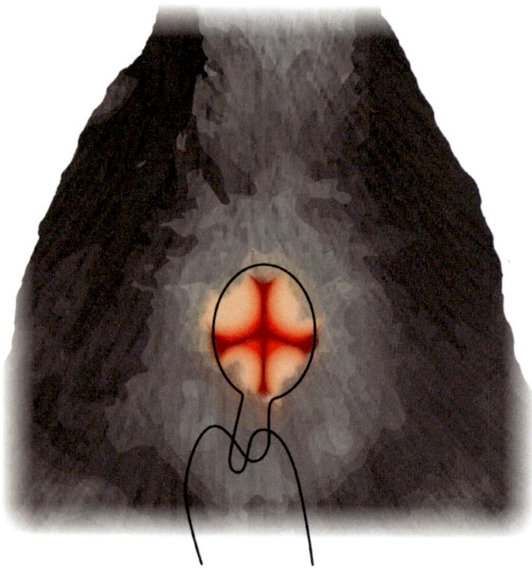

Figure 15. Purse-string suture around the anus.

It is imperative that any packing material and purse-string suture used to temporarily close the rectum is recorded on the patient's records and/or surgical safety checklist to ensure their removal at the end of the procedure (Further discussion of surgical safety checklists follow in Chapter 6). Purse-strings and packing material should be easily removable at the end of surgery, prior to patient recovery.

Patient Clipping

Hair acts like a filter that traps bacteria and dirt and produces a microclimate at skin level. This is ideal for harbouring microorganisms, and for this reason, hair should be removed to prevent contamination of the surgical site with foreign material and allow for effective skin disinfection.

Removal of hair the day before surgery and/or some time prior to anaesthesia induction is associated with an increase in the risk of surgical site infection. Therefore, this is discouraged, although may be unavoidable for abdominal surgery where ultrasound is performed as part of the diagnostic investigation prior to surgery (Renburg, 2012 and Brown, et al., 1997). Clipping damages the surface of the skin allowing bacteria to embed and proliferate over time. For this reason, **patient clipping should be performed ideally after, or no more than, one hour prior to inducing anaesthesia.** If possible, the patient should be bathed with mild pH friendly shampoo 24-hours before surgery, such as in the case of elective surgeries.

Hair should not be removed using razors or hair removal creams as these damage the surface of the skin through physical means and results in microbial colonisation and bacterial infection (Olson et al., 1986). Hair removal creams also case skin irritation, which subsequently cause patient interference and possibly self-mutilation.

The recommended means of surgical hair removal for veterinary patients is using **well-maintained, sharp clippers,** as they cause less trauma to the skin and subsequently their use is associated with fewer surgical wound infections than other forms of hair removal. Clipping is generally recommended **using electric clippers and a size 40 clipper blade.**

When clipping and prepping the skin, **a disposable apron and gloves should be worn** to prevent contamination of the operator's scrub suit which might then result in contamination of the operating theatre environment.

It is **imperative to clip the patient in a separate, designated area,** away from the operating theatre, to prevent contamination of the operating environment. Unless the hair is extremely short, **the hair should be clipped using a two-stroke technique to avoid skin abrasions.** This is evident when long hair is clipped with a single stroke against the lay of the hair because the hair drags the surrounding skin surface into the clipper blades.

- **Two-stroke technique:** the bulk of the hair should be removed by clipping in the direction of the hair, followed by a closer clip against the direction of the hair. This ensures a close clip with minimal trauma.

A wide area should be clipped around the proposed incision site to allow for draping to overlap the incision site, with a minimum 15 cm border of clipped skin.

When preparing the patient for an orthopaedic procedure, the entire limb should be clipped as well as areas used for bone graft harvesting (such as the wing of the ileum or proximal humerus. Depending on the orthopaedic procedure, the distal limb should be covered with an impermeable material (also known as draping out).

To avoid contamination, **any area required for an additional procedure** (which is not the main surgical procedure) **should be prepped at the same time,** e.g. exploratory laparotomy and oesophageal feeding tube placement. The two different surgical sites should be prepared prior to surgery commencing.

Special care is required when clipping around open wounds to prevent contamination of the wound with loose hair. This is achieved by covering the wound with saline soaked gauze swabs or aqueous sterile gel.

A vacuum (with a fine filter which is changed regularly) should be used to remove all fur/hair debris from the patient and surrounding area. Once the area is free from loose hair/fur, the person involved in the patient's skin prep should change their scrub top/apron or remove the protective lab/surgical coat, to prevent contamination of the surgical area being prepared.

Clipping Technique

Clippers must be maintained, and good clipping technique used to prevent skin damage through skin nicks, lacerations, and skin abrasion (clipper rash).

Damaged skin exposes bacteria from the deeper skin layers and hair follicles, which can then colonise these lesions. Furthermore, damaged skin also encourages the patient to lick and or self-mutilate the area around the incision site, increasing bacterial numbers.

Cross contamination between patients should be prevented by using a new blade each time. Coarse blades are ideal to remove the bulk of the hair, and fine blades (e.g. size 40) for the final clip. To prevent skin creases being caught by the clipper blades, one hand should be used to gently pull the skin taut during clipping. For clipping small, delicate areas (e.g. toes, inside ears, over prominent areas) a smaller width clipper with a fine blade should be used.

When clipping large areas, **the clipper blades become hot and therefore should be changed regularly** during the clipping procedure. This prevents skin damage resulting from a hot clipper blade and a loss in the efficiency of the clip due to blunt clippers which results in tissue damage. Ideally, cooling sprays should be avoided as these contain solvents which remove the oil that prevents friction and therefore heat. They also contain chemicals in an aerosol which require PPE for their use.

During clipping **if there is any evidence of pyoderma (skin infection) the veterinary surgeon should be notified** as this may affect wound healing and increase the risk of a surgical site infection, particularly if the pyoderma is near the incision site. For elective surgeries the patient may be recovered from anaesthesia and the surgical procedure rescheduled to a time when the pyoderma has resolved. This is at the discretion of the veterinary surgeon and depends on the type of surgical procedure planned and patient's clinical condition. For example, elective orthopaedic surgeries involving placement of surgical implants are of the greatest concern for surgical site infection as this may result in catastrophic surgical failure due to implant loosening and/or failure of bone healing.

Clipper Maintenance

Proper clipper and clipper blade maintenance is important to ensure a good working machine, and to prevent cross contamination and damage to the patient's skin.

Particularly during a longer clip time, proteins and lipoproteins from the skin and hair will coagulate and adhere to the clipper edges of the blade producing a dull cutting surface. This results in hair being snagged on the blades, thus causing skin abrasions, also known as clipper rash.

Mandatory blade cleaning and maintenance is imperative. Tissue debris should be removed from the fine edges of the blade to restore the fine cutting edges. This can only be achieved with a solvent-based solution. Typical examples include **blade wash** (e.g. Oster Blade Wash™, Andis Blade Care Plus™), whereby running blades are dipped into the solution and dried afterwards, before being lubricated with a lubricating spray. (Because blade wash is a solvent it also removes any lubrication oil previously applied to the clipper blade).

Clipper blades should be oiled at least every 10 minutes, particularly during operation, to prevent friction between the cutting and guard blade and subsequently prevent the blade from becoming hot. A hot blade burns hair and dander, which deposit on the blades. Subsequently the blade will snag on the patient's skin, not clip efficiently, and reduce the life of the clipper motor.

Clipper oil should not be dropped along the teeth because this causes hair to catch between the clipper teeth, causing them to jam and nick the patient's skin. Instead, **oil should be placed within the running rails of the blades,** by sliding the bottom cutter plate to the side, and placing one drop of oil onto each running rail. (Figure 16).

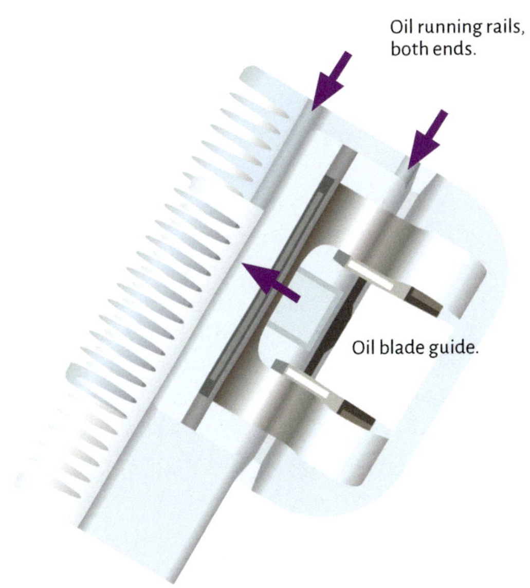

Figure 16. Lubricating positions.

To prevent cross contamination, a new or freshly cleaned clipper blade should be used for each patient. Some patients may require more than one blade per clip, depending on the area to be clipped.

Daily Maintenance

Unplug and Clean

The clipper should be unplugged, cleaned and hair removed from the blades and the head of the clipper with a toothbrush including all vents and places where hair can become trapped.

Tissue debris can be removed with blade wash to restore the fine cutting edge of the clipper. A small amount of blade wash should be poured into a container. With the blade attached to the clipper it should be submerged in the blade wash solution before turning on the clipper for approximately 5–8 seconds, then thoroughly dried with a paper towel.

Inspect and Replace

- The **lever/blade drive assembly:** this causes the blade to move back and forth to create the cutting action. When the lever/blade drive assembly is worn, it should be replaced.
- The **motor carbon brushes:** these are located on the lower portion of the clipper housing. If the clipper begins to run slower than usual, the brushes should be checked for wear. When clipper brushes are worn to half their original length it is time for replacement.
- **Blade latch:** if clipper blades seem to be loose or released during cutting, the latch may need to be replaced or tightened and should be sent for repair.

Weekly Maintenance

Remove and Examine

The blade can be removed from the latch by pushing the blade latch release in using the thumb. The blade socket and rail guide should be examined for wear and the cutter and comb inspected for proper alignment.

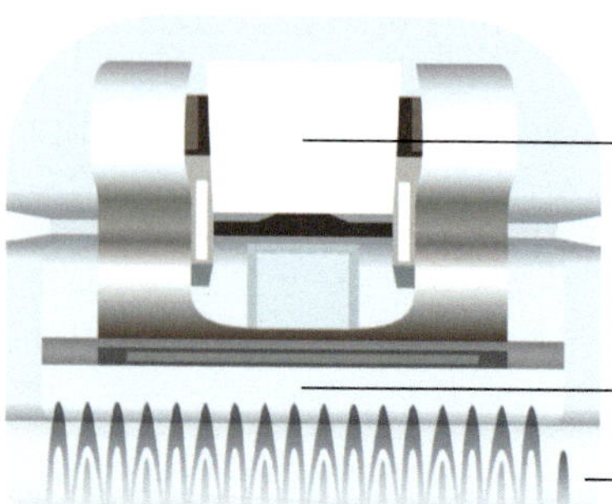

Figure 17. Surgical clipper blade.

Clean

Excess dirt and hair should be removed with a bristle brush. Only the clipper blade should be submerged in a bowl of blade wash solution and the clipper run for five to eight seconds. The blade should then be removed from the clipper and laid on a towel to dry.

Oil and Disinfect

Once dry, the clipper blade can be held side down and sprayed with a disinfectant spray. A few drops of clipper oil can be applied between the upper and lower blades while the motor is running. As it is running, the excess oil and hair will run off the clipper blade. The clipper can then be turned off and the blade dabbed with a paper towel or dry cloth.

Some blade washes such as Andis blade care plus™ also contain lubricating components. It is important to read the manufacturers data sheet.

Blades require sharpening; however repeated sharpening increases the risk of the blade causing clipper rash. Repeated sharpening results in a reduced distance between the cutting points and guard blade which consequently allows the oscillating blade to come into contact with the skin.

Sharpening results in the round edges of the guard blade becoming pointed in shape, which, with careless clipping, dig into the skin causing skin lacerations. It is therefore important that blades are inspected regularly for:

- excessively sharp points on the guard blade
- damage e.g. broken teeth
- a reduced gap between the tip of the guard and cutting blade.

Blades showing any of the above signs should be discarded.

New blades have a protective coating applied to prevent rust. This protective coating adheres to hair and dander subsequently leading to clipper rash. Before any new blade is used, it should be cleaned with blade wash by placing the clipper blade flat into the blade wash and turning the clipper on. A low-pitched sound is heard, and this sound becomes higher pitched when the rust protector has been removed. The blade should then be wiped and oiled correctly before use.

Skin Preparation

Initial skin preparation should take place before the patient is transferred into the operating theatre. This is to ensure that gross dirt and skin debris are removed, eliminating transient bacteria, as well as starting to reduce the patient's resident bacteria within the deeper layers of the skin.

An ideal antiseptic skin preparation solution should be:
- economical
- non-irritating to skin and other tissues
- destroy microorganisms with minimal contact time
- lather to remove dirt and grease
- have broad spectrum bactericidal, fungicidal, virucidal, and sporicidal activity.

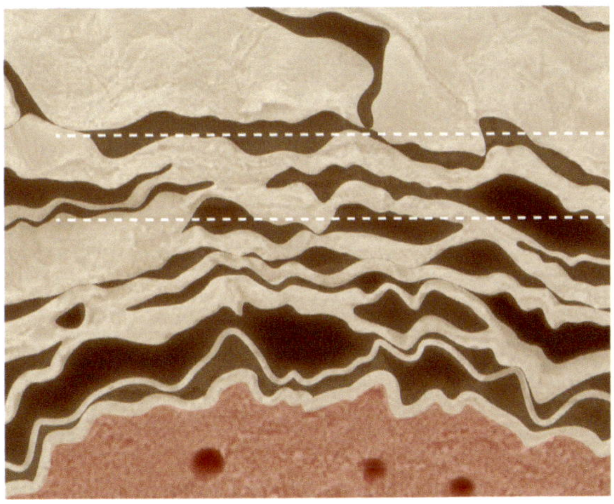

Figure 18. Magnification of skin (© Invicta™).

Skin is the patient's largest continuous protective barrier against infection, and **20% of residual microorganisms reside in the deeper layers of the skin and are therefore inaccessible to skin disinfectants.** Therefore, it is impossible to remove all microorganisms from the patient's skin.

Furthermore, skin is not a continuous simple flat surface and veterinary patients have many hair follicles which can harbour microorganisms; these microorganisms can be spread via the oral-faecal route during patient grooming (Swales et al., 2017).

Preparing the skin prior to a surgical procedure is imperative to prevent surgical site contamination with residual microorganisms.

Skin Disinfection

The purpose of aseptic skin preparation is to:
- remove soil and transient microorganisms from the skin
- decrease the number of resident microorganisms to below pathogenic levels with minimal tissue damage
- inhibit rapid rebound growth of microorganisms.

There are a variety of antiseptic skin preparation solutions used in practice which have a varied mode of action and properties. (Table 8).

Table 8. Antiseptic skin preparation solutions used in practice.

Skin disinfectant	Examples	Mode of action	Properties	Contact time	Residual activity
Iodophors	· Medidine™ · Pevidine™ · Vetasept™ povidone iodine	Penetrates bacterial cell walls and replaces intracellular molecules with free iodine via oxidation resulting in cell death.	· Broad spectrum (including viruses, fungi, and spores). · Organic matter reduces level of activity. · Increased risk of causing skin irritation.	Contact time for bacterial decontamination is 2 minutes. A minimum of 15 minutes is required for sporicidal action.	Minimal residual action. Note: Povidone iodine is tolerated by epithelium but not endothelium.
Chlorhexidine gluconate (Bisbiguanides)	· Hibiscrub™ · Medihex™ · Vetasept™ chlorhexidine	Disrupts bacterial cell walls and membranes and precipitates intracellular proteins resulting in cell death.	· Broad spectrum (less effective against Gram -ve and Gram +ve organisms). · Virucidal. · Reduced fungal activity. · Good residual activity. · Less inhibited by organic matter.	Minimum contact time of 3 minutes. 3–5 minutes recommended for good residual activity.	Binds to the stratum corneum (outermost layer of epidermis) = good residual activity. Note: Chlorhexidine is irritant to the cornea and is ototoxic.
Alcohol-based solutions	· Exidine™ · ChloraPrep™	Synergistic effects through combining alcohol and chlorhexidine.	· Broad spectrum due to combining different modes of action.	Minimum 2 minutes before evaporation for maximum bactericidal effect.	Moderate. Note: Not to be used on open wounds, mucous membranes, cornea. Is also ototoxic due to the chlorhexidine component.
Alcohol	· 70% Isopropyl alcohol	Denatures cell wall proteins, DNA, RNA, and lipids.	· Broad spectrum activity (including fungi and fungi spores). · Rapid onset of action.	Minimum 2 minutes before evaporation for maximum bactericidal effect.	No residual activity. Note: Alcohol must not be used on open wounds or mucous membranes. Care must be taken with its use and pooling must be avoided in a surgical setting particularly where electrocautery is used as it is highly flammable.

The most widely used and recommended skin antiseptic is **4% chlorhexidine gluconate** as it has a longer residual activity time and excellent efficacy against Gram positive and negative bacteria.

Any gross contamination should be removed prior to surgical skin preparation. Detergent within the antiseptic chemical makeup aids in dissolving grease and dirt via its lathering properties, especially as its efficacy is not altered with organic matter unlike povidone iodine. Examination gloves should be worn to prevent contamination of the surgical area and protect the skin of surgical personnel from aseptic solutions.

It is imperative to correctly dilute the antiseptic solution. For example, 4% chlorhexidine is diluted to a ratio of 50:50. For any chemical, the go to documentation on how to use the chemical correctly and its safety precautions are in the manufacturer's instructions.

In some dilute antiseptic solutions, it is known that Gram-negative bacteria (e.g. *Pseudomonas spp.*) can multiply. For this reason, **a fresh skin preparation solution should be used for each individual surgical patient** (Gasson, 2007).

Skin Disinfection Technique

The correct technique used when applying a skin preparation solution can significantly reduce microorganisms on the skin's surface. Traditionally the circular technique has been used within veterinary practice for preoperative skin preparation. However, recent research has shown that the **back-and-forth method, traditionally used in human medicine, is more effective at reducing microbial numbers** (Reynolds et al., 2019 and CareFusion, 2010).

Lint-free non-woven soft swabs or sponges should be used for the initial scrub. Linting swabs leave particles on the surgical site and are considered a form of contamination. Some veterinary personnel prefer to use cotton wool as it is less abrasive. This should be balled up to minimise the risk of fibres being left on the skin. It, however, still leaves some fibres, and therefore contamination.

When using **gauze swabs, each one should be folded into quarters** by bringing the four corners together and then holding them by the corners. This produces a smaller contact area that is easier to control and limits the chance of personnel fingers touching the patient.

Overzealous scrubbing should be avoided as this can bring microorganisms from the hair follicles to the surface, plus cause irritation and small abrasions to the skin's surface, which are then colonised with bacteria.

Starting at the proposed incision site, the gauze is moved in a back-and-forth action for approximately 15 seconds. It is the back-and-forth action that is responsible for most of the cleaning. The skin scrub should begin at the incision site working away from it in a circular anticlockwise pattern. (Figure 19).

- Gradually movement is made from the incision site outward via the back-and-forth motion and regular swab changes.
- A dirty swab should never be returned to the incision site.
- A pattern of L and C-shapes enables the back-and-forth action to be maintained, whilst enabling the skin to be scrubbed from the centre out.

Wiping in a single direction (a.k.a. target or bullseye pattern, also called a concentric pattern) does not have the same mechanical action and is less effective than the back-and-forth motion. Once the fur, or any other dirty or contaminated area has been touched with the gauze, the gauze must never return to the incision site or be placed back into the scrub solution.

The process is repeated until the surgical site looks clean and or complete removal of all visible organic material from the prepared area is achieved; **on the average patient this generally requires a minimum of three passes over each site/area.**

Limbs should be suspended, and skin preparation solution applied in a distal to proximal direction. Nail beds harbour a significant number of bacteria and are very challenging to disinfect appropriately via the skin preparation technique. Therefore, **if paws are part of the surgical field they should be covered with impermeable material.**

Paws that are required to be within the surgical field must be effectively disinfected. This can easily be achieved by placing them inside a glove that contains a 50:50 solution of 4% chlorhexidine and massaging the solution around the clipped nail beds. This process needs to be repeated up to three times depending on the level of contamination.

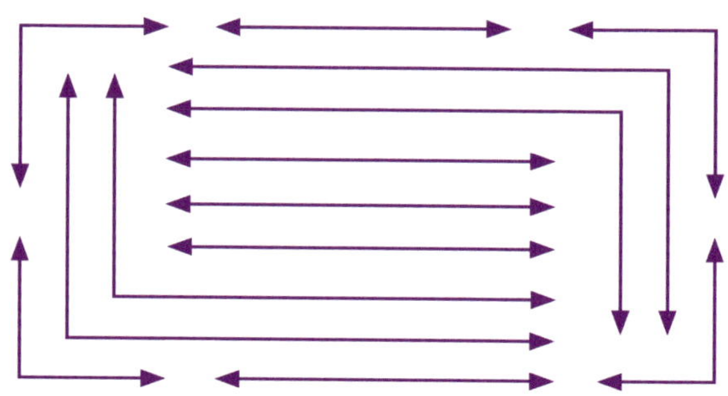

Figure 19. Direction of skin preparation.

For male dogs undergoing abdominal procedures, the prepuce should be flushed with an appropriate diluted antiseptic solution prior to skin preparation. Similarly, the vulva should be flushed on bitches that undergo perineal surgery.

Ideally, the clean surgical site should be aseptically covered with a sterile drape while the patient is transferred to theatre and positioned.

Following patient positioning in the operating theatre, a final surgical paint should be performed using sterile materials. **The solution should contain 70% isopropyl alcohol,** as when added to 2% chlorhexidine gluconate (non-detergent version), this combination has superior antimicrobial activity than other skin preparation solutions (Adam et al., 2005). Alcohol is used to remove the detergent residue from the initial surgical scrub and is also effective against Gram-negative bacteria.

It is **imperative that the same active ingredient is used in the second sterile surgical paint** preparation as was used for the initial surgical scrub. Solutions used with a different chemical makeup may inactivate one another (Williams, 2000).

Pooling of the solution should be avoided (particularly in the inguinal area), especially if diathermy is to be used, due to the solution's flammable properties. Likewise, the rapid evaporation of alcohol is detrimental to the patient due to heat loss. Pooling can be avoided using surgical paint devices.

Chloraprep™ is a surgical paint device which contains 2% chlorhexidine and 70% isopropyl alcohol that comes with or without dye, and in various volumes of solution for coverage of different areas of surgical field.

Each applicator consists of a glass ampoule containing the antiseptic solution of 2% chlorhexidine and 70% isopropyl alcohol inside a protective outer case. The patented design ensures surgical personnel do not come into contact with the contents or the patient's skin, thus preventing contamination of the surgical site. It is single use, easy to apply, and a sterile system applicator all in one.

The way in which the solution is applied to the skin is as important as the solution itself. Studies show the most effective way to apply ChloraPrep™ is with a back-and-forth scrubbing movement because this gives a lower microbial count on the skin than using other application methods. Before the patient is draped, time should be allowed for the surgical site to dry thoroughly.

Skin preparation solutions should not be made up in bulk as there is evidence this may be a contributing factor to antimicrobial resistance. Contaminated chlorhexidine has been linked to multiple hospital acquired infections (Weber et al., 2007). This is in association with using contaminated water and the reusing of bottles with decanted solutions without adequate cleaning and disinfection between refills. Most of these outbreaks were linked to solutions containing 2% chlorhexidine, however up to 4% solution was also involved.

Surgical Preparation of the Eye

Preparation of the surgical ophthalmic patient aims to reduce perioperative infection and **ensure minimal irritation of the periorbital and orbital area** which could lead to postoperative inflammation and discomfort.

No clipping is required for intraocular surgical procedures to limit inadvertent trauma to the eyelid.

For periorbital surgeries, the periorbital area should be clipped carefully **using a small clipper. The eye should be protected using sterile aqueous ocular gel** and or covered with a damp non-woven gauze swab which is removed prior to surgery.

Surgical scrub solutions should not be used periorbitally as they are irritant to the cornea (Mac Rae et al., 1984). As chlorhexidine is also irritant to the cornea **a 10% povidone iodine solution should be used at a dilution of 1:10 to 1:50 using 0.9% sodium chloride.**

Non-woven gauze swabs are used for peri-orbital preparation and cotton buds soaked in the solution are used to prepare the conjunctival fornix, taking care not to come into contact with the cornea.

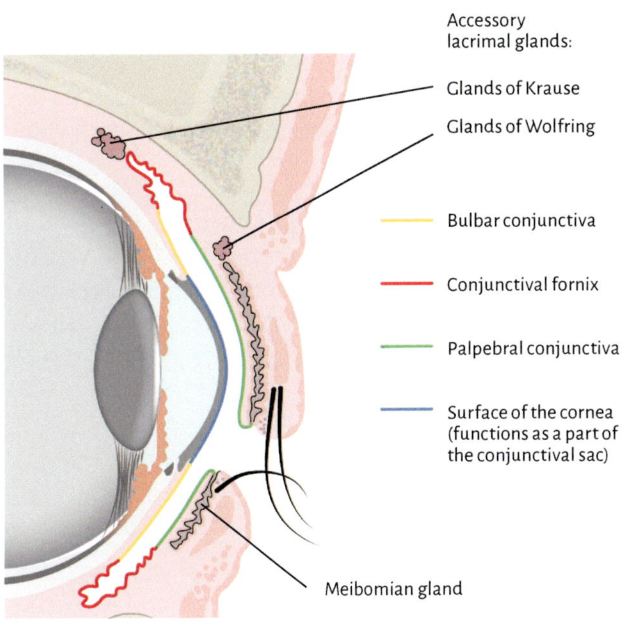

Figure 20. The eye.

The ocular surface should be gently flushed using a 5% povidone iodine solution, followed with 0.9% saline. External pressure on the globe should be avoided to prevent the intraocular pressure being raised and subsequent globe rupture or ocular cardiac bradycardia (ocular cardiac reflex, resulting in severe bradycardia). **Use of any antiseptic solution should be avoided if corneal rupture is suspected.**

Patient Positioning

Correct patient position for the surgical procedure is imperative for optimal surgical outcome and the prevention of surgical site infection by maintaining aseptic technique during surgery. Isolating the surgical site from environmental and patient-based contaminants by adequate patient draping is key to maintaining a sterile surgical field.

Positioning Aids

In theatre, patient positioning depends on the surgical procedure, and aims to ensure the surgical site is accessible to the surgeon and facilitate manipulation where required by the surgeon. The patient must remain in a stable position during the procedure.

The surgical patient's position should be **comfortable for both the patient and the surgeon,** and must prevent compromising superficial nerves, peripheral circulation, and respiratory ventilation, whilst allowing access for anaesthesia monitoring. Consideration of a patient's comorbidities such as joint disease is essential to prevent injury, e.g. by forcing the hips of a dog with severe hip osteoarthritis into extension for a prolonged surgery.

The patient's position is maintained with the use of position aids to prevent movement during the surgical procedure which could break asepsis, reduce the surgeon's field of view, and be detrimental to the patient during delicate surgical interventions. There are a variety of different positioning aids available on the veterinary market:

Sandbags

Ideally sandbags should be colour coded, and specific ones only used for surgical procedures, whilst others are reserved for radiographic positioning etc. They must be **easy to clean and inspected regularly for damage.** Damaged sandbags should be replaced.

Rope Ties

These come in a variety of different lengths and colours. Again, **specific coloured rope ties must only be used for surgical procedures,** with alternative colours for use in other settings. Ropes should be washed between surgical procedures and inspected for damage (such as fraying), and they should ideally be made of polypropylene for easy cleaning.

Troughs

The V-trough should be easy to clean. They are made from either rigid or non-rigid materials and come in various sizes. Ideally, a foam insulated wedge should be used for long surgical procedures to prevent patient discomfort.

Vacuum Beds

These come in a range of sizes and can either use manual or in-line suction for vacuum activation. They gently conform to the patient's body enabling a secure position whilst ensuring patient comfort. They must be easy to clean and inspected for damage daily. **Vacuum beds also conserve the patient's body heat due to their insulation composition and are the ideal patient positioner.**

Adhesive Tape

Comes in various sizes and materials. Care must be taken when using adhesive tapes not to impair the patient's circulation/ventilation. Some patients may be allergic to the adhesives used.

Foam Wedges

These come in various sizes and should be easily cleanable. Specific sets of positioning foam wedges should be reserved for surgery and inspected for damage. Covering them with a plastic sheet improves ease of cleaning and disinfection.

Patient Positioning for Surgical Procedures

The surgical procedure determines how the patient is positioned.

For example:

Thoracic Surgery

The thoracic cavity can be entered by intercostal thoracotomy (between the ribs), median sternotomy (cutting the sternum lengthways), rib resection, and trans-sternal thoracotomy (cutting across the sternum). **The most common approaches are intercostal thoracotomy and median sternotomy.**

Intercostal Thoracotomy and Rib Resection Thoracotomy

The patient should be placed in **lateral recumbency.**

Intercostal thoracotomy is used when exposure of a specific region of the thoracic cavity is required (Monnet, 2005) but **restricts the surgeon to one hemithorax.** Intercostal thoracotomy gives access to approximately one third of the left or right side of the thoracic cavity, and the subsequent mediastinal structures (Charlesworth, 2011).

These procedures are performed with the patient in lateral recumbency. Forelimbs should be pulled in a cranial direction and secured to allow access to the most cranial intercostal spaces if required. The entire lateral thorax (from the scapula) and cranial half of the abdomen are surgically clipped from the ventral midline to close to the dorsal midline. This is necessary to allow palpation and counting of the ribs and to allow for intercostal nerve blocks and thoracic drain placement, plus the surgical procedure itself.

Median Sternotomy

This is the only approach that **allows access to the entire thoracic cavity.** This approach is used to explore the thoracic cavity or for removal of large masses.

The patient should be placed in dorsal recumbency with the patient's forelimbs pulled cranially and secured. Sandbags or a vacuum-based surgical positioning device can be used to help secure the patient and stop them from rolling off the table. The entire thorax should be clipped.

Upper Airway Surgery

Procedures on the upper airway are performed to remove, repair or bypass areas of pathophysiology, obstruction, or injury.

Surgery of the Soft Palate

The patient should be placed in sternal recumbency with their head gently elevated and supported. The patient's position is secured with positioning aids (sandbags/vacuum bed with their head restrained using adhesive tape. The mouth can be opened with bandage which is secured to a drip stand either side of the patient or ideally a specially designed head bar. The tongue is gently pulled and fixed in a rostral position. Alternatively, specifically designed positioning aids or mouth gags may be used.

Tracheostomy

The patient should be placed in dorsal recumbency. The entire ventral aspect of the neck is clipped and aseptically prepared, with the neck supported from underneath.

Laryngeal Tie-back (for laryngeal paralysis)

For arytenoid lateralisation the patient is placed in lateral recumbency with a sandbag, rolled towel, or a 1 l-fluid bag placed under its neck to elevate the laryngeal area towards the surgeon. The forelimbs should be retracted caudally and tied securely.

Abdominal Surgery

The patient should be placed in dorsal recumbency with the forelimbs pulled cranially and hindlimbs caudally, and gently secured. If needed a vacuum cushion, V-shaped trough, or sandbags on either side of the patient can be used to help secure them in position.

Spinal Surgery

Positioning patients for spinal surgery is crucial for optimal operating conditions and operation-site exposure.

Cranial and Mid-thoracic Spine

Generally, a dorsal approach is indicated for the thoracic spine. Reasons for surgery include removal of tumours and stabilization/decompression of congenital vertebral anomalies (e.g. laminectomy).

The patient is placed in sternal recumbency with the forelimbs pulled cranially. **It is imperative the spine is straight and level;** if necessary, the head can be elevated to allow the spine to sit straight.

Lumbosacral Spine

The surgical approach to the lumbosacral region of the spine is via a dorsal approach with bilateral elevation of the sacrocaudalis muscles from the dorsal spinous processes and the dorsal lamina of the vertebrae (Jarram, 2013).

The patient should be positioned in sternal recumbency with the pelvic limbs in a squatting position (or pulled cranially), which provides a more normal standing position with flexion and dorsal opening of the lumbosacral space.

Again, it is imperative the spine is straight and parallel to the surgical table. The patient's head should be elevated as necessary and supported to achieve the desired operating patient position.

Cervical Spine

The most widely performed surgical procedure on the cervical spine is the ventral slot technique (ventral decompression). The patient should be placed in dorsal recumbency with the forelimbs pulled caudally and secured and the neck in mild linear traction and supported under the cervical spine as needed with a sandbag, or vacuum bed.

Other procedures involving the cervical spine include cervical laminectomy and hemilaminectomy via a dorsal approach. The patient is placed in sternal recumbency with the head gently flexed in a neutral position and supported with either a vacuum support or rolled up towel.

Orthopaedic Surgery

The orthopaedic procedure will dictate the patient's position. The patient is either placed in lateral or dorsal recumbency, with the affected limb elevated during skin preparation and draping. It is often helpful to support the patient's fractured limb in a hanging position from the ceiling during preparation, as this results in stretching of the muscles which have contracted at a fracture site and hence facilitates surgical reduction of the fracture during surgery.

Ophthalmic Surgery

Generally ophthalmic surgery is performed by specialist veterinary ophthalmic surgeons, however there are some surgical procedures which are performed without specialised training and equipment (e.g. enucleation, conjunctival flap, and third eyelid flap).

It is important that the endotracheal tube is secured adequately, as it is difficult to reach during surgery and there is a risk of increased movement due to the surgical site position.

Depending on the surgical position, and the surgeon's preference, the patient should be placed in either lateral or sternal recumbency. Care should be taken to ensure there is no pressure on the non-surgical eye when the patient is placed in lateral recumbency to avoid increased intraocular pressure. Similarly, to reduce hydrostatic pressure and thus increased intraocular pressure, the patient's head should be elevated above the rest of the body via positioning aids or by tilting the table (Thomson, 2010).

Surgery of the Perineum, Rectum, and Anus

Surgery of the perineum, rectum and anus is indicated for:

- rectal biopsies
- anal sac disease
- perineal hernia
- rectal perforation
- perineal fistulae
- rectal prolapse
- rectal neoplasia
- faecal incontinence.

For a rectal approach, the patient is placed in sternal recumbency with the pelvis elevated and the tail fixed cranially. It is important the cranial aspect of the hind limbs is appropriately padded to prevent femoral nerve and circulatory damage.

For patients in all positions:

- Anaesthetic monitoring devices and fluid extension lines should be carefully attached to the patient, who is placed on a controlled and monitored heat pad (e.g. Hotdog™) or blanket (Bair hugger™) which is on top of the padded operating table. (Check monitoring devices prior to draping the patient.)
- Monopolar diathermy grounding plates should be adequately lubricated and placed underneath the patient and ensured that they are correctly earthed.

Correct patient positioning requires knowledge of the procedure. This is to anticipate the parts of the patient the surgeon requires access to, position of the surgeon and assistant(s) and the instrument trolley(s).

Draping the Surgical Patient

Surgical Drapes

Once the patient is positioned and a second sterile skin preparation has taken place, the patient is ready to be draped. This may be performed by the scrub nurse, surgical assistant, or the surgeon.

Surgical drapes are used to isolate the surgical site from contamination from the surrounding area and maintain a sterile operative field. The drapes serve as a barrier to endogenous and exogenous sources of contamination, in particular endogenous contamination (patient's skin flora as the source).

Apart from the surgical field, **all parts of the patient should be draped to include full coverage of the operating table.** This is to create a physical barrier which must be maintained throughout the procedure, particularly, if the drape becomes wet via lavage fluid and or blood.

The material used for draping requires the following properties:

- economic

- easy to sterilize
- water-resistant
- non-irritant for the patient
- durable, but flexible
- be able to be cut
- resist ignition from sources such as lasers and electrosurgery.

Drapes can be made of cloth, paper, or of non-woven materials, synthetic and/or natural origin, possibly combined with chemical treatment as well as adhesive plastic. They can also be reusable or disposable and come in various shapes and formations. Some drapes also come with adhesive strips to maintain their position on the patient.

Cloth

Cloth drapes are the easiest to position and use, but the initial purchase cost and continuing maintenance costs are high due to damage with use and laundering. Cloth drapes should be made from surgical sheet fabric where the thread count is of 270 or 280 per square centimetre. Cloth drapes are made of cotton muslin.

Ideally **cloth drapes should be avoided** because they do not maintain a sterile barrier as they wick bacteria through from below when they become wet and hence should always be covered with an impervious layer.

Paper

Paper drapes are convenient, easy to customize and sterilize, and relatively inexpensive, but can be **troublesome to keep in position during surgery as they do not conform to the contour of the patient's body.**

Synthetic and Waterproof

Composed of polyethylene, these drapes can be used either with or without aerosol adhesives.

They are chemically treated to increase the protective barrier of the drape and are **single use.**

Adhesive Plastic

Adhesive plastic drapes adhere to the skin to produce a second skin. The incision is made through the drape and skin. For the drape to adhere the skin must be dry however **these types of drapes tend not to adhere well to animal skin** and research has found these types of drapes do not affect the rate at which bacteria contaminate surgical wounds particularly in clean procedures (Webster et al., 2007).

The advantages of these types of drapes are that they prevent fluid from leaking under the edges of the drape and increase the efficiency of forced air warmers by preventing loss of warm air via open parts of the drape.

Adhesive drapes also come impregnated with antiseptics such as povidone iodine, and so **care should be taken when disinfecting the skin to ensure the same antiseptic** is used to ensure efficacy.

Draping Technique

The technique used to drape the surgical patient is key to establishing a sterile field. The draping technique used will depend on the surgical procedure and the location of the surgical site. The aim is to choose the technique that minimises bacterial contamination to the surgical field/site.

To minimise contamination **a two-glove approach should be used,** whereby the personnel draping the patient wears two pairs of sterile gloves and removes the outer layer once patient draping is complete.

To maximise the physical barrier between the surgical site and surrounding environment a two-layer draping technique is used.

The initial layer isolates a central area which contains the proposed incision site and is achieved by the square-off or four-quarter draping technique (Figure 21).

The four-quarter technique involves placing four separate drapes which are overlapped then secured at each field corner with a Backhaus towel clamp.

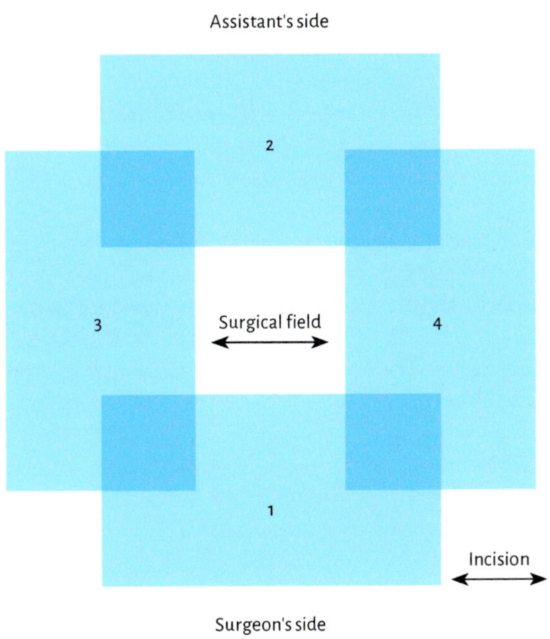

Figure 21. Square-off draping technique.

Drapes with adhesive strips prevent tissue trauma caused by towel clamps and are also indicated when intraoperative imaging requires minimal metallic surgical instruments in the operative field.

The patient's skin should be dry prior to draping and all drapes handled as little as possible. Drapes should not be fanned, flipped, or shaken out as this creates air currents which increase cross contamination of the surgical site. Scrubbed personnel should ensure the area surrounding the operating table and patient is free of equipment to prevent contamination of the drapes during placement.

During the draping procedure, scrubbed personnel should:
- stand away from the operating table
- carry the drape to the operating table
- not lean over the patient or reach across the table.

The first drape is opened and folded along one edge to create a 5–10 cm area of double thickness. The fold is said to be toward the patient as this creates a neater edge. However, in the author's experience placing the fold towards you is more efficient and ensures a more aseptic technique when placing the drape onto the patient.

The surgeon pinches the corners of the folded drape with his/her thumb and forefinger and inserts their fingers into the edge of the folded drape; thus, preventing the scrubbed personnel's gloves from touching the patient's skin.

The drape is then placed aseptically onto the edge of the proposed sterile field firstly at the surgeon's side of the table. The process is repeated for the opposite side and then the opposing adjacent sides. Once the drapes are in place they should not be moved and are secured with atraumatic towel clamps. In male dogs if the incision site extends to the pubis, prior to draping the prepuce should be clamped to one side with a sterile atraumatic tissue clamp.

Single use drapes may contain an adhesive strip. For this reason, only the corners of the drape are folded around the surgeon's fingers to prevent a break in aseptic technique. These drapes tend not to require towel clamps to secure them however sometimes this may be necessary as the adhesive does not adhere to animal skin.

The initial drapes are then covered with one large drape (through which a fenestration is cut) which covers the whole of the operating table and the patient.

For orthopaedic surgical procedures, if the distal limb is not required within the surgical field, then it should be covered with an impermeable layer (e.g. glove, plastic drape) followed by a sterile adhesive bandage, (once sterile draping has been completed around the affected limb).

Even though the non-prepared part of the patient is covered with a physical barrier, there is still a risk of the wound becoming contaminated from resident bacteria within the hair follicles via the skin incision or by being punctured via a towel clamp. The skin is therefore said to not be sterile, and it is important to **remember that a used towel clamp should not be placed back onto the sterile trolley or reused.**

Nursing the Surgical Patient

The Recovery Period

The recovery period is defined as **the return to normal after general anaesthesia and surgery, including the patient's requirement for close monitoring to ensure that its return to normal is uneventful** (Crompton, 2011).

In 2006, Brodbelt et al. examined perioperative small animal fatalities in one of the largest prospective studies in veterinary medicine, known as the Confidential Enquiry into Perioperative Small Animal Fatalities (CEPSAF). (Table 9).

Brodbelt et al. concluded that **a lack of continuous monitoring in the recovery period resulted in unnecessary mortality.**

Table 9. Percentages of perioperative deaths (Brodbelt et al., 2006).

	Dog	Cat	Rabbit
Premedication	1%	1%	0%
Induction	6%	8%	6%
Maintenance	46%	30%	30%
Recovery	**47%**	**61%**	**64%**
Total	100	100	100

The main aims in the immediate postoperative period are:

- **Successfully recover the patient from anaesthesia.**
- **Prevent and manage postoperative complications.**
- **Provide ongoing treatment for pre-existing disease.**
- **Identify any new issues quickly and treat appropriately.**
- **Promote rapid recovery by supporting the patient's physiology.**
- **Ensure patient welfare is maintained.**

These aims are achieved **by close patient monitoring and regular assessment** which alert the veterinary surgeon to the patient's changing needs and allow for intervention in a timely manner.

A specific nurse/technician (primary nursing) or team of recovery nurses/technicians (team nursing) may be responsible for monitoring surgical patients in the immediate postoperative phase.

In the postoperative phase, primary nursing is more beneficial as the single nurse/technician is aware of the complete recovery history. Critical events are noticed earlier as the nurse/technician is familiar with the patient's expected postoperative complications and recorded observations.

The patient's vital signs should be recorded until they are normal, and this is a legal requirement in the UK (RCVS, 2010).

Hypothermia

Hypothermia can be classed as:

- mild: body temperature falls between 32 and 35 °C
- moderate: body temperature falls between 28 and 32 °C
- severe: body temperature falls below 28 °C.

Hypothermia is a preventable complication in the postoperative surgical patient and can have an adverse effect on several body systems. (Table 10)

Table 10. Effects of hypothermia on body systems.

System	Dysfunction
Cardiovascular	Thermoregulatory dysfunction resulting in arterial vasodilation, increased blood viscosity, decreased cardiac output, increased cardiac dysrhythmia, coagulopathies, hypotension, bradycardia.
Respiratory	Decreased respiratory rate, minute volume, and tidal volume.
Neurological	Disrupted cerebral autoregulation and cerebral blood flow.
Immune	Impaired wound healing and increased risk of infection.
Metabolic	Decreased metabolism, leading to drug overdoses and prolonged recoveries.

Alterations in the patient's normal thermoregulatory response may be caused by:

- anaesthetic agents
- changes to hypothalamus function during anaesthesia
- disturbances to the body's ability to distribute heat
- heat loss during surgery.

There are four mechanisms that result in patient heat loss:

Radiation

This is the **most common form of heat loss** in the surgical patient. Heat is exchanged between the environment and the patient via infrared waves, particularly if the patient is vasodilated. Heat then dissipates away from the body to the cooler surrounding air.

Convection

Convection is the second most common form of heat loss in the surgical patient (Feller, 2009). This occurs when body heat is transferred to circulating air over the body's surface. Therefore, the larger the body surface area to volume ratio the more risk of the patient experiencing hypothermia. The process of **heat exchange via confection is exacerbated in patients who undergo extensive clipping and skin preparation.**

Conduction

This occurs when the body touches a cooler surface resulting in body heat being transferred to the cooler surface.

Evaporation

Hypothermia due to evaporation occurs when body heat is lost by moisture evaporating from the body surface or via the respiratory tract. Careful drying of the patient after a surgical procedure can reduce heat loss via evaporation.

When a patient's core body temperature decreases by 1.0 °C their metabolic rate decreases by approximately 10% (Dugdale, 2012). **A decreased metabolic rate results in reduced drug metabolism and elimination subsequently causing drug overdose and a prolonged recovery.**

Reduced metabolism also results in decreased cellular sodium pump activity and cell oedema. Hyperkalaemia and acidosis may result from electrolyte and pH imbalances.

Hypothermia also increases blood viscosity and packed cell volume due to splenic contraction. An increase in the viscosity of the blood increases the workload on the myocardium and hypocoagulability due to an increase in prothrombin time (PT) and partial thromboplastin time (PTT) (Dugdale, 2016).

Mild hypothermia initiates the body's automatic survival response to produce heat, resulting **in an increase in the patient's oxygen demand by up to 300%.** This is also at a time when the delivery of oxygen to the tissues has also been compromised by the depressant effect on the cardiopulmonary system caused by anaesthesia (Holden, 1999).

Body temperatures below 35 °C (95 °F) do not result in thermoregulatory shivering and peripheral vasoconstriction is replaced with active vasodilation promoting core body heat loss. **Active vasodilation leads to hypotension** and reduced sensitivity of baroreceptors results in decreased cardiac output (Oncken, 2001).

Oxygen supplementation should be provided to patients; particularly in those who are suffering from respiratory compromise and have hypothermia. It is therefore imperative that patients are **actively warmed until a body temperature of 37 °C** is reached (Hamilton, 2003).

Methods of warming patients include:

1. **Forced air warmer**
   - continuous active warming with a low risk of patient burning
   - expensive
   - blankets can become soiled
   - varied patient compliance.
2. **Inline intravenous fluid warming**
   - warm fluid entering the patient may initiate vasodilation
   - can be inexpensive
   - minimal effects if used alone
   - warm fluids enter the patient preventing the patient cooling.
3. **Blankets/insulating materials** (bubble wrap/space blankets)
   - reduced risk of overheating the patient
   - not active warming
   - prevents further heat loss via conduction, convection, and radiation.
4. **Heat mat**
   - active warming of the patient
   - increased risk of burning if the patient is recumbent or unconscious
   - waterproof.

Hypoxia

Hypoxia may develop when the patient is **extubated too early** when not adequately conscious.

Cats are at potential risk where laryngospasm is a factor and thus there are various opinions within the veterinary field as to when to extubate cats. Delay in removing the endotracheal tube may cause irritation or spasm to the larynx, particularly in the feline patient. Similarly, if extubating the feline patient is left too late the patient may bite down or chew on the ET tube making extubating difficult and exacerbating laryngeal sensitivity.

Unlike in dolichocephalic and mesocephalic canine patients, the ET tube can be removed when the swallow reflex returns. However, in brachycephalic canine breeds, the endotracheal tube can be left in situ to the point when the patient can no longer tolerate it. Thus, ensuring a patent airway until the patient is fully recovered due to a higher risk of upper respiratory airway obstruction.

Patients with higher risk of respiratory complications postoperatively should be placed in sternal recumbency with their head and neck extended during recovery. This is to allow full expansion of the thoracic cavity and maximise cervical airflow.

It is imperative that reintubation equipment is at hand in an organised fashion to allow for the quick reintubation of these patients if required.

Similarly, **the patient's ventilation status should be assessed at the end of anaesthesia prior to extubating.** This can be achieved via capnography and provides information on the patient's expired carbon dioxide levels identifying if the patient is hypocapnic or hypercapnic (Crompton, 2011).

These patients should be provided with fresh oxygen supplementation until they are able to ventilate normally. Oxygen supplementation can be provided via:

- flow by
- nasal prongs
- nasal catheter
- oxygen tent
- oxygen hood.

Postoperative Monitoring

All postoperative patients must be closely monitored, and this should include the following:

- the cardiovascular system
- respiratory system
- pain management
- thermoregulatory system.

Observations should include (with reference to the patient's American Society of Anaesthesiologists (ASA) grade/surgical procedure):

- analgesia requirements
- expired carbon dioxide concentrations
- oxygen saturation
- intravenous fluid administration
- lung auscultation
- respiratory rate
- capillary refill time
- mucous membrane colour
- temperature
- blood pressure

– peripheral pulse palpation
– heart rate and rhythm.

General Nursing Considerations

Postoperative Nursing

The veterinary surgeon should perform **a physical examination at least twice daily,** however, the frequency is dependent on the patients' requirements.

The first daily physical examination should be undertaken before the daily treatment plan is written so ongoing fluid therapy and analgesia can be adjusted appropriately. If the vet cannot carry out a physical examination with the desired frequency, then this must be undertaken by another member of the veterinary team with clear written guidance on when to contact the veterinary surgeon and or initiate intervention. This can be achieved **by a hospitalisation record, which specifies assessment parameters and set boundaries** as a guide as to when to call the veterinary surgeon. Remember, **veterinary nurses/technicians work under the direction of the veterinary surgeon and hence must not initiate new treatments** unless discussed and directed to do so by the veterinary surgeon.

To achieve the best nursing care, careful patient planning is an integral part of holistic veterinary nursing in practice.

It is important to understand the difference between the terms **care planning and care plan.**

- **Care planning** is the process of recognising a patient's actual and potential problems and thus selecting interventions to assist in reducing them.
- **A care plan** is a written record of the planning process which is used as a tool to facilitate and document the care of an individual patient.

The **advantages of planning a patient's care** are:

- facilitate comprehensive preparation
- set measurable treatment goals for the individual patient
- the written record of the planning process subsequently generates a care plan.

Hospitalisation Record

In the legal world, **"If it's not written, it didn't happen".** Hospitalisation forms are an important part of patient documentation and should be maintained in a manner such that other veterinary clinical staff could, by reading the record, proceed with the proper care and treatment of the patient.

The clinical personnel responsible must note and initial every treatment or observation for a patient on the record. This includes every offering of food and water, every toilet trip including the nature of what was produced, every catheter inspection and care etc. If an intervention is not recorded, then legally it is assumed it never took place. Understanding the importance of a hospitalisation record is paramount for a gold standard level of patient care and veterinary practice.

A standard approach to formulating a hospitalisation record is to **introduce a charting system such as SOAP (subjective, objective, assessment, and planning).**

- **Subjective:** includes patient information (history) that cannot be measured which is not repeatable such as the physical examination and the patient's demeanour. E.g. "was greeted by the patient when approached to their kennel, bedding soaked in urine, however a water bowl also spilled"; "soft abdomen with no patient reaction on abdominal palpation".
- **Objective:** includes quantifiable information (**information that can be graded/scored**). This includes **patient parameters** (temperature, weight, respiration rate, heart rate, pulse rate as well as laboratory data such as PCV/TP, modified Glasgow pain scores etc.).
- **Assessment:** this is the **assessment/interpretation of the patient** based on both the subjective and objective information above, on which a differential diagnosis or diagnosis by the veterinary surgeon can be based.
- **Planning:** the **plan for the patient,** which is categorised into three components:
  - the treatment plan
  - the diagnostic plan
  - the client communication plan.

The Royal College of Veterinary Surgeons' (RCVS) code of conduct sets out clear instructions relating to maintaining clinical and client records. **These include ensuring any notes recorded are clear, legible, accurate, appropriately detailed, and factual, and stored in a secure and confidential manner.**

The main source of veterinary nurses/technician's record keeping is **via the hospitalisation records,** which come in a variety of forms. Hospitalisation forms are dependent on the patient's condition and the individual practice's caseload and may be paper based or electronic.

1. **Electronic:** electronic hospitalisation forms allow several different observations and treatments to be selected from a list, tailoring the hospitalisation record to each individual patient.
2. **Paper based:** when using paper forms, it is beneficial to have a standard hospitalisation sheet, and a critical

or high-dependency patient sheet for patients requiring more frequent observations and treatment.

It is important all hospital sheets clearly display:

- **patient name**
- **owner contact details**
- **patient's problem list**
- **a plan for the day**
- **a list of concerns or notifiers.**

This is so that nursing staff are clear as to when to contact the primary clinician about a problem with the patient and that the contact information can be found quickly in the event of a patient emergency.

The day of each recording and the day of admission should also be recorded, and it is advisable each patient's hospitalisation sheet is numbered to easily track duration of hospitalisation and to refer to previous records quickly when hospitalisation is prolonged.

As a minimum a patient hospitalization record should contain information and monitor the following:

- client name
- patient name
- primary (and secondary) veterinary surgeon in charge of the case
- primary nurse (and secondary) veterinary nurse in charge of the case
- patient species
- patient age
- signalment
- weight, temperature, heart rate, respiration rate, CRT, mucous membrane colour
- resuscitation status
- nutritional support
- date
- laboratory information
- procedures which are required that day
- medications to be administered along with time, route and dose which should be clearly identified by the person who administered the medication
- information on fluid, blood pressure and IV catheter placement and monitoring
- important patient information, such as allergies, warnings, toilet commands
- voiding information and recording (e.g. urination, vomiting, defecation etc.).

Space should be available for **arterial blood pressure measurements,** including space to record the cuff size, location, and measurement method. Similarly, space should be assigned for **pain assessment,** including a scoring system which matches that used in the practice.

There should be **a dedicated section for nutrition** (RER for the day, diet to be offered, and meal size/frequency, and volumes consumed), water intake, urination (including measurement of urine output where required), defecation, vomiting, nausea and regurgitation, scheduled walking or bed checks/kennel cleans, fluid therapy (volumes administered in ml/kg/hr and ml/hr, type of fluid, daily re-assessment of fluid rate, and intravenous catheter care) and bathing/grooming and TLC.

Ensure there is space to record prescribed medications, and other miscellaneous treatments (e.g. feeding tube care or blood sampling).

Critically ill patients typically require more frequent observations, monitoring, and interventions than stable ones. (Box 2).

Box 2. An Intensive Care Hospital Sheet Allows at Least Hourly Recordings of:

- **pulse and respiratory rates**
- **temperature**
- **blood pressure.**

Additional space should be included for further monitoring of parameters such as:

- **ECG rhythm assessment**
- **SpO_2 measurement**
- **fluid therapy instructions**
- **fluids-in and fluids-out monitoring**
- **blood product transfusion administration therapy and blood type**
- **constant rate infusions**
- **feeding and walking instructions**
- **medications.**

A large space is required to record free text observations. Useful additions include modified Glasgow pain score, modified Glasgow Coma score, phlebitis scoring, calculation space for resting energy requirement, and resuscitation codes.

A **patient alerts section** on the standard/ICU hospitalisation sheet is advisable and should include instructions or call parameters/notifiers from the veterinary surgeon alongside their contact details.

Another useful section on an ICU or hospitalisation sheet is a space for **recording key blood results** to allow for quick comparison. It is imperative all ward and clinical staff are aware of how to fill in the hospitalisation record correctly and efficiently, to ensure that all patient information is recorded accurately and is easy to interpret.

Nursing Care Plans

The Use of a Nursing Care Plan

The use of nursing care plans encourages the clinical team **to think of the animal as an individual** instead of just a species or disease state and therefore provide holistic care of the patient. They promote planning and re-assessment of care and transfer thinking into clinical practice.

Nursing care plans are a legal document of the care provided; along with the identity of individuals who planned, implemented, and evaluated that care. There are several different plans/models however the **Orpet and Jeffery Ability Model 2007 is the only veterinary-specific nursing care plan currently available.** It is imperative both objective and subjective observations are used to assess the nursing requirements and patient disease state.

Nursing care plans are important as they ensure **consistency of care** is given by all clinical staff. The use of a set nursing plan ensures clear directions and enables clear decision making for the care and treatment of a patient.

There are three main advantages in planning nursing care:

1. They provide a clear **opportunity to prepare the patient** and the environment for the care interventions and to make the necessary adjustments.
2. **Stimulation of a written care plan** which may be used in several ways.
3. **Advantages** for both the patient and veterinary professionals.

Benefits for the Patient

- facilitates holistic care
- improves continuity of care.

Benefits to Veterinary Personnel

- increases professional satisfaction for veterinary nurses/technicians
- improves multidisciplinary team working
- improves public perception of the role of the veterinary nurse/technician
- a valuable education tool
- increases veterinary practice revenue
- documents patient care to support professional accountability.

A nursing model consists of ideas and factors that help make up the nursing care of the patient. It describes what the process of nursing lacks such as 'what to observe when monitoring a patient' or 'what particular interventions may be appropriate for an individual'. Thus, a nursing model involves the theories, beliefs, values, concepts, and the processes involved in the overall nursing care of an individual.

Model Nursing Care Plans

All models of nursing care plans are based on four concepts:

The Individual Patient

Completion of a plan for each individual patient, identifying their specific individual needs. For example, a patient who has had bilateral stifle surgery requires additional nursing support with a sling when walking. Similarly, a deaf or partially sighted patient requires additional support and nursing care specific to their sensory loss.

The Health Status of that Patient

Consideration of the health needs of the patient and their specific requirements.

The Nursing Skills Required

Consideration of nursing skills required along with further guidance for specific skills or advice from other clinical staff. For example, a paraplegic spinal patient requires nursing care involving urinary care and physiotherapy. Is guidance from a physiotherapist required?

The Prevailing Environment

Specific disease states have environmental requirements, along with the species and the individual requirements of the patient. For example, a patient with reduced cardiovascular function and restricted movement may need environmental warming (if not contraindicated).

The Orpet & Jeffery Ability Model (2007) is one of the most useful models used in veterinary practice as it is based on ten abilities the patient can or may complete. The nursing assessment is structured around the abilities of the patient, thus allowing for clear fluidity between the nursing assessment and the development of nursing goals. (Figure 22).

The Nursing Process

The nursing process (Figure 23) involves using a framework to create care plans; this **framework breaks down care plan creation into five key steps.**

Planning the care of a patient allows clear goals to be set:

1. **Nursing assessments:** recording and communicating information with the aim of recognising actual and potential health issues. Assessing the patient involves obtaining the animal's history and the clinical examination. This may include the patient's normal routine (via a client questionnaire) plus subjective and objective examination findings.
2. **Nursing diagnosis:** a diagnosis is made by analysing the data obtained from the nursing assessment. The nursing diagnosis considers the overall patient's health and wellbeing, not just the patient's physical symptoms. The nursing diagnosis should include key parameters such as the patient's ability to:
    - eat and drink
    - urinate and defecate
    - regulate body temperature
    - breathe
    - sleep and rest
    - mobility
    - groom/cleaning
    - pain
    - express normal behaviour.
3. **The plan:** interventions are then planned according to conclusions made in the assessment and diagnosis stages. Planning the care of a patient allows clear goals to be set which should address both actual and potential health issues the surgical patient may face. Therefore, a list of long and short-term goals of nursing care should be developed which prioritise the patient's:
    - physiological requirements
    - safety requirements (environment, infection control)
    - psychological requirements (interaction, stimulation).
4. **Implementation:** involves applying the nursing care plan to the patient. It is important the plan is clearly legible to ensure it is carried out by all members of nursing staff. The plan also requires contingency planning for unforeseen complications such as:
    - developing other problems
    - not responding to treatment
    - developing side effects from the current treatment.

    Hence the plan will change daily. The result of the nursing interventions is recorded on the patient's hospitalisation and treatment forms.

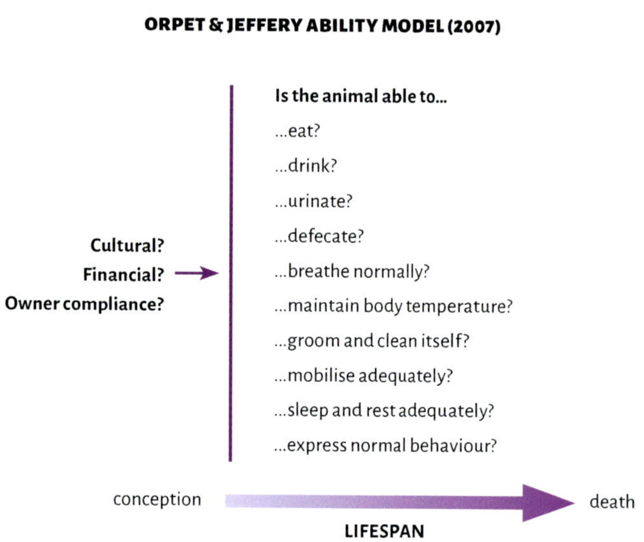

Figure 22. Orpet and Jeffery Ability Model (2007).

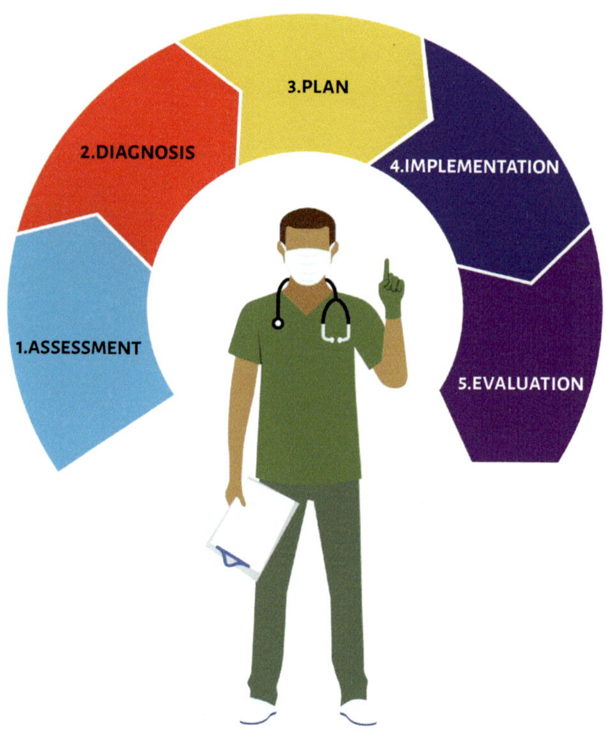

Figure 23. Nursing process.

5. **Assessment and evaluation:** involves evaluating the outcome of the nursing care plan and usually takes place during:
   - the plan's implementation
   - ward rounds
   - staff shift changes.

   Alternatively, an opportunity should be set aside at appropriate daily intervals, for the nursing team to assess the patient's care and evaluate the effectiveness of their nursing interventions. The frequency of the assessments and evaluations depends purely on the individual patient and parameters being monitored. Following the assessment and evaluation, adjustments should be made to the patient's care and an appropriate reassessment time scheduled.

Using a nursing model is helpful to ensure all points are noted and recorded when more than one member of staff is dealing with a patient.

The Orpet & Jeffery Ability Model 2007

In 2007, Orpet and Jeffrey introduced a novel ability model of nursing which was specifically designed for veterinary nursing. Their care plan model encourages veterinary nurses to **move away from a medical model and embrace the holistic approach** and encourages gold standard care for hospitalised veterinary patients.

The Orpet and Jeffrey ability model 2007 considers the Animal Welfare Act 2006 (UK) which states that those temporarily responsible for patients are legally responsible for assuring the five needs of welfare are met.

The five needs of welfare are:

- **Need for a suitable environment.**
- **Need for a suitable diet.**
- **Need to be able to exhibit normal behaviour patterns**
- **Need to be housed with or apart from other animals (as species appropriate).**
- **Need to be protected from pain, suffering, injury, and disease.**

The Orpet and Jeffrey ability model is designed to guide veterinary nurses/technicians through the nursing process framework and away from simply providing medical treatments under the direction of the veterinary surgeon, towards a process of developing their own assessment and gathering specific nursing information from both the patient and their owner (Ballantyne, 2018).

The ability model encourages veterinary nurses/technicians to **use client questionnaires based on ten abilities,** with the priority being to establish what is normal for that individual patient. **The ten abilities are identified as the fundamental elements of the patient's requirements to function and demonstrate its normal behaviour.**

Nutrition and the Surgical Patient

Appropriate nutritional support plays an important part in the recovery of the patient in the perioperative period. Nutritional support recommendations are based on the patient's metabolic response to injury.

Nutrition in the Perioperative Patient

The nutritional status of the patient is a major factor affecting surgical outcome and should be monitored daily, with early intervention if needed. Veterinary nurses have an integral role in the perioperative nutritional care of a surgical patient. This includes everything from obtaining an accurate dietary history, to understanding the metabolic effects of anaesthesia and the appropriate implementation of assisted feeding or diet recommendations.

For surgical patients that are at risk of hyporexia or malnutrition, **an appropriate feeding protocol should be implemented** as it can significantly influence patient recovery and mortality.

When assessing the patient's nutritional requirements body weight, body condition score, muscle condition score and disease processes should be considered. The patient's daily resting energy rate (RER) should be calculated, and an estimate made as to whether the patient is voluntarily consuming the requirement.

Techniques to ensure consumption of the required RER include **appetite stimulants or assisted feeding techniques** such as feeding tube placement.

Ensuring adequate nutrition is vital in the surgical patient and should be initiated as early as possible in the hospitalised patient. Tubes should be managed as per the clinic standard operating procedure to prevent the risk of complications such as infection.

Presurgery Fasting and Anaesthesia

Preoperatively, veterinary nurses and technicians must **confirm the time of the surgical patient's last meal** to ensure appropriate fasting has occurred to decrease anaesthetic risks.

Gastro-oesophageal reflux is well documented, with occurrence rates between 17 and 50% in pre-, peri-, and postoperative patients (both canine and feline patients) (Savvas et al., 2009).

Gastrointestinal complications due to anaesthesia occur because of the drugs which are used to sedate and or anaesthetise the patient. These drugs reduce or eliminate the patient's protective reflexes which protect their airway and normally prevent regurgitation and gastric contents entering the respiratory system. Consequently, intraoperative gastro-oesophageal reflux (GER), could potentially cause aspiration pneumonia or oesophagitis and in severe cases lead to oesophageal stricture.

Gastro-oesophageal reflux often occurs unnoticed during anaesthesia. The incidence of gastro-oesophageal reflux occurring is related to several factors:

During anaesthesia gastro-oesophageal reflux may occur due to:

- surgical manipulation of the stomach and intestinal tract
- patient breed: brachycephalic breeds commonly suffer from hiatal hernias and reduced tone in the lower oesophageal sphincter
- patient age
- drugs used for premedication and induction of anaesthesia
- volume and acidity of gastric contents
- length of fasting time prior to anaesthesia.

The aim of preoperative fasting is to ensure that the stomach is empty, with patients commonly being fasted for at least 12 hours prior to premedication and anaesthesia induction. However, recent studies conclude that **extensive fasting time may be detrimental to patients** as prolonged starvation may lead to accumulation of gastric secretions and increase the risk of GER.

Paediatric patients, i.e. those less than 4–6 months old, should certainly not undergo protracted periods of starvation prior to anaesthesia.

"Increased preoperative fasting times, in animal and human patients, are associated with an increased volume and acidity of gastric contents at induction of anaesthesia." (O'Dwyer, 2016).

A study by Savvas et al. (2009), found that dogs fed two to four hours prior to the induction of anaesthesia, had no increased incidence of reflux. However, patients fasted for 12, 18, or 24 hours had an increase in gastro-oesophageal reflux from 14.8 to 26.9%, respectively.

In the patient group that was **fed two to four hours before the induction of anaesthesia, the pH of the gastric contents remained more neutral.** This benefits the patient, as a more neutral gastric pH reduces gastro-oesophageal reflux during anaesthesia and the risk of oesophagitis if reflux does occur.

Therefore, a fasting time of around six hours may be more beneficial to veterinary patients. Patients likely to have their procedure later in the day should therefore be considered. It is recommended these patients receive a small volume of food, one teaspoon or tablespoon depending on the size of the patient, on the morning of surgery; with **water available up to the time of premedication.**

Intraoperative Nutrition

During anaesthesia, the **response to insulin is impaired in both the healthy and diseased patient, particularly if isoflurane and sevoflurane** are used. This subsequently contributes to hyperglycaemia during and following surgery (Kim et al., 2016).

Catabolic hormones increase blood glucose concentrations and minimise the effects of insulin. Therefore, the normal mechanisms for maintaining glucose homeostasis become ineffective during the perioperative period. Blood glucose concentration increases due to the metabolic stress caused by surgical trauma, this is due to glycogenolysis and gluconeogenesis. The level of response is dependent on the patient and the severity of trauma caused.

Postoperative Nutrition

The metabolic response to injury/disease is complex and increases the risk of malnutrition to the patient, which will have a detrimental effect:

- alterations in energy and substrate metabolism
- reduced immune response
- impaired wound healing
- increased risk of postoperative complications.

When the adequate energy substrates, protein, essential fatty acids, and micronutrients are provided the patients' body is better able to support:

- wound healing
- immune function
- tissue repair.

In some cases, metabolic imbalances may trigger lean body tissue catabolism, and commonly lead to food refusal. This predisposes patients to a negative energy balance, which can be reversed with nutritional support.

Ileus (loss of intestinal motility) is a postoperative complication and is most common in patients that have undergone abdominal surgery. Research indicates gastro-intestinal contractions within the stomach, duodenum, and jejunum/ileum decrease following a 12–24-hour fasting period (Cox, 2019) and can cause:

- vomiting
- abdominal tenderness
- abdominal distention
- nausea
- delayed bowel movements
- flatulence
- depression.

There are several nutritional challenges when managing hospitalised patients, requiring optimum nutritional support. These include:

- nausea
- inappetence
- gastrointestinal motility disorders (i.e. ileus)
- vomiting
- diarrhoea.

Patients with poor appetite may require appetite stimulants, such as mirtazapine or diazepam. However, it is important to note that **appetite stimulants rarely ensure the patient consumes their full nutritional daily requirement** and can increase the risk of complications such as sedation.

It is therefore important to ensure that the patient obtains their full nutritional requirements using the most appropriate diet for their condition. This is achieved by implementing more effective means of nutritional support such as enteral and parenteral nutrition.

- Enteral feeding: intake of nutrition via the gastrointestinal (GI) tract.
- Parental feeding: intravenous infusion of nutrition via the bloodstream.

It has been shown that **early enteral feeding regimes improve recovery times and reduce septic complications** particularly in the post GI tract surgical patient.

Hospital records must be kept accurate and up to date to ensure that the surgical patient receives optimum nutritional support, and timely feeds to prevent in-hospital starvation. Records must be written so that they include: the patient's total RER requirements, when and how much to feed and via which method. Record keeping becomes even more important if there are regular staff changes as inadequate intake may go unnoticed.

The patient's body weight and body condition score should be monitored daily during their hospital stay and the patients' energy intake adjusted accordingly to maintain stable body weight and prevent protein-calorie malnutrition.

To prevent in-hospital starvation, these four basic rules for in-patient feeding should be adhered to:

- Patients **should be fed as soon as is possible** following an investigation or surgery, including patients recovering from GI surgery and pancreatitis (unless contraindicated).
- **The need for nutritional support should be anticipated,** rather than waiting until the patient is debilitated. By which time, the detrimental effects of malnutrition are present, such as impaired immune system and death of enterocytes within the gut wall (malabsorption).
- **Fluid and electrolyte imbalances should be corrected** prior to starting nutritional support.
- **Assisted nutritional support** should be considered if:
    - **The patient has lost >10%** (since onset of clinical signs) of their body weight, which is not due to dehydration or fluid shifts (i.e. diuresis). This is particularly important in the obese and or sick patient as weight loss will be from lean body mass. Weight loss and anorexia in an obese cat is a concern as they are at high risk of developing hepatic lipidosis.
    - **They have been anorexic for three or more days** (including partial and full anorexia.) Prolonged inadequate intake defined as <75% of RER requirement for >5 days. Thus, keeping adequate patient records of how much the patient was offered and how much of that the patient ate is important.
    - **The patient is already in a catabolic state** or is at risk of overt malnutrition.
        - Does the patient have injuries or a disease process that increase its risk of protein loss? These may include pyothorax, draining sepsis, malabsorption, protein losing enteropathy (PLE) etc.
        - Does the patient show evidence they are not in a catabolic state (no weight loss or no loss in lean body mass)?

Other proposed risk factors include:

- **Physical signs:**

- non-healing wounds
- poor hair
- poor skin quality
- muscle wasting.

– **Dietary deficiencies:**
- long term use of unbalanced diets deficient in macro-and/or micronutrients (e.g. taurine deficiency in cats).

– **Chronic malabsorption** digestive disease
- chronic diarrhoea
- steatorrhoea
- EPI
- lymphangiectasia
- IBD
- infiltrative neoplasia.

Nutritional Intake and Resting Energy Requirement (RER)

To determine the individual patient's daily food intake requires calculation of their resting energy requirement (RER).

RER corresponds to the number of daily calories required by the patient to meet their basic needs. The RER is then compared to the quantity of calories the patient consumes per day.

Studies show that trauma, disease, sepsis, or major surgery in dogs is not associated with an increase in energy requirement (Walton et al., 1998; Chan, D 2015).

The RER can be used as a baseline for the recommended energy required in hospitalised patients, regardless of the disease process or surgery.

The simplest method to calculate RER is via the following equations:

Resting Energy Requirement

- **Patients >2 kg: 30 × bodyweight (kg) + 70**
- **Patients <2 kg: 70 × bodyweight (kg) $^{0.75}$**

The patient's bodyweight should be recorded at least once a day. **The day's resting energy requirement (RER) should be calculated based on that weight rather than their weight when admitted.** The RER is then divided by the caloric density of the chosen diet to calculate the amount to be fed.

It is important not to base nutritional calculations on the patient's ideal weight, as this can be associated with over-feeding and refeeding syndrome. For this reason, illness factors are no longer included in nutritional requirements.

It may be necessary to contact the manufacturer to obtain the caloric density of the food as this may not be shown on the food label due to regulation laws which are particularly evident in the EU. Although illness factors are not relevant, **the RER should be adjusted based on the patient's life stage.** (Table 11).

Table 11. RER adjustment based on the patient´s life stage. (Source: Ohio State University, 2020).

Life stage	Corresponding factor
Puppy 0–4 months	3 x RER
Puppy 4 months to adult	2 x RER

Source: Ohio State University, 2020

It is also important the patient's daily protein requirements are met.

- **Protein requirement for dogs:**
5–7.5 g protein per 100 kcal fed.

- **Protein requirement for cats:**
6–9 g protein per 100 kcal fed.

Cats are obligate carnivores and use protein for energy. They also require certain amino acids such as taurine, which they can only get from food. A cat's metabolism breaks down amino acids at a higher rate, which means they require more protein (which is animal-based).

Amount Fed

The RER is the starting point, and the amount fed is adjusted for the patient's needs and life stage. The amount fed requires adjustment when:

– the patient cannot tolerate the full amount and vomiting occurs; and
– the patient continues to lose lean body weight. The amount fed may need to be increased appropriately.

The volume of food offered should be weighed, and the volume consumed measured and recorded. This is to follow the percentage of RER that the patient consumes daily.

When less than 85% of the patient's RER is consumed each day within the hospital environment, consideration should be given to providing nutritional support.

The patient's body condition score (BCS) and muscle condition score (MCS) should also be monitored to identify trends in body and muscle mass appearance. These can give an indication of a catabolic state, particularly in patients with chronic disease or receiving long-term steroids.

The feeding schedule is dependent on the individual patient and how long since they have not received their full nutritional requirement. **Calculated food intake requirements should not be given immediately but introduced slowly over 2–3 days to prevent refeeding syndrome** and to allow the patient's metabolism and GI tract to adapt.

This is important during enteral feeding regimes as the stomach's capacity can reduce by half after two days of anorexia. Anorexia can also result in reduced gastric tone and emptying. Time also needs to be given for the natural microflora and metabolic changes to adapt to the new diet.

Refeeding Syndrome

Refeeding syndrome (Figure 24) is a potentially fatal complication of nutritional rehabilitation in patients with severe anorexia. It occurs in significantly malnourished patients when a diet of increasing calories is initiated orally, or by enteral or parenteral administration.During periods of reduced nutritional intake, the body adapts by reducing its metabolic rate as well as the functional reserves of organ systems. These include:

- GI motility
- cardiac output
- renal concentration capacity
- haemoglobin levels.

A malnourished patient has decreased levels of serum glucose. This is because **the body goes into a catabolic state by the process of gluconeogenesis,** using triglycerides and protein to create glucose.

Gluconeogenesis results in:

- reduction in lean body mass
- reduction in body mass
- reduction of the total body stores of phosphate
- reduction of the total body stores potassium
- reduction of the total body stores magnesium.

The introduction of nutrition via refeeding causes **a shift in the patient's state from catabolic to anabolic** whereby the preferred energy source is carbohydrate and not protein. This stimulates the release of insulin, which subsequently results in major shifts in serum electrolytes from the extracellular space to the intracellular space. (e.g. potassium, phosphorus, and magnesium). Insulin also promotes intracellular update of glucose and phosphorus so that glycolysis can occur.

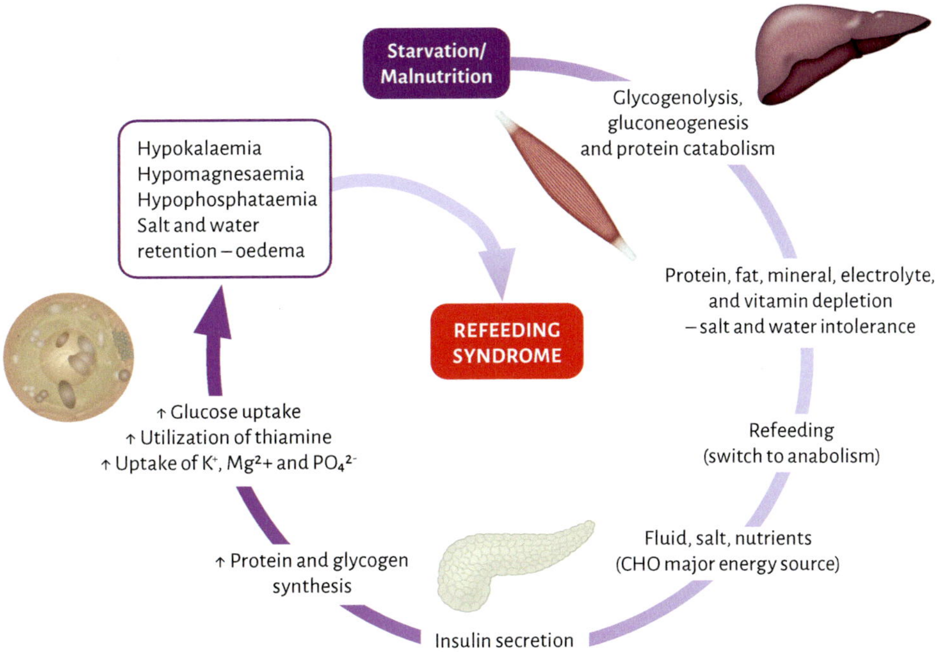

Figure 24. The process of refeeding syndrome.

The fast electrolyte uptake from extracellular space to the intracellular spaces results in **hypophosphataemia, hypokalaemia, and hypomagnesaemia.**

Hypophosphataemia is the main characteristic of refeeding syndrome. Phosphate is used in the following body processes:

- kidney function
- muscle contractions
- normal heartbeat
- nerve signalling
- fluid balance
- bone formation
- structural role in nucleic acids and cell membranes
- required to produce adenosine triphosphate (ATP) in energy production
- for oxygen affinity to haemoglobin.

Hyperphosphataemia has the following effects:

- haemolysis
- muscle weakness (myopathy)
- leukocyte dysfunction
- a reduction of levels in 2,3-diphosphoglycerate in red blood cell, thereby reducing oxygen delivery to tissues
- mental dysfunction
- seizures
- impaired glucose metabolism
- impaired phospholipid synthesis.

Hypokalaemia results in muscle weakness and arrhythmia. Hypomagnesaemia results in arrhythmias, tremors, tetany, and weakness, and potential secondary causes such as hypokalaemia and hypocalcemia.

Due to acid-base effects, fluid overload (if the patient is on IV fluids) and fluid retention can occur. Clinical signs associated with fluid overload and or fluid retention include:

- weight gain
- dyspnoea
- tachypnoea
- pulmonary crackles
- chemosis
- serous nasal discharge.

Typically, refeeding syndrome is noticed within five days after the reintroduction of nutrition and is mostly seen in patients which are critically ill and or are in the late life stages. Similarly, **in patients with a 20% reduction in phosphorus, potassium, or magnesium levels refeeding syndrome should be suspected.**

Careful monitoring is required for patients that are at a higher risk of developing refeeding syndrome. When refeeding syndrome is suspected, the rate of feeding should be reduced immediately by 50–75%. A change of diet to a lower amount of carbohydrate may be considered with the careful supplementation and monitoring of potassium, phosphorus, and magnesium (Sumner, 2021).

Nutritional Planning

A successful nutritional plan takes the patient's diagnosis and treatment into account, and the nutritional support provided by an appropriate route.

Enteral Feeding

Enteral feeding is **any method that delivers part or all of the patient's calories via the gastrointestinal tract.** It includes offering the patient's normal oral diet or the use of nutritional supplements in a liquid form which provide part or all of the patient's daily requirements via a feeding tube.

As a guide:

- Using the gastrointestinal tract for feeding is preferred; thus, if the 'gut works use it'.
- If only part of the GI tract is functional, then that part should be utilised the non-functional proximal portion bypassed.
- If enteral feeding is used, the simplest and most effective route should be chosen so as to prevent patient stress.

The intestinal mucosa needs glutamine and other nutrients for its maintenance. Without this nutrition the **gut is a less effective immunological barrier** and potentially allows bacterial translocation and endotoxin absorption, particularly in critical patients. Enteral feeding ensures the enterocytes within the gastrointestinal mucosa receive their required nutrition directly from the food that passes by them. This maintains:

- the gastrointestinal protective barrier against bacterial translocation and sepsis
- normal intestinal bacterial flora to aid digestion.

Enteral Nutritional Support

There are several techniques which can be used to provide assisted enteral feeding, and many factors that influence the chosen method, for example:

- nature of the disease
- length of time nutritional support is required
- equipment available
- patient's suitability to general anaesthesia.

It is imperative that whichever method is selected, feeding should not be stressful to the patient as this can result in food aversion. There are various methods of enteral nutrition with the method chosen influenced by the patient's health status.

Food aversion is a tendency to avoid or have a negative association with food that has been eaten just before becoming ill or a negative experience.

Oral/Coaxed Feeding

Patients with a reduced, but still present, appetite (hyporexia) may benefit from being enticed with a highly palatable diet. **The diet's palatability can be increased by wetting and or warming and choosing a diet with a strong aroma.** This is particularly important with the feline patient, as stimulation of their olfactory senses may stimulate them to eat.

Some patients may only **eat their normal, home diet.** This should be discussed with the owner who can then provide some of this food. However, care should be taken with raw food, as this may be an infection control risk within the hospital environment for staff and other patients.

Some patients may **respond to owner feeding** (in the case of dogs) and benefit from hand feeding with encouragement. Providing a privacy area is also beneficial to some patients, such as cats. Some patients have feeding patterns, especially cats whereby some are grazers and others dusk/twilight feeders (normal feline feeding habits).

Chemical Stimulation

Appetite stimulants are drugs that increase a patient's appetite.

The hormone ghrelin is essential for survival and is produced primarily in the stomach, but also in the small intestine, pancreas, and brain. Ghrelin is the primary trigger within the centre of the hypothalamus (orexigenic) which triggers the stimulation of food intake and food seeking behaviours. **Cortisol and thyroxine are also important regarding food seeking behaviours.**

There are several off-label drugs that are used as appetite stimulants in both canine and feline patients, however the desired outcome is unpredictable. The **ghrelin agonist class of drugs has been shown to be the most effective.** Examples include Capromorelin; Entyce™, and Mirtazapine (Mirataz™).

Force Feeding

In the author's opinion, **force feeding by syringe causes food aversion and should be avoided,** especially as it is poorly tolerated and stressful to the patient, particularly in cats.

If attempted, care should be taken to avoid food aspiration especially in very depressed patients. Inadvertent food aspiration may result in aspiration pneumonia. Syringe feeding should not be used in the following cases:

- comatose patients
- moribund patients
- patients with neuromuscular disease
- patients with oropharyngeal disease
- dyspnoeic patients.

As this method has an increased risk of resulting food aversion, it should not be used for introducing a new diet, especially one required for long-term management.

In patients who have been hyporexic or anorexic for 48 hours or are not expected to eat for a 48-hour period, then placement of an enteral feeding tube should be considered.

Enteral Tube Feeding

This method is usually safer and less expensive than parenteral nutrition (see later) as it aids in the maintenance of the structure of the GI tract and its function.

Many patients with feeding tubes can be discharged from hospital with their feeding tube in place for their recovery to continue at home. This often allows a quicker recovery as they are not in a hospital environment with its risk and stress factors. However, this is only appropriate with adequate client education, good home care, and client compliance.

Early assessment of the patient to determine if they require a feeding tube is advisable, as this may mean the tube placement can be combined with other procedures and undertaken under a single anaesthetic.

Feeding tubes are indicated in patients with:

- anorexia (total or partial) for >5 days
- significant weight loss (>10%)
- increased nutritional losses
- increased nutritional requirements beyond that which they can consume orally
- a need to bypass specific parts of the alimentary tract e.g. mandibular fractures.

Feeding tubes are likely to be required in patients:

- undergoing surgery that is expected to result in postoperative anorexia (e.g. major gastrointestinal surgery)
- which have increased nutritional requirements but a poor appetite e.g. patients with extensive effusive wounds.

Some types of enteral tube feeding are contraindicated, for example in patients with persistent vomiting, a severe malabsorption condition, or the inability to protect their airway (e.g. coughing/gag reflux).

There are various feeding routes, including:

- naso-oesophageal (NO)/nasogastric (NG)
- oesophagostomy (O)

- gastrostomy (placed either endoscopically (PEG) or surgically by laparotomy (G))
- jejunostomy (J).

Each tube type has advantages and disadvantages, and the selection of which type of tube to use depends on various factors:

1. **The aim should be to utilise as much of the functioning GI tract as possible.** For example, a feline patient with a jaw fracture should be supported with an oesophagostomy tube, whereas a patient with an oesophageal injury should be supported with a gastrostomy tube.
2. **The anticipated duration for which the tube will remain in situ.** Patients requiring short term support may be supported with a naso-oesophageal tube, whereas long term use is best supported with an oesophagostomy or gastrostomy tube (due to the discomfort caused by the presence of NO tubes and their propensity to become obstructed due to their narrow lumen size). It is important to assess the surgical patient's nutritional needs and plan prior to the surgical procedure as long-term feeding tubes can be placed under the same anaesthesia preventing unnecessary costs for the client and additional anaesthetic risks to the patient.
3. **Complication risks.** Gastrostomy and jejunostomy tubes are at risk of developing dehiscence and leakage with imperfect healing round the internal stoma, which might result in septic peritonitis. These risks are amplified if the tube is displaced by the patient. External wound infection at the stoma site is the most common complication. However, this is easily treated, and the patient can still be fed whilst receiving medical antimicrobial treatment.
4. **The type of food used with the tube.** The diameter of the tube governs what type of diet can be used/administered through it. Naso-oesophageal and jejunostomy tubes usually require complete liquid diets, which may require constant infusions of food to provide adequate patient nutrition. Placement of larger gauge tubes results in a greater choice of diet and ability to feed boluses of food. Some diets, however, may need to be liquidized and the addition of water required; this then lowers the caloric density of the diet.

Feeding tubes should not pass through the lower oesophageal sphincter (cardiac sphincter) due to the risk of reflux oesophagitis.

Naso-oesophageal Tube Feeding

Naso-oesophageal (NO) feeding tubes should only be used for up to seven days and therefore are only for short-term use. They are easily placed and do not require anaesthesia and can therefore be placed by the competent veterinary nurse/technician.

NO tubes are made of soft flexible PVC or silicone. The diameter and length of NO feeding tube used depends on the patient's size. Usually, 3.5–5 Fr are used for feline patients and 3.5–8 Fr for canine patients. **The diameter of the tube is determined by the size of the patient's nostrils.** This means liquid food must be of a suitable consistency to prevent the tube from becoming blocked.

- **Advantages:**
  - **Inexpensive**
  - **Quick**
  - **Non-invasive**
  - **No need for anaesthesia.**
- **Disadvantages:**
  - **Small tube size, so liquid diets**
  - **Not all patients tolerate them**
  - **Short term only (up to a week).**

Naso-oesophageal feeding tubes should be placed such that the tip is located within the caudal oesophagus, as opposed to naso-gastric tubes where the tip is located within the stomach. This creates an opening within the cardiac sphincter which may lead to gastric reflux and subsequently oesophagitis. Additionally, an increase in vomiting may occur which may lead to aspiration pneumonia.

When using a naso-oesophageal tube it is important to **check its position prior to each feed,** as it is possible for it to be regurgitated and either chewed off or inhaled.

Placement of a Naso-oesophageal (NO) Feeding Tube

Naso-oesphageal feeding tubes are easy to place and can be placed by competent veterinary nurses/technicians. Equipment and materials required include:

- lubricating gel
- single use local anaesthetic proxymetacaine
- super glue/surgical stapler
- syringes (5 ml)
- cloth tape (e.g. Elastoplast 2.5–5)
- buster collar
- permanent marker
- sterile water for injection
- suitable size oesophageal feeding tube.

Proxymetacaine topical ocular local anaesthetic is administered into both nostrils and the eye (to anaesthetise the rostral and caudal aspects of the nose).

One of the issues when placing NO tubes is inadequate anaesthesia. When administering the local anaesthesia ensure the patient's head is elevated so the local anaesthetic is in contact with the entire surface of the nasal passage. It is also important to leave sufficient time, around five minutes, to allow correct local anaesthesia before placement. If necessary, the local anaesthetic should be administered twice.

The tube should be measured from the 7–9th rib (for a NO tube) and marked, with permanent marker, where it lies next to the entrance of the nostril; the aim is for the end of the tube to sit in the distal oesophagus.

When placing the tube, the tube should be gripped so that only a short section is held, thus maintaining some rigidity when passing the tube into the nostril. The tube should be lubricated and directed **ventrally and medially** threading it rapidly once past the sensitive parts of the nasal passage, the turbinates. Patients swallow when the tube passes the larynx which shows the tube is in the correct position. Correct positioning of the tube should be confirmed by attaching a syringe and aspirating: if negative pressure is present, it is likely the tube is in the oesophagus. If large volumes of air are returned, the tube may be in the airway and requires replacement. If the tube is in the stomach, gastric contents may be aspirated.

Once tube placement is checked, the tube can be secured with a friction (roman sandal) suture, or butterfly tape and suture, staple, or skin glue. It should be secured either to the side of the face, or along the bridge of the nose, **out of the line of sight** to avoid patient removal.

Correct positioning may then also be confirmed using $ETCO_2$ measurement (this should be zero, with the absence of a capnograph trace unless the tube is in the airway). Radiography may also be performed to confirm appropriate placement.

Once a naso-oesophageal feeding tube is in place; they require little maintenance as there is no surgical incision; however, regular checking and cleaning of the nose is recommended, to remove any crusting or discharge causing reduced airflow. It is imperative the tube position is confirmed each time ahead of feeding.

First, the tube should be checked for negative pressure, then flush with 2–5 ml of sterile water for injection (warmed to body temperature). The patient should be observed for signs such as coughing, which can indicate incorrect positioning. If this occurs, feeding should not take place and tube placement confirmed with a radiograph.

After confirming the tube is correctly placed, the patient can be fed with an appropriate liquid diet. This can be via a constant rate infusion where the patient is constantly observed throughout the administration (with prompt intervention if tube movement is detected) or as intermittent bolus feeds (author's preferred method).

The size of each feed should not exceed gastric volume (10 ml/kg), and **a minimum of four hours should be scheduled between feeds,** to allow sufficient time for gastric emptying.

Feeds should be administered slowly, over around 20 minutes, and the patient observed for signs of nausea (e.g. lip-licking, retching). If these are present, the feeding duration may need to be prolonged, or the volume reduced.

Following feeding, the tube should be flushed with a small volume (2–5 ml, depending on the priming volume of the tube) of lukewarm tap water.

Due to the high risk of tube obstruction, **crushed tablets, powders, or viscous liquid medications should not be administered down narrow-bore nasal feeding tubes.**

Naso-oesophageal tubes should not be used if there is:

- rhinitis
- facial injuries involving the nares
- persistent vomiting
- the patient is unconscious
- abnormalities of the pharynx/larynx/oesophagus
- in patients with clotting disorders.

Oesophageal Feeding Tubes

Oesophagostomy tubes have a wider diameter than naso-oesphageal tubes, which allow thicker foods to pass through and are useful in cases requiring short-to-medium term feeding, **however general anaesthesia is required for placement.**

Oesophagostomy tubes are **placed into the mid-cervical oesophagus on the left side** and are well tolerated. There are minimal complications, with the most common being:

- infection at the entry site, which can be prevented by good stoma care
- haemorrhage at the time of placement (jugular puncture)
- Horner's syndrome due to damage to the sympathetic nerves in the neck
- cellulitis.

There are two techniques for oesophagostomy feeding tube placement. The size of tube used depends on the size of the patient; **oesophagostomy feeding sizes range from 8–18 Fr.**

According to Schedule 3 of the Veterinary Surgeons Act (UK), **veterinary nurses/technicians cannot independently place oesophagostomy tubes,** however, are invaluable with assisting with their surgical placement.

Percutaneous Placement

The patient should be placed in right lateral recumbency, and the insertion area prepared aseptically. An introducer needle with a peel away sheath (Van Noort system) should be used.

The metal introducer should be placed into the oesophagus and palpated through the skin; a needle is placed through the skin into the hollow tube at the end of the introducer, then withdrawn leaving the peel-away sheath in place. A premeasured tube should be inserted into the sheath, the sheath removed, and the introducer withdrawn.

Surgical Placement (preferred method)

The patient should be placed in right lateral recumbency, and the insertion area prepared aseptically. Long curved artery forceps (e.g. Carmalt forceps) should be passed into the oesophagus and palpated through the skin, making a skin incision over the tips of the forceps, and subsequently forcing the tips up through the incision. Then either a small stylet to increase the rigidity of the tube can be used and placed directly down the oesophagus, between the open jaws of the forceps. Alternatively, the tip of the tube can be grasped in the forceps and drawn back up into the mouth, where the tip is reversed and inserted back down the oesophagus.

Following placement, the position should be confirmed radiographically, prior to securing the tube in place.

Oesophagostomy feeding tubes should not be used in patients with:

- persistent vomiting
- problems with oesophageal function motility
- laryngeal problems
- gastric outflow obstruction (functional or physiological).

Oesophagostomy tube feeding instructions are the same as nasal feeding tubes, however larger flush volumes may be required depending on the size and length of the tube. Some oesophagostomy tubes can be cut to a shorter length if required, and the syringe adapter moved further down the tube, to minimise priming volumes.

As oesophagostomy tubes are surgically placed it is imperative that the stoma at the incision is managed aseptically. The stoma site should be inspected daily for:

- tube dislodgement/movement
- suture security
- discharge
- redness
- swelling.

To prevent complications at the stoma site, it should be cleaned with diluted chlorhexidine (0.005%) solution and redressed twice daily. Using antimicrobial dressings impregnated with polyhexamethylene biguanide or iodine reduce the risk of infection and for ease of dressing, premade washable Kitty Kollars® can be used around the tube, avoiding the need for a neck bandage.

- **Advantages:**
  - **Inexpensive**
  - **Larger bore tube than naso-oesophageal**
  - **Brief general anaesthesia**
  - **Tolerated well, can be used for months**
  - **Minimal surgical skill involved.**
- **Disadvantages:**
  - **Invasive**
  - **Small risk of infection/fistula**
  - **Needs to be dressed to prevent interference.**

An advantage of oesophagostomy tube placement is the wider bore tubing, which means that crushed tablet or powdered medications, as well as thicker liquid preparations of more calorically dense diets (i.e. >1.3 kcal/ml), can be administered. However, care should be taken to avoid tube blockage; if blockage occurs, a small volume of carbonated water can be used to dislodge this. Patients can also be **discharged with the tube in place for at-home feeding,** with the correct client education and nursing support.

Gastrostomy Tubes

Gastrostomy tubes are suitable for providing **medium to long-term nutritional support.** The tube must be left in place for a minimum of seven days if placed endoscopically to allow a stoma to form and can remain for months or longer if they are correctly managed. Surgically placed gastrostomy tubes are sealed in position at surgery and so earlier removal is possible, however these are often left in place longer prior to removal to avoid disruption of the surgical site and pain during the inflammatory phase of wound healing.

A wider diameter tube can be used because the feeding tube is placed directly into the patient's stomach, and therefore allows for thicker, more highly calorific food such as gruel-consistency foods; for example, the patient's own wet food which has been blended, without the risk of the tube becoming blocked. Additionally, medications can be crushed and administered via the gastrostomy tube. Typically, **gastrostomy tubes used are between 14–20 F.**

Indications for the placement of a gastrostomy tube are when the upper gastrointestinal tract must be bypassed, such as:

- oesophageal stricture
- oesophagitis
- long term anorexia due to trauma
- systemic disease (neurological disease such as myasthenia gravis).

There are **three techniques for gastrostomy tube placement,** all of which require general anaesthesia.

Surgical (at ventral midline laparotomy or via a flank incision)
Involves **placing the tube during laparotomy** and is indicated if laparotomy is planned for other procedures such as exploratory surgery or biopsies (e.g. liver).

A Bard-Pezzer mushroom tip catheter style gastrostomy tube is used. The end of the feeding tube is brought into the abdomen through the body wall. A purse-string suture is placed within the stomach wall and the gastrostomy tube placed through a stab incision which is made in the centre of the purse-string. The stomach is then sutured to the body wall to form an airtight seal around the gastrostomy tube.

Omentum may be wrapped around the gastropexy side between the stomach and the peritoneum to help protect and seal the gastropexy.

Externally the tube is secured to the skin with a friction suture.

Percutaneous Endoscopic Placement (PEG)
Is a minimally invasive technique performed using gastroscopy to guide and place the tube. This technique is advantageous as the oesophagus and stomach can also be viewed and biopsied during the same procedure.

The patient should be placed in right lateral recumbency and an area of 10–15 cm caudal to the last rib prepared aseptically. The gastroscope is passed into the stomach which is inflated with air. The endoscopic light marks the incision point. An assistant inserts the cannula that comes with the PEG kit to which a double suture thread is passed into the gastric lumen. This suture is then grasped with endoscopic graspers and withdrawn so that the suture exits the mouth.

The gastrostomy tube with the internal fixation disk is then tied to the suture via a double thread and loop to loop knot. The end of the gastrostomy tube has a dilator to allow it to stretch the tissue in order for it to exit from the stomach.

The suture thread is then pulled by an assistant who advances the tube down the oesophagus and into the stomach.

The cannula which is in the stomach is then withdrawn and pulled through the body wall, with the dilator portion widening the exit point. The tube is advanced until the mushroom tip is in contact with the stomach wall.

The gastrostomy tube is then anchored at the body wall via the external fixation device. It is important to avoid excessive pressure under the fixation device to prevent tissue necrosis. The mushroom shape of the catheter is the only restraint preventing displacement of the tube from the stomach with this technique, so there is a risk of septic peritonitis with tube displacement.

Blind Percutaneous Placement
There are various types of commercial equipment available, most involving a long hollow rigid stylet (orogastric tube) which is passed into the stomach via the oesophagus. This technique involves a high risk of complications due to limited visualisation of the anatomy. Complications include damage to the oesophagus, stomach wall, and spleen.

For all techniques it is important to **confirm tube placement is correct,** either endoscopically or radiographically. Also, the area should be cleaned with dilute 0.005% chlorhexidine, an impregnated antimicrobial dressing applied, as well as a stockinette vest to protect and anchor the tube to the patient's body.

For non-surgically placed tubes, a stoma must have time to form to avoid peritonitis and the tube should not be used for the first 24-hours. During the first 24-hour period only sterile water flushes should be used, in order to maintain tube patency and flush any gastric contents from the tube. Surgically placed tubes can be used immediately following patient recovery from anaesthesia.

Feeding Via Gastrotomy Tube
The gastrostomy tube should be aspirated prior to each feed to check the residual volume of gastric contents. If greater than 20% of the previous feed volume remains because of delayed gastric emptying or ileus, the meal should be delayed, and the aspiration repeated two hours later. **The next feed should only be given if the residual volume is <20%.**

If issues of delayed gastric emptying persist, a veterinary surgeon should further assess the patient to **consider initiating the use of gastric prokinetics such as ranitidine or metoclopramide.**

Prefeed flushes can be performed with lukewarm tap water (as the risk of tube dislodgement and airway contamination is not an issue with abdominal feeding tubes) and priming volumes are generally larger, so a greater flush volume is needed.

The feed is administered in a similar manner to other tubes, though thicker, more calorie-dense diets can be used. It is imperative that the **administration is at a slow regular pace and takes between 10–20 minutes.** This is dependent on the volume of food to be administered, patient size, and tube used. **The ideal rate of administration is around 1 ml over 1–2 minutes** (Bloor, 2019).

As with oesophagostomy tubes, site checks and dressing changes should be undertaken twice daily. The application of an adhesive dressing around the tube entry site (e.g. a Primapore™ over an antimicrobial dressing) is recommended, followed by a string vest over the abdomen. The remaining tube length can be curled and placed under the vest, with swabs placed around the area for padding.

Tubes placed non-surgically, should not be removed for 7–14 days post-placement, to allow sufficient time for stoma development and avoid complications such as peritonitis.

Advantages of gastrotomy tubes:
- larger diameter tubes with less of a risk of blockage
- liquidised tinned food can be fed
- easy to maintain
- can be left in situ for long periods of time
- patients can be sent home with the tube in situ
- patient interference +/- dislodgement is rare
- allows gastric decompression after gastric surgery
- calorically dense diets can be used (i.e. >1.3 kcal/ml).

Disadvantages of gastrotomy tubes:
- general anaesthesia required for placement
- specialist equipment required to place them (e.g. PEG)
- must stay in situ for at least 14 days if placed non-surgically
- risk of peritonitis if not managed correctly.

Jejunostomy Tube/Enterostomy Tubes

Enterostomy tubes are not commonly used. The procedure is used to bypass the stomach, pancreas, and biliary tract and tubes are most often placed via a laparotomy or a celiotomy surgical procedure through the right side of the abdomen. Due to the risk of peritoneal leakage these tubes are often placed through a gastrostomy tube via a J-through-G technique.

The J-through-G technique allows decompression of the stomach while also being able to administer feeds distal to the stomach.

Food administered through a jejunostomy tube bypasses the stomach and duodenum therefore incomplete digestion occurs. Subsequently highly concentrated liquid diets are used and as they are administered at this point in the small intestine can cause problems such as osmotic overload and diarrhoea.

A jejunostomy tube has a smaller diameter (5–8 F) than a gastrostomy tube and therefore the rate of food administration is required to be slower. For this reason, food is administered via a constant rate infusion (CRI).

Medications should not be administered via a jejunostomy tube since they require transport through earlier portions of the gastrointestinal tract. Feeding should be delayed for 24-hours after tube placement, with sterile water flushes only during this time. Site care and dressing change requirements are identical to oesophageal and gastrostomy tubes.

Complications include peritoneal and subcutaneous leakage due to premature removal and tube induced jejunal perforation (Seimm, 2004).

- **Advantages:**
  - **Distal to the stomach/pancreas/biliary tract**
  - **Well tolerated.**
- **Disadvantages:**
  - **Cost**
  - **Longer general anaesthesia**
  - **Peritonitis risk**
  - **Narrow tube size**
  - **Remain in place for at least 14 days.**

Feeding Tube Complications

There are a variety of possible tube related complications. These include:
- dislodgement of the tube; whereby the seriousness depends on the location of the feeding tube (i.e. naso-oesphageal, gastrostomy before stoma formation);
- dislodgement resulting loss in feeding access;
- refeeding syndrome: (hyperglycaemia, hypophosphataemia, haemolytic anaemia) plasma phosphate and potassium should be monitored. Supplementation may be required;
- diarrhoea: caused by increased gastric emptying if diet is cold, fed too much, and too quickly;
- stoma site infections; and
- aspiration pneumonia.

During each feed, the patient should be monitored closely for signs of nausea, regurgitation, and vomiting. If signs occur feeding should be suspended. A common issue with feeding tubes is blockage. If the tube becomes blocked, **3 ml of a fizzy drink such as cola or soda water can be instilled in the tube and left for 15–20 minutes to aid in the dislodgement of the blockage.** Alternatively, a small amount of pancreatic enzyme powder with carbonated water can be used with care. It is crucial to feed food of the right consistency to prevent obstructions.

Tubes should be cleaned with an appropriate antiseptic skin solution and appropriately dressed to prevent contamination of the stoma site which could result in infection. If infections occur the tube may need to be removed, particularly if systemic infection is suspected.

Parental Nutrition (PN)

Parenteral nutrition is administered when food administration via the gastrointestinal tract is not possible. **PN involves**

administration of the three macronutrients: lipids, carbohydrates (dextrose) and amino acids in conjunction with electrolytes and trace elements directly into the bloodstream. Parenteral nutrition is more expensive than enteral feeding.

It is mainly used for cases such as:
- protracted vomiting
- acute pancreatitis
- severe malabsorption disorders
- severe ileus
- patients with reduced consciousness/recumbency.

There are two types of parenteral nutrition:
- **Total parenteral nutrition (TPN):** delivered via a central line catheter providing all the patient's energy requirements.
- **Partial parenteral nutrition (PPN):** delivered via a central line but also a peripherally inserted central catheter (PICC) line and only provides 40–70% of the patient's energy requirements and is thus intended for short term use.

Formulation of a parenteral nutrition solution requires calculation of the patient's protein and energy requirements, whilst ensuring the volume of lipids, proteins and dextrose are not excessive.

Generally, commercial products such as Kabiven® (TPN) and Perikabiven® (PPN) (both are Fresenius-Kabi products) feature a three-chamber bag with compartments providing a combination of amino acids, lipid, glucose, and electrolytes. This ensures appropriate nutrition for most patients in a single bag in a convenient time and cost-saving formulation. Both forms come in a range of volumes depending on the size of the patient (Fresenius-Kabi).

Parenteral Nutrition Preparation

Parenteral nutrition (PN) is generally only used in a specialist setting, as the solutions must be **administered through a central venous catheter.** This is because the glucose content of the PN solution (which is usually 11%) causes high osmolarity, causing phlebitis when administered through a peripheral vein.

The PN solution must prepared aseptically with the use of sterile gloves, maintaining the sterility of the administration lines. Sterile gloves should also be worn whenever handling the bag, lines, or central venous catheter.

The bag (Figure 25) comes in a clear over pouch allowing for quick visual inspection to confirm the bags integrity. The inner bag is composed of the three chambers which contain:
- lipids
- amino acids and electrolytes
- dextrose.

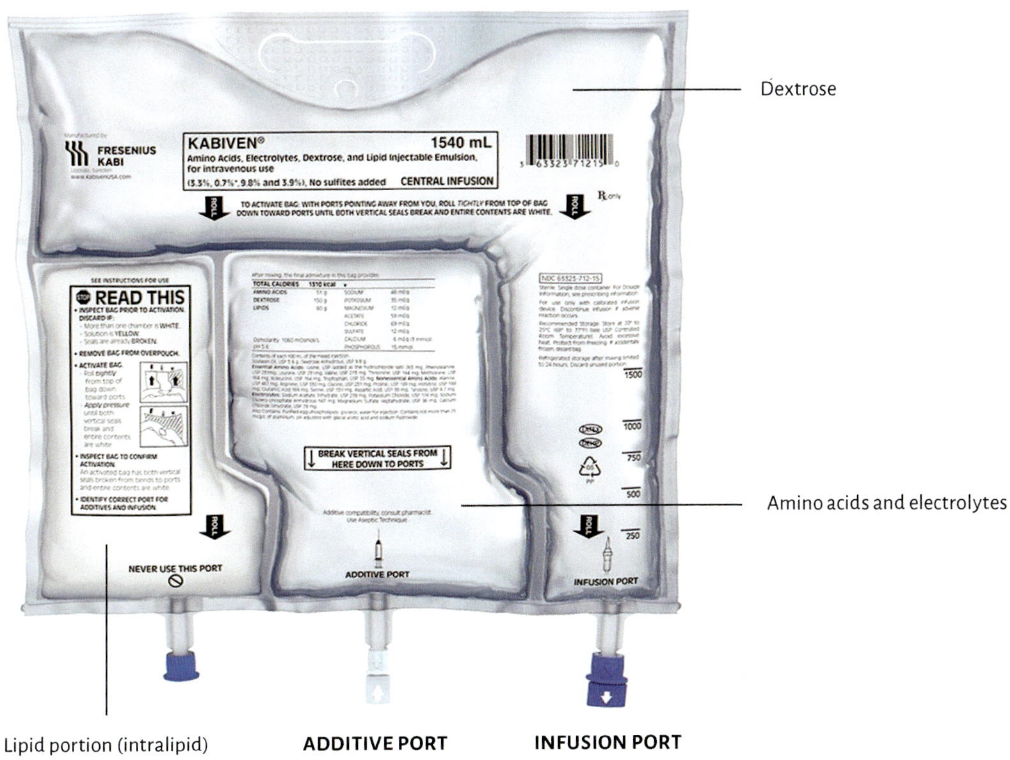

Figure 25. A parenteral nutrition bag.

The three chambers are separated by a horizontal and two vertical seals which aim to enhance stability for storage and prolong the shelf-life.

The bag also has **three ports clearly labelled:**

- **Do not use it:** far left and is a blind port.
- **Additive port:** white and has an arrow pointing towards the bag.
- **Infusion port:** blue and has an arrow pointing away from the bag.

All the ports are protected with tamper evident caps which are sterile and self-sealing.

The bag is contained in an over-pouch which protects the inner bag containing the parenteral nutrition. Prior to activating the bag's contents, the bag should be inspected as per the manufacturer's instructions.

The chamber on the left containing the lipid portion should be white and the other two chambers clear and colourless. The bag must be discarded if the:

- over-pouch is damaged or opened
- more than one chamber is white in colour
- clear solutions are yellow in colour.

Bag Activation Process

1. The bag should be placed on a clean, flat surface with the text side up and the ports facing away from the clinical personnel.

2. The bag should be tightly rolled from the top towards the ports, ensuring application of pressure until both the vertical seals are broken, and the entire contents are white in colour.

3. Ensuring that the two vertical seals are fully broken, the contents should be thoroughly mixed by inverting the bag, a minimum of three times. (Note that an activated bag has the vertical seals broken from the bends to the ports.)

4. Additions such as trace elements, vitamins and additional electrolytes are added to the parenteral nutrition bag after it has been activated via the white additive port, using an aseptic technique. The port should not be used more than ten times. After each addition, the bag must be adequately mixed and labelled with the additional additives. Additives used must be compatible with the solution.

The solution must be run through an in-line 1.2-micron lipid filter, to prevent lipid emboli entering the circulation. Alcohol or chlorhexidine-soaked swabs can be wrapped around connections in the line/ports to provide additional antimicrobial activity and prevent disconnection.

There is an increased risk of bacterial contamination due to the makeup of PN solutions (i.e. lipid component) therefore, strict aseptic technique is required when handling catheter lines. Additional, intravenous catheter lines should not be disconnected, except for once every 24-hours when the bag and line are discarded and replaced with a new set.

The administration rate is calculated based on the patient's RER and the calorie content (kcal/ml) of the fluid bag. When administering these solutions intravenously, the fluid rate of other fluids administered to the patient must be considered and may need to be reduced, to avoid fluid overload.

Complications

Parenteral nutrition is associated with several risks, as all parenteral nutrition must be administered via a specifically placed intravenous catheter and strict aseptic technique used.

Patients receiving parenteral nutrition require 24-hour monitoring and careful aseptic technique when handling them and their parenteral nutrition line, as the solution contains no preservative, which makes an ideal environment for bacteria to colonize.

Complications with parenteral nutrition include:

- mechanical complications of the IV catheter and line
- sepsis
- thrombophlebitis
- metabolic disturbances such as hyperglycaemia and electrolytes disturbances.

Patients should be continually reassessed to ensure early problem identification and that prompt action is initiated. The patient's vital signs should be monitored at least twice daily; catheter sites checked, and aseptically maintained and routine biochemistry and electrolytes monitored regularly to identify metabolic complications which include:

- hyperglycaemia
- glycosuria
- hypokalaemia
- hypophosphataemia
- lipaemia
- hyperkalaemia.

It may be necessary to adjust the ratio of nutrients, administration rate, administer insulin (if hyperglycaemia occurs), supplement potassium (if hypokalaemia develops), or give phosphate (in the face of hypophosphataemia).

As parenteral nutrition does not provide direct nutrition to enterocytes, with prolonged use this can cause compromise to the gastrointestinal barrier, risking bacterial translocation and sepsis.

If required, patients should receive partial parenteral nutrition, in addition to any amounts administered by enteral feeding. Patients should be gradually transitioned off parenteral nutrition.

Nutritional Calculations

One of the most important considerations in the perioperative management of the surgical patient is the patient's nutrition. It is imperative veterinary nurses and technicians understand the role that nutrition plays in a surgical patient's recovery and can determine the patient's resting energy requirement (RER) and nutritional administration requirements.

Nutritional Planning

To provide complete patient care, nutritional support should be part of the therapeutic plan. Providing nutrition accomplishes several goals:

- **minimize metabolic derangements**
- maintain hydration
- reduce/prevent acid-base and electrolyte disorders
- reduce/prevent electrolyte disturbances
- provide disease-specific nutrients
- **provide nutrients to aid recovery**
- suppress an increased metabolic response
- restore or reverse protein catabolism
- maintain gastrointestinal tract integrity and function
- optimize immune function
- **maintain lean body mass and body weight**
- promote further lean muscle production
- **avoid complications associated with refeeding:** prevent surges in insulin and thus hypokalaemia, hypomagnesaemia, and hypophosphataemia.

The diet chosen depends on a variety of factors such as availability and cost, however the patient's medical condition must be the main reason for the specific choice of diet with the overall aim of providing the patient with calories.

First, it should be established if the patient is willing to eat. By tempting the patient with a gastrointestinal diet and then moving on to something like cocktail sausages, rice, chicken, or scrambled egg this helps to determine the patient's willingness to eat.

Care must be taken to avoid to certain human foods such as baby foods as these foods may contain toxic ingredients such as onion and garlic.

Feeding tubes also influence the choice of diet. Typically, small bore tubes require the use of a liquid enteral diet that meets the nutritional requirements of the patient.

Critical care diets are typically high in protein and fat, and low in carbohydrate. They are high energy, calorie dense diets and therefore, the volume of food administered is lower:

- **High in protein:**
  - **maintenance of muscle mass**
  - **highly digestible, good quality protein**
  - **amino acids: L-carnitine and glutamine.**
- **High in fat:**
  - **high energy, calorie dense**
  - **protein sparing**
  - **omega 3 fatty acids.**
- **Low in carbohydrate:**
  - **aid in glucose intolerance in stress starvation**
  - **aids in insulin resistance in critical patients.**

Not all diets marketed for enteral tube feeding use are nutritionally complete and balanced, therefore prior to feeding the enteral diet should be checked to determine if it meets the patient's needs (Parker, 2013). Commercially available life stage or therapeutic diets can be made into blended foods with the addition of an equal amount of water and then straining the diet to remove large particles, before administering through a feeding tube.

Calorie Requirement

The number of calories provided over a 24-hour period should be sufficient to sustain body functions such as:

- immune function
- wound repair
- cell division and growth.

The use of mathematical formulas is the only practical means of estimating the patient's daily caloric requirement. Historically, illness factors were added to account for a presumed increase in the patient's energy requirements associated with the patient's specific condition/injury.

To avoid overfeeding and its associated complications (e.g. gastrointestinal complications, hepatic dysfunction, increased carbon dioxide production) a more conservative energy estimate is calculated using the patient's resting energy requirement (RER).

RER is defined as **"The amount of energy (calories) required to maintain homeostasis in the fed state in a thermo-neutral environment"** (Haskey, 2019).

Resting Energy Requirement

The amount fed is calculated from the caloric density of the diet (a diet with the desired caloric density should be chosen) and the patients' resting energy requirements.

The diet should be introduced slowly to prevent problems due to hyperosmolarity. If patients have not had a period of malnutrition, then they can be offered 50% of their RER on day one to start with and then this can be increased to 100% RER on day two.

To reduce the risk of refeeding syndrome, anorexic patients should be fed using the guidelines shown in Table 12.

Table 12. Guidelines to feed anorexic patients.

Period of malnutrition	Percentage of RER fed			
	Day 1	Day 2	Day 3	Day 4
<3 days	50%	100%	–	–
3–5 days	33%	66%	100%	–
>5 days	25%	50%	75%	100%

Feeds should be split equally into 4–5 meals per day, with 4–6 hours between meals. Usually, the first day is divided into 6–8 feeds and if the patient then tolerates this then the total volume of food is split between 4–6 meals on day two. It is imperative that the volume fed per meal does not exceed the total stomach capacity of the patient. The maximum capacity of the feline stomach is estimated to be 20 ml/kg to ensure that the stomach does not become overextended. However, the gastric capacity of both feline and canine patients can be 45–90 ml/kg retrospectively.

As the normal volume of feline and canine stomachs reduces during periods of anorexia, gastric distention during food reintroduction may result in nausea, regurgitation, and vomiting. Individual meals should therefore not exceed 50% of the total stomach capacity of the patient and thus **the volume of food per meal should not exceed 10–15 ml/kg during the reintroduction phase.**

Maintenance water requirements are administered in the same number of feeds. However, care should be taken to prevent gastric distention. Daily water requirements are usually met with the water used to flush the feeding tube prior and post feeding, dilution of the food, the moisture content of the diet and or from voluntary intake/intravenous fluid therapy.

Recording and Calculation of Amount Fed

It is important to record each meal along with any complications, and all clinical staff should be aware of the patient's nutritional plan. This can be achieved by an enteral feeding chart.

An example of formulation of a feeding plan using the chart on Figure 26 is shown for the patient below.

Many patients will voluntarily drink or receive IVFT if they are unable to or to treat dehydration. Water administered by the above routes is therefore deducted from the nutritional calculation.

Example 1: Alfie

Alfie is a 2-year-old male neutered Devon Rex weighing 4 kg who has undergone maxilla surgery following a fracture. An oesophagostomy tube was placed at the time of surgery and Alfie has not eaten properly for two days. Alfie is currently being administered Hartman's solution intravenously at a rate of 8 ml/hr (maintenance rate) which the veterinary surgeon would like to continue for at least three days. A specific liquid enteral diet will be chosen. In this case the diet chosen is Royal Canin Recovery Liquid™ (1 kcal/ml).

Calculate Alfie's RER

RER formula used:

Patient is >2 kg = 30 × Body Weight (kg) + 70
= 30 × 4 + 70
= 190 kcal/24 hr

Calculate the amount to be fed in a 24-hour period

RER = 190 kcal/24 hr

Energy density of feed is 1 kcal/ml

Amount fed = RER (kcal/24 hours)/energy density of feed (ml)

Amount fed = 190 = 190 ml/24 hr

Enteral Feeding Chart

Weight at admission: **5** kg Diet chosen for enteral feeding: **Waltham Support**

BW <2 kg RER (Kcal/day) = body weight $^{0.75}$ × 70

BW >2 kg RER (Kcal/day) = 30 × body weight + 70

For both calculations please ensure that the patients´actual weight is used and not their "ideal" weight.

RER = **200** Kcal/day. Divide by the caloric density of selected food.

Caloric density of fook = **1.3** Kcal/ml

Total Kcal/day (ml) = RER/Caloric density of selected food = **190** Kcal/day (ml)

Total daily feed volumen	Day 1: Feed 1/3 total daily volumen	= **66.7**	ml/day
	Day 2: Feed 2/3 total daily volumen	= **133**	ml/day
	Day 3: Feed total daily volume	= **200**	ml/day
Daily water requirement	48 ml/kg/day (2 ml/kg/hr)	= **210**	ml/day

Day and date	**Body weight (kg)** Record daily to ensure changes are noted	**Time of feed**	**Food** (as made up, in ml)	**Water (ml)**	**Flush (Pre) 5 ml**	**Flush (Post) 5 ml**	**Comments** Any residual food on aspiration (record volumen), any complications noted during feeding (e.g. swallowing, lip smacking, nausea, regurgitation)
Day 1	5	08:00	13.3	29.9	5	5	
		12:00	13.3	29.9	5	5	
		16:00	13.3	29.9	5	5	
		20:00	13.3	29.9	5	5	
		24:00	13.3	29.9	5	5	
Day 2	5	08:00	26.6	19.8	5	5	
		12:00	26.6	19.8	5	5	
		16:00	26.6	19.8	5	5	
		20:00	26.6	19.8	5	5	
		24:00	26.6	19.8	5	5	
Day 3	5	08:00	40	9.6	5	5	
		12:00	40	9.6	5	5	
		16:00	40	9.6	5	5	
		20:00	40	9.6	5	5	
		24:00	40	9.6	5	5	

Figure 26. Enteral feeding chart.

As Alfie has not eaten for at least two days the total amount will be slowly introduced over a 3-day period. Feeding 1/3 on day 1; 2/3 on day 2 and the full amount on day 3.

Calculating total amount on day 1

Total amount to be fed is 190 ml. As 1/3 of this amount is being fed, this should be multiplied by 0.33 (33/100 = 33%) or 1/3 = 0.3.

Total volume to be fed on day 1 = 190 x 0.33 = 62.7 ml

This volume is then divided into 6–8 meals. In this case the volume to be fed is divided into 6 meals.

Therefore 62.7/6 = 10.4 ml per meal

Calculate the total amount required for day 2

Total amount to be fed is ⅔ RER of 190 ml.

Therefore, the total volume to be fed on day 2 = 190 × 0.66 = 125.4 ml/24 hr

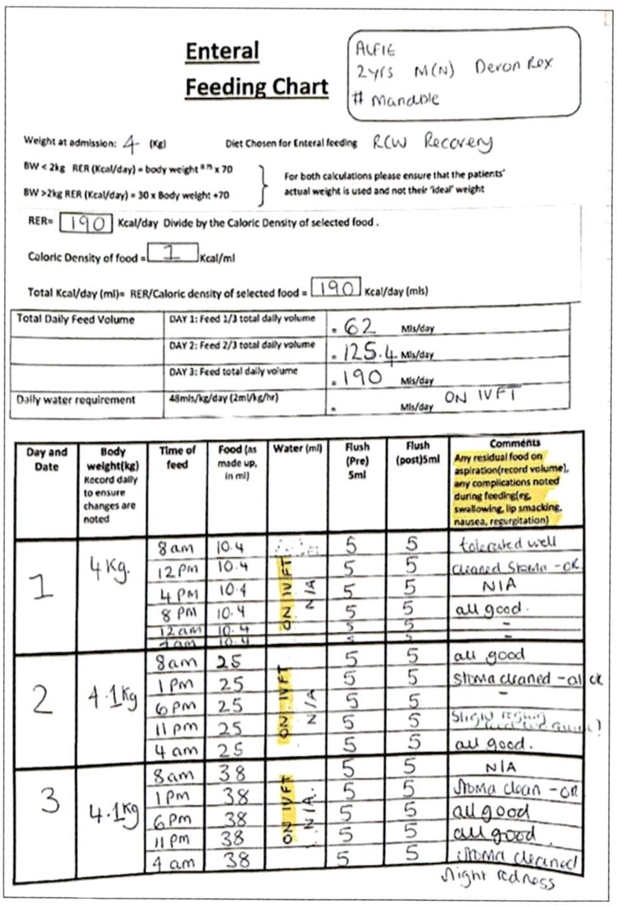

Enteral Feeding Chart

ALFIE
2yrs M(N) Deron Rex
Mandible

Weight at admission: 4 (Kg) Diet Chosen for Enteral feeding RCW Recovery

BW < 2kg RER (Kcal/day) = body weight $^{0.75}$ x 70
BW >2kg RER (Kcal/day) = 30 x Body weight +70
For both calculations please ensure that the patients' actual weight is used and not their 'ideal' weight

RER= 190 Kcal/day Divide by the Caloric Density of selected food.

Caloric Density of food = 1 Kcal/ml

Total Kcal/day (ml)= RER/Caloric density of selected food = 190 Kcal/day (mls)

Total Daily Feed Volume	DAY 1: Feed 1/3 total daily volume	= 62 Mls/day
	DAY 2: Feed 2/3 total daily volume	= 125.4 Mls/day
	DAY 3: Feed total daily volume	= 190 Mls/day
Daily water requirement	48mls/kg/day (2ml/kg/hr)	= Mls/day ON IVFT

Day and Date	Body weight(kg) Record daily to ensure changes are noted	Time of feed	Food (as made up, in ml)	Water (ml)	Flush (Pre) 5ml	Flush (post)5ml	Comments Any residual food on aspiration(record volume), any complications noted during feeding(eg, swallowing, lip smacking, nausea, regurgitation)
1	4 Kg.	8 am	10.4	ON IVFT N/A	5	5	tolerated well
		12 PM	10.4		5	5	cleaned Stoma - OK
		4 PM	10.4		5	5	N/A
		8 PM	10.4		5	5	all good.
		12 am	10.4		5	5	–
		4 am	10.4		5	5	–
2	4.1Kg	8am	25	ON IVFT N/A	5	5	all good
		1 PM	25		5	5	stoma cleaned - all ok
		6 PM	25		5	5	–
		11 pm	25		5	5	Slight [illegible]
		4 am	25		5	5	all good.
3	4.1Kg	8am	38	ON IVFT N/A	5	5	N/A
		1 PM	38		5	5	Stoma clean - OK
		6 PM	38		5	5	all good
		11 PM	38		5	5	all good
		4 am	38		5	5	stoma cleaned slight redness

Figure 27. Enteral feeding chart for Alfie.

Presuming Alfie tolerates tube feeding well on day 1 this volume can then divide into 4–5 meals. In this case the volume to be fed will be divided into 5 meals.

Therefore 125.4/5 = 25 ml/per meal

Calculate the total amount fed per meal on day 3

The total volume to be fed is 100% RER of 190 ml.

This volume is then divided into 5 meals.

Therefore 190/5 = 38 ml per meal

Example 2: Rosie

Rosie, a 5 kg Dachshund that is not receiving IVFT and not voluntarily drinking. She requires a feeding plan for an oesophageal tube placement as she has been anorexic for four days. The food of choice is Royal Canin Waltham Convalescence Support instant feed.

Calculate Rosie's RER

RER = 30 × BW + 70
= 30 × 5 + 70 = 220 kcal/day

Calculate the volume of feed per day

The 50 g sachet of food requires reconstituting with 150 ml of water to make a 200 ml feed, which has an energy density of 1.1 kcal/ml (indicated by the packet).

Therefore: RER/calorific energy density of food
= 220/1.1 = 200 ml/day

Calculate the volume of food required per meal per day and the daily water requirement

For day 1. 1/3 of the RER will be fed.

So: **200 x 0.33 = 66 ml per 24 hrs**

For day 2. 2/3 of the RER will be fed.

So: **200 x 0.66 = 132 ml per 24 hrs**

For day 3. **The full RER amount is fed = 200 ml/24 hrs**

Presuming Rosie tolerates tube feeding well on day 1 this volume is then divided into 4–5 meals. In this case the volume to be fed will be divided into five meals.

Daily water requirement: 50 ml/kg/day = 50 x 5 = 250 ml/day

Table 13. Rosie´s daily feed and water requirement.

Total daily volume to feed	Day 1	Day 2	Day 3	Daily water requirement
= RER/ Caloric density of diet	Feed 1/3 daily feed volume	Feed 2/3 daily feed volume	Feed total volume of daily RER requirement	50 ml/kg/day
= 220/1.1 = 200 ml/day	66 ml/day	133 ml/day	200 ml/day	250 ml/day
Volume of food fed per meal	13.2 ml (66/5)	26.6 ml (133/5)	40 ml (200/5)	–

Calculate the volume of water to administer with each feed

Firstly, the moisture content of the chosen diet should be calculated. To reconstitute the pack 200 ml of water needs to be added.

But the unconstructed moisture content which is 4% (as stated on the 50 g packet) should also be consulted on the packet. Therefore, to calculate the volume of water contained in a non-reconstituted packet multiply the unconstructed moisture content by the weight of the packet.

4% is the same as 4/100 = 0.04

0.04 x 50 g = 2 ml of water is part of the moisture content of a 50 g packet

However, 150 ml of water was required to reconstitute the packet. So, we need to add this to the moisture content of the packet. Therefore, 152 ml of water is provided via the food.

So, for each 50 g packet that is reconstituted to make 200 ml of food what is the volume of water per ml?

152 ml/200 ml = 0.76 ml of water per reformulated diet.

Then the total volume of water provided by the diet per day should be calculated (Table 14). To calculate this, multiply the total volume of feed required per day by the volume of water per reformulated diet.

Table 14. Total volume of water provided by the diet.

	Total volume of feed	Volume of water per reformulated	Total volume of water provided by the diet
Day 1	66	0.76 ml	**50 ml**
Day 2	133	0.76 ml	**101 ml**
Day 3	200	0.76 ml	**152 ml**

Now the volume of additional water to add to the feed should be calculated.

The total volume of water the patient requires per day is 250 ml. For this example, look at day 1.

On day 1 the volume of water provided by the diet is 50 ml. So, by subtracting this volume from the total volume per day the volume of water to add to the feed can be calculated.

250-50 ml = 200 ml required

The volume of flush used before and after feeding should also be considered.

In this case 10 ml in total is used per feed (5 ml pre- and 5 ml postfeed) over five feeds.

Therefore, 10 ml x 5 feeds = 50 ml total flushing volume

The total flushing volume should then be subtracted from the total volume added.

200-50 ml = 150 ml

This total volume is then divided into the number of meals. In this case 5, which results in the total volume of water which is required to be added to each meal

150/5 = 30 ml

Therefore, if the above calculation is applied to day 2 and 3 then:

Table 15. Calculations for total volume of water to be added to food based on five meals per day.

Total daily volume of food	Total volume of food per 5 meals	Total daily volume of water	Total volume of water to be added to food per 5 meals
66	13.2 ml	150 ml	30 ml
133	26.6 ml	99 ml	20 ml
200	40 ml	48 ml	9.6 ml

It is important each meal is recorded along with any complications and that all clinical staff are aware of the patient's nutritional plan. This can be achieved by an enteral feeding chart.

The patient should be tube fed until they are voluntarily eating over 85% of their daily RER and then withdrawn gradually over 2–3 days so that metabolic and gastric adjustments can occur. Ensuring the patient receives adequate nutritional requirements is more important than simply the period of transition to voluntary feeding and thus withholding tube feeds so that the patient becomes hungry is not appropriate in most cases.

If the patient is not tolerating bolus feeds, then another option is to place the patient on a continuous rate infusion of food via a drip pump or syringe driver. In these situations, the daily RER is calculated and divided by 24 to obtain a rate per hour for administration. It is imperative the patient is closely monitored to prevent complications such as tube displacement which may result in aspiration pneumonia in the case of oesophageal feeding tubes. CRI food administration is therefore not recommended for these types of feeding tubes.

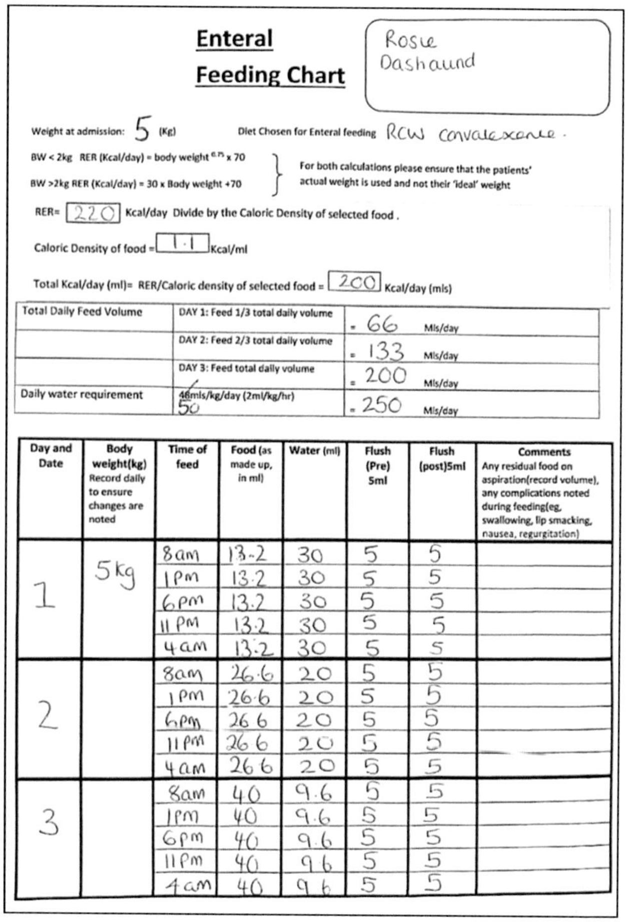

Enteral Feeding Chart

Rosie
Dashaund

Weight at admission: 5 (Kg) Diet Chosen for Enteral feeding RCW convalescence.

BW < 2kg RER (Kcal/day) = body weight $^{0.75}$ x 70
BW >2kg RER (Kcal/day) = 30 x Body weight +70
For both calculations please ensure that the patients' actual weight is used and not their 'ideal' weight

RER= 220 Kcal/day Divide by the Caloric Density of selected food.

Caloric Density of food = 1.1 Kcal/ml

Total Kcal/day (ml)= RER/Caloric density of selected food = 200 Kcal/day (mls)

Total Daily Feed Volume	DAY 1: Feed 1/3 total daily volume	= 66 Mls/day
	DAY 2: Feed 2/3 total daily volume	= 133 Mls/day
	DAY 3: Feed total daily volume	= 200 Mls/day
Daily water requirement	48mls/kg/day (2ml/kg/hr) 50	= 250 Mls/day

Day and Date	Body weight(kg) Record daily to ensure changes are noted	Time of feed	Food (as made up, in ml)	Water (ml)	Flush (Pre) 5ml	Flush (post)5ml	Comments Any residual food on aspiration(record volume), any complications noted during feeding(eg, swallowing, lip smacking, nausea, regurgitation)
1	5kg	8am	13.2	30	5	5	
		1pm	13.2	30	5	5	
		6pm	13.2	30	5	5	
		11pm	13.2	30	5	5	
		4am	13.2	30	5	5	
2		8am	26.6	20	5	5	
		1pm	26.6	20	5	5	
		6pm	26.6	20	5	5	
		11pm	26.6	20	5	5	
		4am	26.6	20	5	5	
3		8am	40	9.6	5	5	
		1pm	40	9.6	5	5	
		6pm	40	9.6	5	5	
		11pm	40	9.6	5	5	
		4am	40	9.6	5	5	

Figure 28. Enteral feeding chart for Rosie.

Parenteral Nutrition

Calories can be provided by a balance of:

- fat
- amino acids
- dextrose.

The selection of lipid to dextrose ratio should take into consideration parenteral nutrition solutions and the patient's hepatic state (metabolic state). As with enteral feeding, **a high percentage of lipids are chosen because free fatty acids provide the main fuel** in the patient in a catabolic state.

The recommended amount of protein in parenteral nutrition solutions ranges from 3–6 g/100 kcal and the amount of protein used depends on the patient's ability to discard products formed from protein breakdown (i.e. nitrogenous waste). This ability is diminished if the patient shows signs of renal or hepatic dysfunction. The diet should also be selected to meet the protein requirements of the patient.

Solutions used for total parenteral nutrition (TPN) have electrolytes added within the amino acid solution and are generally higher in osmolarity, whereas solutions used for partial parenteral nutrition (PPN) have no added electrolytes to the amino acid solution and therefore have a lower osmolarity. (A solution with a low osmolality has fewer solute particles per litre of solution. A solution with a high osmolarity has more solute particles per litre of solution.)

As TPN solutions have a higher osmolality (very hypertonic) and have an osmolality of >1500 mOsm/l they must be administered via a central line (be administered into a large central vein) to reduce the risk of thrombus formation and phlebitis.

A PPN solution has a lower osmolarity and can therefore be administered via a periphery vein safely and therefore reduces the risk of periphery phlebitis. The osmolality of PPN solutions should be less than 600 mOsm/l. The patient's risk of developing thrombophlebitis depends on the rate of infusion and the solutions osmolality.

Calculating Parenteral Nutrition Administration

Calculating the administration rate of a parenteral infusion is based on combining a fluid therapy calculation and a RER calculation.

The following calculation is based on a commercial parenteral nutrition diet.

- calculate kcal/ml of PN
- calculate RER (or % of RER to feed that day if less)
- calculate the ml per day required of PN using RER/kcal/ml
- calculate the administration rate in ml/hr using ml/day/24 hrs
- adjust other IV fluid rates as needed to prevent overload

Example 1: Indigo

Indigo a 5-year-old F(N) Golden Retriever weighing 25 kg is to be placed on TPN. The veterinary surgeon has chosen a particular commercial premade solution and has asked you to calculate the administration rate for a 24-hour period for day 1. Indigo has been anorexic for five days.

Calculate the kcal/ml of PN

In this example the TPN solution contains 1200 kcal in 1920 ml. So, using a simultaneous equation:

1200 kcal/1920 = 1920 ml/1920

0.63 kcal = 1 ml

Calculate Indigo's RER

Using the formula 30 x BW (kg) + 70

30 x 25 + 70 = 820 kcal/24 hrs

As the aim is to prevent refeeding syndrome, parenteral nutrition will be slowly introduced. Therefore, only 33% of the patient's RER is required on day 1.

Therefore:

RER x 0.33 = 820 x 0.33 = 270 kcal/24 hrs

Calculate the ml per day required of PN using RER/kcal/ml

Total ml of PN required per day = RER/kcal/ml

= 270/0.63 = 178.2 ml

Calculate the administration rate in ml/hr using ml/day/24 hours

Total number of ml per hour = 24 hrs/ total number of ml per day

178.2/24 hours = 7.4 ml/hr

Example 2: Cliff

Calculate the PN administration rate for day 2 for Cliff a 40 kg M(N) German Shepherd. The veterinary surgeon has asked you to use a commercial premade parenteral nutrition which has 1400 kcal in 1920 ml.

Calculate the kcal/ml of PN

So, using a simultaneous equation:

1400 kcal/1920 = 1920 ml/1920

0.73 kcal = 1 ml

Calculate Cliff's RER

30 x 40 + 70 = 1270 kcal/24 hrs

The calculation is for day 2 so only requires 66% of the patients full RER.

1270 x 0.66 = 838 kcal/24 hrs

Calculate the ml per day required of PN using RER/kcal/ml

Total ml of PN required per day = RER

kcal/ml = 838/0.73 = 1148 ml

Calculate the administration rate in ml/hr using ml/day/24 hours

Total number of ml per hour x 24 = Total number of ml per day

47.8 ml/hr over 24 hrs = 1148 ml

References

■ Adams, D., Quayum, M., Worthington, T., Lambert, P. and Elliott, T. (2005) Evaluation of a 2% chlorhexidine gluconate in 70% isopropyl alcohol skin disinfectant. *Journal of Hospital Infection*, 61 (4), 287-290.

■ Armitage Chan, E.A., O'Toole, T., and Chan, D.L. (2006) Management of prolonged food deprivation, hypothermia, and refeeding syndrome in a cat. *Journal of Veterinary Emergency and Critical Care*, 16, S34-S41.

■ Baines, S. (1996) Surgical asepsis: principles and protocols. *In Practice*, 18(1), 23-33.

■ Brown, D.C. (2012) Wound infections and antimicrobial use. *Veterinary Surgery, Small Animal. Elsevier Saunders, Missouri*, 135-139.

■ Chan D. (2015) *Estimating Energy Requirements of Small Animal Patients. Nutritional Management of Hospitalised Small Animals*. Chapter 2. Wiley Blackwell, pp. 10–12.

■ DeAvilla, M.D. and Leech, E.B. (2016) Hypoglycemia associated with refeeding syndrome in a cat. *Journal of Veterinary Emergency and Critical Care*, 26 (6), 798–803.

■ Dugdale, A. (2010) Hypothermia: Consequences and prevention. In: *Veterinary Anesthesia Principles to practice.* Wiley-Blackwell, p. 179.

■ EClinPath (2020) Cornell University College of Veterinary Medicine. Available from: https://eclinpath.com/

■ Ehrhart, N. (1998) Principles of tumor biopsy. *Clinical Techniques in Small Animal Practice*, 13 (1), 10–16.

■ Elliott, D.A. (2004) Parenteral Nutrition, *World Small Animal Veterinary Association World Congress Proceeding.* https://www.fresenius-kabi.com/us/products/parenteral-nutrition

■ Fusion, C. (2010) ChloraPrep. *Patient Preoperative Skin Preparation CHL089a* Available from: www.chloraprep.co.uk [Accessed 13 June, 2012].

■ Gasson, J. (2007) Theatre Practice course notes. *Improve International Ltd: Swindon.*

■ Greenwell, C.M., Epstein, S.E., and Brain, P.H. (2014) Influence of needle gauge used for venipuncture on automated platelet count and coagulation profile in dogs. *Australian veterinary journal*, 92 (3), 71–74.

■ Gwaltney-Brant, S.M. (2021) Nutraceuticals in hepatic diseases. In *Nutraceuticals*. Academic Press, pp. 117–129.

■ Hayton-Lee, E. (2015) How to provide nursing care to the surgical ophthalmic patient. *The Veterinary Nurse*, 6 (1), 41–45.

■ Jackson, K. (2011) An introduction to magnetic resonance imaging. *Veterinary Nursing Journal*, 26 (11), 390–392.

■ Keane, M., Paul, E., Sturrock, C.J., Rauch, C., and Rutland, C.S. (2017) Computed tomography in veterinary medicine: Currently published and tomorrow's vision. *Computed Tomography-Advanced Applications*, 271–289.

■ Lumbis, R. H. (2017) How to place commonly used feeding tubes in dogs and cats. *Veterinary Nurse*, 8 (2), 104–115.

■ Mazzaferro, E.M. (2009) Arterial Catheterization. *Small Animal Critical Care Medicine.* St. Louis, Elsevier Saunders, pp. 206–208.

■ Mazzaferro, E.M. and Hauser, C. (2012) Arterial puncture and catheterization. In: *Advanced monitoring and procedures for small animal emergency and critical care*, 69–81.

■ McMillan, S. (2014) An evidence-based approach to infection control in the operating theatre. *The Veterinary Nurse*, 5 (4), 194–200.

■ Merrill, L. ed. (2012) *Small animal internal medicine for veterinary technicians and nurses.* John Wiley & Sons.

■ Mosing, M. (2016) General principles of perioperative care. In: T. Duke-Novakovski, M. de Vries and C. Seymour, ed., *BSAVA Manual of Canine and Feline Anaesthesia and Analgesia*, 3rd ed. Gloucester, BSAVA, p. 21.

■ O'Dwyer, L. (2016) Nursing notes: presurgery fasting and anesthesia. *Vet Times*, 16 (12), p. 19. https://www.vettimes.co.uk

■ Owen, L. (2007) Surgical wound infections: controlling contamination. *Veterinary Times*, pp. 14–15.

■ Renberg, W.C. (2012) Preparation of the patient, operating team, and operating room. *Veterinary Surgery Small Animal.* St. Louis, MO: Elsevier Saunders, pp. 164–170.

■ Reynolds, H. and Nichols, A. (2019) Which skin preparation technique is most effective to minimise bacterial contamination? *The Veterinary Nurse*, 10 (3), 162–166.

■ Savvas, I., Rallis, T. and Raptopoulos, D. (2009) The effect of pre-anaesthetic fasting time and type of food on gastric content volume and acidity in dogs. *Veterinary Anaesthesia and Analgesia*, 36 (6), 539–546.

■ Seim, H.B. (2004) Feeding Tube Placement, *World Small Animal Veterinary Association World Congress Proceedings.*

■ Sirois, M. (2020) *Laboratory procedures for veterinary technicians.* 7th Ed. St. Louis, Missouri, p. 433.

■ Solbak, S., Epstein, S.E. and Hopper, K. (2019) Influence of needle gauge used for venipuncture on measures of hemostasis in cats. *Journal of feline medicine and surgery*, 21 (2), 143–147.

■ Sumner, C. (2021) *Refeeding syndrome.* MSPCA Angell West. Available from: www.angell.org/emergencyemergency@angell.org

■ Thomovsky, E., Backus, R., Reniker, A., Mann, F.A. and Dodam, J.R. (2007) Parenteral nutrition: formulation, monitoring, and complications. *Compend Contin Educ Vet*, 29 (2), 88–102.

■ Villiers, E. and Blackwood, L. (2015) *BSAVA Manual of canine and feline clinical pathology*, 2nd ed. Gloucester, British Small Animal Veterinary Association,

■ Warner, C. (1988) Skin preparation in the surgical patient. *Journal of the National Medical Association*, 80 (8), 899–904.

■ Williams, M. (2000) Aseptic skin preparation revisited. *British Journal of Perioperative Nursing* 10 (7), 364–72.

■ Weber, D.J., Rutala, W.A. and Sickbert-Bennett, E.E. (2007) Outbreaks associated with contaminated antiseptics and disinfectants. *Antimicrobial agents and chemotherapy*, 51 (12), 4217–4224.

■ Yokoyama, M., Nakahara, K., Kojima, M., Hosoda, H., Kangawa, K. and Murakami, N. (2005) Influencing the between-feeding and endocrine responses of plasma ghrelin in healthy dogs. *European journal of endocrinology*, 152 (1), 155–160.

Test

Answers on Page 140

1. Brick red mucus membranes are an indication of early shock, sepsis and or systemic inflammatory response syndrome (SIRS).

a. True.
b. False.

2. What is paradoxical respiration?

a. Abnormal movement of the diaphragm during respiration.
b. Short and shallow breath sounds.
c. Loud breath sounds.
d. Normal movement of the diaphragm.

3. In paradoxical respiration, the chest moves outwards during inspiration and inwards during expiration.

a. True.
b. False.

4. A 4% solution of chlorhexidine is made by making a 40:100 solution.

a. True.
b. False.

5. How often should clipper blades be oiled during operation?

a. Every 10 minutes.
b. Every 30 minutes.
c. Every 60 minutes.
d Every 24 hours.

6. What are the 5 key steps that make up the framework of the nursing process?

a. Assigning, Diagnosis, Planning, Implying, Evaluation.
b. Analysis, Deciding, Planning, Investigation, Evaluation.
c. Assessment, Diagnosis, Plan, Implementation, Evaluation.
d. Analysis, Diagnosis, Plan, Implementation, Evaluation.

7. The Ability Model is based on establishing how many patient abilities?

a. 5.
b. 10.
c. 12.
d. 15.

8. What is the physiological reasoning why padding the cranial aspect of the hind limbs appropriately is important during perineal surgeries?

a. Prevents femoral nerve damage.
b. To raise the patient.
c. To secure the patient's positioning.
d. To insulate the patient.

9. Parenteral nutrition provides direct nutrition to the enterocytes.

a. True.
b. False.

10. Horner's syndrome is a common complication following oesophagostomy placement.

a. True.
b. False.

Correct answers

1. a
2. a
3. b. In paradoxical respiration, the chest moves inward during inspiration, and outward during expiration.
4. b. A 50:50 solution using 4% chlorhexidine will give a solution of 4%.
5. a
6. c
7. b
8. a
9. b
10. a

Notes

Anaesthesia

Nicki Grint

Chapter Summary:

- **Blood products, fluid replacement options, and acid/base balance.**
- **Fluid administration calculations.**
- **Understanding and completion of client consent forms, patient anaesthesia records.**
- **Familiarity with the pros and cons of different preanaesthetic, induction, and maintenance agents.**
- **Types of endotracheal tubes and their uses, basic intubation techniques, and difficult intubations.**
- **Basic to advanced monitoring techniques, including pulse oximetry and capnography waveforms.**

Preanaesthesia Considerations

Consent for Anaesthesia or Sedation

In veterinary practice it often **falls on the nurse to gain the owner's consent for anaesthesia,** sedation, and medical or surgical procedures. This consent can be oral or written, although written is preferred in case of a future dispute.

There are two different types of consent:
1. **Implied: by the owner's cooperation during the consultation or physical examination of the patient.**
2. **Express: the owner is made aware of material risks and gives permission to proceed.**

Whether the consent is oral or written, it must be informed, which means the owner must understand:
- the nature of the proposed procedure or treatment
- the financial implications
- the principal risks and side effects.

The consent form should:
- specify all likely procedures
- carry an estimate of costs
- contain a reference to any unauthorized or unlicensed medications likely to be used
- include the owner's contact telephone number, where they can be contacted urgently to discuss treatment options
- provision for the vet or veterinary nurse to act without the client's consent, if necessary, in the interests of the patient
- consent (where appropriate) for preanaesthetic blood tests.

Preanaesthetic Blood Tests

The Association of Veterinary Anaesthetists advise that **a thorough history and clinical exam are an essential part of the preoperative risk assessment,** but the routine use of preanaesthetic blood tests is not necessarily beneficial for low-risk patients (Hall et al., 2001).

So, in general, **if the patient is young, fit and healthy, with no abnormalities on clinical exam or history, then preanaesthetic bloods are not indicated.** If a problem is identified from the patient's history, clinical exam, or signalment (this includes advanced age), owners should be guided by the vet's recommendation and advised of the likely costs involved.

Anaesthesia Risks

Data collected by Brodbelt et al., (2008) during the CEPSAF (The Confidential Enquiry into Perioperative Small Animal Fatalities) survey indicate that the risk of perianaesthetic death varies depending on species and health status (Table 1).

Table 1. Risk of death associated with anaesthesia in the dog and cat.

	Dog	Cat
ASA 1-2 (healthy)	0.05%	0.11%
ASA 3-5 (diseased)	1.33%	1.4%

Where possible, a copy of the consent form should be given to the person signing it. **The signed consent form becomes part of the clinical record,** and any subsequent amendments should be made in ink, initialled, and dated, with a note of subsequent conversations recorded on the clinical records. Consent forms must be kept in a locked cabinet or, if scanned, in a password protected database.

Anaesthetic Records

The anaesthetic record is often the sole documentation of an anaesthetist's interaction with their patient. Anaesthetic records are:

- a medical record and communication tool
- a template which facilitates the anaesthetist's efficient documentation of patient care
- a way to "tell the story" from preinduction period to recovery period
- a method of communicating the care given and complications encountered to other staff
- legal documents which can provide evidence in a variety of settings
- useful for research and quality assurance purposes.

Preanaesthetic Medication

Preanaesthetic medication (premed) is used for a variety of reasons:

- **anxiety reduction:** making the patient more amenable to handling for intravenous catheterisation and subsequent anaesthesia induction
- **smoother anaesthesia induction** which means a reduced dose of anaesthetic agent
- **smoother maintenance phase of anaesthesia,** with reduction in the percentage of volatile agent required
- **smoother recovery from anaesthesia**
- **preemptive analgesia**
- provides muscle relaxation.

Drugs are usually injected, either by subcutaneous, intramuscular, or intravenous injection. **The route of drug administration influences the speed of onset of the drug** and the intensity of the drug's effects, hence why the oral route is rarely used for premedication. Once the drug is administered, the animal should be left undisturbed for the time it takes for the drug to achieve its peak effect. However, during this waiting time, animals should be monitored unobtrusively.

Different drug combinations have different effects and are selected according to what premedication need to achieve, such as heavy sedation in a vicious dog or calming a brachycephalic animal whilst avoiding excessive sedation. The drugs below are those most commonly used in veterinary practice but can be combined for greater effect. Opioids are commonly used premeds and can be added to any of the drugs below, however, they are discussed more fully in the analgesia chapter.

Phenothiazines

Acepromazine (ACP) is a drug belonging to the phenothiazine drug group. It is most commonly administered with opioids. Acepromazine causes sedation and some anxiolysis. There is no antagonist for this drug.

Once absorbed, ACP affects several different receptors and has several actions:

- antiadrenergic (α-1 adrenoceptor blockade) which causes vasodilation
- antidopaminergic
- anticholinergic
- antihistaminic
- antiserotonergic
- antithrombotic.

Phenothiazines are highly protein bound. They undergo hepatic metabolism and are then excreted in urine and bile.

The dose of acepromazine should be reduced in the following scenarios:

- age: the very old and very young
- renal disease
- hepatic disease
- hypovolaemia
- congestive heart disease
- brachycephalic animals.

α-2 Adrenergic Agonists

Medetomidine (1 mg/ml) and dexmedetomidine (0.5 mg/ml) (medetomidine's active isomer) are α-2 adrenergic agonists.

These injectable drugs can be administered intravenously, intramuscularly, or subcutaneously. They can be combined with opioids and with ketamine for more profound sedation. When these drugs bind to the α-2 adrenoceptors in an animal's central nervous system, they produce anxiolysis, profound sedation, and analgesia. Other effects include:

- muscle relaxation
- bradycardia
- blood pressure effects: initial hypertension, then reduction in blood pressure to near normal blood pressure
- emesis
- reduction in gastrointestinal tract motility
- increases in uterine activity
- diuresis.

Atipamezole (Antisedan®) is an antagonist, specifically for the antagonism of medetomidine and dexmedetomidine. In dogs, an equal volume of atipamezole to that of the medetomidine used is administered, whereas in cats, half the volume is used. Intramuscular administration is the most commonly used route.

α-2 adrenergic agonists are relatively contraindicated or used at much reduced doses in the following cases:

- neonates
- elderly patients
- renal disease
- hepatic disease
- hypovolaemia
- congestive heart disease
- brachycephalic animals.

Benzodiazepines

Diazepam (5 mg/ml) and midazolam (5 mg/ml) are commonly used for veterinary anaesthesia in small animal species. Midazolam is twice as potent as diazepam and shorter acting. These drugs provide no analgesia, but are used for the following reasons:

- anticonvulsant
- anxiolysis
- sedation in certain animals
- skeletal muscle relaxation.

At clinical doses, benzodiazepines cause few cardiovascular or respiratory effects. They can be used as premedicants, especially in very young or very old animals, and combined with opioids for more profound sedation. Benzodiazepines are a useful adjunct to ketamine anaesthesia, to reduce the muscle rigidity which occurs when ketamine is used alone. They can also be used as co-induction agents, i.e. as an intravenous injection just before the induction agent, to reduce the amount of induction agent required. As premedicants in fit, healthy animals, they have the potential to cause excitement, as animals become disinhibited.

Benzodiazepines bind to benzodiazepine binding sites associated with GABA receptors (γ-aminobutyric acid).

Flumazenil and sarmazenil are the specific antagonists available for benzodiazepines.

Oxygen Supplementation

The normal percentage of oxygen in normal atmospheric air is 21% (or 0.21). For animals suffering from respiratory, cardiac, or neurological pathologies, or after trauma, it can be beneficial to increase the concentration of oxygen in inspired air (FiO_2). This aims to improve or prevent hypoxaemia (an abnormally low oxygen content in the blood) and there are several techniques to do this.

Ideally, techniques should:

- increase FiO_2
- not be stressful
- not cause accumulation of CO_2 or humidity
- not dry the airways.

Flow by Oxygen

This technique involves ducting oxygen from a cylinder (e.g. from an anaesthetic machine) through tubing to near the animal's nose and mouth. This is useful if the animal resents a face mask being placed over its nose/mouth and the ensuing struggle further compromises its clinical condition. This technique is wasteful and requires a member of staff to be constantly present.

Face Mask

Face mask, which fits snuggly over the animal's nose and mouth, delivers oxygen via tubing or a breathing system, to a the mask.

Oxygen Hood

A makeshift oxygen hood can be made using an Elizabethan collar placed over the animal's head, with clingfilm covering the open mouth of the collar. Oxygen can be delivered into the hood via tubing or a breathing system attached to an oxygen cylinder. In an emergency the clingfilm can be omitted, as high oxygen flow rates delivered near the animal's nose/mouth still increases inspired oxygen levels above that of room air.

Oxygen Cage

These are appropriate for use in cats and small dogs. Incubators are capable of providing an oxygen enriched environment, although many only deliver inspired oxygen percentages up to a maximum of 40%. Many practices now use collapsible oxygen tents. These have a variety of venturi devices which will deliver different FiO_2 depending on the oxygen flow and the aperture of the device. A makeshift oxygen cage can be created by placing a cat carrier inside a plastic bag into which a high flow of oxygen is delivered.

Nasopharyngeal Catheters

A nasopharyngeal catheter allows oxygen to be delivered into the pharyngeal area. At flow rates of 200 ml/kg/min, FiO_2 can be increased to almost 50% by this means, and even up to 80% with flow rates of 500 ml/kg/min, although the exact inspired oxygen concentration depends on the size of the tube, the oxygen flow rate, the position of the tube tip within the nasopharynx, and the breathing pattern of the animal.

Soft feeding (naso-oesophageal) tubes are preferred, and placed, with the aid of local anaesthetic, into the ventral nasal meatus so that the tip lies in the nasopharynx.

Trans-tracheal

Trans-tracheal oxygen delivery via a needle or catheter is a technique reserved for emergency situations where there is marked upper respiratory obstruction. The needle or catheter is attached to the barrel of a 2 ml syringe which in turn is attached to a breathing system via a 7.5 mm endotracheal tube connector (Figure 1).

Oxygen Humidification

Oxygen directly from a cylinder is cold and dry. When breathed for long periods of time (over a few hours), especially when the upper respiratory tract is bypassed (the nasal passages help warm and moisten inspired air), the oxygen should be humidified. This is easily achieved by bubbling the oxygen through a chamber containing sterile water. Not doing so leads to mucus desiccation and compromise of the airway's mucociliary escalator function.

Oxygen Toxicity

Breathing an oxygen percentage >60% for prolonged periods of time can lead to lung damage due to the generation of free radicals, with subsequent attack of the alveoli. Thus, oxygen therapy with an FiO_2 >60% should only be provided when absolutely necessary, and FiO_2 should be reduced as soon as possible to a level sufficient to prevent hypoxaemia.

Induction of Anaesthesia

Anaesthesia is induced, once the premed has taken effect, with the aim of facilitating endotracheal intubation ready for the maintenance phase of the anaesthetic.

Anaesthesia can be induced via:

- injectable: intravenous
- injectable other: usually intramuscular
- inhalational.

The relative pros and cons of each method are detailed in Table 2.

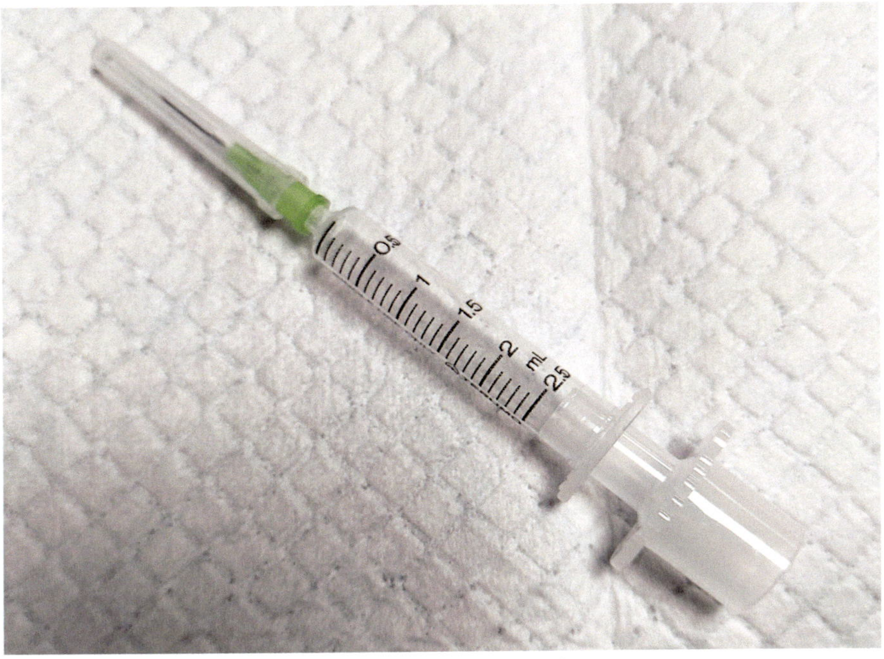

Figure 1. Image of a 2 ml syringe with a 7.5 mm endotracheal tube connector.

Table 2. The pros and cons of different methods of anaesthetic induction.

Intravenous	Intramuscular	Inhalation
Can be titrated to effect.	Whole dose given, unable to give to effect.	Can be titrated to effect.
Effect usually shorter.	Effect usually longer.	Effect usually shorter.
Needs intravenous access.	No special equipment needed.	Volatile agent, mask and oxygen needed.
No pollution potential.	No pollution potential.	Environmental pollution potential.
Rapid induction.	Slower induction.	Slower induction.
Accurate weight needed.	Accurate weight needed.	Accurate weight not needed for induction.

Anaesthetic Agents

Propofol

Propofol is a substituted phenol and is for **intravenous use only.** It is not irritant if injected outside the vein, but may occasionally cause pain on injection. It is formulated in an emulsion consisting of soya bean oil, glycerol, and egg phosphatide. There are formulations with no preservatives where the remainder in the bottle should technically be immediately discarded once opened. Newer formulations contain preservatives, which means once breeched the bottle can be kept for 28 days.

Propofol acts on GABA receptors and is highly protein bound (98%). The drug provides no analgesia. A combination of myocardial depression and dilation of peripheral veins produces hypotension. Splenic engorgement also occurs. Post-induction apnoea may be observed.

In the dog, propofol undergoes rapid hepatic metabolism, primarily through the glucoronidation and hydroxylation pathways. Cats lack the glucoronidation pathway and therefore recovery from propofol anaesthesia is not as rapid. There may also be some sites of metabolism which are not the liver, e.g. the lungs.

In the dog, the drug is not cumulative and can therefore be used to maintain anaesthesia. The drug is not licensed in species other than the dog or cat although is used off licensed in other small animals.

Alfaxalone

Alfaxalone is solubilised in cyclodextrins (sugar ring molecules) and is licensed for use in the cat, the dog and the rabbit, although it has been used off license in several other species.

Alfaxalone can be administered either by intravenous or intramuscular injection (not currently licenced for this route in UK), as it is non-irritant. Preserved (28 day discard) and non-preserved (immediate discard) versions of alfaxalone are available. The drug produces anaesthesia by binding to GABA receptors. It is not highly protein bound (30%). After anaesthesia induction, apnoea is often observed. Reflex tachycardia often occurs in compensation for a decrease in blood pressure (Rodriguez et al., 2012). It is metabolised by the liver and is non-cumulative. It can be infused to maintain anaesthesia.

Ketamine

Ketamine is a member of the phencyclidine group and produces dissociative anaesthesia, Dissociative anaesthesia is characterised by:

- profound analgesia
- light sleep
- amnesia
- trance-like immobility
- poor muscle relaxation
- hypersensitivity to noise
- active cranial nerve reflexes (i.e. palpebral and swallowing reflexes persist)
- occurrence of salivation and lacrimation
- nystagmus which is commonly seen in horses.

Because it causes muscle rigidity and hypersensitivity, ketamine is rarely used alone. However, these effects are offset when ketamine is combined with α-2 adrenergic agonists or benzodiazepines. The drug can be administered intravenously or intramuscularly (often in cats and exotics), although intramuscular injections often sting. The onset of action of this drug is slower than other induction agents and can be up to 1–2 minutes.

Recovery from anaesthesia depends on both hepatic metabolism and redistribution, although the drug is excreted unchanged in the cat. Overall, effects on the cardiovascular system are mildly stimulatory with an increase in heart rate and blood pressure. Occasionally irregular respiratory patterns are observed.

Induction

Inhalational Induction

There are a variety of techniques which facilitate the patient inhaling a volatile agent to induce anaesthesia. However, independent of the technique used, the time taken to intubation is longer than for intravenous induction, and so where possible the latter is preferred.

Chamber Induction

Chamber inductions can be used to induce anaesthesia in cats and other small animals. These chambers can be specially constructed or made from plastic boxes (Figure 2). The box should have a tight seal with an entry portal for fresh gas flow from the anaesthetic machine and exit portal to attach the scavenger hose.

Once the patient is inside the chamber, high flow oxygen can be introduced to acclimatize them to the environment and the volatile agent can be added incrementally. The higher the fresh gas flow, the faster the changes in the percentage of volatile agent are made. The volatile agent should be administered until the animal loses their righting reflex, then turned off and disconnected. The chamber should then be flushed with oxygen, and the animal removed. If required, further volatile agent can be administered by face mask.

Mask Induction

Small animals may be suitable for mask induction, although this technique produces the most environmental pollution. Clear plastic masks with a good fitting rubber seal help to minimize this pollution. Occasionally, patients exhibit involuntary excitement as they progress through the stages of anaesthesia, this can be reduced by a small dose of intravenous induction agent.

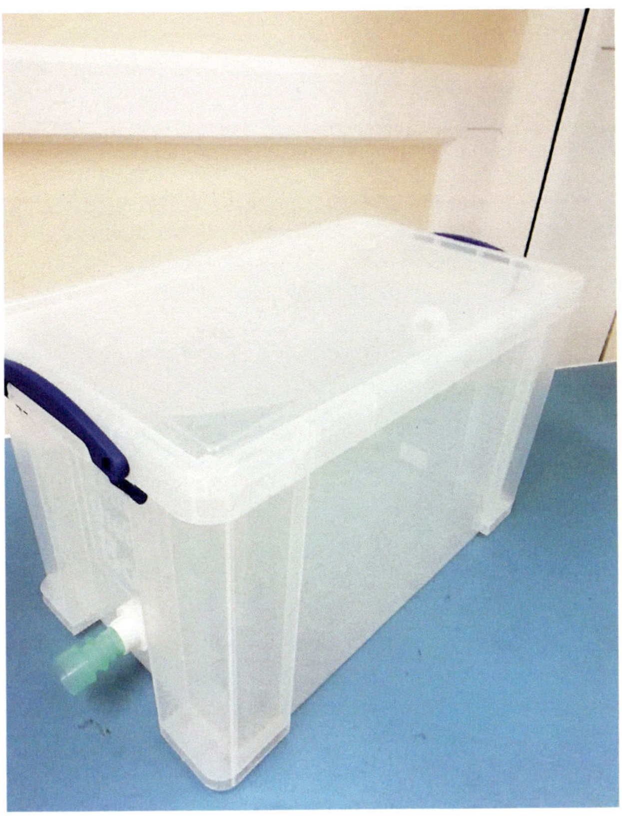

Figure 2. Chamber induction made from a plastic box.

Volatile Agent Choice for Induction of Anaesthesia

An inhalational induction is stressful for the patient, but adequate premedication can help to alleviate this anxiety. All volatile agents can be used for inhalation induction, but the ideal agent has the following properties:

- non-irritant
- nice tasting
- lacking in respiratory depression
- no arrhythmias produced if adrenaline is released
- fast onset of action.

Sevoflurane is the most suitable volatile agent for anaesthetic induction.

Positioning for Induction

Most small animals are held in sternal recumbency for induction, and then intubated in either sternal or lateral recumbency. There are a couple of scenarios where alternative positions are preferable.

Head-up Inductions

This is where the nurse restrains the patient with their head up and keeps it elevated above the level of the thorax until the trachea is intubated and the cuff inflated. This position uses gravity to prevent regurgitation of stomach contents, and is used in patients which haven't been starved, or have a history of regurgitation (e.g. megaoesophagus) or delayed gastric emptying.

Head-flat Inductions

Head flat inductions are useful for animals with neck pain, as it avoids potentially wrenching their neck when held for intubation. It is very important to use this position for any suspected cases of cervical vertebral fractures or dogs with Wobbler syndrome. With this technique, the head is held flat on the table during tracheal intubation. It is technically more demanding due to the more awkward angle, and so it is beneficial to preoxygenate the patient using a mask and use a laryngoscope to aid visualisation.

Endotracheal Intubation in the Dog and Cat

Endotracheal intubation is the process of placing a tube, either via the nose (nasotracheal) or more usually via the mouth (orotracheal), into the trachea.

Endotracheal intubation is performed during general anaesthesia for a variety of reasons:

- to ensure a patent airway in unconscious animals and prevent respiratory obstruction
- to act as a conduit for oxygen, volatile agents and other carrier gases to reach the patient's lungs, and to remove waste gases, i.e. carbon dioxide
- to facilitate intermittent positive pressure ventilation of the patient's lungs
- to protect the animal's airway from aspiration of foreign material
- to protect personnel from exposure to volatile agents.

Endotracheal tubes come in a variety of sizes and materials, including red rubber, PVC, and silicone tubes. The features of these different materials are included in Table 3.

Most tubes have cuffs with pilot balloons attached to them. These cuffs are inflated to create a seal between the tube and the tracheal wall. The purpose of this cuff is to:

- prevent dilution of inspired gases with room air
- prevent pollution of room air with anaesthetic gases
- prevent aspiration (inhalation into the lungs) of fluid or debris.

Over-inflation of the cuff places too much pressure on the tracheal wall mucosa and can cause ischaemia, leading to tissue necrosis. To prevent this, after intubation the nurse should listen for leaks by the patient's mouth, as the reservoir bag is squeezed, until the sound of the leak just disappears.

Some tubes, especially smaller ones, are uncuffed. These tubes are often used in cats, as cases of tracheal rupture in cats due to endotracheal intubation with cuffed tubes have been reported in veterinary literature.

Endotracheal intubation is usually performed in dogs and cats with the vet or vet nurse directly visualizing the larynx. This is aided by a laryngoscope, which is used to depress the tongue and shine a light into the oral cavity.

Before endotracheal intubation, the following equipment should be prepared:

- appropriate sizes of endotracheal tube: one above and one below the predicted size (see Table 4 for sizing guide), in addition:
    - cuff inflation should be checked and the cuff left inflated;
    - cleanliness and patency of tube should be checked;
    - tubes should be lubricated if appropriate (silicone based spray or K-Y jelly);
- the laryngoscope should be checked to ensure it is functioning and is of appropriate size;
- a cuff inflation syringe and bandage to secure the tube in place should be prepared.

Table 3. Features of different types of endotracheal tubes. (Adapted from Hughes. Chapter 5 in BSAVA Manual of Canine and Feline Anaesthesia and Analgesia, 2016).

Feature	Red rubber	PVC	Silicone
Durability	Can be reused but may perish over time	Disposable	May be reused
Repair	No	No	Yes
Sizes	2–16 mm ID	2–11 mm ID	2–16 mm ID
Autoclave	Yes	No	Yes
Withstands kinking	No	Better than red rubber	Better than red rubber
Irritant	Yes	No	No
Expensive	Moderate	Least	Most
Blockage visible	No	Yes	Perhaps
Curved or straight	Curved	Curved	Straight
Ease of insertion	Easy	Easy	May require stylet
Self-sealing pilot balloon	No	Yes	Yes
Cuff type	LV HP	LV HP HV LP	LV HP

HV: high volume, LP: low pressure, LV: low volume, HP: high pressure.

Table 4. Estimates of sizes of endotracheal tubes for different body weights of dogs and cats.

Internal diameter (mm)	Approximate lean body weight (kg)
2.0, 2.5, 3.0	1–2.5
3.5, 4.0, 4.5	2.5–5
5, 6	4–9
7, 8	7–15
9, 10	15–25
11, 12	25–45
14, 16	>40

At the end of an anaesthetic the patient is extubated. In the dog, this is when the dog starts to swallow. If any debris or haemorrhage is present in the mouth, ahead of extubation, this should be removed by swabbing or suction and the cuff left inflated until the swallowing is brisk. At this point the cuff should be partially deflated before extubation. Patients with raised intra-cranial pressure concerns benefit from an early extubation (at first swallow) to avoid them coughing or gagging on the endotracheal tube.

Due to cats increased mucosal sensitivity and predisposition to laryngospasm, the tube should be removed slightly earlier than in the dog; when a brisk palpebral movement, ear twitching or any movement is noted.

Maintenance of Anaesthesia

Anaesthesia is maintained using injectable drugs or inhalational agents.

Injectable Agents

Propofol, alfaxalone, and ketamine are commonly used agents capable of maintaining anaesthesia. Drugs are administered intravenously by top up, intermittent bolus injections, or by a constant rate infusion (CRI). If these drugs are the sole maintenance agents (i.e. no volatile agents are used) this is called TIVA (total intravenous anaesthesia).

Volatile Agents

Volatile agents are converted from a liquid state into a gas (using a vaporiser), which is added to the oxygen in the anaesthetic machine. This gas mixture is delivered through a breathing system to the patient, either via a mask or an endotracheal tube. When inhaled into the lungs, volatile agents (e.g. isoflurane, sevoflurane and desflurane) produce and maintain anaesthesia in all species. These agents all produce similar effects and side effects on the physiological processes of the body, although to differing degrees. See Table 5.

Table 5. Characteristics of different volatile agents.

	Isoflurane	Sevoflurane	Desflurane
Respiratory depression	++	++	++
Vasodilation	++	++	++
Myocardial depression	+	+	+
Arrhythmogenic	-	-	-
Blood gas solubility	Low (++)	Low (+)	Very low
MAC	1.3%	2.5%	7.2%
Liver metabolism	0.2%	2%	0.02%
Odour / taste	Unpleasant	OK	OK
Hepatic blood flow	++	+	+

Key = - : reduced, + : increased, MAC: minimum alveolar concentration.

Blood Gas Solubility

This property dictates how **quickly or slowly the volatile agent takes effect.** The lower an agent's blood gas solubility, the faster its onset of action, the quicker the changes in the depth of anaesthesia, and the faster the patient recovers from anaesthesia.

MAC

MAC stands for minimum alveolar concentration. This is the end tidal concentration of an agent at which 50% of patients fail to respond to a standard noxious stimulus (e.g. skin incision). MAC is an indicator of potency. The lower the MAC of an agent, the more potent it is (i.e. it causes an effect at a lower percentage).

Nitrous Oxide

Nitrous oxide (N_2O) is an anaesthetic gas, usually used as a carrier gas, alongside oxygen. **It cannot be used as a sole anaesthetic agent,** as its MAC is greater than 100% The benefits of use are that it is a potent analgesic and reduces the MAC of the other volatile agents used.

Nitrous oxide should not be used in certain clinical situations. Including this gas as a carrier gas decreases the percentage of oxygen inspired by the patient, which may be detrimental to some patients with respiratory disease. Nitrous oxide also diffuses very quickly into air filled spaces, and increases their volume substantially. Nitrous oxide should be discontinued five minutes before the patient is disconnected from the oxygen supply to prevent diffusion hypoxia. Due to nitrous oxide's environmental effects as a greenhouse gas, the use of this gas in clinical practice is diminishing.

Intravenous Fluid Therapy

Fluid Compartments

Water makes up 60% of an adult's total weight, whilst total body water is divided into **extracellular and intracellular fluid** (ECF and ICF respectively) (see Figure 3).

Extracellular fluid generally occupies two regions of the body; as plasma in the blood (intravascular volume) and as fluid which bathes the cells in the rest of the body (interstitial fluid).

There is an additional category of transcellular fluid, e.g. synovial and CSF (cerebrospinal fluid), which only comprises a very small percentage of the total body water and is therefore not considered further.

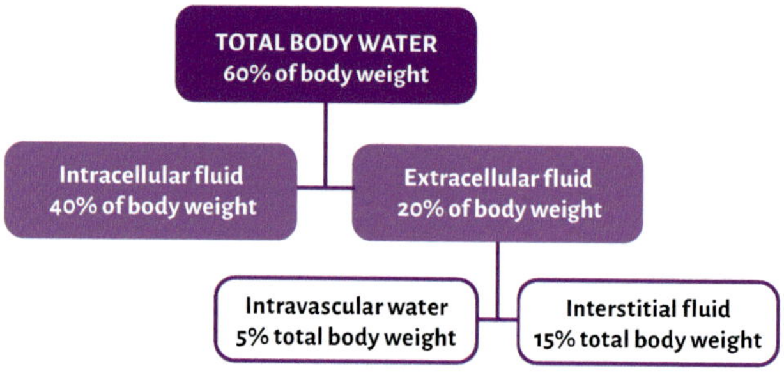

Figure 3. Total body water is subdivided between intracellular and extracellular fluid.

Types of Fluid Losses

Sick or injured animals can suffer fluid loss from one or more of the fluid compartments listed:

Whole Blood Loss

- **Possible cause:** severed superficial arteries or large veins.
- **Compartment lost from:** intravascular compartment.
- **Components of fluid lost:** water, colloidal particles, red cells and electrolytes, platelets, clotting factors etc.

Extracellular Fluid Loss

- **Possible causes:** vomiting, diarrhoea, diuresis.
- **Compartment lost from:** interstitial compartment and intravascular compartment.
- **Components in fluid lost:** Na^+, Cl^- and water.

Protein Rich Extracellular Fluid Loss

- **Possible causes:** some pleural/peritoneal effusions, protein losing enteropathies, burns.
- **Compartment fluid lost from:** interstitial compartment and intravascular compartment.
- **Components in fluid loss:** Na^+, Cl^-, water and proteins.

Pure Water Loss

- **Possible causes:** high respiratory rate or primary water deprivation.
- **Compartments lost from:** water is lost from all compartments as pure water loss, since water moves freely across all compartments.

Fluid Therapy Plans

The fluid requirements of each patient vary depending on:
- the type of fluid lost
- the volume of fluid lost
- the duration of fluid loss, and whether it is acute or chronic.

Knowing the compartment from which the fluid was lost and what the components of the fluid are, helps answer the first question which should be asked: "What type of fluid has been lost?"

For example:

1. **Pure water losses are usually replaced with crystalloids (lower sodium fluids are best but should be infused slowly so that plasma sodium concentrations do not change rapidly).**
2. **Vomiting and diarrhoea cause the loss of extracellular fluid composed of water, sodium, and chloride. These are best replaced by isotonic crystalloids (containing water and electrolytes including sodium and chloride).**

What are Hypo-, Iso- and Hypertonic Fluids?

The tonicity of a fluid is a way comparing the concentration of solutes (such as sodium or other electrolytes) **in one solution compared to another solution.** Two solutions of the same concentration are said to be isotonic, whilst a "stronger" solution (a higher concentration of electrolytes) is hypertonic, and a "weaker" solution is hypotonic.

Sodium is usually considered the main electrolyte as it is the major extracellular cation (positive ion) and is therefore commonly referred to as the osmotic skeleton of the ECF.
- Hypotonic: Na^+ concentration is lower than plasma e.g. 0.18% NaCl with 4% glucose.
- Isotonic: Na^+ concentration is similar to plasma e.g. Hartmann's solution or 0.9% NaCl.
- Hypertonic: Na^+ concentration is higher than plasma e.g. 7.2% NaCl.

These solutes or electrolytes cannot pass through semipermeable membranes, but water can and tries to follow solutes to even out concentrations. For example, infusing hypertonic (7.2%) saline intravenously pulls water from the interstitial space into the intravascular space, which increases blood volume and blood pressure. This is because the water from the interstitial space is following the solute to even out the concentrations between the intravascular and interstitial fluid compartments.

Types of Fluids

Crystalloids

Crystalloid refers to any solution of crystalline solids (the solute) **dissolved in water** (the solvent). The crystalline substance can be sodium or dextrose based. When the electrolyte composition of the solution is similar to extracellular fluid, then the fluid is known as **a balanced electrolyte solution.**

Crystalloids are divided into extracellular fluid volume replacers and maintenance solutions.

Extracellular Fluid Volume Replacers

If the concentration of sodium in the fluid is similar to the ECF sodium concentration, then this fluid will remain in the extracellular compartment and is a good option for replacing extracellular fluid loss.

These fluids can be infused rapidly as they will not induce changes in electrolyte composition, especially of sodium ions. It is important not to change serum sodium concentrations too quickly. The rate of change of sodium should be no faster than 1 mmol/hr.

After IV administration the fluid redistributes between the intravascular and interstitial compartments; thus, for every 1 litre of fluid administered IV, only about 250–300 ml remain in the intravascular space after 1–2 hours.

Two examples of ECF volume replacers are Hartmann's solution (also known as Lactated Ringers) and normal saline:

- **Hartmann's: ~131 mmol Na^+, 5 mmol K^+, 111 mmol Cl^-, 1.4 mmol Ca^{2+}, 29 mmol lactate.**
- **Normal saline (0.9% NaCl): ~150 mmol Na^+, ~150 mmol Cl^-.**

Maintenance Solutions

In addition to supplying water, a maintenance fluid should deliver electrolytes. Crystalloid often have lower sodium and chloride concentrations compared to ECF, and to meet specific daily requirements supplementation may be required. For example, many patients on maintenance fluids are inappetant, and since food is the main source of potassium, potassium supplementation may be needed.

Hypotonic solutions cannot be used, as they would **cause red blood cells to lyse** (burst). Maintenance solutions work because they are isotonic, and it is the addition of dextrose, +/- the small amount of sodium, which makes them isotonic. Once the dextrose is metabolised and is no longer osmotically active, only water remains which can distribute freely throughout the three fluid compartments. Note that the amount of dextrose in the solution provides negligible energy at the concentrations used.

Because the sodium concentration is very different from that of the ECF, these fluids should not be given at fast rates, but slowly infused over 24 hours. These fluids are no use for restoring circulating volume but are ideal for treating primary water loss.

Examples of maintenance fluids:

- **4% glucose with 0.18% sodium chloride, (supplemented with 20–30 mEq/l of potassium for maintenance).**
- **5% dextrose (supplemented with 20–30 mEq/l of potassium for maintenance).**

Hypertonic Saline

Hypertonic saline can be used in shocked animals. It causes an increase in blood pressure by several mechanisms, the main one being that it **draws water out of the interstitial space.** However, the beneficial effect of hypertonic saline is transient and it should be followed by the administration of isotonic crystalloids to replace borrowed water. The use of hypertonic saline also carries potential side effects such as hypernatraemia/hypokalaemia, haemolysis, ventricular arrhythmias, potential for re-haemorrhage.

Colloids

Colloids are fluids in which large molecular weight particles are suspended but not visible. **Colloids contain large molecules that cannot pass through the vascular endothelium.** They increase the colloid osmotic pressure of the plasma and in addition to each litre of fluid which remains in the intravascular compartment, they also pull water from the interstitial space into the intravascular space. To avoid dehydrating the interstitium, crystalloids should be used concurrently or just after the colloid, to pay back the fluid borrowed from the interstitial space.

Colloids remain in the intravascular space for several hours, compared to an hour for crystalloids. Therefore colloids are also called **plasma volume expanders** and used in any case where rapid improvement of circulating volume is necessary. As a general rule **no more than 25% (usually 20 ml/kg in the dog) of circulating volume of an animal** should be administered as a colloid at any one time (usually within a 24-hour time frame), otherwise haemodilution dilutes out clotting factors etc. Colloids can be used intraoperatively to help maintain blood pressure or if an animal has a total protein of less than 35 g/l in order to prevent extravasation of fluid.

Some disadvantages of colloids include volume overload, anaphylactic reactions, and clotting problems. Large scale studies in the human field have identified potential side effects especially due to the starches. These results prompted a reduction in starch production in the human medicine field and this in turn has affected supplies available to the veterinary sector.

Calculations for Intravenous Fluid Therapy

An animal's maintenance requirement is defined as the amount of water and electrolytes required to replace those lost through normal physiological processes, i.e. through respiration, perspiration, and excretion via the alimentary and urinary tracts.

Maintenance fluid therapy rates used to be calculated at 2 ml/kg/hr but more recent thinking suggests maintenance rates differ between species and sizes of animal.

An individual's fluid therapy rate (total volume over 24 hours) can be calculated using the following formulae (Davis et al., 2013):

- **Cat: 80 x body weight (kg)$^{0.75}$ (Rule of thumb = 2–3 ml/kg/hr).**
- **Dog: 132 x body weight (kg)$^{0.75}$ (Rule of thumb = 2–6 ml/kg/hr).**

Clinical Signs of Dehydration

If an animal is admitted with a preexisting degree of dehydration this deficit needs to be factored in and compensated for in the fluid therapy plan.

Firstly, animal's level of dehydration should be assessed using a combination of clinical signs and laboratory data.

Clinical signs to check include:

- Moistness of mucous membranes: when patients become dehydrated their mucous membranes can become tacky.
- Skin turgor: i.e. the result of tenting the skin on the back of the neck.
- Sunken eyes: the fat pad behind the orbit can shrink when dehydrated and the eyes appear to sink back into the skull.

Findings when assessing these signs should be used to estimate the degree of dehydration using Table 6.

Table 6. Clinical signs of dehydration

Percentage dehydration	Clinical signs
4%	· no clinical signs
5%	· semi dry oral mucous membranes · normal skin turgor · moist eyes
6–7%	· dry oral mucous membranes · moist eyes · mild loss of skin turgor
8–10%	· dry oral mucous membranes · eyes retracted · considerable loss of skin turgor · signs of hypoperfusion
10%	· very dry mucous membranes · severe eyeball retraction · eyes dull · complete loss of skin turgor · altered consciousness · greater signs of hypoperfusion
12%	· as 10%, moribund
12–15%	· as 10% but dying

Fluid Deficits

The percentage dehydration value from Table 6 indicates the amount of water lost as a percentage of body weight. **To find out how much fluid has been lost, or the fluid deficit, this percentage should simply be multiplied by the animal's body weight.**

Fluid to restore this deficit, depending on the severity of the animal's dehydration, can be given over 12–24 hours. In more acute situations, deficits need addressing more quickly, with 30% of the fluid deficit front loaded in the first few hours and the rest administered over the rest of the 24 hour period. If the animal is in a shocked state, the full fluid deficit should be administered in a shorter time frame e.g. 1–4 hours. When considering how quickly to administer the fluid deficit, the time taken for the patient to lose the fluid should be considered.

In addition to restoring the fluid deficit, **if the animal is not eating or drinking, then maintenance needs to be provided** during the time frame that the fluid deficit is being replaced.

If a patient is dehydrated from vomiting or diarrhoea, it is common for these losses to continue even once the patient is hospitalised. Additional boluses of fluids for each episode of vomiting or diarrhoea the animal has whilst hospitalised should be included. Equal volumes to those lost should be administered, but measuring this accurately is often difficult (and unpleasant!) so some texts suggest 4 ml/kg per episode.

In a dehydrated patient, water has been lost from all compartments and therefore when using a crystalloid (where water is the solvent), water will distribute freely across all compartments to restore the fluid deficits. If rapid restoration of the fluid deficit is necessary, then a balanced ECF volume replacer such as Hartmann's should be used, as the sodium composition is more similar to plasma than a maintenance crystalloid, and is thus safer to infuse at faster rates. The use of maintenance crystalloids should be considered for primary water deprivation cases when the fluid deficit is repaid over a longer period of time, e.g. 24 hours.

Fluid Therapy Rates for Anaesthesia

Correcting dehydration, as above, helps stabilise the patient for an anaesthetic, but they still need fluid therapy during anaesthesia. Even fit, healthy animals undergoing a procedure under anaesthesia (such as a bitch spay) require fluid therapy in excess of maintenance rates. This is because anaesthetic agents tend to produce hypotension, either via vasodilation or decreasing myocardial contractility. Therefore, in addition to required "maintenance" for each animal, supplementary fluids help support blood pressure. Also, in the case of the bitch spay and similar procedures, fluid losses may occur from blood loss and evaporative fluid losses from the open abdomen.

Current recommendations from the American Animal Hospital Association (AAHA) (Davis et al., 2013) suggest that **normal healthy dogs should start with a crystalloid fluid therapy rate of 5 ml/kg/hr and cats with 3 ml/kg/hr and then every hour these rates should be reduced by 25% until maintenance is reached.**

If under anaesthesia, hypotension (mean blood pressure <60 mmHg) develops, the AAHA recommends fluid boluses (even when initial crystalloid and colloid boluses were used) and administering positive ionotropic or sympathomimetic treatment as warranted (Figure 4).

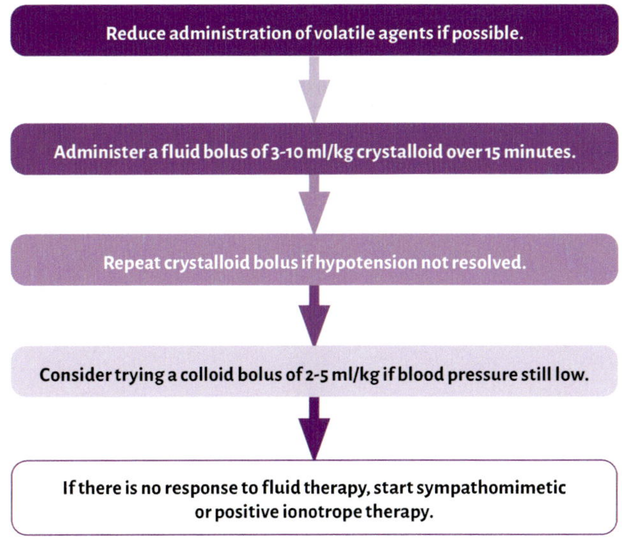

Figure 4. Hypotension flow chart.

Blood Products

There are several different blood products available in the UK for use in canine patients. Currently there are no stored blood products for cats, but feline donations of whole blood are an option. Depending on the clinical presentation, different blood products are suited to different patients.

Whole Blood

Whole blood contains red blood cells, white blood cells, clotting factors, platelets, and plasma proteins amongst other components. One unit is approximately 450 ml in volume for dogs and 45 ml in cats. Whole blood is the best way of transfusing platelets into another patient, although the number of active platelets is not significant. Platelets continue to lose viability over the first 1–3 days.

Blood can be stored for up to three weeks at between 1 and 4 °C (refrigerator), provided a closed system is used for collection. Whole blood should be transfused as soon as possible after collection. The risk of transfusion reactions increase the older the blood is.

Packed Red Cells

Canine whole blood can be separated out into packed red cells and plasma. The packed red cells are washed with saline and re-suspended in minimal saline and SAGM (Saline, Adenine, Glucose and Mannitol) nutrient solution. The packed cell volume (PCV) of packed red cells is significantly higher than whole blood, often between 60–80%. If the PCV is very high, the packed red cells can be further re-suspended in sterile normal saline to facilitate administration. A sample should be taken aseptically from the packed red cells to ascertain the actual PCV.

A typical canine unit of packed red cells is approximately 200–250 ml in volume. The unit must be stored in the fridge between 2 and 6 °C and used within 42 days of production.

Fresh Plasma

When plasma is separated from the packed red cells (by centrifugation) and transfused within six hours after harvesting, this is termed fresh plasma. It is very rich in clotting factors and platelets. However, in most situations the plasma is frozen to create fresh frozen plasma.

Fresh Frozen Plasma

When whole blood is centrifuged and plasma harvested and frozen to -180 °C within 6 hours this is termed fresh frozen plasma (FFP). It is rich in clotting factors and also contains immunoglobulins, lipids, albumin, and electrolytes. This product can be stored for up to one year below -18 °C; but after thawing should be given within six hours.

A unit of canine FFP is approximately 200 ml in volume.

If FFP is stored at -18 °C for 1–5 years, this is classed as frozen plasma. The product still contains non-labile clotting factors (such as II, VII, IX and X), immunoglobulins, albumin, lipids, and electrolytes.

Cryoprecipitate and Cryosupernatant

If fresh frozen plasma is partially thawed and then centrifuged, the cryoprecipitate is a plasma fraction which is separated from fresh frozen plasma. It is a concentrated product containing the labile clotting factors fibrinogen (factor I), factor VIII and Von Willebrand factor. The remaining fraction is the cryosupernatant, containing plasma proteins including albumin and vitamin K dependant clotting factors II, VII, IX, and X. It can be stored at -18 °C or below for up to one year.

Whole Blood Donation in a Dog

A canine blood donor should ideally be:
- friendly
- clinically normal
- aged between 1–8 years-old
- large breed dogs (at least 25 kg lean weight)
- easily accessible veins
- a universal donor blood type (see below).

The following attributes mean a dog is not suitable as a donor:
- recent bite wounds
- acute vomiting or diarrhoea
- fever
- currently pregnant
- dogs who have been vaccinated within the last 10–14 days
- dogs with a foreign travel history
- dogs with a parasite burden
- dogs on medication
- dogs that have previously received a blood transfusion.

The donor should undergo a clinical examination and pre-donation bloods should be taken. For the later, the **bare minimum is a PCV/total protein,** but a routine complete blood count and biochemistry panel are preferred. This is to check for any underlying pathological conditions, including anaemia, which would make the dog unsuitable as a donor. In addition, part of the sample is used to **ascertain the dog's blood group.**

Blood groups are defined by inherited antigens present on the surface of the red blood cell. If there is an antibody directed against a blood group antigen, this results in haemolysis.

Canine blood groups are defined by **dog erythrocyte antigens (DEA).** Of the DEAs, DEA 1, and 7 are the most important.

Dogs rarely have naturally occurring allo-antibodies, so the first transfusion is unlikely to cause problems even if blood was not of the same blood group. However, it is still advisable to blood type both recipient and donor to check for incompatibility as the life span of the red blood cells may be shortened once transfused into the donor. In addition, if antibodies are generated from an incompatible transfusion, the potential for future transfusions is limited. Dogs must be cross matched for second and any subsequent transfusions.

Box 1 details the process of taking a canine, whole blood donation.

Feline Whole Blood Donation

A feline blood donor should ideally be:
- friendly: although sedation is usually still required
- clinically normal: a predonation exam must be conducted to ensure they are healthy)
- The Pet Blood Bank recommends all donors have an echocardiographic examination to check for occult heart disease
- aged between 1–8 years old
- a large cat, ideally at least 5 kg lean weight
- a high PCV (>30%) donor is preferred
- pregnant queens should not be used: but previous pregnancy does not exclude a queen from donating blood
- ideally an indoor cat
- tested for FEL, FIV, and FIP
- cats should be free from for *Haemobartonella felis*, and *Bartonella*, *Dirofilaria*, and *Babesia*.

Feline Blood Groups

- Group A = dominant to AB, and most common.
- Group B = thought to be common in some breeds, e.g. Persian, British Shorthair.
- Group AB = recessive to A, co-dominant with B.

Box 1. Procedure for Taking a Whole Blood Donation from a Dog

- Hands should be washed and clean examination gloves worn.
- The dog should be restrained in lateral recumbency by an assistant. The jugular vein is most easily visualised if the chin is tilted up and the forelimbs gently pulled caudally.
- A square of hair (5 cm x 5 cm) should be clipped over the jugular vein and the site aseptically prepared (with a final Surgical Spirit™ application). A fenestrated sterile drape should be used to improve sterility.
- An assistant, wearing a clean pair of examination gloves, should remove the collection bag from its plastic storage bag and place it on the scales.
- The scales should be positioned at a level lower than the dog and the weight set to zero once the bag is on the scales.
- If an in-line clamp is provided on the kit, it should be closed off. Alternatively, a haemostat can be clamped approximately 5 cm from the needle on collection tubing.
- A sterile pair of gloves should be used.
- The jugular vein should be raised with the non-dominant hand.
- Venipuncture should be performed with the bevel of the needle facing upwards.
- The haemostat or clamp should be released.
- Blood should flow easily from the collection line to the bag.
- As soon as the blood starts to enter the collection bag, the bag should be rocked gently to mix the blood with the anticoagulant. This should be repeated regularly (approximately four times a minute) during collection.
- The weight of the bag should be checked intermittently. One full unit is 450 ml. Once the unit has been collected, the vein no longer needs raising and the collection bag can be clamped.

Box 2. Procedure for Taking a Whole Blood Donation from a Cat

- Sedation is usually required, with the protocol selected based on the cat's temperament and health status. The author has previously used alfaxalone intramuscularly or sevoflurane by mask. Others suggest α-2 adrenergic agonist-based protocols although this class of drugs prevents compensatory tachycardia as a response to a loss of blood volume.
- For all sedated cats, flow-by oxygen by mask should be used, in addition to anaesthetic monitoring, and lubrication of the eyes.
- **A typical unit of cat blood is 45 ml;** but no more than 12 ml/kg per donation should be taken.
- A ratio of 1 ml of anticoagulant (drawn in a sterile manner from the bag of anticoagulant) to 7 ml of whole blood should be prepared.
- The area over the jugular vein should be clipped and prepared aseptically.
- Sterile gloves should be worn.
- The butterfly catheter and three-way tap should be attached to the 60 ml syringe (containing anticoagulant amount described above) and the anticoagulant injected through the three-way tap into the butterfly needle.
- The jugular vein should be raised and the butterfly catheter inserted into the vessel, with the bevel facing upwards and blood should be gently aspirated into the syringe. The blood should be aspirated at a rate of 5 ml/min or greater.
- Once the desired volume has been collected in the syringe, the three-way tap should be turned off from the butterfly needle and the needle removed from the vessel.
- Apply pressure to the venepuncture site.
- Demeanour, heart rate, mucous membrane colour, and pulse quality should be checked. If the donor is showing any signs of hypovolaemia, such as tachycardia or pale mucous membrane colour, then crystalloid fluid therapy should be administered (at three times the volume removed) intravenously.

Cats are born with naturally occurring allo-antibodies to other cats' blood groups and there is no universal donor group in cats, so cross matching should always be performed – even if compatibility of blood types has been checked between donor and recipient. A more recently identified red blood cell antigen (Mik) is a potential cause for such non-AB incompatibilities. A step-by-step guide to taking a whole blood donation in the cat is shown in Box 2.

Usually, the whole blood is used immediately, but if storage is required, this should be in a fridge (1–4 °C) for up to three weeks assuming the donation was taken in a sterile manner. If sterility was compromised, the blood must be used immediately (and certainly within 24 hours). When stored in the fridge, the bag or syringe should be agitated every 2–3 days to ensure mixing of contents.

Giving a Blood Transfusion

Prior to use, red cell products must be warmed gradually, either by allowing them to reach ambient temperature or by placing them in a warm water bath <37 °C.

A giving set with an in-line filter must be used with all blood products (to filter out any debris and micro-thrombi). Smaller volume whole blood donations (e.g. for cats and small dogs) may be delivered via a syringe driver, and therefore an in-line filter used between the syringe and intravenous catheter.

Blood should not be administered through lines that contain Hartmann's, or other calcium-containing solutions. Citrate (part of the anticoagulant in the blood collection bag) binds to calcium in the blood and calcium is required for the coagulation cascade, therefore the citrate stops the blood clotting. Hartmann's contains calcium, so adding extra calcium will cause blood clots to form where the two fluids mix.

Monitoring the Transfusion

Before starting the transfusion, the recipient's baseline temperature, pulse, and respiration (TPR) should be recorded. This makes it easier to spot reactions when monitoring the transfusion.

If the patient is stable, the initial transfusion rate should be 0.5 ml/kg/hr, for the first 15 minutes to check for acute reactions. During this first 15 minutes, the patient must be continuously monitored and further TPR recordings taken every five minutes.

After the initial 15 minutes, if there are no signs of a transfusion reaction, the infusion rate can be increased to 5–20 ml/kg/hr.

The author suggests further recordings of TPR continuing every 15 minutes for the first hour, then half hourly observations for the next hour, and then hourly observations until the end of the transfusion. Ideally, the transfusion should be completed within four hours.

In the dog a small (100 ml) bag of 0.9% saline can be used following the transfusion to ensure that blood product is not lost in the drip tubing. Alternatively, in the cat, sufficient saline can be flushed through the administration line to flush all remaining whole blood into the catheter.

In a patient with acute hypovolaemic anaemia, the benefit of a fast infusion rate may outweigh the risks of a transfusion reaction.

A post-transfusion blood sample should be taken to check how successful the transfusion has been e.g. if the reason for transfusion was anaemia, PCV/TP should be rechecked, if the reason for transfusion was hypoalbuminaemia, albumin should be rechecked. This should be repeated after a further 12 hours.

Transfusion Reactions

These can be immunological or non-immunological.

Immune-mediated Transfusion Reactions

Signs associated with an immune mediated response include:

- agitation/restlessness/change in attitude
- nausea, vomiting, salivation
- urticaria with or without pruritus
- anaphylaxis
- pyrexia
- tachypnoea/dyspnoea
- tachycardia
- hypotension
- seizures
- haemolysis, jaundice, haemoglobinuria.

Non-immune Related Transfusion Reactions

Non- immune related reactions include:

- hypocalcemia: due to too much citrate binding blood calcium
- circulatory overload
- hypothermia: blood not warmed prior to infusion
- transmission of infectious diseases.

If a transfusion reaction is suspected the infusion should be stopped and the vet contacted. The vet may decide to dampen down the immune response by using corticosteroids. They may also administer antihistamines if appropriate. Dependent on the cost/benefit ratio, if a mild reaction is suspected the transfusion may continue but at a much slower rate under close monitoring. Otherwise, in the case of a more severe reaction, no more of the blood product transfusion should be given.

Monitoring Anaesthesia

Animals under anaesthesia must be continuously monitored, and in some cases this monitoring starts once the patient has had their premed medication. It should also continue well into the recovery from anaesthesia since it is during this period that the majority of peri-operative fatalities occur (Brodbelt et al., 2008). Monitoring equipment is described hereinafter, but it is important to remember **that the nurse is the most important monitor of all with so-called "hand and eye" monitoring** (Figure 5).

Tools for Monitoring Anaesthesia

Hand and Eye Monitoring

Hands and eyes provide much vital information about the patient's state and should also be used to check what monitors are telling you.

Only hands and eyes can:

- **Feel pulses.**
- **Assess mucous membrane colour and capillary refill time.**
- **Watch the bag and chest movements.**
- **Monitor the eye position and palpebral reflex.**
- **Check the pedal reflex.**
- **Assess jaw tone.**
- **Check levels of volatile agent in the vaporiser, and gases in the cylinders.**
- **Monitor for blood loss in the surgical field.**

Assessing Anaesthesia Depth

The veterinary nurse must give the surgeon accurate information about whether or not the patient is adequately anaesthetised. The aim is to prevent the animal being anaesthetised too lightly and aware of surgical pain or too deeply with anaesthetic agents having a profound effect on their physiological system. The signs used to assess anaesthesia depth include:

- Heart and respiratory rate: these usually increase as a patient gets lighter, but this may not be the case when the patient is hypercapnic.
- Palpebral reflex: should be very sluggish but present.
- Corneal reflex: often used in avian anaesthetic monitoring with a dampened cotton bud.
- Eye position: should be ventro-medially rotated in a surgical plane of anaesthesia.
- Nystagmus: may be present at very light or very deep planes of anaesthesia.
- Lacrimation: may be observed in very light planes of anaesthesia.
- Salivation: may be observed in very light planes of anaesthesia.
- Tongue curl: may be observed in very light planes of anaesthesia.
- Laryngeal/pharyngeal reflexes: may be observed in very light planes of anaesthesia. May be retained when ketamine-based anaesthetics have been used.
- Anal reflex: can be useful if the surgeon is working at the head end of the patient.
- Jaw tone: should be relaxed in a surgical plane of anaesthesia.
- Pedal reflex: regular assessment of this is not recommended as it can caused postoperative discomfort.

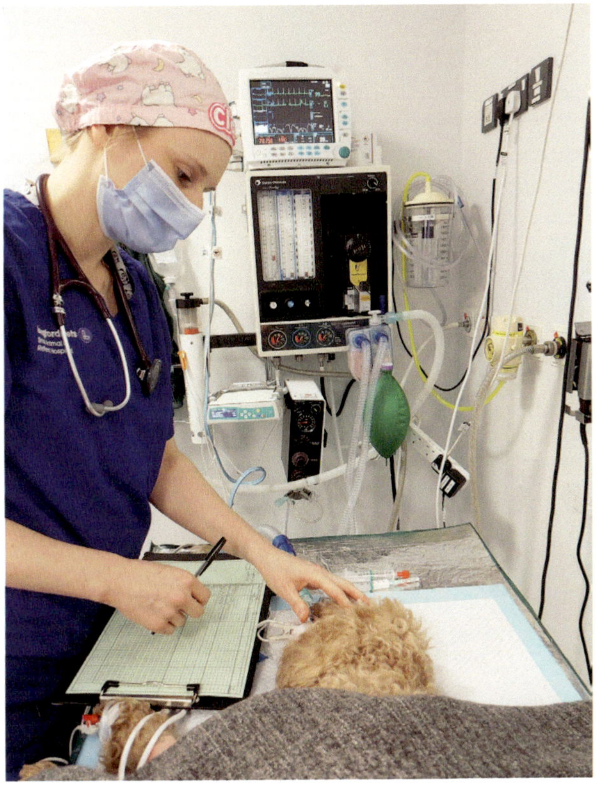

Figure 5. Monitoring an anaesthetic.

Capnometry

Capnometry monitors the partial pressure or concentration of carbon dioxide in respiratory gases breathed out by the patient. Capnometry is an indirect monitor of carbon dioxide, which may not be as accurate as arterial blood gas analysis (the gold standard), but is non-invasive and can be used continuously during an anaesthetic. The monitor detects carbon dioxide exhaled by the patient through an attachment placed between the endotracheal tube and the breathing system.

The partial pressure of carbon dioxide in respiratory gases is continuously measured by a capnometer using infrared light absorption. There are two types of analysers: sidestream and mainstream.

- A sidestream analyser aspirates gas from a connector between the endotracheal tube and the breathing system, to be analysed in the main body of the monitor.
- A mainstream system performs the analysis at the site between the endotracheal tube and the breathing system.

The relative advantages and disadvantages of these systems are listed in Table 7.

Table 7. Comparison of sidestream and mainstream analysers.

Sidestream	Mainstream
There is a time lag before the CO_2 value is demonstrated on the screen, as the gas sample must be aspirated up a length of tubing to reach the monitor.	As the sensing part of the monitor is in between the breathing system and endotracheal tube, there is no time delay between sampling and display of CO_2 values.
The sampling tubing is prone to blockage.	No sampling lines are needed, and therefore the inherent blocking of sampling lines is avoided.
Sampling tubing and water traps need to be replaced.	As the sensor is nearer to the patient's respiratory tract, it is more frequently affected by respiratory secretions.
Very few machines using sidestream analysers divert the gas into the scavenge system, and so waste gases are vented to the atmosphere.	There is no diversion of gases to a remote site and therefore atmospheric pollution is not an issue with this type of machinery.
Connector produces less increase in dead space to a mainstream analyser.	The connector represents an increase in breathing system dead space to the patient.
The main monitor (and most expensive part of the equipment) is remote from the patient's mouth (and teeth!).	The most expensive part of the equipment is next to the patient's mouth and is therefore prone to damage.

Table 8. Potential causes for hypercapnia and hypocapnia.

End tidal CO_2 change	Potential cause
Zero level from beginning of anaesthesia	possible endo-oesophageal intubation
Sudden decrease to zero	· airway obstruction · airway disconnection · ventilator failure · capnograph malfunction · obstructed aspirating tube · apnoea · cardiac or respiratory arrest
Hypocapnia	· airway leaks · severe cardiovascular disturbance · hyperventilation · hypothermia · vasoconstriction · low aspirating flow rates · fresh gas contamination · large physiological dead space · small tidal volume
Hypercapnia	· hypoventilation · increased rate of metabolism · rebreathing

Carbon dioxide values are displayed simply as numbers, usually in pressure units (mmHg or kPa). However, the most useful display on a capnometer is the capnograph.

The usual wave form of a capnograph has four distinct phases (see Figure 6). The end tidal CO_2 value ($ETCO_2$) is the value displayed on all capnometers and is defined as the value at the end of the alveolar plateau.

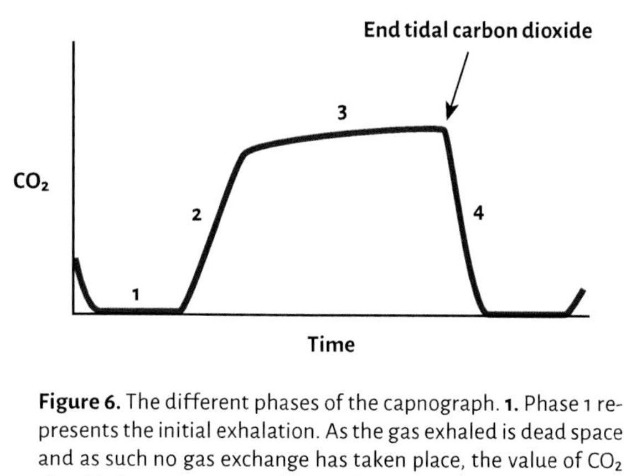

Figure 6. The different phases of the capnograph. **1.** Phase 1 represents the initial exhalation. As the gas exhaled is dead space and as such no gas exchange has taken place, the value of CO_2 should always be zero. **2.** Phase 2 is a steep slope representing the increased levels of CO_2 as exhalation continues. The gas is now from parts of the respiratory tract where gas exchange has taken place. **3.** Phase 3 is the alveolar plateau where the alveoli continue to empty of CO_2. **4.** Phase 4 is a downward slope indicating inspiration. The CO_2 levels are decreased due to dilution from the fresh gas flow.

Carbon dioxide (CO_2) is produced as a by-product of metabolism and eliminated from the body by the lungs. **A capnograph therefore provides information about CO_2 production, perfusion of the lungs, alveolar ventilation, respiratory patterns, and elimination of CO_2 from the breathing system.**

Normocapnia (i.e. normal $ETCO_2$ values) is 35–45 mmHg, with hypercapnia and hypocapnia indicating higher than normal or lower than normal CO_2 values respectively. $ETCO_2$ values represent a balance between CO_2 production and CO_2 elimination. Common reasons for hypo- and hypercapnia are listed in Table 8. One of the occasions when capnography is invaluable in anaesthetic monitoring is in the case of cardiac arrest, as this is often the first monitor to identify a problem. If circulation slows or stops, then the blood cannot deliver carbon dioxide (which is a waste product from cells) to the lungs to be eliminated, and so a sudden decrease in CO_2 levels should prompt an assessment of the animal's pulse.

Note the marked oscillations in phase 4 (Figure 7), which are in phase with the patient's heart rate. This can be a normal variation in a capnograph when the patient's respiratory rate is slow.

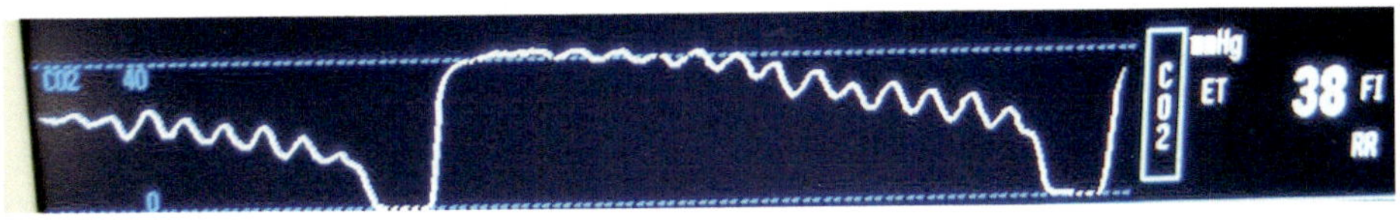

Figure 7. Cardiac oscillations can be seen in phase 4.

The failure of phase 1 to return to baseline indicates that CO_2 is present in the inhaled (and thus dead space) gas. This suggests rebreathing (Figure 8), which may be due to exhausted soda lime, a valve which has become stuck in a circle system, or insufficient fresh gas flow in the case of a non-rebreathing system.

Bronchospasm (for example in asthma) or obstruction of the endotracheal tube (Figure 9) causes a slanting and prolonged phase 2, and an increased slope in phase 3.

Oesophageal Stethoscope

This simple and relatively cheap piece of monitoring equipment is **used to monitor heart rate, although respiratory sounds are also often heard.** A stethoscope head piece is attached to a long tube of soft plastic. After premeasuring the length of the tube to the point of the elbow, it is passed down the oesophagus in the anaesthetised patient (whose trachea has already been intubated). When passed to the premeasured point, its tip should lie just over the heart base and transmit heart sounds through the ear pieces.

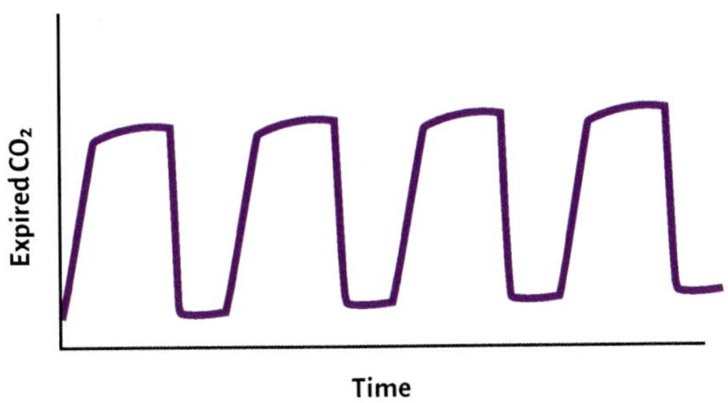

Figure 8. Failure of the trace to return to baseline indicates rebreathing.

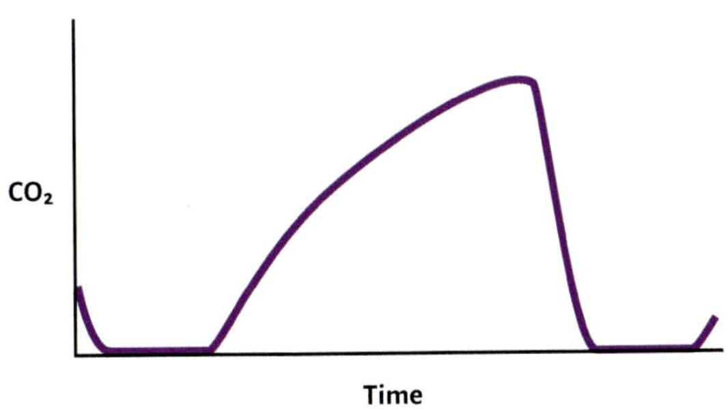

Figure 9. Capnograph shape which can suggest obstruction of the endotracheal tube.

Blood Pressure Measurement

Measurement of arterial blood pressure is one of the most useful measures of cardiovascular function available in clinical practice. **Arterial blood pressure is measured either invasively (directly) or non-invasively (indirectly),** the relative advantages and disadvantages of which are summarised below.

Table 9. The advantages and disadvantages of different blood pressure measurement techniques.

Direct blood pressure	Indirect blood pressure
invasive technique	non-invasive technique
moderate skill required to place arterial line	some skill required for placement of cuff (+/- Doppler probe)
complications associated with arterial line placement	no complications associated with arterial line placement to consider
measurements are accurate, even at low blood pressures	measurements are less accurate, especially at lower blood pressure
arterial blood gas samples can be drawn from the catheters	no catheter for arterial blood gas analysis
continuous data is displayed giving "beat to beat" indication of blood pressure	data displayed intermittently

Direct Measurement

Direct arterial blood pressure measurement requires the placement of an intra-arterial catheter. In dogs and cats, the typical site is the dorsal pedal (also known as metatarsal artery), although auricular artery catheterisation in the ear is another possibility. The catheter and attachments must be placed aseptically and secured well, as dislodgment of any part results in a large haematoma formation, air embolism, or severe blood loss.

The catheter is connected via saline-filled extension tubing to a pressure transducer device, which converts the pulsatile pressure signal into a numerical value. Pressures are measured against a reference level and devices to record pressure need to be zeroed (at the level of the heart). Electronic transducers convert the numerical values into wave forms.

Non-invasive Blood Pressure Measurement

These techniques utilise a cuff to occlude blood flow to an appendage by increasing the inflation pressure to greater than that of systolic blood pressure. As the cuff is gradually deflated, the resumption of the arterial blood flow is detected by a variety of methods. The width of a cuff should be 40% of the circumference of the appendage (limb or tail) to which it is fitted.

Doppler blood pressure monitors use sound waves emitted from a Doppler probe. When the sound waves are reflected back by a moving structure (e.g. arterial wall or blood cells) then an audible signal (a whoosh) is heard.

Oscillometric Blood Pressure

Oscillometric blood pressure monitors are automated and can be programmed to measure blood pressure at set intervals, and display the results digitally, alongside a pulse rate. The cuff usually has an arrow indicating which part of the cuff to position over the pulse.

Electrocardiogram (ECG)

The ECG is a useful tool for monitoring during an animal's anaesthetic, especially if they have cardiac or respiratory pathology, or electrolyte imbalances. The ECG indicates the electrical activity of the heart but gives no information as to whether or not the heart is beating satisfactorily.

The ECG electrodes need to triangulate over the heart. In small animals they are usually placed on the two front limbs and the left hind limb. They are attached using crocodile clips or sticky pads, using spirit or gel to improve conductance of the electrical signal.

Central Venous Pressure

Central venous pressure (CVP) measurements represent the pressure in the intra-thoracic vena cava. Central venous pressure is a measure of the relative ability of the heart to pump the blood returning to it and is a useful tool if a degree of heart failure is suspected. It is also an estimate of the relationship between blood volume and blood volume capacity, and as a monitor can be used to tailor fluid therapy in hypovolaemic animals. Normal CVP in small animals is between 0–10 cm H_2O. Generally, low value ranges indicate relative hypovolaemia, and if the value is raised, this indicates relative hypervolaemia, and the heart's inability to cope with venous return.

Central venous pressure measurement requires placement of a central catheter, usually a jugular catheter.

Temperature Monitoring

Hypothermia is a common problem in small animal anaesthesia, leading to problems such as delayed recovery. Whilst rectal thermometers are commonly used in veterinary practice, this reflects more of a peripheral reading. Temperature probes inserted into the nasopharynx or oesophagus are thermistor based, and oesophageal readings reflect the temperature of the heart which is a core temperature.

Urine Output

To ensure a patient's kidneys are being perfused sufficiently, urine output is monitored. This is performed by placing an indwelling urinary catheter into the animal's bladder and attaching it to a closed system. Intermittently, (every 1–4 hours) the volume of urine collected is measured. Urine output should be at least 1–2 ml/kg/hr but may be more if fluid therapy or diuretics are used.

Pulse Oximetry

Pulse oximetry is a non-invasive, continuous monitor of arterial haemoglobin oxygen saturation. Oxygen is carried in the blood either dissolved in the blood or bound to haemoglobin, with the vast majority (97%) bound. The percentage saturation of haemoglobin bound with oxygen is known as SpO_2.

Pulse oximetry is based on the absorption of light transmitted through a pulsatile vascular tissue bed. The probe on a pulse oximeter, which can be of several types, has a light emitting diode on one side and a photodetector (which detects light) on the other side. There are different pulse oximeter probe designs.

Haemoglobin fully saturated with oxygen (oxyhaemoglobin) and haemoglobin with no oxygen bound to it (de-oxyhaemoglobin) absorb light differently, and so the amount of light transmitted through the tissue bed (e.g. the tongue) and reaching the photodetector on the other side depends on the proportions of oxyhaemoglobin and de-oxyhaemoglobin present.

A pulse oximeter indicates two things: the haemoglobin oxygen saturation (SpO_2) as a percentage and the pulse rate in beats per minute. Pulse oximetry is not an indicator of whether an animal is breathing or ventilating adequately (this assessment requires use a capnograph to measure end-tidal carbon dioxide). A pulse oximeter can also indicate that there is sufficient peripheral perfusion for the machine to detect a pulse.

All animals should have an oxygen haemoglobin saturation of at least 95%. A value of below 95% is considered moderate hypoxia, a value of below 90% is considered profound hypoxia and in both of these circumstances action should be taken.

Arterial Blood Gas Analysis and Acid Base Balance

Arterial blood samples can be drawn from an indwelling arterial catheter or via a needle stick. The blood sample is then run through a blood gas analyser.

Blood gas analysis is useful in the diagnosis, prognosis, and monitoring of several conditions in small animal clinical practice. It provides information on the respiratory system, perfusion, acid base, and electrolyte balance of the patient.

There are two main components to acid base analysis: respiratory and metabolic.

- **Respiratory:** this looks at the efficiency of ventilation. If the ventilation is inadequate, then carbon dioxide accumulates. Extra CO_2 molecules combine with water to form carbonic acid, which makes the pH more acidic.
- **Metabolic:** when normal metabolism is impaired, acid forms, e.g. lactic acid from poor perfusion. The acid is not from a respiratory source so is termed metabolic.

Usually, patients that are clinically unwell present with an acidic pH, the following is a step-by-step guide to determine what is happening:

1. **Look at the pH of the blood** to tell whether there is acidaemia or alkalaemia. The normal blood pH is approximately 7.35–7.45. Less than 7.35 suggests acidaemia, >7.45 suggests alkalaemia. The next step is to work out why there is too much/too little acid/alkali in the blood.
2. **Look at the respiratory component:** indicated by the pCO_2 (the partial pressure of carbon dioxide in the blood). If the pH is acidic, and the pCO_2 is raised (normal is 35–45 mmHg) this suggests acidaemia with a respiratory cause, therefore a respiratory acidosis. There are occasions, where in addition there is acid created by metabolic causes, which is an example of a mixed respiratory/metabolic acidosis.
3. **Evaluate the metabolic component** by looking at the base excess (BE) whose normal range is -5 to +5 mmol/l. If the blood is acidaemic and the BE is below -5 mmol/l, this suggests the cause is metabolic. (Again, if the pCO_2 is also elevated, then this would be a mixed metabolic and respiratory acidosis.) If the BE is above +5 mmol/l then this suggests a metabolic alkalosis (either through a loss of acid or a gain of base).

Usually, the body makes an effort to compensate for any acid base abnormalities. The compensation is made by the unaffected system, so for example, the respiratory system compensates in response to a metabolic disturbance (e.g. an animal trying to lower its CO_2 to shift the pH back to normal after a metabolic acidosis). It is less common to see metabolic compensation for a respiratory disturbance, as usually the change in ventilation is too rapid for metabolic compensation to occur.

Indices of oxygenation

- **PaO_2 in mmHg is the partial pressure of oxygen dissolved in arterial blood.**
- **SaO_2 (%) is the saturation of haemoglobin with oxygen as measured by arterial blood gas analysis. It is equivalent to SpO_2.**
- **PaO_2 <60 mmHg or SaO_2 <90% = severe hypoxaemia.**
- **PaO_2 60–80 mmHg or SaO_2 90–95 % = moderate hypoxaemia.**
- **PaO_2 should be approximately 5 x fraction of inspired oxygen (FiO_2), e.g. when breathing room air (21% FiO_2), the PaO_2 should be 5 x 21 = 105 mmHg.**

Anaesthesia for Thoracic Surgery

When the thoracic cavity is open, negative pressure in the pleural space is lost which means that even though the ribs still move up and out, the lungs are unable to inflate. **Therefore, from the moment the chest cavity is opened, intermittent positive pressure ventilation (IPPV) is needed to inflate the lungs.**

Intermittent Positive Pressure Ventilation

Intermittent positive pressure ventilation (IPPV) can be manual or mechanical. Manual IPPV involves closing the breathing system's APL (Adjustable Pressure Limiting) valve and giving the reservoir bag a squeeze to inflate the patient's lungs, a little bit more than for a normal spontaneous breath, and then open the valve to allow the patient to exhale fully. However, mechanical ventilation can maintain more constant respiratory variables and free the anaesthetist for monitoring and other tasks.

Monitoring during Thoracic Anaesthesia

Out of all anaesthetics, thoracic anaesthesia requires the most extensive monitoring because so many body systems are affected by the anaesthetic technique, primary disease, or the surgery.

Capnography

Capnography provides information about the end tidal carbon dioxide, which in turn indicates the efficiency of ventilation and lung excursions. It can indicate disconnection from the ventilator and any obstruction of the endotracheal tube with blood, pus etc. End tidal carbon dioxide is often altered if lungs are packed out of the way by the surgeon during a thoracotomy.

Pulse Oximetry

Pulse oximetry helps detect poor blood-oxygen content and is mandatory where lung pathology is expected. SpO_2 may drop if there is obstruction of large airways with debris or the lung is packed away.

Electrocardiogram

An ECG is useful during thoracic anaesthesia as there are several nerves which run through the thoracic cavity, which may generate arrhythmias when tweaked. During cardiac surgery, arrhythmias occur when the surface of the heart is touched, and if the animal is hypercapnic or hypoxic, arrhythmias may also be seen.

Blood Pressure

Some thoracic surgeries carry the potential for massive blood loss. At the start of ventilation, blood pressure often decreases, and the vena cava may be compressed by the surgeon which alters venous return to the heart. Blood pressure measurement can be direct or indirect. When available, arterial blood pressure measurement is preferable as it gives a beat to beat indication of blood pressure, and an arterial blood sample can be taken from the arterial line to look at blood gases. Central venous pressure monitoring may also be useful.

Pain Management of Thoracic Surgeries

Multi-modal analgesia should be used, preemptively where possible.

A base opioid can be used for premedication and often CRIs of more potent opioids, such as fentanyl or alfentanil, are used to supplement opioid analgesia intraoperatively. The benefit of these opioid CRIs are that they may cause respiratory depression/apnoea which decreases the animal's attempts of moving their chest wall in between ventilated breaths.

Ketamine can be used as a CRI or as bolus injections especially for thoracic opening and closure as it is a very good analgesic for somatic pain (i.e. that arising from skin and the thoracic wall). Ketamine does have some cardiovascular side effects and so the patient should be cardiovascularly stable for this drug to be used.

Non-steroidal anti-inflammatory drugs can be used if the animal is normally hydrated, has normal renal function, no gastrointestinal disease, and no cardiovascular disease. These drugs should be avoided in surgeries if blood loss or hypotension is a possible consequence, or administration held until the end of surgery. In dogs, paracetamol can be used as an alternative if typical NSAIDs are contraindicated.

α-2 adrenergic agonists, if used in preanaesthetic medication, can also be continued as a CRI and contribute to multi-modal analgesia. **Nitrous oxide is generally contraindicated in thoracic surgery.** Often patients with lung pathologies have a requirement for higher concentrations of inspired oxygen, in addition, if there is air in the pleural space, nitrous oxide rapidly expands a pneumothorax.

Other drugs administered to the patient in the long term contribute to analgesia including gabapentin, maropitant, tramadol etc.

Local anaesthetic techniques are strongly indicated for thoracic surgery. For a lateral thoracotomy the use of intercostal nerve blocks, interpleural analgesia, wound diffusion catheters, and high epidurals with morphine should be considered. For sternotomy approaches, interpleural blocks can be used alongside incisional infiltration (either as a one off at the end of surgery or via a wound diffusion catheter) and a high epidural with morphine is also appropriate.

Conditions of the Thorax

Thoracic Trauma

Trauma cases which need immediate surgical intervention include flail chest (multiple adjacent ribs are broken in multiple places, separating a segment, so one part of the chest wall moves independently from the rest of the chest wall), punctured thorax, or uncontrolled intrathoracic bleeding. Minimal stabilisation may be possible if these are emergency surgeries. Animals are in pain, therefore analgesia should be provided, usually with opioids such as methadone, as soon as possible. In addition to welfare concerns, analgesia makes the animal easier to handle and improves ventilation if they have chest wall pain. Blood loss may be severe, and volume of blood loss should be quantified if possible.

It is important to gain control of ventilation as soon as possible, i.e. once the animal is anaesthetised – not when the thoracic cavity is about to be opened. The only relative contraindication to this is if the patient has a tension pneumothorax, as this is worsened with ventilation.

As the patient's chest wall has suffered trauma, there may be **concomitant injuries** e.g. pulmonary contusions and cardiac contusions. Pulmonary contusions are bruises of the lung, caused by chest trauma, and as a result of damage to capillaries, blood and other fluids accumulate in lung tissue. The excess fluid interferes with gas exchange, potentially leading to hypoxia. Cardiac contusions are bruises in the heart muscle and represent focal damage to the heart which can cause life-threatening arrhythmias.

Diaphragmatic Hernias

Diaphragmatic hernias may be traumatic or congenital and, acute or chronic. Some animals may be dyspnoeic, some asymptomatic. The abdominal organs that enter the chest cavity most commonly are the liver and the small intestine. Wherever possible, the patient should be stabilised before continuing with anaesthesia, using fluids, analgesia (non-emetic opioid usually), and oxygen. If the stomach has entered the thorax, it can distend with air quickly and require more urgent surgery.

Drug choice is affected by which organ is in the chest, it is essential to remember that certain drugs make some organs (e.g. spleen) increase in size, which further compromises tidal volume. The animal should be constantly monitored after premedication. Oxygen supplementation should be attempted as long as it is stress free. The lungs should be ventilated from anaesthetic induction, rather than waiting until the abdominal cavity is open. The tidal volume of the lungs is compromised by abdominal content in the chest, so to compensate a small tidal volume should be used but at an increased respiratory rate to maintain minute ventilation. This pattern is called a **high frequency, low volume** ventilatory pattern. It is also important not to overinflate lungs that have been atelectatic for a while, as it may predispose to pulmonary oedema once the ruptured diaphragm is corrected.

Once anaesthetised, **the animal should be tipped so abdominal contents fall caudally;** a foam pad (used for radiography positioning) is useful for this. The animal should be clipped in both lateral recumbencies if possible, and should not be positioned in dorsal recumbency until the last minute as this will cause the patient to desaturate. Monitoring should be from preanaesthetic medication onwards until recovery.

Thymoma

Thymomas are the most common tumour of the thoracic cavity. They are a remnant of the thymus, an organ that usually disappears when an animal is young, but sometimes it persists and becomes neoplastic. Physical effects of the tumour, include their size which compromises tidal volume, and compression of the trachea and vena cava. **Thymomas can wrap around large blood vessels and cause major blood loss upon dissection.**

Thymomas often cause myasthenia gravis, an autoimmune reaction to acetylcholine receptors. Often myasthenia gravis patients are treated with anticholinesterases, these drugs alter the duration of action of opioids and the response to neuromuscular blockers (so very low doses should always be used to start with). Myasthenia gravis causes megaoesophagus through weakness of the oesophageal muscular wall. **This makes animals prone to regurgitation** and possibly aspiration pneumonia. Therefore, animals should be preoxygenated and induced in a head up fashion (Figure 10), with suction available.

Persistent Right Aortic Arch

A persistent right aortic arch forms a restrictive lesion around the oesophagus. It is usually paediatric patients that are anaesthetised for treatment of this condition. It is usually recognised when the animal is weaned, as whilst milk can fit past the restrictive lesion, solid food cannot. Therefore, paediatric anaesthetic considerations should be taken into account, in addition to the patient being in poor body condition. As the oesophagus has a restrictive lesion, animals are prone to regurgitation and head up inductions and suction should be used. They may also have aspiration pneumonia and therefore preoxygenation, monitoring SpO_2, and oxygen supplementation during recovery is warranted.

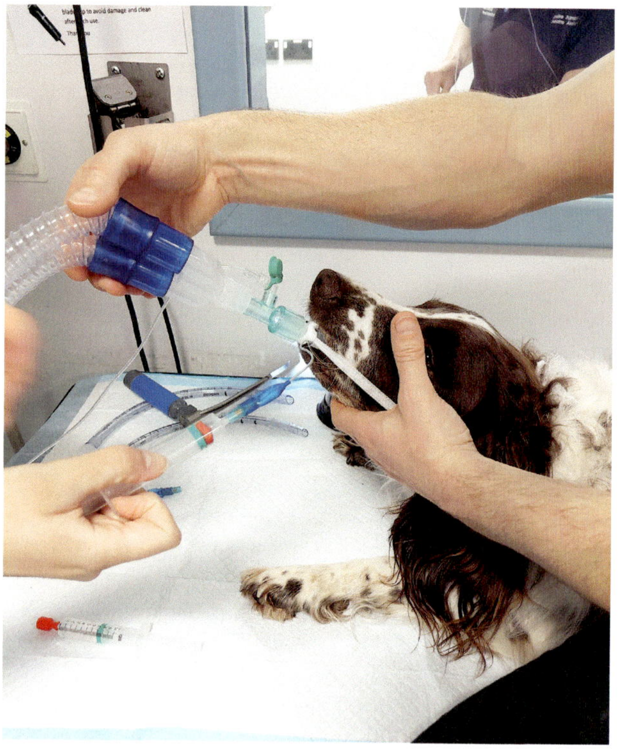

Figure 10. Head up induction.

Pulmonary Lesions

Examples of pulmonary lesions include abscesses, tumours, and foreign bodies and surgery may consist of localised resection, lung lobectomy or even a lungectomy (removal of either the right or left side of the lung). Oxygenation is often compromised, so preoxygenation is recommended, along with use of 100% oxygen during anaesthesia and supplemental oxygen in recovery. The surgeon often packs the lung (including healthy lung) out of the way, causing alterations in blood pressure, carbon dioxide, and SpO_2. If the surgeon is performing a resection, the airway gases may be released into the atmosphere so TIVA should be considered to reduce atmospheric contamination.

When certain types of lesions (e.g. abscesses, tumours with necrotic centres) are disturbed, they release pus into the airways. Bronchial blocker tubes are helpful to avoid airway contamination with pus.

Pericardiectomy

This surgery is used to relieve pericardial effusion (where fluid is trapped between the pericardial sac and the heart muscle). If a large volume of blood accumulates in the pericardial sac it causes cardiac tamponade and the blood must be drained (usually under ultrasound guidance) before attempting anaesthesia.

The effusion may be associated with a heart base tumour, and therefore the vet will have staged the tumour prior to anaesthesia. Fluid therapy is needed to maintain venous return. Volatile agents produce significant myocardial depression and therefore MAC sparing drugs are warranted, to reduce the percentage of volatile agent used.

Bradycardia should be avoided as this blunts the compensatory tachycardia which is often present. This is because the animal is trying to maintain cardiac output, as the stroke volume ejected by the heart with every beat, is limited. Arrhythmias are to be expected when surgical instruments touch the epicardium. These are usually self-limiting, but the vet may use an antiarrhythmic drug such as lidocaine if they persist.

There may be major blood loss. Blood-soaked swabs and the suction bottle (Figures 11 and 12) should be monitored, whilst performing blood loss calculations to inform the vet when taking fluid therapy decisions.

Patent Ductus Arteriosus (PDA)

Patent ductus arteriosus (PDA) is a hole between the aorta and pulmonic artery, and represents a shunt between pulmonary and systemic circulation. It is often found and treated in young

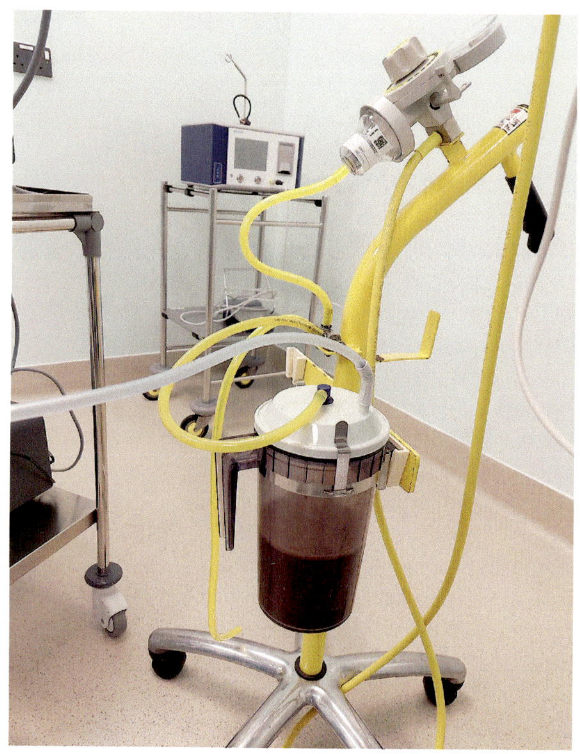

Figure 11. Blood in suction.

animals (therefore the paediatric factors affecting anaesthesia should be considered) but there may be left ventricular enlargement in cases not recognised until later. Diastolic pressure is often low (because of the connection of the systemic circulation with the much lower pressure respiratory circulation) and so the aim should be to maintain blood pressure during anaesthesia.

Thoracotomy or interventional cardiology (implanting a metal plug in the PDA via the femoral artery) can be used. When performing a surgical ligation, there is often reflex bradycardia (Branham's sign) as a response to the increase in blood pressure (especially diastolic). If bradycardia persists, anticholinergics such as atropine can help. This is less likely to occur with the implant technique. The dissected area is often very vascular; with a small chance of sudden, major blood loss.

Thoracoscopy

Thoracoscopy is a minimally invasive procedure that allows surgeons to examine the pleural lining of the lungs and the surface of the lungs. It may be for diagnostic purposes or surgery.

It usually involves placement of a thoracoscope in the thoracic cavity, whilst inflating the pleural space with gas to aid visualisation. This insufflation of the pleural space can influence blood pressure, oxygenation and tidal volume. Positive pressure ventilation is still needed. Thoracoscopy is usually less painful than thoracotomy, but if CO_2 is used as the insufflation gas, this can produce a stinging sensation. One lung ventilation using a special ETT can be performed to isolate one lung, and cause the other to collapse.

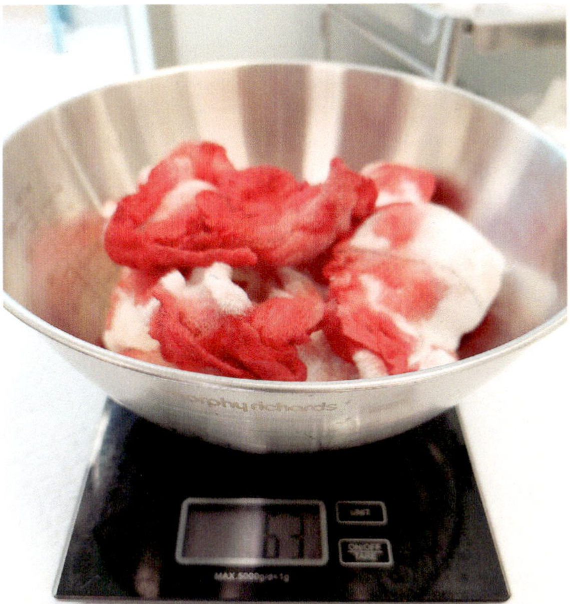

Figure 12. Blood soaked swabs.

Anaesthesia for Head and Neck Surgery

Anaesthesia for head and neck surgery is complicated by a need to protect the airway whilst allowing the surgeon adequate access. Another consideration is ensuring the endotracheal tube is well secured when it may not be possible to secure with a tie around the head. It may even be necessary to direct the ETT away from the surgical site or indeed use an alternative airway.

The choice of breathing system also needs consideration, choosing a system with less drag (in case the ETT is not well secured), and the APL valves and scavenge mounts positioned well away from the head.

Alternative Airways

The standard endotracheal intubation is orotracheal intubation i.e. through the mouth. However, the surgeon may decide to use an alternative airway in cases where standard intubation is inappropriate for the proposed dental treatment or oral surgery. In two of these alternative airways the endotracheal tube still goes into the trachea through the larynx but comes out via the pharynx (pharyngostomy intubation) (Smith, 2004) or at the level of the first molar tooth over the mandible (mylohyoid intubation) (Soukup & Snyder, 2015) instead of the mouth.

A third alternative airway is the tracheostomy, which is more invasive and requires careful consideration, because of complications and the fact that postprocedural care is more intense. This time, the tube bypasses the larynx and enters the trachea through tracheal rings in the neck.

Difficulty with Oral Access

Some patients have a limited gape, either due to pain or functional difficulty opening the mouth. It is important to assess if this will cause a problem through history taking and conscious examination to assess the extent of the gape.

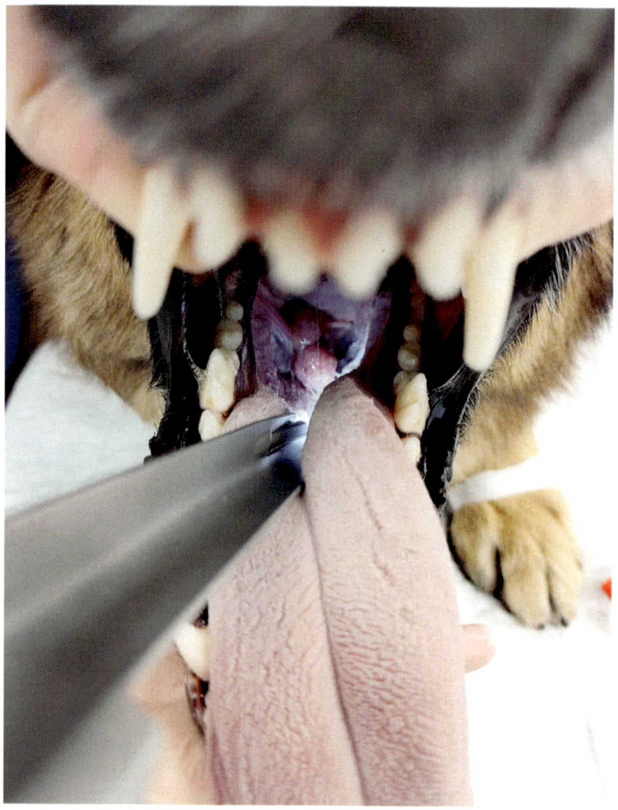

Figure 13. A tonsillar mass is lying in front of the larynx, making endotracheal intubation more difficult.

When a limited gape is suspected, it should be ensured that effective analgesia is included in the premed +/- benzodiazepines for improved muscle relaxation. Preoxygenation and setting up for a difficult intubation is also worthwhile. This is also the case for suspected oral tumours (see Figure 13), where the extent of any potential obstruction is assessed before induction, with preoxygenation and preparation for a difficult intubation as standard.

Preparation for a difficult endotracheal intubation (Figure 14):

- **preoxygenation by mask for five minutes;**
- **a range of endotracheal tube sizes, plus stylet/ urinary catheter should be prepared;**
- **laryngoscope with working light and appropriate length blade;**
- **suction;**
- **ensure easy access to trans tracheal oxygen;**
- **ensure easy access to a tracheostomy kit.**

Airway Protection

During head surgeries (e.g. jaw surgeries, dentals) it is vital to protect the airways from the aspiration of water, saline, blood, tartar, pus, or other cellular debris. One of the main ways to do this is the use of a cuffed endotracheal tube.

Endotracheal tubes are not efficient at protecting the airway if the cuff is leaky. It is important to check cuffs before use, by inflating them and leaving them inflated for several minutes to check for slow leaks. The cuff profile should also be checked when inflated to see if it is normal rather than eccentric (suggesting a weakness in one part of the cuff).

Dental anaesthetics are implicated in a high incidence of tracheal rupture in cats, usually due to over-inflation of the endotracheal tube cuff. When using cuffed tubes in cats, great care should be taken when inflating the cuffs and sufficient air should be added to the pilot balloon to only just stop a leak being heard when the reservoir bag of the breathing system is squeezed. In addition, endotracheal tubes and breathing systems should be disconnected when turning an anaesthetized patient.

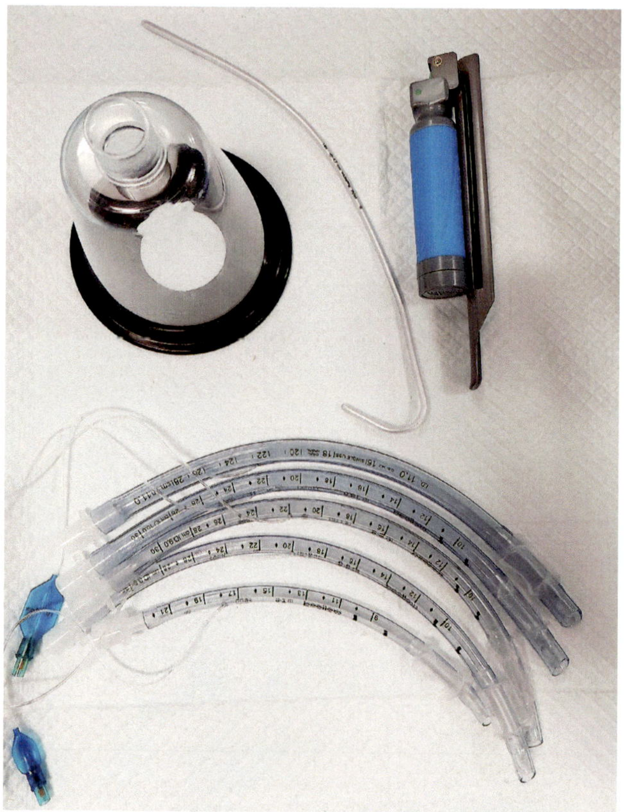

Figure 14. Difficult airway kit.

As well as using cuffed endotracheal tubes, suction may be used at different points of anaesthesia (induction, during anaesthesia, and immediately before extubation) to aid in airway protection.

Pharyngeal packs (Figure 15) are used during some jaw or dental procedures to aid airway protection. These soak up liquid and produce a barrier against solid debris. These can be either sponge or swab types and placed at the back of throat around the ETT once in place. **The packs should be attached to the ETT to ensure they are removed at the end of anaesthesia.**

Staff involved with performing head and neck procedures are at an increased risk of exposure to volatile agents escaping from the oral cavity. To reduce this incidence, the following approach should be used:

- use of cuffed endotracheal tubes;
- the vaporiser should not be switched on until the cuff is inflated;
- total or partial intravenous anaesthesia (TIVA or PIVA) should be considered;
- ensure high rates of ventilation in the work space and scavenging systems are well maintained and regularly serviced;
- low fresh gas flow rates should be used;
- at the end of the procedure, the patient should be kept attached to the breathing system until the majority of the volatile agent has been exhaled.

Positioning for Certain Head and Neck Investigations and Treatments

In certain head and neck investigations and surgeries, special positioning is required (flexed, extended, or rotated) but this can pose problems for the anaesthetist. Whenever a change of position is made, the head and neck must be stabilised when any forces are applied. There is an increased risk of airway obstruction, breathing system disconnection, and inadvertent extubation.

To prevent shearing forces on the tracheal mucosa from the endotracheal tube cuff, **the tube should be disconnected from the breathing system when the patient's position is changed.**

Good ETT security is needed to prevent endotracheal tubes coming out as a patient is moved or positioned. Monitoring of

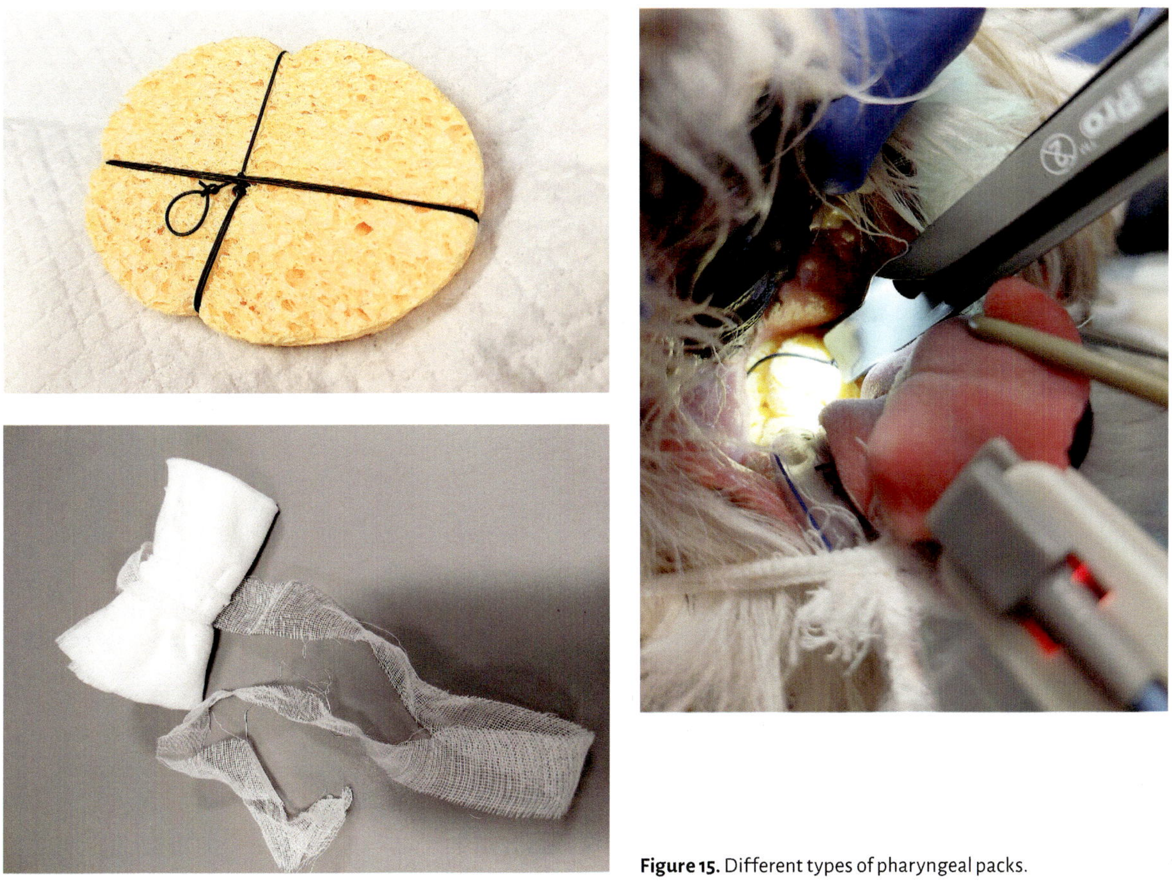

Figure 15. Different types of pharyngeal packs.

capnography helps to identify accidental disconnection. There is evidence that red rubber ETTs are more prone to kinking than silicone or plastic if the head and neck are flexed substantially (Campoy et al., 2003). An armoured ETT is an alternative where this is anticipated as a problem, as armoured ETTs have a spiral of metal in the wall to resist kinking. There are some disadvantages to these types of tubes as they are more floppy to hold and more difficult to place, their internal diameter is smaller than a regular ETT given the thickness of the wall, and they cause distortion to images on an MRI scan of the brain.

Mouth Gags

There are several publications of potential consequences of using mouth gags in cats for dental procedures. This is a particular issue in the cat, whose cerebral blood supply comes solely from the maxillary artery (whereas other species have additional routes of supply). Spring-loaded gags generate a constant force which can contribute to bulging of soft tissue between the mandible and tympanic bulla, decreasing maxillary blood flow. **The decreased cerebral blood flow usually manifests as postprocedural blindness.**

Specific Considerations

Dentals

Dentals are usually performed in older animals, with geriatric anaesthetic considerations to take into account. Airway protection is important to prevent fluid and tartar inhalation, and this consists of cuffed ETT and pharyngeal packs.

Animals should be stabilisated prior to general anaesthesia; this could include intravenous fluid therapy in dehydrated patients or those with concurrent chronic renal failure. Also, antibiosis in cases with evidence of infection and feeding up patients whose appetites have decreased.

It is important to keep the patient warm as they may become hypothermic with the fluid used for the dental procedure, however care should be taken when mixing electrical cables and water.

Analgesia should be multi-modal and preemptive and include local nerve blocks if extractions are anticipated.

Pharyngeal Stick Injuries

If the injury occurred some time ago, the patient may have sequelae which complicate anaesthesia. For example, the dog may be dehydrated from an inability to eat/drink or debris may be present in the pharynx which makes intubation difficult. Other potential concerns include pneumothorax, pneumomediastinum, and subcutaneous emphysema.

Once under anaesthesia, problems may occur when the stick is removed (e.g. arrhythmias, blood loss) as there are large blood vessels and nerves (vagus and sympathetic nerves) running through the neck. Postoperatively, pharyngeal swelling is a possibility.

Jaw Fractures

Jaw fractures usually happen as a result of a trauma, and other injuries must be carefully assessed (e.g. head trauma and raised intra-cranial pressure). Also, whether the animal has been eating and drinking, and whether it is dehydrated should be assessed.

It is wise to preoxygenate by mask and prepare for a potentially difficult intubation. Special attention should be paid to protecting the airway and a plan made of how to share the airway with the surgeon if necessary. There may be further blood loss during surgery, so blood in swabs, suction etc should be monitored and the veterinary surgeon notified when 10%, 15% and 20% total blood volume is lost. Analgesia is also paramount; a multi-modal approach including local anaesthetic techniques should be used.

Some jaw fracture repairs require wiring, which impairs the ability to open the mouth. On recovery constant monitoring is required, in case of complications such as the patient vomiting but being unable to open the mouth. Scissors (for suture closures) or wire cutters (if wire is the closure material) should be kept close at hand next to the kennel.

Jaw Surgery for Neoplasia

This surgery requires airway protection (due to presence of blood and tumour tissue including pus if there is a necrotic centre). Blood loss should be anticipated especially for maxillectomies. Sharing an airway with the surgeon is also a requirement.

When anaesthetising a patient with neoplasia, any metastasis must be taken into account. Sites of local expansion (especially maxillary tumours) and sites of metastasis (especially to pulmonary sites) should be considered, in addition to paraneoplastic syndromes due to the production of chemical signalling molecules (such as hormones or cytokines produced by tumour cells), or by an immune response against the tumour.

Such paraneoplastic syndromes include hypercalcaemia of malignancy, anaemia, clotting dysfunctions, and cancer cachexia.

Excellent analgesia is essential, including local anaesthetic techniques as long as these do not seed tumour cells.

Laryngeal Paralysis

Laryngeal paralysis often occurs in older dogs, and geriatric anaesthetic considerations apply. In this condition, one or both sides of the larynx is paralysed, producing an obstruction to breathing. The dog may present with stridorous sounds, with or without respiratory distress/cyanosis. Dogs are often stressed, which worsens their breathing, which becomes a vicious cycle.

The patients often present hypoxic, hypercapnic, and hyperthermic; all of which make the animal prone to arrhythmias if not stabilised before anaesthesia. These dogs may need sedation or a short general anaesthetic to stop the vicious cycle or indeed they may need general anaesthesia for surgical correction (elective or emergency), colloquially called a tie-back procedure.

If the patient is cyanotic, hyperthermic, and stressed, then time should be taken to cool, calm, and oxygenate. An intravenous catheter should be placed (and ideally a blood sample should be taken in geriatric patients) and fluid therapy started to cool the patient and support any renal compromise. Other cooling therapies include fans, cold towels, and spirit on paws. Body temperature should be monitored and cooling stopped once it is one degree centigrade above the optimal temperature as there will always be some over-swing.

Preanaesthetic medication helps calm the patient; a non-emetic opioid should be used as there is less laryngeal function to protect the airway from vomitus. Acepromazine at a low dose is often included as the drug is an antiemetic and it reduces body temperature (through vasodilation and re-setting the thermoregulatory centre of the brain). Low doses produce mild sedation, which is sufficient for cases with potential airway obstruction.

Oxygen should be provided during stabilisation via mask, nasopharyngeal prongs, or flow by; whichever option is the least stressful to the patient. Sedation alone may break the vicious cycle but sometimes it is necessary to administer a general anaesthetic and then allow the patient to recover slowly once their temperature is corrected (if not performing surgery). Whilst under this anaesthetic, the vet may elect to perform diagnostics such as examining laryngeal function at induction and also taking chest radiographs.

For stable patients the following are considerations when planning their anaesthetic:

- premedication includes a non-emetic opioid +/- acepromazine;
- preoxygenation by mask.

Anaesthesia is induced with intravenous propofol or alfaxalone. The vet will give sufficient induction agent to achieve a light plane of anaesthesia so as to examine laryngeal function. If a greater dose of induction agent is given, this inhibits laryngeal movement making it impossible to know if this was the effect of the drug or the laryngeal paralysis.

Once the endotracheal tube is in place, there should be very few respiratory problems during anaesthesia, as the disease causes upper respiratory tract obstruction (which is now bypassed). Sharing the airway with the surgeon is not so much of an issue as the surgery is performed via an approach through the left lateral neck. However, the surgeon may request endotracheal extubation and reintubation towards the end of surgery to check laryngeal abduction.

Airway protection is a concern, and with limited laryngeal function there is a high risk of aspiration pneumonia. In recovery, the animal should be monitored closely for postoperative swelling; the vet may consider administering NSAIDs or steroids (but should check their renal function before NSAID administration).

Brachycephalic Obstructive Airway Syndrome

Brachycephalic obstructive airway syndrome (BOAS) involves:

- elongated soft palate
- everted laryngeal ventricles
- stenotic names
- hypoplastic trachea.

Dogs with BOAS are prone to regurgitation and should therefore be induced with their head up until the endotracheal tube is placed and the cuff inflated. If the dog is a known regurgitator, intravenous omeprazole is recommended the night before and the morning of anaesthesia. Preoxygenation by mask should be undertaken and preparation undertaken for a difficult endotracheal intubation with a wide range of endotracheal tubes (a hypoplastic trachea means the tracheal lumen is narrower than expected for the size of dog). Eye care is important as these dogs often have bulbous eyes prone to exposure keratopathy.

The tube is usually directed out of the side of the mouth but most of the surgery can be done with the endotracheal tube in place. Endotracheal extubation may be required for laryngeal ventricle resection. Postoperative monitoring should be constant (Figure 16) until the animal is fully recovered from anaesthesia. An airway kit should be kept next to the patient's recovery kennel.

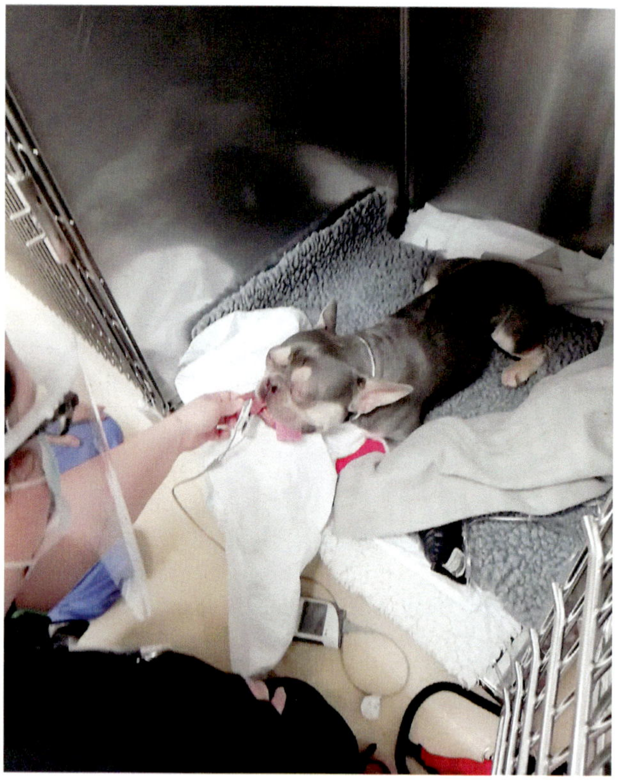

Figure 16. Patients with confirmed BOAS should be monitored closely in recovery.

Anaesthesia for Abdominal Surgery

Analgesia

An abdominal surgical procedure usually means the patient experiences both somatic and visceral nociception. Somatic pain comes from the skin, muscles, and soft tissues, while visceral pain comes from the internal organs. Different analgesics work well for somatic pain (e.g. ketamine) and visceral pain (e.g. intravenous lidocaine).

Open vs Laparoscopic Surgery

The vast majority of abdominal surgical procedures are performed via an open laparotomy. Certain interventions can be performed using a laparoscopic technique, also known as key-hole surgery, which from an anaesthesia standpoint creates less nociceptive input and causes less heat loss during surgery, both of which are beneficial.

Even when a laparoscopic approach is planned, it is important to be prepared for conversion to an open approach, both in terms of clipping the area and also for analgesic provision. The surgeon may also request altered body positions to access different abdominal organs e.g. the patient tilted with the head up and hind limbs down position (e.g. for liver biopsy), the main complications of this position are hypotension and an increased risk of venous air embolism. The head down position (e.g. for ovariohysterectomy) means the weight of the abdominal viscera further reduces functional residual capacity and increases atelectasis.

To increase the visibility of the abdominal contents, insufflation gas is used which is usually CO_2 as it does not support combustion. Gas embolism is a risk, and when CO_2 is used there may be an increase in end tidal CO_2 and $PaCO_2$. This is because gas distending the abdomen reduces the tidal volume and therefore the animal's ability to ventilate, but also because CO_2 is absorbed across the peritoneum into the blood stream. Insufflation pressure should be limited, otherwise venous return may be compromised. Carbon dioxide can produce a stinging sensation during insufflation, which may produce a noxious response.

Stomach

Gastrotomy

A gastrotomy may be required to resect neoplasia or remove a foreign body. It is likely there is a history of regurgitation, and where this is a concern then starvation time should be longer than the recommended 4–6 hours (Grubb et al., 2020) to allow for gastric emptying. If an animal has been regurgitating, then aspiration pneumonia should be anticipated as a potential sequela. The particular risk times for anaesthesia are at induction after the patient loses their protective reflexes but the airway is not yet protected. Inducing the patient in a head up position until the trachea is intubated and the cuff of the tube inflated, utilises gravity to try and prevent regurgitation. Omeprazole, the evening before and the morning of anaesthesia, should be administered intravenously.

As the stomach tissue will be incised, NSAIDs should be avoided (although paracetamol in the dog is a potential alternative) as these drugs can affect gastrointestinal mucosal healing.

Analgesia should cover both somatic and visceral pain; lidocaine CRIs may be beneficial, as in addition to visceral analgesia, anti-inflammatory, antiendotoxic, and prokinetic (preventing ileus) effects are seen.

Gastric Dilatation and Volvulus

This is a true emergency in small animal practice. Dogs are usually in shock for multiple reasons:

- hypovolaemia from third space losses and possible blood loss (if splenic torsion)
- distributive from release of endotoxins
- obstructive from compression of vena cava
- cardiogenic from ventricular arrythmias.

These patients require high volume fluid therapy and gastric decompression prior to general anaesthesia. The fluid used could be isotonic crystalloids, colloids, or hypertonic saline. Often, colloids or hypertonic saline are used for initial stabilisation as greater blood volume and pressure support can be achieved with smaller volumes and therefore in a shorter time frame, however, this should be followed up with isotonic fluids as water is drawn from the interstitial space into the intravascular space. Before fluid therapy is commenced, a minimum database (PCV, total protein, glucose and urea), lactate and electrolytes should be measured. These form a baseline for repeated measurement and lactate is also a prognostic indicator.

Patients suffering from dilatation and volvulus are prone to arrythmias, usually of a ventricular origin. If this is recognised on ECG, lidocaine should be administered via boluses or a CRI. Systemic lidocaine also contributes to visceral analgesia. Multimodal analgesia is recommended, although nitrous oxide should be avoided because it diffuses into the air distended stomach rapidly increasing its volume.

The distended stomach can have major effects on ventilation, limiting tidal volume and FRC. Therefore, oxygen supplementation is recommended and IPPV may be necessary.

In addition to monitoring ECG, capnography, and pulse oximetry, blood pressure should be monitored since blood pressure support (e.g. vasopressors or positive inotropes) may be needed. Because of the high chance of hypotension, NSAIDs should be avoided but paracetamol is appropriate. Central venous pressure (CVP) could also be measured if a jugular catheter has been placed, which helps when planning fluid therapy. At the beginning of anaesthesia, the CVP is often high due to the rotated stomach, but as the stomach decompresses and de-rotates, the CVP drops significantly, especially if insufficient fluid loading has taken place.

Intestinal Surgery

Anaesthesia may be required for enterotomy or enterectomy, for either neoplastic reasons or to remove a foreign body. If for neoplastic reasons, metastasis to the lungs should be considered as well as the effects of anaesthetic drug choices on metastasis.

The patient may present with signs of intestinal obstruction, due to a foreign body or a mass. This can cause dehydration, acid base changes, sepsis, and aspiration pneumonia (through repeated vomiting or regurgitation).

For analgesia, a multi-modal approach should be used. **Insufficient analgesia may lead to ileus** as intestinal motility is governed by the parasympathetic nervous system (and if an animal is in pain, the sympathetic nervous system is upregulated, and the parasympathetic nervous system downregulated).

Analgesics to consider include:

- lidocaine CRI: in addition to analgesia, this provides prokinetic, anti-inflammatory, and antiendotoxic effects
- opioids
- paracetamol (in the dog)
- ketamine for abdominal opening and closure.

As prostaglandins are integral in the maintenance of the gut lining, the use of NSAIDs is not advised in these cases.

Monitoring should be thorough, especially at the time of intestinal manipulation as vagal reflexes may affect the heart rate.

Splenectomy

Splenectomy is often undertaken for neoplastic or trauma reasons. If it is performed for neoplastic reasons, secondary or metastatic sites should be considered (e.g. right atrium which may cause arrythmias or the lungs, which may affect oxygenation). If splenectomy is required because of trauma, potential comorbidities including thoracic trauma should be considered.

These patients usually present with a history of haemorrhage and may be anaemic. Blood transfusions should be considered, but unless severely anaemic, the transfusion can be delayed until after the spleen is removed. This is firstly because the blood may be lost straight into the abdominal cavity, but also, aggressive fluid therapy increases blood pressure and pops off the clots which are trying to form to stop the bleeding. The concept of **delayed fluid resuscitation** is to give sufficient fluids to stabilise the patient (e.g. bringing heart rate down and improving pulse quality) followed by anaesthetising the patient for the surgeon to remove the bleeding spleen, and then the rest of the fluid deficit (potentially including blood) is paid back.

These cases are prone to arrythmias; therefore, the ECG should be monitored closely. Lidocaine CRIs may be antiarrhythmic and also contribute to analgesia.

As always, an individual plan should be made for the patient, but in general, drugs causing splenic engorgement should be avoided, as should NSAIDs because of the possibility of intraoperative haemorrhage and thus hypotension.

Liver

The liver has many functions and if it is not working properly, anaesthesia can be affected in several ways, which are identified by biochemical and haematological blood analysis:

- Hypoproteinaemia: this may result in ascites (compromising ventilation), oedema (including pulmonary oedema), lower plasma oncotic pressure, and affect drug binding.
- Anaemia: if moderate to severe, this affects oxygen carrying capacity, the ability to visualise cyanosis, and drug binding.
- Hypoglycaemia: may cause systemic effects such as neuronal damage, immunosuppression, and muscle weakness.
- Tendency to hypothermia as the liver is very exothermic.
- Prolonged clotting times as the liver is a site of clotting factor production.
- Raised blood ammonia as the liver detoxifies ammonia from the blood. This leads to dullness, depression, hepatic encephalopathy and potentially seizures.
- Increased risk of bacteraemia because the liver filters out bacteria from the blood stream, which can lead to an increased risk of infections.
- Jaundice obscures other mucous membrane colours, e.g. paleness.
- Hepatomegaly (usually seen with a mass) may reduce the ability of the animal to ventilate and oxygenate properly. Predisposing to hypoxia and hypercapnia.

Importantly, the liver is the site of biotransformation of many anaesthetic drugs, and so their metabolism may be slowed. If giving pro-drugs, consideration should be given to the fact that the formation of the active drug is delayed.

Porto-systemic Shunts

This condition is often congenital (and carries paediatric considerations for anaesthesia). An aberrant blood vessel diverts the blood coming back from the intestine around the liver rather than into it. Medical stabilisation is usually required which incorporates:

- lactulose
- antibiotics
- appropriate diet.

Shunt ligation is usually undertaken via an exploratory laparotomy although interventional coil placement is an option.

- As the liver is not functioning correctly, concerns regarding liver dysfunction above should be considered. The vet should use anaesthetic drugs with a short duration of action or with an alternate route of elimination.
- Endogenous benzodiazepines are implicated in hepatic encephalopathy and therefore exogenous benzodiazepines should be avoided.
- Central venous pressure is a useful monitoring tool. The CVP value may drop significantly as the shunt is ligated.
- Intestinal blood flow can be affected, and abdominal crises are sometimes observed postligation.

Liver Lobe Resection

This is usually performed to resect neoplasia, therefore the implication of metastasis at other sites should be considered. There is often a history of haemorrhage and the animal may be anaemic. In this situation, delayed fluid resuscitation should be considered. Liver function may be affected. One of the major risks of these anaesthetics is the possibility of intraoperative haemorrhage and vena cava compression. Therefore, direct blood pressure monitoring is preferable, with blood products readily available.

Pancreas

Insulinomas

This is a tumour of the pancreas which releases high levels of insulin. Patients often present with signs of hypoglycaemia including collapse/seizures. An exploratory laparotomy is required to resect the tumour from the pancreas. Starving the night before surgery may lead to life threatening low blood glucose levels therefore a short starvation time should be employed and blood glucose checked before preanaesthetic medication.

The vet may consider using an α-2 adrenergic agonist if the patient is cardiovascularly stable enough. This class of drugs inhibit insulin which produces higher blood glucose levels and therefore less intervention for low blood glucose during anaesthesia is required. (Guedes & Rude, 2013).

Blood glucose should be monitored every 15 minutes during anaesthesia. The frequency of testing should increase when the pancreatic mass is being handled.

Nephrectomy

This may be to remove a neoplastic or otherwise diseased kidney. Because of the anatomical location of the kidneys, good muscle relaxation is required. As the surgeon works to remove the kidney, aorto-caval compression may be observed, reducing venous return and decreasing cardiac output. Blood pressure monitoring (ideally direct) is recommended.

When removing one kidney, it is vital to maintain the health of the remaining kidney under anaesthesia by ensuring:

- **adequate blood pressure**
- **normal oxygen and carbon dioxide**
- **appropriate depth of anaesthesia**
- **avoiding NSAIDs.**

Adrenals

The paired adrenal glands sit next to their respective kidneys, but one may need to be removed in an adrenalectomy. Again, because of their anatomical location, the surgeon requires good muscle relaxation and may cause aorto-cava compression whilst gaining access to them. Unfortunately, many adrenal masses have invaded the vena cava and therefore blood loss is a distinct possibility.

Adrenal tumours may produce different substances, e.g. either producing excessive amounts of cortisol (producing Cushingoid signs) or excessive amounts of catecholamines (pheochromocytoma).

Bladder

A cystotomy may be required as a divert for urinary tract trauma. These animals may be experiencing postrenal failure, i.e. an increase in urea and creatinine because they cannot void urine. They may also be uraemic and have acid base and electrolyte changes (primarily metabolic acidosis and hyperkalaemia). They need stabilisation before anaesthesia is attempted. Fluid therapy is usually the first line in stabilising these patients. If fluid therapy alone does not correct potassium, glucose +/- insulin or calcium gluconate may be required.

In addition to postrenal failure there is a possibility the patient has intrinsic renal failure and therefore NSAIDs should be avoided until volume status and blood parameters have normalised.

Uterus

Pyometra

In this disease process inflammatory cells, bacteraemia, and secretions accumulate in the uterus. **The patient may present with endotoxaemia and possible septic peritonitis.**

Mild signs include polyuria and polydipsia, but more severe signs include lethargy, anorexia, fever, dehydration, tachycardia and tachypnoea. *E.coli* endotoxins leads to antidiuretic hormone (ADH) insensitivity and diuresis and permanent renal tubular damage can occur.

Preanaesthetic bloods may highlight the following abnormalities:

- **albumin (low)**
- **urea/creatinine (high)**
- **hepatic enzymes (high)**
- **glucose (low or high)**
- **chloride (low).**

Stabilisation with IVFT (crystalloids+/-colloids) and continued fluid therapy intra- and postoperatively is recommended. The anaesthetic protocol used depends on the severity of clinical signs. Mildly affected patients may be anaesthetised with a standard bitch spay protocol, although NSAIDs should be avoided (because of the possible renal tubular damage). However, sicker patients need a much-altered anaesthetic protocol, avoiding drugs with more profound cardiovascular effects.

Caesarean Section

The physiological changes in the third trimester of pregnancy involve multiple body systems.

Cardiovascular System

Cardiac output and blood volume increase with an increase in both plasma volume and red cell mass. Systemic vascular resistance decreases due to vasodilation. Hypotension can occur because of this vasodilation and the pressure of a gravid uterus on the aorta and vena cava.

Respiratory System

Minute volume and oxygen consumption increases and functional residual capacity decreases, therefore oxygen supplementation is recommended.

Gastrointestinal

The gravid uterus places pressure on the stomach and the oesophagus is kinked by an altered position. Together with an increase in serum progesterone, this means animals are more prone to regurgitation.

Whilst the aim is to produce live puppies or kittens, the safety of the dam or queen is the priority. That said, an attempt should be made to maintain placental delivery of oxygen and placental blood flow until the foetuses are delivered. Short acting drugs or drugs which do not cross the placental barrier should be used when possible.

Whether or not to premedicate the patient is a contentious issue. The dam is often exhausted and may not require much preanaesthetic medication. Any preanaesthetic medication drug is passed to the offspring, but preanaesthetic medication decreases the amount of other drugs e.g. induction agent. Analgesia (such as an opioid) included in the preanaesthetic medication also provides preemptive analgesia. Other ways of providing analgesia include the use of local anaesthetic line blocks and paracetamol (in the dog).

As much of belly as possible should be clipped before induction. Intravenous catheter access should be secured, to administer drugs and provide isotonic crystalloid fluid therapy. If possible the animal should be preoxygenated to maintain placental oxygenation and because patients are more prone to desaturation.

A head up induction should be used as animals are prone to regurgitating. A cuffed ET tube should be used (both due to the chance of regurgitation and the possible need to perform IPPV). Low solubility volatile agents produce a fast recovery from general anaesthesia for both mother and offspring. Minimum alveolar concentration (MAC) in pregnant animals is decreased i.e. lower dial volatile agent concentrations should be used.

Anaesthesia for Spinal Cases

Imaging is often required to investigate spinal pathology. There are several modalities available, most requiring the patient to be anaesthetized rather than sedated:

- radiography: plain or myelogram
- computed tomography +/- myelogram
- magnetic resonance imaging.

Intravenous access is recommended in all cases, no matter which imaging modality. Fluid therapy is recommended. Preanaesthetic medication is required but differs between cases. Analgesic drugs are required if the patient is painful or surgical treatment is anticipated. Calming the patient with preanaesthetic medication facilitates safe moving of the patient, which may be vital in certain patients with unstable spines.

Induction of anaesthesia is usually performed using intravenous agents such as propofol or alfaxalone, given slowly to effect. Cervical spinal cases benefit from a head flat endotracheal intubation (Figure 17) following preoxygenation.

Maintenance of anaesthesia is usually under volatile agent anaesthesia (+/- analgesic continuous rate infusions). During spinal surgery, ventilation of the lungs may be useful.

Magnetic Resonance Imaging (MRI) Scanning

Anaesthesia in the MRI environment poses challenges to the anaesthetist (Figure 18). The animal lies in a long narrow tube and is not easy to access, and the MRI facility is often some way from the clinic's ICU in cases of emergency.

The presence of a strong magnetic field attracts ferromagnetic objects (ranging from laryngoscopes, scissors and oxygen cylinders to anaesthetic machines) potentially turning them into fast moving projectiles. Therefore, all anaesthetic equipment which enters the MRI space must be MRI compatible. Small amounts of ferromagnetic substances e.g. the spring in the pilot balloon of an endotracheal tube can cause anomalies on the MRI scan. Intravenous contrast medium can be nephrotoxic, cause anaphylactic reactions and lighten the plane of anaesthesia.

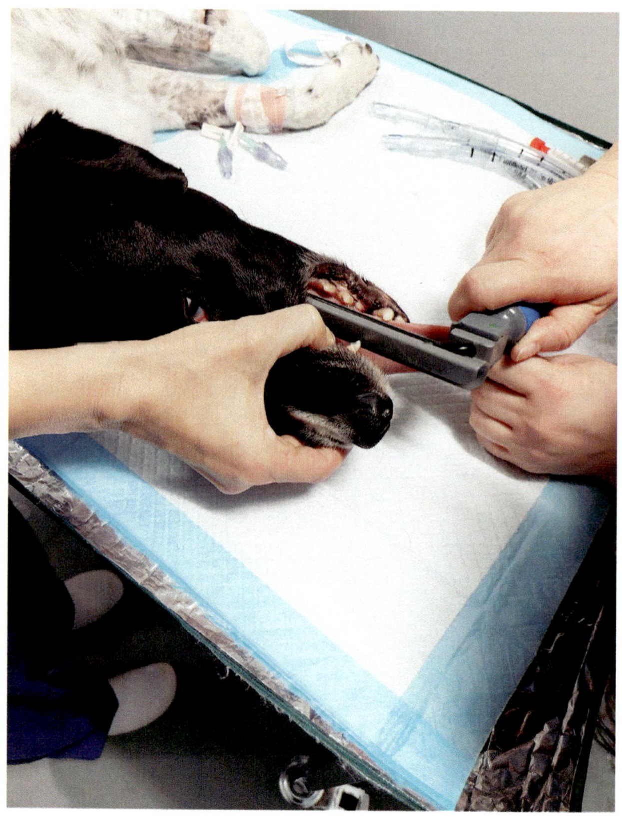

Figure 17. A head flat induction and endotracheal intubation is indicated for patients with unstable cervical spines.

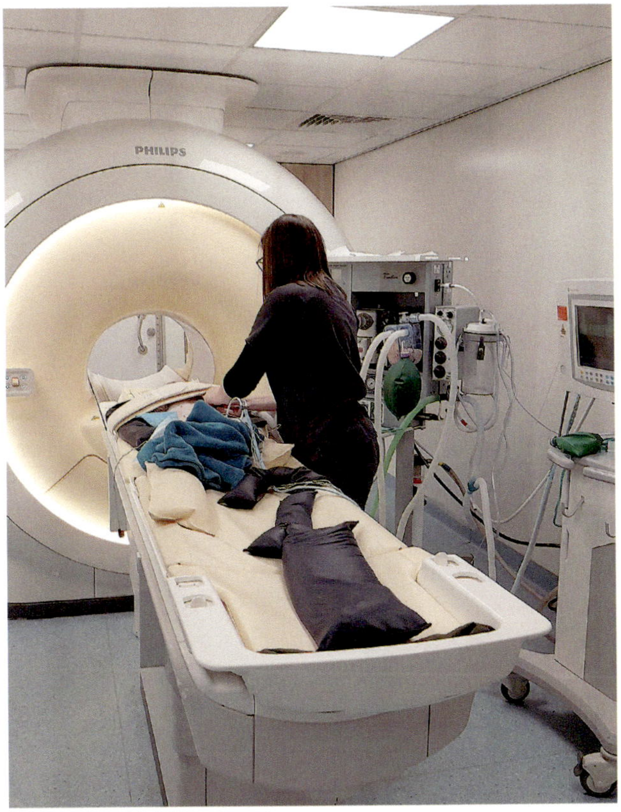

Figure 18. Monitoring anaesthesia in the MRI scanner can be difficult because of a lack of access to the patient.

References

- Brodbelt et al. (2008) *Veterinary Anaesthesia Analgesia.* 35, 365–373.
- Campoy et al. (2003) *Journal of Small Animal Practice.* 44, 3–7.
- Davis et al. (2013) *Journal of the American Animal Hospital Association.* 49(3), 149–159.
- Grubb et al. (2020) *Journal of the American Animal Hospital Association.* 56, 59–82.
- Guedes & Rude (2013) *Veterinary anaesthesia and analgesia.* 40(5), 472–481.
- Hall et al. (2001) *Veterinary Anaesthesia.* UK, Saunders.
- Hughes (2016) Chapter 5: Breathing systems and ancillary equipment. In: *BSAVA Manual of Canine and Feline Anaesthesia and Analgesia*, pp. 45–64.
- Rodriguez et al. (2012) *Veterinary anaesthesia and analgesia.* 39(4), 357–365.
- Smith M. M. (2004) *Journal of veterinary dentistry.* 21, 191–194.
- Soukup & Snyder (2015). *Veterinary surgery.* 44, 432–436.

TEST

ANSWERS ON PAGE 178

1. When gaining consent for a procedure requiring general anaesthesia or sedation, the type of consent should ideally be:

a. Implied and verbal.
b. Implied and written.
c. Explicit and verbal.
d. Explicit and written.

2. Which of these drugs is a benzodiazepine?

a. Acepromazine.
b. Glycopyrrolate.
c. Midazolam.
d. Alfaxalone.

3. What action does acepromazine have on α receptors to produce vasodilation?

a. α-1 agonism.
b. α-1 blockade.
c. α-2 agonism.
d. α-2 blockade.

4. For which group of drugs is flumazenil an antagonist?

a. α-2 adrenergic agonists.
b. Phenothiazines.
c. Opioids.
d. Benzodiazepines.

5. What type of capnograph trace would endo-oesophageal intubation cause?

a. No trace on the capnograph.
b. A prolonged upward slope in phase 2.
c. Oscillations in phase 4.
d. A lack of return to baseline in phase 1.

6. What PaO_2 reading should a patient breathing an inspired oxygen fraction of 50% have?

a. 50 mmHg.
b. 100 mmHg.
c. 250 mmHg.
d. 500 mmHg.

7. Which of the following is a clinical sign of a non-immune mediated transfusion reaction?

a. Urticaria.
b. Hypocalcemia.
c. Angioedema.
d. Haemolysis.

8. What piece of monitoring equipment can be used to provide information about a patient's ventilation?

a. Pulse oximetry.
b. Blood pressure.
c. Central venous pressure.
d. Capnography.

9. An animal suffering from insulinoma usually has:

a. Increased levels of insulin and increased levels of glucose.
b. Increased levels of insulin and decreased levels of glucose.
c. Decreased levels of insulin and decreased levels of glucose.
d. Decreased levels of insulin and increased levels of glucose.

10. What rate do current recommendations from the American Animal Hospital Association (AAHA) suggest as a starting rate for crystalloid fluid therapy at the beginning of anaesthesia in normal healthy dogs?

a. 5 ml/kg/hr.
b. 6 ml/kg/hr.
c. 10 ml/kg/hr.
d. 4 ml/kg/hr.

Clinical Case

A 3 kg cat is presented out of hours with inappetence. The vet palpates an abdominal mass and suggests an exploratory laparotomy, planned for in 10 hours' time. On clinical exam, the cat has the following signs of dehydration:

- semi dry oral mucous membranes
- normal skin turgor
- moist eyes.

1. How dehydrated is the cat?

2. What does this percentage represent?

3. What is the fluid deficit in this cat?

4. The fluid deficit needs to be restored before surgery as well as providing maintenance fluid therapy over this time frame, as the patient is not eating. What is the maintenance rate for this cat?

5. Using the information above, what is the fluid therapy plan to rehydrate the cat before general anaesthesia?

6. The next morning the cat's hydration status is checked again; the cat is weighed and is now 3.15 kg and the vet feels the cat is now normally hydrated and the fluid deficit has been restored. You are going to anaesthetise the cat for the exploratory laparotomy, but what fluid rate should the cat be on during anaesthesia?

7. Based on the American Society of Anesthesiologists (ASA) classification of the cat, what risk of perianaesthetic mortality should the vet give to the owner when getting anaesthetic consent?

8. What top three pieces of monitoring equipment would you choose for this anaesthetic. Justify your choices.

Correct Answers:

Test

1. d
2. c
3. b
4. d
5. a
6. c
7. b
8. d
9. b
10. a

Clinical Case

1. How dehydrated is the cat?
5%

2. What does this percentage represent?
The percentage of bodyweight lost as water.

3. What is the fluid deficit in this cat?
5/100 x 3 kg = 0.15 kg = 0.15 l = 150 ml
(Remember the density of water is 1 g/ml)

4. What is the maintenance rate for this cat?

- In the cat, the formula is 80 x bodyweight (kg) 0.75 and this gives the total volume of maintenance fluid for 24 hours.
- Maintenance over 24 hours = 80 x 30.75 = 182 ml over 24 hours

This is the maintenance requirement over 24 hours, but we are interested in how much we need to give over 10 hours as this is the time frame for the fluid therapy plan in question i.e. up until the point of the exploratory laparotomy.

10/24 x 182 ml = 76 ml over 10 hours

5. What is the fluid therapy plan to rehydrate the cat before general anaesthesia?

Pay back the 150 ml fluid deficit during the 10 hours plus 76 ml maintenance. Then these should be added together:

150 + 76 = 226 ml over 10 hours = 22.6 ml/hr

6. What fluid rate should the cat be on during anaesthesia?

Following AAHA guidelines, a starting rate of 3 ml/kg/hr should be used for the first hour then reduced by 25% every hour until the maintenance rate is reached. With the cat's new weight, maintenance is 80 x 3.15 x 0.75 = 189 ml over 24 hours.

189/24 = 7.9 ml/hr and as the cat now weighs 3.15 kg, this is 2.5 ml/kg/hr.

So the anaesthesia fluid therapy should be started at 3 ml/kg/hr but dropped to 2.5 ml/kg/hr after 1 hour because this is the cat's maintenance rate and a drop of 25% every hour is used, until maintenance is reached, and the maintenance rate is higher than the 25% reduction.

7. What risk of perianaesthetic mortality should the vet give to the owner when getting anaesthetic consent?

This cat would be considered as an ASA 3, therefore the risk of perianaesthetic death is 1.4%.

8. What top three pieces of monitoring equipment would you choose for this anaesthetic.

Several pieces of monitoring equipment are justifiable, even if your choices are not included in the top three here, as long as you can justify the reason, then that is fine.

Temperature monitoring: the cat is small and its abdomen will be open, both predisposing to hypothermia. Heart rate, either via ECG or stethoscope: there is a possibility of a vagal response when gut is handled. Blood pressure: many animals are prone to hypotension under anaesthesia.

NOTES

Analgesia

Nicki Grint

Chapter Summary:

- **The pathophysiology of pain.**
- **Pain scoring methods in different species.**
- **Different classes of analgesia and their pharmacology: including opioids, NSAIDs, and local anaesthetics.**
- **Preemptive and multi-modal analgesia.**
- **CRI infusion: appropriate agents, monitoring, and CRI calculations.**
- **Local anaesthetic techniques and appropriate case selection.**
- **The safe administration of local anaesthetics via transcutaneous electrical nerve stimulation.**

Physiology of Pain

The International Academy for the Study of Pain (IASP) updated their definition of pain in 2020. The revised definition is: "an unpleasant sensory and emotional experience associated with, or resembling that associated with, actual or potential tissue damage".

The sensory component alone is nociception. For the term pain to be used there must be an emotional component as well.

Types of Pain

Nociceptors

When tissue (skin, ligaments, viscera) is damaged this activates nociceptors (pain receptors). **Nociceptors respond to different noxious stimuli;** some respond to extremes of temperatures (thermoreceptors), some respond to extremes of pressure including incisions (mechanoreceptors) or chemicals (chemoreceptors). Some nociceptors are **unimodal** (i.e. only respond to one set of stimuli), and some nociceptors are **polymodal** and respond to more than one type of stimuli.

Nociceptors have a **firing threshold,** which is the threshold that triggers an electrical stimulus. The threshold might be a certain temperature or a pressure. **When tissue is damaged, this releases inflammatory mediators** such as prostaglandins and leukotrienes to form an inflammatory soup. These inflammatory mediators lower the firing thresholds and make nociceptors respond to less intense stimuli. **This lowering of the firing threshold contributes to the phenomena of allodynia and hyperalgesia.** In addition, silent nociceptors (usually dormant/inactive) can be recruited by the inflammatory soup.

Somatic and Visceral Pain

- **Somatic pain** is that arising from skin or muscle.
- **Visceral pain** is that arising from internal organs.

Visceral nociceptors are often polymodal C fibres. They are sparsely distributed when compared to those in the skin (approx. 1:100). This means **visceral pain is difficult to localise because it is a diffuse sensation.** Visceral nociceptors also respond to different stimuli than those in the skin e.g. sharp incisional stimuli is more painful for skin than viscera. **Stretching and distension** are often the major stimuli for visceral pain.

The Pain Pathway

The pain pathway is illustrated in Figure 1.

The conversion of a noxious stimulus (such as an extreme temperature or pressure) into an electrical stimulus is called **transduction,** and this is the first part of the pain pathway.

These electrical signals pass up nerves (either A-δ or C fibres) to a part of the spinal cord called the dorsal horn. This part of the pain pathway is called **transmission.**

- **A-δ fibres** are fast conducting, small fibres which are myelinated for sharp, mechanical pain.
- **C fibres** are slow conducting, unmyelinated fibres for longer lasting or dull, burning pain.

At the dorsal horn of the spinal cord, several things happen, including a reflex arc which makes the motor nerves (if the animal is conscious) move the muscles to remove the part of the body affected away from the noxious stimulus.

Also at the dorsal horn, a decision is made whether to pass the signal up the spinal cord to the brain, or not. This decision making is called **modulation.** When the signal is passed up to the brain and arrives at the cerebral cortex, this is when the animal becomes aware of the pain (**perception**).

Acute vs Chronic Pain

- **Acute pain** is sudden onset and usually the result of a clearly defined cause such as an injury or surgery. Acute pain resolves with the healing of its underlying cause and is alleviated by analgesic drugs.
- **Chronic pain** persists for weeks or months, well past the course of the disease. Chronic pain is seldom totally alleviated by analgesics.

Box 1. Physiological Consequences of Pain

- **Increased sympathetic tone.**
- **Increased systemic vascular resistance and preload.**
- **Increased stroke volume.**
- **Increased myocardial work.**
- **Increased metabolic rate.**
- **Altered clotting function.**
- **Decreased gastrointestinal and urinary tone.**
- **Increased ACTH, cortisol, ADH, renin, angiotensin.**
- **Hyperglycaemia.**
- **Increased protein muscle metabolism.**
- **Retention of Na^+ and water.**
- **Hypoventilation.**

Physiological Consequences of Pain

As well as being a welfare issue, animals should not be allowed to remain in pain, several physiological consequences occur which are listed in Box 1.

Pain Assessment

In 2020, the International Academy for the Study of Pain (IASP) updated their definition of pain and added an addendum: "Verbal description is only one of several behaviours to express

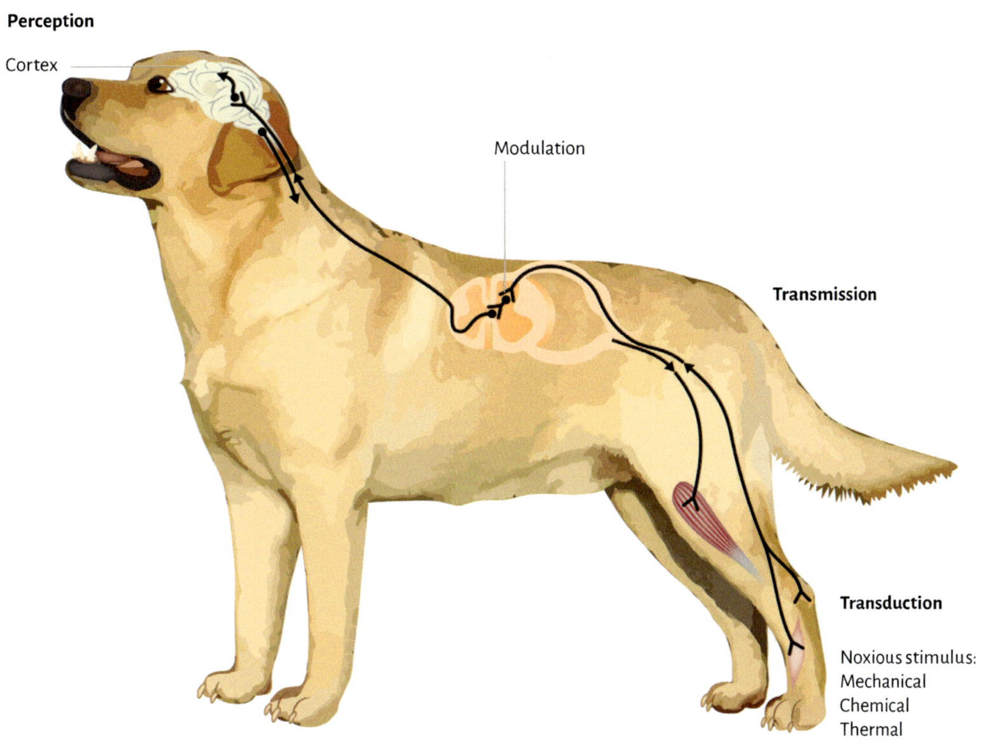

Figure 1. The pain pathway.

pain; inability to communicate does not negate the possibility that a human or a nonhuman animal experiences pain."

This encapsulates **the difficulty in assessing pain in animals as they cannot verbalise their pain** and we have to rely on behavioural clues. The difficulty in assessing pain in animals results in one of two outcomes. Either analgesics are withheld because the animal is not showing overt signs of pain, or an assessor is overly anthropomorphic and assumes that because a human undergoing the same surgery requires a certain level of analgesia, the animal requires the same, and may administer excessive analgesics.

There is no gold standard pain assessment system; and **all rely on the interpretation/ recognition of behaviours and so have a large subjective component** which is prone to observer error and bias. More objective measures such as physiological data (Box 2) can be used as part of pain assessment (e.g. the University of Melbourne Pain Scale (dogs) and Botucatu Scale (cats)) but are not reliable, as these are not specific enough to differentiate pain from other stressors e.g. anxiety, fear, or other pathologies.

Box 2. Physiological Signs Associated with Pain (Adapted from Muir & Gaynor, 2002)

- Tachypnoea or panting.
- Tachycardia.
- Dilated pupils.
- Hypertension.

Difficulties in Pain Assessment

To recognise pain behaviours in an individual animal, it is **useful to know what the animal's normal behaviour is,** which is knowledge gained from the veterinary nurse's interaction with the patient in the kennels preoperatively. However, animals hospitalised away from their owner often do not exhibit normal behaviours in a strange environment. Small mammals housed in close proximity to their predators will also not exhibit normal behaviour. Difficulties in interpretation also stem from how different species exhibit different signs of pain behaviour. Even within a species, different breeds and individuals respond to pain in different ways. The obvious and well quoted example is the comparison of the Labrador still wagging its tail with a broken leg, compared to a Greyhound that screams during the premedication injection.

Postoperative pain scores are also be confused by concomitant drug therapy. Just because an animal is sedated, it does not necessarily mean its analgesia is adequate. Take for example the drugs dexmedetomidine, medetomidine, and morphine, where it is thought that the sedation caused by these drugs outlasts the analgesia. Observer variation also plays a part with some observers scoring consistently higher than others. This can to some extent be minimised if all observers use the same systematic approach to pain scoring.

A Dynamic and Interactive Approach

Whatever the pain scoring system, the observer must employ a dynamic and interactive approach. In any assessment it is not enough to merely observe the patient to assess pain, but **must be interactive which means using palpation.** Firstly, the observer approaches the animal from outside the kennel to take note of any signs such as abnormal postures, restlessness, and attention to any wounds (e.g. licking, biting or chewing). The observer then opens the cage door and attracts the animal to the front of the cage, noting the animal's willingness to interact and move, and their general demeanour. Finally, the animal should be allowed out of the cage (if their condition allows) to move around. Observers should watch for signs such as reluctance to move, and lameness. Then, importantly, the animal's painful focus (e.g. the surgical site) should be gently palpated and the animal's response (which watch out – could include turning and biting) noted (Figure 2). **All of this information should be considered together when**

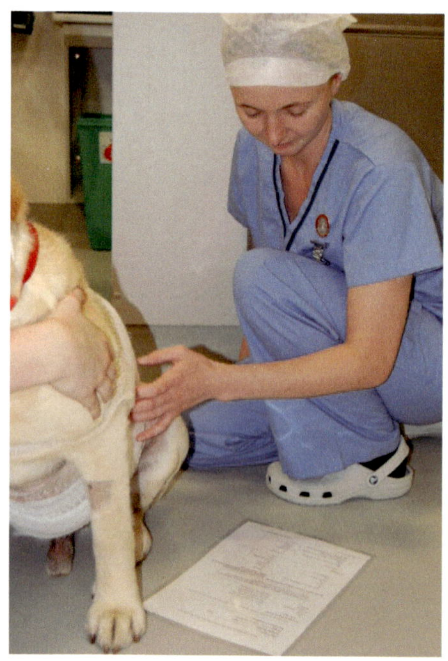

Figure 2. Nurse performing pain score.

assigning a pain score. Some published pain scoring systems suggest that if there is no painful focus, the palpation of a stifle for consistent comparison.

Different Types of Pain Scoring Systems

The three main types of pain scores are known as visual analogue scales (VAS), numerical rating scales (NRS), and simple descriptive scales (SDS) as described in Table 1.

The scales can be used to assign an overall pain score or used to compile composite scores (also known as categorical or multi-factorial). **A composite score is where there are multiple scales for different aspects of pain behaviour.** Scores are assigned in categories such as vocalisation and posture, and then added together to create a total score. Using composite scales often reminds the observer to look at several aspects of the animal's behaviour before assigning the pain score.

How to Use Pain Scoring Systems

Pain scales usually have an intervention level which guides the user as to when the animal requires additional analgesia. If the nurse's clinical opinion is the animal is uncomfortable, but the pain score has not reached the intervention level, analgesia should not be withheld for this reason.

Pain Assessment in Dogs

Table 2 includes behaviours to look for in dogs that are indicators of pain.

Table 2. Some pain related behaviours observed in dogs.

Behavioural aspect	Dog
Vocalisation	Howls, barks, groans, whimpers, growls.
Facial expression	Furrowing of brow, fixed stare.
Self-awareness	Looks at painful area, licks, chews, or bites at it.
Locomotion	Limping or non-weight bearing on a painful limb.
Activity	Restless, slow to rise, reluctant to move.
Attitude	Poor response to owner with weak tail wag or can become aggressive with tendency to escape.
Appetite	Decreased, picky or absent.
Urination and bowel movements	Urine retention and constipation.
Grooming	Reduced.
Response to palpation	Vocalisation, aggression, withdrawing.
Posture	Abnormal positions may include dropped head, hunched, tucked in abdomen, "praying" position.

There are several published pain scores that are validated in dogs, but the one in common place use is the **Glasgow Composite Measure Pain Scale.** It is a composite simple descriptive scale with six categories:

- posture
- activity
- vocalisation
- attention to wounds
- demeanour
- mobility
- response to touch.

The maximum score is 24, but where it is not appropriate to make the dog rise and leave the kennel, the maximum score is 20. **The analgesic intervention level is 6/24 or 5/20.**

Table 1. Visual analogue scales (VAS), numerical rating scales (NRS), and simple descriptive scales (SDS).

	VAS	NRS	SDS
Description	· Semiobjective scoring system. · A 100 mm straight horizontal line anchored with two phrases. · The observer places a mark on the line corresponding to the degree of pain.	· Semiobjective scoring system. · Pain score is assigned as a whole number. · Typically 0-10 is used.	· Semiobjective scoring system. · 4 or 5 categories of pain intensity. · Each descriptor is assigned a number
Example	No pain ⊢X———⊣ Worst possible pain (100 mm)	No pain 0 1 2 X 3 4 5 Worst possible pain	1. No pain 2. Mild pain 3. Moderate pain X 4. Severe pain

Pain Assessment in Cats

Pain assessment in cats has lagged behind that of dogs. Cats tend to conceal pain more than dogs, which may be a reason analgesia is often suboptimal in this species.

When performing a dynamic and interactive assessment of the cat, there are three main phases of pain assessment: observation of the cat in the cage, interaction with the cat, and palpation of the painful area. The interactive portion of the assessment is often not be feasible in feral cats. Table 3 includes what to look for during pain assessment.

Table 3. Some pain related behaviours observed in cats.

Behavioural aspect	Cat
Changes	This could be an absence of a normal behaviour or a presence of a new one.
Facial expression	Fear slope, muzzle tension, orbital squeezing/ eye squinting, hanging head, furrowed brow.
Posture	Hunched position or tense abdomen, shifting of weight or lying in an abnormal position.
Attention to wounds	Licking, chewing or scratching.
Vocalisation	Crying, hissing or growling or unusually quiet.
Response to palpation	Swish tail, flatten ears, cry, hiss or growl, bite or lash out.

There are three pain scoring systems validated in cats:

- Glasgow Composite Measure Pain Scale for cats (Glasgow CMPS).
- UNESP Botucatu Multidimensional Composite Pain Scale.
- Feline Grimace Scale (University of Montreal).

The Glasgow CMPS is a composite simple descriptive scale. Several of the categories have questions regarding presence or absence of behaviours but also include caricatures of two aspects of facial expression (ear position and muzzle tone). **The authors suggest an analgesia intervention level of 5 out of 20.**

UNESP Botucatu Scale is a composite descriptive scale. It has been validated in Portuguese and English. It includes several categories including objective (blood pressure measurement) and subjective evaluations. **The authors suggest an intervention level of ≥8 out of 30.**

The Feline Grimace Scale concentrates solely on the cat's face. It scores five facial action units: whisker position, orbital tightening, ear position, head position, and muzzle tension. Each facial action unit is scored from 0 to 2. The score is then added up and divided by the total possible score (i.e. if that facial action unit cannot be scored, it is left out). **The intervention level is >0.39 out of 1.0.** This would be the equivalent of a total of 4 out of 10 unit scores.

Pain Assessment in Small Mammals

Some behavioural signs associated with pain in small mammals include:

- **Rabbits: hide, face back of cage, may become aggressive or docile, reduced appetite and grinds teeth.**
- **Guinea pig: hide, lie recumbent, quiet, terrified, repetitive squealing, reduced appetite with increased respiratory rate.**
- **Rats: hiding or hunched, back arched and stretching (abdominal pain), aggressive or docile, reduced appetite, self-trauma, eating bedding, piloerection, lack of grooming, porphyrin staining (reddish-brown staining around eyes and nose). (Adapted from Grant, 2007).**

Much work has been done on facial action units in various species (e.g. Feline Grimace Scale). Researchers at the University of Newcastle have published posters detailing pain assessment using facial expressions in rats, mice, and rabbits.

Nociceptive Threshold Testing

The majority of pain assessment techniques are subjective. However, veterinary research has looked at nociceptive threshold testing as an objective tool to quantify an animal's nociceptive thresholds and see how they change after surgery and/or analgesia.

The technique involves application of a mechanical or thermal stimulus. For example, the mechanical test is the application of a blunt ended pin to a site next to the surgical site. The blunt ended pin is attached to a force or pressure metre. The blunt ended pin is then applied until the animal's reaction suggests they find it a noxious stimulus e.g. flinching, growling, snapping, lifting a leg. The force or pressure at which this occurs is the animal's nociceptive threshold. A baseline value is obtained before surgery. After surgery, if analgesia is insufficient the threshold goes down (i.e. the patient tolerates less stimulus before reacting). If analgesia is administered, the threshold increases.

This technique used to be used under Home Office licence, however, it is now legal for it to be used in clinical practice.

However, it is best used in addition to pain scoring, rather than to replace it.

Preemptive Analgesia

To produce effective analgesia, **the aim should be to use a preemptive approach. The concept of preemptive analgesia is to have the analgesic agents on board before the painful stimulus starts.** Theoretically preemptive analgesia blocks the afferent input to the nervous system in order to prevent peripheral and central sensitisation. This decreases the amount of analgesia required postoperatively and also prevents long term problems associated with surgery such as abnormal sensitivity of the wound (allodynia and hyperalgesia).

Peripheral sensitisation is defined as the increased responsiveness and reduced threshold of nociceptive neurones in the periphery to the stimulation of their receptive field. This is initiated when nociceptors are exposed to noxious stimulus, which releases an inflammatory soup in the damaged tissues. These inflammatory mediators result in a lowered activation threshold and thus an increase in responsiveness of nociceptors.

Central sensitisation is defined as an increased responsiveness of nociceptors in the central nervous system to either normal or sub-threshold afferent input resulting in:

- hypersensitivity to stimuli
- responsiveness to non-noxious stimuli
- increased pain response evoked by stimuli outside the area of injury and expanded receptive field.

Theoretically, administering analgesia before the noxious input should result in lower pain scores postoperatively and less requirement for analgesia, compared to the patient that receives analgesia after the noxious input.

Lots of studies have been done in human and veterinary fields to see whether preemptive analgesia is more effective. All of the studies are preincisional versus postincisional (i.e. two groups of patients having the same surgery, with one group getting an analgesic drug before surgery and one group getting the same drug after surgery). The postoperative pain scores and analgesic requirements are then compared between the groups and theoretically the preincisional groups would have lower pain scores and postoperative analgesic requirements.

The evidence in human anaesthesia literature is equivocal, i.e. some studies show the preincisional group had lower pain scores, some studies the postincisional group had lower pain scores, and in some studies there was no real difference.

What could be the explanation for these equivocal results?

- **Types of surgeries and type of analgesia used in the studies, and if the degree of afferent block (analgesia) is sufficient.**
- **Use of analgesia control groups: in human analgesia studies control groups with no analgesia cannot be used as this is unethical. Nor can human studies include doing a thoracotomy with just a paracetamol tablet for analgesia. People undergoing thoracotomy would have opioids, local blocks, CRIs of other analgesics etc. This may make differences between preincisional and postincisional paracetamol less clear.**
- **How is postoperative pain monitored? In human studies, levels of postoperative pain are measured by self-reported pain scales and patient demands for analgesia. However, there are groups of people that are very stoic and do not want to ask for analgesia, nor report how much pain they are in, and then on the other hand, people who have low pain thresholds and report higher pain scores and require more analgesia. This could really confound results.**

There have also been discussions surrounding what is termed as preemptive analgesia. It is not enough just to have drug bound before the noxious stimulus starts, but it is important to continue drugs bound to receptors throughout the primary and secondary phases of tissue injury (Box 3).

Box 3. The Primary and Secondary Phases of Injury

- **Primary phase of injury = noxious stimulation of the incision.**
- **Secondary phase of injury = release of chemicals and enzymes from damaged tissues.**
  - **This secondary phase extends well into the postoperative period.**

However, several veterinary studies appear to prove the effectiveness of preemptive analgesia in dogs, cats and rats using various drug groups including NSAIDs, ketamine, and opioids. This was a real breakthrough in the field of pain research. The differences between the veterinary studies and the human studies, which means they may be a more valid investigation of this concept is that:

- the types of surgery and the afferent nerve block (i.e. degree of analgesia) were better matched;
- in earlier studies, "no analgesia" control groups were allowed, although as soon as animals were seen to be in pain, intervention analgesia was given;
- in these studies, usually one analgesic drug (often just the study drug) is used, and the drugs used for the anaesthetic protocol (e.g. preanaesthetic sedation and induction drug) are not inherently analgesic. Therefore, the effects of the timing of the analgesic drugs are seen more clearly;
- pain scoring and therefore postoperative analgesia provision is performed by one trained observer in each study, who is unaware of the treatment groups.

Other benefits of providing preemptive analgesia include that many analgesics are also sedative and contribute to preanaesthetic medication. This calms and sedates the animal, facilitates intravenous catheter placement, and reduces amount of induction drug needed. Having centrally active analgesics on board during surgery smooths the anaesthetic and reduces the amount of volatile agent required.

There are occasional situations where it is more appropriate to give a specific analgesic drug after anaesthesia and surgery. Examples include:

- **Emetic drugs in the preanaesthetic medication if vomiting is contraindicated for the patient's clinical situation, e.g. fragile eye, pharyngeal stick injury, gastric dilatation-volvulus. The drugs could be given intraoperatively as once the patient in unconscious they are not able to vomit.**
- **Non-steroidal anti-inflammatory drugs. These should be left until the patient has recovered from anaesthesia if hypotension or hypovolaemia through blood loss is a possibility during the anaesthetic.**

However, it is important to remember, that even if one of these drugs was omitted from the preemptive analgesia plan, there should be other analgesic drugs in the multi-modal approach to provide sufficient preemptive analgesia.

Multimodal Analgesia

The pain pathway is complex, involving multiple neurotransmitters and receptors. It is therefore extremely difficult to achieve effective analgesia by using a single class of analgesic drug alone. There are several drug groups that have analgesic properties, and it is good practice to try and include a drug from several different groups to optimise analgesia when anaesthetising a patient who is in pain or who is undergoing a painful surgery (Figure 3).

Using several drugs that target the pain pathway at several points mean it is possible to use lower doses of drugs to achieve the same or better effect than one very large dose of a drug such as an opioid. The benefit of using lower doses of drugs means a reduced risk of inducing the side effects of those drugs.

There may be a little overlap between parts of the pain pathway (e.g. α-2 adrenergic agonists when administered via an epidural have a local anaesthetic type effect) but in general, different analgesic drug groups act on the following parts of the pain pathway.

Transduction

Non-steroidal anti-inflammatory drugs (NSAIDs) reduce the formation of prostaglandins, part of the inflammatory soup which sensitizes nociceptors and lowers their firing thresholds.

Transmission

Local anaesthetics when injected peri-neurally. A local anaesthetic binds to the sodium channel and blocks the influx of sodium ions. This block stops nerve conductance and prevents further signals reaching the dorsal horn of the spinal cord.

Modulation

Modulation is a decision-making process in the dorsal horn of the spinal cord (and also in the brain stem) which decides the output from the dorsal horn. This output is dependent on various spinal mechanisms which either increase or decrease the activity of dorsal horn neurons. Such mechanisms include local excitatory and inhibitory inter-neurones, N-methyl-D-aspartate receptor activation (remember ketamine is an antagonist here), and descending influences from the brainstem, which can be both inhibitory and excitatory in nature and involve both opioid receptors and α-2 adrenergic receptors.

Perception

There are opioid, α-2 adrenergic agonists and NMDA receptors in the cerebral cortex of the brain so when drugs bind to these receptors, they produce analgesia (and often sedation).

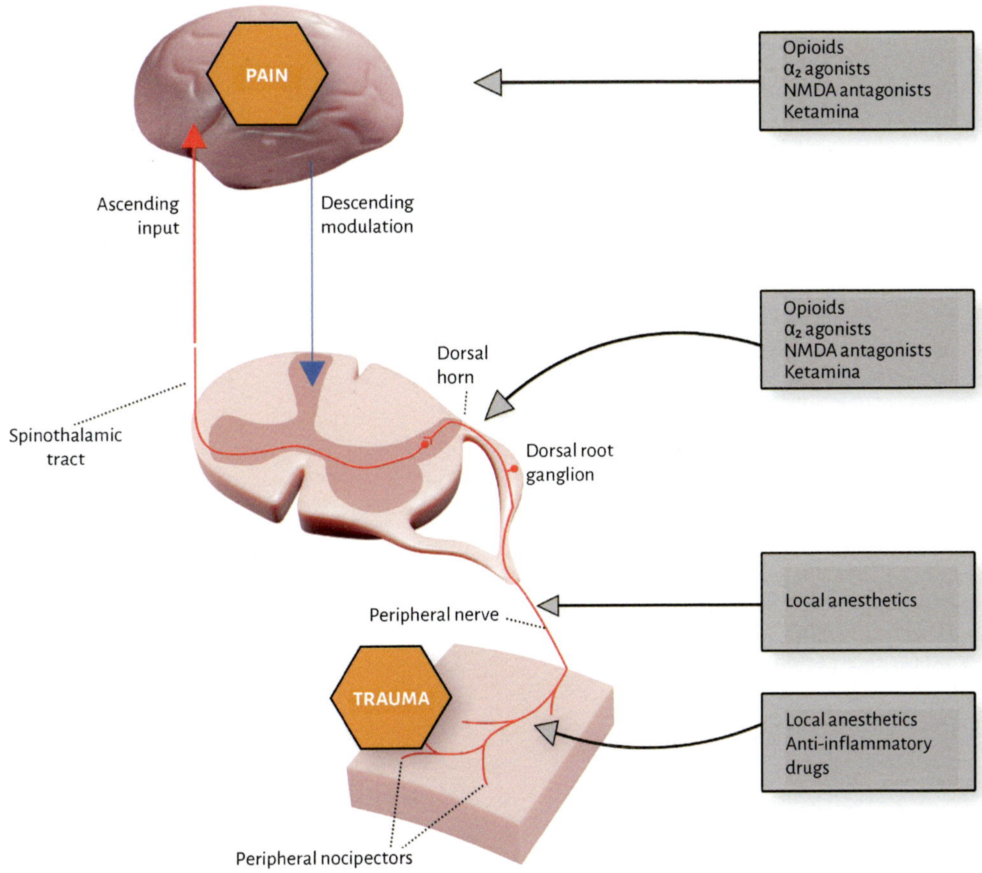

Figure 3. Points of action of drugs on the pain pathway.

Analgesic Drugs

Opioids

Opioids are commonly used in small animals, and include morphine, pethidine, methadone, buprenorphine, butorphanol, fentanyl, and alfentanil. They provide analgesia at modulation and perception sites on the pain pathway. These drugs all work on opioid receptors, of which there are several subtypes, including μ (mu), κ (kappa), and δ (delta). Different opioids act at different receptors, with the most effective analgesics being pure μ-agonists such as morphine, methadone, and pethidine. Buprenorphine is a partial μ-agonist, and butorphanol is a κ-agonist and a μ-antagonist. Figure 4 demonstrates the difference between full and partial agonists.

The drugs are usually given in injectable form, and can be given intravenously (except pethidine), intramuscularly, subcutaneously, and epidurally. Some drugs are also readily absorbed across the mucous membranes. They are metabolized in the liver and excreted in the urine.

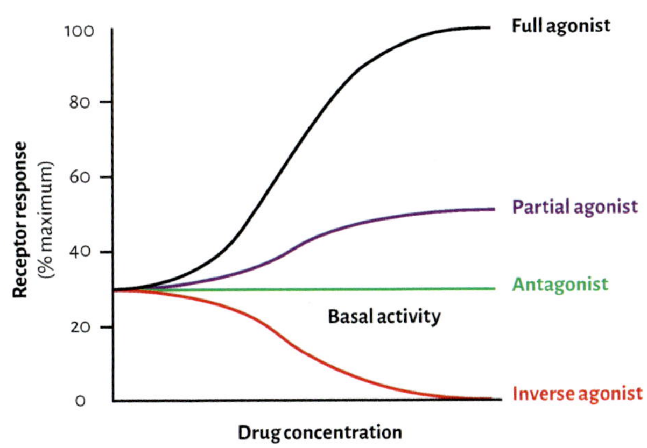

Figure 4. How full agonists compare against partial agonists.

- Morphine, pethidine, buprenorphine, methadone, and butorphanol are commonly used for preanaesthetic medication, either by themselves, because they have good sedative properties, or in combination with acepromazine, the α-2 adrenergic agonists or benzodiazepines.
- Injectable fentanyl, alfentanil, and remifentanil tend to be used for analgesia when an animal is already anaesthetized, because they can have more profound effects on an animal's physiology. Patches containing either fentanyl or buprenorphine are available to stick on to animal's skin, so the drug releases slowly across the skin over a period of a few days.

Most opioids decrease heart rate (especially fentanyl and alfentanil). This is of little clinical relevance with morphine, methadone, and buprenorphine, and pethidine tends to increase heart rate somewhat. At normal clinical doses, the opioids (except fentanyl, remifentanil and alfentanil) cause minimal respiratory depression. Some opioids are emetic (especially morphine) and vomiting may be contraindicated in certain clinical scenarios.

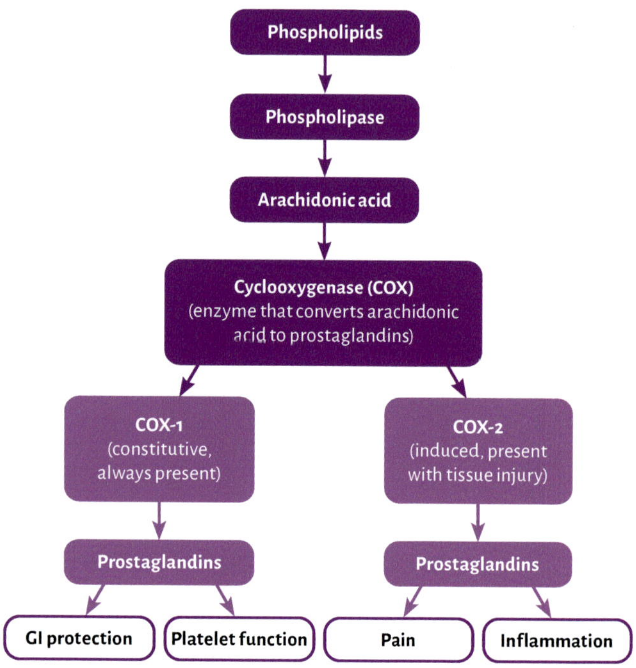

Figure 5. The COX pathway.

Box 4. Non-steroidal Anti-inflammatory Drugs (NSAIDs).

NSAIDs work by blocking cyclooxygenase enzymes (COX). COX enzymes convert arachidonic acid to substances called prostaglandins (Figure 5). These prostaglandins are one of several substances which accumulate in areas of tissue injury and make the tissue – red, swollen, warm and painful. By blocking these enzymes, NSAIDs provide analgesia by affecting the transduction part of the pain pathway.

As well as analgesia, other beneficial actions of NSAIDs include:

- anti-inflammatory
- antipyretic (decreases body temperature)
- anti-endotoxaemic.

Non-steroidal anti-inflammatory drugs should not be used in certain clinical situations:

- when a steroid has been used
- in renal failure
- hypovolaemic patients
- hypotensive patients
- evidence of gastro-intestinal ulceration, vomiting or diarrhoea
- animals with a clotting dysfunction.

The rationale behind many of these reasons is that prostaglandins not only play a role in the inflammatory soup (post tissue damage) but are also part of the kidney and gut's homeostatic mechanisms. In times of poor perfusion to these organs (e.g. if animals are hypotensive or hypovolaemic) these prostaglandins help maintain function, and blocking them leads to serious consequences including intestinal ulceration and kidney dysfunction. Non-steroidal anti-inflammatory drugs can also have an effect on clotting as thromboxane A2 is a factor which helps in clotting and is also blocked when NSAIDs are administered.

α-2 Adrenergic Agonists

This class of drugs provide good analgesia, mainly by affecting the modulation and perception part of the pain pathway. They can be given via the epidural route to provide analgesia, which helps alter pain transmission. Often, these drugs are given as part of the animal's preanaesthetic medication, although they are also suitable for use as CRIs either intraoperatively or whilst the animal is conscious.

Medetomidine (1 mg/ml) and dexmedetomidine (medetomidine's active isomer) (0.5 mg/ml) are α-2 adrenergic agonists used in small animal practice. These drugs are available in injectable form, and can be administered intravenously, intramuscularly, or subcutaneously. They are also readily absorbed via the mucous membranes.

These drugs bind to the α-2 adrenoceptors in an animal's central nervous system, to produce anxiolysis, deep sedation, and analgesia, along with some profound physiological effects. The drugs are metabolised in the liver and excreted in the urine. Atipamezole is an antagonist specifically for the antagonism of medetomidine and dexmedetomidine. However, when the sedative action of α-2 agonists is antagonized, this also stops any analgesia they provide. Also, the sedation α-2 agonists provide outlasts the analgesic effect, so just because an animal appears sedated does not mean they are pain free.

Ketamine

Although ketamine is a widely used induction agent, at subanaesthetic doses, it is a very effective analgesic. Because these doses are much smaller than those required to induce anaesthesia, the side effects of this drug are also limited. Ketamine works well in animals which have chronic pain (i.e. a painful condition which has lasted a long time), and may not be alleviated by normal doses of analgesic drugs. Its effectiveness against chronic pain is based on its action as an antagonist at NMDA (N-methyl D-aspartate) receptors which are involved in the development of central sensitisation. Ketamine is also a useful analgesic for somatic pain (i.e. that associated with superficial tissues, skin etc.).

For analgesia ketamine can be given intramuscularly, subcutaneously, or intravenously. It is suitable for CRIs and can also be given by epidural injection. It is not very highly protein bound (30–50%). In the dog and horse, ketamine undergoes hepatic metabolism, and renal excretion. In the cat, it is excreted unchanged in the urine.

Local Anaesthetics

These drugs are the only ones which can produce a total absence of pain, all other drugs just reduce pain to a more tolerable level. These drugs block pain because they stop the nerves conducting the pain signals and work on the transmission part of the pain pathway.

To stop the transmission of the electrical impulses along nerves, the drugs block the sodium channels in the nerve fibres. Both sensory and motor nerves can be affected, so areas of the body are desensitised, but may also experience temporary loss of function and movement of that part of the body if the motor nerves are affected.

Examples of drugs in this class include lidocaine, bupivacaine, ropivacaine, mepivacaine, and procaine. Local anaesthetics are subdivided into two groups depending on their chemical structures; lidocaine, bupivacaine, mepivacaine and ropivacaine all belong to the amide linked group, which undergo hepatic metabolism. Procaine belongs to the ester linked group; these drugs are broken down in the blood by enzymes.

Lidocaine, bupivacaine, and ropivacaine are most commonly used in small animal practice.

- **Lidocaine has a short onset of action (5–10 minutes) but also lasts for a limited amount of time (up to 1 hour).**
- **Bupivacaine has a longer onset (30 minutes) and duration (6–8 hours).**
- **Ropivacaine also has a similarly long onset and duration of action as bupivacaine, but often produces less motor blockade.**

Local anaesthetic can be applied topically, such as in creams to desensitise the skin or drops for eyes to prevent corneal sensation. They can be injected subcutaneously to create a wheal, through which an instrument or catheter can be placed without the animal feeling it. They can also be injected into joints (intra-articular). Infiltration of local anaesthetic around specific nerves (peri-neural analgesia) supplying certain areas of the body can also be performed, e.g. intercostal nerve blocks, brachial plexus blocks, nerve blocks for dental extractions. Local anaesthetics can be injected into the epidural space to desensitise hind limbs, abdomens, tails etc. They can also be injected into the pleural cavity in the chest and are a useful adjunct to provide pain relief for indwelling chest drains. Lidocaine only can also be used to provide analgesia when given intravenously as an infusion. Other benefits of lidocaine CRIs include potential anti-endotoxic, anti-inflammatory and prokinetic effects.

Care must be taken not to overdose local anaesthetics, as both central nervous system and cardiac complications may ensue.

Chronic Pain Drugs

The Pain Ladder

Figure 6 shows the WHO (World Health Organisation) ladder for chronic pain relief in people.

In dogs and cats, a similar approach is taken, **escalating the class of drugs as the severity of pain worsens.** Licensed products should always be used where possible, however, many drugs used to treat chronic pain in small animals are off-licence.

- **Mild pain: non-opioid (NSAIDs) +/- adjuvant.**
- **Mild to moderate pain: weak opioid +/- non-opioid +/- adjuvant.**
- **Moderate to severe pain: strong opioid +/- non-opioid +/- adjuvant.**

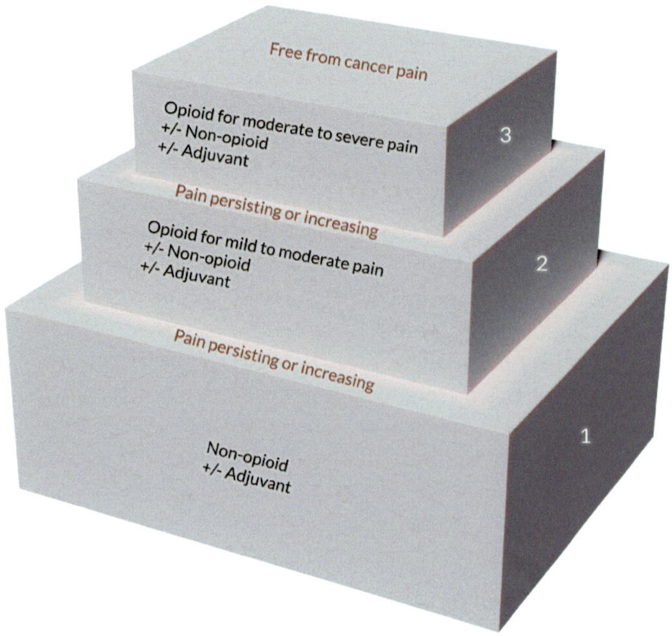

Figure 6. The World Health Organisation (WHO) pain ladder.

Commonly Used Drugs

Non-steroidal Anti-inflammatory Drugs

Non-steroidal anti-inflammatory drugs are used in cases of mild chronic pain, especially if there is an inflammatory component to the pain. Some animals need long term administration of NSAIDs.

To avoid side effects the following guidelines should be adhered to:

- **Not to be used with concurrent steroids or other NSAIDs.**
- **To wean down to the lowest effective dose.**
- **To allow a sufficient wash out period before switching to another NSAID.**
- **To ask owners to monitor for gastrointestinal upsets and cease treatment pending veterinary advice if any seen.**

In 2018, a new drug, grapiprant was released indicated for use in osteoarthritis pain in dogs. Unlike classic NSAIDs, it works as an antagonist at the EP4 receptor for PGE2, which means it can provide analgesia for osteoarthritis without affecting housekeeping enzymes.

Paracetamol (Acetaminophen)

This is a non-acidic NSAID which acts at the level of the spinal cord on COX enzymes, the opioid, serotoninergic, and cannabinoid systems. It is also antipyretic and can be used more safely on animals where COX inhibition is a concern (e.g. renal failure patients) than traditional NSAIDs, in dogs at a dose rate between 10 mg/kg (IV) up to 30 mg/kg (PO) BID or TID. Pardale V is the licensed product in dogs, in which 400 mg paracetamol is combined with 9 mg codeine. In this formulation is it licensed for five days.

Use in the cat is contraindicated.

Pregabalin and Gabapentin

These drugs were originally produced as antiepileptics. Their mechanism of action seems to be by binding to calcium channels in the CNS, reducing the production of pronociceptive inputs and facilitating descending inhibitory pathways. They are useful for chronic and neuropathic pain in people. Usually, they are started in conjunction with an NSAID or opioid but are often used as a sole agent in the long term. Their major side effect is sedation. As they are metabolized in the liver and excreted by the kidneys, care should be taken in animals with dysfunction of these organs. These drugs are well tolerated long term, although in humans, a gradual tapering of dose is suggested to prevent status-epilepticus. This has not been documented in veterinary species so far.

Opioids

If NSAID type drugs are inadequate in controlling pain, opioids such as tramadol and oral transmucosal buprenorphine may be used. Tramadol works at the μ-opioid receptors, 5HT receptors, and noradrenaline receptors. Tramadol needs to be metabolized to the active metabolite to exert analgesic effects at the μ-opioid receptor, and in acute pain models using nociceptive threshold testing, tramadol was shown to produce minimal analgesia in dogs which was likely due to the low levels of metabolite produced. The analgesic effect of tramadol in chronic pain may be through the non-opioid based mechanisms and therefore it may still be of use in these situations. Side effects include vomiting, diarrhoea, sedation, dysphoria, and lack of palatability (in cats).

Buprenorphine can be administered oral transmucosally in dogs and cats. It is particularly useful in cats, in which the bioavailability is very high. It can be used in dogs, but due to a lower bioavailability higher dose may be needed for sufficient effect. Case selection is important, both in terms of the lay people administering the drug at home, and the size of patient, as use in larger patients is expensive.

NMDA Antagonists

Amantidine is the main drug used in this group for chronic pain. It decreases central sensitization and is particularly useful in cases with neuropathic pain. It is not licensed in dogs or cats but has been used successfully in combination with NSAIDs for osteoarthritis pain.

Tricyclic Antidepressants

The supposed analgesic mechanisms for these drugs include blocking serotonin and noradrenaline reuptake in the CNS, increasing endogenous opioids, and altering the binding of substances at NMDA receptors. These drugs are particularly good at treating neuropathic pain. The drugs require hepatic and renal function to metabolise and eliminate them, and therefore care must be taken in patients with reduced function of these organ systems. Side effects include sedation, excitability, vomiting, weight gain, and arrythmias.

Monoclonal Antibodies

More recently, bedinvetmab (Librela) was released for the alleviation of pain associated with osteoarthritis in dogs. It contains the active substance bedinvetmab. It is a solution for injection to be given subcutaneously once a month. Bedinvetmab is a monoclonal antibody designed to recognise and attach to a protein called nerve growth factor (NGF). Once attached, it prevents NGF from attaching to its receptors on nerve cells and interrupts the transmission of pain signals. A drug with a similar mechanism of action (frunevetmab) is available for use in cats.

Adjunctive Therapies

In addition to drugs, other therapies such as **acupuncture and physiotherapy** (including massage and hydrotherapy) can be incorporated into treatment plans. Acupuncture is an act of veterinary surgery in the UK. By inserting solid needles into either trigger points (painful knots in the muscle) or specific acupuncture points, pain relief is produced, mediated by endorphins and other opiates, and the suppression of transmission of signals along C fibres. Electroacupuncture is a more intense alternative to the basic needling technique, where a low electric current is passed through paired acupuncture needles.

Physiotherapy adjuncts can be added to a treatment plan under the direction of a registered physiotherapist to maintain and restore function.

Environmental modifications can be suggested to owners of patients with chronic pain, both to facilitate activities during daily living without causing discomfort and to improve the animal's affective state (mood).

Local Anaesthesia

The 2020 AAHA guidelines on dog and cat anaesthesia recommends that: **local anaesthetics should be used, insofar as possible, with every surgical procedure.** Local blocks are useful because they are the only class of analgesics which completely block pain sensation. In contrast, the drugs considered as analgesics, e.g. opioids and non-steroidal anti-inflammatory drugs are technically "hypoalgesics" in that they reduce pain sensation to a tolerable level.

For most of the blocks described, no specialist equipment is required, other than a syringe, needle, and the local anaesthetic. For perineural injections of local anaesthetics, nerve location equipment can be used as a guide so long as a motor nerve accompanies the sensory branch.

Table 4 lists the maximum doses of local anaesthetic; however, many local nerve blocks also have a maximum volume of injectate. These are suggested volumes for average sized doliocephalic dogs, and these should be reduced appropriately according to the size of the dog or cat.

Table 4. Dose ranges of commonly used local anaesthetic drugs.

Drug	Dose range	Onset of action	Duration of action
Lidocaine	2–4 mg/kg	10 min	1–2 hours
Bupivacaine	1–2 mg/kg	20–30 min	2–6 hours
Ropivacaine	0.1–2 mg/kg	2–20 min	2–6 hours

When performing a block, blood drawback should always be checked for by aspirating prior to injecting, as local anaesthetics (with the exception of lidocaine in certain circumstances) should never be given intravascularly. Intravenous administration or overdose of local anaesthetics can cause cardiotoxic (peripheral vasodilation, hypotension, decreased myocardial contractility, and arrythmias) or neurotoxic (sedation, disorientation, ataxia, convulsions) side effects. **In addition, care should be taken not to insert the needle through infected tissue or into tissues containing with tumour cells.**

Head Blocks

Many of these blocks are used for dentals, mandibular and maxillary surgery. For the surgical removal of masses from the skin on the head or gums, these blocks provide excellent analgesia. Instead of injecting a wheal around the mass, which may disseminate tumour cells, the injection site is remote from the mass. When deciding which block to perform, remember the structures rostral to the injection site will be blocked. Infraorbital and mental nerve blocks may not desensitise teeth, unless the needles are inserted into the canals, however teeth are blocked if more caudal blocks (maxillary and mandibular) are performed.

Infraorbital Nerve Block

The infraorbital foramen is midway between the rostrodorsal border of the zygomatic arch and canine root tip. Local anaesthetic injected here blocks the upper lip and nose (nasal planum and roof of nasal cavity), and skin rostroventral to the infraorbital foramen. Running a needle or catheter further up the infraorbital canal may block deeper structures. The maximum injection volume is 3 ml, although if resistance to injection is felt, then no more local should be injected as this suggests the infraorbital canal has been filled. Brachycephalics and cats have very short infraorbital canals and therefore premeasurement or just injecting local anaesthetic at the entrance to the canal should be used in these patients. (Figures 7 and 8).

Maxillary Nerve Block

Local anaesthetic is injected into the pterygopalatine fossa, between the rostral alar foramen and the maxillary foramen (entrance to the infraorbital canal). The nerve is blocked by inserting a needle under the rostral portion of the zygomatic arch directing it towards the maxillary foramen. This block desensitises the maxilla rostral to the block on the side of the injection. The maximum injection volume is 3 ml. This block can also be performed from an intraoral approach, by injecting caudal to the dental arcade and palate on the relevant side (Figures 7 and 8).

Mental Nerve Block

This nerve is blocked where the middle mental nerve exits the middle mental foramen (see Figures 7 and 8). The middle mental foramen is biggest in dogs and carries the largest of the mental nerves. It is usually not possible to run a needle into the mental canal therefore the local anaesthetic is infiltrated where the nerve exits the foramen. This injection blocks the lower lip/chin rostral to the site of the block but not any teeth. The maximum volume of injection is 2 ml.

Mandibular Nerve Block

To block this nerve, the non-dependent hand should be placed inside the mouth to palpate the mandibular foramen (on the inside of the mandible). Then, the needle inserted percutaneously at the lower angle of the jaw, and advanced against the medial side of the mandible and directed towards the foramen. Often the needle can be guided whilst feeling the foramen and nerve from inside the mouth on the medial surface of the mandible. Local anaesthetic deposited here blocks the lower teeth, mandible, skin and mucosa of the lower lip. The maximum volume for injection is 2 ml. (See Figures 7 and 8).

Retrobulbar Block

The retrobulbar block is another head block which is useful for ocular surgery. The retrobulbar block involves injecting local anaesthetic behind the globe. The injection blocks cranial nerves II, III, IV, V (ophthalmic and maxillary branches), and VI, which desensitises the globe, lids, conjunctiva, and much of the upper face, and also blocks the extra-ocular muscles and therefore produces a central eye. Some eyelid tone may remain from palpebral (cranial nerve VII) innervation.

There is a chance the globe can be punctured and so the author tends to reserve this block for enucleation surgeries. Even in these cases, a retrobulbar block is contraindicated if tumour and overt infection is the reason for enucleation, as the needle may disseminate tumour cells or infection to the back of the eye. Retrobulbar injections may produce traction on the optic nerve and therefore the technique is often avoided in shallow orbited cats, whose optic nerves (both in the injected eye and the contralateral one) may be affected by this tension.

A needle is inserted at 10 o'clock and 5 o'clock sites. The author uses a 21–23G needle, and slightly bends it whilst keeping it sterile before injection. The tip of the needle is bounced off the orbit until the tip sits behind the globe (Figure 9). Aspiration should be performed prior to injection, to check for blood but also for cerebrospinal fluid.

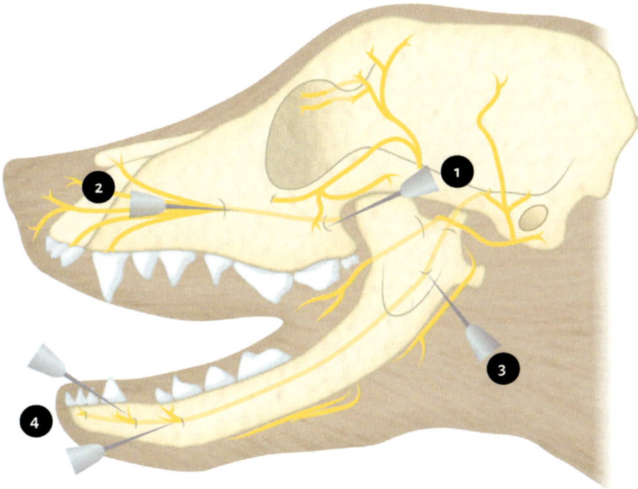

Figure 7. Maxillary (1), infraorbital (2), mandibular (3) and mental (4) nerve block in the dog.

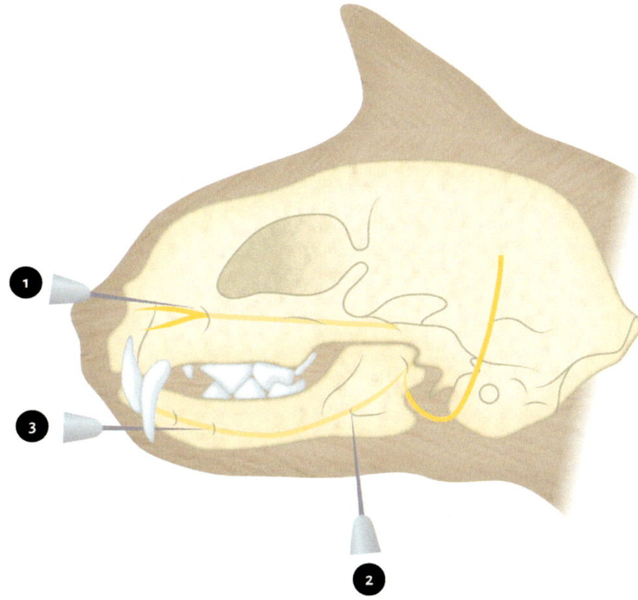

Figure 8. Infraorbital (1), mandibular (2) and mental (3) nerve block in the cat.

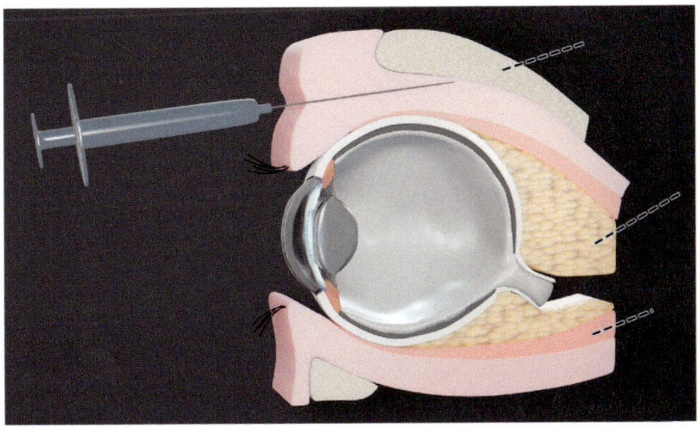

Figure 9. Retrobulbar block.

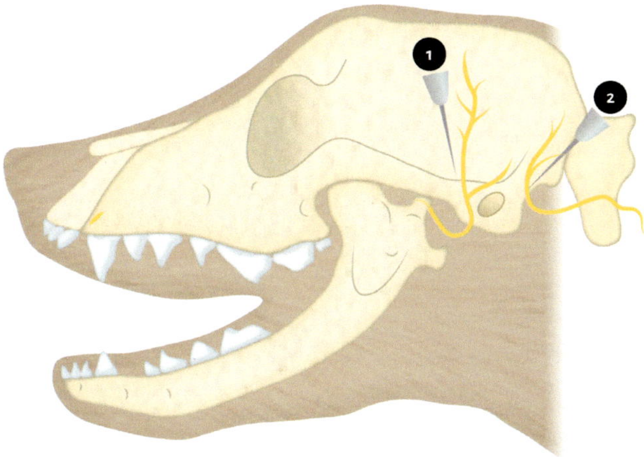

Figure 10. Greater auricular and auriculotemporal nerves can be blocked to provide analgesia for ear surgery. Auriculotemporal (1) and greater auricular (2).

Auriculotemporal and Great Auricular Nerve Block

Blocking the auriculotemporal and great auricular nerve desensitizes the inner surface of the auricular cartilage and the external ear canal, which is ideal for ear surgeries such as total ear canal ablation. The auriculotemporal nerve is blocked by inserting a needle rostral to the vertical ear canal and directing it towards the base of the "V" formed by the caudal aspect of the zygomatic arch and the vertical canal (Figure 10). The great auricular nerve is blocked by inserting a needle ventral to the wing of the atlas and caudal to the vertical ear canal and directing it parallel to the vertical canal (Figure 10). An alternative to this block is a splash block where local anaesthetic is squirted down the ear canal during surgery or injected around the surgical site prior to closure.

Limb Blocks

As orthopaedic surgery becomes more common place in general practice, most aspects of limbs can be desensitized with one of the following blocks.

Intra-articular Analgesia

This is a simple local anaesthetic block which can be done before or after any surgery involving a joint, including arthroscopy.

As with all local anaesthetic blocks, it must be performed in a strictly aseptic manner to avoid introducing infection into the joint. Current recommendation is that this is performed as a one-off shot rather than a continuous infusion. As with all analgesia, preemptive administration is best, and so ideally the drug should be injected before surgery (often this can be performed once a joint tap has been performed with the same needle in place). Alternatively, it can be injected at the end of surgery just before the joint is closed, ensuring that saline flush is not performed immediately afterwards, otherwise the local analgesia is washed out of the joint.

Ropivacaine is the local anaesthetic of choice, but in animals with chronic joint disease, morphine can be added to the local anaesthetic. This is because with chronic joint inflammation, synovial opioid receptors are upregulated, and morphine should improve the quality and the duration of the analgesia.

Ring Block

Local anaesthetic agents can literally be injected to encircle the area of interest, e.g. a distal limb. **Local anaesthetics containing adrenaline should not be used,** as this may compromise the blood supply to the distal area. The local anaesthetic solution may be diluted to provide an easier volume to inject and reduce the risk of causing toxicity. It is important not to inject through inflamed or infected tissue as this may disseminate infection and is less effective due to altered pH of the tissue.

Intravenous Regional Analgesia

Intravenous regional analgesia (IVRA) is often used to desensitise distal limbs. Only lidocaine (without adrenaline) should be used with this technique, as it is the least cardiotoxic of the local anaesthetics. Local anaesthetic is injected distal to a tourniquet which is in place to keep the lidocaine in a discrete area (including the surgical site). The local block works for as long as the tourniquet is in place, as the drug does not return to the liver to be metabolised. **The tourniquet should not be left in place for more than 60–90 minutes.** An added bonus of this technique is that if the limb is exsanguinated, there is a bloodless field for surgery.

The step-by-step method for performing IVRA (using the exsanguination method) is outlined in Box 6.

Box 5. A step-by-step Guide to Performing IVRA (with exsanguination)

- **Clip and prep area of interest and place IV catheter (facing downwards).**
- **Exsanguinate limb from toe upwards by wrapping some cohesive bandage from the toe upwards, tying a tourniquet at the top, and then unwinding the bandage from the toe upwards.**
- **Inject lidocaine into catheter (up to 4 mg/kg and flush), then the catheter can be removed.**
- **Wait five minutes before starting surgery.**
- **Do not remove the tourniquet until at least 15 minutes after the local anaesthetic is injected. If removing earlier than this, the ECG should be monitored.**

Digital Nerve Block

This block is useful for any pad or digital surgery, including digit amputation. The author often uses this block with sedation to suture pads, and without sedation to pull torn nails. A short needle should be inserted in the gap between the digits. This needs to be done in the inter-digital space either side of the affected digit. After aspiration to check for blood, inject a maximum volume of 0.5 ml on either side.

Epidural

Epidural (or extradural) analgesia is the administration of analgesic drug (including local anaesthetic) into the epidural space surrounding the spinal cord or cauda equina. Epidural injections are usually injected into the lumbo-sacral space (L7–S1) but the epidural space can be accessed at other points including more cranially, and between the coccygeal vertebrae. The remainder of this section pertains to lumbo-sacral epidurals.

Epidural analgesia is used to provide peri-operative analgesia for hind limb surgery, perineal, and tail surgery, as well as abdominal and thoracic surgery. Other drugs in addition to local anaesthetics which can be used include opioids (usually morphine), α-2 adrenergic agonists, and ketamine. The author uses opioid epidurals for thoracic surgeries, but often uses local anaesthetics for other surgical indications.

Relative contraindications for epidurals are given in Box 5. The volume of epidural injections should be reduced in the following cases:

- **obese animals:** the epidural space is only the same size as a lean dog, and therefore doses should be based on lean weight;
- **pregnant animals:** the increased intra-abdominal pressure and engorged epidural vessels promote forward flow of the injectate; and
- **elderly animals:** sclerosis of the intervertebral foramina reduces lateral flow of the injectate and therefore promotes forward flow.

Box 6. Some Relative Contraindications to Epidural Injections

- **Obesity – difficult to find landmarks.**
- **Pelvic injuries and fractures – if the anatomy is distorted and the lumbosacral space cannot be identified.**
- **Coagulopathies.**
- **Preexisting neuropathies.**
- **Infection/dermatopathy of the skin over the injection site.**

For hindlimb surgery and abdominal surgery, 0.5 ml/kg volume should be used in the dog, and the author recommends a total of 0.5 ml per cat.

To locate the epidural space, first the craniodorsal iliac spines should be identified. An imaginary line can be drawn between these, which should intersect the dorsal spinous process of L7. Slightly caudal to this line is a dip between the L7 dorsal spinous process and the smaller sacral dorsal processes, i.e. the L7–S1 interspace. (Figure 11).

In most dogs the spinal cord terminates at about L6–7, whereas in cats it terminates at S1–3, and hitting CSF is more likely.

For epidurals the animal should be sedated or under anaesthesia. The animal should be placed in either sternal or lateral recumbency, but **it is important the animal is straight.** If in sternal, then the L7–S1 interspace is easiest to palpate with the legs frog-legged beneath the animal. Once the space is located, then the hind legs can be drawn forwards underneath

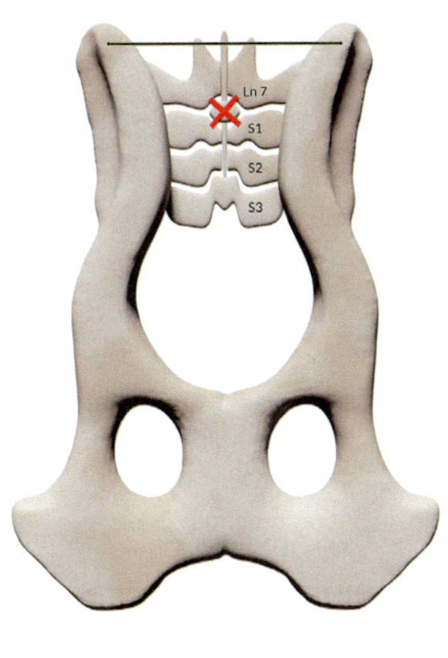

Figure 11. The cross indicates the palpable dip when locating the lumbosacral space.

the animal as this tenses the dorsal ligaments allowing a better popping sensation to be felt as the ligamentum flavum is penetrated. Other techniques to check for correct placement of the needle are suggested in Box 7.

Box 7. Checks Ensuring the Needle is in the Correct Space

- **A "popping" sensation is felt when advancing the needle.**
- **Lack of resistance to injection of a test injectate (air/saline).**
- **Air bubble technique (an air bubble at the top of the syringe should not compress when the drug is injected).**
- **Hanging drop technique (the stylet is removed from the needle after it has been passed through the skin and a drop of saline or drug is placed on top of the needle. As the needle advances into the epidural space, the negative pressure should "suck" the fluid in.**

The landmarks should be located, and a scalpel blade then used to make a nick in the skin. A spinal needle should be introduced through the skin nick with bevel facing forward, at 90° to skin. The needle should be advanced until a popping sensation is felt. The stylet should be withdrawn, and the needle stabilised. The vet should aspirate to check for blood or cerebral spinal fluid. If aspiration is negative, then the drugs can be injected slowly.

Depending on the viscosity of the solution injected, many anaesthetists move the animal into lateral recumbency which means the affected leg is dependent, encouraging a denser block on the affected side.

Saphenous, Common Peroneal, and Tibial Nerve Blocks

Blocking these nerves (see Figure 12) provides analgesia for surgeries and injuries distal to the stifle. They are more commonly performed with a peripheral nerve stimulator.

- The saphenous nerve (branch of femoral nerve) is palpated in the femoral triangle on the medial aspect of the thigh. Pulsation of the artery helps guide needle placement, as injections should be aimed cranial to the artery.
- The common peroneal nerve (branch of the sciatic nerve) is blocked by injecting distally to the fibular head.
- The tibial nerve (branch of the sciatic nerve) is blocked by placing a needle deep to the medial and lateral heads of the gastrocnemius.

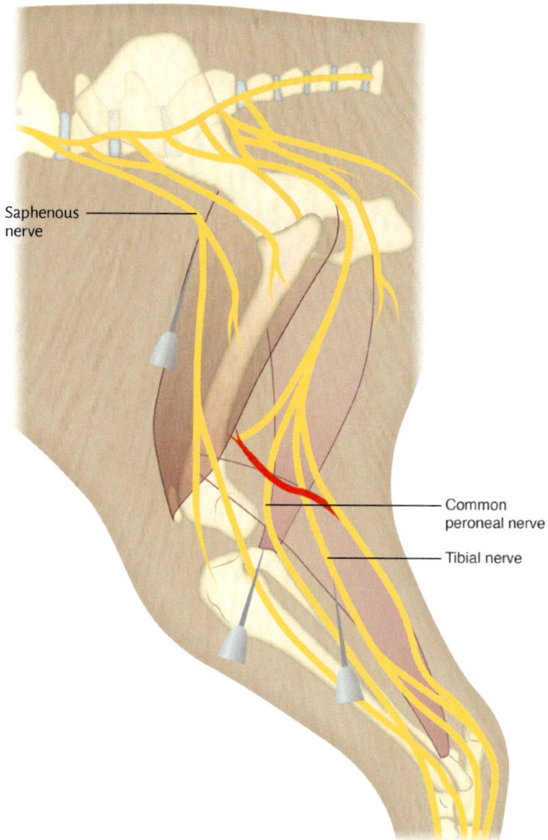

Figure 12. Saphenous, tibial, and common peroneal nerve blocks.

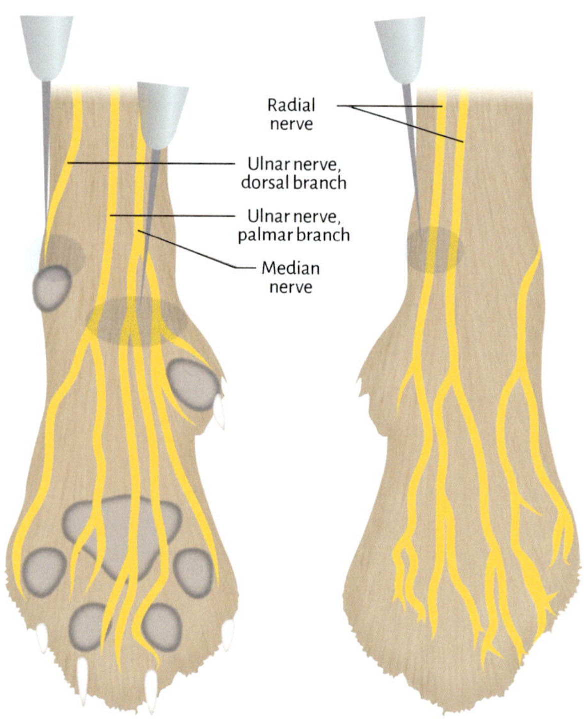

Figure 13. Radial, ulnar and median blocks in the cat.

Radial, Ulnar, and Median Nerve Blocks

Blocking these nerves desensitises the distal forelimb. Peripheral nerve stimulation can help identify the individual nerves.

In the cat, blocking the median, ulnar and radial nerves desensitizes the fore paw (Figure 13). The radial nerve can be blocked by placing the needle subcutaneously dorsomedial to the carpus proximal to the joint. The median and ulnar nerves are blocked by injecting medially and laterally to the accessory carpal pad on the palmar surface of the paw.

Blocking the radial, ulnar, median and musculocutaneous nerves (Figure 14) in the dog will desensitize the forelimb distal to the elbow.

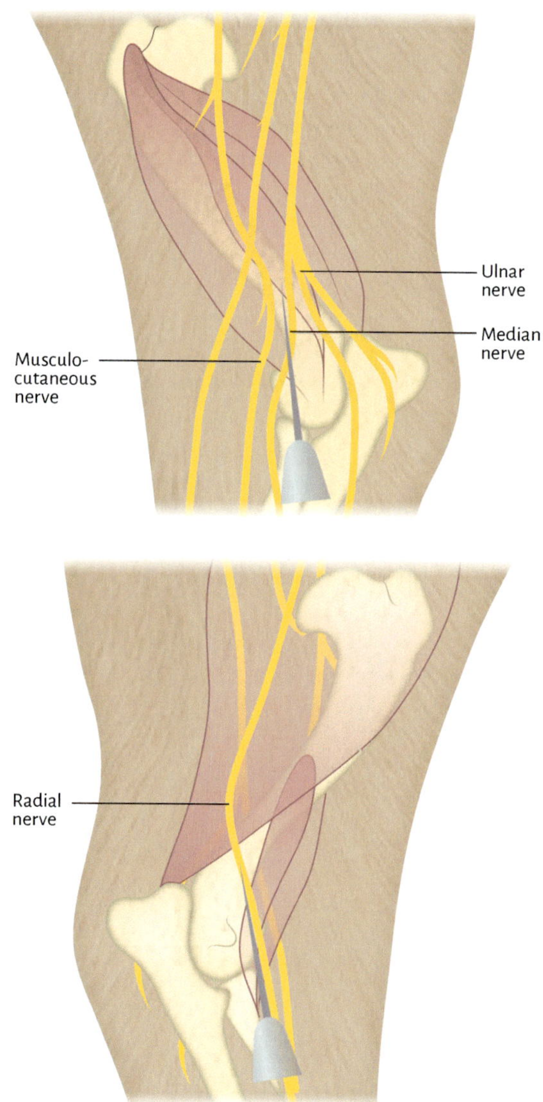

Figure 14. Blocking the radial, ulnar, median and musculocutaneous nerves in the dog will desensitize the forelimb distal to the elbow.

The radial nerve can be blocked by injecting proximal to the lateral epicondyle of the humerus and directing between the brachialis and lateral head of the triceps. The ulnar, median and musculocutaneous nerves are blocked by injecting proximal to the medial epicondyle of the humerus and directing between the biceps brachii and the medial head of the triceps.

Brachial Plexus Block

Blocking the nerves of the brachial plexus provides excellent analgesia for some forelimb surgeries and fracture repairs. The traditional brachial plexus block, injecting approximately 10–15 ml of local anaesthetic (for a 25 kg dog) into the axillary space at the level of the point of the shoulder blocks the lower forelimb, but not the shoulder or the proximal humerus (Figure 15).

The paravertebral brachial plexus technique produces a more complete blockade, including more proximally. Local anaesthetic is injected so the nerves of the brachial plexus are blocked as close as possible to the intervertebral foramina.

The scapula should be shifted caudally to expose the large transverse process of the sixth cervical vertebrae and the first rib.

The ventral branches of C6 and C7 should be blocked as they cross the dorsal surface of the transverse process of the sixth cervical vertebrae. This is done by inserting a needle dorsal to the process and directing it towards the caudal and cranial margins.

The ventral branches of C8 and T1 can be blocked on the lateral surface of the first rib by directing the needle to the cranial and ventral border of the dorsal part of the first rib.

Pneumothorax is a potential complication of both of these blocks and aspiration to check for air should be performed before each injection. Bilateral blocks should be avoided due to potential blockade of the phrenic nerve.

Thoracic Blocks

Intercostal Nerve Block

Intercostal nerve blocks are a useful analgesic adjunct for lateral thoracotomy surgeries but are also used to good effect to provide pain relief for rib fractures and chest tube placements.

The intercostal nerves are closely associated with the caudal borders of the ribs. For the chest wall there is much overlap of innervation, which means at least two blocks (cranial and caudal to the intercostal site that requires analgesia) (Figure 16).

To do this the needle should be aimed perpendicular to the body wall, sliding the needle through the skin and then off the caudal border of the rib and proximal to the incisional site. Injection should be as close to the intervertebral foramen as possible, as high up the intercostal nerve as possible so as to block the maximum number of branches. Aspiration should then be used to check the needle tip is not in the vascular component of the neurovascular bundle. ¼–1 ml should be injected per site, depending on the animal's size.

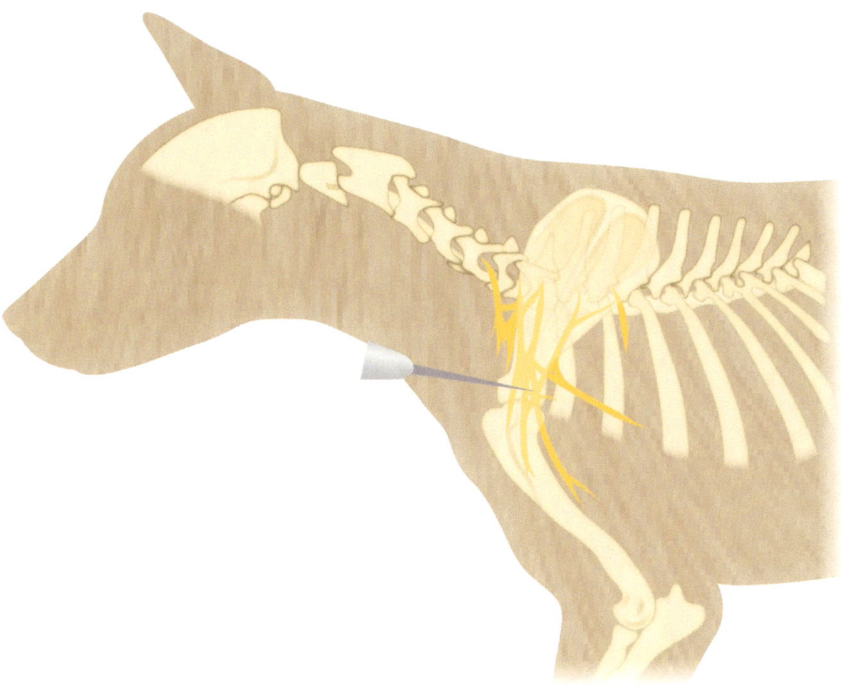

Figure 15. Brachial plexus block in the dog.

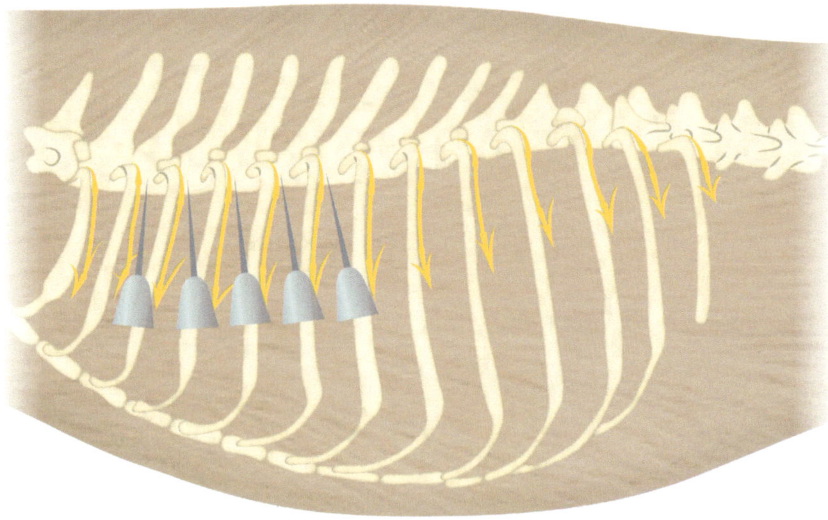

Figure 16. Intercostal nerve blocks are sited on the caudal edge of the ribs.

Interpleural Analgesia

Interpleural analgesia is also useful post thoracotomy (lateral thoracotomy or sternotomy). This can be achieved by instilling local anaesthetic down an in-dwelling chest drain. Otherwise, a catheter can be placed into the pleural space percutaneously or under direct view before closure of a thoracotomy incision.

The author tends to instil the local anaesthetic down the chest drain whilst the animal is still under anaesthesia, and then rolls the animal so that the drug bathes the affected area (as long as this does not compromise the animal's ventilation). Interpleural anaesthesia can also provide pain relief for animals with indwelling chest drains. Analgesia of cranial abdominal organs and cranial mammary glands is also produced with local anaesthetics injected interpleurally, due to the stellate ganglion in the thorax which provides innervation to these organs.

Local Anaesthetic Techniques for Neutering

For ovariohysterectomy, local analgesia can be a line block (either before first incision or during abdominal wall closure) and intraperitoneal administration of a local anaesthesic in an aseptic manner just before abdominal closure. Local anaesthetics can also be applied to the ovarian ligaments and cervix before ligation.

Intratesticular injections of local anaesthetic may be of use if administered early enough in the surgical preparation to allow for diffusion into the spermatic cord. Additional sites for local anaesthetic injection include the prescrotal site for the skin incision and the spermatic cord just before clamp application.

Wound Soaker Catheters

These catheters can be implanted in any closed incision to provide excellent postoperative local analgesia. They are loosely tacked into place in the subcutis before skin closure and secured to the skin using a roman sandal suture. They are easily removed by pulling once the roman sandal suture is cut. Local anaesthetic is injected into the catheter and diffuses through a bacterial filter system (included in the catheter set) and injected in bolus doses or as a continuous rate infusion via an extension set to a syringe driver.

Transcutaneous Electrical Nerve Stimulation (TENS)

Local anaesthetic is placed using anatomical landmarks, whereas electrical nerve locators/stimulators are used to aid placement of regional nerve blocks, where the nerves have a motor component (i.e. muscle twitches are seen in areas served by the nerve).

TENS equipment uses an insulated needle (the insulated area allows for safe handling), which is longer than conventional hypodermic needles. The stimulator is set to deliver a repeated stimulus at 1 mA current. The needle is moved towards the anatomical location of the nerve until the greatest muscle twitching is observed distally, which suggests the tip of the needle is in the proximity of the nerve bundle. At this point the current is gradually reduced to 0.4 mA, and if the needle is close enough to the nerve bundle, muscle twitches are still be seen. A very low current (<0.4 mA) check ensures the tip of the needle is not inside the nerve bundle itself before injecting the local anaesthetic.

If the nerve locator needle is left in place, reduced or absent twitches are observed a few minutes after local anaesthetic deposition.

Ultrasound guidance can be used to locate nerve trunks, because they usually run alongside arteries and veins, which are easily visualised.

Constant Rate Infusions (CRIs) for Analgesia

Continuous or constant rate infusions (CRIs) are used to provide analgesia both intraoperatively and perioperatively for small animal patients. **The reason that some drugs are given continuously is to avoid the peaks and troughs in plasma levels which occur with repeat bolus injections (Figure 17).** This is especially important if the drug has a narrow therapeutic window, as the up-swings and down-swings associated with bolus dosing may produce toxic levels (at the peak of the upswings) or non-therapeutic levels (at the trough of the down swing).

CRIs for analgesia are useful because the nurse does not have to wait to see signs of pain (as the previous dose wears off) before administering the next dose. Also, the patient's wellbeing is improved because the drugs are administered through an indwelling intravenous catheter, instead of disturbing the patient every four hours to repeat an intravenous injection, or even worse to repeatedly inject drugs into the muscle.

Often, before starting a constant rate infusion a loading dose of the particular drug is given. This is to quickly get plasma levels of the drug close to therapeutic levels (Figure 18). If the infusion is relied on solely, it takes approximately five half-lives of the drug before therapeutic levels are reached. (Half-life = Time taken for the plasma concentration to fall to 50% of its initial value (see black line on Figure 19).

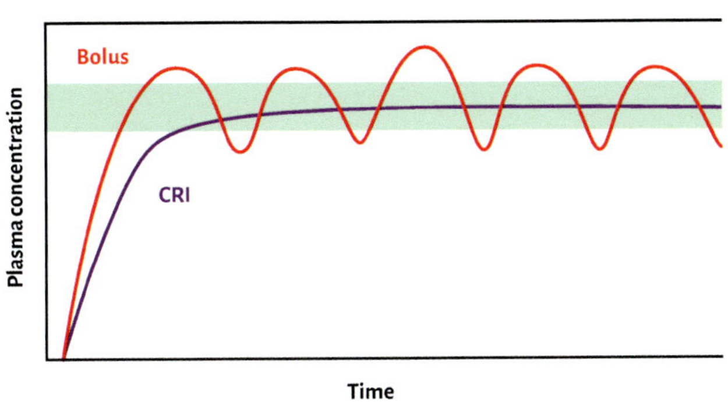

Figure 17. CRI versus bolus dose.

To maintain a therapeutic plasma level, infusion of the drug should be started to establish a steady state (Figure 20).

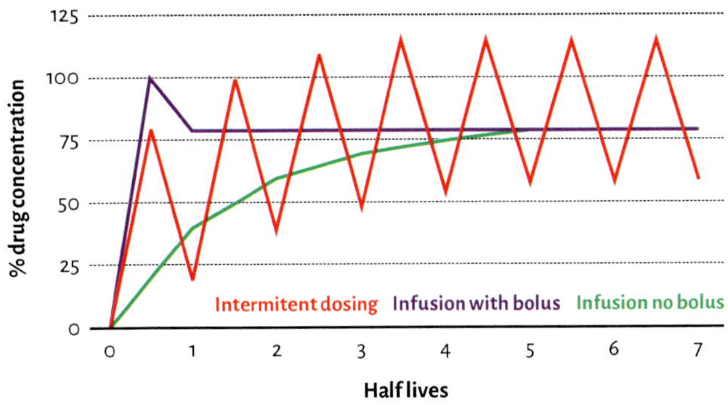

Figure 18. Plasma concentration of drug X after different methods of administration. Giving a loading dose means that therapeutic concentrations are reached more quickly.

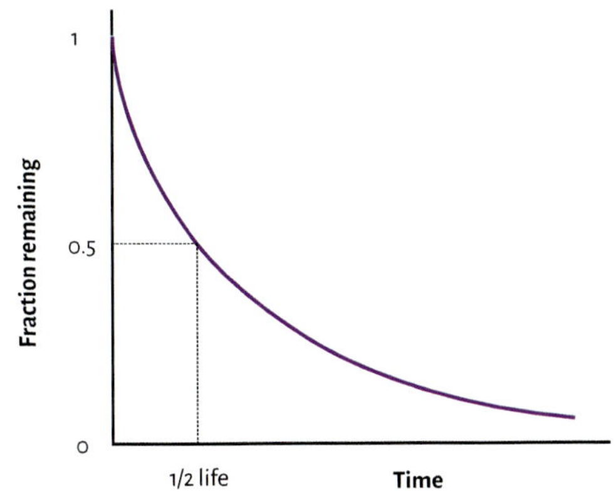

Figure 19. The half-life is the time taken for the plasma concentration to fall to 50% of its initial value.

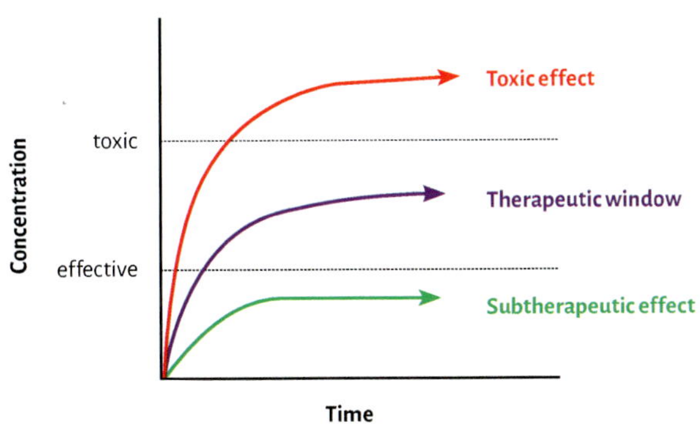

Figure 20. Administering an infusion at a steady state avoids toxic side effects or subtherapeutic levels.

A steady state is where the rate of the drug administration is equal to the rate of drug elimination, so the levels in the blood do not accumulate or drop out of the therapeutic range.

Intravenous infusions require a well-secured intravenous catheter placed after aseptic preparation. A peripheral vein is usually appropriate for an analgesic CRI, although some CRIs of other drugs, e.g. high glucose content or total parenteral nutrition, require a larger bore central venous catheter.

The drug to be administered is usually dissolved in a crystalloid solution, either 0.9% sodium chloride or Hartmann's solution. The dose rate must be carefully controlled and therefore an infusion pump or a syringe driver is needed to ensure accurate administration. Finally the drug in question needs to be drawn up after first checking the concentration of the solution and ensuring the solution's sterility.

Most importantly, a suitably qualified member of staff should monitor the patient, either under anaesthesia or in a ward situation. Infusions of these drugs alter how the animal responds to anaesthesia; and may alter their heart rate or their ability to ventilate. When the animal is conscious, attention needs to be paid to the catheter, to make sure that the animal is receiving the analgesics, and that rate is not too low (and the animal is still painful) or too high (and the animal is experiencing side effects).

Table 5 details some commonly used analgesic CRIs in small animal patients.

Table 5. Commonly used CRI rates for small animal analgesia.

Drug	Loading dose (slowly over 2–3 minutes IV)	Infusion rate (check whether per hr or per min)
Ketamine	0.5 mg/kg	10–20 µg/kg/min
Morphine	0.3 mg/kg	0.1–0.2 mg/kg/hr
Lidocaine	2 mg/kg	50–100 µg/kg/min
Fentanyl	1–5 µg/kg	2–5 µg/kg/hr
Alfentanil	0.5–1 µg/kg	0.5–1 µg/kg/min
Remifentanil	1 µg/kg	0.1–0.2 µg/kg/min
Medetomidine	5 µg/kg	1–2 µg/kg/hr
Dexmedetomidine	2 µg/kg	1 µg/kg/hr

NB: There are 1000 µg (micrograms) in a mg (milligram).

It is common to see combinations of some of the different analgesic drugs, such as morphine, lidocaine, and ketamine. These combinations are profoundly MAC sparing under anaesthesia, and postoperatively cause profound sedation. The author suggests running these combinations as separate infusions, so that the veterinary surgeon can turn one up or down without necessarily altering the others.

Many rates suggested in books are on a ml per kilogram basis, with instructions provided of how to make up the bag. Sometimes this is a wasteful approach, if say for example, the infusion is only required for a couple of hours.

To calculate a rate from scratch, the following information is required:

- animal's weight
- the infusion rate
- the drug concentration
- duration of infusion
- whether or not the fluids making up the infusion also constitute the animal's intravenous fluid therapy.

All infusions should be fully and clearly labelled once made up, including drug added, amount of drug added, infusion rate, patient's name, date drawn up, and by whom. If for any reason, the animal's fluid therapy demands change, then the infusion should be discontinued and swapped for another fresh bag of crystalloids, whilst the deficit is corrected (e.g. it may need a bolus of fluids). If the overall rate changes, then this should be drecalculate and the infusion redrawn.

1. The rate for the patient's weight should be calculated:

- Weight (kg) x infusion rate (mg/kg/minute) = mg/minute

2. Then converted from milligrams per minute to milligrams per hour (as this is what most syringe drivers or infusion pumps work in):

- Dose rate (mg/min) x 60 = dose rate (mg/hour)

3. It should be decided how long the infusion is to continue:

- Dose rate (mg/hour) x number of hours = dose (mg)

This is the dose required to add into the bag or syringe of fluids.

4. To calculate the volume of drug the following formula can be used:

- Dose/concentration = volume

This shows how much drug needs to be added.

If this infusion is just piggybacking the animal's fluid therapy (an adjunct), i.e. via a separate line, then the drug can be added to a known volume (e.g. 500 ml bag or a 20 ml syringe of crystalloid).

If the drug volume is large, then the equivalent volume of fluid should be withdrawn from the bag or the syringe before adding in the drug.

5. The infusion rate to dial up on the syringe driver or fluid pump should be calculated:

- Volume of bag/syringe (ml)/number of hours (hr) = infusion rate (ml/hr)

6. Where the infusion is also the patient's fluid therapy, their required fluid therapy rate should be calculated:

- Fluid therapy rate (ml/kg/hr) x weight (ml/hr) = fluid therapy rate (ml/hr)

7. How many hours' worth of infusion that a bag will supply should be calculated:

- Volume of bag (ml)/fluid rate (ml/hr) = number of hours of infusion (hr)

This number of hours should be inserted into equation 3) to calculate the total dose needed for a particular bag, and then equation 4) for the volume. This volume of drug should be injected into the bag and the fluid administered at the fluid therapy rate chosen for the animal.

References

- Grant, D. (2007) *Pain management in small animals. A manual for veterinary nurses and technicians.* Elsevier.

Test

Answers on Page 204

1. Which of the validated feline pain scales includes a physiological category?
- a. Glasgow Composite Measure Pain Scale for cats.
- b. Feline Grimace Scale.
- c. Botucatu Pain Scale.
- d. Melbourne Pain Scale.

2. When using a peripheral nerve locator for a local block what is the low current limit that should be checked to ensure the tip of the needle is not inside the nerve bundle itself before injecting the local anaesthetic.
- a. <0.2 mA.
- b. <0.4 mA.
- c. <0.6 mA.
- d. <0.8 mA.

3. When performing an intercostal nerve block, where should you aim for?
- a. The cranial aspect of the rib as dorsal as possible up the rib.
- b. The caudal aspect of the rib as dorsal as possible up the rib.
- c. The cranial aspect of the rib as ventral as possible down the rib.
- d. The caudal aspect of the rib as ventral as possible down the rib.

4. The Glasgow CMPS for dogs is an example of what type of pain scale?
- a. Visual analogue scale.
- b. Numerical rating scale.
- c. Simple descriptive scale.
- d. Grimace Scale.

5. What three facial action units are featured in the Feline Grimace Scale but not the Glasgow CMPS for cats?
- a. Ear position, orbital tightening, whisker position.
- b. Head carriage, orbital tightening, muzzle tone.
- c. Whisker position, head carriage, ear position.
- d. Head carriage, whisker position, orbital tightening.

6. Which technique used to verify correct lumbosacral epidural needle placement is dependent on negative pressure being present in the epidural space?
- a. The "popping sensation" technique.
- b. Lack of resistance technique.
- c. Air bubble technique.
- d. Hanging drop technique.

7. The standard brachial plexus block (injected into the axilla) would be an appropriate local anaesthetic technique to desensitize the limb for what type of surgery?
- a. Elbow fracture repair.
- b. Bone graft taken from the humerus.
- c. Forequarter amputation (including scapula removal).
- d. Metatarsal plating.

8. A local analgesic injected perineurally works on which part of the pain pathway?
- a. Transduction.
- b. Transmission.
- c. Modulation.
- d. Perception.

9. Ketamine works as an antagonist against which receptor?
- a. α-2 adrenergic.
- b. μ-opioid.
- c. Serotoninergic.
- d. N-methyl D-aspartate.

10. Which opioid is classed as a partial μ-agonist?
- a. Methadone.
- b. Pethidine.
- c. Buprenorphine.
- d. Butorphanol.

Clinical Case

A cross breed dog is being anaesthetised for an exploratory laparotomy to remove an intestinal foreign body. The dog has been vomiting for the past three days and a radiopaque foreign body is identified within the small intestine on radiography.

The vet plans a preanaesthetic medication of dexmedetomidine and methadone, anaesthetic induction with alfaxalone, and maintenance with isoflurane in oxygen. They request an intramuscular injection of ketamine just before the start of surgery, a paracetamol intravenous injection and a lidocaine continuous rate infusion.

1. **From the protocol listed above (preanaesthetic medication), identify the drugs which are considered analgesic, and specify what drug groups they belong to/which receptors they work on.**

2. **You have been asked to calculate and draw up the lidocaine CRI using the following parameters:**
   Body weight = 10 kg.
   Lidocaine CRI rate = 25 µg/kg/min.
   Concentration of lidocaine = 20 mg/ml.
   Duration of CRI = 5 hours.
   What volume of lidocaine is needed for this CRI?

3. **What are the benefits of lidocaine as a CRI for this particular case?**

4. **How else could local anaesthetic techniques be applied to this case – ensuring you respect the top doses for local anaesthetics?**

5. **Why do you think the vet chose paracetamol instead of a typical NSAID (e.g. meloxicam or carprofen)?**

Correct Answers:

Test

1. c
2. b
3. b
4. c
5. d
6. d
7. a
8. b
9. d
10. c

Clinical Case

1. **From the protocol listed above (preanaesthetic medication), identify the drugs which are considered analgesic, and specify what drug groups they belong to/which receptors they work on.**
   Dexmedetomidine = α-2 adrenergic agonist.
   Methadone = pure μ-opioid agonist.
   Ketamine = NMDA antagonist.
   Paracetamol = atypical NSAID.
   Lidocaine = local anaesthetic.

2. **What volume of lidocaine is needed for this CRI?**
   Convert µg into mg.
   1000 µg in 1 mg therefore CRI rate is 25/1000 = 0.025 mg/kg/min.
   10 x 0.025 mg/kg/min = 0.25 mg/min.
   0.25 mg/min x 60 mins = 15 mg/hr.
   15 x 5 hrs = 75 mg over 5 hours.
   75 mg/20 mg/ml = 3.75 ml lidocaine required for the CRI.

3. **What are the benefits of lidocaine as a CRI for this particular case?**
   As well as providing systemic analgesia, a lidocaine CRI is also prokinetic, anti-inflammatory and anti-endotoxic which may all be useful for patients having intestinal surgery.

4. **How else could local anaesthetic techniques be applied to this case – ensuring you respect the top doses for local anaesthetics?**
   A line block, either infiltrated preincision or as the surgeon closes the linea alba could be used. A wound diffusion catheter could be used to similar effect and maintained to continue local analgesia in recovery. Intra-peritoneal local analgesia could also be considered by instilling local anaesthetic into the abdominal cavity at the end of surgery.

5. **Why do you think the vet chose paracetamol instead of a typical NSAID (e.g. meloxicam or carprofen)?**
   The prostaglandins that typical NSAIDs block are important in maintaining gut mucosal integrity and gut healing, and therefore not indicated for use around gut surgery. Also, the patient has been vomiting for several days and may be dehydrated, another contraindication for NSAID use.

Notes

Imaging

Barbara Gomes

Chapter Summary:

- **Radiographic techniques. Principles and use in specific situations.**
- **Radiographic contrast studies.**
- **Radiographic interpretation.**
- **Ultrasonography techniques. Point of care ultrasound (POCUS).**
- **Ultrasound guided interventional techniques.**
- **Echocardiography in cats and dogs.**
- **Interventional radiology.**
- **Advanced diagnostic imaging techniques.**

Radiology

Wilhelm Conrad Roentgen discovered X-rays in 1896 (Figure 1). Since then, X-rays have revolutionised the field of diagnostic imaging in both human and veterinary medicine. Radiography was one of the first modalities to be developed in the field of radiology (which includes other modalities that use radioactive compounds, electromagnetic radiation, or sound waves for imaging purposes).

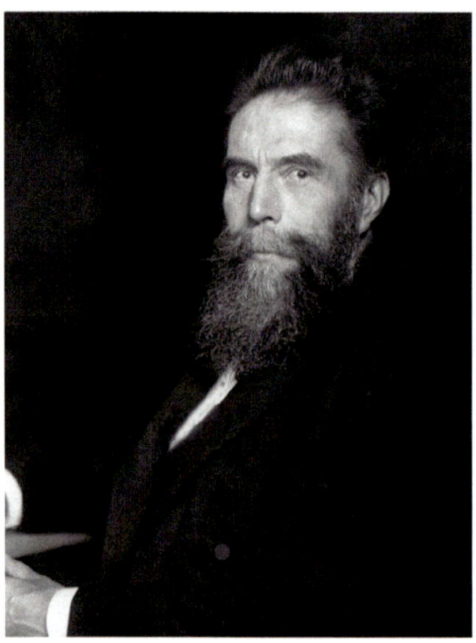

Figure 1. Photo of Wilhelm Conrad Roentgen.

Types of Radiography

Conventional Film Screen Radiography

Conventional film screen radiography was a major innovation for veterinary medicine, however its use has now been **superseded by digital radiography.**

Conventional film screen radiography consists of a film emulsion layer sandwiched between two fluorescent intensifying screens located inside a light tight cassette (Figure 2). The front of the cassette is made of a low atomic number material (e.g. plastic) to allow the X-rays in. The back of the cassette is made of a high atomic number material (e.g. lead) to reduce backscatter.

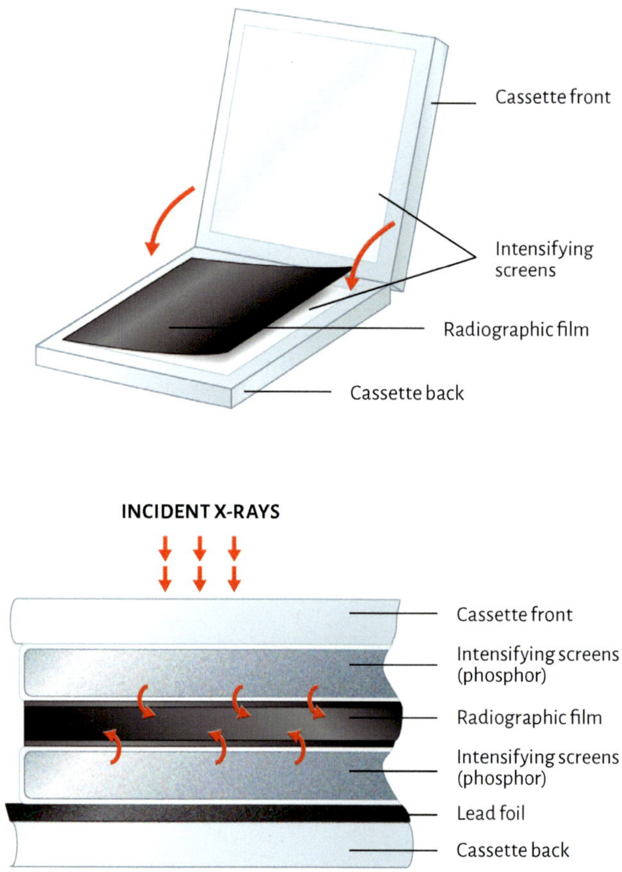

Figure 2. Composition of conventional screen film cassette.

Conventional radiography image formation and processing differs from digital radiography. The radiographic image is created by the number of X-ray photons passing through the patient and the light emitted by the intensifying screen which **exposes the radiographic film.** The latent image in the film only becomes visible after **chemical film processing.** The structure and processing of the film affects the optical density (blackness) of the image. Once the film is processed and the radiographic image formed, **further manipulation of the image is not possible.**

The contrast and spatial resolution depend on the combination of **film screen and film type.**

Intensifying screens have a much higher absorption efficiency for X-ray photons and convert the X-ray photon energy to visible light. The use of an intensifying screen results in a lower radiation dose to the patient, but the disadvantage is that it creates blur.

Advantages of film screen radiography:
- higher spatial resolution

Disadvantages:
- radiographic image is fixed
- narrow dynamic range and latitude: promotes exposure error (overexposure and underexposure)
- difficult to store and archive
- processing images is time consuming and expensive

Digital Radiography

Digital radiography consists of an imaging acquisition process that **generates an electronic image which is viewed and manipulated on a computer.**

There are **two types** of digital radiography, which differ in the way the X-ray photon pattern is converted to an electrical digital signal. These are:
- computed radiography (CR)
- direct digital radiography (DR).

Computed Radiography (CR)

CR systems are **cassette based systems,** but instead of containing conventional film the image plate is coated with a photostimulable phosphor (PSP) (Figure 3). The X-ray attenuation pattern of the patient is stored temporarily as a latent image in the PSP, and used in the same way as film screen cassettes but requires a plate reader following exposure to obtain the image.

Direct Digital Radiography (DR)

DR systems consist of a technology that produces an almost instantaneous image. These systems provide a major advantage over CR systems and film screen radiography because they produce images more quickly (Figures 4 and 5).

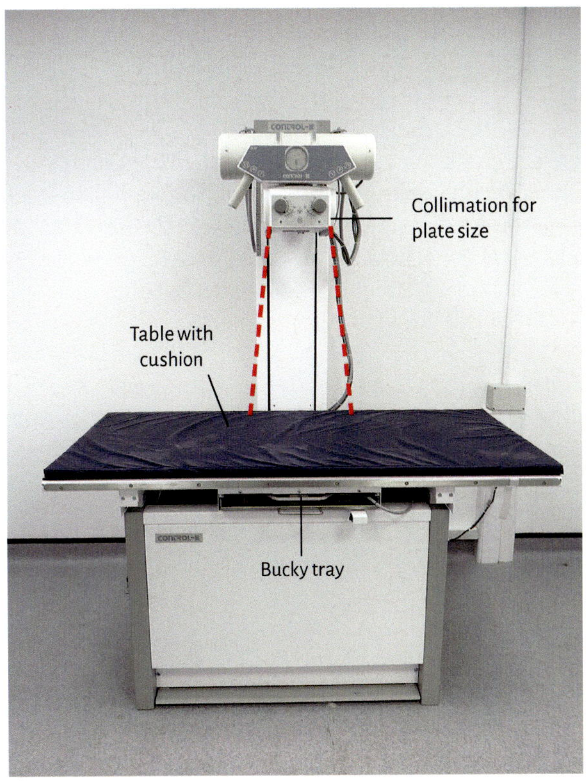

Figure 4. X-ray unit, DR system.

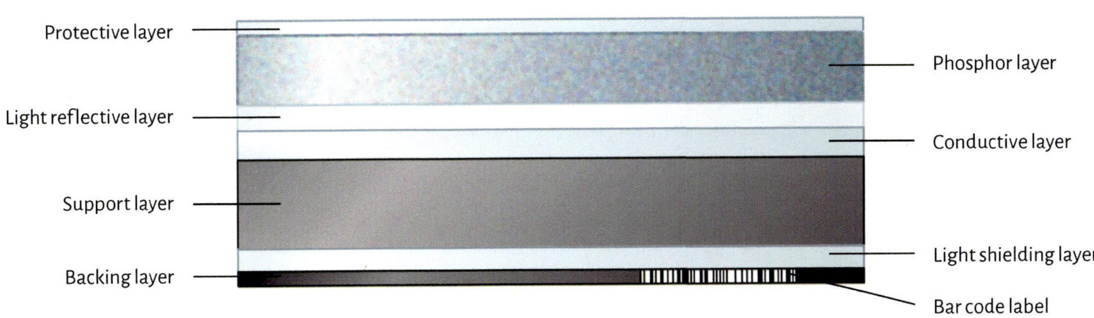

Figure 3. Composition of a CR cassette.

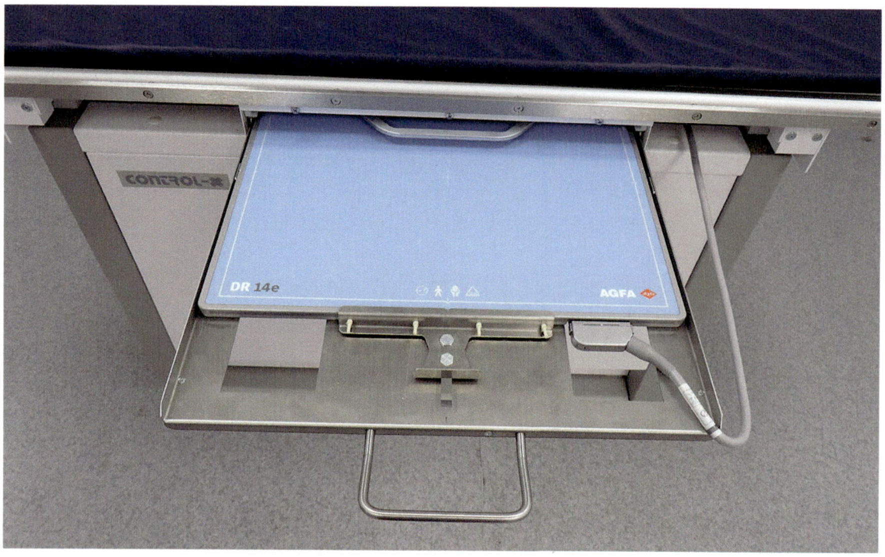

Figure 5. DR cassette.

There are three main types of DR systems (Figure 6). Some systems directly convert the X-ray photons into electrical energy (direct digital radiography) whereas others produce an electrical signal through an intermediate light phase (indirect digital radiography).

- **Direct flat panel detector system:** direct conversion of the X-ray photons into an electrical charge using a photoconductor. This charge is then read directly by the thin film transistor array, processed, and converted to an electronic file.
- **Indirect flat panel detector system:** indirect conversion of the X-ray photons into an electrical signal. There is an intensifier screen built into the flat panel detector which converts X-ray energy emerging from the patient into visible light. An array of tiny photodiodes layered in the intensifying screen converts visible light emitted into an electronic signal which is then read by a thin film transistor array into an electronic file, creating an image.
- **Charged coupled device (CCD):** CCD chips are commonly used in video and digital cameras. In humans, CCDs are used to image small areas (i.e. dental radiography and mammography), however their use in veterinary medicine is uncommon.

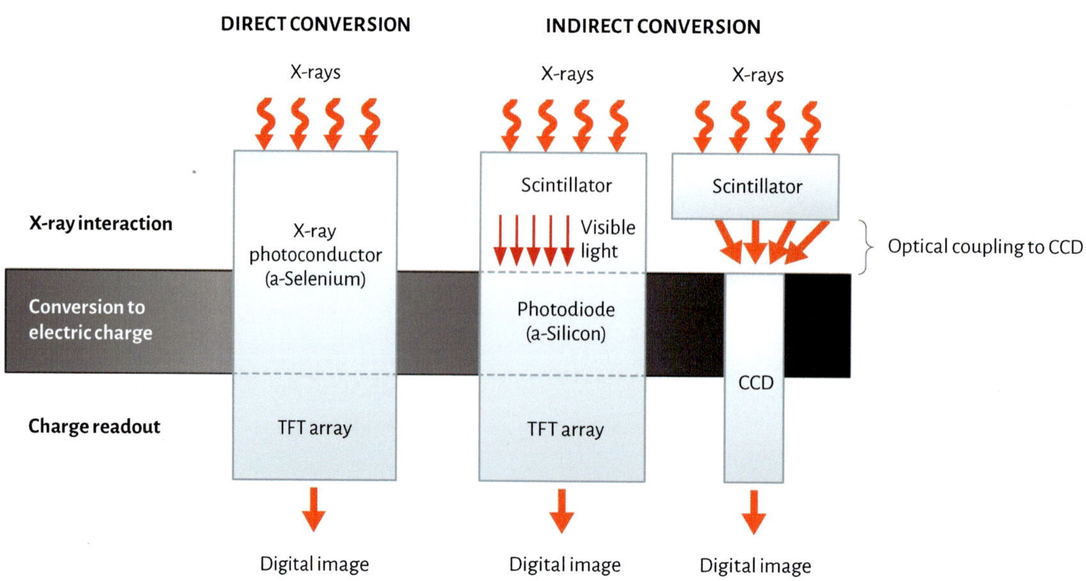

Figure 6. Illustration showing the three types of DR systems.

Advantages:

- no dark room, chemicals, or film required
- wide dynamic range/exposure latitude allowing a larger range of exposure factors
- ability to manipulate image after acquisition (window level and window width; rotate; zoom)
- improved image accessibility and storage using PACS (picture archiving and communication system).

Disadvantages:

- inferior spatial resolution to conventional film screen radiography
- in some systems, horizontal beam projection with the fixed intable DR system may not be possible
- initial setup cost is expensive

Despite the great advantages of the DR system, radiographic repeats due to poor positioning or patient movement, do not go away. All practitioners still need to have good technical knowledge and skills to produce good quality radiographs.

Patient and Room Preparation

Patient and room preparations are required prior to some elective studies, these may include:

- withholding food for 12 hours, especially if chemical restraint is used
- allowing the animal to urinate and defaecate prior to the study
- removing the collar and harness
- identifying all required radiographic projections, preparing supplies and equipment, before sedating or placing the animal on the X-ray table.

Careful planning and preparation (Figures 7–10) reduces the total time needed for patients to remain in position on the X-ray table.

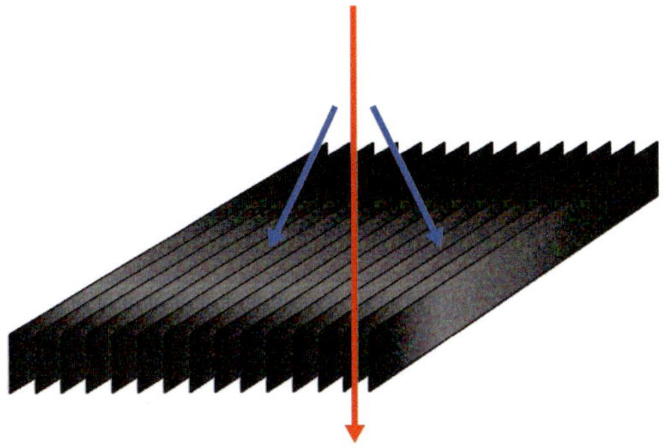

Figure 8. Radiographic grids reduce scatter radiation reaching the cassette and improve image quality.

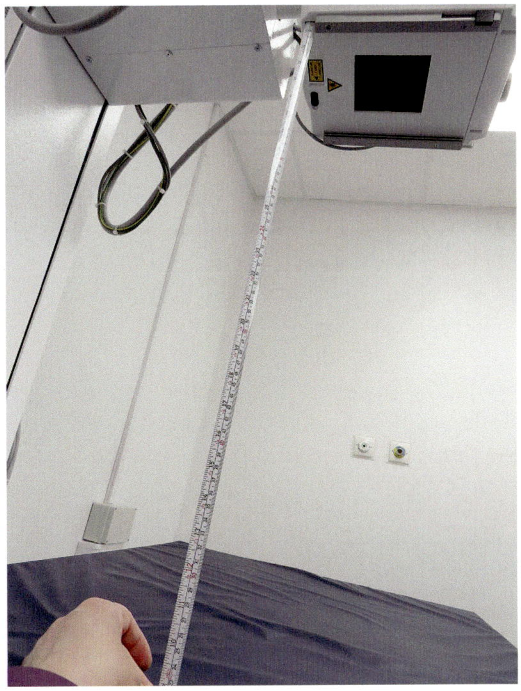

Figure 9. X-ray calliper used to measure the thickness of the area being radiographed.

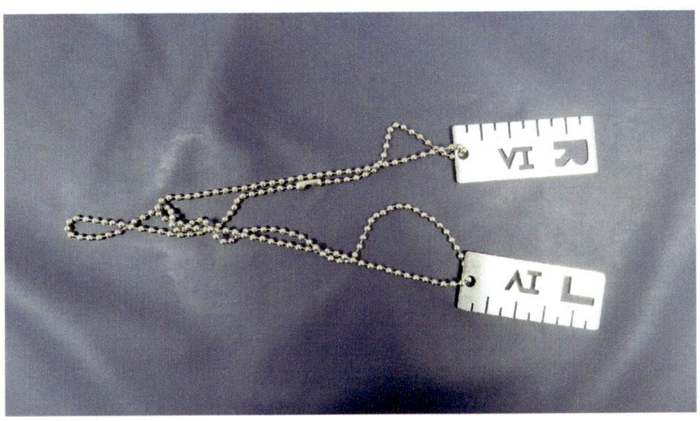

Figure 7. X-ray marker used to accurately identify the side of the patient (right or left).

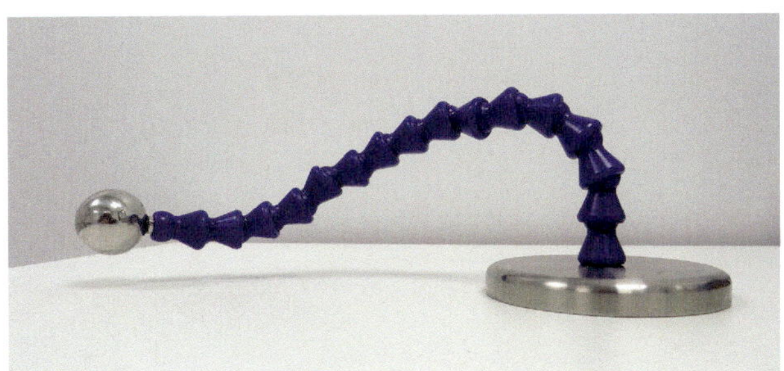

Figure 10. Radiographic reference ball used for radiographic calibration, to reduce scaling errors when templating for implants or examining structures. Supplied with a stable base with a flexible neck, allowing positioning at the same level as the area of interest.

Patient Restraint and Positioning Aids

The use of **positioning aids and restraint techniques** are necessary for appropriate patient positioning and increase the likelihood of obtaining good quality radiographs. Furthermore, they improve safety for both patient and personnel by decreasing the need for manual restraint, reducing exposure to ionising radiation and the number of radiographs taken due to poor patient positioning.

Appropriate patient positioning **requires the patient to be immobile:**

- **chemical restraint** (general anaesthetic or sedation)
- **mechanical restraint** (positioning aids)
- **manual restraint** by personnel should be avoided and only be used in exceptional circumstances. As per Ionising Radiation (Medical Exposure) Regulations (IRMER) 2018, The Ionising Radiations Regulations 1999 (IRR99), Ionising Radiations Regulations 2017 (IRR17) and local rules:
  - The person manually holding the patient must wear appropriate PPE and be as far away from the primary X-ray beam as possible (IRR99).
  - No hands with or without lead gloves should be in collimated area.

Intensity of the radiation follows Newton's inverse square law: the intensity is inversely proportional to the distance from the source (Figure 11).

Positioning Aids

The Guidance Notes for the Safe Use of Ionising Radiations in Veterinary Practice (BVA, 2002) state that **"No animals should be held unless there are good clinical reasons why they cannot be restrained by other means".**

Positioning aids should be used with care as they may cause harm to the patient if used inappropriately.

- A sedated restrained animal should never be left unattended.
- General anaesthesia or sedation helps produce well positioned, diagnostic radiographs, and increase patient comfort, whilst also allowing the handler to step away from the patient during the procedure.

When manual restraint is needed, **positioning aids assist the handler in maintaining the animal in the correct position.** Positioning aids should be small and lightweight to allow ease of use and storage. The full weight of the aid should never rest on sensitive areas such as the airways. Commercially available positioning aids include sandbags (Figure 12), foam wedges or blocks (Figure 13), trough (Figure 14), rope or gauze ties (Figure 15 and 16 A), and tape (Figure 16 B).

Advantages:

- improved patient comfort, whilst also providing support
- minimised rotation
- aid appropriate restraint
- minimised manual restraint:
  - lowers risk of radiation exposure for personnel usually lightweight
- easy mobility and storage appropriate materials easily cleaned.

Disadvantages:

- most positioning aids leave some density shadows:
  - should not be placed over or under the area of interest
  - should be aware of radiopacity before use

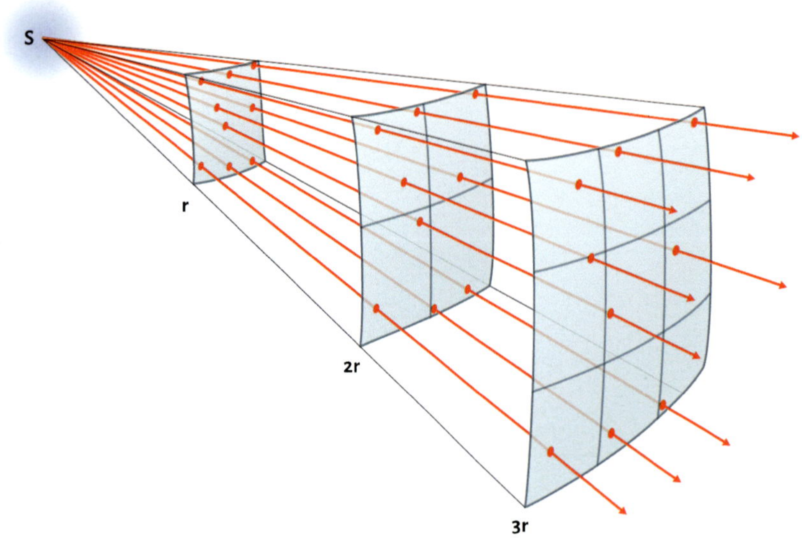

Figure 11. Diagram illustrating the field intensity is inversely proportional to the square of the distance from the source. This is the principle of dose reduction as the distance from the source increases.

– initial purchase costs
– contamination/act as fomites:
  - cleaning necessary between patients.

General Radiographic Principles

Divergence

The patient should always be positioned with the region of interest at the centre of the X-ray film; being a few millimetres off centre can be critical for accurate projection of a joint space.

In the spine, divergence results in increasing oblique projections of the vertebral end plates, which means the intervertebral spaces are obscured away from the film's centre. Thus, in all but the smallest patients, it is preferable to **expose narrow areas (collimation),** initially chosen according to the clinical signs, rather than attempting to cover the whole spine in one exposure.

The specific anatomical structures to be included on radiograph **are identified by surface landmarks.** These are fixed areas on the patient's body which can be seen or palpated. For example, the last rib, the angle of the mandible, and the scapula are useful palpable landmarks.

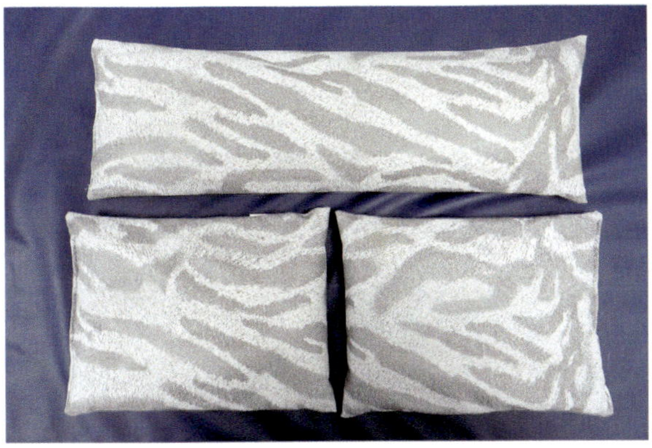

Figure 12. Sandbags.

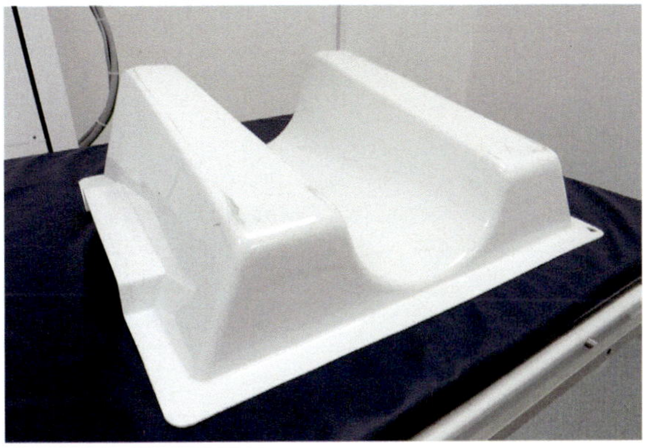

Figure 14. Trough.

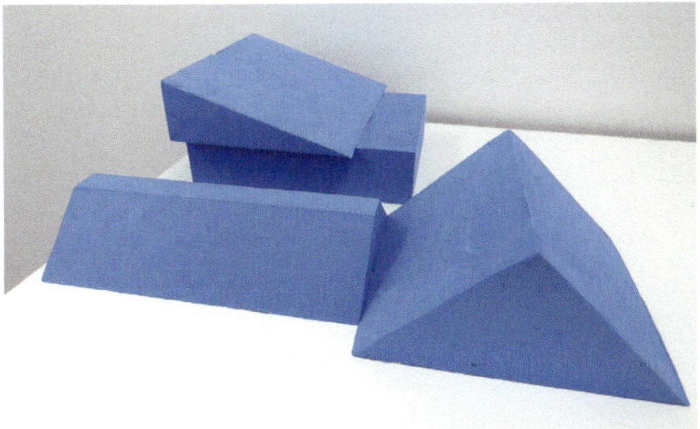

Figure 13. Foam pad and wedges.

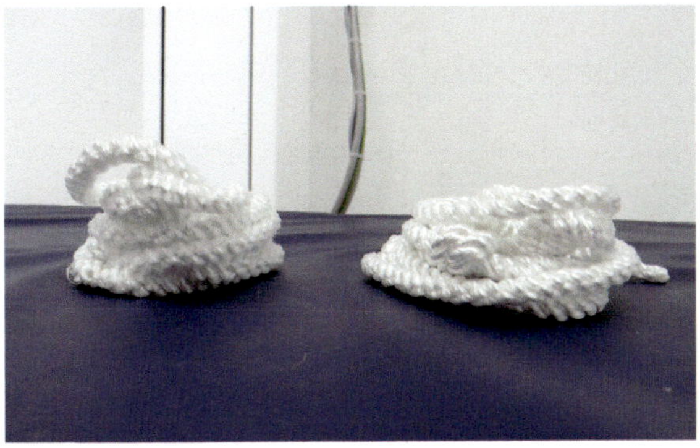

Figure 15. Rope.

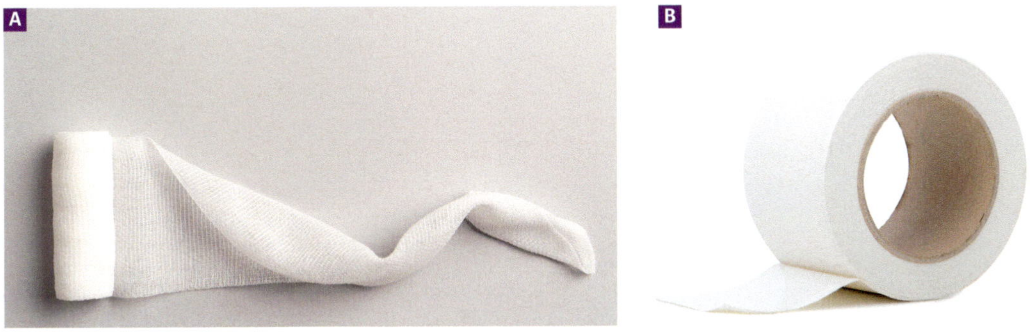

Figure 16. Roll gauze (**A**) and adhesive tape (**B**).

Film Focal Distance (FFD)

Focal film distance (FFD) is the distance between the centre of the anode of the X-ray tube (the focal spot) and the film (top of cassette). This distance should be approximately 100 cm (Figure 17).

The greater the FFD distance, the less the magnification and therefore better detail.

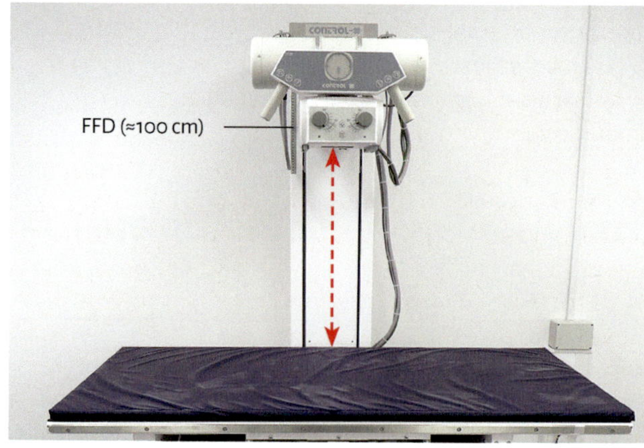

Figure 17. Film focus distance (red arrow).

Object Film Distance (OFD)

Object film distance is the distance between the patient and the film.

The shorter the OFD:
- the sharper the image and detail
- the less distortion and magnification
- the less penumbra effect is created.

Patient Positioning

Patients are usually positioned with the **area of interest as close to the X-ray** cassette as possible; this decreases magnification and increases detail.
- When the area of interest is parallel to the cassette, and perpendicular/central to the X-ray beam this creates less distortion.
- Distortion occurs at the margins of a radiograph.

Correct positioning maximises image interpretation (Figures 18 and 19).

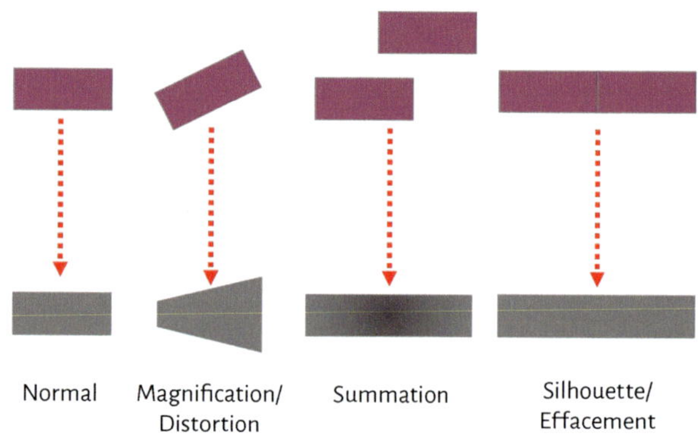

Figure 18. Effects of positioning. Magnification: production of an image larger than the object being examined; Summation effect: superimposition of different organs (e.g. ribs and lung vessels) results is a summation image representing areas of increased opacity; Effacement/silhouetting effect: loss of normal borders between structures of similar opacity (e.g. pleural effusion and cardiac silhouette).

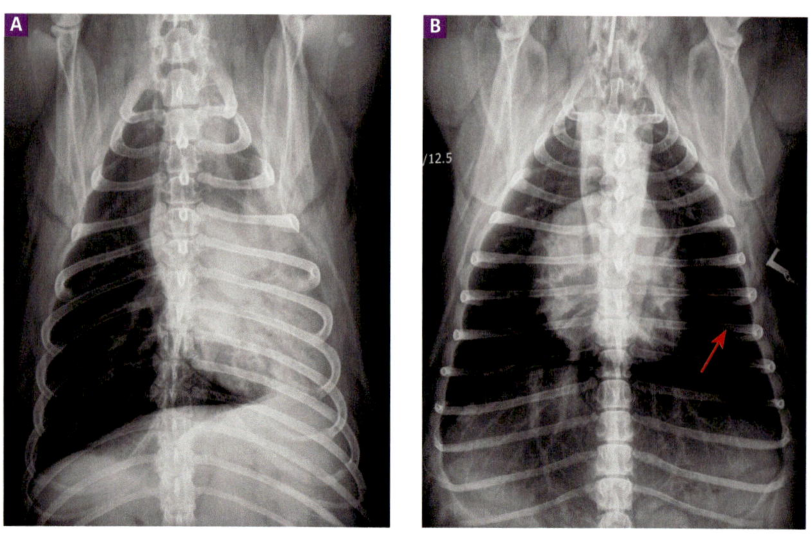

Figure 19. VD radiographic projection of the thorax. Image **A** shows atelectasis of the left hemithorax causing effacement/silhouetting the pulmonary nodule that has similar soft tissue opacity. Image **B** is after intermittent positive pressure ventilation (IPPV) to inflate the lungs. The pulmonary nodules (red arrow) become more evident. Courtesy of Gawain Hammond.

Collimation is essential for all radiographs and should be kept as close as possible to the area of interest. Good collimation improves image quality and helps radiation safety by reducing scatter radiation.

Poor collimation often occurs due to uncertainty of the central point and an inclination to enlarge the collimation to include as much of the patient as possible on the radiograph (Figure 20). **Poor collimation contributes to poor image quality** due to increased scatter, penumbra, geometric distortion, and magnification.

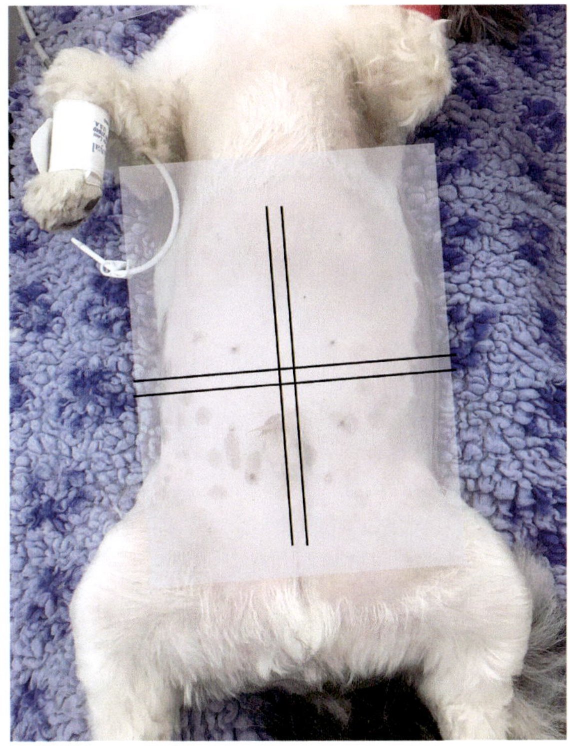

Figure 20. Collimation of the abdomen. Image showing the collimation of the abdomen for a ventrodorsal projection.

Exposure

The correct exposure setting allows clear visualisation of all anatomical parts with detailed trabecular bone pattern and clear distinction between soft tissue and fat.

Digital systems have greater latitude than conventional screen film systems, which means a wider range of exposure factors that contribute to a diagnostic image. **Radiographic exposure is created by a combination of milliampere second (mAs) and kilovoltage (kV) factors.**

- **Milliampere seconds (mAs):** mA x time = mAs. The number of X-ray photons produced by the X-ray tube at the setting selected (quantity of X-rays). Time is how long the exposure lasts.
- **Kilovoltage peak (KVp):** the peak potential applied to the X-ray tube, which accelerates electrons from the cathode to the anode. The power and strength of the X-ray beam (quality and penetration of the X-rays).
  - **kVp controls the penetrating strength of an X-ray beam** (beam quality). the X-rays must be energetic (strong enough) to penetrate the area of interest. Therefore, kVp is selected based on how thick the body part is and what type of tissue will be exposed.
  - **kVp also controls the amount of contrast** (the difference between whites and blacks). The amount of contrast visible in an image is referred to as grey scale. In a high contrast image, there will be white and black areas on the film, but very few greys in between. Low contrast images will have numerous shades of greys.
  - As kVp goes up, radiographic contrast goes down.

The mAs and kV are altered to optimise radiographic contrast.

The abdomen has an inherent low contrast. To maximise the difference in soft tissue in the abdomen a combination of low kV (45–70) and high mAs (8–20) are necessary to maximize contrast.

The converse applies to the thorax. **The thorax has a high inherent contrast** due to air filled lungs. To compensate this high contrast a combination of high kV and low mAs are used, which also reduce the risk of motion blur.

15% rule

Increasing the kV by 15% doubles the film density; therefore, is similar to doubling the mAs:

- **to maintain the equivalent radiographic density, the mAs are halved; and**
- **equally, decreasing the kV by 15% is equivalent to reducing the mAs by half.**

Radiographic Techniques

Good radiographic technique is crucial to acquire high quality, diagnostic radiographs.The primary goal is to obtain good quality radiographs which accurately represent the anatomy of the patient, with good contrast and without distortion, blur, or artefacts.

The radiographer should ensure all equipment is available, appropriately prepared, and be familiar with radiographic projections.

- There is superimposition of the structures along the path of the X-ray photon. Therefore, to localise a structure, two projections are required at 90 degrees of one another, these are called orthogonal projections.
- Two orthogonal projections should always be taken (Figures 21 and 22).

Poor patient positioning (Figure 23) causes:

- poor quality radiographs
- inaccurate interpretation of the radiograph
- incorrect diagnosis (false positives and false negatives).

The following rules apply when taking radiographs:

- a minimal **object film distance** (OFD) should be maintained
- it is important to ensure there are no overlying structures (i.e. cables, IV fluid tubing)
- **parallel placement** of the patient and plate/cassette:
  - the area of interest must be placed parallel to the X-ray plate
- correct **labelling:** L or R (left or right)
- accurate centring/**collimation:**
  - region of interest (ROI) close to the centre of the primary beam
  - cathode side: the anode heel effect can be used to

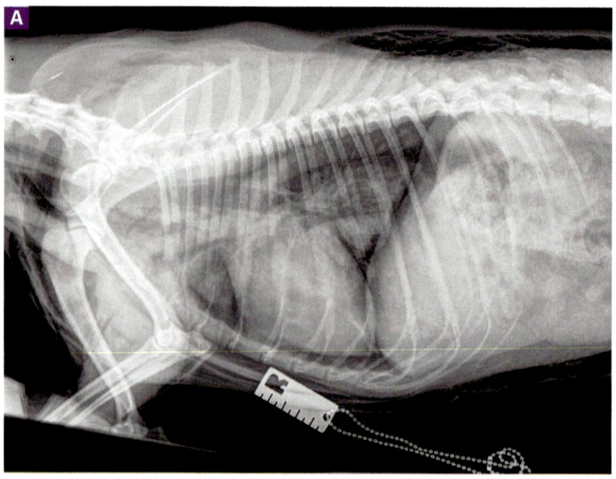

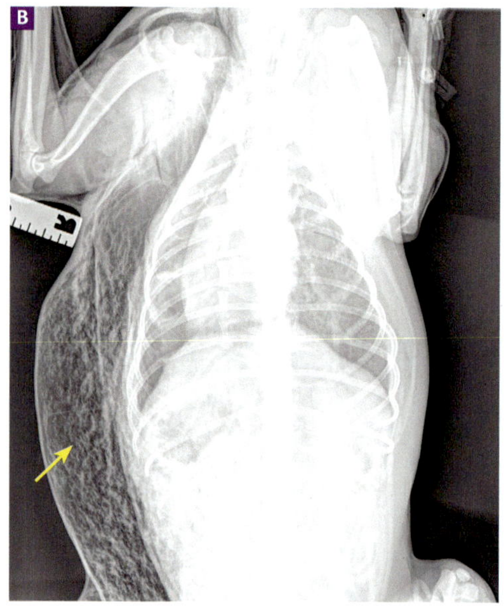

Figure 21. A. Right lateral (RL); **B.** Dorsoventral (DV) thoracic radiographs. Note that the marked subcutaneous emphysema on the right side of the thoracic wall (yellow arrow) seen on the DV projection cannot be appreciated on the right lateral projection.

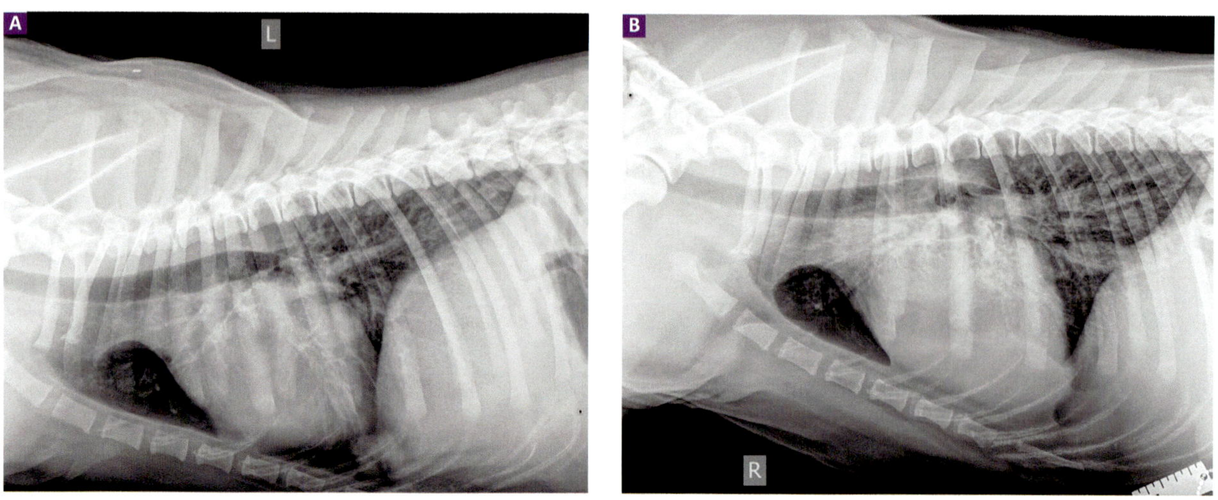

Figure 22. Thorax radiographs. Mass lesion in the right middle lung lobe seen on the left lateral projection (**A**), superimposed on the cardiac silhouette and not seen on the right lateral projection (**B**).

advantage when the anatomical parts have unequal thickness and densities
  - scatter can be reduced +/- grid (>6–10 cm width)
- **appropriate exposure settings** should be used, as per thickness, region, density, FFD (measurements using callipers).

The anode heel effect refers to the variation of radiation intensity along the anode cathode axis of the X-ray tube, decreasing towards the anode (Figure 24).

Patient positioning varies for the anatomical area under evaluation and depends on specific protocols. In this chapter the axial and appendicular system, thorax, and abdomen of the surgical patient are considered, in addition to presurgical, postsurgical, and follow up radiographs of the skeletal system.

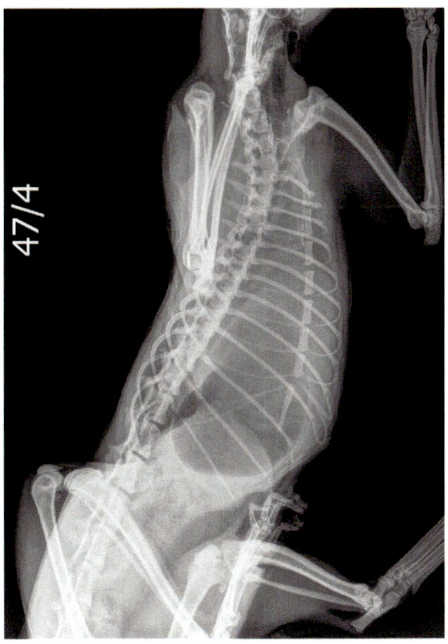

Figure 23. Bad positioning and orientation of the thorax of a cat. Courtesy of Mark Coia.

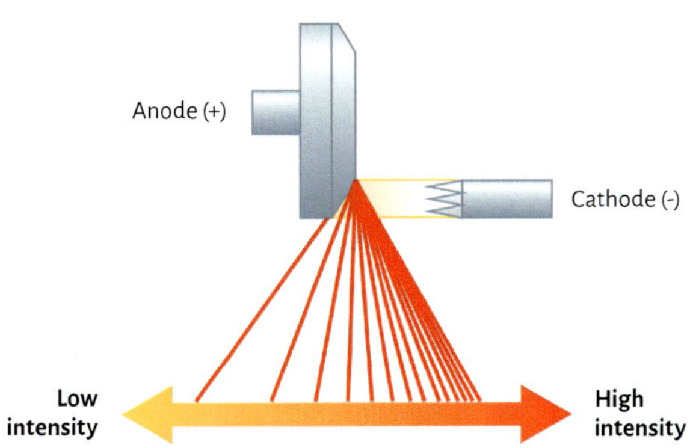

Figure 24. Anode heel effect.

Radiographic Terminology

The following table describes the terminology used in radiology and the abbreviations which are normally utilised to identify the radiographic projections. (Table 1).

Table 1. Terminology and abbreviations used in radiography.

Full description	Abbreviation	Direction of the primary beam
Left or Right	**L or R**	The practice of describing the dependent side or the side in question of the patient
Dorsal	**D**	Describes the front of the lower limbs (bellow carpus or tarus) or top of the trunk
Ventral	**V**	Underside of the animal
Cranial	**Cr**	Towards the head (cranium)
Caudal	**Cd**	Towards the tail
Rostral	**R**	Towards the nose
Medial	**M**	Inside surface of the leg (more axial surface)
Lateral	**L**	The outside surface of the leg (more abaxial surface)
Proximal	**Pr**	The higher end of a bone or anatomical part
Distal	**Di**	The part of a bone or limb furthest from the main body
Palmar	**P/Pa**	The back edge of the lower forelimb (below the carpus). NB: think of the aspect being your palm
Plantar	**Pl**	The back edge of the lower hindlimb (below the tarsus)
Oblique	**O**	An oblique projection is similar to a "skyline" which will help outline a lesion with minimal superimposition. Radiographic projections taken with the primary beam entering at < or > 90° to the anatomical area of interest but usually wary from 35–60° angles
Dorsoventral	**DV**	Dorsal (towards the spine) surface and exits the ventral (sternal) surface of the patient
Ventrodorsal	**VD**	Opposite to DV: ventral-dorsal surface
Craniocaudal	**CrCd**	Cranial surface to caudal surface. This relates to extremities proximal to the level of tje carpus or tarsus
Caudocranial	**CdCr**	Opposite direction of the CrCd. Caudal to cranial passage of the primary beam through the anatomical region
Dorsopalmar/ Dorsoplantar	**Dpa/DPl**	Distal to the carpus. Dorsal to palmar direction. Distal to the tarsus. Dorsal to plantar, respectively
Palmardorsal/ Plantardorsal	**PaD/PlD**	Palmar to dorsal. Plantar to dorsal surface of the body, respectively

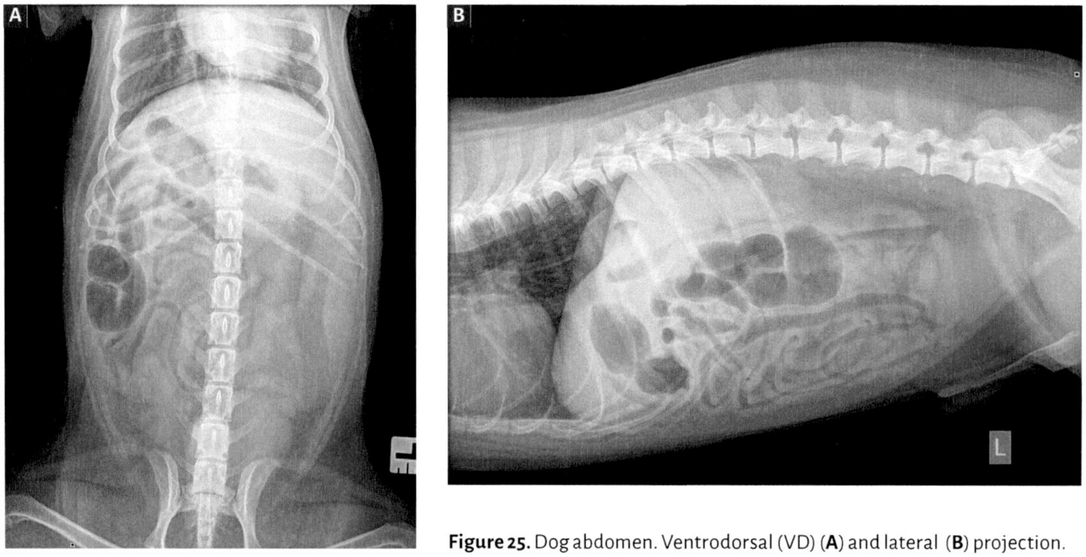

Figure 25. Dog abdomen. Ventrodorsal (VD) (**A**) and lateral (**B**) projection.

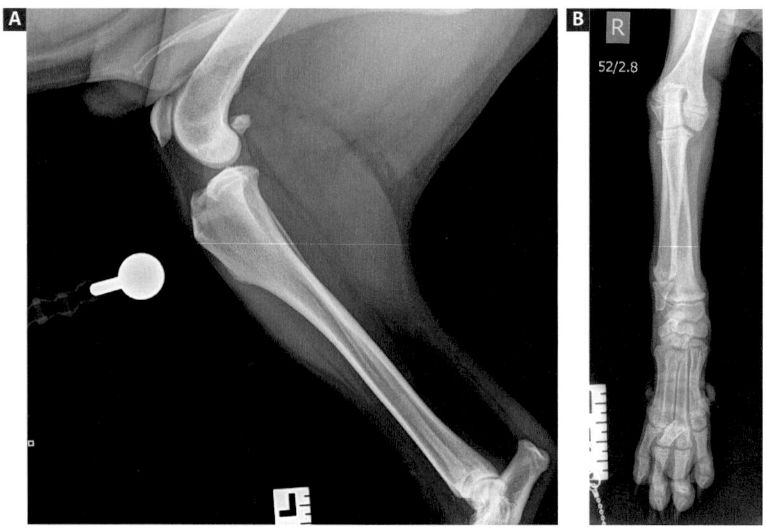

Figure 26. Mediolateral projection (**A**) of a dog's stifle. Dorsopalmar projection (**B**) of the carpus/manus.

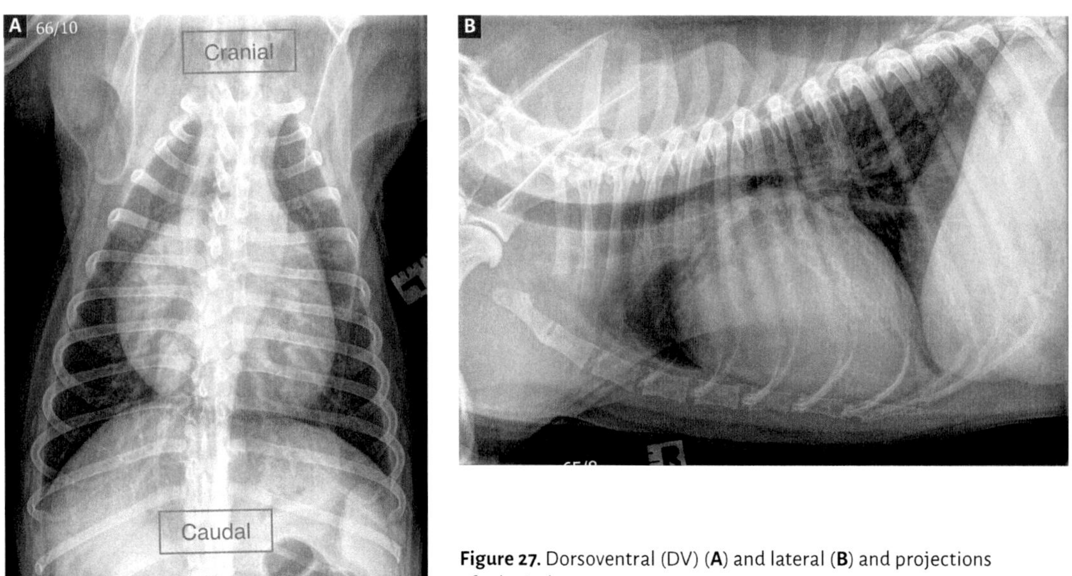

Figure 27. Dorsoventral (DV) (**A**) and lateral (**B**) and projections of a dog's thorax.

Thoracic radiographs

Common views:

- ventrodorsal projection (VD)
- dorsoventral projection (DV)
- right lateral projection (RL)
- left lateral projection (LL).

Lateral Projection

The lateral view (Figures 28 and 29) is often a more stable and comfortable position for an animal to lie in and, therefore, there is less resistance to manipulation. A sandbag is often required over the neck and the lumbar spine to help keep the animal lying down.

Exposure during expiration increases space between the organs.

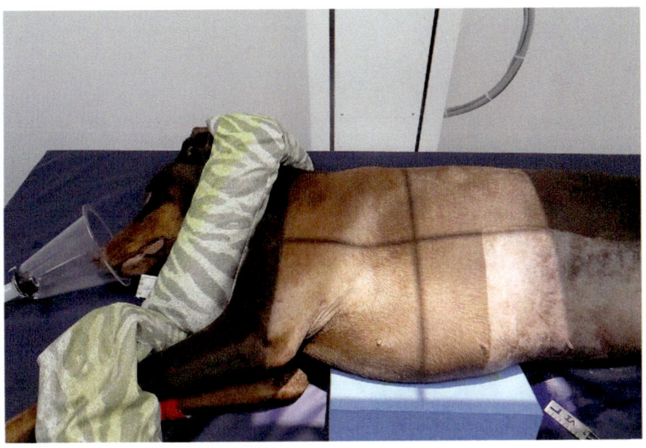

Figure 28. Dog in correct position for right lateral thorax radiograph.

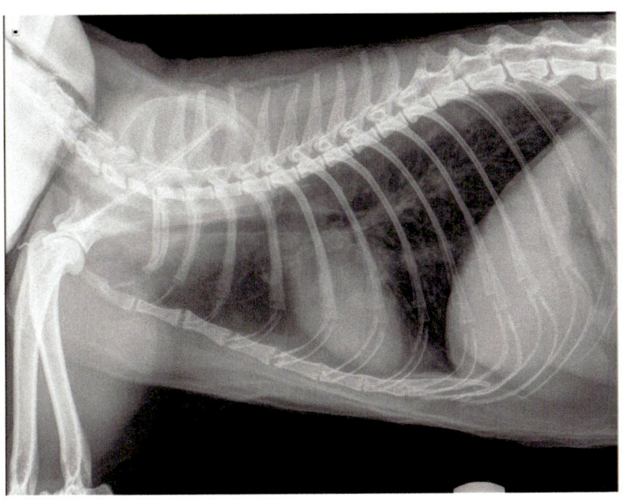

Figure 29. Right lateral radiograph of the thorax of a cat.

Positioning

- right lateral recumbency is preferred as this allows assessment of the cardiovascular system;
- forelimbs should be extended cranially and hindlimbs caudally;
- a foam pad should be placed under the sternum to avoid rotation and to maintain horizontal alignment of the sternum and spine;
- it is important to check the neck is in a natural position.

Centring

- caudal dorsal border of scapula.

Collimation

- entire rib cage within collimated area
- cranial border: thoracic inlet
- dorsal border: spinous processes of spinal column
- ventral border: xiphoid process
- caudal border: last rib.

Important features:

1. The limbs should not be superimposed on the cranial thorax.
2. The costochondral junction should be level.
3. Inspiratory film: the triangle should be identified. The triangle is formed by the ventral border of the vena cava, the caudal border of the heart and the diaphragm, and should be as large as possible indicating an inspiratory timed exposure.

A positive pressure of 10–12 cmH_2O using the breath hold technique may be considered when fully inflated lung radiographs are needed under general anaesthesia.

Labelling

- right or left markers should be within the collimated area, ensuring the marker does not obscure anatomical structures;
- the identification label should be in the caudal region within the collimated area.

Technique

- measurements should be taken at the highest point of the ribs and a grid used if this distance >10 cm;
- wedges should be used under the sternum to keep the sternum spine plane parallel to the cassette/plate;
- the radiograph should be acquired at peak inspiration;
- sandbags should be used to pull the forelimbs forwards. Ideally sandbags should not be in the collimated area.

Other considerations

- broad chested animals may not require foam padding for positioning;
- large/giant breeds may need two radiographs, one of the cranial and one of the caudal thorax.

Dorsoventral Projection

Positioning

- sternal recumbency (Figures 30 and 31);
- the forelimb should be extended slightly cranial with carpus at level of ears;
- the head should be resting on the tabletop;
- the hindlimbs should be in a natural flexed position;
- the spine should be superimposed over the sternum (Figure 30).

Centring

- caudal border of scapula.

Collimation

- cranial border: thoracic inlet
- lateral borders: body wall.

Labelling

- right and left markers should be placed caudal to the axilla within the collimated area;
- the identification label should be in the caudal region within the collimated area.

Technique

- measurements should be taken at the highest point (usually the last rib).

Other Considerations

- the alignment of the sternum and spine should be maintained;
- this position may also be used for horizontal beam X-ray;
- sandbags should not be used directly against the chest to push the chest into a straight position, a radiolucent foam block/wedge should be placed between the chest and sandbag;
- covering the eyes of some animals with paper tissue or cloth prevents them from seeing the operator leaving the table to go and press the exposure button.

Ventrodorsal Projection

Positioning

- dorsal recumbency;
- forelimbs should be extended cranially with the nose between the forelimbs;
- the head should be resting on the tabletop;
- hindlimbs should be extended caudally;
- a V trough should be used to superimpose the sternum and spine (Figure 32).

Centring

- the caudal border of the scapula should be centred on the midline.

Collimation

- cranial border: thoracic inlet
- V trough entirely within collimated area
- lateral borders: body wall.

Labelling

- right and left markers should be cranial to the axilla within the V trough;
- the identification label should be in the cranial or caudal region within the collimated area.

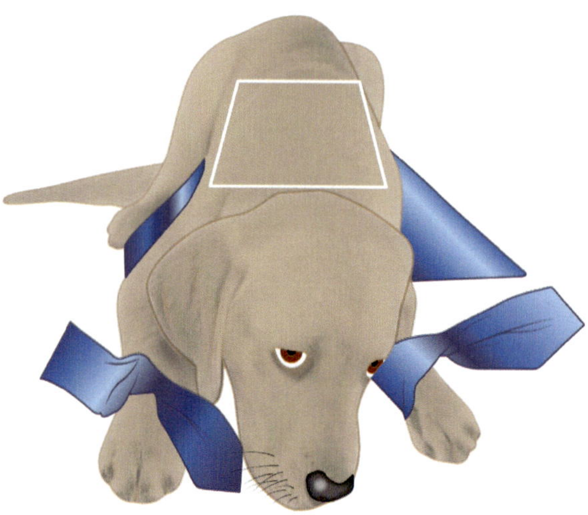

Figure 30. DV positioning.

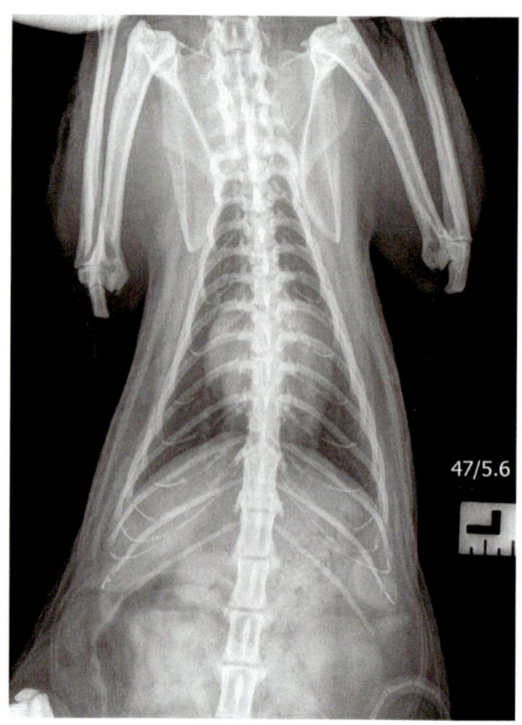

Figure 31. DV thoracic radiograph of a cat. Note that the sternum is aligned with the thoracic vertebrae.

Technique

– measurements should be taken at the highest point (usually the last rib).

Other Considerations

– foam pads help maintain alignment of the sternum and spine and avoid rotation;
– this position may also be used with horizontal beam X-ray and is referred to as the lateral decubitus view.

Surgical Cases

The thorax is rarely evaluated by the orthopaedic surgeon but is an important area for soft tissue surgeons. Evaluation of the thorax can be crucial when the decision is taken as to whether the patient needs surgery (i.e. diaphragmatic hernia, Figure 33), to explain respiratory distress (i.e. pneumothorax or pleural effusion), to follow up on pulmonary changes (i.e. aspiration pneumonia), or to check if an oesophageal tube is correctly positioned after surgery (Figure 34).

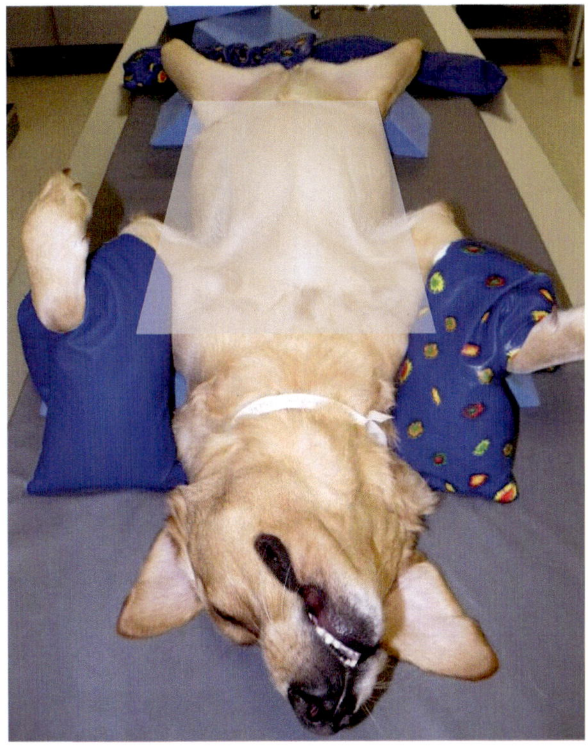

Figure 32. VD projection of the thorax of a dog. Courtesy of Gawain Hammond.

Table 2. Differences between DV and VD radiograph projections.

Dorsoventral	Ventrodorsal
Allows evaluation of cardiovascular system	Allows evaluation of full lung field
Diaphragm (cupula) – rounded appearance	Diaphragm (cupula) – flatted with the characteristic "Mickey mouse" ears pattern
Less stressful for the patient	Not recommended in a distressed patient
Safer during respiratory distress	Atypical appearance of the cardiac silhouette → elongated

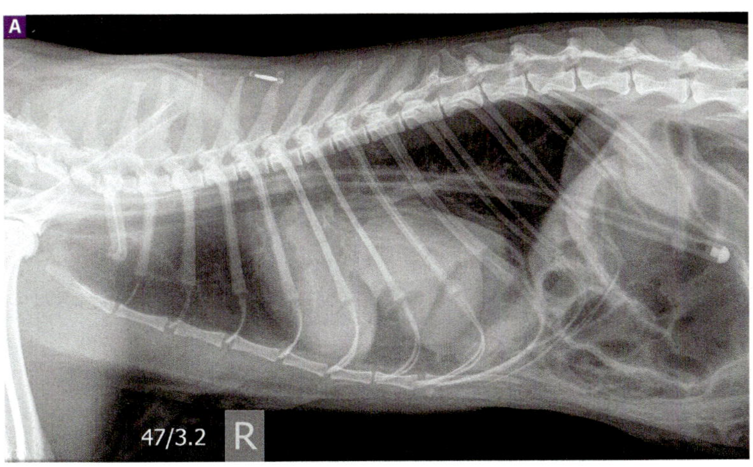

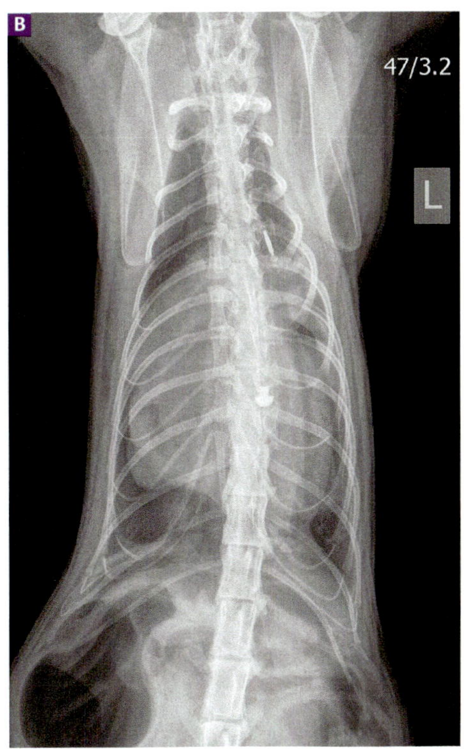

Figure 33. Right lateral (**A**) and DV (**B**) projections of a feline thorax. Demonstration of a pericardial peritoneal diaphragmatic hernia (PPDH) with falciform fat and the liver seen in the thorax within the pericardial sac just caudal to the cardiac silhouette. Gastric tube is in place.

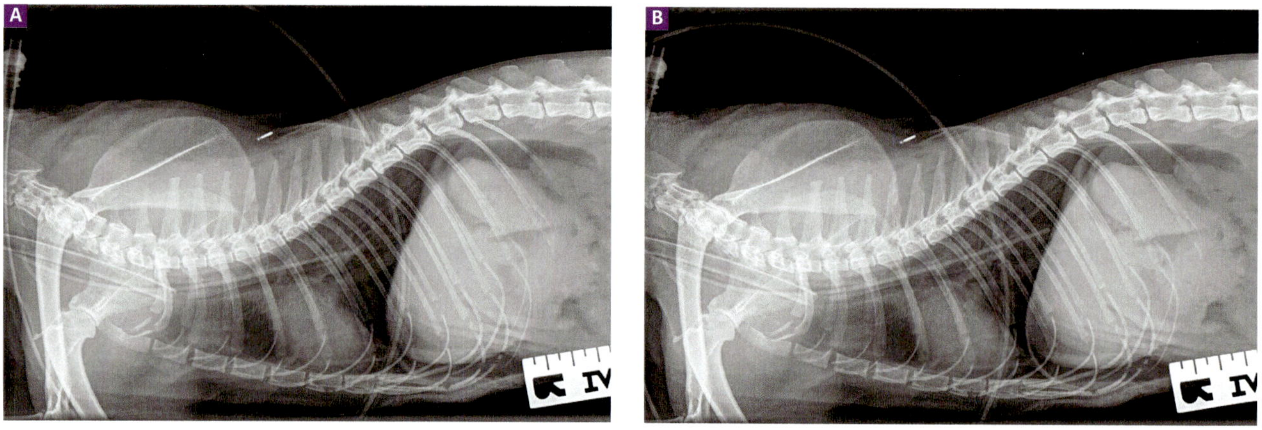

Figure 34. Right lateral projection of the thorax of a cat. Checking positioning the oesophageal tube. **A.** Tube correctly positioned, **B.** Tube too long.

Abdominal Radiographs

Abdominal radiographs have a short scale of contrast, with high mAs and low kVp required for imaging.

Common views are:

- lateral projection (right and left)
- flexed leg lateral projection
- ventrodorsal projection
- left lateral decubitus projection: horizontal beam
- dorsoventral projection.

Lateral Projection

Positioning

- the forelimbs should be extended cranially (Figures 35 and 36);
- the hindlimbs slightly retracted caudally. Overextension of the hindlimbs can tighten the abdominal wall and compress the viscera, making interpretation more difficult;
- rotation should be avoided, using foam wedges under the sternum and ventral abdomen if necessary.

Centring

- in dogs the radiograph should be centred just caudal to the caudal border of 13th rib, midway between dorsal and ventral skin surfaces;
- in cats this should be approximately two finger widths further caudal.

Collimation

- cranial border: 2.5 cm cranial to the tip of the xiphoid of the sternum
- caudal border: the greater trochanter.

Labelling

- right or left markers should be used;
- the identification label should be cranial or caudal to the region within the collimated area.

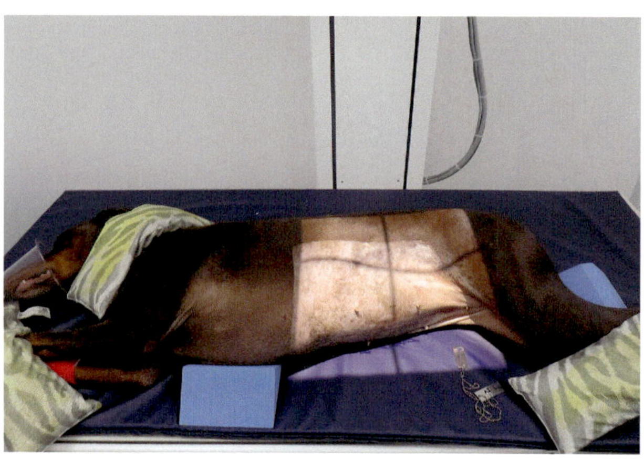

Figure 35. Lateral abdomen projection patient positioning.

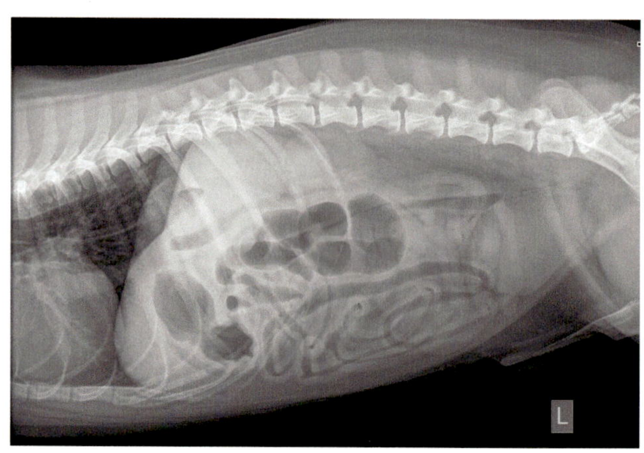

Figure 36. Lateral abdomen projection of a dog.

Technique

- measurements should be taken at the highest point. Usually, the ribs are measured laterally, 2.5 cm caudal to the tip of the xiphoid of the sternum.

Other Considerations

- foam pads can be used between the femurs and under the sternum to maintain alignment of the sternum and spine, and avoid axial rotation;
- this projection may be used with horizontal beam X-ray and is referred to as the lateral decubitus view.

Ventrodorsal Projection

(Figures 37 and 38)

Positioning

- the pelvic limbs should be in a neutral frog legged position;
- the thorax should be placed within a positioning trough/cradle to prevent rotation;
- pads under the thighs can help to reduce tilting;
- rotation should be avoided, foam wedges can be used under the sternum and ventral abdomen if necessary.

Centring

- in dogs the radiograph should be centred just caudal to the caudal border of 13th rib, midway between lateral skin surfaces;
- in cats this should be approximately two finger widths further caudal.

Collimation

- cranial border: 2.5 cm cranial to the tip of the xiphoid of the sternum
- caudal border: the greater trochanter.

Labelling

- right or left markers should be used at the cranial end of the radiograph;
- the identification label should be placed in the cranial or caudal region within the collimated area.

Technique

- measurements should be taken at the highest point;
- usually, the ribs are measured laterally, 2.5 cm caudal to the tip of the xiphoid of the sternum.

Other Considerations

- the sternum and spine should be superimposed.

Flexed Leg Lateral Projection

This technique is used for evaluation of the urethra and retrograde urethrograms.

Positioning

- the forelimbs should be extended cranially;
- the sternum and spine should be parallel to each other and equidistant from the tabletop;
- the hindlimbs should then be hyperextended cranially towards the abdomen to allow visualisation of the urethra;
- the projection should be acquired on expiration.

Centring

- caudal abdomen (Figure 39).

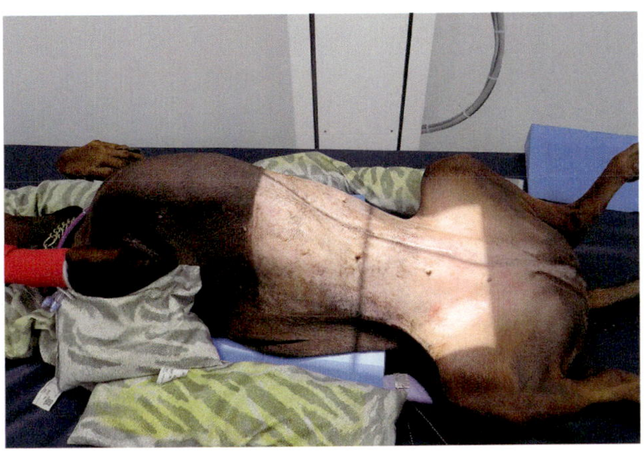

Figure 37. VD projection patient positioning.

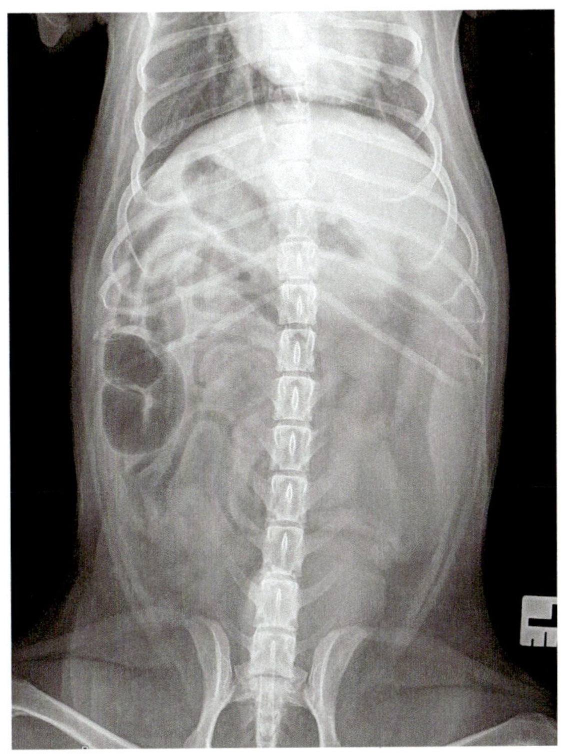

Figure 38. VD abdominal projection.

Collimation

- cranial border: mid abdomen
- caudal border: perineum.

Labelling

- the right/left marker should be placed dorsally on the radiograph.

Technique

- measurements should be taken at the highest point at mid abdomen.

Other Considerations

- sandbags are necessary for cranial hyperextension of the hindlimbs;
- Figure 39 highlights the importance of the flexed projection for the evaluation of the urethra in male dogs.

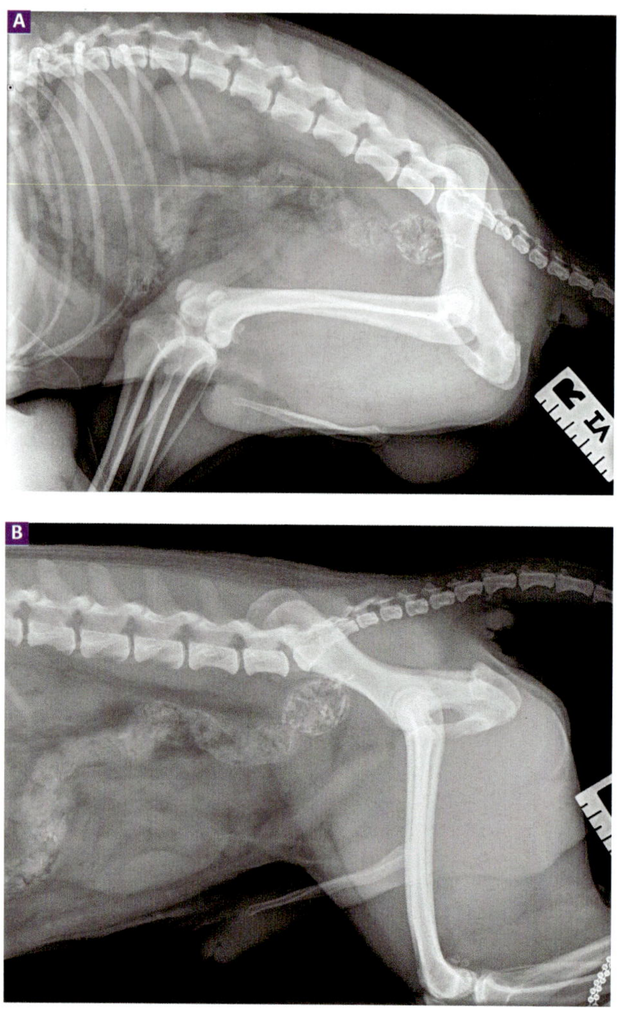

Figure 39. A. Lateral projection of caudal abdomen with flexed legs; **B.** Lateral projection of caudal abdomen with the legs in neutral positioning.

Left Lateral Decubitus Projection (Horizontal Beam)

Horizontal beam radiographs allow for orthogonal views without patient movement and are especially useful for patients with severe dyspnoea or spinal injuries. However, they are dependent on the room infrastructure and X-ray machine, as some equipment is static which means horizontal beam cannot be performed.

Positioning

- horizontal beam: safety issues, care should be taken with the other side of the wall;
- wedges/sandbags should be used to support the cassette;
- the FFD should be maintained;
- a grid should be used if needed;
- the X-ray should be lined up by eye;
- this technique is useful when looking for free gas within the abdomen.

> - **Horizontal beam X-rays can be taken with the patient in lateral, dorsal, or ventral recumbency. This technique detects small volumes of free gas in the peritoneal cavity and pleural effusion in the thorax.**
> - **Horizontal views can also be considered to obtain a standard lateral thorax or abdominal projection in unstable patients.**

Dorsoventral Abdomen

This projection is not indicated for evaluation of the abdomen (Figure 41) as there will be crowding of the organs and prominent skin folds preventing accurate interpretation. If a VD projection cannot be obtained, then two lateral projections of the abdomen should be taken rather than a DV projection.

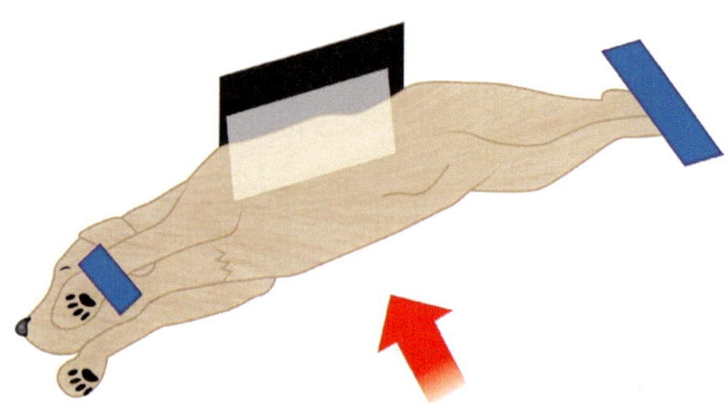

Figure 40. Diagram demonstrating positioning for a lateral decubitus radiograph of the thorax/abdomen.

Abdominal Radiographs in Surgical Cases

Abdominal radiographs are essential to detect abnormal patterns where the treatment is surgical, such as bladder stones, foreign body, abdominal masses etc. (Figures 41–43).

The order in which abdominal radiographs are taken is crucial in the search for gastrointestinal tract obstruction. The left lateral projection should be taken to start with, which makes gas in the gastrointestinal tract rise and move into the pylorus and duodenum. Then VD and right lateral projections should be acquired as the gas in the duodenum remains and highlights any intra luminal foreign bodies.

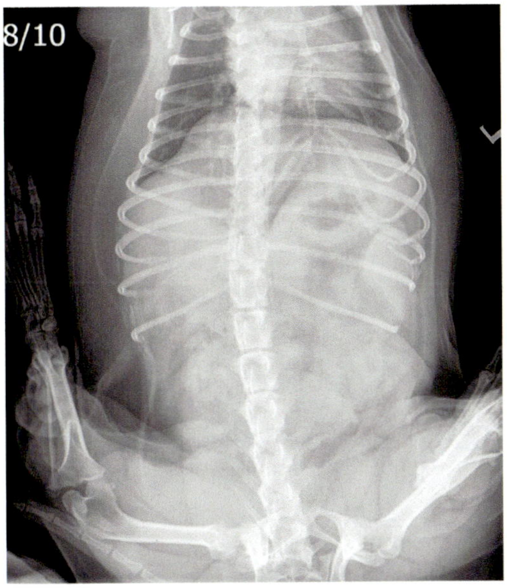

Figure 41. DV projection of the abdomen of a dog.

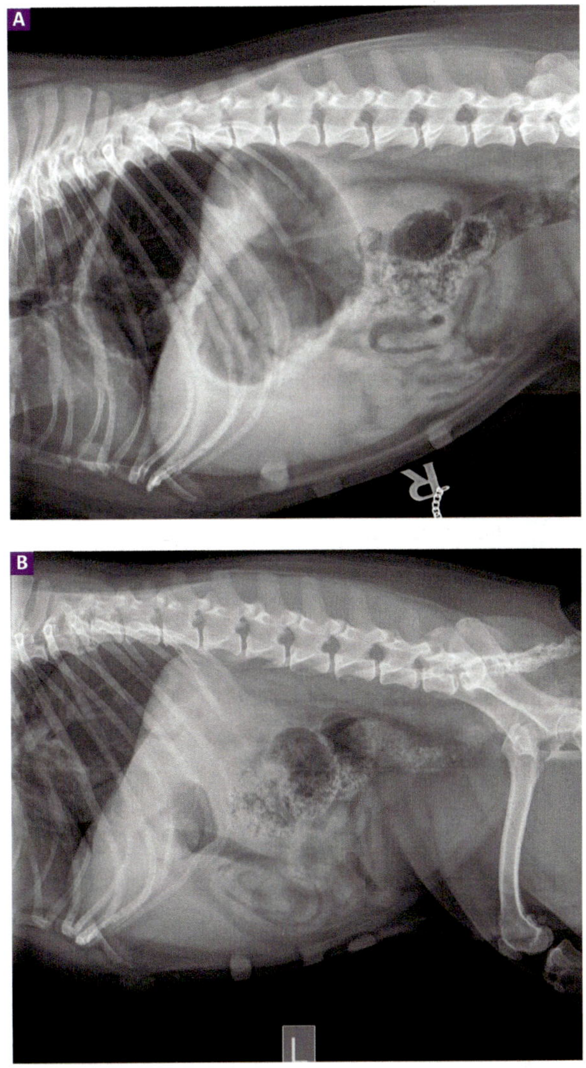

Figure 42. Dog with a type IV hiatal hernia. Right (**A**) and left (**B**) lateral projections of the abdomen.

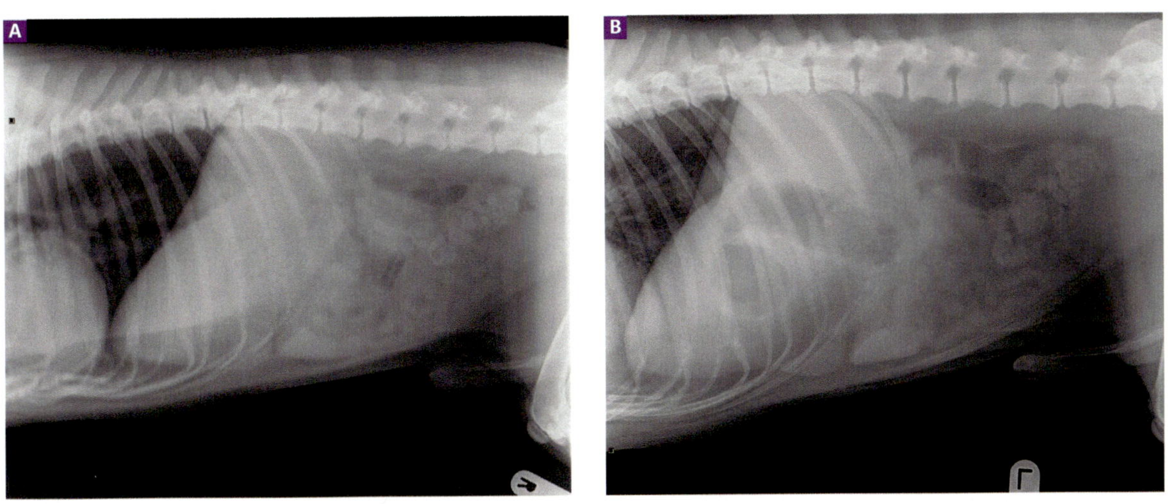

Figure 43. Dog with a duodenal foreign body. Highlighting the importance of using both right lateral (**A**) versus left lateral (**B**) projections.

Appendicular System Radiographs

Commonly imaged regions include:

- pelvis: lateral and VD (extended/frog legged) projections
- stifles: mediolateral (ML), caudocranial (CdCr)
- carpi/tarsi: ML, dorsopalmar/plantar (DP)/palmarodorsal/plantarodorsal (PD), stressed, or oblique
- shoulder: lateral, CdCr
- elbow: ML (neutral or flexed), craniocaudal (CrCd).

Appendicular radiographs are routinely used in first opinion and referral practice due to the common occurrence of hip, joint disease, and trauma cases. Presurgical radiographs are taken for surgical planning and the same radiographs are repeated 6–8 weeks postsurgery, depending on the age of the patient. In most cases, these are routine radiographic projections.

Pelvis: Ventrodorsal (VD) Frog Leg

Positioning

- dorsal recumbency (Figures 44 and 45);
- the forelimbs should be extended cranially;
- the hindlimbs should be in a natural flexed position; in most normal patients, the femurs naturally assume an angle of approximately 45° to the spine. In some large dogs, the femurs may naturally assume an angle of 90° angle to the spine;
- a V trough should be used with foam pads on the lateral aspect of body wall to superimpose the sternum and spine.

Centring

- midline between the left and right ischial tuberosity.

Collimation

- cranial caudal border: cranial to the wing of ilium to caudal border of ischium.
- lateral border: to include proximal third of femur.

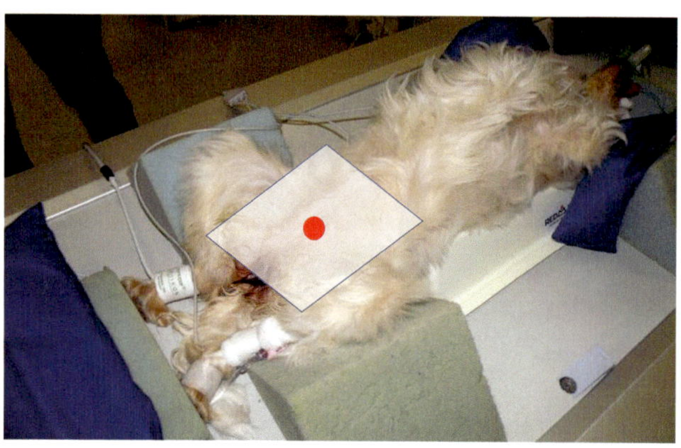

Figure 44. Positioning of a patient for a VD frog leg projection of the pelvis. Courtesy of Gawain Hammond

Labelling

- right and left markers should be within the collimated area away from bony areas; and
- identification labels should be positioned in the caudal region.

Technique

- measurements should be taken at the widest part of the pelvis.

Other Considerations

- sandbags should be placed outside the collimated area on the tarsus or can be used to maintain symmetry.

Hip: VD Extended

Positioning

- dorsal recumbency (Figures 46 and 47);
- the forelimbs should be extended cranially and evenly with the nose between them;
- the hindlimbs should be extended caudally and evenly into full extension;
- V trough should be used with foam pads on the lateral aspects of the body wall to superimpose the sternum and spine;
- femurs should be rotated medially so they are parallel to one another and the X-ray table, and the patella is centred within the patellar groove over the stifle and taped in place;
- the tail should be aligned with the spine.

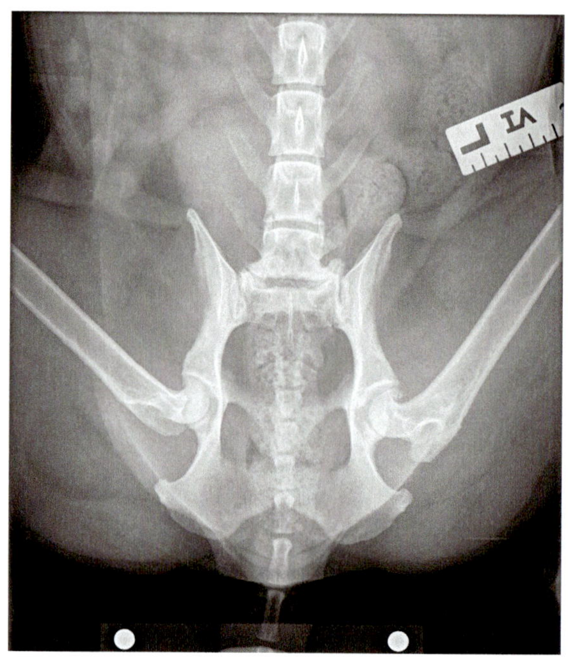

Figure 45. VD radiographic projection of the pelvis in a dog in the frog leg position.

Centring

– midline between the left and right ischial tuberosity.

Collimation

– cranial caudal border: cranial to the wing of ilium and distal to the stifle joint
– lateral borders: lateral to the ischium.

Labelling

– right and left markers should be within the collimated area away from bony areas.

Technique

– measurements should be taken at the widest part of the pelvis.

Other Considerations

– hindlimbs should be extended evenly so that digits on both feet are even with each other;
– a long piece of tape should be used to keep the femurs rotated by applying tape sticky side up under the stifles, excluding the tail. A triangular wedge should be positioned to support the tarsus and pes and a sandbag used to keep them in position.

Key Points

– femurs should be parallel (Figure 48);
– dorsal spinous processes should be seen in the middle of the vertebrae;
– patellae should be centred over the middle of the femurs;
– obturator foraminae symmetrical;
– if asymmetric "large hole is higher", the larger foramen is further from the plate and that side needs to be rotated down;
– distortion with increased object film distance (OFD).

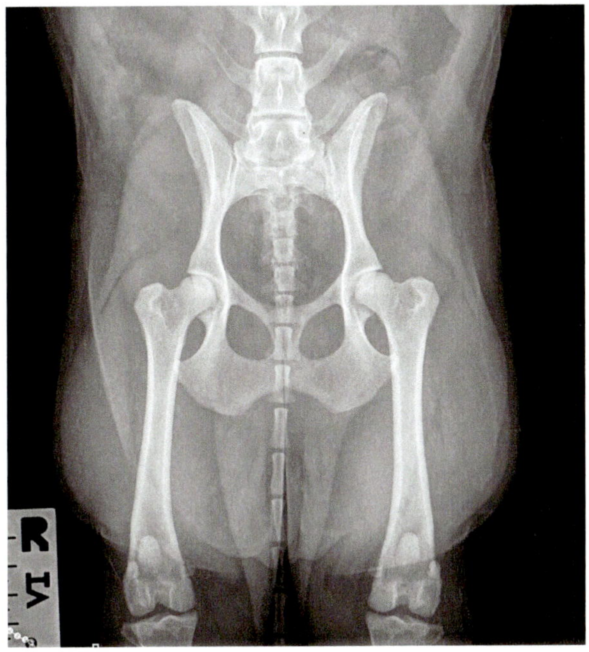

Figure 47. VD projection of the pelvis of a dog.

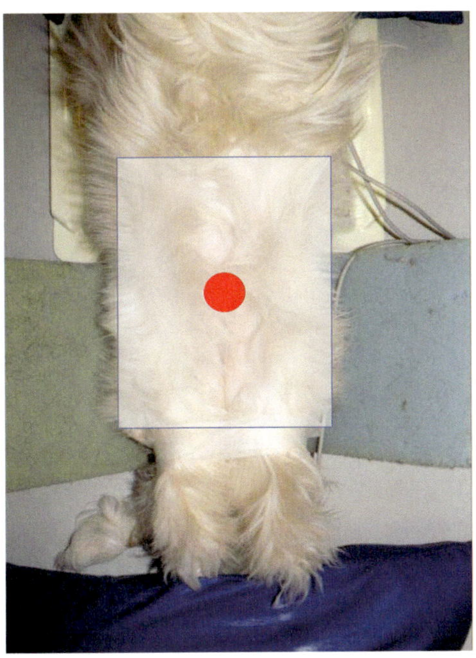

Figure 46. VD extended positioning. Courtesy of Gawain Hammond.

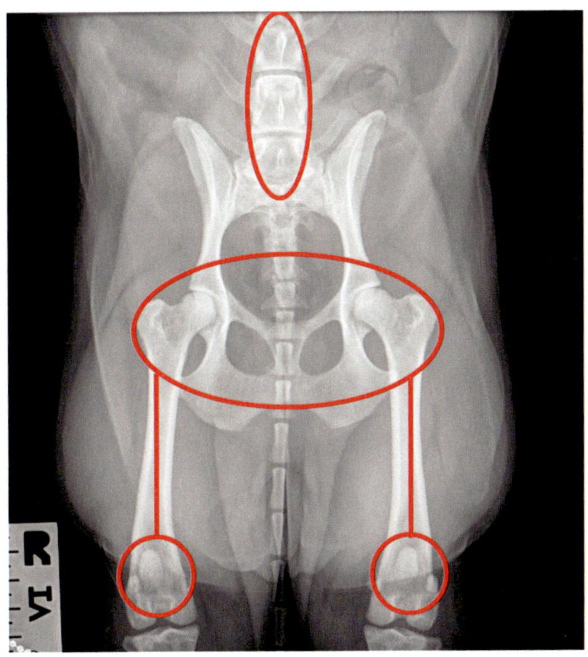

Figure 48. VD projection of the pelvis. Red landmarks demonstrate accurate positioning and symmetry of the lumbar spine, obturator foramen, femurs, and patella.

Pelvis: Lateral Projection (Figures 49 and 50)

Positioning

- right or left lateral recumbency (side of interest should be closest to the cassette);
- a foam wedge should be placed between the hindlimbs to superimpose both sides of the pelvis;
- alternatively, the bottom leg can be extended cranially and the top leg extended caudally (scissor position).

Centring

- greater trochanter of the femur.

Collimation

- cranial edge of ilium to caudal border of ischium
- dorsal border: dorsal to the wing of the ilium.

Labelling

- right or left marker should be used to indicate which limb is closest to the cassette;

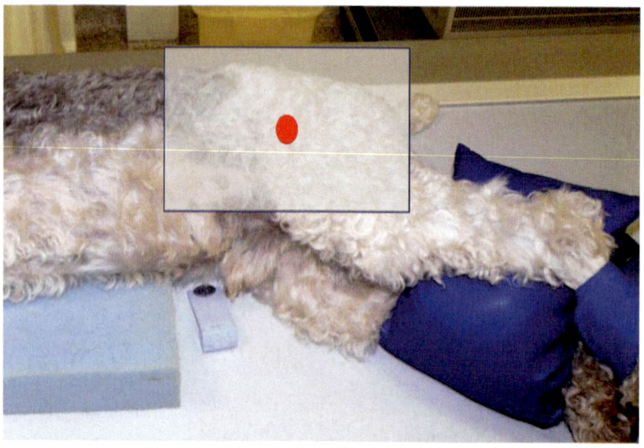

Figure 49. Positioning for lateral radiograph of the pelvis. Courtesy of Gawain Hammond.

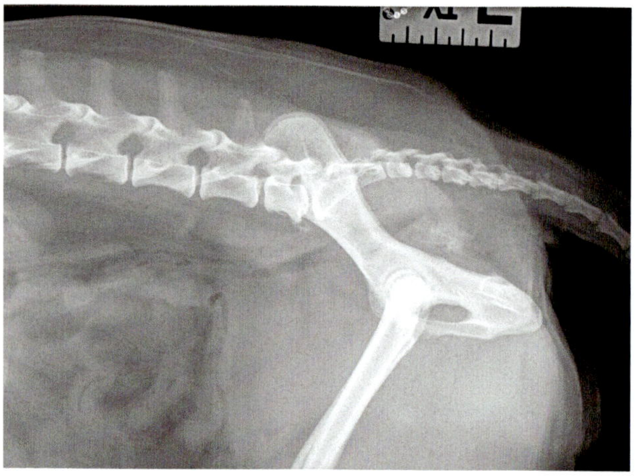

Figure 50. Left lateral projections of the pelvis.

- identification labels should be placed in the right cranial region or left caudal region within the collimated area to avoid overlapping with bone.

Technique

- measurements should be taken at the highest area at the level of the trochanter.

Other Considerations

- the limb furthest from the cassette is magnified.

Key Points

- sides of pelvis and hips are superimposed;
- the higher side is magnified;
- the transverse processes of the spine are at same level.

Elbow: Mediolateral Projection

Positioning

- the patient should be in lateral recumbency with the affected limb underneath (Figures 51 and 52);
- the affected limb should be extended cranially;
- the unaffected limb should be pulled caudodorsally.

Centring

- the humeral condyles should be palpated and used to centre the radiograph.

Collimation

- distal third of the humerus to the proximal third of the radius and ulna.

Labelling

- labels should be positioned cranial to the joint.

Technique

- measurements should be taken at the thickest part of the joint.

Other Considerations

- placement of a sponge under the shoulder may be necessary dorsally to assist with ensuring the patient is lateral;
- an alternate image includes the CrCd supinated position, which is used when evaluating for the presence of elbow dysplasia, which requires a 10–15° oblique view;
- the mediolateral hyperflexed projection uses a similar technique to the neutral positioning. By hyperflexing the elbow, the joint angle is reduced. This projection is used to assess the anconeal process.

Key Points

- there should be a clear view of the joint space.

Elbow: Craniocaudal Projection

(Figures 53 and 54)

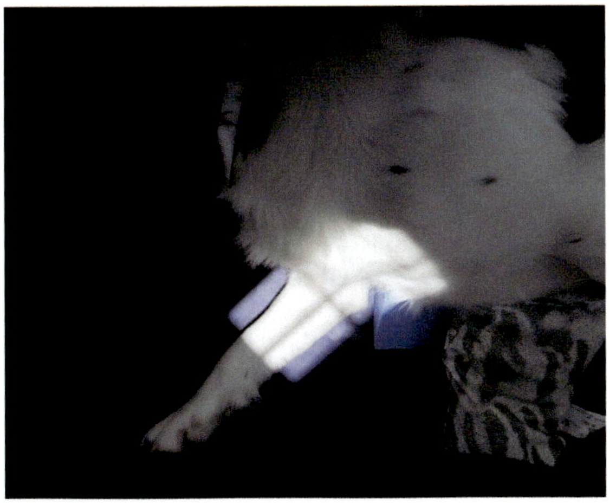

Figure 51. Radiographic positioning for a ML projection of the elbow in a neutral position.

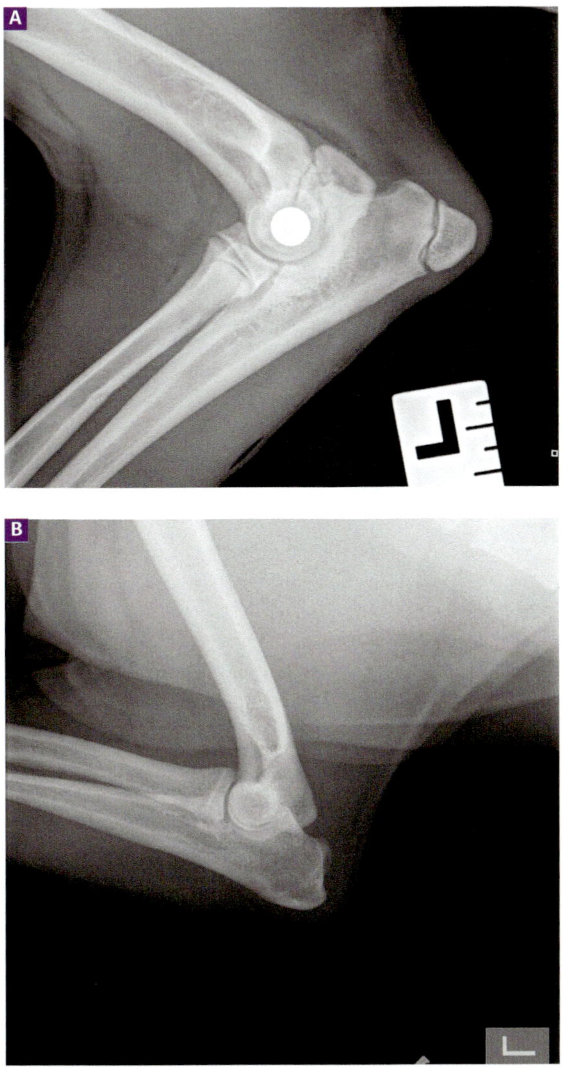

Figure 52. ML elbow projections. Neutral (**A**) vs flexed (**B**).

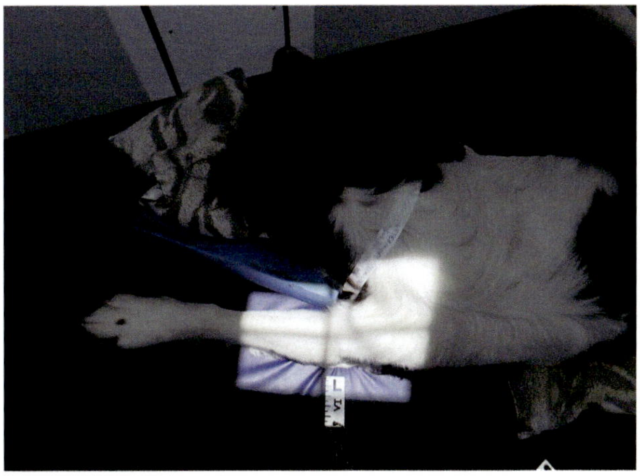

Figure 53. Radiographic positioning for a CrCd projection of the elbow.

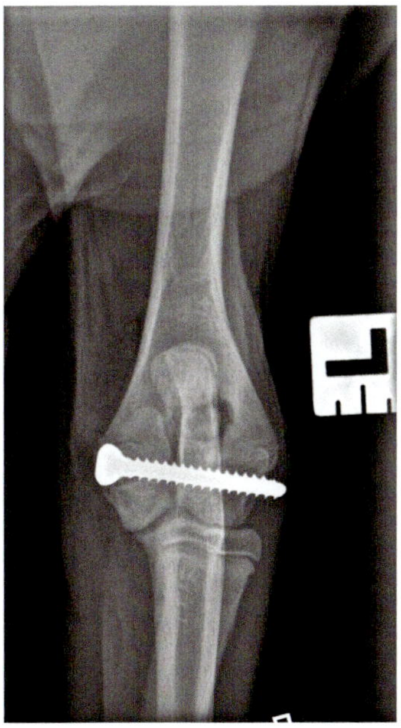

Figure 54. CrCd projection of the elbow.

Positioning

- the patient should be in sternal recumbency;
- both front legs should be extended forward individually;
- the head should be extended laterally to the opposite side of the affected limb and stabilized with tape or a sandbag;
- a V trough can help stabilize the caudal half of the body;
- the back legs should be extended caudally to assist in keeping the spine straight.

Centring

- the humeral condyles should be palpated and used to centre the radiograph.

Collimation

– from the distal third of the humerus to the proximal third of the radius and ulna.

Labelling

– labels should be placed laterally.

Technique

– measurements should be taken at the thickest part at the centre of the joint.

Key Points

– there should be a clear view of the joint space (Figures 53 and 54);
– the radius/ulna and humerus should be aligned;
– there is superimposition of the olecranon and humerus.

Stifle: Mediolateral Projection

Positioning

– the patient should be in lateral recumbency with the affected limb underneath;
– the unaffected limb should be taped around the stifle and tarsus and pulled up and out of the way.

Centring

– the radiograph should be centred on the stifle joint.

Collimation

– proximal to the distal third of the femur and distal to the proximal third of the tibia.

Labelling

– label should be placed cranial to the joint.

Technique

– measurements should be taken at the centre of the joint. The indentation of the joint (fat pad) should be palpated on the dorsal aspect of the stifle. The radiograph should be centred on the indentation (Figures 55 and 56).

Other Considerations

– it is important to include the soft tissues on the caudal aspect of the stifle joint to visualize the fascial stripe which runs proximally and distally. When this stripe is absent, it is a sign of joint effusion.

Key Features

– there should be a clear view of the joint space; and
– there is superimposition of the femoral condyles.

Stifle: Caudocranial Projection

Positioning

– the patient should be positioned in a V trough in ventral recumbency;
– both hindlimbs should be pulled behind the patient and a band of tape placed around the femurs just proximal to the stifles and the femurs pulled together to bring the patellas straight over the distal femurs;
– alternatively, the unaffected limb can be flexed up next to the body if the patient is more comfortable.

Centring

– the radiograph should be centred on the stifle joint.

Collimation

– proximal to the distal third of the femur and distal to proximal third of the tibia.

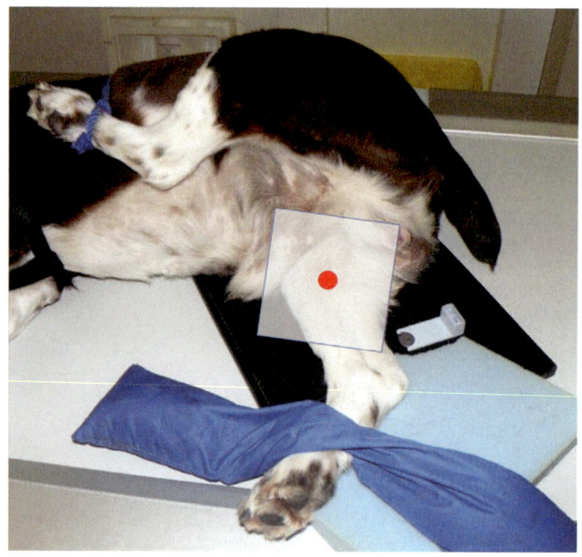

Figure 55. Radiographic positioning for a ML projection of the stifle. Courtesy of Gawain Hammond.

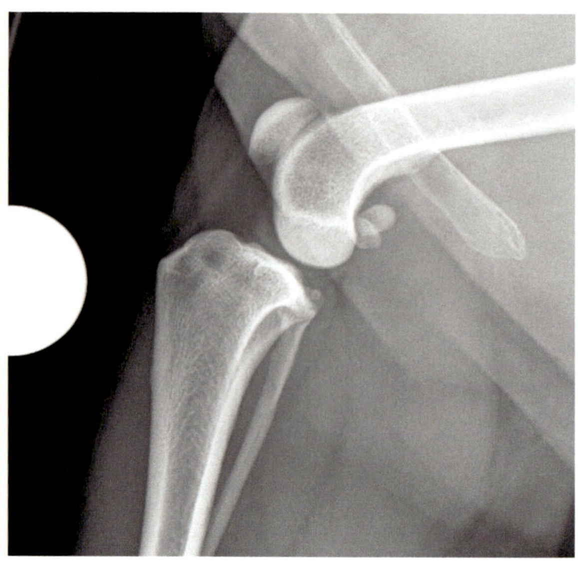

Figure 56. ML projection of the stifle.

Labelling
- labels should be placed lateral to the joint.

Technique
- measurements should be taken at the centre of the joint.

Key Points
- the patella should be in the midline of the femur (Figures 57 and 58);
- the fabellae should be in a symmetrical position;
- there should be a clear view of the joint space.

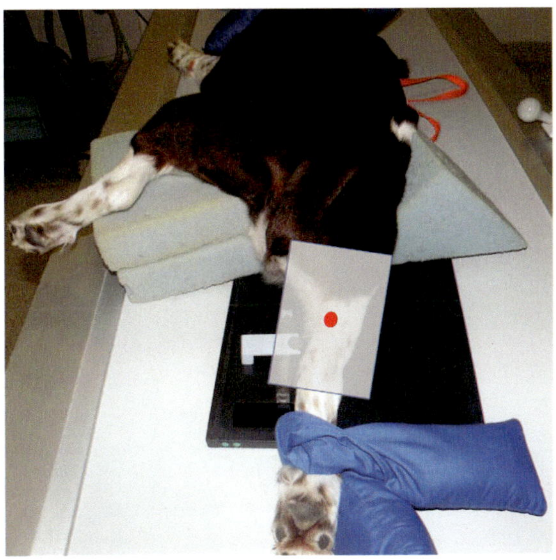

Figure 57. Radiographic positioning for CdCr projection of the stifle. Courtesy of Gawain Hammond.

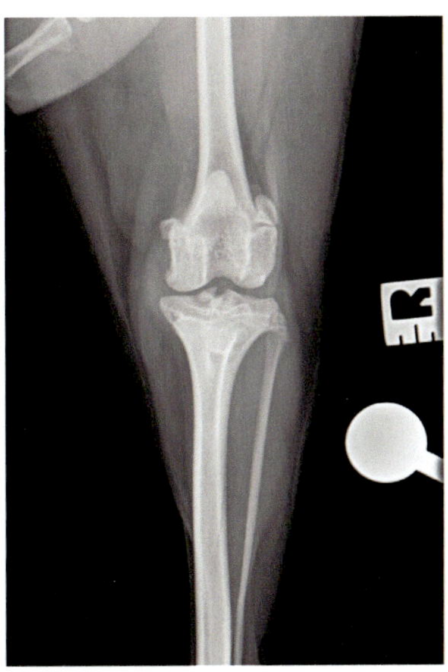

Figure 58. CdCr projection of the stifle.

Shoulder: Lateral Projection
Positioning
- the patient should be in lateral recumbency with the affected limb closest to the cassette/plate;
- the affected limb should be pulled cranially and ventrally, while pulling the other forelimb caudally;
- the head and neck of the patient should be extended slightly to avoid superimposing the trachea on the joint.

Centring
- the radiograph should be centred on the shoulder joint.

Collimation
- proximal mid distal scapula and distal to proximal half of the humerus.

Labelling
- labels should be placed cranial to the joint.

Technique
- measurements should be taken at the centre of the joint.

Shoulder: Caudocranial Projection
Positioning
- the patient should be placed in dorsal recumbency;
- the forelimbs should be extended cranially. To avoid an oblique projection of the shoulder, rotation of the humeri should be avoided.

Centring
- the radiograph should be centred on the shoulder joint (Figure 59).

Collimation
- proximal mid scapula and distal to proximal half of the humerus.

Labelling
- labels should be placed cranial to the joint.

Technique
- measurements should be taken at the centre of the joint.

Stifles: Tibial Plateau Levelling Osteotomy (TPLO)/ Tibial Tuberosity Advancement (TTA) Radiographs
Radiographic techniques are used for surgical planning in patients with cruciate disease. Collimation for these projections is slightly different (Figures 60 and 61) to the standard mediolateral projection.

The same point is used to centre the radiograph, but the collimation is from the proximal third of the femur up to the tarsus, including the joint. This allows the surgeon to measure for implant placement.

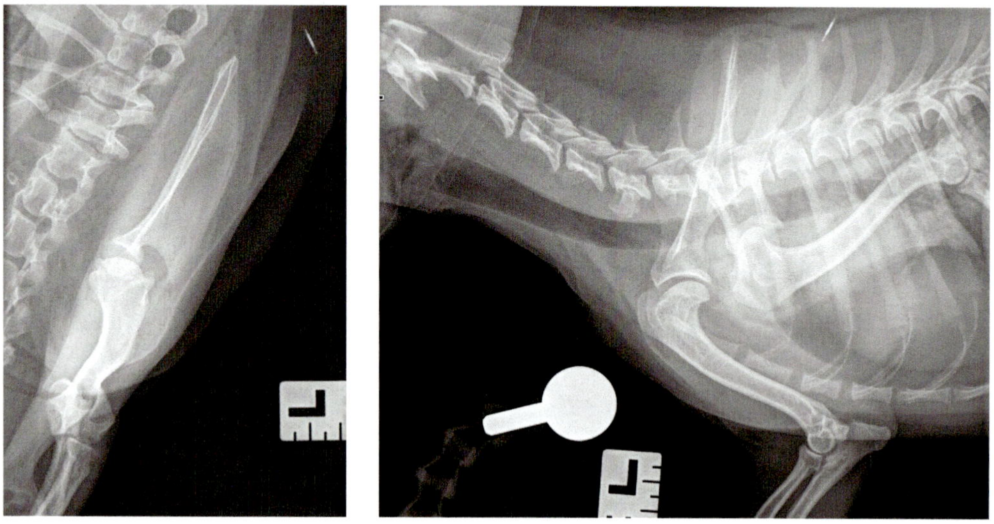

Figure 59. CdCr (**A**) and lateral (**B**) projections of the shoulder.

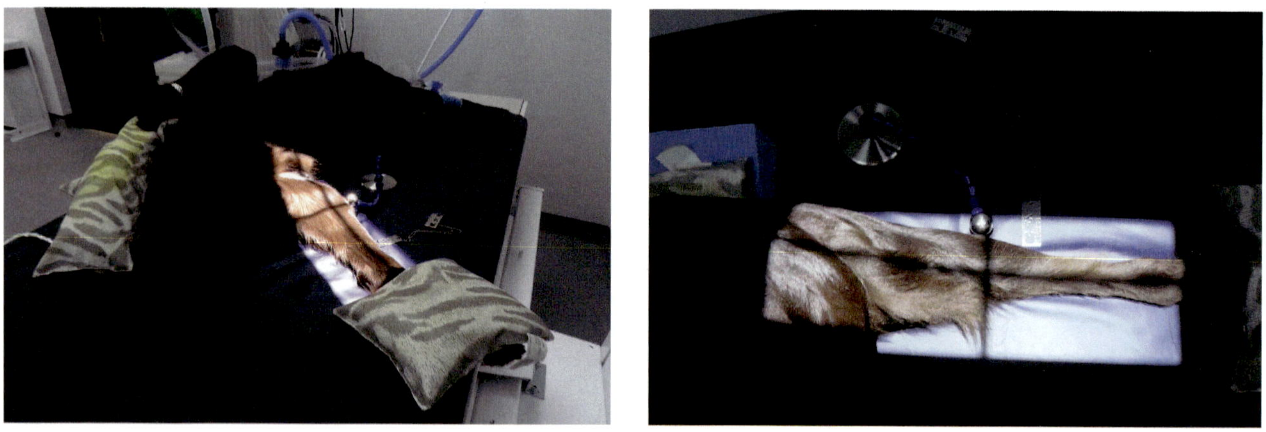

Figure 60. Radiographic positioning for ML (**A**) and CdCr (**B**) projections.

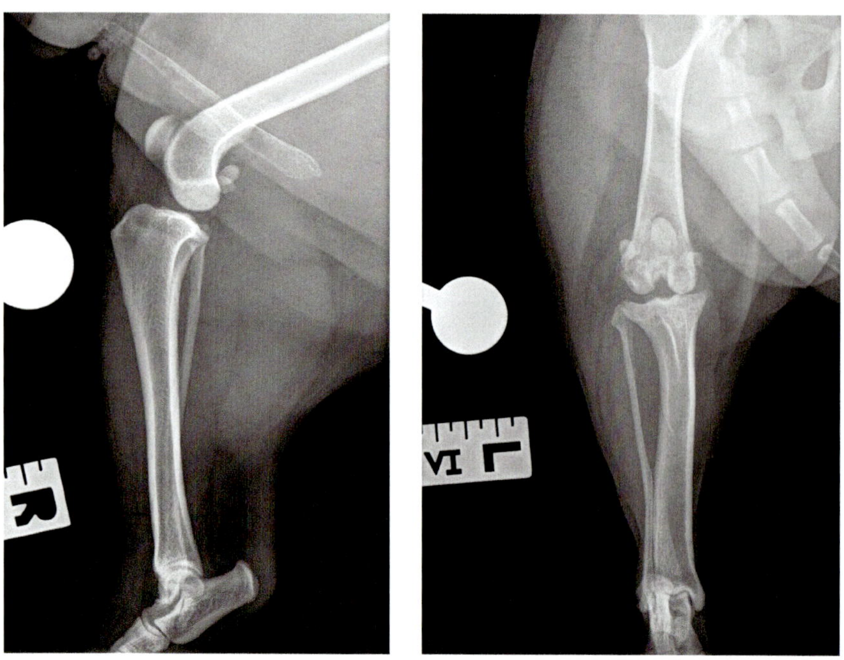

Figure 61. ML and CdCr projections of the stifle for TPLO surgical planning.

Hip and Elbow Scoring

The projections necessary for hip scoring vary with the company responsible for assessing the radiographs. However, the standard projection is the VD extended hip projection. The patient should be placed in dorsal recumbency with the hindlimbs extended and parallel to each other. Stifles should be rotated medially and it should be ensured that the pelvis is symmetrical. Collimation is from the cranial aspect of the wings of ilium up to the stifle joint. The patellae must be in the trochlear ridges, well aligned and symmetrical.

For the elbow, the patient should be placed in lateral recumbency with the elbow under evaluation closest to the cassette. Radiographs should be acquired with the elbow in an extended position at about 110° and with the elbow in a flexed position at about 45°.

> **Hip/Elbow Scheme requirements for BVA/KC:**
>
> - **The dog must be at least one year old, but there is no upper age limit.**
> - **The dog must be permanently and uniquely identified by way of a microchip or tattoo.**
> - **The dog's KC registration certificate and any related transfer certificates must be available so that the appropriate details can be printed on the radiographs.**
> - **Microchip/tattoo numbers must also be printed on the radiographs.**
> - **The owner should sign the declaration (first part) of the certificate, to verify the details are correct and grant permission for publication of the results.**
> - **Radiographs of non-registered dogs may also be submitted to the ED scheme. (just for the elbow scheme).**

The above technique is often used for the Orthopaedic Foundation for Animals (OFA) and British Veterinary Association (BVA). PennHip request additional radiographs such as compression and distraction frog leg VD projections to evaluate joint laxity.

Total Hip Replacement Projections

When preparing a patient for a total hip replacement, an additional view is required beside the standard extended hip and frog leg projections. Additional radiographs include a lateral projection and craniocaudal projections of the femur (Figure 62).

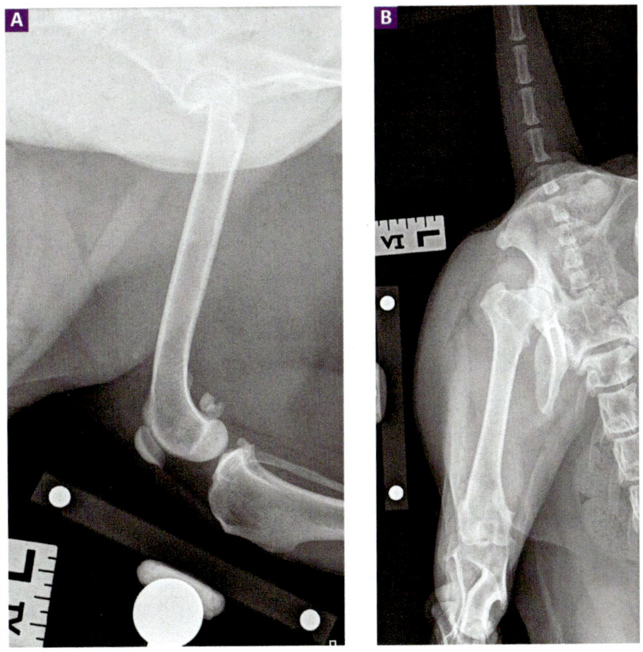

Figure 62. Lateral (**A**) and craniocaudal (**B**) projections of the femur.

Stressed Radiographs

These are usually applied at a joint, most commonly the carpi or tarsi. A rope should be applied proximal and distal to the joint, held at the other end by a sandbag on opposite sides to apply opposing forces proximal and distal to the joint. This technique is used to confirm joint instability. Care should be taken when performing these techniques not to make the instability worse.

Axial System Radiographs

Head Radiographs

The head has a complex anatomy which causes a lot of superimpositions of structures, leading to difficult interpretation. Skull radiographs are rarely performed nowadays because they have been superseded by computed tomography (CT) imaging. Yet, it is possible to obtain good head radiographs.

Radiographic projections of the head:

- lateral projections with the mouth open or closed
- lateral oblique projections with the mouth open or closed
- dorsoventral/ventrodorsal projections
- oblique 20° ventrodorsal projection of the maxilla
- intraoral dorsoventral and ventrodorsal projections
- skyline rostrocaudal projection of the frontal sinus with the mouth closed.

Intraoral radiography is necessary to evaluate the teeth. To assess the temporomandibular joints and tympanic bullae a lateral 20° rostral to caudal projection with the mouth open is needed for each side. Brachycephalic dogs require a greater elevation of the nose at 30°. To complete investigation of tympanic bullae an additional projection should be considered. This is a rostral caudal open mouth projection with a 90° flexion of the head. In cats a 10° rostrocaudal projection is used instead.

Next to the usual dorsoventral or ventrodorsal intraoral projection an additional open mouth 20° ventrodorsal projection can be performed to further assess the nasal cavity.

To assess the frontal sinuses the patient can be placed in dorsal recumbency with a 90° flexion of the head and a caudal angle to the nose of 10°. This is the correct positioning for a rostrocaudal projection.

Spine Radiographs

Obtaining straight projections is a challenge when it comes to the spinal column, and yet they are crucial for accurate interpretation. **Orthogonal projections** should be performed e.g. lateral and ventrodorsal projections. Oblique projections can be acquired for better evaluation of the intervertebral foramen but are rarely performed. The open mouth rostrocaudal projection described to evaluate the dens of C2 should not be performed due to the risk of damaging the spinal cord. Dynamic studies (extension, flexion, and traction) of the neck are usually performed with myelography.

It is important not to radiograph the entire spine at once to avoid beam divergence which can alter the intervertebral spaces. Correct collimation should be applied to each area; cervical, thoracic, and lumbar spine.

Centring

- cervical: C2–C3, C5–C6
- thoracic: T1–T8, T13–L1
- lumbar: L3–L4, L7–S1.

Spinal radiographs are indicated when there is a suspicion of disc protrusion/extrusion (mineralised) with or without myelogram, spinal trauma, or spinal instability. These patients are normally presented as urgent cases and correct investigation is necessary to implement appropriate treatment and avoid permanent damage to the spinal cord. If CT is available, most of the time radiographs are skipped and CT is performed because of its speed, specificity, and sensitivity in the detection of these types of lesions.

Key points when taking radiographs:

- careful positioning is important to minimise rotation;
- centring and collimation should be accurate;
- use of the other leg should be considered for comparison:
    - left and right markers should be in the collimated area of the primary beam
- a grid should be used if tissue thickness is >10 cm;
- radiograph quality should be assessed:
    - exposure, collimation, labelling, position, etc.

Radiographic Contrast Studies

Contrast Media

Contrast media are widely used in veterinary medicine for **radiographs, computed tomography, magnetic resonance imaging (MRI), and fluoroscopy.** When used in specific procedures the contrast media allows evaluation of normal structures and abnormal structures by altering the contrast of tissues or inside organs.

Types of Contrast Media

Negative Contrast

These agents are radiolucent (less radiopaque than soft tissue) and appear black or darker than soft tissue on the radiograph.

Negative contrast agents are gaseous, with a low physical density and appear radiolucent. A variety of gases are used such as, air, carbon dioxide, nitrous oxide. Carbon dioxide and nitrous oxide are safer for the patient than air due to their greater solubility in plasma, but air is most commonly used.

Negative contrast agents can only be used in the gastrointestinal tract (pneumogastrography, pneumocolonography) and bladder (pneumocystography). Formerly they were also used in the peritoneal cavity (pneumoperitoneography) and the pericardial sac (pneumopericardiography). The latter techniques have been replaced by ultrasonography.

Positive Contrast

Positive contrast agents are more radiopaque than the surrounding tissue and appear whiter than bone (radiopaque). **Positive contrast agents have a higher atomic number and attenuate the X-ray** photons, which results in increased opacity on a radiograph.

Positive contrast media (Figure 63) are divided into two groups:

- **barium** sulphate based
- **iodine** based.

Barium

- atomic number 56
- inert
- relatively palatable
- prepared in suspension
- no osmotic potential
- is not absorbed
- provides a good coating of the mucosa.

Barium sulphate should only be given per os or per rectum and should only be used for gastrointestinal studies. Barium may be mixed with food of various consistencies (liquid, soft and solid food) for pharyngeal, oesophageal, and gastrointestinal studies.

Contraindications

Barium use is contraindicated for the urinary, neurological, and vascular systems, and in the GI tract if perforation is suspected.

Barium Preparations

Barium sulphate (Figure 63) comes in a variety of concentrations **classified by weight to volume (w/v)** (where a weight of barium is added to water to make a specific volume) or weight to weight (w/w) (where a certain weight of barium is added to water to make a specific weight of suspension).

- **Colloidal suspensions:** can be given on their own for gastrointestinal studies or mixed with food which can be eaten or administered by stomach tube or syringe. Colloidal suspensions should be shaken before use (e.g. Baritop®). They facilitate assessment of GI wall thickness and changes to mucosal surfaces and they can be combined with a negative contrast agent to perform double contrast studies in the stomach and colon.
- **Powder:** can be mixed with water or food to make a paste or suspension. The suspension may not be as uniform as a colloidal suspension.
- **Paste:** used for oesophageal studies to assess the mucosa (ulceration).
- **Barium impregnated polyethylene spheres (BIPS):** spheres impregnated with barium (1.5 mm and 5 mm). Either 10 large or 30 small spheres should be used. BIPS are used to assess gastrointestinal obstruction or motility and interpretation of studies where they are used may be difficult and unspecific.

Complications/Contraindications

- may persist indefinitely;
- leakage into the thoracic or abdominal cavities can result in a granulomatous reaction (granulomatous mediastinitis, granulomatous peritonitis) with adhesions and fibrosis;
- aspiration of barium: the severity depends on the volume aspirated. If significant volume is aspirated, it may lead to bacterial infection and aspiration pneumonia (Figure 64);
- when there is a suspicion of oesophageal or **gastrointestinal perforation barium should not be used** and a low osmolar iodinated contrast medium is preferred;
- barium should not be given <24 hours before endoscopy.

Iodinated Contrast Agents

- atomic number 53
- water soluble
- excreted by the kidneys.

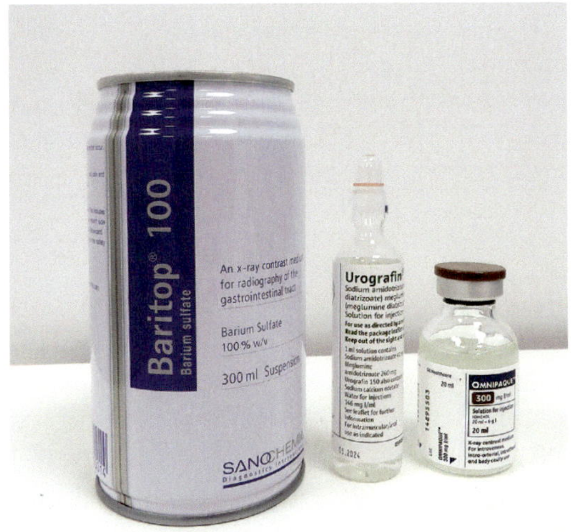

Figure 63. Contrast media. Barium, Urografin® and Omnipaque®.

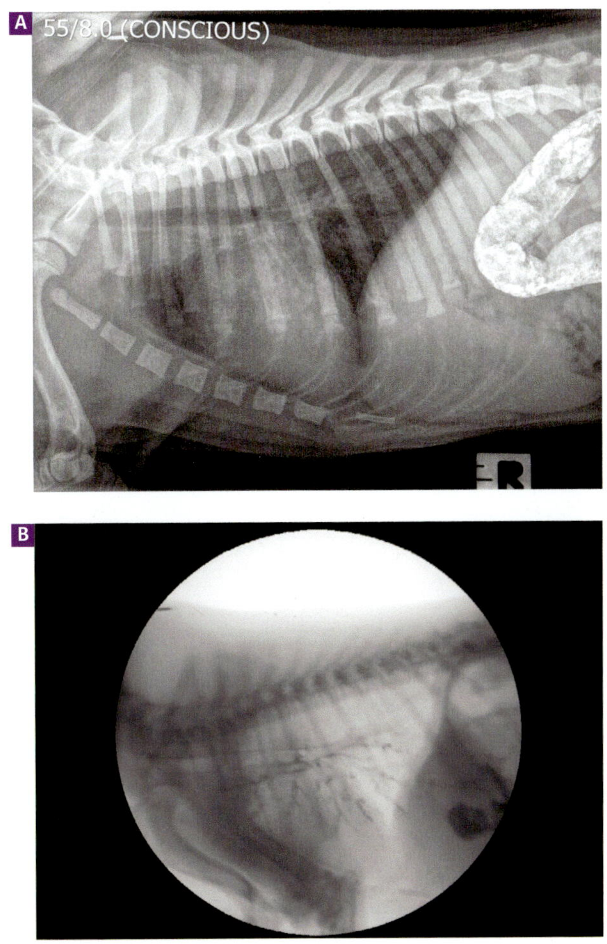

Figure 64. A. Right lateral projection of the thorax. There is an alveolar interstitial pattern in the cranioventral lung lobes consistent with aspiration pneumonia. **B.** Fluoroscopy image demonstrating barium aspirated during a swallowing study. Note the radiopaque barium in the trachea and bronchial tree.

Iodinated contrast agents can be used for:

- intravascular studies
- lower urinary tract
- joints (arthrography)
- salivary glands (sialography)
- lacrimal sac and duct
- sinuses and fistulas
- myelography
- lymphangiography
- gastrointestinal studies.

Iodinated contrast agents are derived from organic tri-iodinated benzoic acid. They are divided into **ionic and non-ionic contrast media** and are further classified by their osmolarity (Table 3).

Ionic Contrast Media

Ionic contrast agents are monomers and contain sodium and/or meglumine salts from iothalamic diatrizoic or metrizoic acids. Sodium salts are more toxic than meglumine salts (less viscous). These preparations are hyperosmolar (1000–2000 mOsm/kg) and can lead to hypertonicity, ionicity and allergic reactions (Conray®, Urografin®, Gastrografin®).

Table 3. Classification of iodinated contrast medium.

Contrast	Commercial name	Osmolality
	Ionic monomers	
Diatrizoate	Gastrographin® Urographin®	
Metrizoate	Isopaque®	High osmolar
Iothalamate	Conray®	
	Ionic dimers	
Ioxaglate	Hexrabrix®	Low osmolar
	Non-ionic monomers	
Iohexol	Omnipaque®	
Ioversol	Optiray®	
Iopamidol	Iopamiro®	
Iobitridol	Xenetix®	
Iopentol	Imagopaque®	Low osmolar
Iomeprol	Lemoron®	
Iopromide	Ultravist®	
Ioxilan	Oxilan®	
	Non-ionic dimers	
Iotrolan	Isovist®	Iso osmolar
Iodixanol	Vispaque®	

Contraindications

- hypotensive or dehydrated patients
- severe renal failure
- ionic contrast agents should never be used for myelography because they are nephrotoxic and induce seizures.

Non-ionic Contrast Media

Non-ionic contrast media do not dissociate in solution and are considered iso-osmolar to blood plasma, therefore, direct chemotoxicity is reduced. They are associated with fewer allergic reactions. In veterinary practice, the most widely used agents are iohexol, ioversol and iopamidol, (Omnipaque®, Optiray®, Iopamiro®). Non-ionic contrast agents are mainly used for myelography and arthrography. They are also used in cardiovascular and urinary tract studies where ionic media is contraindicated (Figure 65).

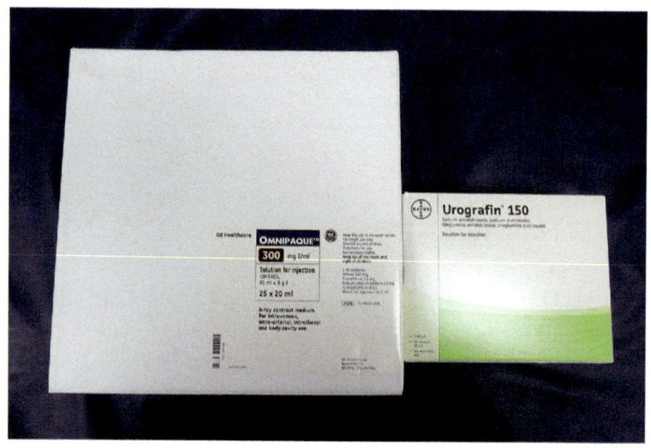

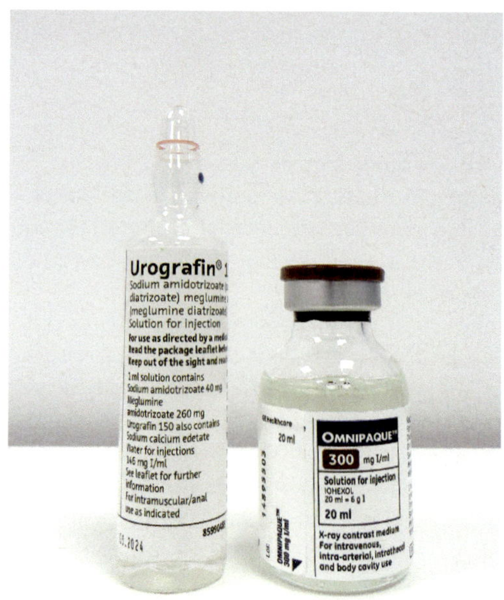

Figure 65. Images of an ionic iodinates and non-ionic contrast medium (Urographin® and Omnipaque®).

Side Effects of Iodinated Contrast Mediums

Idiosyncratic reactions are independent of the dose administered. These represent **anaphylactic or allergic type reactions** and may be acute (5–10 minutes from administration) or delayed. The most severe reactions are cardiovascular or respiratory in nature.

Non-idiosyncratic reactions are dose dependent and associated with hyperosmolarity and ionicity. Therefore, these reactions are more severe for ionic agents than non-ionic ones.

- Contrast induced nephrotoxicity is associated with renal vasoconstriction, renal hypoxia, and direct toxic effect on the renal tubular epithelial cells. Predisposing factors include dehydration, hypotension, and preexisting renal disease. Renal failure is not a contraindication for the use of the contrast media, however, it is a risk factor, and their use is contraindicated in cases of severe renal failure.
- Ionic contrast agents are hyperosmolar and should not be administered orally to dehydrated patients as they can lead to hypovolaemic shock.
- Cardiovascular effects include bradycardia, hypertension, and hypotension.

Gastrointestinal Contrast Studies

Nowadays these studies are rarely performed in veterinary practice because endoscopy and ultrasound have superseded the use of radiographic contrast studies for evaluation of the gastrointestinal tract. Also, radiographic barium follows through studies are expensive, time consuming and provide a limited diagnostic yield compared to the other techniques.

Contrast Agent

- barium sulphate is preferred:
  - barium should never be administered orally to an anaesthetised animal
- iodinated contrast media: should only be used if perforation is suspected:
  - water soluble ionic iodinated contrast material (sodium meglumine diatrizoate oral solution) at a dose of 3 ml/kg can be used
  - non-ionic iodinated contrast medium, such as iohexol or iopamidol can be used. They should be diluted (1:1) with water prior to administration and then used at a dose of 13 ml/kg. Dilution leads to a reduction in opacity as they transit the intestine.

Patient Preparation

- food should be withheld for 12–24 hours;
- an enema can be used to remove contents from the stomach, small intestine, and large intestine;
- the animal should be offered the opportunity to void and empty the bladder;
- sedation can be necessary but may delay gastric emptying and increase the risk of regurgitation and aspiration pneumonia. If sedation is used, acepromazine and/or butorphanol or buprenorphine is recommended as it causes minimal effects to intestinal motility in dogs. In cats, a combination of diazepam and ketamine cause minimal effects on intestinal motility.

Material

- preparation of the X-ray room for the procedure (Figure 66).

Oesophageal Studies

Material

- food bowl
- 60 ml catheter tip syringes
- palatable food (liquid, soft and hard). Liquid food is indicated when using a gastric tube.

Positive Contrast Oesophagram

Nowadays, the use of fluoroscopy/dynamic studies are preferred instead of radiography.

Indications

- regurgitation
- haematemesis
- suspected oesophagitis
- suspected oesophageal ulcers
- dysphasia
- suspected motility disorders.

Contrast Agent

- 45–85% barium sulphate suspension (60% weight/volume barium sulphate suspension is generally used)
- barium paste/oesophageal cream.

Dosage

- dogs: 15–30 ml, depending on the size of the dog
- cats: 5–7 ml.

Technique

Step 1. Orthogonal survey radiographs should be acquired: lateral projections.

Step 2. Radiographs should be evaluated.

Step 3. The barium should be administered in a suspension, paste or with food. The appropriate barium preparation should be selected based on clinical suspicions. Large volumes of liquid barium are difficult to administer by syringe, so barium paste is usually placed under the tongue and hard palate to ensure it persists long enough to obtain radiographs. 30 ml of liquid barium can be mixed with soft or semi liquid food and the patient allowed to eat.

Step 4. Radiographic projections: lateral projections. Lateral views should be centred in the cervical (including the oropharynx) and thoracic oesophagus (including the thoracic inlet and stomach).

Stomach and Small Intestinal Studies

Material

- food bowl
- 60 ml catheter tip syringes
- orogastric tube
- palatable food (liquid, soft and hard). Liquid food is indicated when using a gastric tube.

Type of Study

- pneumogastrogram
- positive/double contrast gastrogram
- positive contrast upper gastrointestinal studies.

Indications

- haematemesis
- assessment of stomach location
- suspected gastric or intestinal foreign body.

Double Contrast Gastrogram-contrast Media

Contrast Agent

- **barium sulphate** 30–60% weight/volume suspension should be used for a regular gastrogram; or
- high-density barium of 100% weight/volume is preferred for double contrast studies but is not mandatory;
- **negative contrast** gastrogram–air, carbonated soda (7-Up®), effervescent granules or tablet.

Dosage

- small/medium dogs: 6–12 ml/kg
- large dogs: 1.5 ml/kg
  - the high dose/kg is recommended for cats and small dogs while the low dose/kg is recommended for large dogs.

Technique

Step 1. Survey radiographs should be acquired, including VD and left/right lateral projections.

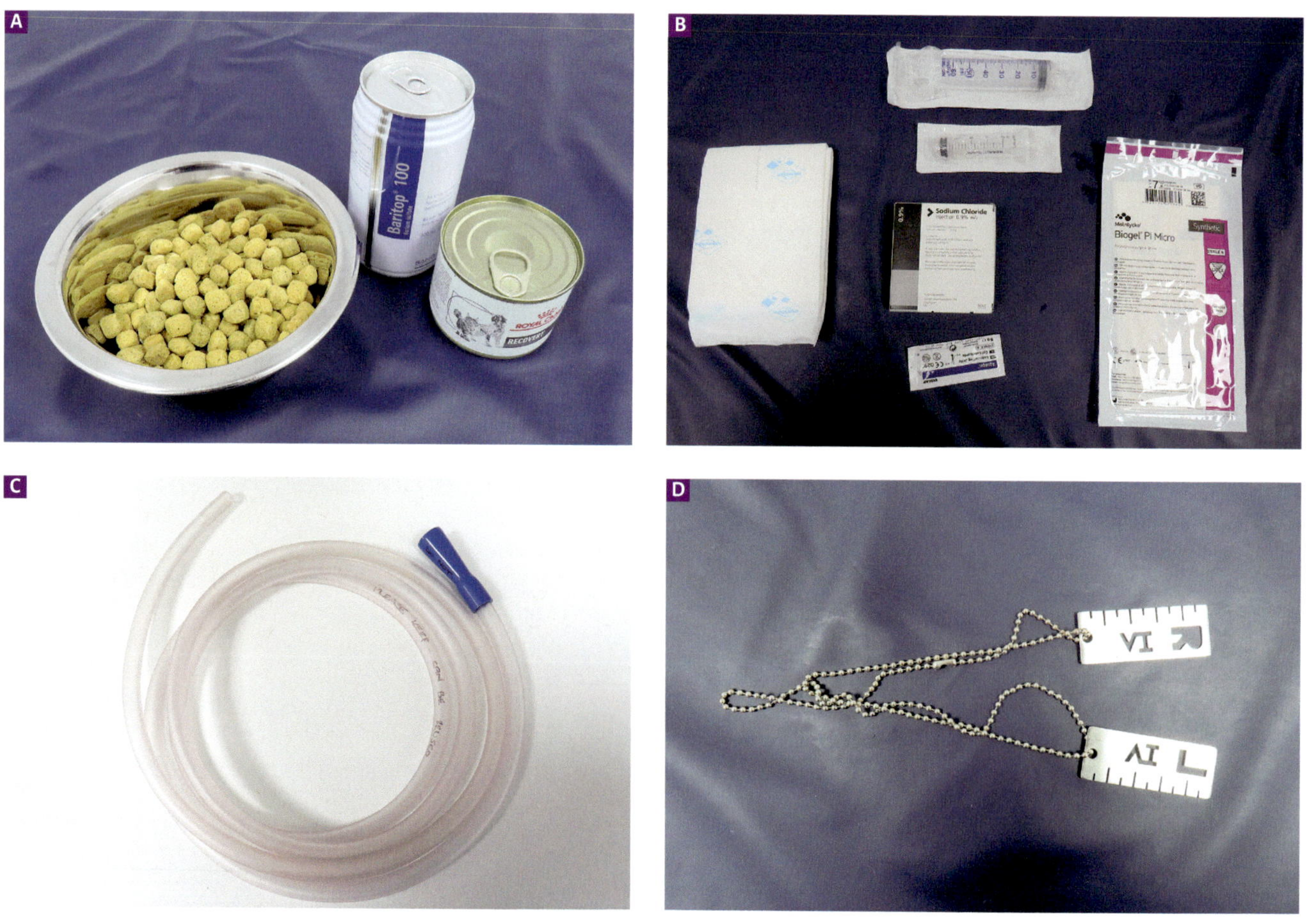

Figure 66. A. Food and barium; **B.** Gloves, syringes; **C.** Gastric tube; **D.** X-ray marker.

Step 2. Liquid barium should be administered via orogastric tube.

Step 3. 20 ml/kg of air should be administered to distend the stomach if doing a double contrast study.

Step 4. The tube should be removed, and the animal rotated multiple times to coat the stomach.

Step 5. VD, right lateral, and left lateral projections should be acquired. If barium coating is inadequate, an additional 1 ml/kg of barium should be added.

Step 6. Air should be removed via the orogastric tube when the study is complete.

Positive Contrast Upper Gastrointestinal Study

Contrast Agent

The most commonly used contrast medium for the stomach is barium.

Dosage

Barium sulphate:

- small and medium dogs: 8–12 ml/kg
- large dog: 5–7 ml/kg
- cats: 12–20 ml/kg
- simple location of the stomach: a low dosage of 1–2 ml/kg.

The stomach has a much greater capacity than 13 ml/kg and the only complication with higher doses is vomiting.

Ionic or non-ionic contrast media:

- Dogs:
  - Ionic: Gastrografin® or MD-Gastroview® 3–5 ml/kg.
  - Non-ionic: Omnipaque® 240 (iohexol) 700–875 mg I/kg, diluted in water for a whole volume of 10 ml/kg. 10 ml/kg 1:2 dilution.
- Cats:
  - Ionic: Gastrografin® or MD-Gastroview® 3–5 ml/kg.
  - Non-ionic: Omnipaque® 240 (iohexol) 600–800 mg I/kg, diluted in water for a whole volume of 10 ml/kg. 10 ml/kg 1:2 dilution.

Indications

- for assessment of luminal diameter and wall thickness
- evaluation of the mucosal surface
- for identification of radiolucent foreign bodies
- to determine the position of the stomach and small intestine
- to evaluate gastric and intestinal transit times.

Technique

Step 1. Orthogonal survey radiographs should be acquired.
- stomach: right and left lateral and ventrodorsal (VD) projections; or
- small intestine: lateral projection and VD.

Step 2. The radiographs should be evaluated.

Step 3. The barium should be administered.
- the appropriate barium preparation should be selected based on clinical suspicion; and
- the barium suspension should be mixed with food in a bowl or syringe or orogastric tube.

Step 4. Subsequently radiographic projections should be acquired.
- stomach: right and left lateral and ventrodorsal (VD) projections; or
- small intestine: lateral projection and VD.

Step 5. Radiographs should be taken at 0 minutes.
- right and left lateral and ventrodorsal (VD) projections.

Step 6. Right lateral and VD projections should also be acquired at 15 minutes, 30 minutes, and 60 minutes after administering the contrast media (Figure 67).

Step 7. Radiographs should be acquired every 30 minutes until the contrast media reaches the colon (Figure 68 and 69).

Step 8. Radiographs should be repeated at 24 hours to demonstrate contrast has reached the colon and there is no retention of contrast in the stomach or small intestine.

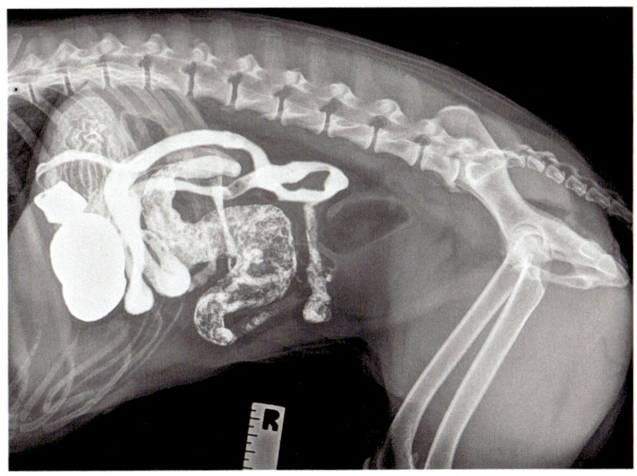

Figure 67. Abdomen right lateral radiograph taken one hour after administering the contrast media.

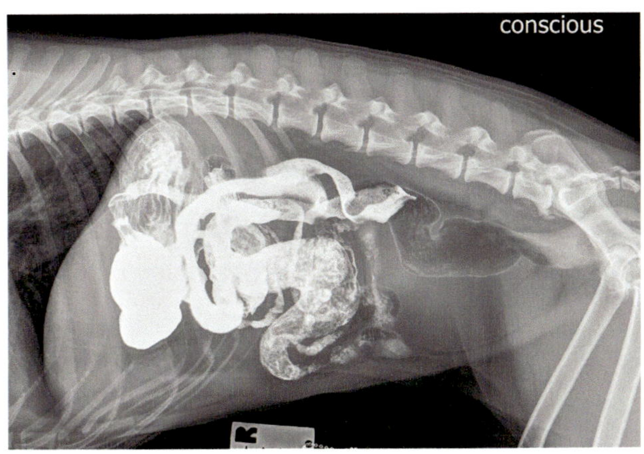

Figure 68. Abdomen right lateral radiograph taken five hours after administering the contrast media.

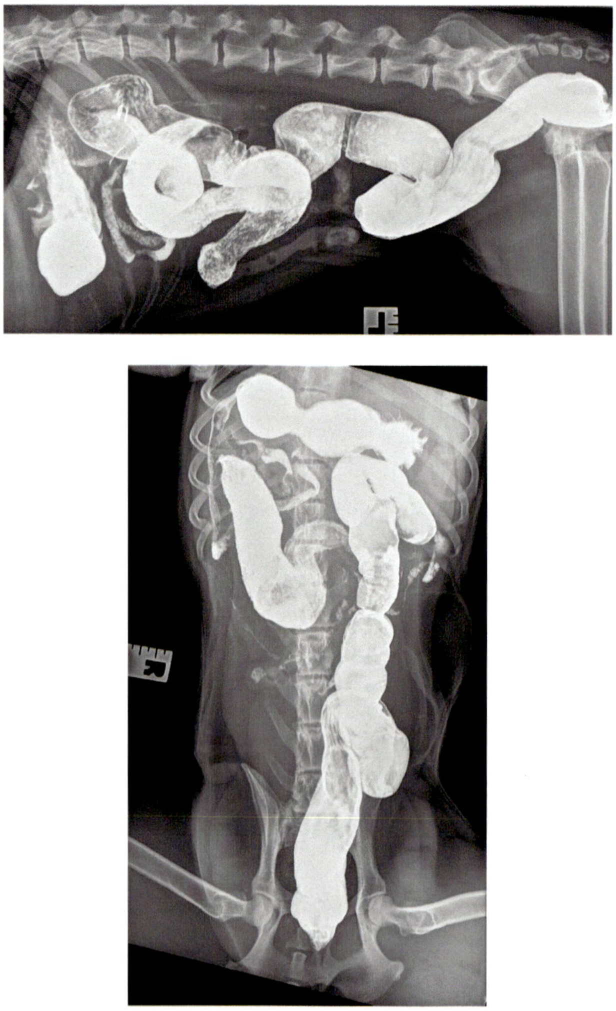

Figure 69. Abdomen left lateral and VD radiographs taken eighteen hours after administering the contrast media.

Intestinal Transit Time

Transit time is usually shorter with iodinate based contrast media than with barium.

- Stomach: gastric emptying starts immediately or at least within 15 minutes. In nervous animals it can take up to 2–3 hours.
- Small intestine: takes 2–4 hours in the dog, with the small intestine being empty within 5 hours. Small intestinal transit is approximately 1 hour in the cat.
- Large intestine: barium should reach the colon within 4 hours of administration and all barium should have reached the colon in 24 hours.

Contraindications

- intestinal dilation and mechanical obstruction are suspected;
- perforation is suspected;
- caution should be exercised when the patient demonstrates aspiration pneumonia. Aspiration of ionic iodinated contrast medium causes fulminant pulmonary oedema which is usually fatal;
- ionic iodinated contrast media should not be used if the animal is very young or debilitated. The fluid drawn into the intestine may lead to dehydration. Non-ionic iodinated contrast medium has less osmotic effect is the safest alternative to barium.

Barium Impregnated Polyethylene Spheres (BIPS)

BIPS have limited applications and cannot be recommended as an alternative to positive contrast intestinal radiographic study.

- The smaller spheres should move through the intestinal tract at the same speed as ingesta. This provides an indication of intestinal transit time.
- The larger spheres can be used for assessment of suspected obstruction (partial/complete). If there is an obstruction, they may accumulate proximal to the obstruction site if the lumen is sufficiently narrowed or occupied by material.

Technique

Step 1. Orthogonal survey radiographs should be acquired, including right and left lateral and VD projections.

Step 2. Radiographs should be repeated around 24 hours after administration of the BIPS, at this point the BIPS should be in the colon.

Large Intestine Studies

Endoscopy is the diagnostic method of choice to evaluate the colon, and therefore radiography is rarely used nowadays.

Material

- Foley balloon tip catheter
- "Christmas tree" adaptor
- Luer tip syringe
- examination gloves
- lubricant
- 60 ml syringes.

Type of Study

- pneumocolon
- positive contrast or double contrast enema.

Indications

- tenesmus
- haematochezia or melaena
- chronic diarrhoea
- colonic stricture
- suspected colonic mass
- evaluation of colon position.

Contrast Media

- dogs/cats: 15–30% weight/volume barium sulphate or iodinated contrast.

Dosage

Positive barium enema:

- canine: 8 ml/kg rectally.

Negative contrast enema:

- dogs/cats: 5–8 ml/kg of air is administered rectally.

Double contrast barium enema:

- 4–6 ml/kg of 20–25% weight/volume barium sulphate should be administered in dogs and cats and administration of air should follow this.

Pneumocolon

Step 1. Rectal examination should be performed by the clinician.

Step 2. A warm enema should be performed several hours before the procedure.

Step 3. Orthogonal survey radiographs should be acquired, including lateral and VD projections. If patient preparation is inadequate, the enema should be repeated (2–3 warm water).

Step 4. The procedure should ideally be performed under general anaesthesia.

Step 5. A Foley catheter with the a "Christmas tree" adaptor for a Luer tip syringe should be put into place. The lubricated foley catheter should be inserted and the balloon gently inflated. If there is any leakage of air a purse-string suture can be used.

Step 6. The colon should be inflated with approximately 5–8 ml/kg of air (volume will vary depending on whether cat or dog). The colon should be palpated, and more air added, if necessary, based on the radiographs.

Step 7. Lateral and VD radiographic projections should be acquired. Oblique projections can be obtained to better evaluate the intrapelvic region.

Positive Contrast Study: Barium Enema

Step 1. Rectal examination should be performed by the clinician.

Step 2. A warm enema should be performed several hours before the procedure.

Step 3. Orthogonal survey radiographs should be acquired, including lateral and VD projections. If patient preparation is inadequate, the enema should be repeated (2–3 warm water).

Step 4. The procedure should ideally be performed under general anaesthesia.

Step 5. A Foley catheter with the a "Christmas tree" adaptor for a Luer tip syringe should be put into place. The lubricated foley catheter should be inserted and the balloon gently inflated. If there is any leakage of air a purse-string suture can be used.

Step 6. The colon should be inflated with 8 ml/kg of a 20–25% weight/volume barium solution. Colloidal suspension is preferred to barium powder.

Step 7. Lateral and VD radiographic projections should be acquired. Oblique projections can be obtained to better evaluate the intrapelvic region.

Step 8. Barium should not be administered if perforation is suspected.

Genitourinary Contrast Studies

To **evaluate the urogenital tract,** the most common procedures used are cystography, retrograde vagionourethrography and urethrography.

Patient preparation:

- Prior to a contrast study, a urine sample should be collected for urinalysis, culture, and sensitivity.
- Food should be withheld for 24 hours. An oral bowel cleansing solution should be administered the day before the procedure. Alternatively, a warm enema the day before and 1–2 hours prior to the contrast study can also be used.
- Before the procedure patients should be offered the opportunity to void.

Intravenous Excretory Urography

Contrast Media

Iodine contrast agents should be administered at a dose of 600–800 mg/kg. This is approximately 2 ml/kg of a solution containing 300/400 mg I/ml. Both ionic (Conray® or Renografin®) and non-ionic (Ultravist®, Isovue®, Optiray®, Omnipaque®, or Visipaque®) are suitable for this procedure. For patients with preexisting conditions, non-ionic contrast agents should be used.

Urinalysis and culture should be performed prior to contrast medium administration. The contrast agent can affect the measurement of specific gravity and inhibit the growth of some bacteria. Urinalysis results are not accurate for at least 24 hours after contrast medium administration.

The first phase of the excretory urogram is the nephrogram, which occurs when contrast medium is present in the terminal glomerular renal vessels and the renal tubules. Peak opacity occurs at 10–30 seconds. The intensity and duration of the opacity of the kidneys, depends on the dose of the contrast agent, renal perfusion, glomerular filtration of the contrast medium, tubular resorption of water, and the patency of the renal outflow tract.

The nephrogram usually lasts for approximately two minutes. Following this, the second phase occurs, this is termed the pyelogram, which may last for two or more hours after contrast medium injection.

Indications

- haematuria
- urinary incontinence (suspected ectopic ureters)
- suspected uroabdomen
- renal evaluation: size, shape, and localisation.

Contraindications

- anuria
- dehydration
- previous or known hypersensitivity to the contrast agent.

Side Effects

- administration of ionic iodinated contrast agents is safe in most patients, but mild to severe adverse reactions may occur due to the hypertonicity of the contrast agent.

Material

- intravenous catheter with injection cap/t connector
- 2–50 ml syringe depending on patient size
- needles
- emergency drug kit
- kidney dish
- urinary catheter.

Technique

Step1. General anaesthesia is required as it allows better patient positioning, improves patient safety, and avoids artefacts.

Step 2. Cleansing enemas should be performed two hours prior to the procedure

Step 3. Survey radiographs should be acquired including VD and right lateral abdominal projections. The colon should be checked for any faecal material. If necessary, another enema can be given and the colon rechecked an hour later.

Step 4. A negative contrast cystogram can be performed following survey radiographs if ectopic ureters are suspected. This gives a mild double contrast cystogram and highlights the uretrovesicular junctions point of entry.

Step 5. The patient should be placed in a VD recumbent position.

Step 6. The contrast media should be injected as a rapid intravenous bolus.

Step 7. A VD projection should be taken immediately post injection (5 seconds). A right lateral projection may be required if a lesion is identified and requires assessment on a lateral projection.

Step8. Subsequent exposures should include VD projections at one and five minutes. After five minutes the patient can be turned to lateral recumbency for lateral and VD projections at 10, 15, 20 and 40 minutes.

Step 9. Oblique views (45° lateral oblique projections) of the abdomen may be necessary to overcome superimposition of the structures.

Step 10. Additional projections may need to be taken at 45, 60, or 90 minutes if there is a delay in contrast enhancement of the renal system.

Step 11. The timing and correct labelling should be typed onto each radiograph for interpretation.

Positive Contrast Cystography

Contrast Media

- water soluble ionic or non-ionic contrast agents: 120–400 mg/ml.

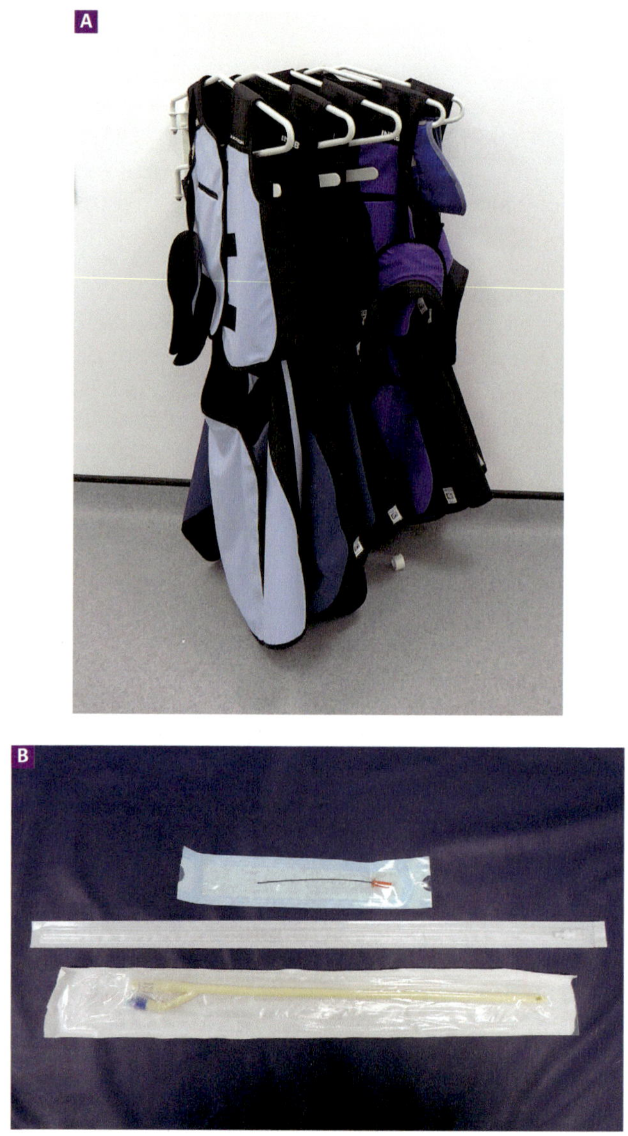

Figure 70. A. Leads aprons; **B.** Urinary catheter/Foley catheter.

Dosage

- contrast should be diluted to 25% (1 part contrast to 3 parts sterile water or saline):
  - dogs: 5–10 ml/kg
  - cats: 2–5 ml/kg: approximately 25 ml in total.

Material

- urinary catheter/Foley catheter
- sterile "Christmas tree" adapter
- 3 way tap connector
- syringes
- sterile lubricant
- germicidal soap and water preparation
- gauze
- sterile gloves
- vaginal/otoscope speculum (female patients)
- kidney dish/measuring jug
- incontinence pads
- sterile saline.

Technique

Step 1. General anaesthesia is required as it allows better patient positioning, improves patient safety, and avoids artefacts.

Step 2. Cleansing enemas should be performed two hours prior to the procedure.

Step 3. Survey radiographs, including VD and right lateral abdominal projections should be acquired. The colon should be checked for any faecal material, and another enema given if necessary, and then rechecked after an hour.

Step 4. Orthogonal radiographs should be acquired, including right lateral and VD projections (centred in the caudal abdomen).

Step 5. Bladder size can be assessed by palpation, the bladder should be emptied to avoid over distension and rupture.

Step 6. The external area surrounding the urethra should be cleaned with soap solution.

Step 7. The patient should be catheterised aseptically using sterile lubricant and the bladder emptied.

Step 8. The catheter should be prefilled with sterile saline to avoid introduction of air bubbles into the bladder.

Step 9. The contrast medium should be injected slowly. The bladder can be palpated during injection to avoid overdistension.

Step 10. Radiographs should be acquired, including right lateral, VD, and oblique projections if necessary (Figure 71).

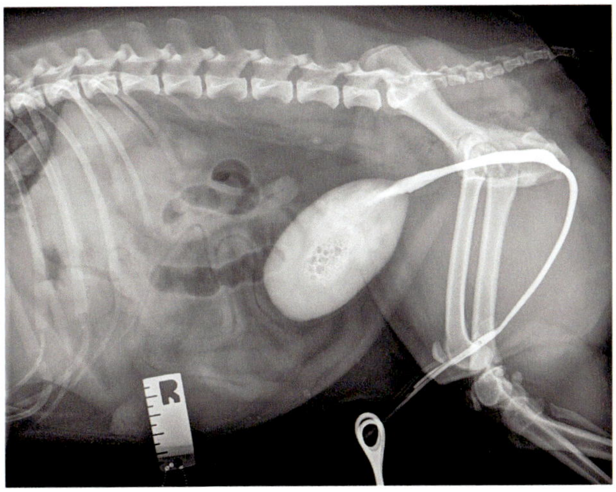

Figure 71. Positive retrograde urethrocystogram. Stones can be appreciated inside the bladder.

Pneumocystography

Pneumocystography is rarely used as a sole imaging technique.

Contrast Media

- air/soluble gas (e.g. carbon dioxide, nitrous oxide).

Dosage

- **dose is patient dependent.** Palpation of the bladder is recommended while administering the gas to prevent rupture or overdistension of the bladder.
  - large dogs: 50–300 ml
  - small dogs and cats: 35 ml.

Indications

- evaluation of bladder size and identification of radiopaque calculi.

Material

- urinary catheter/Foley catheter
- sterile "Christmas tree" adapter
- 3 way tap connector
- syringes
- sterile lubricant
- germicidal soap and water preparation
- gauze
- sterile gloves
- vaginal/otoscope speculum (female patients)
- kidney dish/measuring jug
- incontinence pads
- sterile saline.

Technique

Step1. General anaesthesia is required as it allows better patient positioning, improves patient safety and avoids artefacts.

Step 2. An enema should be performed two hours prior to the procedure.

Step 3. Survey radiographs should be acquired, including VD and right lateral abdominal projections (Figure 72). The colon should be checked for any faecal material and if necessary, another enema given and then rechecked in an hour.

Step 4. Orthogonal radiographs, including right lateral and VD (centred in the caudal abdomen) projections should be acquired.

Step 5. Bladder size should be assessed by palpation. The bladder should be emptied to avoid over distension and rupture.

Step 6. The external area surrounding the urethra should be cleaned with soap solution.

Step 7. The patient should be catheterised aseptically using sterile lubricant and the bladder emptied.

Step 8. The gas should be injected slowly, palpating the bladder during injection to avoid overdistension or rupture.

Step 9. The tip of the catheter should be withdrawn to the urethra to avoid artefact.

Step 10. Radiographs should be taken, including right lateral, VD, and oblique projections if necessary.

Double Contrast Cystography

This technique combines the advantages of both negative and positive contrast cystography. The first phase is usually a pneumocystogram, followed by a small volume of positive contrast medium providing the double contrast, resulting in distension of the bladder with negative contrast medium and a small pool/puddle of positive contrast medium centrally. Nowadays, ultrasonography has superseded cystography, however this technique is still useful.

Contrast Media

- air or soluble gas
    - large dogs: 50–300 ml
    - small dogs and cats: 35 ml
- water soluble ionic or non-ionic contrast agents
- contrast should be diluted to 25% (1 part contrast to 3 parts sterile water or saline)
    - small dogs and cats: 1–2 ml
    - large dogs: 2–10 ml.

Indications

- assessment of bladder wall and mucosa
- differentiation between cystoliths and blood clots.

Materials

- urinary catheter/Foley catheter
- 3 way tap connector
- syringes
- sterile lubricant
- germicidal soap and water preparation
- gauze
- sterile gloves
- vaginal/otoscope speculum (female patients)
- kidney dish/measuring jug
- incontinence pads
- sterile saline.

Technique

Step 1. General anaesthesia is required as it allows better patient positioning, improves patient safety, and avoids artefacts.

Step 2. A cleansing enema should be undertaken two hours prior to the procedure.

Step 3. Survey radiographs should be acquired, including VD and right lateral abdominal projections. The colon should be checked for any faecal material and if necessary,

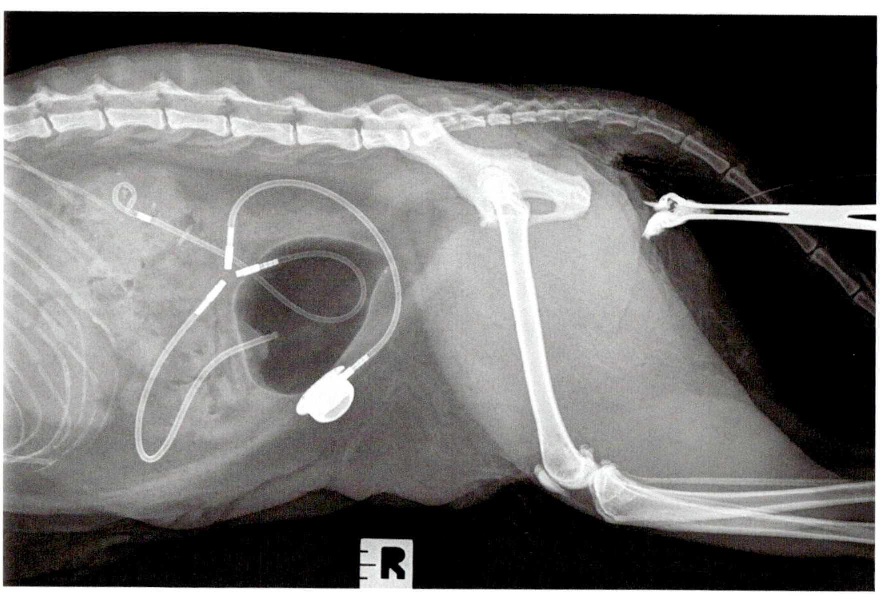

Figure 72. Right lateral radiograph of the abdomen. Pneumocystogram in a cat with a SUB (subcutaneous ureteral bypass) in place.

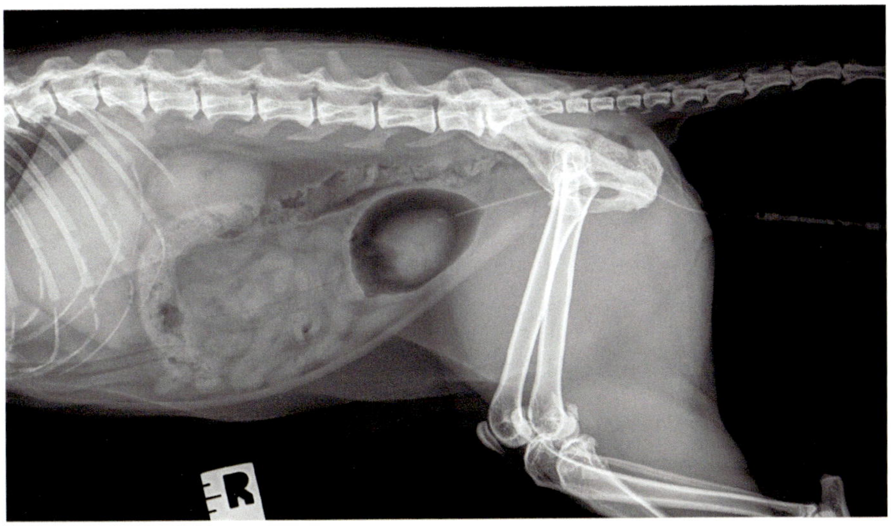

Figure 73. Lateral radiograph demonstrating a double contrast cystogram.

another enema given and rechecked an hour later.

Step 4. Orthogonal radiographs should be acquired, including right lateral and VD projections (centred on the caudal abdomen).

Step 5. Bladder size should be assessed by palpation. If necessary, the bladder should be emptied to avoid over distension and rupture.

Step 6. The external area surrounding the urethra should be cleaned with soap solution.

Step 7. The patient should be catheterised aseptically using sterile lubricant and the bladder emptied.

Step 8. The catheter should be prefilled with sterile saline to avoid air bubbles entering the bladder.

Step 9. The contrast mediums should be injected slowly. The bladder should be palpated during injection to avoid overdistension. The positive contrast medium should be injected into the bladder, followed by gas. The gas is injected slowly to avoid formation of gas bubbles. If the positive contrast cystogram is performed after pneumocystography, the patient should be rolled to ensure contrast medium coats the bladder wall. If double contrast cystography is to be performed after intravenous urography, the bladder must be empty of the contrast medium and gas, and reinflated. Additional positive contrast medium should not be necessary as the kidneys continue to excrete the contrast into the bladder.

Step 10. Radiographs should be taken, including right lateral (Figure 73), VD, and oblique projections if necessary.

Retrograde Urethrography

Contrast Media

Water soluble ionic or non-ionic contrast agents should be used. Dilution may be necessary to reach the adequate concentration (1:2 dilution).

Dosage

- cats: 5 ml
- small dogs: 10 ml
- medium dogs: 20 ml
- large dogs: 30 ml.

Indications

- haematuria
- dysuria
- urinary incontinence/ectopic ureters
- lower urinary tract obstruction
- prostatic disease
- disease of the urethra or os penis
- trauma to the urethra.

Material

- urinary catheter/Foley catheter
- 3 way tap connector
- syringes
- sterile lubricant
- germicidal soap and water preparation
- gauze
- sterile gloves
- kidney dish/measuring jug
- incontinence pads
- sterile saline.

Technique

Step 1. General anaesthesia is required as it allows for better patient positioning, improves patient safety, and avoids artefacts.

Step 2. A cleansing enema should be undertaken two hours prior to the procedure.

Step 3. Survey radiographs should be acquired, including VD and right lateral abdominal projections. The colon should be checked for any faecal material and if necessary, another enema given and rechecked an hour later.

Step 4. The preputial fold and external area surrounding the penis/urethra should be cleaned with soap solution.

Step 5. The patient should be aseptically catheterised using sterile lubricant and the bladder emptied.

Step 6. Occasionally, a full bladder is preferred for better distension of the urethra.

Step 7. Orthogonal survey radiographs should be acquired, including right lateral and VD projections (centred on the caudal abdomen).

Step 8. The patient should be positioned for the radiographs, starting with right lateral projection with the legs pulled forwards, to better visualise the urethra between the ischial arch and the caudal aspect of the os penis. Then a right lateral projection should be acquired with the legs pulled caudally to assess the pelvic and prostatic urethra. VD and oblique projections should also be acquired if necessary.

Step 9. The catheter should be prefilled with contrast medium to avoid introducing air bubbles into the bladder.

Step 10. The catheter should be introduced into the tip of the penile urethra and gently clamped across with the preputial fold just before the penis using bowel clamps. This helps to keep the catheter in place and avoids leakage of contrast medium.

Step 11. Contrast mediums should be injected slowly and radiographs taken during the final part of the injection. Appropriate PPE is required.

Retrograde Vaginourethrography

Contrast Media

Water soluble ionic or non-ionic contrast agents should be used. Dilution may be necessary to reach an adequate concentration of 150–200 mg/ml.

Dosage

1 ml/kg should be used to fill the vagina and then overflow into the urethra, with overall dose varying according to size and species:

- cats: 5 ml
- small dogs: 10 ml
- medium dogs: 20 ml
- large dogs: 30 ml.

Indications

- haematuria
- dysuria
- urinary incontinence/ectopic ureters
- lower urinary tract obstruction
- vaginal stenosis
- trauma to the urethra or vagina.

Material

- Foley catheter
- sterile "Christmas tree" adapter
- 3 way tap connector
- syringes
- sterile lubricant
- germicidal soap and water preparation

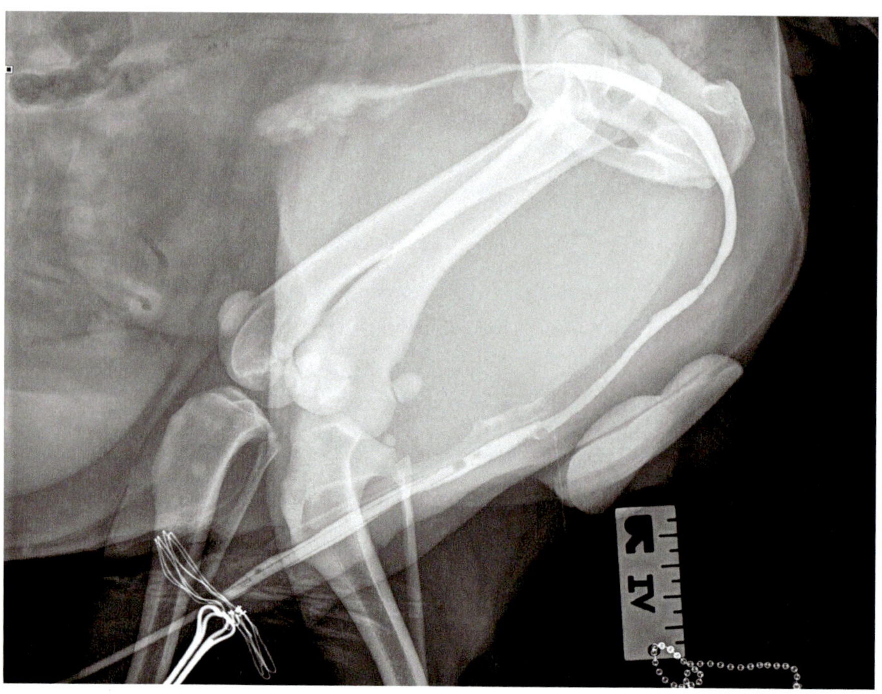

Figure 74. Right lateral projection demonstrating a retrograde urethrogram. Note some gas bubbles in the penile urethra. Likely due to some air in the syringe or if the catheter was not prefilled before the procedure.

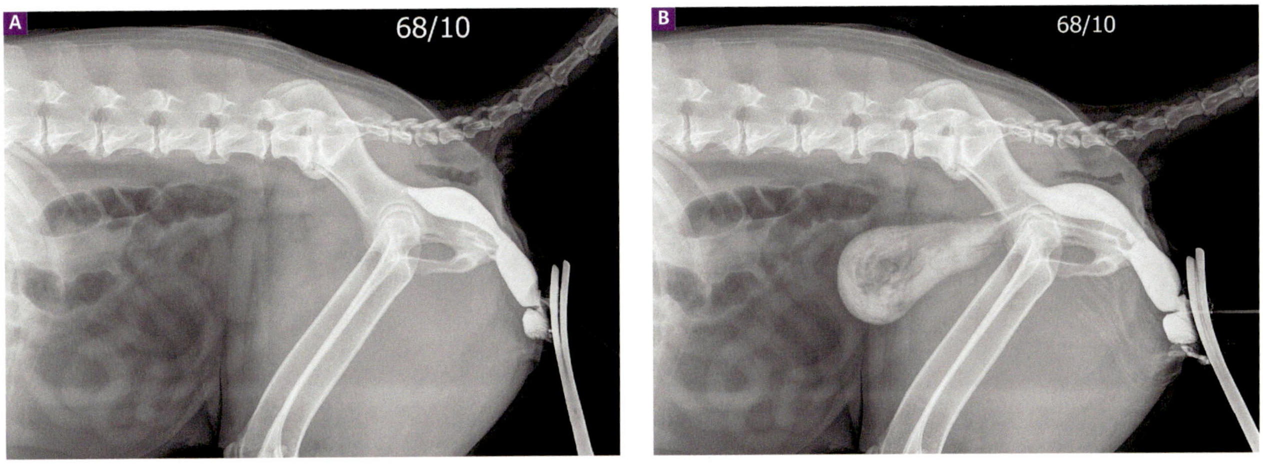

Figure 75. A. Lateral projection demonstrating a positive vaginogram;
B. Lateral projection demonstrating a positive vaginourethrogram.

- gauze
- sterile gloves
- vaginal/otoscope speculum
- kidney dish/measuring jug
- incontinence pads
- sterile saline.

Technique

Step 1. General anaesthesia is required as it allows for better patient positioning, improves patient safety and avoids artefacts.

Step 2. A cleansing enema should be undertaken two hours prior to the procedure.

Step 3. Survey radiographs should be acquired including VD and right lateral abdominal projections. The colon should be checked for faecal material and if necessary, another enema given and rechecked an hour later.

Step 4. The vulva and external area surrounding the entrance to the urethra should be cleaned with soap solution.

Step 5. The patient should be catheterised aseptically using sterile lubricant and the bladder emptied.

Step 6. Occasionally, a full bladder is preferred for better distension of the urethra.

Step 7. Orthogonal radiographs including right lateral and VD projections (centred in the caudal abdomen) should be obtained.

Step 8. The catheter should be prefilled with contrast medium to avoid introducing air bubbles into the bladder.

Step 9. The Foley catheter should be introduced into the vulva and the cuff inflated just inside the vestibule.

Step 10. The contrast medium should be injected to adequately fill the vagina.

Step 11. Radiographs should be acquired, including a right lateral projection at the end of the injection, followed by VD and oblique views if necessary. Appropriate PPE is necessary if close to the primary beam.

Axial and Appendicular Arthrography Contrast Studies

The study most commonly performed is of the shoulder joint.

Contrast Medium

- non-ionic contrast medium (e.g. Omnipaque®).

Dosage

- 1–5 ml of a non-ionic contrast agent diluted to 100–150 mg I/ml should be used for the shoulder joint;
- 0.4 ml/kg of a contrast agent diluted to 100 mg I/ml should be used for the bicipital groove;
- non-ionic contrast agents should be diluted to one part contrast agent to two parts isotonic sterile saline.

Material

- 21–23 gauge needle (5/8 to 1.5 inch)
- 2 ml syringes
- Surgical Spirit™
- diluted Hibiscrub®
- sterile gloves
- clippers
- sterile swabs
- EDTA and heparin collection tubes.

Technique

Step 1. General anaesthesia is usually required; however the procedure may be tolerated with heavy sedation.

Step 2. Orthogonal survey radiographs should be acquired, including mediolateral (ML) and CdCr (caudocranial) projections. An additional projection, the skyline (cranioproximal craniodistal) projection can be used to evaluate the bicipital groove.

Step 3. The lateral aspect of the shoulder joint should be clipped and the area scrubbed aseptically.

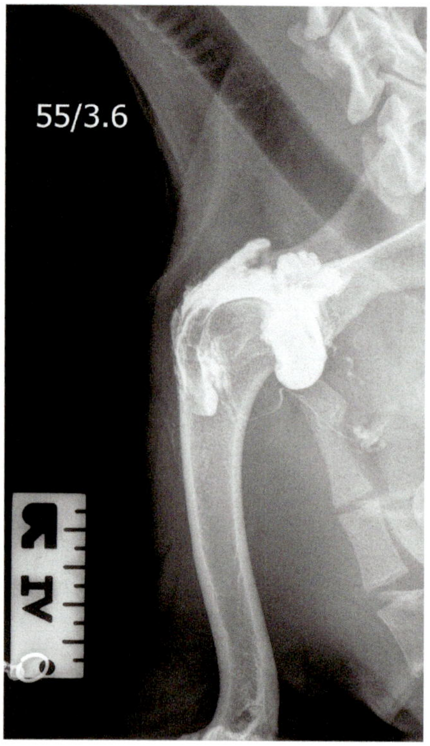

Figure 76. Lateral projection demonstrating a positive contrast arthrogram.

Step 4. The patient should be placed in lateral recumbency with the joint being examined uppermost.

Step 5. Synovial fluid should be withdrawn, keeping the needle in place and injecting 1–5 ml of diluted (100–150 mg I/ml) non-ionic water soluble contrast medium.

Step 6. The joint should be flexed and extended to distribute the contrast in the joint space.

Step 7. Radiographs should be acquired, including mediolateral (ML) and CdCr (caudo cranial) projections. An additional projection, the skyline (cranioproximal craniodistal) projection and oblique views can also be taken if needed.

Myelography

MRI and CT have largely replaced myelography, as they are more sensitive and specific at identifying spinal cord pathology.

Indications

- ataxia, paresis, paralysis due to spinal pathology or compression
- spinal pain.

Contrast Media

- iohexol (Omnipaque® 240 mg I/ml) or iopamidol (Isovue® 200 mg I/ml) should be used; and
- only non-ionic iodinated contrast agents with an iodine concentration of 200–300 mg I/kg are approved for intrathecal use.

Dosage (Cats and Dogs)

- cisternal injection:
  - cervical spine: 0.3 ml/kg
  - thoracolumbar spine: 0.45 ml/kg
- lumbar injection:
  - cervical spine: 0.45 ml/kg
  - thoracolumbar spine: 0.3 ml/kg
- the recommended dosage should not be exceeded.

Material

- spinal needles 20–22 gauge
- clippers
- surgical scrub
- sterile gloves
- EDTA and plain tube for CSF sample.

Technique

Step 1. The patient must be anaesthetised and either the cisternal or lumbar injection site clipped.

Step 2. Orthogonal survey radiographs of the entire spine should be acquired, including right lateral and VD projections.

Step 3. The site of injection should be scrubbed aseptically.

Step 4. The clinician should aseptically place the spinal needle into the subarachnoid space and collect CSF for cytology analysis.

Step 5. Needle placement should be verified by injecting 0.2–0.5 ml of contrast followed by a right lateral radiograph centred on the region of injection to confirm proper placement. This step can be skipped if the clinician is content with needle positioning.

Step 6. The contrast agent should be injected slowly over one minute.

Step 7. Radiograph projections should be acquired, including a right lateral projection at the end of the injection confirming adequate filling of the subarachnoid space.

Step 8. The needle should be removed. It may be necessary to tilt the animal's body to facilitate better filling of the subarachnoid space.

Step 9. Radiograph projections which should be acquired include the following:

- cervical spine: lateral and VD projections. Oblique, flexion and extension and traction lateral projections are acquired only if the clinician requests;
- thoracolumbar spine: lateral and VD projections. Oblique projections are acquired if the clinician requests;
- lumbar spine: lateral and VD projections. Oblique projections are acquired if the clinician requests.

Step 10. If fracture is suspected (this should be looked for on the survey radiographs), a lateral projection and

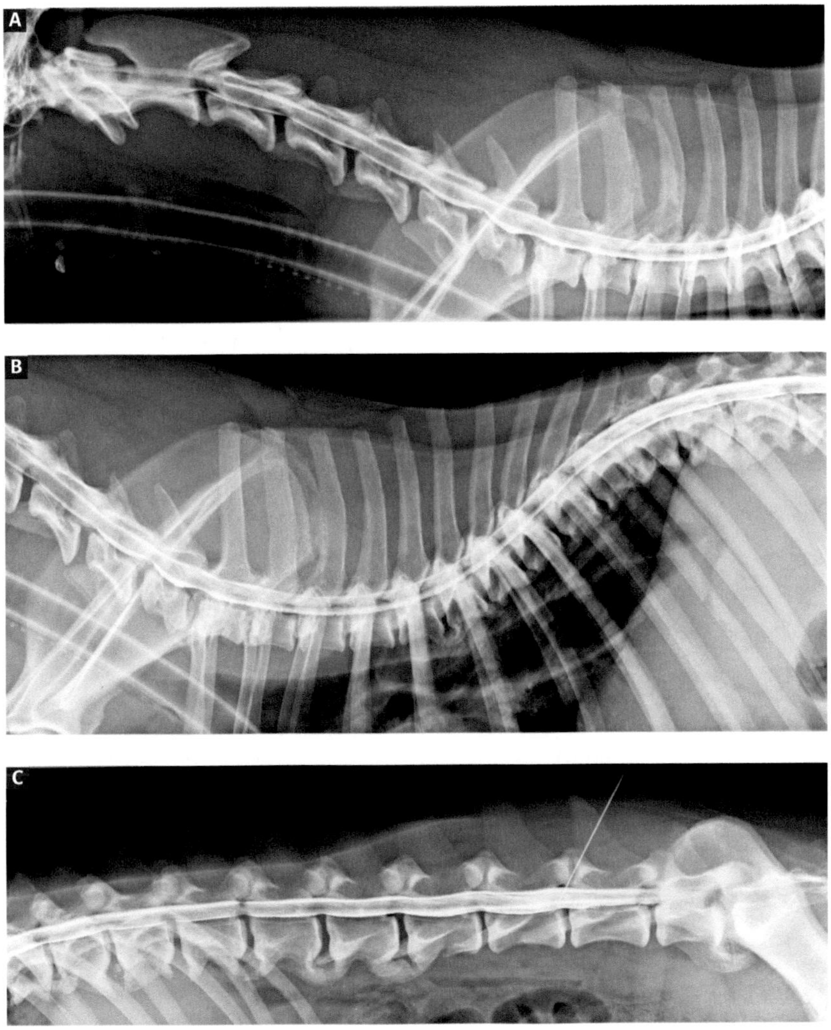

Figure 77. Myelogram of cervical spine (**A**), thoracic spine (**B**) and lumbar spine (**C**).

horizontal beam to obtain a VD projection may be necessary (equipment dependent).

Radiograph Interpretation

Overview

The best approach to radiographic interpretation is to be consistent and **use a systematic examination pattern which allows for better recognition of normal versus abnormal anatomy.**

Radiographic stations must be quiet and dark, with at least two viewing monitors or light boxes. Radiographs should always be viewed with a dark adapted eye, meaning an eye that has been allowed to adjust in order to view objects in a dim light.

Radiographs should be positioned on the viewer in a consistent manner:

- lateral projections: the head should be placed to the left side of the screen (Figure 78);
- dorsoventral/ventrodorsal projection: the left of the animal should be positioned on the right side of observer and head at the top;
- radiographs of extremities: the proximal aspect should be positioned at the top and the cranial/dorsal aspect towards the left side.

Assess Radiographic Technique

Radiographic technique should be assessed for:

- correct labelling (left/right marker, patient details)
- radiographic projections
- quality
- artefacts.

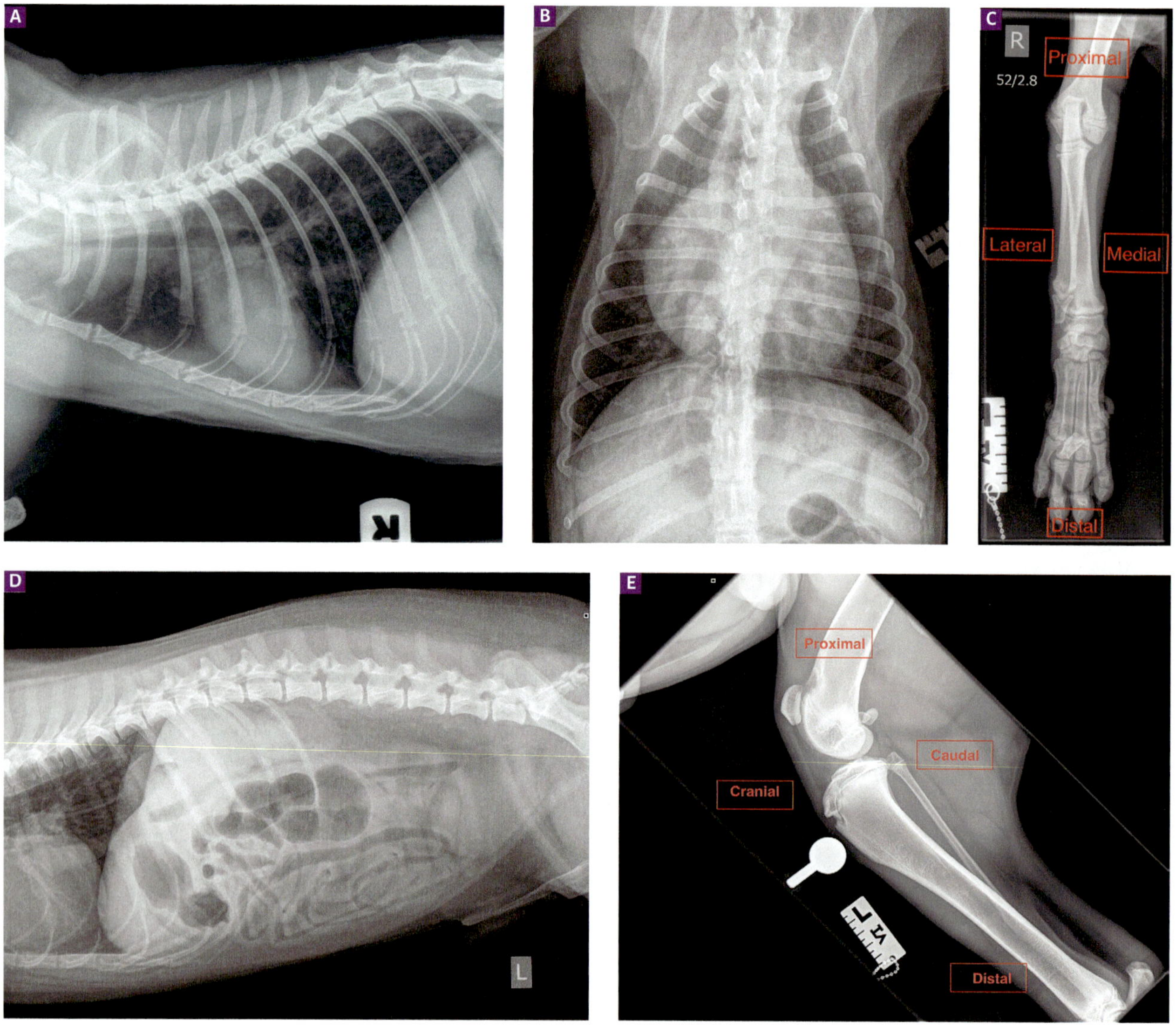

Figure 78. Example of radiographic orientation. Thorax lateral (**A**) and thorax DV (**B**), DP carpus (**C**), lateral abdomen (**D**), ML stifle (**E**).

Systematic Approach

A systematic approach is essential when interpreting radiographs. Each observer should develop their own preferred approach to avoid missing an inconspicuous lesion or getting distracted.

Radiographic evaluation can be performed per cavity using an organ or area/circle approach (concentric/eccentric circles).

Three Dimensional (3D) Concept

When viewing radiographs, the viewer must mentally create a three dimensional image from a radiograph that only has two dimensions. A minimum of two radiographic projections, taken at right angles to one another, are necessary to create a three dimensional perspective.

Standard projections:

- orthogonal views (perpendicular/90° to one another)
- 3D impression achieved
- a minimum of two projections should always be taken (Figure 79).

When patients are not positioned properly, this can lead to inaccurate interpretation of the radiograph which may lead to an incorrect diagnosis.

When taking or evaluating radiographs, the operator must be aware of the standard nomenclature. Nomenclature means

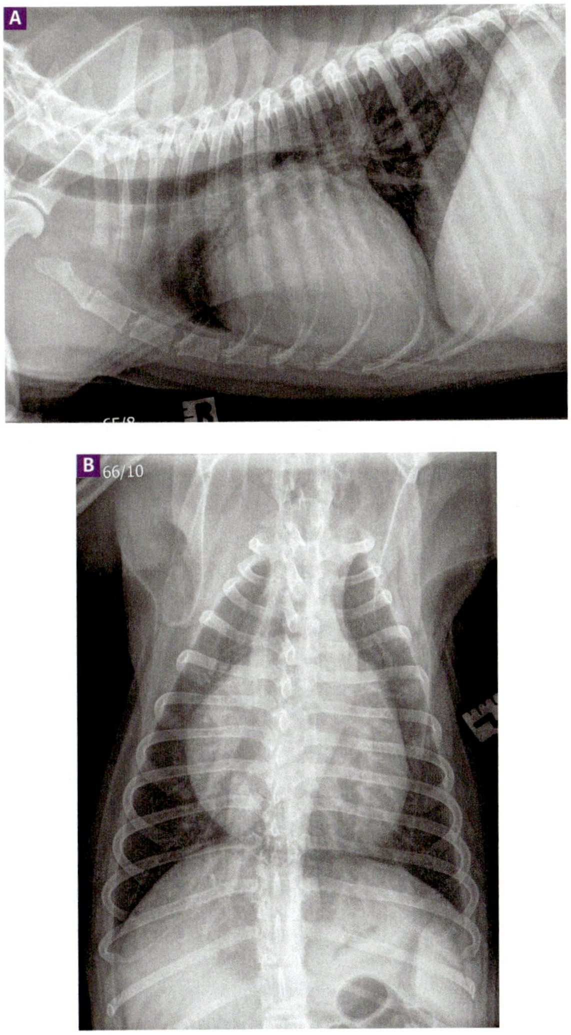

Figure 79. Lateral (**A**) and DV (**B**) thorax.

the terminology used, in this case, to describe radiographic positioning.

Radiographic projections should be named according to the direction of the X-ray beam:

- point of entrance → point of exit
- e.g. dorsoventral:
    - point of entrance = dorsal aspect
    - point of exit = ventral aspect.

However, lateral projections of the thorax and abdomen are described as the patient is positioned, rather than the X-ray beam direction, e.g. left lateral view = left side of the body closest to the plate.

A similar method is used for body parts. All body parts have appropriate directional terminology that is used when interpreting radiographs. (Figure 80).

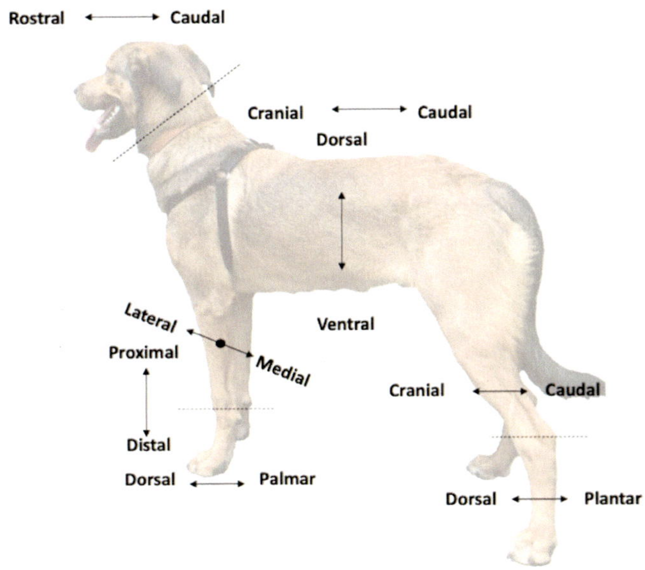

Figure 80. Nomenclature image.

Anatomical Landmarks

Anatomy and radiology textbooks and skeletons are helpful as aids in radiographic interpretation. To recognize an abnormality, it must be looked for and to see it, a deep knowledge of normal radiographic anatomy is essential. (Figure 81).

Roentgen Signs

Roentgen signs is the method used for describing radiographic abnormalities.

Roentgen signs:

- **Size:** changes in size of an organ or structure.
- **Shape:** variation in shape.
- **Location:** change in position of an organ or structure.
- **Number:** variation in number of organs or lesions.
- **Margination:** serosal surface definition.
- **Opacity:** alteration in the normal opacity of an organ.

Radiographic Opacities

Attenuation of X-ray photons results in reduction in the intensity of the X-ray beam as it passes through matter, due to absorption or scatter or a combination of both. **Each type of matter has a different attenuation coefficient.** Every X-ray has a fixed range of attenuation through tissue. **Radiopacities depend on the atomic number, physical opacity, and thickness of the area being radiographed** (Figures 82 and 83).

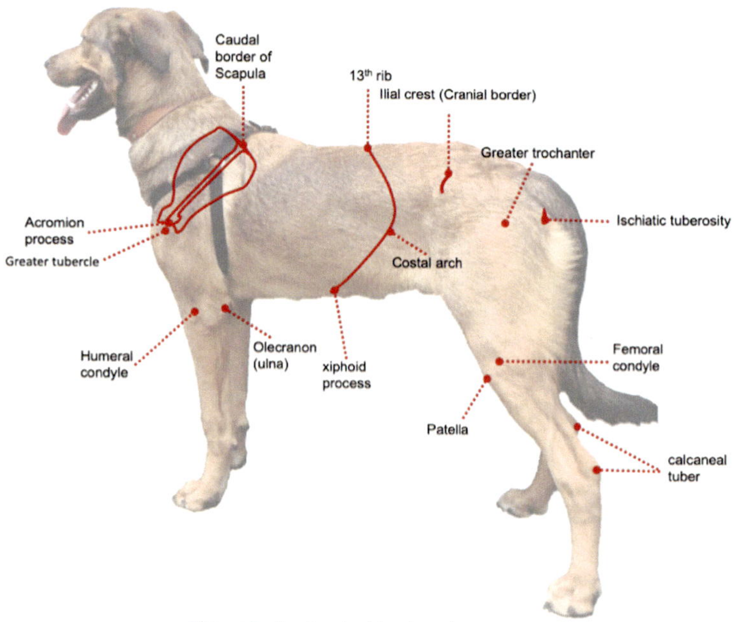

Figure 81. Anatomical landmarks.

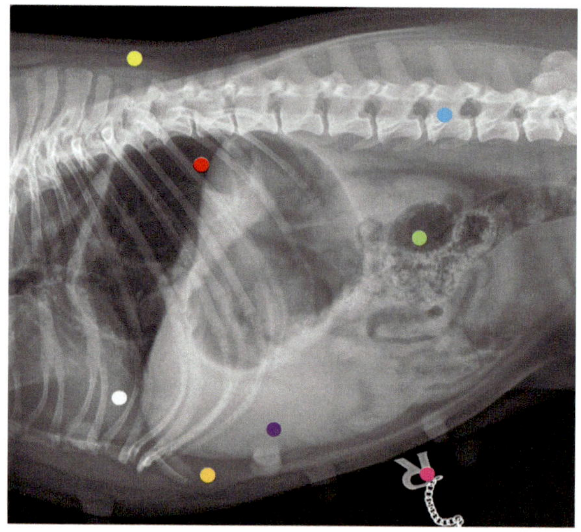

Figure 83. Examples of air, fat, soft tissue, bone and metal opacities. Yellow: fat opacity; Red: gas opacity; Blue: bone opacity; Purple: soft tissue; Pink: metal opacity; Orange: fat opacity; White: soft tissue opacity; Green: air.

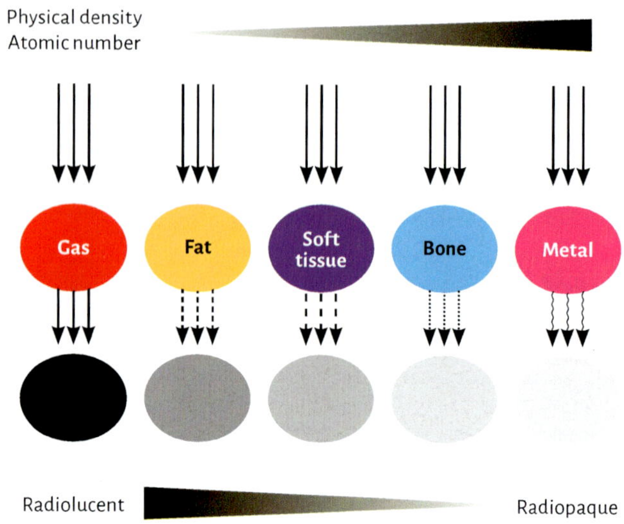

Figure 82. Radiopacities.

There are five basic radiographic opacities: air, fat, soft tissue, bone, and metal. Air attenuates a minimal amount of the X-ray beam, allowing nearly the full X-ray beam to expose and blacken the X-ray film. Conversely, bone and metal attenuate a larger proportion of the X-ray beam than other tissues (air, fat, or soft tissues) and as a result bone appears more radiopaque (whiter) on the film even when superimposed on other tissues.

The patient's thickness should also be considered because it increases the opacity of the radiograph.

Interpretation errors can occur regardless of expertise of the person interpreting; bias and answer satisfaction can lead to judgment errors (i.e. under and overinterpreting and faulty reasoning).

Good radiological interpretation depends on:

- practice
- good radiographic technique
- recognising good radiographic quality
- understanding different radiographic opacities
- knowledge of radiographic anatomy
- thorough review of the radiograph
- application of the findings with the clinical signs.

Radiographic Artefacts and Faults

An artefact is an unwanted feature in the image and should be avoided as it may compromise image interpretation (Figures 84–87). All diagnostic imaging modalities are prone to imaging artefacts; these are more often encountered with screen film but can also occur with both CR and DR.

In general artefacts can be divided into three types:

- incorrect choice of **exposure factors**
- inappropriate **acquisition, centring, collimation, or use of a grid**
- incorrect/**faulty processing.**

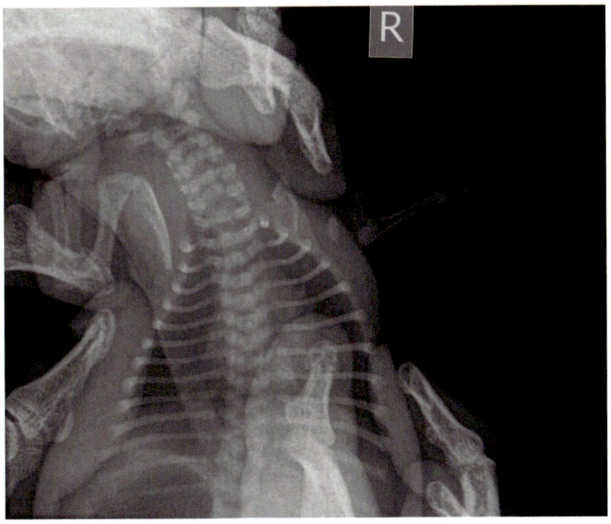

Figure 84. Manual restraint of a patient. This radiograph demonstrates poor patient positioning and restraint, making the radiograph of poor diagnostic quality. The local ionising radiation guidelines and rules about manual restraint should be referred to. Courtesy of Gawain Hammond.

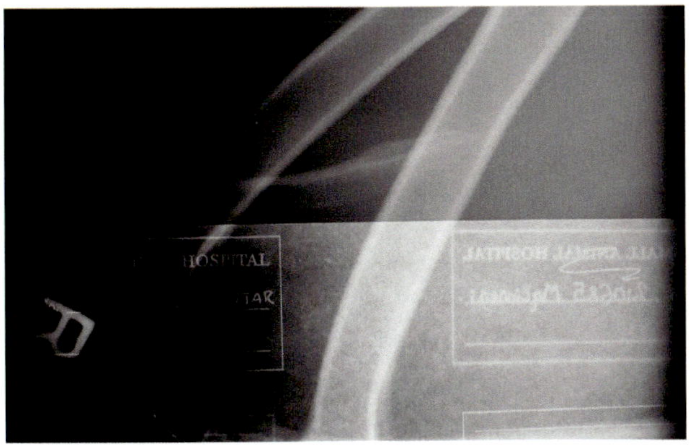

Figure 85. Hospital label left inside the cassette. Courtesy of Gawain Hammond.

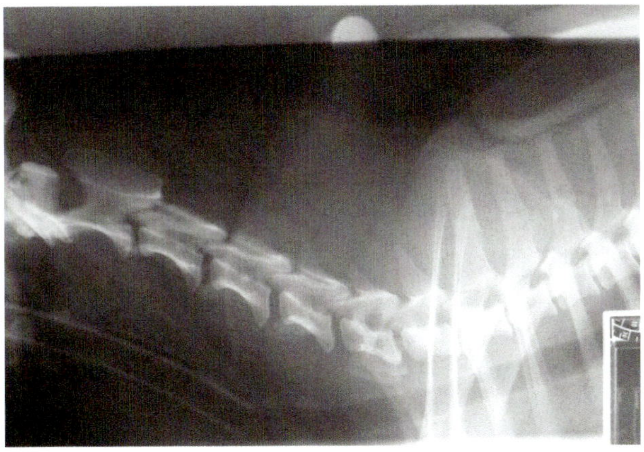

Figure 86. Skin fold artefact. Breeds with excessive skin should be positioned carefully to make sure their skin does not ruche and create a skin fold artefact. Courtesy of Gawain Hammond.

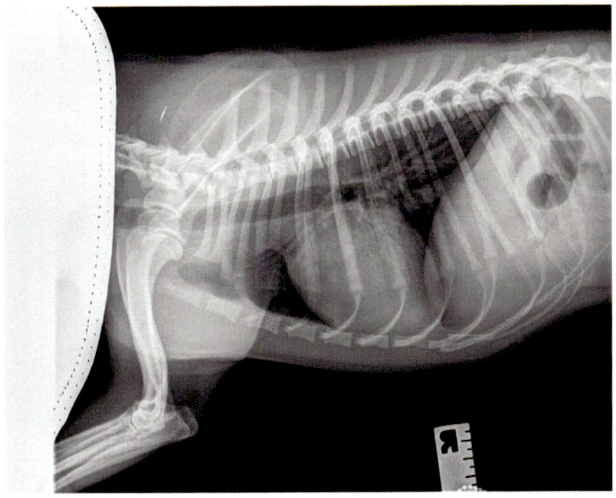

Figure 87. Lead glove in the primary beam. Lead personnel protective equipment (PPE) does not provide protection against primary radiation.

Preexposure Artefacts

Preexposure artefacts, as the name suggests, occur before the radiographic exposure is taken and tend to be related to storage and handling of X-ray cassettes.

Storage Scatter (Convectional Film and CR)

Conventional cassettes and CR imaging plates are more sensitive to scatter. This can occur due to incorrect storage of the imaging plate. All imaging plates should be kept outside the X-ray room during radiographic acquisition. Erasure of the plates before use is recommended to eliminate storage scatter.

Cracks (Conventional Film, CR and DR)

Imaging cassettes and CR plates are prone to damage and should always be handled with care. Cracks in the imaging plate can appear as white line or dots and are usually located at the periphery of the image.

Partial Erasure (CR)

Incomplete erasure of the latent image by the laser light; there is a faint image superimposed on the most recent radiograph. Bright visible light is most commonly used for erasure of the plate. Ultraviolet light can be used additionally for a more thorough erasure.

Phantom/Ghost Artefact (CR)

Faint superimposition of a latent image from the previous radiograph. This occurs due to prolonged time between the erasure of the cassette and subsequent exposure.

Exposure Artefacts

These are less common, but not excluded from CR and DR systems, due to the wide range of exposures.

Underexposure (Conventional Film, CR and DR)

An underexposed radiograph appears too light overall. This occurs due to either too few photons reaching the film (mAs), insufficient energy of the photons (kV), or a combination of both. **In the digital system, underexposure can be seen as grainy or noisy due to insufficient photons reaching the detectors** (Figures 88 and 89).

252

Overexposure (Conventional Film, CR and DR)

An overexposed radiograph appears too dark and bones may or may not be visible. If the bones are visible and the unexposed parts of the film are white, the mAs should be halved. If the film is too black and the bones are indistinct, the kV should be reduced by 10–15% and the mAs halved (Figures 90 and 91).

In the digital system, overexposure is well tolerated and diagnostic quality radiographs can still be produced. In extreme overexposure, there is some detail visible, but areas of low density may be displayed as completely black without anatomical discernibility.

Underexposure and overexposure may be indicated by the exposure index on each radiograph; an optimal range should be provided by the manufacturer. **Increasing or decreasing the kV by 15% is a good starting point for correction of the exposure.**

Double Exposure (CR and DR)

This occurs when a radiographer accidentally takes multiple radiographs without erasing the cassette (Figures 92 and 93).

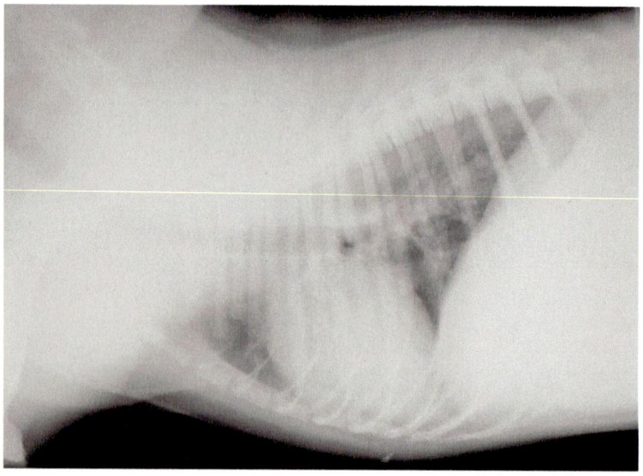

Figure 88. Underexposure (CR) of thoracic radiograph. Courtesy of Gawain Hammond.

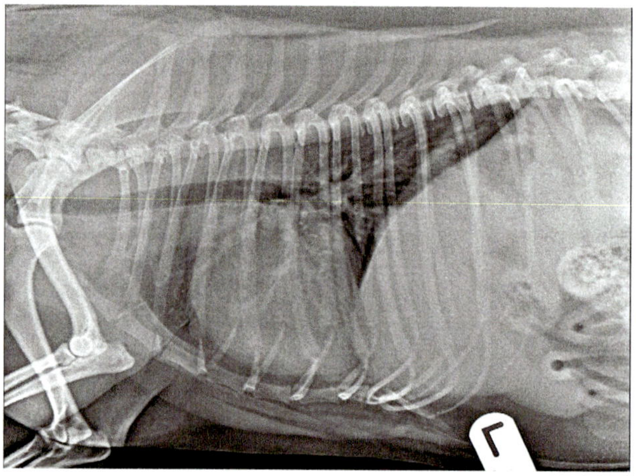

Figure 89. Thoracic radiograph (DR) demonstrating an underexposed radiograph. The radiograph is grainy, consistent with a quantum mottle artefact.

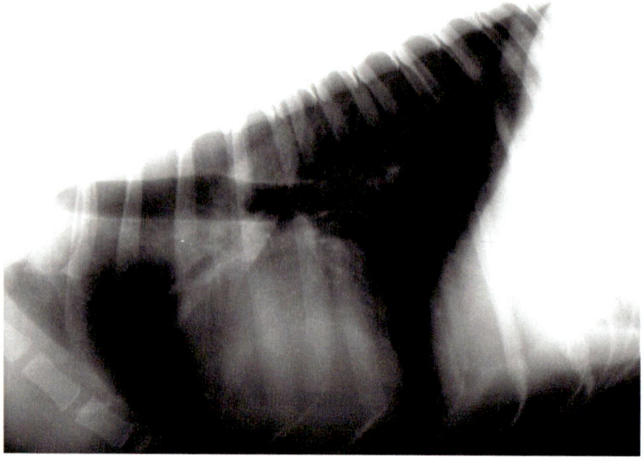

Figure 90. Overexposed thoracic radiograph (CR and DR). Courtesy of Gawain Hammond.

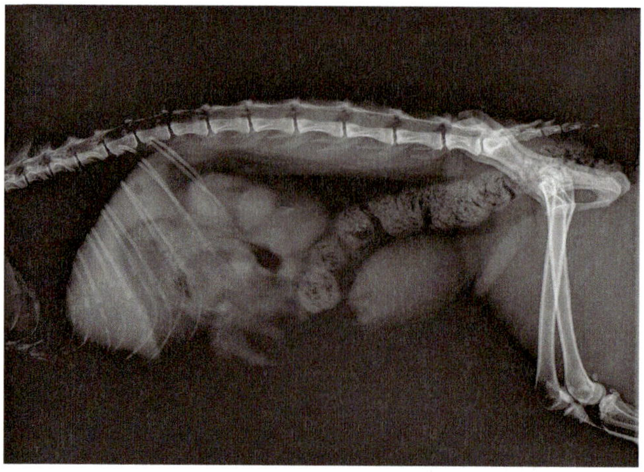

Figure 91. Overexposed abdominal radiograph (DR).

Uncollimated Images (CR and DR)

The image plate is sensitive to scatter radiation. **An uncollimated radiograph has increased fogging and decreased image quality.** Thus, the importance of collimating the area of interest.

Planking (DR)

Rectangular areas of different intensities due to variation in signal amplification as a result of high levels of exposure. Reduction of the exposure and recalibration of the plate detectors helps correct this artefact.

Upside Down Cassette (CR)

Exposure performed with the cassette upside down. A pattern consistent with the back of the cassette appears on the radiograph. The correct use and orientation of the cassette corrects this artefact.

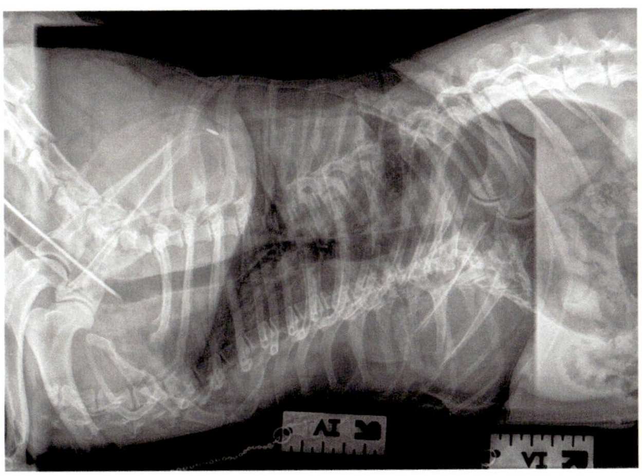

Figure 92. Double exposure artefact. Courtesy of Gawain Hammond.

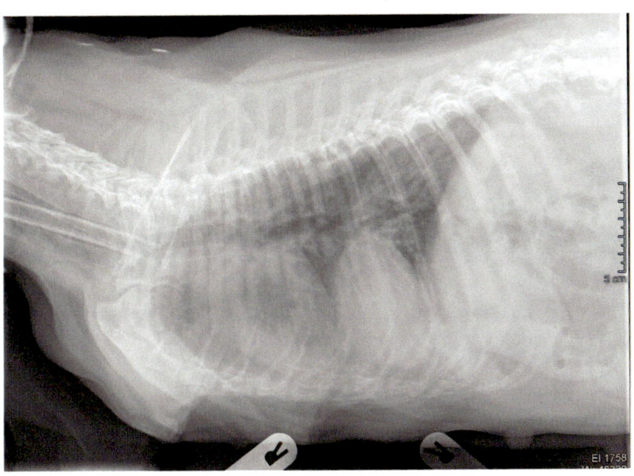

Figure 93. Double exposure artefact. Courtesy of Naomi Earley.

Motion Artefact (CR and DR)

When there is **movement of the patient, cassette or tube moves during the exposure creating a blurry image** (Figure 94). The patient's breathing contributes to this artefact, therefore reducing exposure time as well as proper patient positioning/restraint are essential to minimise this artefact.

Dirt Artefact (CR and DR)

This is a common CR system artefact and results from dirty plates/cassettes and cassette reader. These appear as white marks (focal white spots or linear white marks) which are visible in multiple radiographs (Figures 95 and 96).

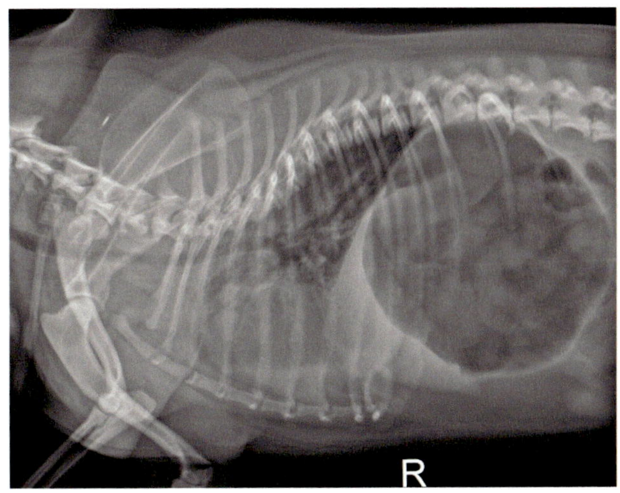

Figure 94. Thoracic radiograph with motion artefact. Courtesy of Naomi Earley.

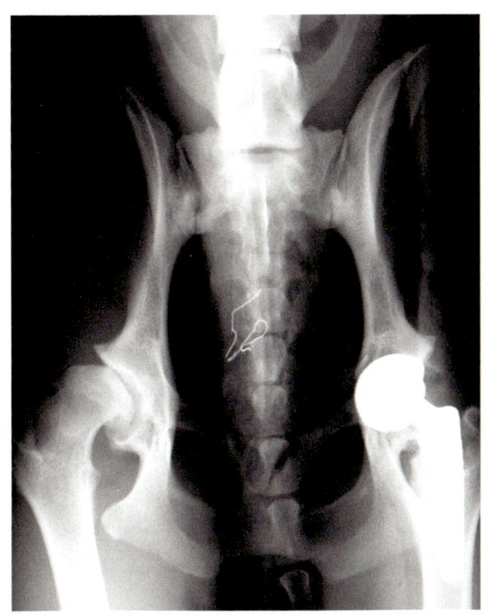

Figure 95. Dirt artefact. Pelvis radiograph with a thread on the screen. Courtesy of Gawain Hammond.

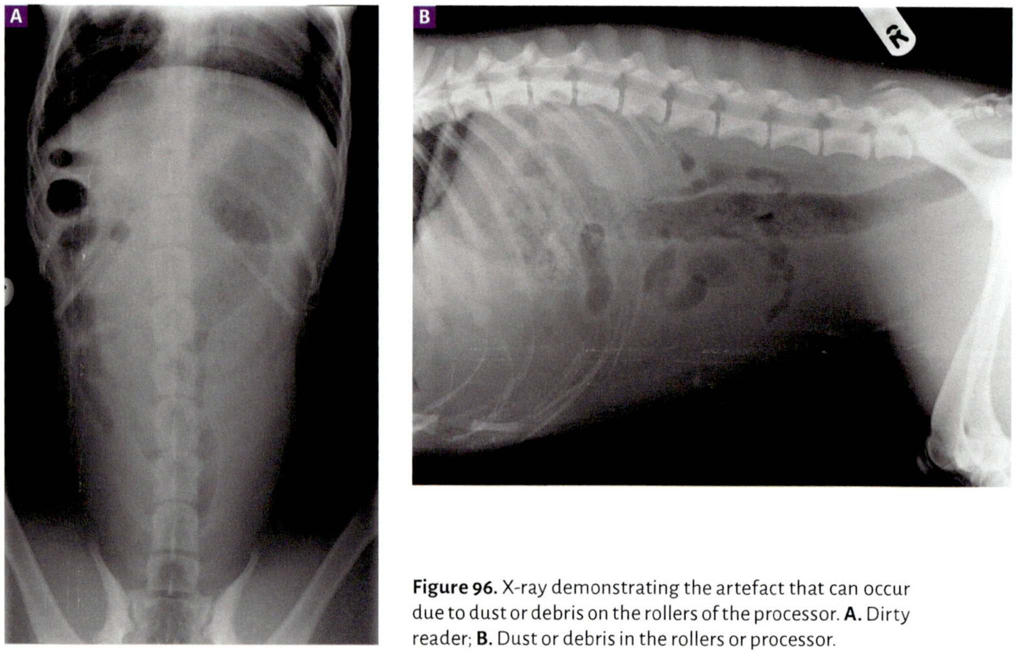

Figure 96. X-ray demonstrating the artefact that can occur due to dust or debris on the rollers of the processor. **A.** Dirty reader; **B.** Dust or debris in the rollers or processor.

All imaging plates/cassettes should be handled with care and stored away from heat, humidity, and any source of radiation. The radiographic readers should be kept clean as per the manufacturer's guidance.

Backscatter (Conventional Film and CR)

Conventional cassettes and CR imaging plates are more sensitive to scatter. This can occur due to incorrect collimation and the X-ray reaching a distant object and returning to expose the imaging plate. Backscatter can increase with increased object thickness, field of view, and kV peak. Correction of backscatter is made by using correct exposure times and appropriate collimation.

Postexposure Artefacts

Moire Artefact (CR and DR)

This artefact consists of parallel lines of increased attenuation corresponding to the grid's line density. This occurs because the X-ray beam is not perpendicular to the grid/plate (Figure 97 and 98). Correction of this artefact is made by aligning the X-ray beam and grid, by using an oscillating Potter-Bucky grid or choosing a grid with more than 180 lines per inch.

Überschwinger Artefact (CR and DR)

This is also called **halo artefact or rebound effect,** and results from an imaging processing error (Figure 99). It occurs most frequently between two objects of major difference in density and is most often present at the edge of metallic orthopaedic implants. It can mimic a low grade implant infection or implant loosening. This artefact cannot completely be avoided, however, the software settings can be adjusted to reduce the artefact.

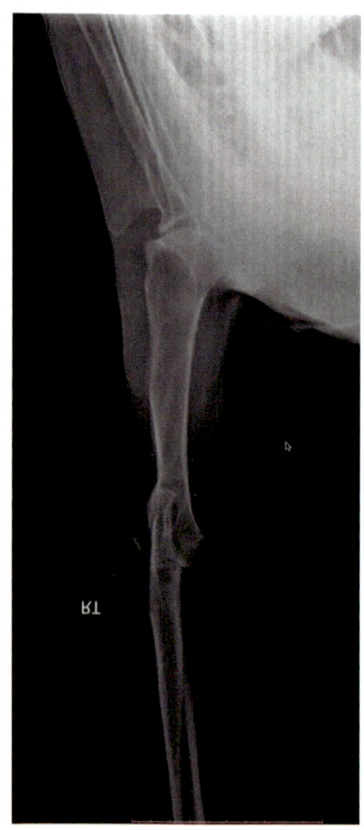

Figure 97. Moire artefact. Note the parallel grid lines. Courtesy of Naomi Earley.

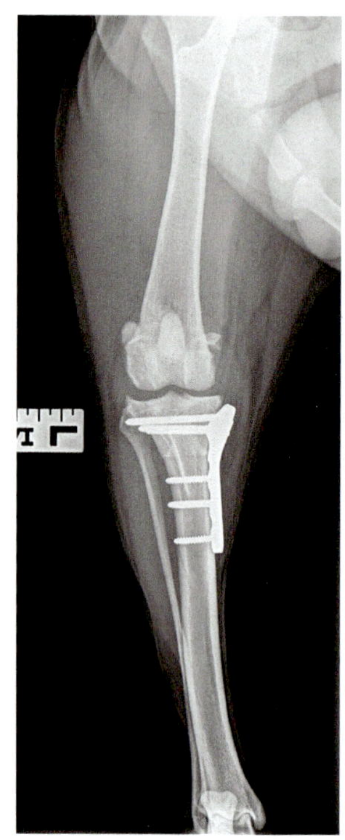

Figure 99. Überschwinger artefact around the screws.

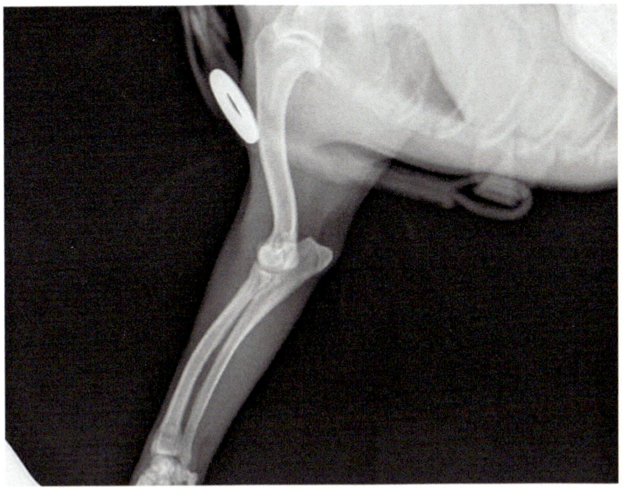

Figure 98. Moire artefact. Note the parallel grid lines. Courtesy of Gawain Hammond.

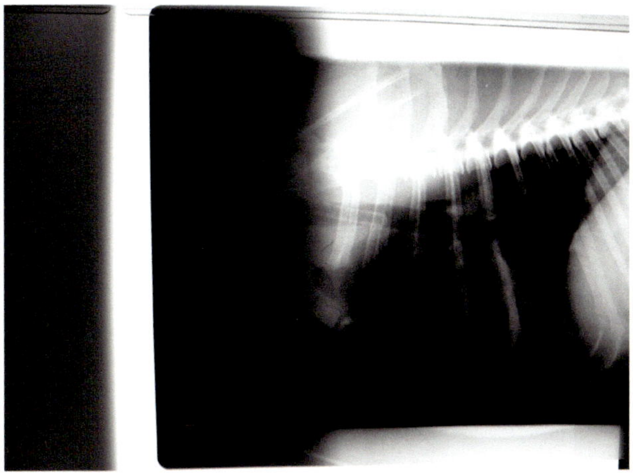

Figure 101. A light leak artefact where the X-ray film has been exposed to light, this is due to improper handling and/or storage. The entire film will be black if completely exposed. Image courtesy of Gawain Hammond.

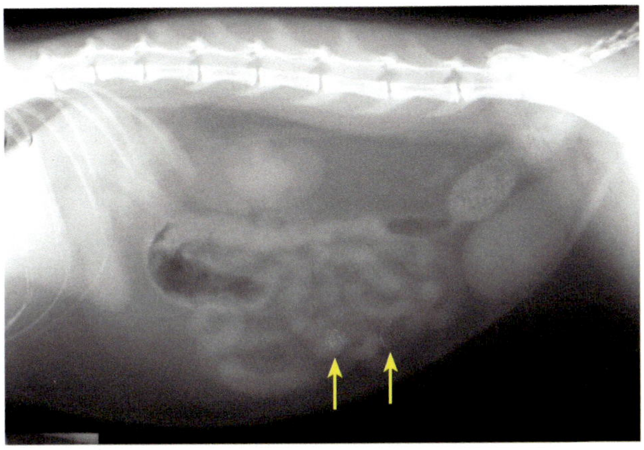

Figure 100. Fingerprint marks on the X-ray film due to improper handling (yellow arrows). Image courtesy of Gawain Hammond.

Conventional Film Artefacts

Conventional film radiography has been largely superseded by CR and DR modalities, therefore many of the artefacts seen with conventional film no longer occur (Figures 100 and 101).

Other conventional film artefacts include:

- white film (too light): underdevelopment
- crescent shaped black lines: fingernail pressure on film or crimp marks form careless handling of the film
- dark or black patches: fixer splashed onto film prior to developing (unprocessed film)
- pale patches: dried splashes of liquid on the intensifying screen, splashes of water or fixer prior to developing.

Point of Care Ultrasound (POCUS)

Veterinary POCUS includes focused assessment sonography for trauma (FAST) ultrasound examination. FAST examination involves the abdominal FAST (AFAST) and thoracic FAST (TFAST).

The objectives of the POCUS and FAST examination are to:

- assess the patient and obtain a rapid answer
- create a problem list
- establish a diagnostic plan
- assist the decision of whether the case is surgical or non-surgical or if it requires additional investigation.

POCUS is a rapid, noninvasive, safe, portable technique which can be repeated even in the unstable patient.

FAST examination is very sensitive and specific at detecting free abdominal fluid and has a high sensitivity and specificity even when performed by no radiologist.

AFAST was developed to target organs and a fluid scoring system and TFAST for pneumothorax, pleural, pericardial effusion, and echo views for cardiac abnormalities; and more recently Vet BLUE (veterinary brief lung ultrasound exam). A basic understanding of ultrasound and, ultrasound artefacts are necessary to perform the examination and understand the findings.

There are multiple indications for the use of POCUS in veterinary patients.

Indications

- all blunt and penetrating trauma
- all anaemic cases
- collapsed cases
- cases of unexplained hypotension, tachycardia, altered mentation
- acutely unwell or unstable patients
- respiratory distress
- acute abdomen or abdominal pain
- postop patient (dehiscence, haemorrhage, infection)
- suspicion of coagulopathy
- suspicion of pleural or peritoneal effusion or pneumothorax
- urinary bladder volume estimation
- other: ileus, pyometra, congestive heart failure, anaphylaxis, patients which are "not quite right" etc.

Equipment

- portable ultrasound (Figure 102)
- small footprint transducer (microconvex)
- frequency (5–10 MHz) with a maximum depth of 12–15 cm

Hair is generally not clipped but parted for the best probe skin contact and/or alcohol based hand sanitiser used as an acoustic coupling agent. Ultrasound gel may be used to enhance the image (Figure 103), but it is important to ensure no air bubbles are trapped between the gel, the coat and the transducer. Alcohol based hand sanitiser has the benefit of being easily wiped off and evaporates quickly compared to isopropyl alcohol. Also, isopropyl alcohol may cause damage to the head of the transducer.

Basic Echogenicities

Hyperechoic: returning sound waves with increased amplitude and appears brighter than the surrounding tissue.

Echogenic: returning sound wases produce grey scale pixel.

Isoechoic: returning sound of similar amplitude and appears equal on greys scale.

Hypoechoic: returning sound with decreased amplitude and appears darker than the surrounding tissue.

Anaechoic: complete absence of returning sound wases. Black.

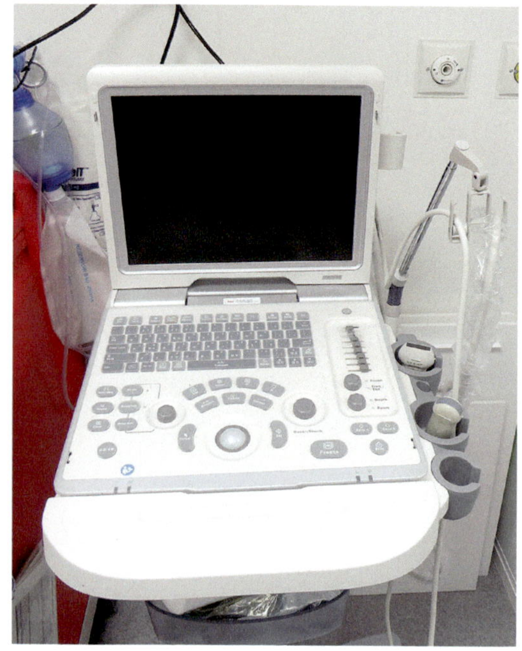

Figure 102. Portable ultrasound machine and transducers.

AFAST (Abdominal Focused Assessment for Trauma)

The AFAST examination involves visualizing the diaphragm, liver, gallbladder, spleen, kidneys, intestinal loops, and urinary bladder for **the detection of free fluid.** Free fluid is anechoic (black) when visualised on ultrasound but depending on the nature of the fluid it may be more or less echogenic. Fluid tends to collect in the most dependent areas as triangles surrounded by organs.

Patient Position

- right lateral recumbency is the preferred position for examination;
- modified lateral sternal recumbency allows the forelimbs to be sternal and the hindlimbs to be moved together laterally;
- standing/sternal;
- in respiratory compromised patients it is important to be aware that the fluid scoring system is not validated;
- dorsal recumbency should never be used as a position during examination. N.B. fluid will move under gravity so diagnosing free fluid is more challenging in dorsal recumbency.

Technique

The transducer is placed longitudinally at four locations with the mark towards the head of the patient. Using different transducer movements such as rocking, rotation, sliding and fanning promotes better visualisation of organs and areas of interest.

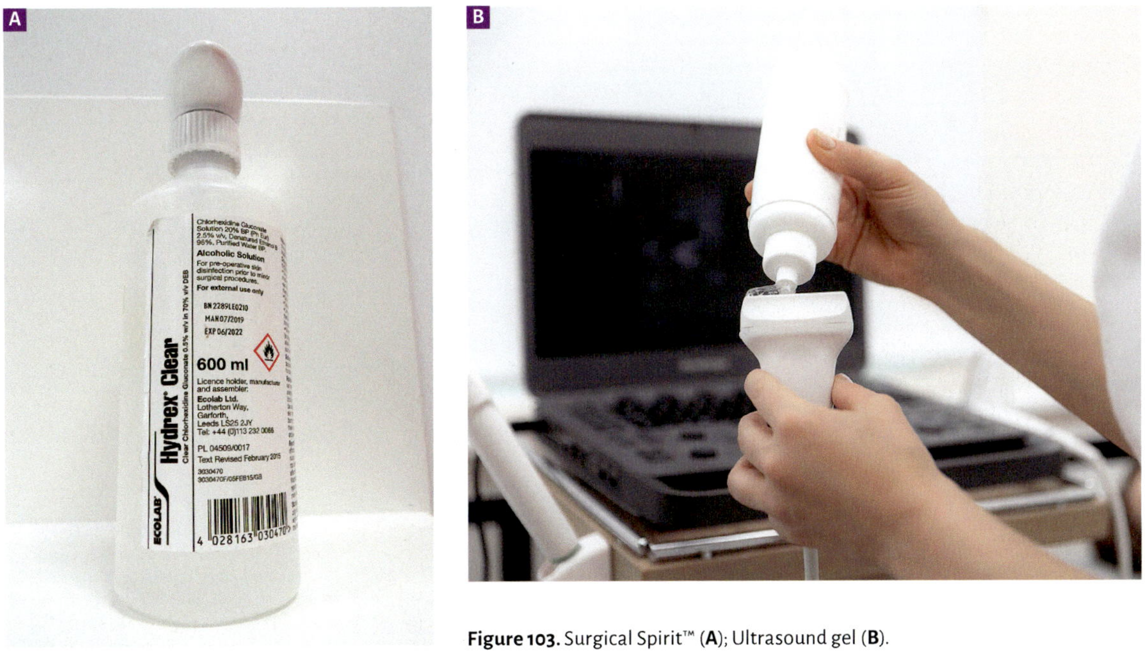

Figure 103. Surgical Spirit™ (**A**); Ultrasound gel (**B**).

The examination is evaluated in a clockwise rotation, from the subxiphoid region, to the nongravity dependent flank, to the bladder, to the gravity dependent flank.

AFAST can be performed with limited scanning planes (Figure 104). At each site, the transducer can be moved a few centimetres in several directions and fanned through an angle of 45° until target organs are identified. Scanning organs in two different planes at a 90° angle to each other (longitudinal and transverse) may be necessary to confirm the presence of free fluid.

The AFAST examination consists of four points which should be scanned. Four windows:

- **DH: diaphragmatico hepatic**
- **SR: splenorenal**
- **CC: cystocolic**
- **HR: hepatorenal.**

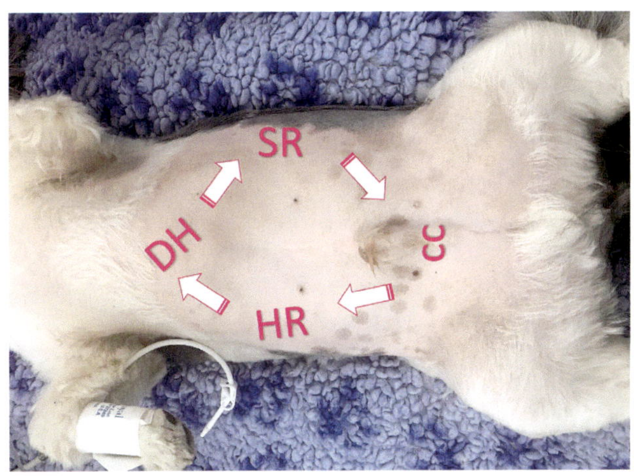

Figure 104. Dog AFAST windows. Please note, the patient should be scanned in lateral recumbency and not dorsal.

Diaphragmatico Hepatic (DH) Window

The subxiphoid view should be used to evaluate the hepato diaphragmatic interface, gallbladder region, pericardial sac, and pleural spaces. The purpose of the DH view is to have a general overview of the gallbladder, cardiac bump, and caudal vena cava:

- the transducer should be placed in the subxiphoid region and rocked cranially;
- the diaphragm is seen as a hyperechoic curvilinear interface;
- the hepatic parenchyma has a course echotexture;
- the transducer should be fanned left right following the diaphragm in a sagittal plane;
- the presence of any anechoic material between the liver and diaphragm or between the hepatic lobes should be identified.

Gallbladder Assessment

The gallbladder (GB) is positioned to the right of the midline between the right medial and quadrate hepatic lobe in the dog and between the right medial hepatic sublobes in cats (Figure 105).

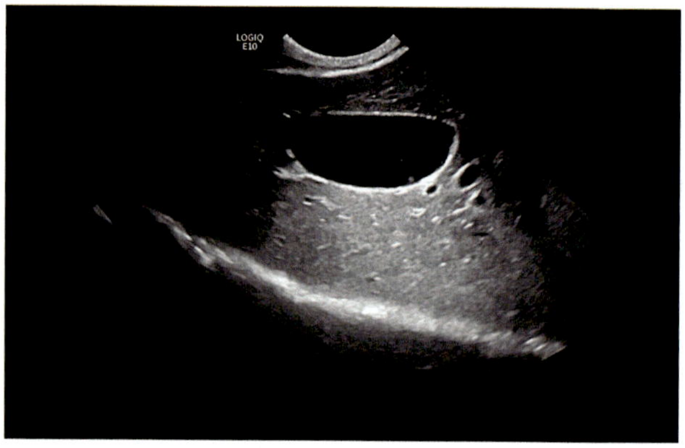

Figure 105. Ultrasound image of the liver and gallbladder.

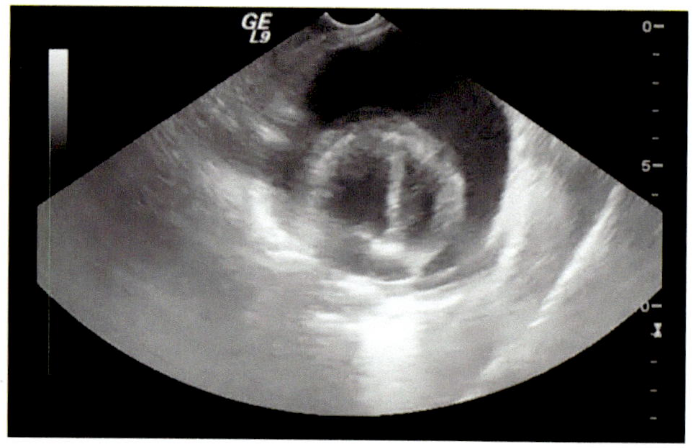

Figure 106. Transthoracic ultrasound demonstrating a pericardial effusion.

The GB appears as a thin walled, ovoid structure formed of anechoic material.

Abnormalities which may be identified include:

- gallbladder leakage, rupture, and peritonitis
- large volume of organized, nonmobile contents
- anechoic surrounding fluid
- hyperechoic adjacent fat (steatitis).

Pericardial Assessment

Pericardial effusion (Figure 106) is seen as anechoic fluid surrounding the cardiac apex surrounded by an outer thin, echogenic interface consistent with the pericardium. Using this window alone, it may not be possible to differentiate between pericardial and pleural effusion; thus, a complete TFAST examination is warranted in dogs or cats when pleural or pericardial effusion is present or suspected.

Splenorenal (SR) Window

A left flank view is used to assess the splenorenal (SR) interface and areas between the spleen and body wall:

- the costal arch should be followed on the left flank caudal to the 13th rib and ventral to the lumbar hypaxial musculature interface between the spleen and the kidney (the kidneys are retroperitoneal and the spleen peritoneal);
- the transducer should be fanned dorsomedial and dorsolaterally to search for the left kidney;
- once identified the transducer should be used to fan through the kidney in both directions until the kidney disappears. Feline kidneys are mobile;
- with the kidney centred, the transducer can be rocked cranially to identify the spleen, which is then examined using the fanning movement. The head of the spleen is fixed to the fundus by the gastrosplenic ligament, and the rest is mobile;
- the presence of any fluid between and adjacent to the kidneys and spleen should be identified;
- when only small volumes are present it may be difficult to distinguish between peritoneal and retroperitoneal effusion.

Cystocolic (CC) Window

A midline bladder view to assess the apex of the bladder (Figures 107 and 108):

- the transducer should be placed caudally along the midline with the marker oriented cranially to create a long axis image;
- the normal urinary bladder is an ovoid structure containing anechoic material, surrounded by a thin echogenic wall with three discernible layers:
  - outer serosa layer (hyperechoic)
  - three smooth muscle layers (hypoechoic)
  - lamina propria submucosal layer (hyperechoic), which parallels the inner mucosal layer (hypoechoic).

The colon is located dorsally to the bladder and generally contains gas and faecal material, which may generate reverberation and distal acoustic shadowing artefacts (clean or dirty shadowing).

Another artefact to watch for is the edge shadowing artefact (pseudo urinary bladder rupture). This is created when the ultrasound wave strikes the edge of a fluid filled structure with a curved surface. Ultrasound waves are reflected to a certain degree and these reflected sound waves do not reach the transducer. As a result, a thin hypoechoic to anechoic area is created lateral and distal to the to the edge of the curved surface (Figure 109). If there is true rupture of the urinary bladder it will be collapsed.

Hepatorenal (HR) Window

A right flank view for assessment of the hepatorenal (HR) interface and the areas between intestinal loops, the right kidney, and the body wall (Figure 110):

- the transducer should be placed under and caudal to the right 13th rib, ventral to the lumbar hypaxial musculature;

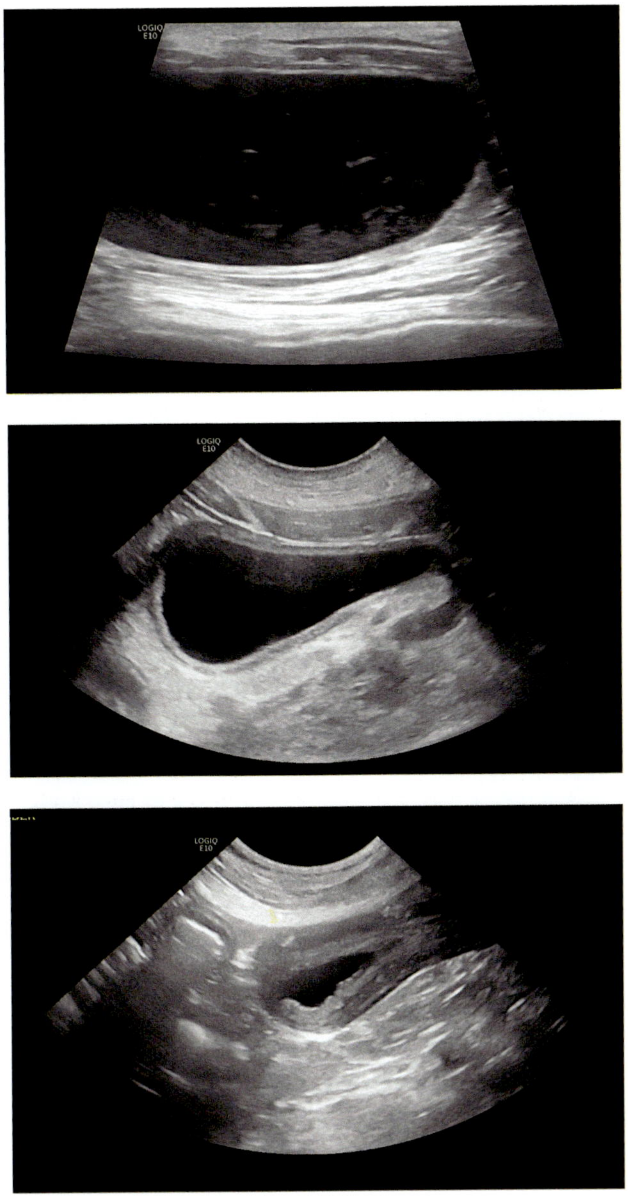

Figure 107. Ultrasound images of the bladder with a variable lumen from full to empty.

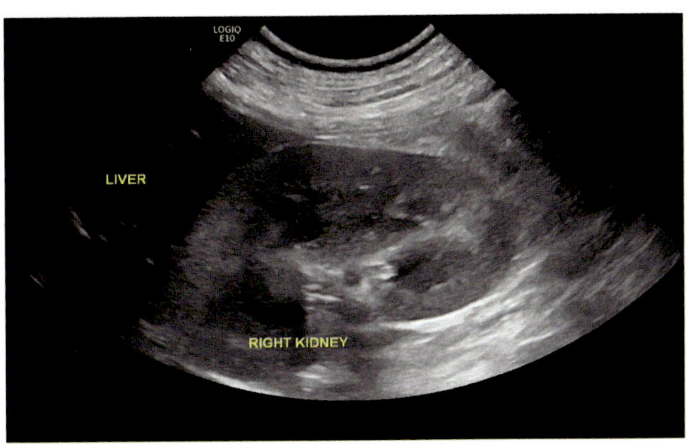

Figure 110. Ultrasound image of the liver and the right kidney.

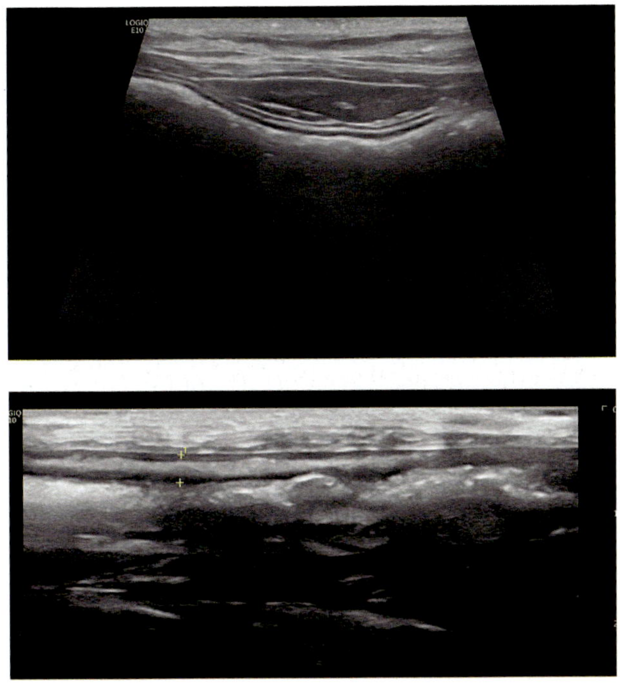

Figure 108. Ultrasound images demonstrating a full colon with faecal content and an empty colon.

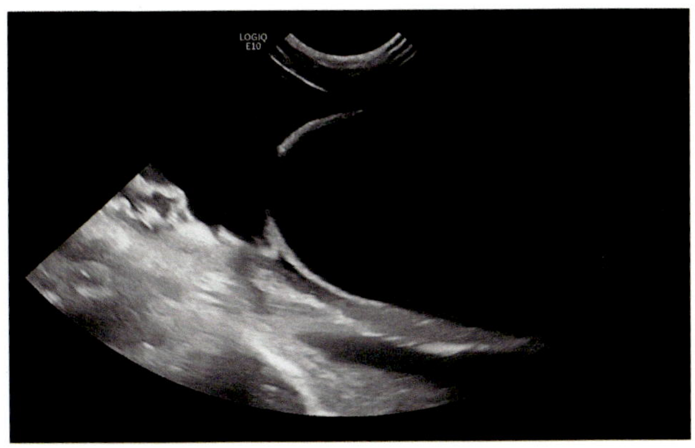

Figure 109. Edge shadow artefact. A refractive artefact that occurs at the edge of a large, curved boundary with a different speed of sound than that of the surrounding tissues. This image demonstrates a discontinuation of the cranial aspect of the bladder wall consistent with the edge shadow artefact.

- the right kidney is located within the renal fossa of the caudate hepatic lobe in dogs;
- in cats it is often surrounded by retroperitoneal fat;
- the right kidney is generally in a more cranial position compared to the left kidney;
- in large breed or deep chested dogs, use of a right dorsal intercostal window between the 11th or 12th intercostal space may be necessary to visualize the kidney;
- anechoic material between the hepatic parenchyma and the kidney may represent retroperitoneal or peritoneal effusion.

Fluid Scoring System

The AFAST applied fluid scoring system is a 4 point scan developed for semiquantification of effusion volume (Figure 111). Abdominal fluid scoring (AFS) follows the below grading system:

- an AFS of 1 is defined as positive in any AFAST view;
- an AFS of 2 is positives in any two views;
- an AFS of 3 is positive in any three views;
- an AFS of 4 (maximum) is positive in all views.

AFS in a bleeding patient:

- AFS 1–2 is characterised by small volume bleeding;
- AFS 3–4 is characterised by large volume bleeding.

A modification of the abdominal fluid scoring system, using maximum dimensions, was developed to better differentiate between small and large volume bleeding. The modified version includes scores 0, ½, and 1. The measurement approach categorises positives as ½ and 1 dependent on the maximum dimensions in each AFAST view.

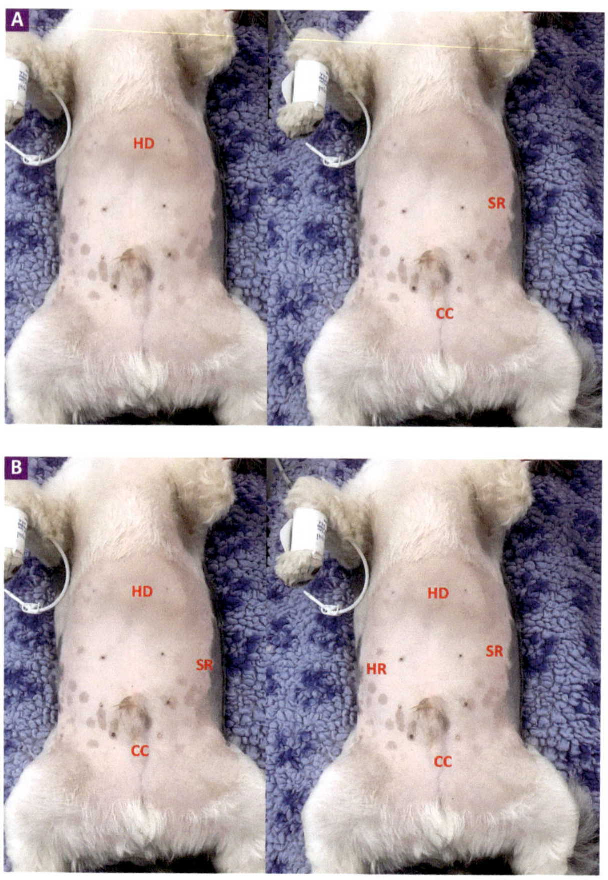

Figure 111. Image illustrating the different grading for abdominal fluid score. AFS 1–2 (**A**) and AFS 3–4 (**B**).

The suggestive classification is based under-over 1 cm (10 mm) in dogs and 0.5 cm (5 mm) in cats. If the volume of fluid measures less or equal to 1 cm (dog) and 0.5 cm (cat), it is scored as ½ and if it is above 1 cm (dog) and 0.5 cm (cat) is scored as 1. The small volume and large volume bleeder principles stay the same. However, the addition of the ½ helps to better semi quantify and categorise the bleeding in dogs and cats.

The modified fluid scoring can also be applied to nonhaemorrhagic effusion. Clinical judgment and patient clinical presentation should also be considered alongside the fluid scoring system.

Serial AFAST with assigned AFS is used to monitor gradual changes before the patient decompensates and small volume turns into large volume, or to monitor ongoing or resolution of haemorrhage or peritoneal effusion. Serial AFAST examinations should be performed every four hours, or more frequently if clinical findings deteriorate.

Urinary Bladder Volume

The CC window can be used for estimating urinary bladder volume in cats and dogs. The urinary bladder estimation formula provides a noninvasive method which is performed during AFAST (Figure 112).

Length x width x height x 0.2 π =
estimated urinary bladder volume (ml)

The volume is calculated over a certain time to estimate urine output (UOP). Urine output (ml/kg/hr) can provide important clinical information for patients receiving IV fluid therapy and reflects kidney function when placed in a clinical context.

Caudal Vena Cava (CVC) Volume (Dogs)

Assessment of intravascular volume status is crucial in the management of critical dogs. The dog should be placed in left lateral recumbency on a standard examination table with ECG pads. Care is needed to avoid collapsing the CVC by excessive pressure on the ultrasound transducer. Three views of the CVC are obtained for volume calculation.

Subxiphoid View

The transducer is placed longitudinally under the subxiphoid process and angled cranially to visualize the diaphragm.

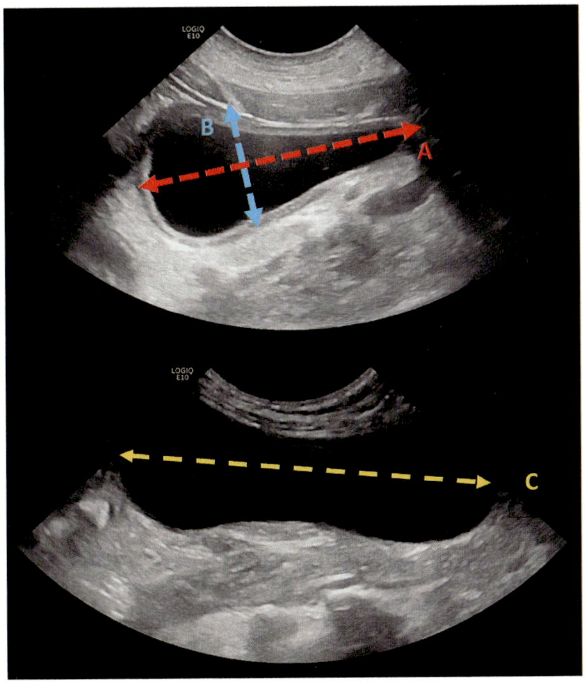

Figure 112. Bladder volume measurements. A: length, B: height, C: width. Ultrasound image of the urinary bladder from the cystocolic view with measurement of the maximal length and height in the longitudinal (sagittal) plane and the maximal width in a transverse orientation.

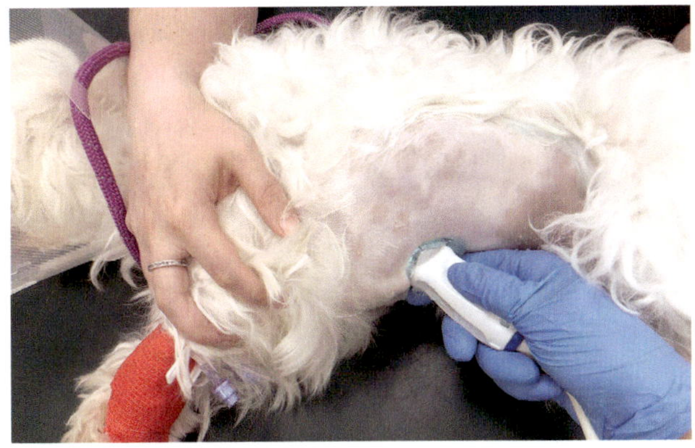

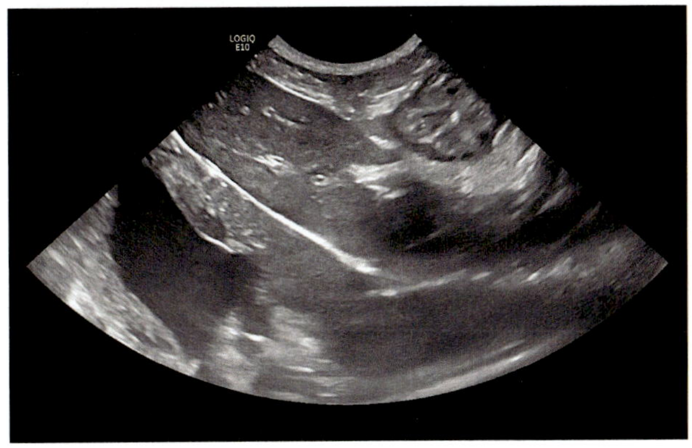

Figure 113. Visualisation of diaphragm using subxiphoid view.

The ultrasound transducer is fanned to the right of midline without excessive pressure until the CVC is identified at the point it crosses the diaphragm. The ultrasound transducer should then be fanned or rotated to obtain the optimal view, where the CVC has a maximal diameter. Maximal diameter of the CVC is seen during expiration. Measurements should be taken where the ventral wall of the CVC crosses the diaphragm perpendicular to its dorsal wall (Figure 113).

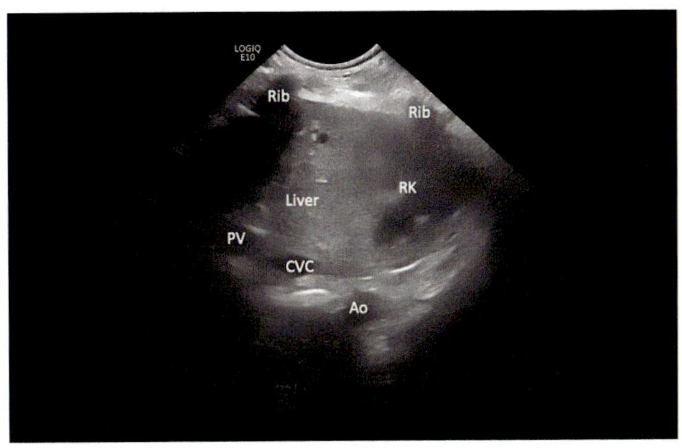

Figure 114. Intercostal view. PV: portal vein; CVC: cauda vena cava; Ao: aorta; RK: right kidney.

Paralumbar View

To obtain this view, the transducer should be placed with the marker pointing cranially and under the last rib, allowing visualization of the right kidney in a longitudinal view. The transducer should then be fanned or moved dorsomedially until the CVC and aorta are identified in a longitudinal cross section.

Intercostal View

The transducer should be placed parallel to the ribs in the upper third of the thorax below the epaxial muscles in the 10th–12th right intercostal space (Figure 114). If aerated lung is encountered, the transducer should be angled caudally or moved one intercostal space more caudally or dorsally over the epaxial muscles and slowly slid ventrally between the ribs until the porta hepatis is identified.

A transverse image of the porta hepatis should then be obtained, where three rounded anechoic structures are seen (portal vein, CVC, and aorta).

The size of the CVC is calculated with measurements in short and long axis using B mode. The maximal CVC area on expiration and the minimal CVC on inspiration are then estimated using the below ellipsoid formula:

$$\pi \times [(\text{CVC short-axis})/2] \times [(\text{CVC long-axis})/2]$$

TFAST (Thoracic Focused Assessment for Trauma) and VetBLUE

This is a useful technique when patients are too unstable for standard radiographs.

Patient Position

- standing or sternal recumbency is recommended;
- right lateral recumbency;
- modified lateral sternal recumbency which allows the patient to ventilate more efficiently when in respiratory distress.

TFAST examination consists of five points or windows which should be scanned (Figure 115):

- CTS: chest tube site (bilaterally)
- PCS: pericardial site (bilaterally)
- DH: diaphragmatico hepatic.

The CTS is best used to exclude pneumothorax and to assess lung pathology, whereas the PCS view is used to detect the presence of pleural and pericardial fluid. Additionally, the right PCS view is used for assessment of the aortic/left atrial ratio. The DH view can be advantageous over the PCS views because of the acoustic window into the pleural and pericardial spaces.

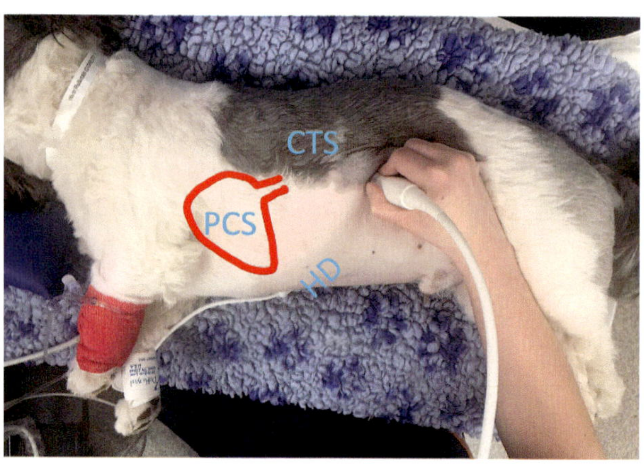

Figure 115. TFAST windows.

The ribs are seen as curved hyperechoic interphases causing marked distal acoustic shadowing. The orientation for the lung ultrasound is known as the gator sign (Figure 116). **The normal motion of the lung sliding along the thoracic wall is called the glide sign** (also known as the sliding sign).

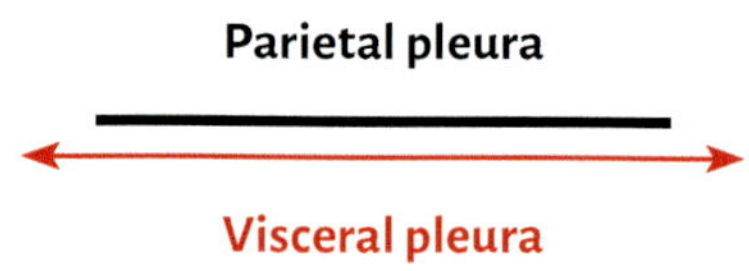

The gliding sign is the to and from respirophasic movement of the parietal and visceral pleura over one and another.

The pulmonary pleural interface (PP line) is not to be confused with the distally positioned equidistant reverberation artefacts or A-lines (air reverberation artefact) which are parallel and extend from the PP line (Figures 117–119).

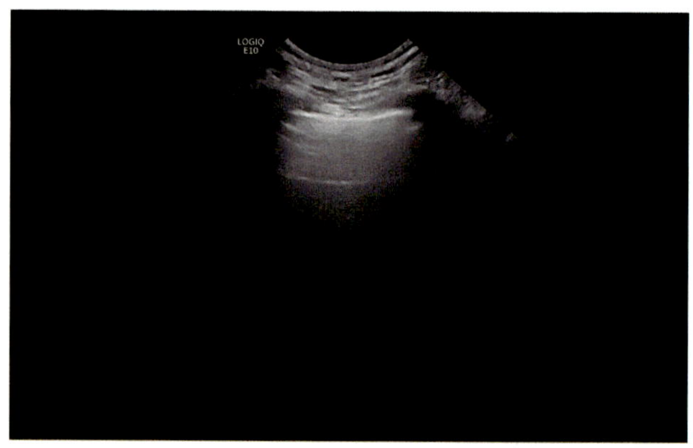

Figure 116. Ultrasound image of the gator sign.

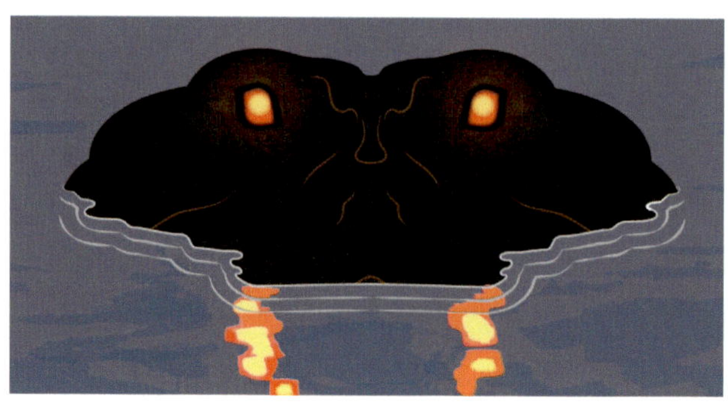

Figure 117. The rounded rib heads seen on the ultrasound are comparable to the eyes of an alligator at night, and the pulmonary-pleural (PP-line) interface to the bridge of its nose (see Figure 116).

A-lines are air reverberation (A stands for air). These are equidistant horizontal lines parallel to the intercostal space extending from the reflective lung surface, which repeat themselves and their equidistant spacing through the distant field.

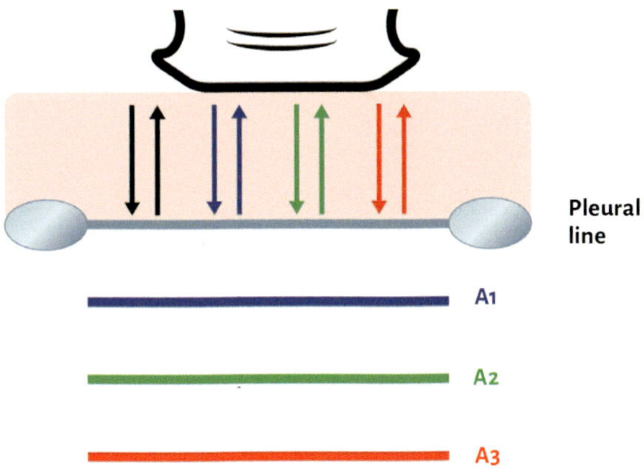

Figure 118. Formation of A-lines.

B-lines are also known as lung rocket, ring down artefacts, and comet tail artefacts (Figures 120 and 121). B-lines are artefacts caused by the high impedance gradient created when there is a fluid air interface which occurs when there are fluid filled alveoli surrounded by air. These appear on ultrasound as hazy hyperechoic discrete narrow based vertical bands that extend from the PP interface to the far aspect of the screen becoming gradually wider, without fading, extending through the distant field eliminating the A-lines. This artefact moves synchronously with the breathing.

Ultrasound is not transmitted through aerated lung and the presence of ultrasound lung rockets (wet lung artefact) primarily represent forms of interstitial pathology.

Some B-lines can be seen in in normal animals. They are only considered pathological if >3 lines are seen in any single view. **The number of B-lines are associated with severity.**

The presence of the glide sign or the presence of rock lines/B-lines excludes pneumothorax. The highest point on the thorax should be scanned to rule out pneumothorax (Figure 119).

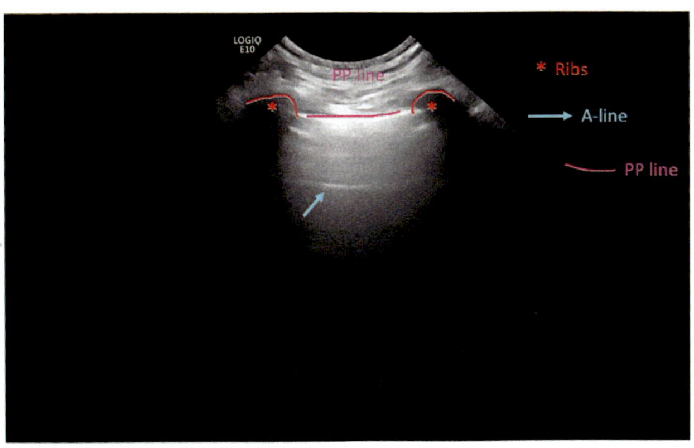

Figure 119. Image showing the "gator sign" demonstrating some A-lines.

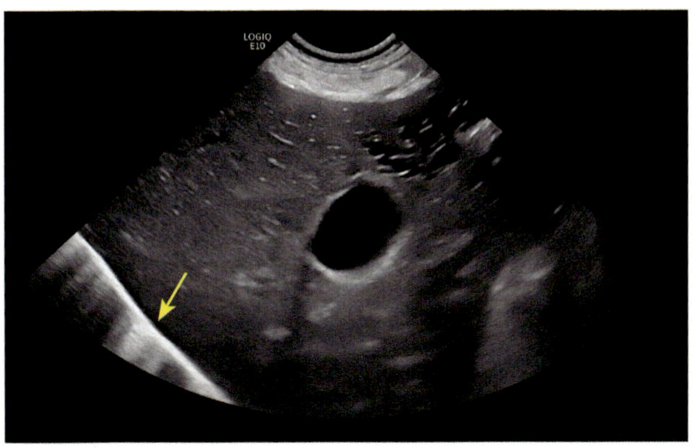

Figure 121. Transabdominal ultrasound image of the liver with some visible B-lines at the diaphragmatic line (yellow arrow) in a dog that had pulmonary metastasis.

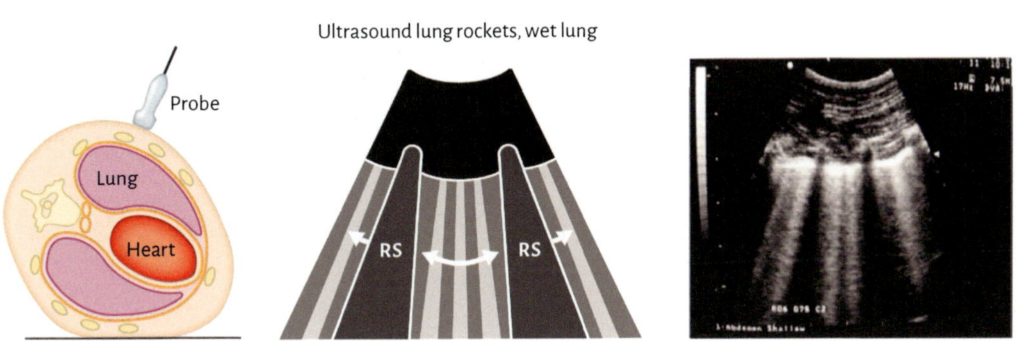

Figure 120. B-lines. Illustration inspired on Boysen & Lisciandro (2013).

Pneumothorax: Partial versus Massive

The degree of pneumothorax is subjectively determined by identifying the location where collapsed lung/lung recontacts the thoracic wall, the so called lung point. To find the lung point several intercostal spaces must be scanned from dorsal to ventral until either the gliding sign or rocket lines are detected. (Figure 122).

The distance from the CTS to the lung point may be used to subjectively assess the degree and progression of the pneumothorax (Figure 123).

Pleural and Pericardial Effusion

PCS views are gravity dependent and used for detecting either type of effusion. The DH view is the most sensitive view because the acoustic window allows visualisation of the pleural and pericardial spaces (Figure 124). Obtaining multiple views provides a more accurate assessment, while lowering the probability of mistaking normal structures for pathology.

The PCS should be assessed between the 5th–6th intercostal space. The transducer should be placed on the ventrolateral thoracic wall between the 5th and 6th rib space.

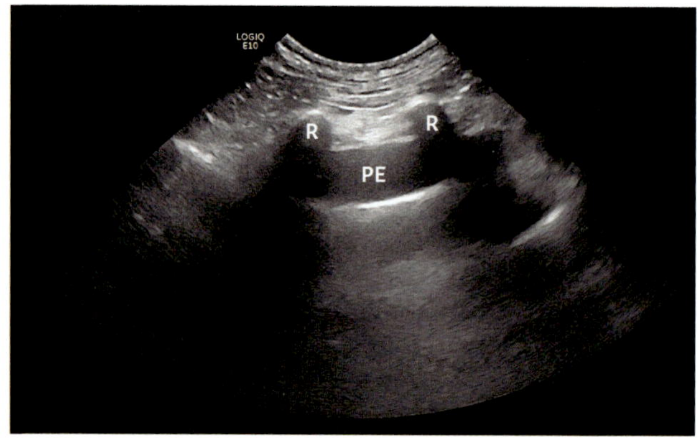

Figure 124. Transthoracic ultrasound image demonstrating a mild pleural effusion. PE: pleural effusion; R: rib.

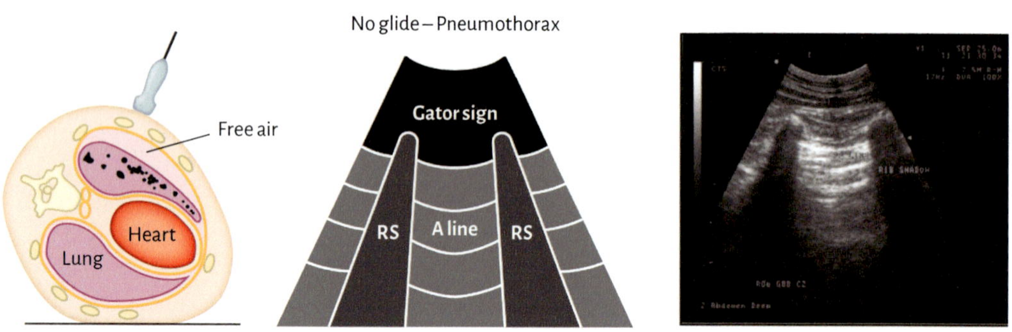

Figure 122. Pneumothorax ultrasound. Illustration inspired on Boysen & Lisciandro (2013).

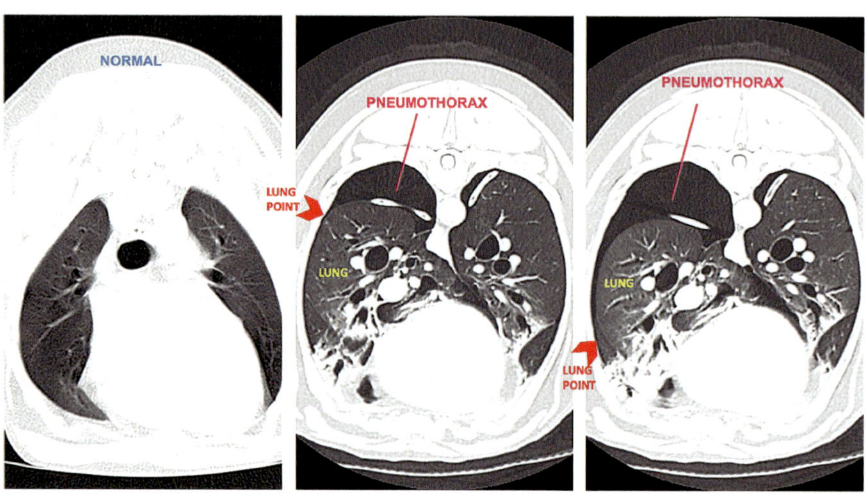

Figure 123. Computed tomography images of the thorax of a normal dog and a dog with a spontaneous pneumothorax (lung window). The red arrows demonstrate the "lung point". Note that in the last image the lung point is very low to nearly nonexistent suggesting progression of the pneumothorax. There is an absence of the gliding sign where the pneumothorax is localised.

Features to look for include:

- absence of normal parenchyma: PP lines
- anechoic/echogenic fluid between the costal wall and lung or heart
- pulmonary atelectasis secondary to pleural effusion, and the collapsed lung parenchyma may look like liver
- hypoechoic/echogenic structures seen floating within the effusion.

The pericardium appears as a thin hyperechoic/echogenic curvilinear wall, maintaining the fluid around the heart. Pericardial effusion consists of fluid surrounding the entire heart contained by the pericardium. The fluid can be anechoic or echogenic. When there is a cardiac tamponade, collapse of the right side of the heart can be appreciated (Figure 125).

Cardiac Tamponade

- elevated intrapericardial pressure within pericardial sac;
- pericardial pressure exceeds intracardiac pressure leading to collapse or inward motion of the right ventricular and right atrial free wall throughout the cardiac cycle; and
- pericardiocentesis is indicated if the animal is haemodynamically unstable.

Vet BLUE

Vet BLUE is a rapid point of care lung ultrasound used in the evaluation of patients in respiratory distress or respiratory compromise. It is based on the concept of wet lung vs dry lung. Vet corresponds to veterinary and BLUE to either cyanosis or bedside lung ultrasound exam or in-an-emergency. **Ultrasound lung rockets or B-lines are infrequently detected in cats and dogs without respiratory disease** and when present, are found in small numbers (1–2).

The use of Vet BLUE is handy for small animal practitioners, because it can be used in unstable patients or when there is a lack of technical radiographic support. If there is a lack or inability to use radiographic techniques, clinical decisions are often made based on the patient history, physical examination, and evaluation/characterisation of the breathing pattern.

Adding Vet BLUE as an extension of TFAST provides additional information in the diagnosis of lung conditions and guides in the treatment decision for the patient.

Advantages:

- rapid scan
- minimal restraint
- radiation sparing
- monitoring by serial examinations.

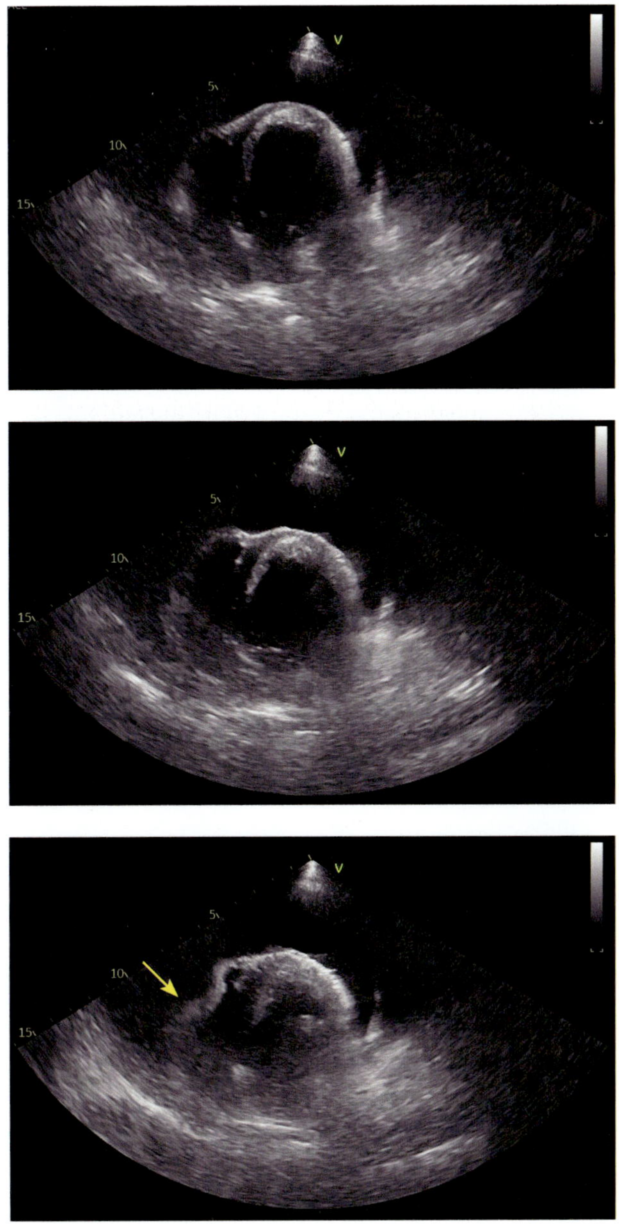

Figure 125. Transthoracic ultrasound demonstrating a pericardial effusion causing cardiac tamponade. The yellow arrow shows collapse of the right side of the heart.

Limitations:

- does not provide a definitive diagnosis;
- lung conditions must reach peripheral anatomy;
- cannot detect lung pathology deep within the lung. These lesions are missed because ultrasound cannot penetrate or image through aerated lung;
- cannot replace X-rays or CT but can be used as an adjunctive diagnostic aid.

Technique

Examination of the acoustic windows (Figure 126) are usually performed from dorsal to ventral and cranial:

Left Cd → Left Ph → Left Md → Left Cr → DH →
Right Cd → Right Ph → Right Md → Right Cr

Starting dorsally allows the presence of a pneumothorax to be ruled out and allows detection of the lung point.

Nine acoustic windows (five views, of which four are bilateral):

- caudodorsal (Cd) lung region, right and left:
  - 9–10th intercoastal space, near the highest point over the pleural cavity with the lung
- perihilar (Ph) lung region, right and left:
  - 6–7th intercostal space, perihilar region on a radiograph
- middle (Md) lung region, right and left:
  - 4–5th intercostal space, lower half of the thorax
- cranial (Cr) lung region, right and left:
  - 1–3rd intercostal space, region caudal to the thoracic inlet and cranial to the heart
- diaphragmatic hepatic (DH) view from the AFAST examination.

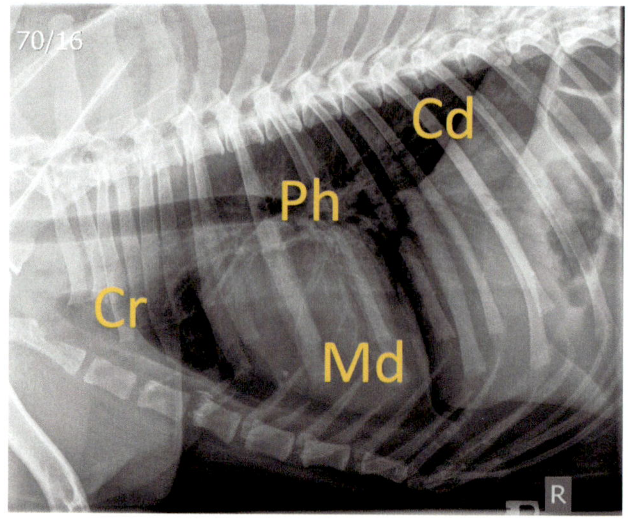

Figure 126. Vet BLUE acoustic windows. Cr: cranial; Ph: perihilar; Cd: caudodorsal; Md: middle.

Terminology

- Dry lung: normal aerated lung surface, A-lines with lung gliding sign. Dry lung is a feature seen with pneumothorax where A-lines are visible but there is an absence of the lung gliding sign.
- Wet lung: alveolointerstitial syndrome, B-lines. There are other causes of wet lung but these are far less common (i.e. pleural thickening from pleural fibrosis).
- Shred sign: air bronchogram. Lung consolidation with hyperechoic foci (air).
- Tissue sign: hepatization. Consolidation more severe than the shred sign without any aeration, thus has the appearance of liver.
- Nodule/mass sign: nodule or mass (mass if >3 cm). Organised consolidation in a shape, oval, or circle which can represent neoplasia/metastasis, granulomatous, or infectious processes. The nodule is often anechoic/hypoechoic with a distant border that is hyperechoic with a pseudo B line.
- Wedge sign: infarct, pulmonary thromboembolism (PTE). This occurs after the shred sign. It has a triangular wedge shape representing lung surface infarction and vascular necrosis of the periphery of the lung.

Wet Lung vs Dry Lung

A-lines with the pulmonary gliding sign represent a dry lung at the surface. A-lines with no gliding sign indicate pneumothorax.

B-lines represent wet lung and are most common with alveolointerstitial oedema. B-lines are not specific in that they do not indicate what type of alveolointerstitial disease is present. Therefore, the presence of B-lines is commonly referred as alveolointerstitial syndrome.

Based on clinical history and Vet BLUE it should be possible to include or exclude:

- lung contusions in a trauma patient
- cardiogenic pulmonary oedema
- noncardiogenic pulmonary oedema.

Patients with left sided congestive heart failure (LCHF) typically manifest pulmonary oedema. Early stages or mild pulmonary oedema may be difficult to identify on radiographs or the patient might not tolerate being positioned for radiographs due to respiratory distress. Also, thoracic radiographs are associated with misinterpretation in patients with early stages of pulmonary oedema. However, point of care lung ultrasound is an effective tool for the diagnosis of LCHF in cats and dogs. In addition, it can be used to differentiate between cardiogenic pulmonary oedema and noncardiac pulmonary oedema (neurogenic causes, electrocution, choking or other causes such as drowning, acute lung injury and respiratory distress syndrome).

In healthy patients ultrasound lung rockets are infrequent and dry lung artefacts predominate. B-lines can be identified in normal healthy dogs (up to 11–31% of dogs with radiographically normal lungs). In these cases, there is a single B line and on most occasions this is confined to a single site or a single B line at two sites without respiratory disease. Based on the application of Vet BLUE in humans, the findings are only significant if there are three or more B-lines. On the other hand, numerous multifocal B-lines have been reported in cardiogenic pulmonary oedema, pneumonia, and pulmonary contusions in dogs and cats.

The presence and number of B-lines vary with mitral valve staging and whether pulmonary oedema is present. Dogs in stage B1 and B2 had absent or rare B-lines in the absence of pulmonary oedema. All dogs in stage C, without radiographic signs of pulmonary oedema, had absent or rare B-lines. Dogs in stage C, with radiographic signs of pulmonary oedema, had numerous or confluent B-lines in 90% of the cases. Lung ultrasound in this study detected pulmonary oedema with a sensitivity of 90% and specificity of 93% in dogs with mitral valve disease.

In CHF, B-lines are located in the caudodorsal and perihilar regions with wet lung and with dry lung in the ventral, middle, and cranial regions. A similar pattern of dry vs wet lung is present with acute noncardiogenic pulmonary oedema, with B-lines predominantly located in the caudodorsal lung lobes. On the other hand, ventral wet lung patterns are more suggestive of pneumonias.

Knowledge of patient clinical history and pathophysiology of most common pulmonary diseases is important before performing TFAST and/or Vet BLUE. For example, considering where a foreign body (FB) will migrate in a patient with a history of acute choking due to a FB; or which lung lobes are most affected in patients with acute suspected aspiration pneumonia (right middle lung lobe, however right cranial and left cranial lung lobes can also be affected) (Figures 127–130).

Lung ultrasound is useful for serial monitoring of pulmonary oedema in humans with LCHF, with B-lines decreasing over several hours and resolving within days of diuretic treatment. There is little information on the application of this method in cats and dogs, nonetheless sequential ultrasound can potentially be useful in animals for monitoring purposes.

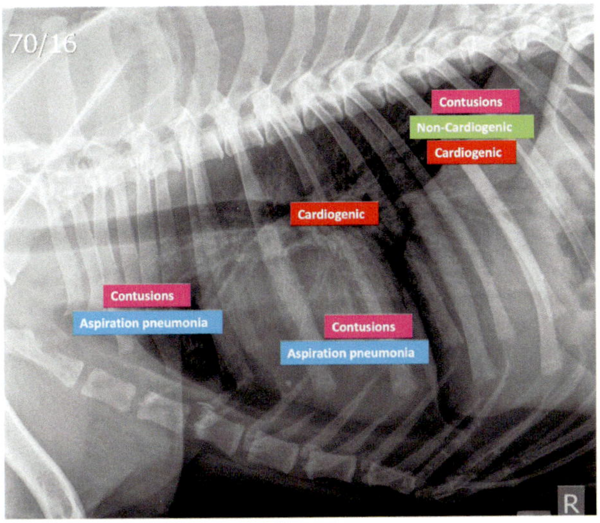

Figure 127. Vet BLUE disease distribution.

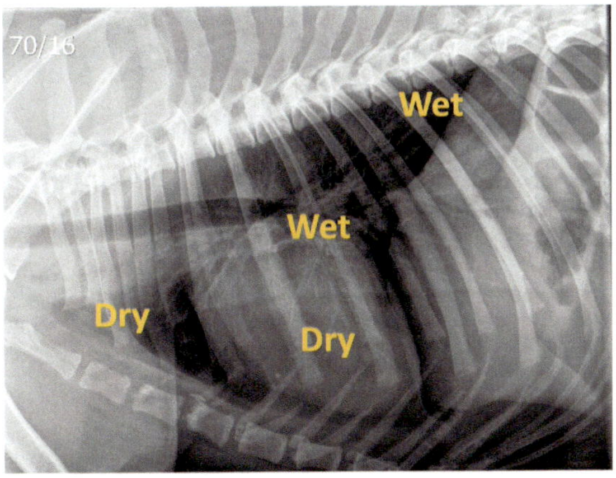

Figure 128. Vet BLUE pulmonary oedema (dry versus wet).

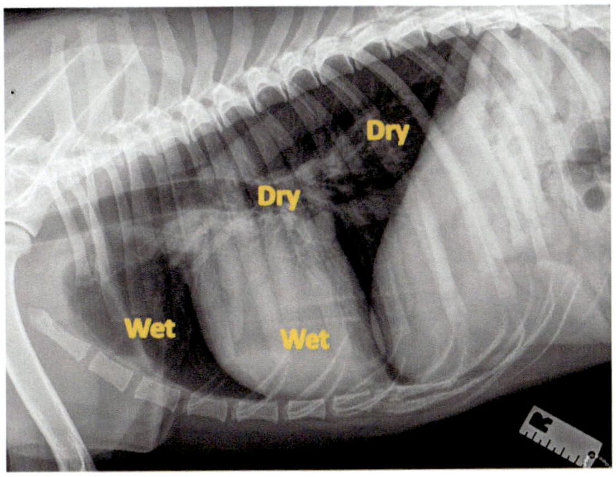

Figure 129. Vet BLUE aspiration pneumonia (dry versus wet).

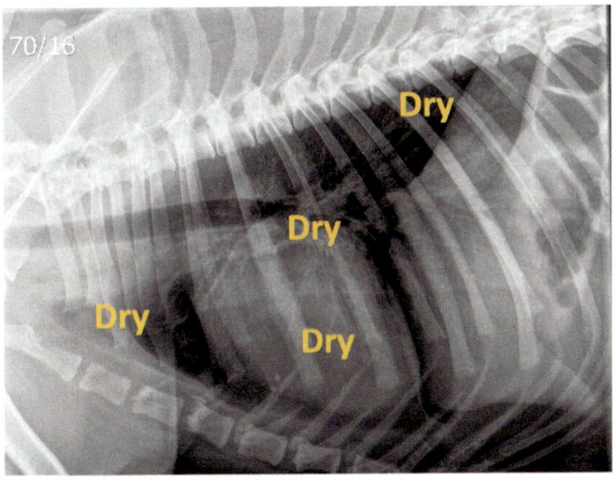

Figure 130. Vet BLUE in a normal patient.

Ultrasound Guided Interventional Techniques

Tissue sampling techniques are an essential tool for sonographers. Ultrasonography is a desired modality due to its noninvasive nature providing guidance as to what is going on with the patient, but it cannot provide an accurate definitive diagnosis. Some diseases have pathognomonic ultrasonographic features, but without more invasive techniques, such as fine needle aspirates or biopsy, a definitive diagnosis cannot be made.

The reason for performing these procedures is because they are minimally invasive and ultrasound provides a suitable and safe route to the area of interest, avoiding large blood vessels, bowel loops or inflated lungs.

Ultrasound guided interventional techniques are classified as indirect, freehand and mechanically guided (Figure 131).

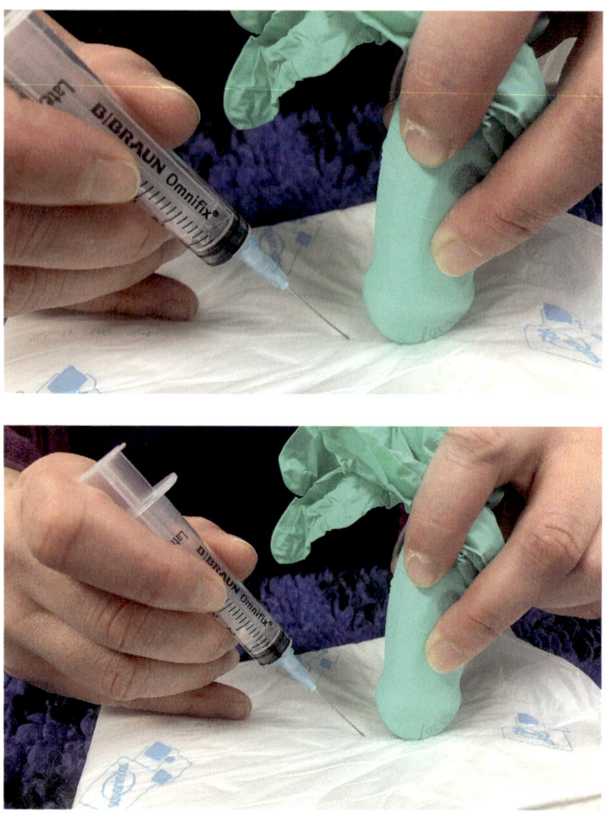

Figure 131. Transducer and needle. It is important to keep the needle in the plane of the ultrasound transducer. This is achieved by angling the needle at 30–50° to the skin. The needle should be inserted 1–3 cm from the side of the ultrasound transducer. It is important to take note of where the needle is being introduced in relation to the transducer marker, so that the operator is aware of where the needle will appear on the screen.

- **Indirect method:** ultrasound is used to determine the location and depth of the target, usually fluid. The needle is not visualized in real time during the procedure. The indirect method is commonly used for pericardiocentesis, thoracocentesis and abdominocentesis.
- **Freehand method:** the location and depth of the target are determined, and real time ultrasound is used to visualize and help guide the needle into the desired target. This provides great flexibility to the sonographer to angle the needle and change its direction avoiding other structures. This is the most preferred method for ultrasound guided sampling procedures. All intervention procedures described in this chapter are based on this method.
- **Mechanical guided method:** a rigid system containing the transducer and an attachment containing a slot helping the needle into the target, cavity, or tissue. The fixed path of the device ensures the needle remains in the plane of the ultrasound beam. This device is not available as standard in veterinary medicine

Cystocentesis

Cystocentesis is an ultrasound guided technique for the collection of a urine without contamination. This is a quick technique which can be performed in a conscious or sedated/anaesthetised patient if the bladder is distended enough.

Material (Table 3)

- 5 ml syringes
- needles:
  - 23 gauge x 1 inch (0.6 x 25 mm) (blue)
  - 23 gauge x 1¼ inch (0.6 x 30 mm) (blue)
  - 21 gauge x 1 inch (0.6 x 25 mm) (green)
  - 21 gauge x 1½ inch (0.8 x 40 mm) (green)
- Surgical Spirit™
- swabs
- protective cover for the transducer (glove finger or cling film) – it is important not to forget to put ultrasound gel between the transducer and the protective cover
- urine containers for analysis and culture
- clippers.

Technique Considerations

- Before the procedure, the region should be cleaned and sprayed with Surgical Spirit™. If the patient is dirty, cleaning the skin with diluted Hibiscrub® is necessary before the Surgical Spirit™ is applied.

- Surgical Spirit™ provides better contact with the transducer and the skin.
- Cystocentesis can be performed in right, left, and dorsal recumbency depending on operator preference.
- Once the sample is collected, the urine should be stored in the appropriate containers for analysis and/or culture.
- The samples should be correctly labelled.

Abdominocentesis

Abdominocentesis is the ultrasound guided technique for collection of free abdominal fluid. A small volume of anechoic free fluid may be physiological in kittens and puppies. Larger volumes are considered abnormal. Small volumes of peritoneal free fluid tend to accumulate around the liver, spleen, and bladder in triangular or sharp angle pockets. If the volume is very small, these areas are very difficult to sample. Finding a pocket of fluid in the mid abdomen is often a lot easier.

This a quick, single technique that can be performed in a conscious or sedated/anaesthetised patient depending on the volume of the fluid. Smaller volumes require the patients to be sedated/anaesthetised for precision, in order for the needle to reach the desired pocket of fluid and to avoid nearby abdominal organs.

Material (Table 3)

- syringes:
  - 2.5 ml for small volumes
  - 5–10 ml
- needles:
  - 23 gauge x 1 inch (0.6 x 25 mm) (blue)
  - 23 gauge x 1¼ inch (0.6 x 30 mm) (blue)
  - 21 gauge x 1 inch (0.6 x 25 mm) (green)
  - 21 gauge x 1½ inch (0.8 x 40 mm) (green)
  - 19 gauge x 1 inch (1.1 x 25 mm) (yellow) – usually used for very large volumes
- Hibiscrub®
- small bowl
- swabs
- Surgical Spirit™
- blood tubes: EDTA and plain
- microscope slides
- slide container
- pencil for labelling the slides
- protective cover for the transducer (glove finger or cling film) with ultrasound gel between the transducer and the protective cover
- clippers.

Technique Considerations

Abdominal ultrasound is necessary as part of the investigation **to ascertain the origin of the peritoneal effusion before abdominocentesis.** This also provides an idea as to where the larger and safe pockets of effusion are located for abdominocentesis. Abdominocentesis may be performed with the patient in right, left or dorsal recumbency and even standing. It should be performed using aseptic technique, clipping and preparing the skin with Surgical Spirit™.

If the needle is not visible ultrasonographically, the transducer should be moved slightly to each side until the needle can be seen. Small needles may be difficult to see, depending on the ultrasound equipment. In these cases, advancing and retracting the needle a few millimetres causes the tissue to move and helps localise the needle.

Cholecystocentesis

Cholecystocentesis or biliary cystocentesis is the ultrasound guided technique for **collection of a bile sample.** This is most often performed to obtain a sample for cytology and culture in cases of suspicion of an infection. A transhepatic approach is recommended, inserting the needle through the liver into the gallbladder. The liver acts as a plug and helps avoid bile peritonitis.

Material (Table 3)

- syringe size depends on gallbladder volume:
  - 5 ml
  - 10 ml
  - 20 ml
- needle type varies with patient size and approach to the gallbladder. The most commonly used type are spinal needles:
  - 22 gauge x 1½ inch; 2½ inch; 3½ inch (0.7 x 38 mm; 63 mm; 90 mm) (black spinal needle)
  - 20 gauge x 1½ inch; 3 inches (0.9 x 38; 75 mm) (yellow spinal needle)
  - 23 gauge x 1¼ inch (0.6 x 30 mm) (blue)
  - 21 gauge x 1½ inch (0.8 x 40 mm) (green)
- swabs
- Surgical Spirit™
- Hibiscrub®
- bowl
- blood tubes: EDTA and plain
- microscope slides
- slide container
- pencil for labelling the slides

- protective cover for the transducer (glove finger or cling film), with ultrasound gel between the transducer and the protective cover
- clippers.

Technique Considerations

- Cholecystocenthesis is performed with the animal in dorsal or left lateral recumbency, using aseptic technique. The skin should be clipped and prepared with diluted Hibiscrub® and then Surgical Spirit™.
- The patient should be heavily sedated or anesthetised. Patient motion and even breathing motion can lead to focal haemorrhage/bile leaks.
- Emptying the gallbladder entirely is recommended as this decreases the risk of leakage. However, this is not always possible.
- Complications are infrequent even if bile is not drained completely. Risks for complications are higher if the gallbladder is largely distended and/or if its wall is diseased. Bile leakage with subsequent peritonitis is a serious complication. Peritoneal haemorrhage is rarely seen.

Ultrasound Guided Fine Needle Aspiration

Fine needle aspiration (FNA) is a minimally invasive method used for aspiration of tissue cells using a needle. This technique is essential for the diagnostic process, especially for tumour staging.

Ultrasound guided FNA can be undertaken to sample any organs or masses in the abdomen (thorax, abdomen, subcutaneous tissue), however, FNA of urinary bladder tumours is contraindicated due to high risk of seeding. Prostatic tumours have similar risk; however, the technique is often performed due to poor cell collection during prostatic washes. This also depends on whether the patient will be receiving treatment (i.e. chemotherapy). If owners decline treatment, then it is better not to increase the risk of seeding and reducing the life expectancy of the patient.

FNA of the pancreas is routinely performed if abnormal. However, in both humans and animals there is the risk of needle tract tumour implantation. Most cases of needle tract seeding are diagnosed within two to six months of the procedure.

Fine needle aspirations can be performed in the conscious patient but are more often performed under sedation or general anaesthesia due to the localisation of the pancreas and the size of the organ/lesion. Another factor which should be taken into consideration is patient temperament and the organ to be sampled.

Material (Table 3)

- syringes: 5 ml
- needles:
  - 23 gauge x 1 inch (0.6 x 25 mm) (blue)
  - 23 gauge x 1¼ inch (0.6 x 30 mm) (blue)
  - 22 gauge x 1½ inch (0.7 x 38 mm) (black spinal needle)
  - 21 gauge x 1 inch (0.6 x 25 mm) (green)
  - 21 gauge x 1½ inch (0.8 x 40 mm) (green)
- Surgical Spirit™
- swabs
- microscope slides (minimum three slides per organ)
- slide container
- pencil for labelling the slides
- protective cover for the transducer (glove finger or cling film) with ultrasound gel between the transducer and the protective cover
- clippers.

Technique Considerations

FNA should be performed using aseptic technique, clipping and preparing the skin with Surgical Spirit™. There are two FNA techniques, FNA with suction versus no suction. The major advantage of the no suction technique is the reduced blood contamination when sampling highly vascular tissues, such as the spleen, kidney, and liver.

The no suction technique has been found to have similar or greater sensitivity when aspirating the spleen and abdominal lymph nodes. Whereas the suction technique has shown an increased diagnostic yield in the liver and pancreas compared to the no suction technique. For the liver, pancreas, and more solid masses FNA with suction should be used.

Suction can be performed using a 5 ml syringe, only displacing the plunger to the 2 ml mark 3–4 times in a row.

For the no suction technique, the needle is moved back and forwards 3–4 times without leaving the target lesion using short, rapid strokes in a swift cutting motion.

The work station should be prepared before performing the FNA. It is important to have the microscope slides ready for direct smear.

As a general rule of thumb three samples should be obtained from each tissue. It is always important to read the laboratory

Table 3. Images of the material used for the different techniques.

Technique	Material	Images
Cystocentesis:	· ultrasound spirit · urine containers · syringes	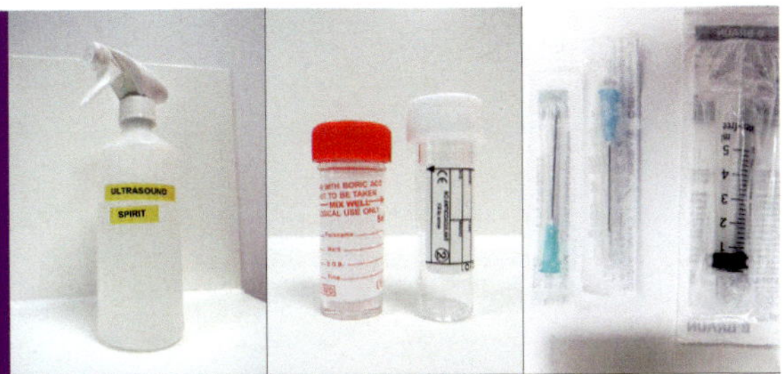
Ultrasound guided fine needle aspiration:	· ultrasound spirit · microscope slides · syringes and needles	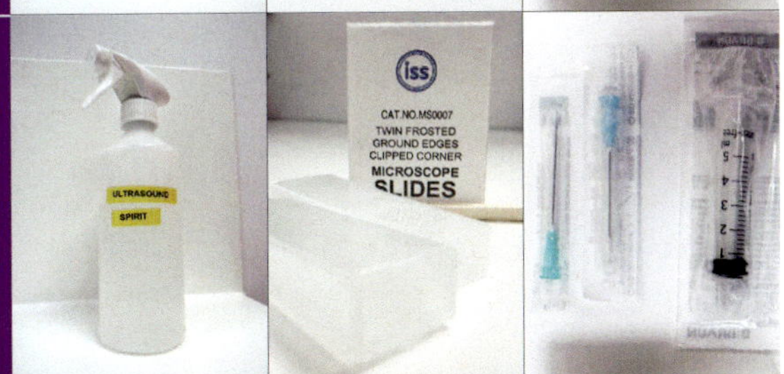
Cholecystocentesis:	· ultrasound spirit · microscope slides · Hibiscrub® dilution · blood tubes · needles	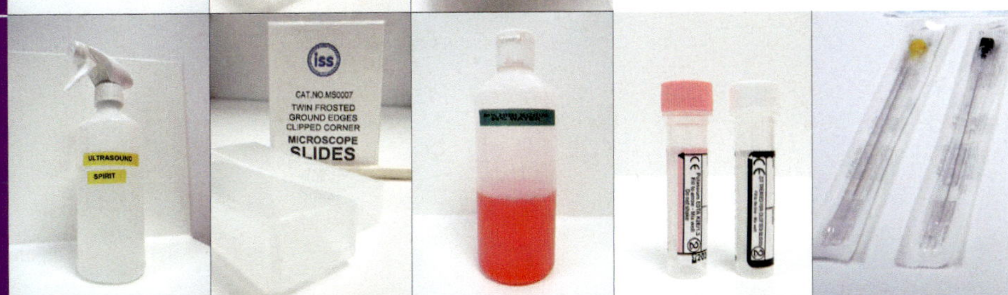
Abdominocentesis:	· ultrasound spirit · microscope slides · Hibiscrub® dilution · blood tubes · syringes · needle	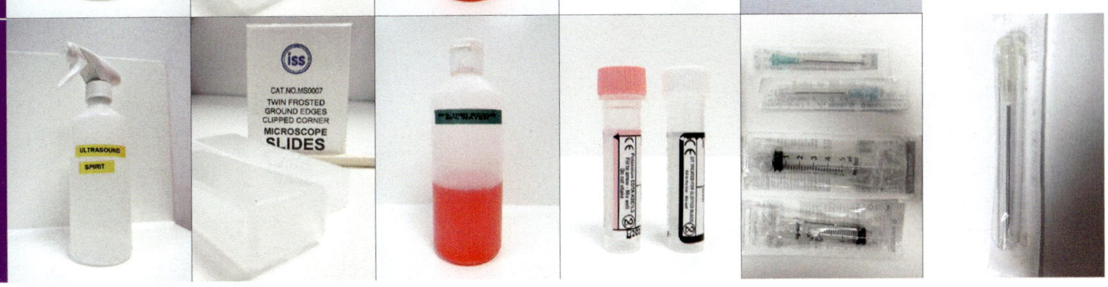

quality evaluation of the slides. If the cell yield is persistently low or there is a high number of damaged cells, the sampling technique should be reconsidered and changed.

FNA should not be performed if the patient is thrombocytopoenic to avoid haemorrhage. The overall bleeding risk is minimal with FNA.

Ultrasound Guided Tru-cut® Biopsy

There are two types of needle core biopsy available: the semiautomated needle biopsy and the automated needle biopsy. The semiautomated needle core biopsy (Tru-cut®) is the most commonly used.

Tissue biopsy harvests more information compared to FNA, as more tissue is sampled. However, it is more invasive and expensive, and there is a slightly higher rate of complications. This technique is usually used to obtain a biopsy of the liver, kidney or abdominal, subcutaneous and intramuscular masses.

Material (Figure 132)

- biopsy device: Tru-cut® 18, 16, or 14 gauge, depending on the target and personal preference
- nº. 11 scalpel blade for the incision
- sterile gloves
- Hibiscrub®
- swabs

- bowl
- Surgical Spirit™
- 10% formalin pot
- pen for labelling
- protective cover for the transducer (glove finger or cling film) with ultrasound gel between the transducer and the protective cover
- clippers
- skin staples
- small bandage.

Technique Considerations

Platelet count and coagulation profile should be evaluated before the Tru-cut® biopsy is performed, due to the increased risk of bleeding; also, general anaesthesia is required.

As with previous procedures mentioned in this chapter, the patient's skin should be prepared aseptically, and in addition a stab incision should be made in the skin before introducing the biopsy device.

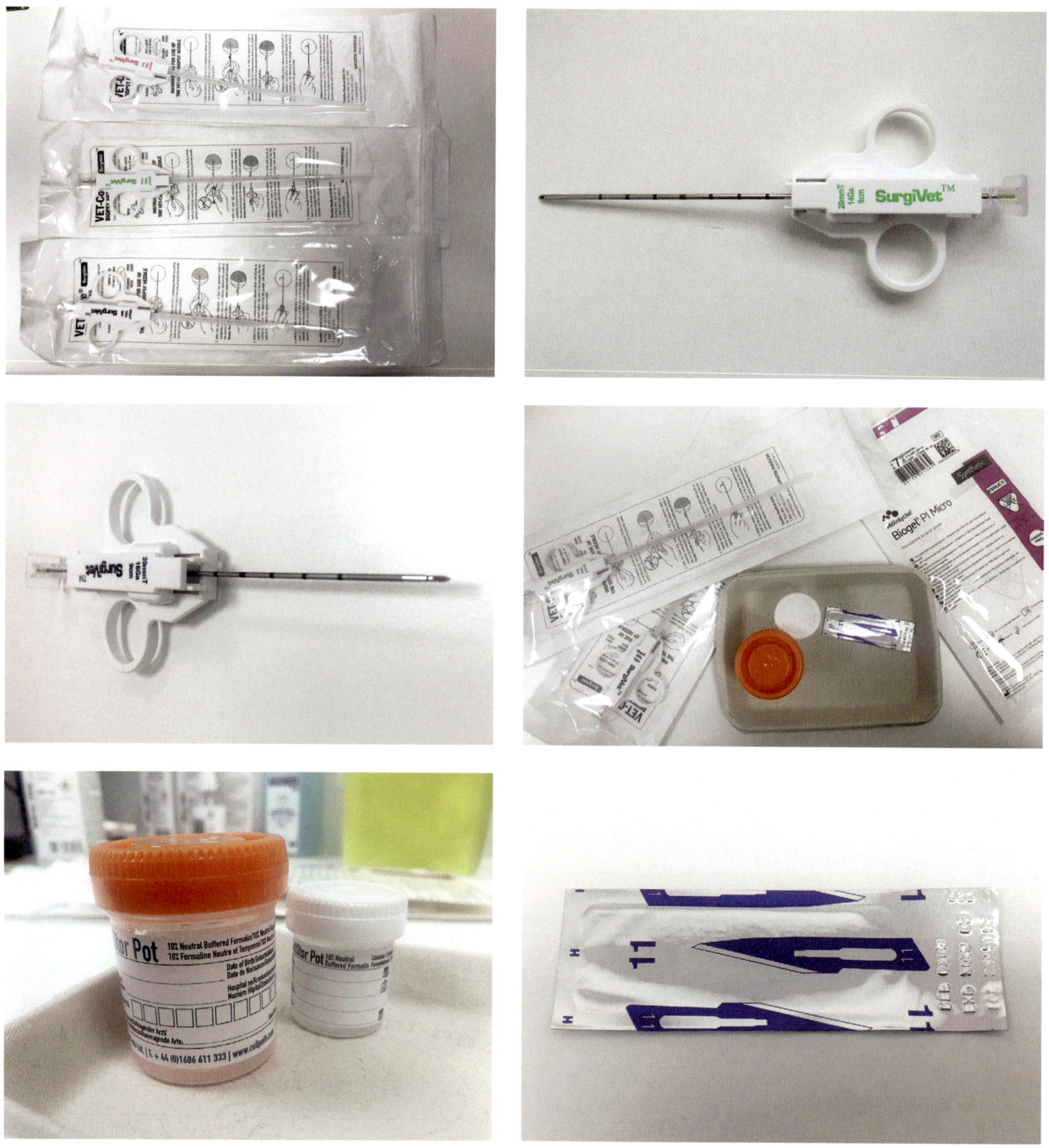

Figure 132. Material used for an ultrasound guided Tru-cut® biopsy.

The tip of the needle should be visualised via ultrasound to ensure the needle is advanced to the correct depth (Figure 133). The device is then fired, and a sample is obtained as the Tru-cut® sheath advances producing a tissue sample with approximately 50–60% of the diameter of the needle core. Once the sample is obtained it should be stored in a 10% formalin pot. After the procedure, the patient should be monitored for complications.

Complications

- Haemorrhage: can occur with FNA of diseased and friable organs such as the liver. Focal haemorrhage can occur following a needle core biopsy and most of the time is self-limiting.
- Bladder rupture: the risk is only significant if the bladder is hard and markedly distended.
- Peritonitis: resulting from a fluid leak, bile or content from a cavitary lesion (e.g. abscess).
- Pneumothorax: can occur after FNA of aerated lung or lung nodules/masses closely associated with aerated lung.
- Haematuria: uncommon complication following cystocentesis.

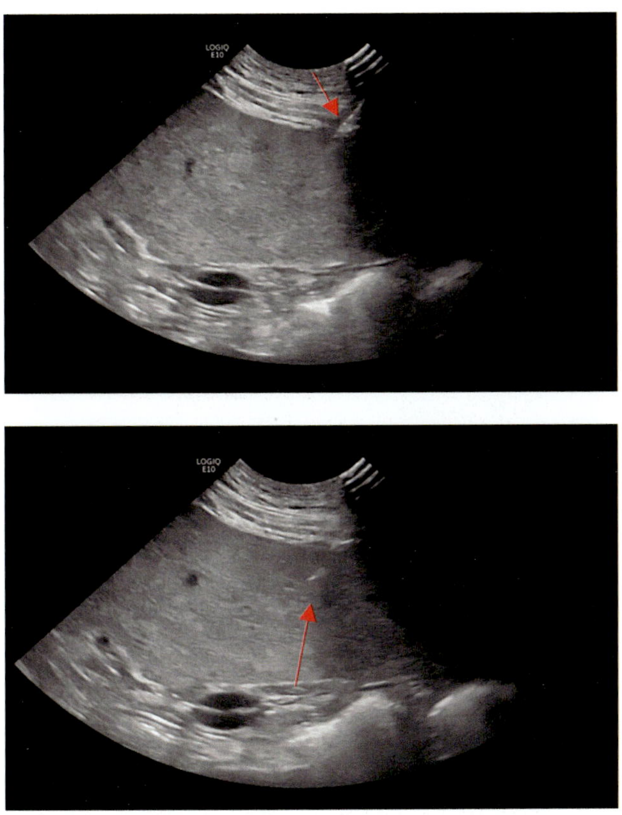

Figure 133. Transabdominal ultrasound of the spleen. The needle is visible crossing the abdominal wall and can be seen in the spleen (red arrow).

Echocardiography in Cats and Dogs

Echocardiography is a commonly used imaging technique to assess the cardiovascular system; it is a noninvasive technique and provides information on cardiac morphology and function.

Perioperative (pre, intra, and postoperative) cardiac complications are one of the most important causes of mortality associated with surgery. These can be better controlled or avoided with intensive patient assessment and preparation prior to surgery. Patients with a heart murmur are at higher risk for perioperative cardiac mortality. This a dilemma for the anaesthetist and leads to increased demand **on anaesthetists to assess the patient prior to a full anaesthetic.** This assessment involves a full physical examination, blood tests, and cardiovascular evaluation in patients with diagnosed or undiagnosed cardiovascular disease.

Echocardiography is currently the gold standard for evaluation of cardiac function and cardiovascular chamber morphology and size, as well as evaluation of the great vessels and valves.

Transoesophageal echocardiography (TEE) is commonly used by anaesthetists as a noninvasive technique to investigate cardiac pathology. This technique is used for perioperative assessment and to establish if cardiovascular risk factors may cause postoperative mortality. The disadvantage of TEE is that it is not widely available and requires good operator training. Focused TTE does not replace the role of the cardiovascular assessment with echocardiography but provides more accurate assessment than physical examination alone.

Thoracic radiography is used as a complementary technique to echocardiography. Radiography allows evaluation of the pulmonary parenchyma and vasculature to assess if the patient has decompensated or is at a higher risk of decompensation due to the cardiac disease.

Indications

All patients with heart murmurs, with undiagnosed or diagnosed cardiovascular disease.

Patient Preparation

Dogs and cats require little preparation and are evaluated whilst conscious. However, not all patients are compliant, and sedation is required to perform the echocardiogram.

If sedation is used, sedatives with minimal effect in the cardiac function are indicated. **Sedatives with the least effect on cardiac function** include, butorphanol, buprenorphine, and acepromazine. These are usually ineffective in a fractious cat, therefore for cats, midazolam, ketamine, and in extreme situations medetomidine or dexmedetomidine can be used. The cardiologist or person performing the echocardiogram must consider the effect these have on the measurements.

Patients are normally examined in **right and left lateral recumbency** because there is less lung interference, providing a better window to the heart and improving image quality. Thoracic radiography is used as a complementary technique to echocardiography. Radiography allows evaluation of the pulmonary parenchyma and vasculature to assess if the patient has decompensated or is at a higher risk of decompensation due to cardiac disease. (Figure 134).

A table with a cut out section is recommended for better positioning of the transducer between the ribs on the dependent aspect of the body wall. As the patient is in lateral recumbency, the dependent side of the lungs collapses (atelectasis) and provide a better acoustic window to the heart.

The patient's hair should be clipped over the left and right precordial transducer locations, where the strongest apex beat is felt. This is usually between the 4th–6th intercostal space. Water should be used to reduce the presence of gas bubbles between small hairs and then ultrasound gel to improve transducer contact.

In a dyspnoeic patient, positioning the patient in sternal recumbency is preferred.

Placement of ECG leads are essential to enable measurements to be taken at the correct phase of the cardiac cycle.

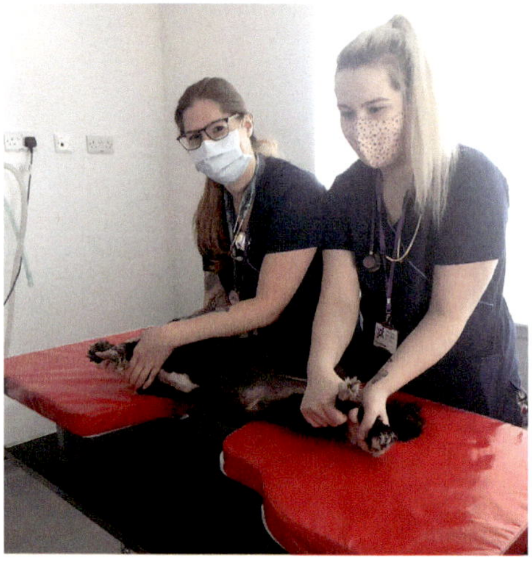

Figure 134. Patient positioning.

Equipment

Ultrasound machines are typically equipped with broadband transducers with several different frequencies. Transducers that generate a fan shaped beam (sector scan) are most practical. (Figure 135).

Thoracic radiography is used as a complementary technique to echocardiography. Radiography allows evaluation of the pulmonary parenchyma and vasculature to assess if the patient has decompensated or is at a higher risk of decompensation due to the cardiac disease. **The highest frequency transducer which can be used in a patient is recommended,** for the best image resolution. However, the higher frequency may not penetrate to an adequate depth so the transducer selected should provide a balance between resolution and penetration (Figure 136):

- large breed dogs: 2.0 and 4.0 MHz transducer
- medium breed dogs: 4.0 and 8.0 MHz transducer
- cats and small dogs (<4 kg): 7.5 and 12 MHz transducer.

Echocardiography Views

Right Parasternal (RPS) View

Standard 2D images from the RPS views include short and long axis views (Figures 137–139).

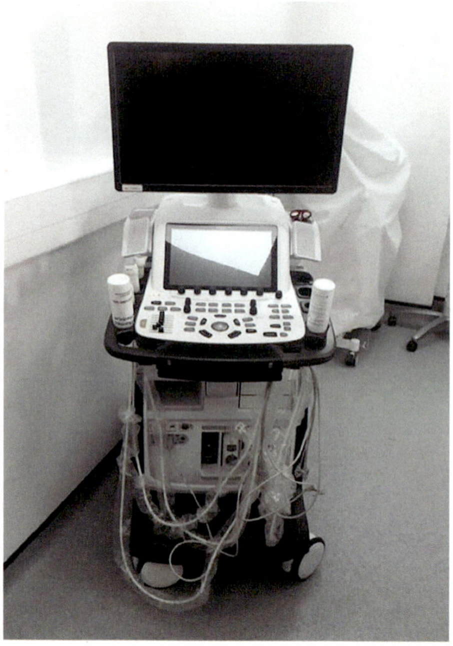

Figure 135. Ultrasound machine.

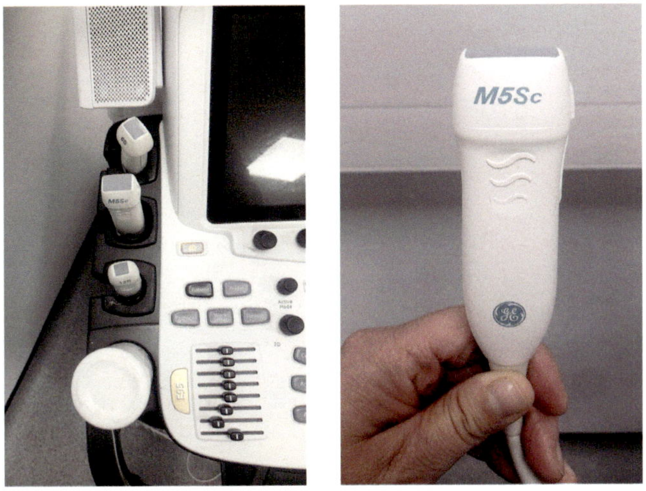

Figure 136. Ultrasound transducers.

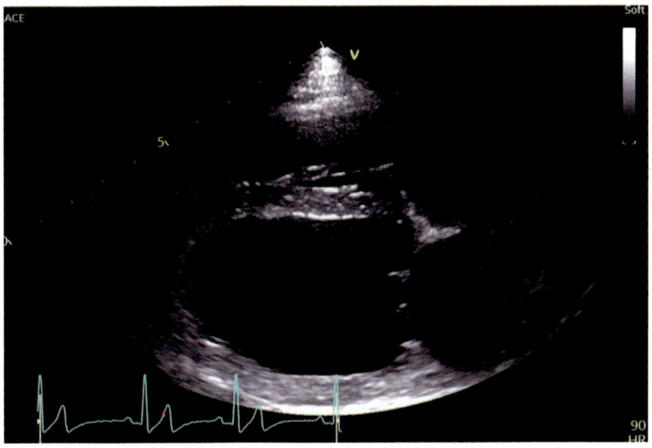

Figure 138. RPS long axis view. Left ventricle and left atrium.

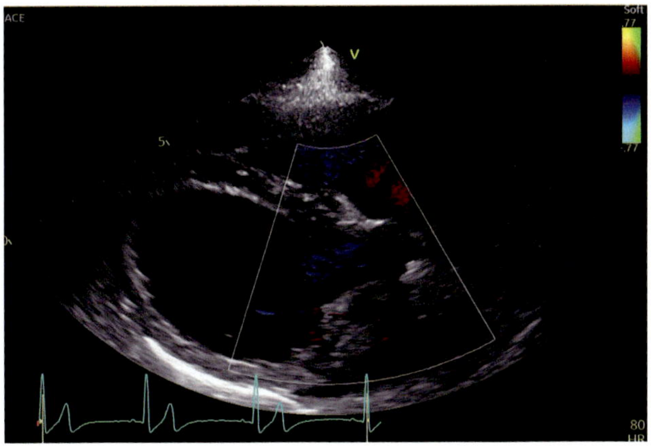

Figure 139. RPS long axis view. Left ventricle and aorta.

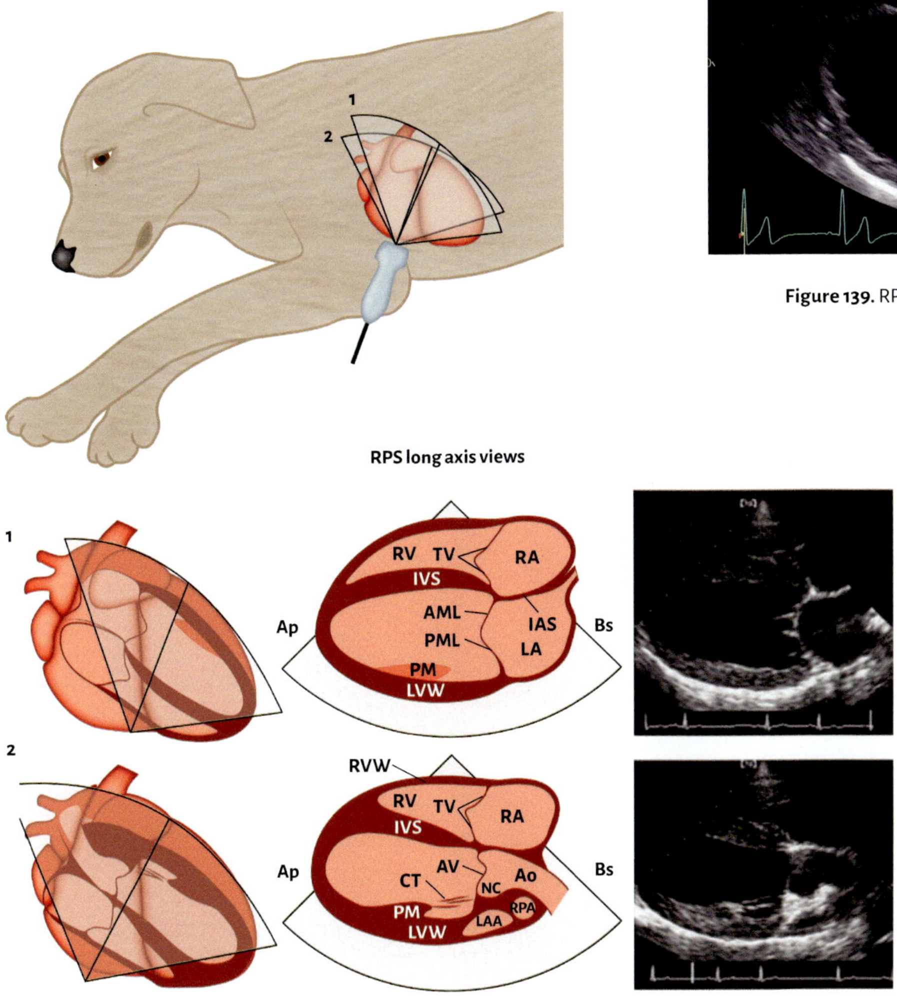

Figure 137. RPS long axis view. Image inspired on Brown, D., Gaillot, H., & Cunningham, S. (2015).

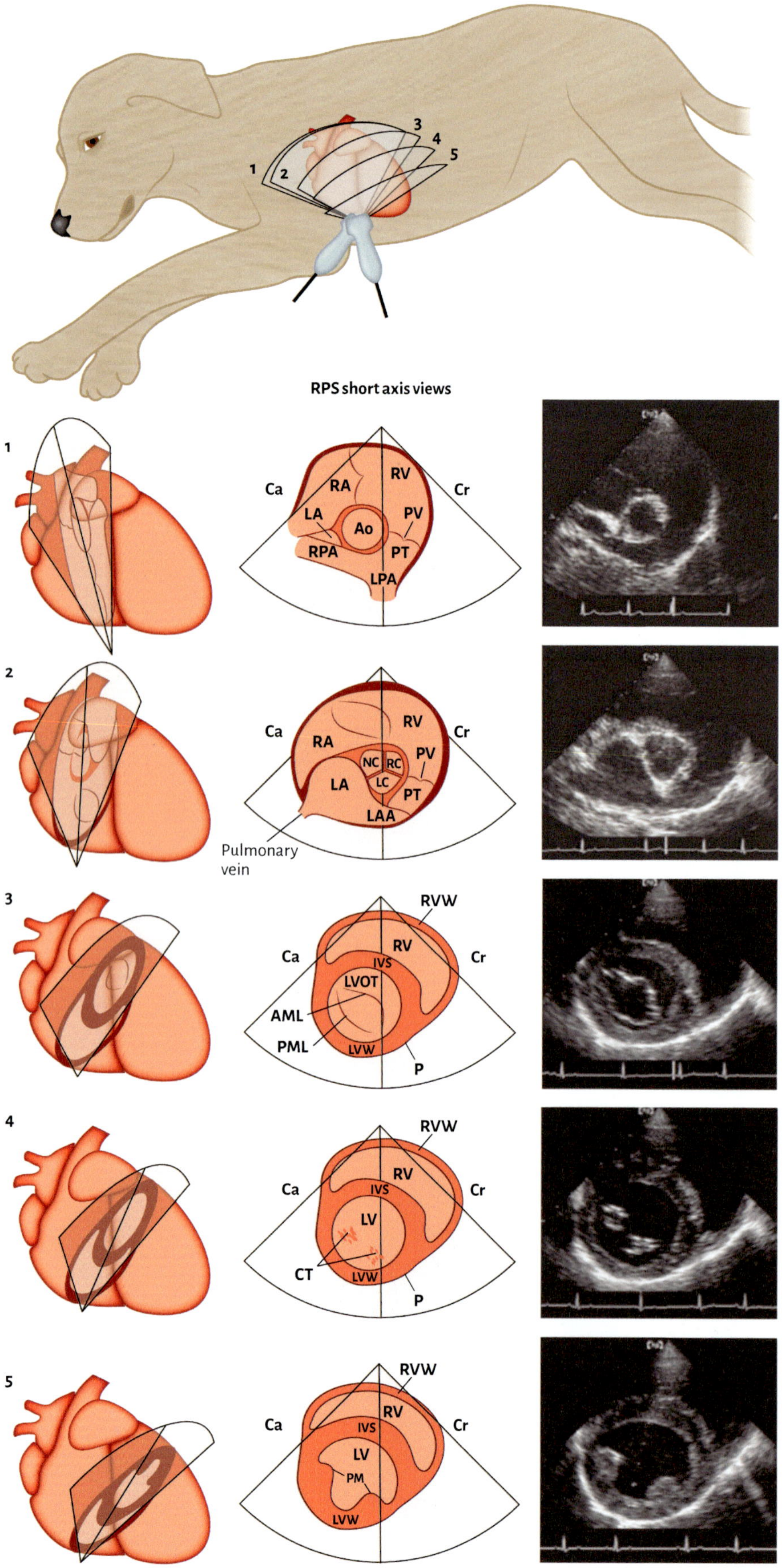

Figure 140. RPS short axis. Image inspired on Brown, D., Gaillot, H., & Cunningham, S. (2015).

The acoustic window is usually around the 4th–5th intercostal space.

RPS long axis views:

- left ventricle and left atrium (four chamber view)
  - chordae tendinae
- left ventricle and aorta (five chamber view).

The transducer should be positioned in the intercostal space, parallel with the ribs at the point of maximal apex beat. The right ventricle and atrium appear in the near field, with the left ventricle and atrium in the far field.

This view assesses cardiac morphology, provides a subjective evaluation of cardiac function and a comparison of right and left sides of the heart. Colour Doppler can be used to evaluate the mitral and tricuspid valves.

- Measurements: LV length, diastolic and systolic volumes, and calculation of ejection fraction (Simpson's rule).

Ejection fraction (%) = [(EDV-ESV)/EDV] x 100

ESV = end systolic volume
EDV = end diastolic volume

A slight anticlockwise rotation of the transducer and a slight tilt cranially are necessary to obtain the five chamber view. This view aims to evaluate the left ventricular outflow tract using colour flow and also allows evaluation of the valves.

RPS Short Axis Views

- left ventricle (LV)
- mitral valve (fishmouth)
- heart base (aorta, pulmonic trunk and left atrium).

To obtain the short axis views the transducer is rotated by 90° anticlockwise from the long axis view. The transducer is then perpendicular to the LV. Angling/fanning of the transducer in the base apex direction and vice versa allows visualisation of RPS short axis views (Figure 140).

LV at Papillary Muscle Level (Figures 141 and 142)

- The left ventricle has a mushroom appearance.
- M mode assessment is used for fractional shortening measurements and for LV wall measurements in cats.

Fractional shortening (%) = [(LVIDd–LVIDs)/LVIDd] x 100

LVID = left ventricular internal dimension
d = diastole
s = systole

- Fractional shortening (FS)% varies with the breed and specie.
- Most normal dogs have a FS of 25–50%, with a value <20% indicative of poor systolic function (such as dilated cardiomyopathy).
- Normal cats generally have a FS of 30–55%.
- Cats should have a diastolic LV thickness <6 mm.

LV Measurement (Cat)

The diagnosis of hypertrophic cardiomyopathy (HCM) in an asymptomatic cat is partly reliant on a cut off value for the left ventricular diastolic wall thickness (≥6.0 mm) (Figure 143). Values of >8.0 mm are considered more severe. However, there is an overlap of measurement between healthy cats versus cats with HCM. Normal cats can have a LV with a wall thickness of ≥6.0 mm and thus be diagnosed as false positive HCM. Or to the contrary, a cat with HCM with a wall thickness <6.0 mm could be diagnosed as a false negative.

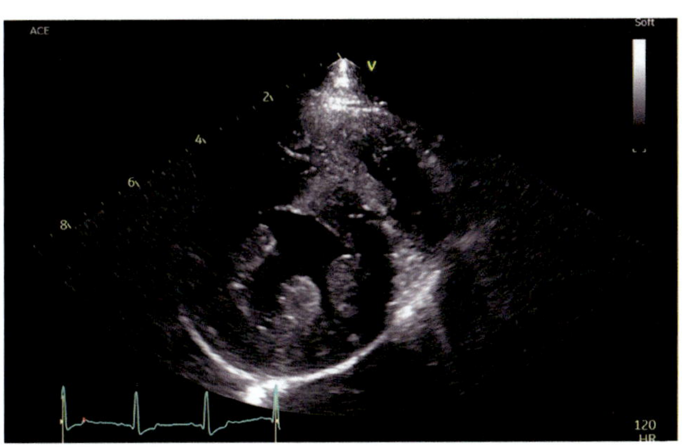

Figure 141. RPS short axis view. Left ventricle (LV) at the level of the papillary muscles.

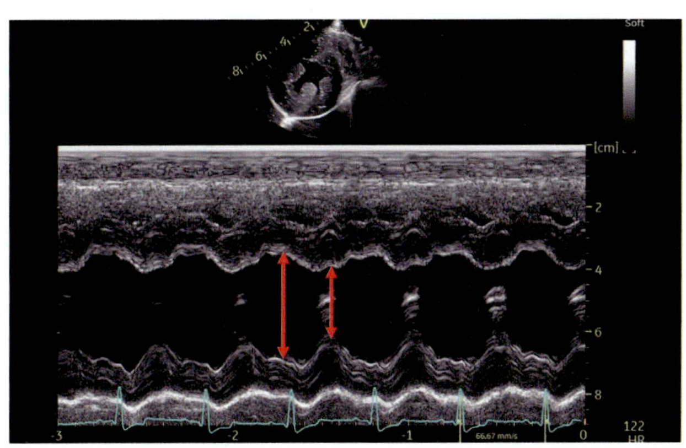

Figure 142. RPS short axis view. M mode at the level of the papillary muscles.

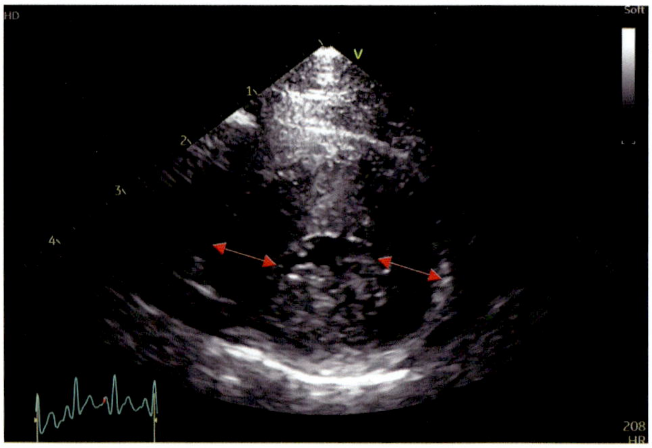

Figure 143. RPS short axis view. Marked thickening of the LV can be seen. Measurement of a severely thickened LV in diastole in a cat with HCM (red arrow).

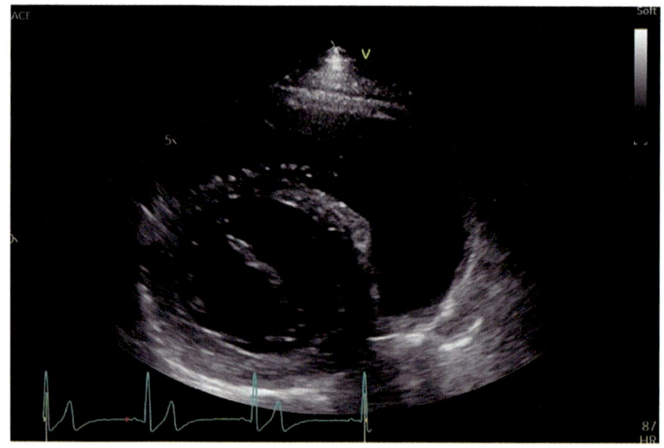

Figure 144. RPS short axis view. Fish mouth view of the mitral valve leaflets.

Fish Mouth View of the Mitral Valve Leaflets

- Shows opening and closing of the mitral valve (Figure 144).
- M mode is used to assess the E point to septal separation (EPSS). A simple but useful assessment for left ventricular volume overload. In dogs EPSS should be <7 mm.

Heart Base, Left Atrium, Aorta, and the Right Heart

The heart base is imaged with the aorta at aortic valve level (Mercedes Benz sign) in the centre of the image. At this level the left atrium to aorta ratio (LA:Ao) can be measured.

At the right ventricular outflow tract (RVOT) (Figures 145 and 146) the pulmonic trunk is seen wrapping around the right side of the aorta. The pulmonic valves appear at nine o'clock to the aorta. Doppler evaluation is used for flow velocities during systole and detection of regurgitant jets.

LA:Ao Ratio

Left atrial to aortic ratio (LA:Ao ratio) can be obtained using a microconvex transducer with a static or portable ultrasound. This measurement is taken from the right parasternal short axis (Figure 147).

- In healthy dogs, this ratio is found to be <1.6 and >1.5 in dogs with LA enlargement. However, a full assessment is needed to consider different echocardiographic views, or a volumetric assessment of the LA for a more comprehensive evaluation of LA size.
- In cats, LA:Ao ratio should be <1.5.

Left Parasternal (LPS) View

LPS views (Figure 148):

- four chamber view
- five chamber view.

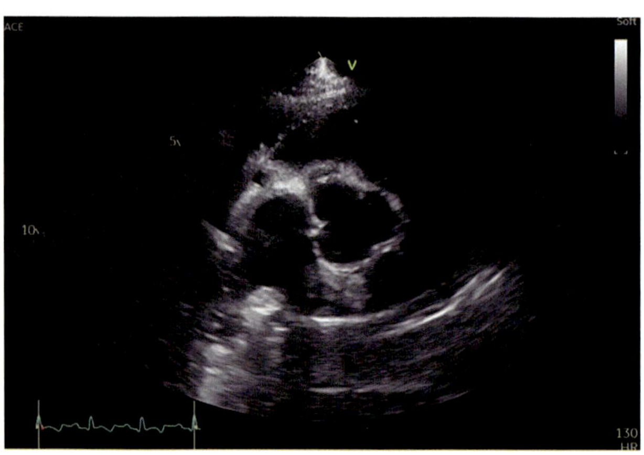

Figure 145. RPS short axis view. At the heart base, left atrium, aorta and the right heart.

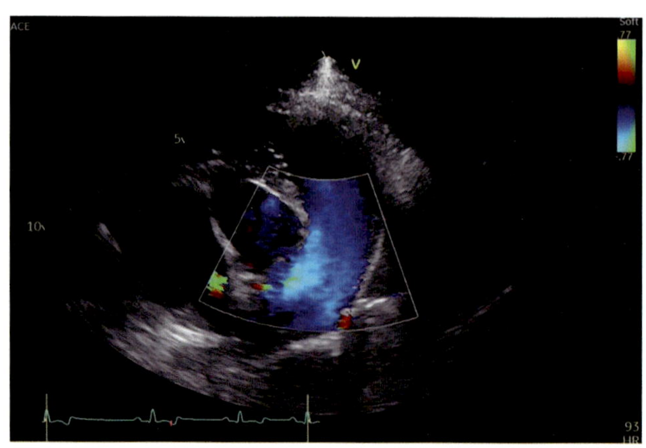

Figure 146. RPS short axis view of the right ventricular outflow tract (RVOT), the pulmonic trunk is seen wrapping around the right side of the aorta with colour Doppler.

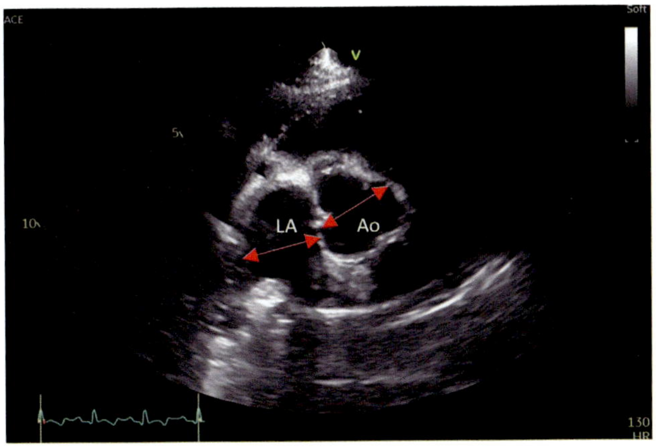

Figure 147. RPS short axis view. LA:Ao measurement.

Four Chamber View (Figures 149 and 150)

The transducer should be positioned with the thumb about 30–45° to the intercostal space, towards the head, angled dorsally. This view is used for colour flow and spectral Doppler studies of the mitral and tricuspid valves, valve regurgitation, assessment of left ventricular length and volume, M mode mitral annulus motion, and power Doppler examination of pulmonary venous flow.

Five Chamber View (Figures 151 and 152)

From the left apical four chamber view, the transducer should be rotated about 10° anticlockwise and angled cranially to visualise the LVOT and aorta.

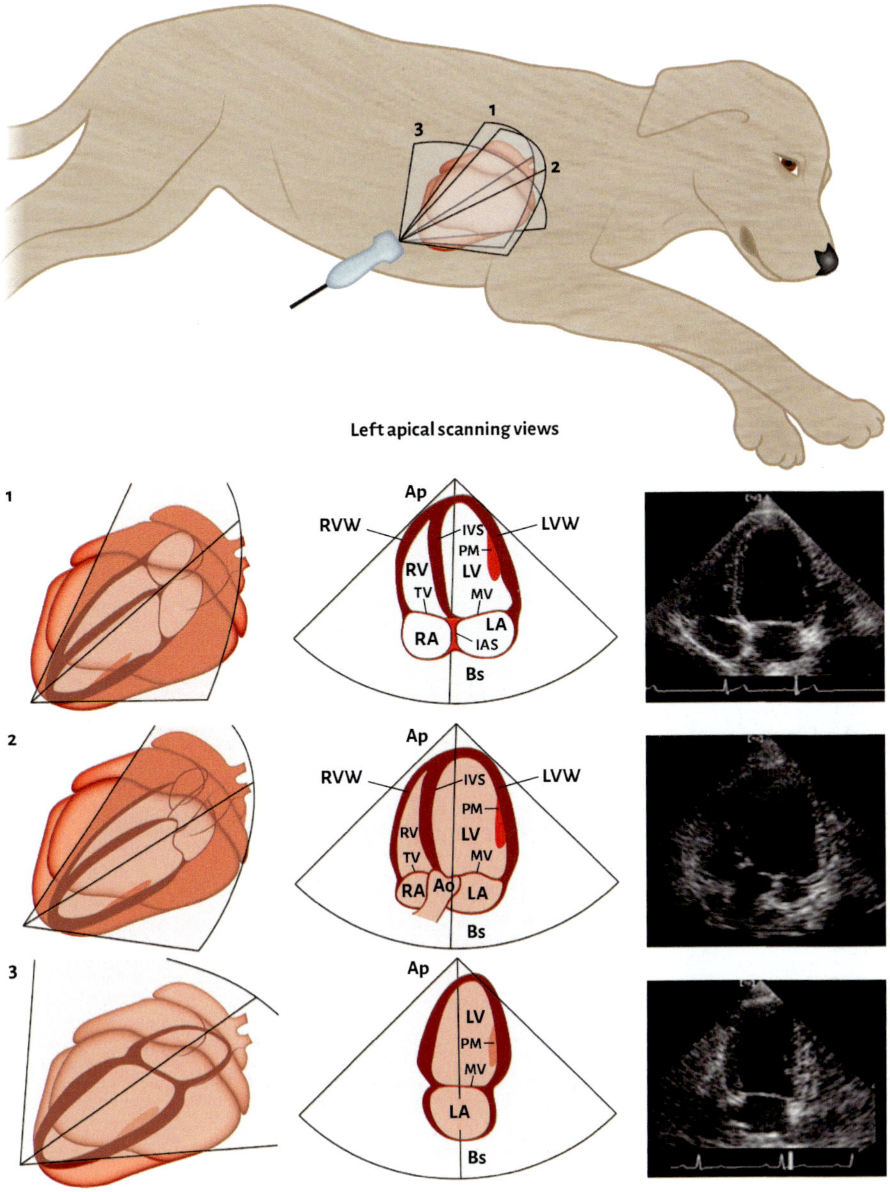

Figure 148. LPS Long axis view. Image inspired on Brown, D., Gaillot, H., & Cunningham, S. (2015).

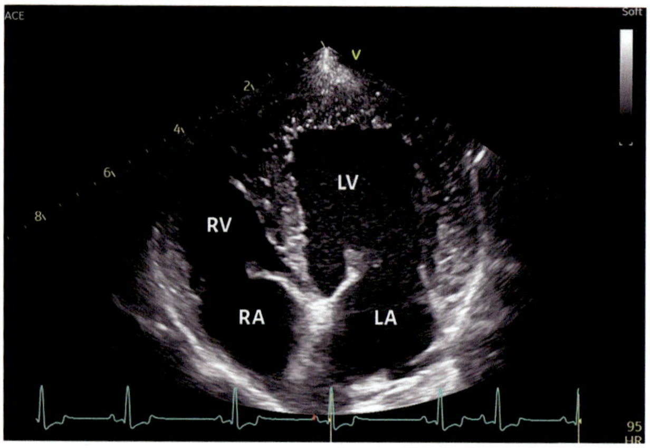

Figure 149. LPS long axis four view. RA: right atrium; RV: right ventricle; LA: left atrium; LV: left ventricle.

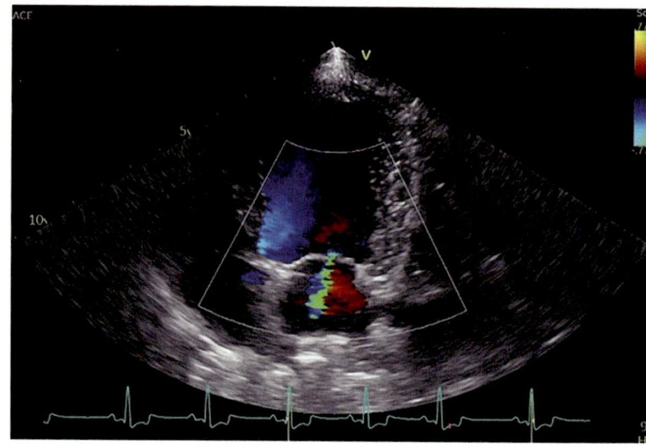

Figure 150. LPS long axis four view. Colour Doppler demonstrated turbulent flow from the left ventricule into the left atrium consistent with mitral valve regurgitation.

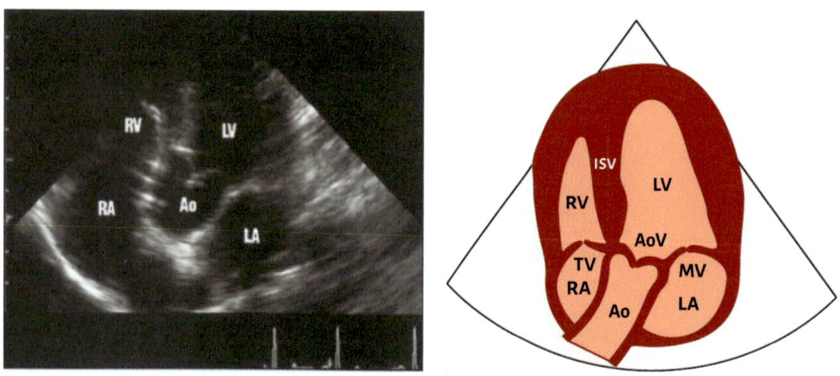

Figure 151. LPS five chamber view. Image inspired on Seiler, G., Dukes-McEwan, J., & Gaschen, L. (2011).

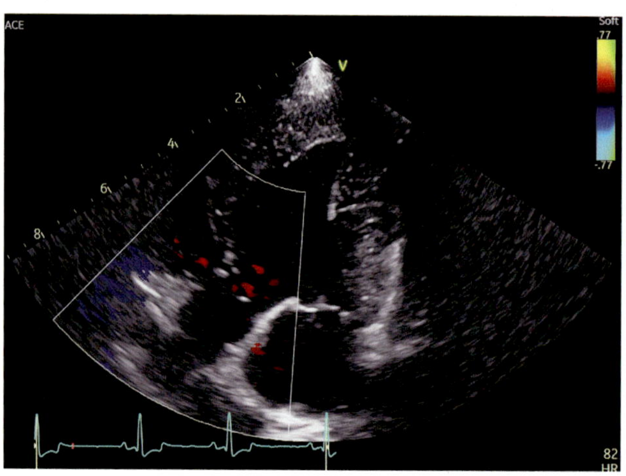

Figure 152. LPS long axis view of the five chambers showing the aortic outflow tract.

Subcostal View (Figure 153)

The transducer should be positioned caudal to the xyphoid process angling and pushing cranially, as if scanning the liver but with more pressure. The depth of field should be increased due to the distance between the heart and the transducer. The view is used to measure aortic outflow velocity.

Standard Doppler Examination

Doppler ultrasound can determine the direction of blood flow (towards or away from the transducer) and blood flow uniformity (laminar versus turbulent) and velocity when the beam is parallel with movement. (Figure 154).

Colour Flow Doppler

Advantages:

- can be used to assess blood flow direction and uniformity:

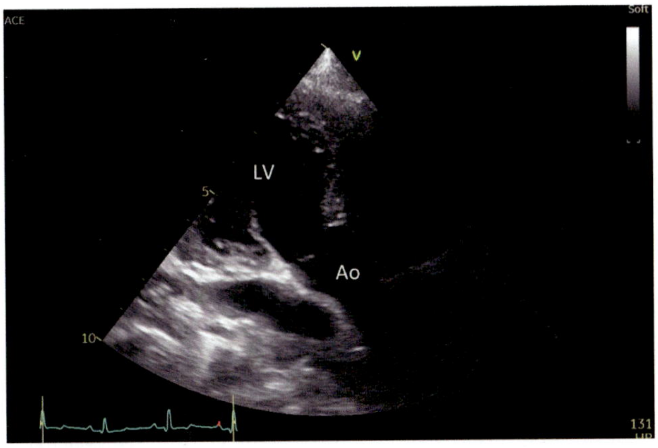

Figure 153. Subcostal view demonstrating the aortic outflow tract. LV: left ventricle; Ao: aorta.

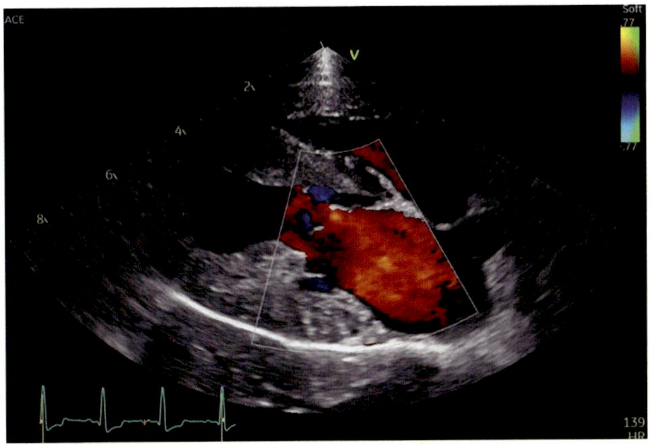

Figure 154. RPS long axis. Colour Doppler over the mitral valve.

flow uniformity can be laminar or turbulent, often appearing green or mosaic
– detection of areas of abnormal flow e.g. regurgitation
– can be used as a guide to pulsed wave spectral Doppler gate placement.

Disadvantages:
– cannot be used to measure velocity of flow.

The simplified Bernoulli equation can be used to estimate pressure difference across valves.

$$\Delta P = 4(V^2)$$
$$p1 - p2 = 4(V^2)$$

V = velocity m/s; P = pressure gradient; p = pressure

Pulsed Wave Spectral Doppler

(Figures 155 and 156)

Used to determine velocity of the mitral/tricuspid valve inflow and aortic/pulmonic outflow.

Advantages:
– can be used to assess flow direction, uniformity, and limited velocity.

Disadvantages:
– cannot measure high velocities: aliasing occurs. To evaluate higher velocities of regurgitant flow, continuous wave Doppler is indicated.

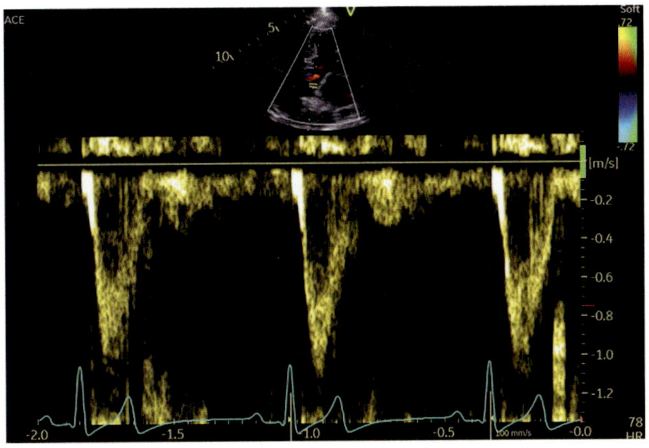

Figure 156. Pulsed wave spectral Doppler of the aorta.

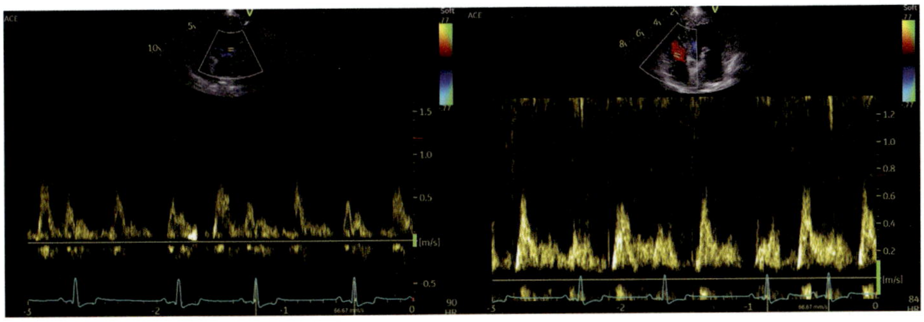

Figure 155. Pulsed wave spectral Doppler of the mitral and tricuspid valves.

Continuous Wave Spectral Doppler

(Figure 157)

Advantages:

- can be used to measure all flows
- determines direction of flow.

Disadvantages:

- does not assess uniformity.

Other left parasternal views can be performed, and many other measurements can be taken to provide a full echocardiography study, which are outside the scope of this chapter. For further information and more details, the BSAVA Manual of Canine and Feline Thoracic Imaging can be consulted.

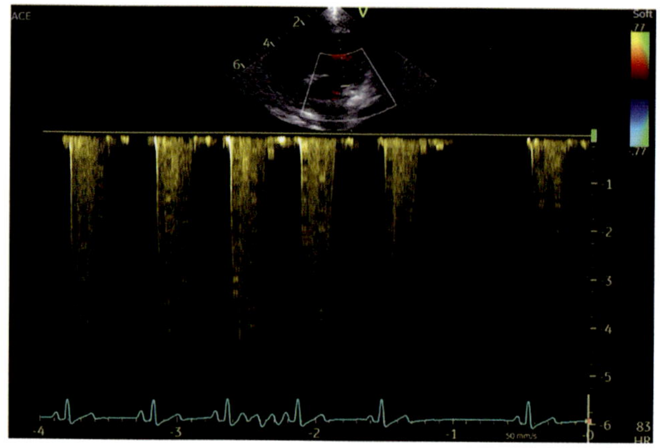

Figure 157. Continuous wave spectral Doppler of mitral valve regurgitation.

Importance of Echocardiography in the Surgical Patient

Nonspecific, incidental clinical findings such as heart murmur, cardiac arrythmias, and abnormal heart sounds should be investigated before and after surgery. Any cardiac findings detected, or untreated cardiac disease require a full cardiovascular investigation to accurately assess anaesthetic risk.

Echocardiography enables preoperative haemodynamic assessment. The basic haemodynamic state can be defined as the interaction between myocardial and vascular function, (left ventricular systolic failure, hypovolaemia, primary diastolic failure, or vasodilation are examples of haemodynamic states). Echocardiography can be used isolated or in conjunction with pressure based information to identify the haemodynamic state, alongside other echocardiography measurements.

Many cats and dogs with cardiac disease have potential haemodynamic changes that are relevant to anaesthesia, due to undiagnosed or investigated diseases or cardiovascular diseases. Depending on the cardiovascular disease the anaesthesia plan will need to be adjusted accordingly to avoid perioperative, intraoperative and postoperative complications (e.g. significant volume overload from fluid therapy).

The cardiovascular investigation includes physical examination, electrocardiogram, blood tests, radiographs, and echocardiography. The latter is an important tool in the cardiovascular investigation; however, it is highly operator dependent and relies on the proper acquisition and interpretation of results. This can be a limiting factor in first opinion practice, limiting evaluation of the patient before surgery. Therefore, other steps can be taken to assist in preanaesthetic assessment before the patient is anaesthetised. Point of care ultrasound imaging facilitates procedures and cardiovascular diagnosis. Instead of a trolley based machine, a portable machine is used to measure the LA:Ao ratio and obtain LV wall measurements.

Echocardiography may also be indicated in cases of splenic mass before a splenectomy is performed. Haemangiosarcoma is a common neoplasm which can originate in or metastasise to the heart base, therefore visualising this area with echocardiography is crucial before surgery. It is important to note that a negative echo does not rule out the presence of cardiac haemangiosarcoma, as masses may be too small to visualise, however this examination should still be performed. In addition to the echocardiography, thoracic radiographs are indicated when haemangiosarcoma is suspected to rule out pulmonary metastasis.

Interventional Radiology

Interventional radiology (IR) is a minimally invasive technique that uses the guidance of imaging (fluoroscopy – Figure 158, computed tomography or ultrasound) to precisely target a region or organ. In veterinary medicine IR procedures are commonly performed under the guidance of fluoroscopy. These techniques are typically associated with lower risks of complications due to their minimally invasive nature. However, it is not a procedure that is readily available in first opinion practice.

These techniques are routinely used in human medicine, however, despite potential applications, they are **not yet widely adopted in veterinary medicine.** There are several IR techniques, but cardiac interventions are some of the most

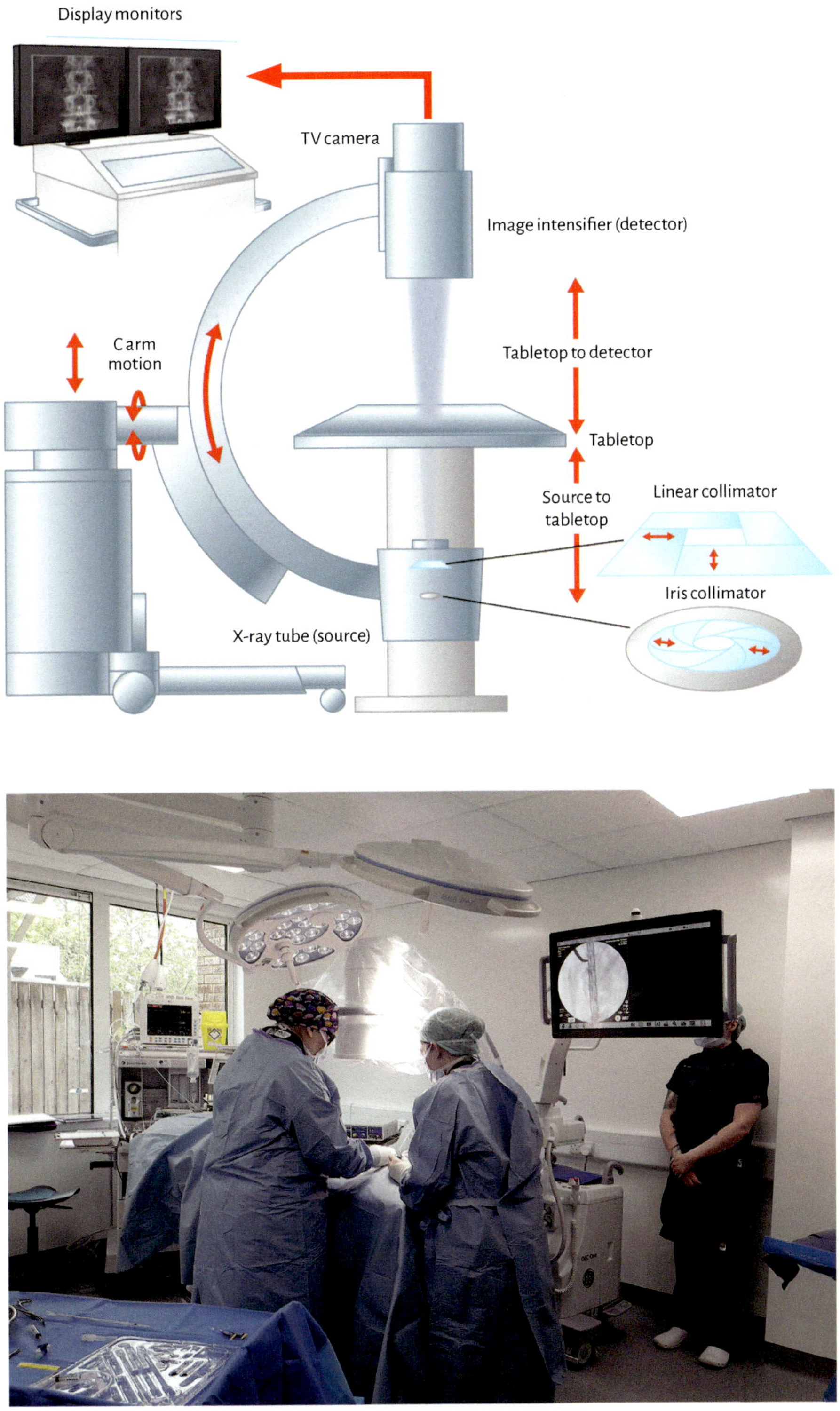

Figure 158. Fluoroscopy equipment.

commonly performed (e.g. pacemaker placement, PDA, pulmonic stenosis etc.), however, there is an increasing use of IR in respiratory (e.g. tracheal or bronchial collapse etc.), hepatobiliary (e.g. portosystemic shunts etc.), urogenital (ureteric or urethral obstruction) and vascular diseases (e.g. thromboembolism etc.) and orthopaedic cases.

Advantages:

- minimally invasive
- reduced perioperative morbidity and mortality
- shorter anaesthetic and hospitalization times
- alternative treatment options.

Disadvantages:

- technical expertise required
- specialized and expensive equipment.

Equipment

The equipment used varies with procedure. Standard equipment includes:

- Fluoroscopy unit (C arm): the latest technology, such as flat panel thin film transistor arrays offer greater capabilities and image quality, while reducing radiation exposure.
- C arm operator to run the fluoroscopy unit. A pedal is also available for use by the clinician. Fluoroscopy operators are classified as radiographers, radiologists, IR trained nurses, orthopaedic surgeons, soft tissue surgeons, and cardiologists.
- Non-ionic iodinated contrast medium/barium: depending on the procedure.
- Power injector for the non-ionic iodinated contrast medium.
- Personnel protective equipment: lead gown and thyroid shield and ring and glasses when hands are close to the primary beam.
- Dosimeter badge underneath the lead gown.
- Crash cart and defibrillator available, this is even more important if the procedure involves the cardiovascular system.
- Surgical kit: soft tissue versus orthopaedic equipment.
- Anaesthetic equipment for patient monitors.

A trained member of staff must also be designated as the C arm operator to run the fluoroscopy unit. This may be via a handset or foot pedal; the latter option is useful if the surgeon needs to control the unit during the procedure. Fluoroscopy operators can be radiographers, radiologists, IR trained nurses, orthopaedic surgeons, soft tissue surgeons, or cardiologists.

Procedural Equipment

- Stents: tubular devices used to maintain luminal patency of a vessel or other anatomic structures (e.g. ureter, urethra, nasopharynx, trachea).
- Coils and occlusion devices: used endovascularly to reduce or obliterate blood flow through vessels, fistulae, or cardiac septal communications.
- Balloon dilation catheters: used to dilate areas of stenosis/strictures from vessels, urethra, nasopharynx, cardiac valves, or ureterovesicular junctions. They are composed of four parts: a double Luer lock, a shaft, the balloon, and the tip. They have radiopaque markers on either end of the balloon to allow for exact positioning of the device under fluoroscopy.
- Angiographic catheters: used to deliver radiopaque contrast media or treatment to a specific location within the body.
- Introducer sheaths: these are used in most angiograms and vascular procedures. They allow the easy and protected passage, and manipulation of various guidewires and catheters through their lumens.
- Access catheters: used to establish vascular access. They have a central lumen, which allows the passage of the guidewire.
- Guidewires: radiopaque guidewires which can be advanced and operated to gain access to a specific location and provide guidance for catheter placement.

Patient Preparation

Most of IR procedures are performed under general anaesthesia.

Radiation Safety

Ionizing radiation exposure is affected by the following three main factors:

- time
- distance
- intensity.

There are no reports of fluoroscopy induced radiation injury in small animals. Nevertheless, when performing IR procedures the aim is to minimise procedure time, use the lowest possible fluoroscopic dose while still getting an adequate image quality to make the procedure safe.

Whilst also using collimation, magnification, and X-ray beam geometry to help limit patient and operator exposure during IR procedures.

Respiratory System

Tracheal collapse is the weakening of the tracheal cartilages causing it to collapse and obstruct on inspiration. Some cases respond to medical management (e.g. weight loss, harness walking only) but severe cases or those that do not respond to treatment, may require stenting. A metal stent is placed under general anaesthesia using fluoroscopic guidance and holds the trachea open to prevent airway obstruction.

Urinary Tract

The occurrence of ureteric obstruction is a frequently diagnosed disease in veterinary medicine, particularly in cats. The most efficient treatment option is surgery, with placement of stents or subcutaneous ureteral bypass systems (SUBs) under fluoroscopic guidance. Medical management has been found to be unsuccessful in moderate/marked ureteric obstructions.

Ureteral stents are commonly used in people to prevent or relieve ureteral obstruction but are not used as commonly in cats and dogs. Ureteral stents are indicated for the treatment of benign and malignant ureteral obstructions and prevention of obstruction following ureteral surgery. Stents result in passive dilation of the ureter, which helps prevent reobstruction from urolithiasis.

Endoscopic or percutaneous placement is commonly performed in the dog, whereas surgical placement is used in the cat.

Stents can be used in the urethra for the following conditions:

- urethral obstruction due to neoplasia
- external urethral compression secondary to lymphadenomegaly due to metastatic spread
- urethral obstruction associated with previous urethral trauma, previous surgery, reflex dyssynergia, and less commonly urethritis.

SUBs are the method of choice for cats with ureteric obstruction and are placed under fluoroscopy guidance. The SUB system utilises a combination of a locking loop nephrostomy catheter attached via a 3 arm Y connector or a 4 arm X connector to a straight cystotomy catheter and a SwirlPort. This port allows for subcutaneous access to the device for flushing and drainage (Figures 159 and 160)

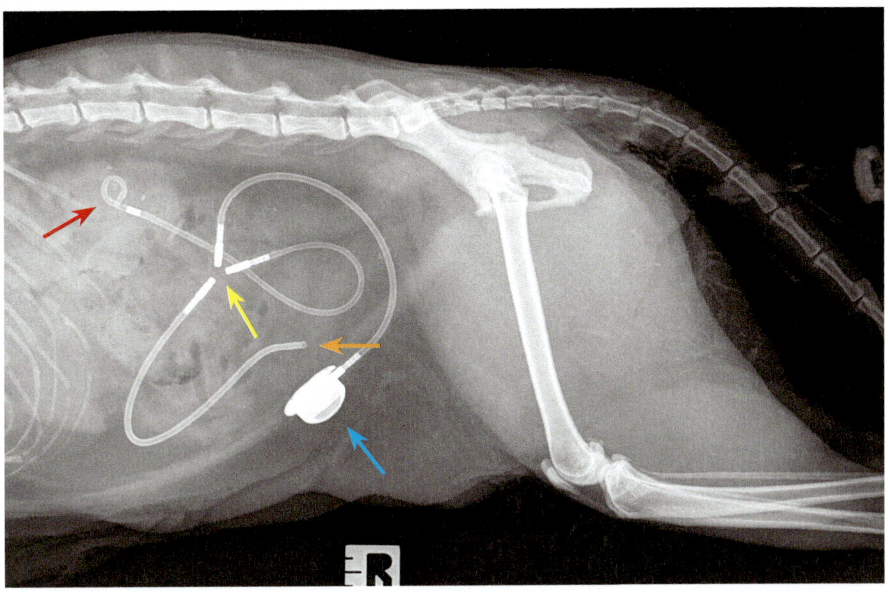

Figure 159. SUB in a feline patient that had a ureter obstruction. The locking loop in the kidney (red arrow), the 3 arm Y connector (yellow arrow) connecting the kidney to the bladder (orange arrow) and the subcutaneous port (blue arrow) can be seen.

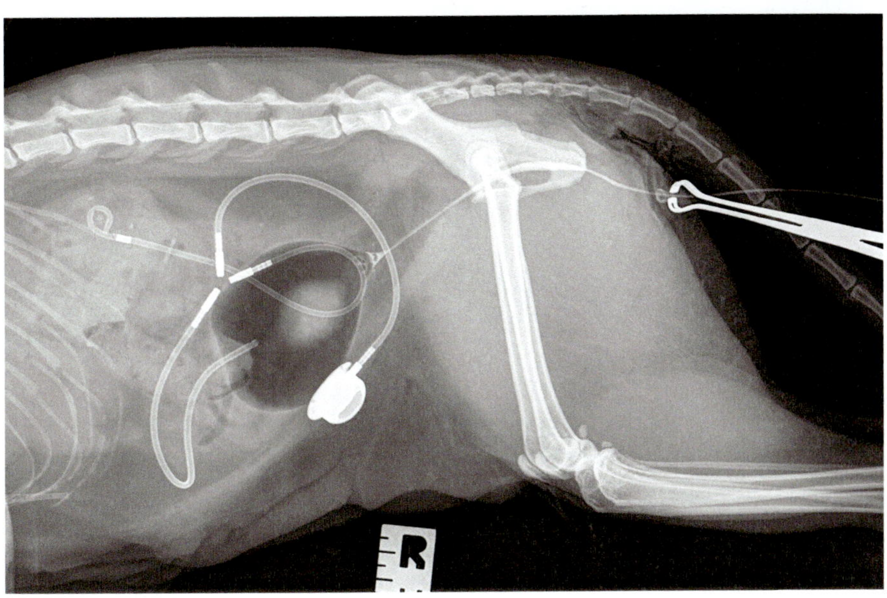

Figure 160. Feline SUB with a pneumocystogram.

Vascular System

Fluoroscopy can assist in the diagnosis and guidance during surgery for an extra or intrahepatic portosystemic shunt. It can also be used for measurement of the portal system and CVC pressure gradient. These procedures are complex and require indepth knowledge of the vascular system.

Skeletal System

Fluoroscopy is frequently used during orthopaedic surgery to assist with implant positioning. (Figure 161).

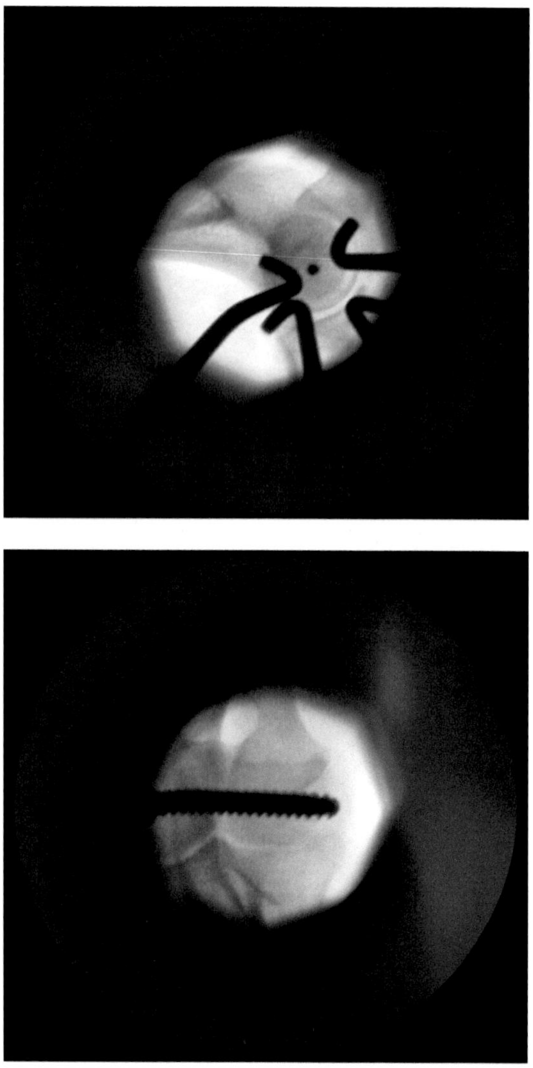

Figure 161. Orthogonal fluoroscopy images of the elbow to check implant positioning (lag screw) in a dog that had incomplete ossification of the humeral condyle.

Advanced Diagnostic Imaging Techniques

Advanced imaging techniques have become essential in veterinary medicine as a diagnostic aid. CT and MR imaging share several characteristics regarding image formation. Each CT or MR image represents a thin slice of the body.

Advantages:

- thin slices, more so CT than MRI
- no superimposition
- CT image reformatting and 3D volume rendering
- CT and MRI both have increased contrast resolution (MRI>>CT)
- provide the ability to distinguish different types of soft tissue.

Disadvantages:

- exposure to ionising radiation: CT
- long acquisition time: MRI.

Computer Tomography (CT)

Computed tomography (CT) is an advanced imaging technique and a superior method over conventional radiography. A CT system is composed of a scanning unit gantry (with a rotating X-ray tube and a detector system), a patient table, and a computer that allows acquisition parameters to be adjusted and image reconstruction. (Figures 162–164).

Nowadays most CT are helical, permitting a body region or the whole body to be scanned, without interruption and at greater speed, eliminating acquisition gaps and reducing motion artefact. Helical scanning is possible because the gantry rotates around the patient, which then creates a continuous scan and produces a large data volume rather than a single slice. CT images can be acquired only parallel to the gantry (transverse). Therefore, images are normally transverse to body parts scanned on the CT table. (Figures 165 and 166).

Image Formation

CT images are composed of pixels (Figure 167) that represent the mean X-ray attenuation corresponding to a voxel. The system reconstructs the data measured from each detector as it rotates around the patient. The concept of X-ray attenuation depends on the electron density of the medium. Attenuation is equivalent to radiopacity in radiography. X-ray attenuation is measured from the fraction of radiation removed in passing through the thickness of a given medium.

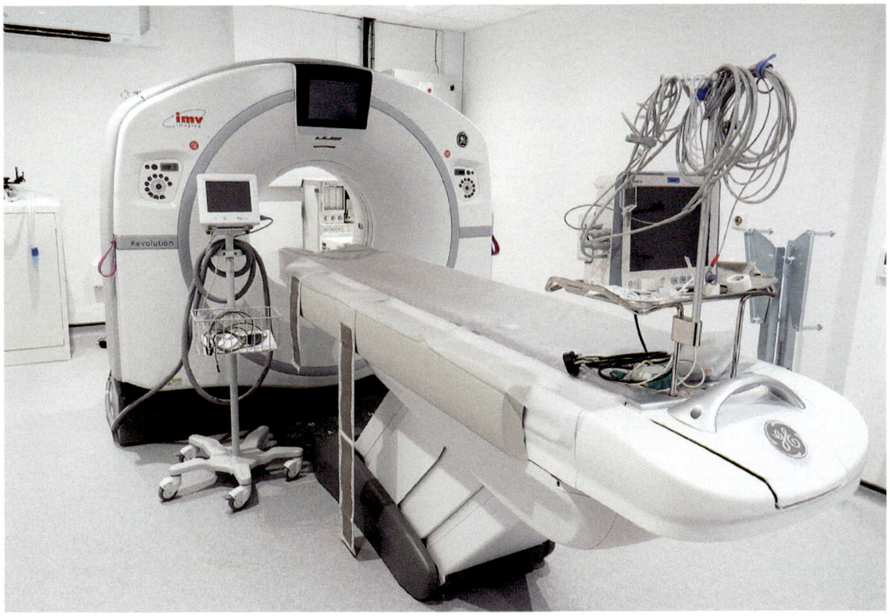

Figure 162. CT unit.

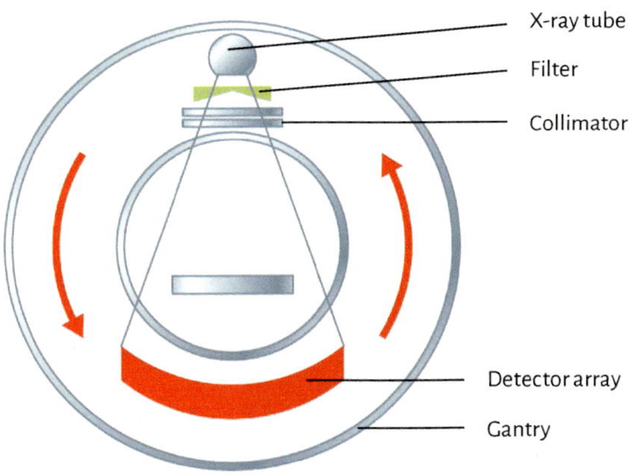

Figure 163. Image illustrates the X-ray tube positioning relative to the detector. These are within the gantry and rotate around the patient as they move through the CT.

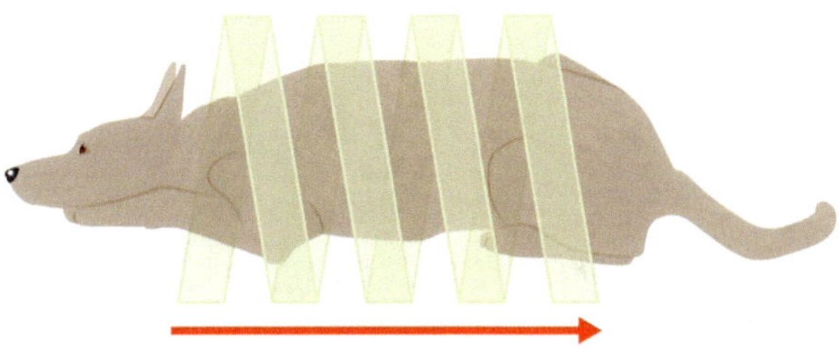

Figure 165. Helical CT. The gantry keeps rotating and continuously releasing X-rays as the patient moves on the table, providing a continuous volumetric image acquisition. Red arrow: continuous table movement during scanning.

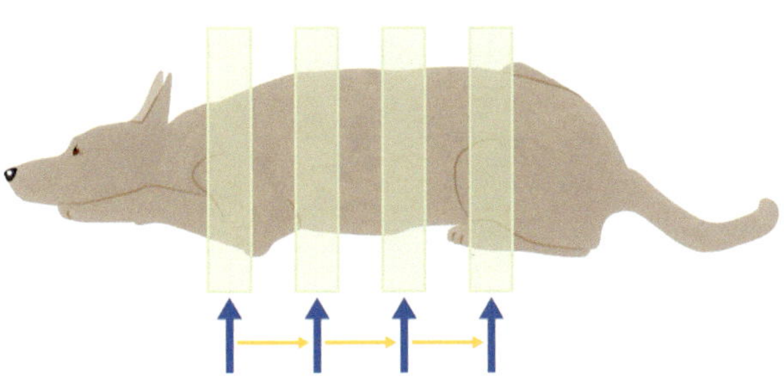

Figure 164. Axial CT scan. Image showing convectional method before helical CT was available. The patient is moved through the CT with short pauses. During those pauses the CT acquires data from a single slice. The image is then reconstructed based on each slice. Blue arrows: table stops for scanning; Yellow arrows: table moves.

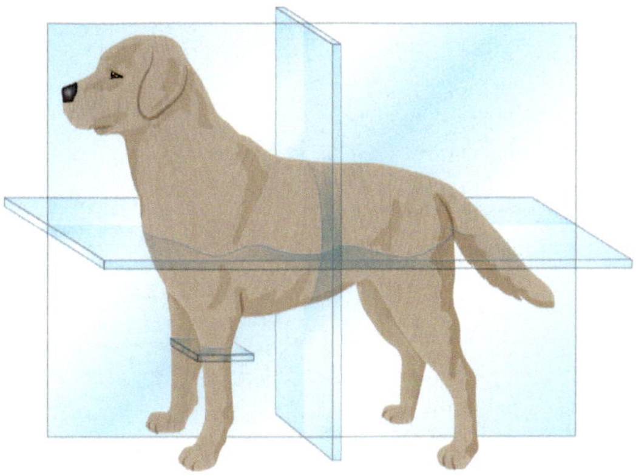

Figure 166. The image demonstrates the different planes of image display. CT image acquisition is transverse, but images can be reformatted in different planes using multiplanar reconstruction (MPR).

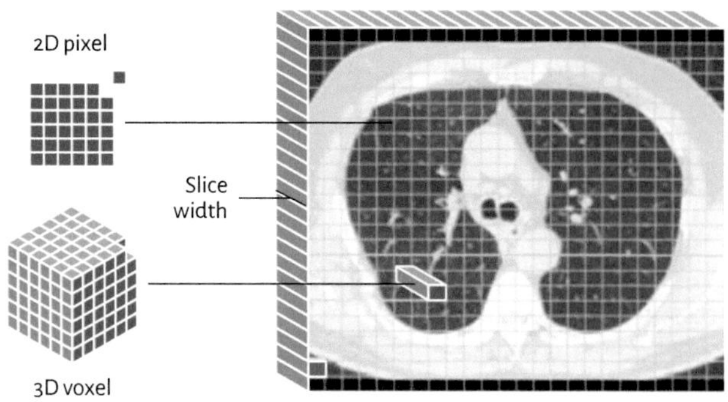

Figure 167. Pixels of a CT image. Voxel (volumetric pixel). Its width is the slide thickness.

The reconstruction process allocates a value (CT number) to each voxel that is linearly related to the attenuation coefficient (μ) of the tissue(s) within a voxel. The attenuation coefficient of the radiation within a tissue is used during reconstruction to produce a greyscale image. CT number is also known as Houndsfield unit (HU), which is then calculated from a linear transformation of the measured attenuation coefficients based on arbitrarily assigned densities of air (-1000 HU) and pure water (0 HU).

HU = 1000 x (μt–μw)/μw

μt = attenuation coefficient of tissue
μw = attenuation coefficient of water

Different tissues have different attenuations (Hounsfield units). The Hounsfield unit (HU) of water is zero and any structure or tissue causing more X-ray attenuation than water have a HU value above zero and vice versa (negative HU). The differentiation between fluid and soft tissue can be made based on their HU value. (Figure 168).

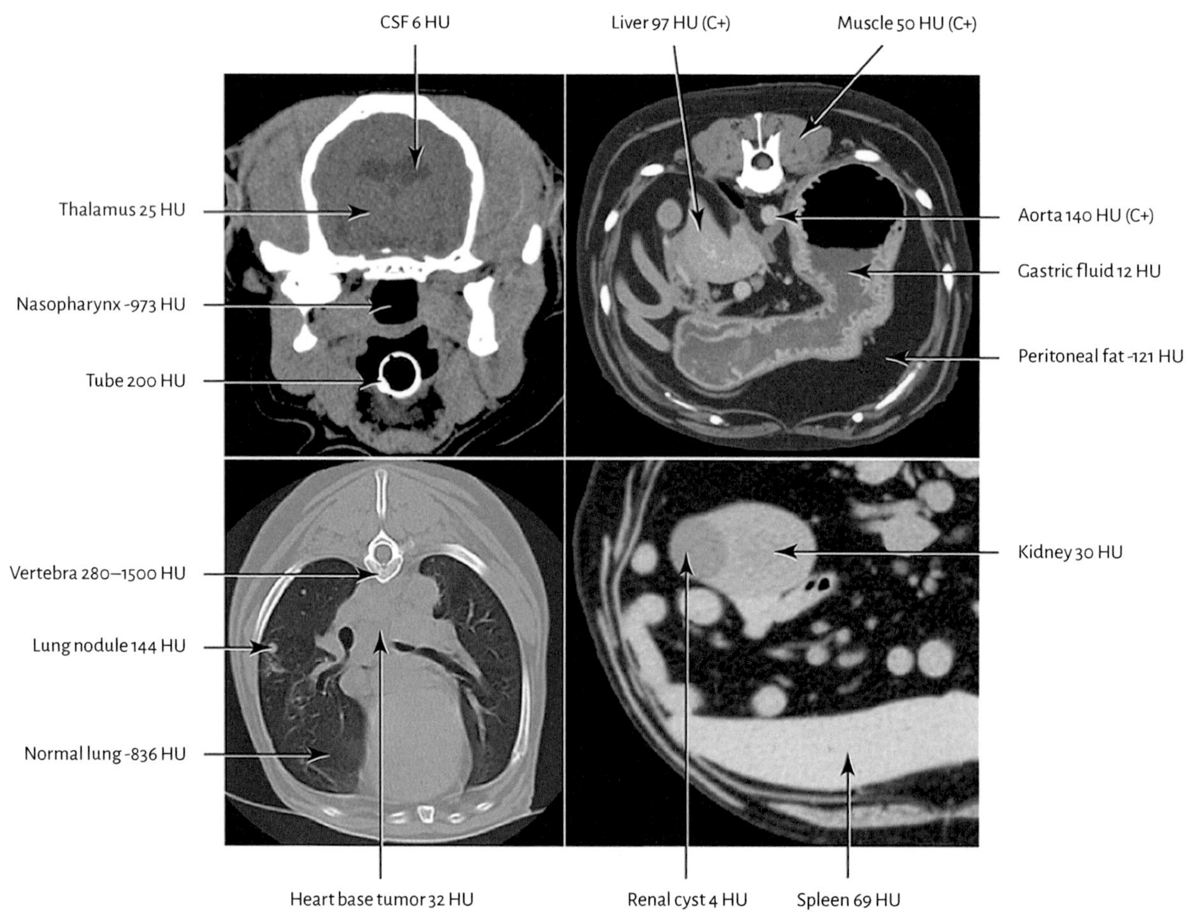

Figure 168. Different attenuations (Hounsfield units) of several tissues.

Image Display

HU values are measured approximately from 1000 to +3095 HU, for a total of 4096 shades of grey (12 bits of greyscale), which cannot be resolved by the human eye. To appreciate such variety of HU in the tissues, the image requires adjustment of the grey scale. The latter can be done by altering the window width (W) and level (L) of the image grayscale according to the area of interest. This is also called windowing.

A lung window (W1500 L700) shows greater detail of the lungs, but almost all other structures appear white with reduced detail. A bone window (W2000 L400) demonstrates a higher detail of skeletal structures, showing clear distinction of bone cortex and trabeculae, and soft tissues have a grey attenuation with little detail and the lungs appear black. A soft tissue window (W350 L40) provides better contrast and shows more detail in soft tissue structures such as the liver, spleen, intestines (Figure 169).

The interpretation of CT images requires a deep knowledge and understanding of anatomy and radiographic opacities. These are usually performed by radiologists on site or reported by radiologists remotely through use of a teleradiology company.

Reformatting

Due to the continuous helical scanning, **CT images can be rearranged, or reformatted, so that transverse images can be displayed in sagittal, transverse, and dorsal planes (multiplanar reformatting).** This allows better, more complete structure recognition and evaluation of tubular or tortuous structures, and of normal or abnormal tissues.

CT software or image viewer software can be used to **generate a 3D representation** through volume or surface rendering methods. This tool is useful for clinicians that are less familiar with tomographic imaging and for showing images to owners or planning for surgery.

The image quality of the reformatted section or 3D images is influenced by the initial image spatial resolution, and slice thickness. For example, thick slice thickness (3–5 mm) generates a step artefact once images are reformatted in sagittal or dorsal planes. Whereas, when images are obtained in thin slices (i.e. 0.5 mm), the images generated have a smoother contour. This level of reconstruction is not always necessary, but it is routinely used by radiologists for a more accurate interpretation and detection of small structures (e.g. bone fragments or lung nodules) (Figures 170 and 171).

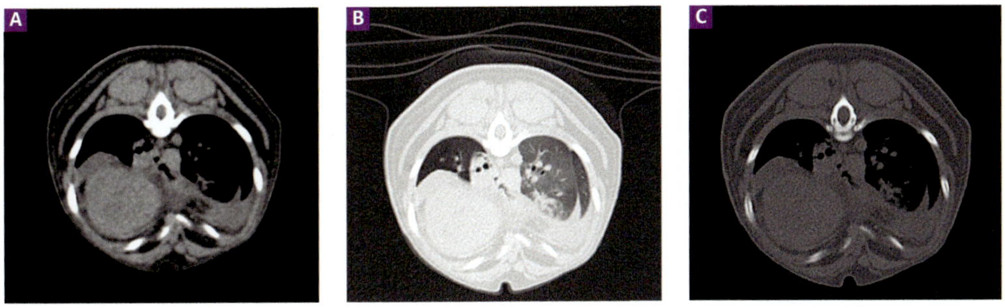

Figure 169. Windows. CT of the thorax illustrating soft tissue (**A**), lung (**B**) and bone windows (**C**).

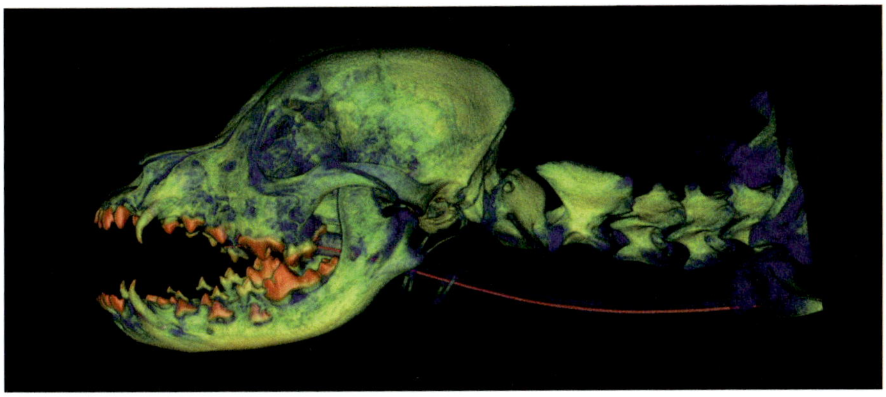

Figure 170. 3D volume rendering of a skull.

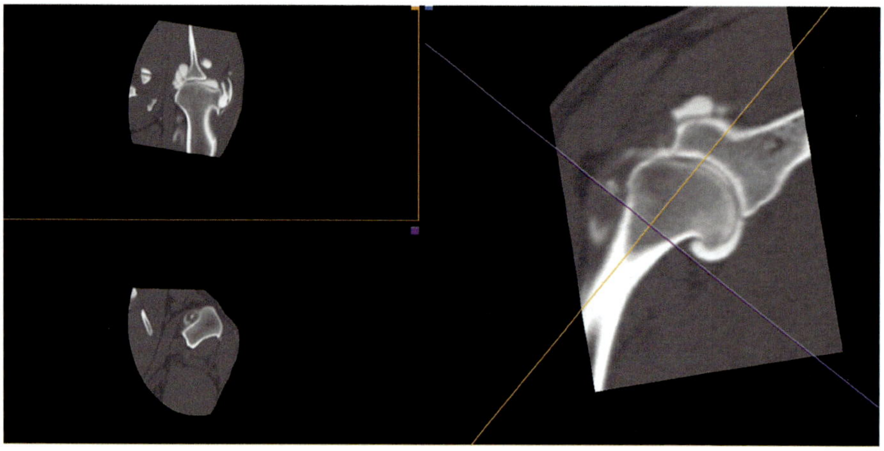

Figure 171. Multiplanar reconstruction (MPR) of a shoulder of a dog with intra-articular contrast medium demonstrating a complete biceps tendon rupture.

Contrast Procedures

The use of **iodinated contrast medium** has become standard for most CT procedures in veterinary medicine. Intravenous injection of contrast medium provides information on the perfusion of tissues and integrity of natural barriers, such as the blood brain barrier. (Figure 172).

Angiography represents another important application of CT imaging. CT is used to obtain images with contrast medium timed according to the vascular phase being examined and its enhancement peak. This is used with a power injector which triggers a remote injection of the contrast medium and monitors the enhancement peak phase. Precise acquisition timing is important when looking for portosystemic shunts or pancreatic insulinomas.

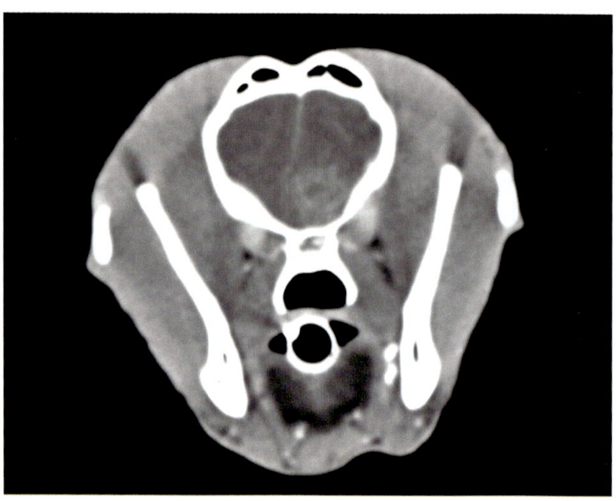

Figure 172. CT image of the head (soft tissue window) demonstrating contrast enhancement of an intracranial meningioma in a cat.

Iodinated contrast medium is eliminated by glomerular filtration, therefore contrast enhanced CT can be used to assess the renal collecting system by obtaining images of the nephrogram and pyelogram phases. Intravenous urography is superior when using CT rather than radiography because superimposition is eliminated, which allows better visualisation and more accurate identification of ectopic ureters.

Even though MRI is the gold standard modality for evaluation of the brain and spinal cord, **CT with non-ionic iodinated contrast medium can be used to detect lesions localised to the forebrain or a section of the spinal cord (when MRI is not available).** CT can be used with intrathecal contrast medium for myelography, confirming disc protrusion/ extrusions, intradural lesions and spinal cord compression due to neoplasms. However, vascular and inflammatory problems and some herniated discs may not be detected on CT.

It is important to obtain pre and post contrast medium sequences when acquiring CT images, because lesions with abnormal vascularity may only be visible after contrast administration. Depending on the lesion, contrast enhancement may be mild to marked or there may be no contrast enhancement at all.

CT Application

CT can be used to image almost any part of the body of cats and dogs. The most common applications are for the **head/ nasal cavity and auditory canal** (due to the lack of structure superimposition) and thorax (high sensitivity in detecting 1 mm metastatic nodules and better characterisation of mediastinal lesions). It is also used to evaluate the spine, brain, extremities, neck, and abdomen.

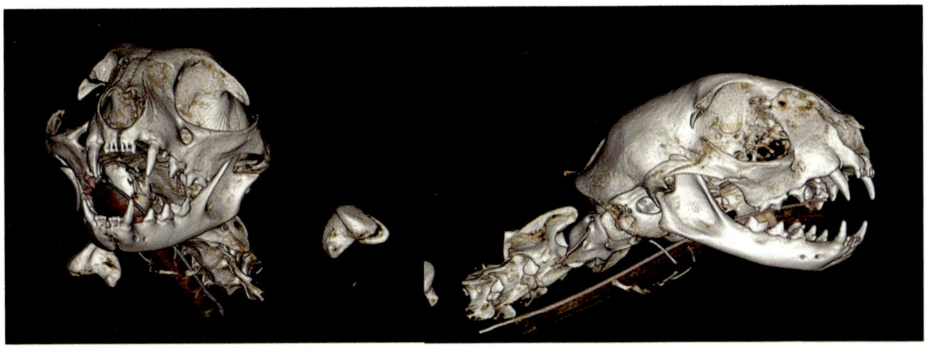

Figure 173. 3D reconstruction of a polytraumatic cat with multiple skull fractures.

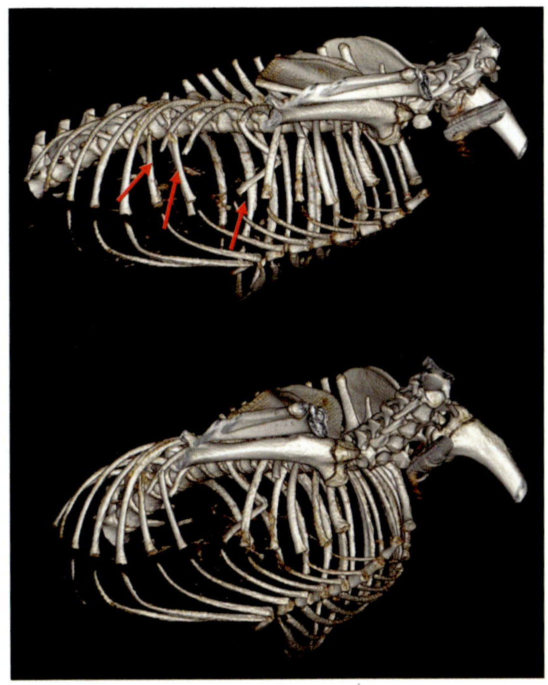

Figure 174. 3D reconstruction of a polytraumatic dog with multiple rib fractures.

CT is a valuable modality when evaluating a **polytraumatic patient** (Figures 173 and 174). The patient can be anaesthetised or conscious using a vet mouse trap. This allows a rapid interpretation of multiple skull or body fractures, or detection of the origin of pneumothorax or haemoabdomen faster than using other multimodalities. CT is the fastest and most efficient modality for detection of acute intracranial haemorrhage and severe brain oedema.

The use of CT is essential in the surgical patient (Figures 175 and 176) **for planning purposes:**

- for demonstration of tissue invasion and mass characteristics
- CT angiogram is useful for the detection of portosystemic shunts and pancreatic masses
- CT of the shoulders and elbows is routinely performed in the investigation of lameness. CT is superior to X-rays in the evaluation of joints due to absence of superimposition.

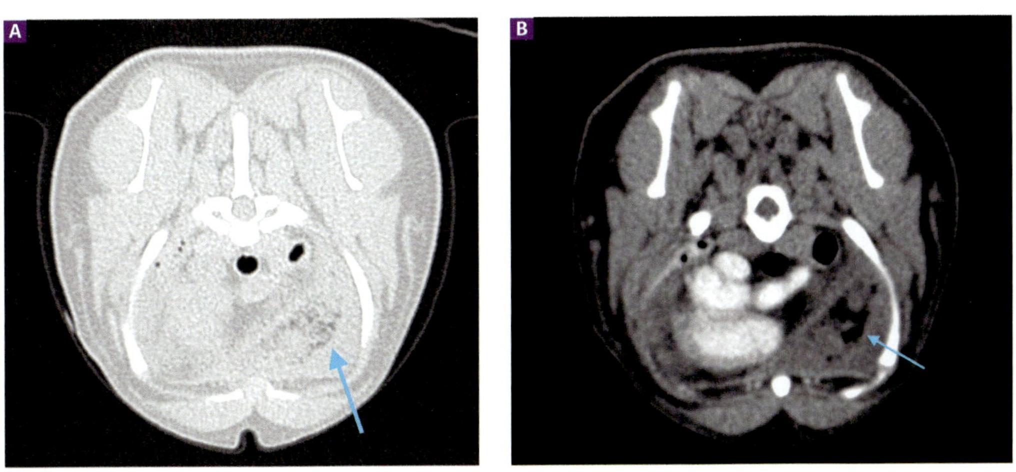

Figure 175. CT images of the thorax (lung window (**A**) and soft tissue window (**B**) of a dog with left cranial lung lobe torsion. The blue arrow highlights the vesicular pattern within the lung.

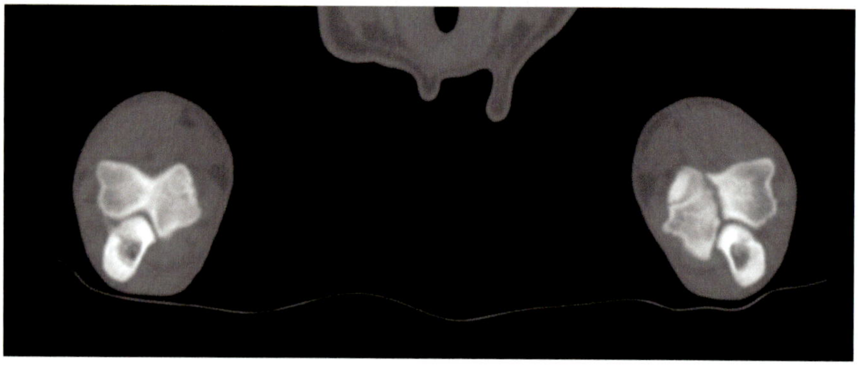

Figure 176. CT image (bone window) of the elbows of a young adult dog with an incomplete ossification of the humeral condyle.

Magnetic Resonance Imaging (MRI)

(Figure 177)

MRI has an inherent high contrast resolution compared to CT, which allows better characterisation of soft tissue. Unlike CT, no ionizing radiation is used in MRI. MRI functionality and contrast resolution revolves around the electromagnetic properties of hydrogen nuclei, which are abundant in body tissues. Hydrogen is universally distributed in the body, essentially in water molecules.

MR images are created from signals arising from excited tissues. The body is made up mostly of millions of hydrogen atoms. The nuclei of the hydrogen atom have an intrinsic spin which when magnetized, align themselves parallel with the magnetic field. Radiofrequency coils are placed around the patient and these are tuned to a particular frequency producing short bursts of radio waves to disrupt the orientation of the atoms. When the radio signal ceases, the atoms realign or precess with the magnetic field and then emit energy. This energy is picked up by the coils and sent to the computer to produce an image of the body. Different tissues (i.e. bone, muscle, nerves etc.) have different resonance characteristics. The different T1 and T2 relaxation times between tissues, or other sequences, can be used to excite and receive signals. Water has long relaxation times, soft tissues are intermediate, and fat has short relaxation times. Sequences are divided into two main groups: spin echo and gradient recalled sequences. There are a wide range of MRI sequences available. Each sequence is selected based on the patient's clinical history and area scanned, emphasising different tissue characterises. By using different MR sequences, these properties can be exploited, and tissues differentiated. (Figure 178).

Signal intensity is used to describe the appearance of the tissue in MRI, based on the radio signal generated by tissues in response to the stimulating radio energy pulse.

MRI has an exceptional contrast resolution in soft tissues and is very sensitive to changes such as oedema and haemorrhage. Bones, ligaments, and tendons appear quite dark on all image sequences because they contain little water and therefore less hydrogen to generate a signal. Nonetheless, MRI provides useful data regarding these structures.

Like CT, contrast medium can be used intravenously to assess vascular perfusion, helping in the detection and characterisation of pathological tissues. The contrast agents used in MRI are based on gadolinium, which alters the local magnetic field and changes signal intensity. (Figure 179).

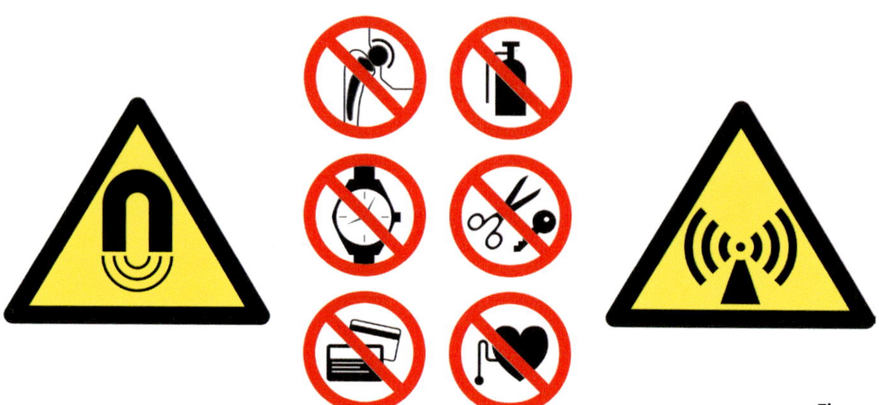

Figure 177. Warning signs for MRI.

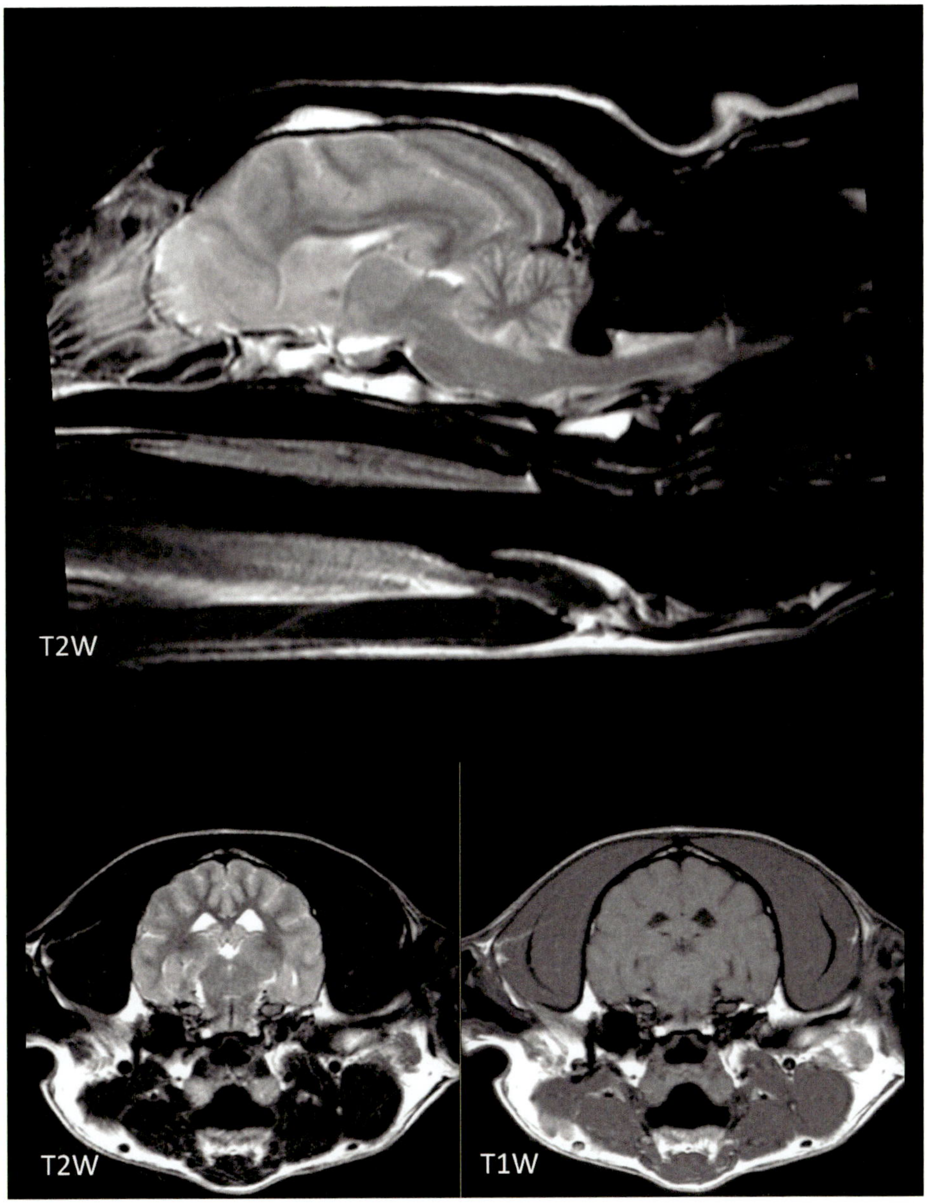

Figure 178. MRI of the brain. Sagittal and transverse T2 weighted images and T1 weighted images of the brain.

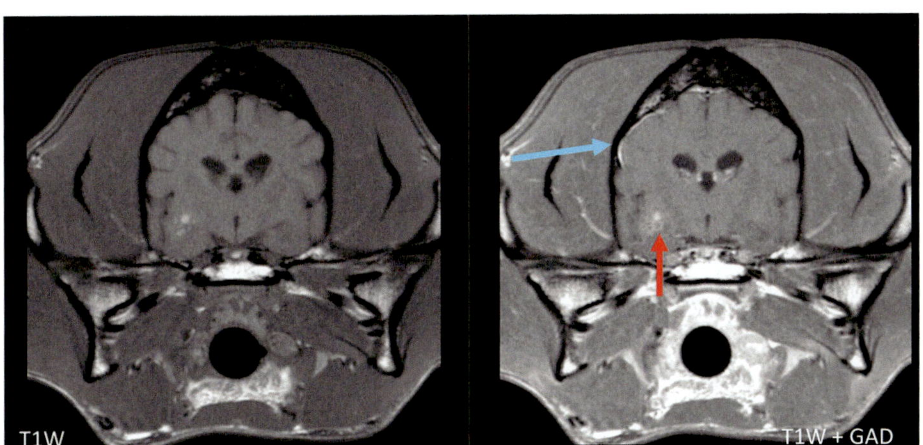

Figure 179. MRI of the brain of a dog. Transverse section of the brain of a T1W weighted imaged pre and post contrast highlighting showing an intraaxial lesion (red arrow) and meningeal thickening (blue arrow).

MRI physics is complex and requires a welltrained radiographer to run the machine and radiologist to interpret the images.

The challenge with MRI is the image acquisition time which increases patient general anaesthetic time. Most procedures are performed as quickly as possible without major deterioration of the image quality. MRI image acquisition usually takes a long time compared to CT (approximately 45 minutes versus 5–10 minutes). This is because each sequence (T1W, T2W, GRE, FLAIR and others) have to be obtained in all planes (sagittal, dorsal, transverse, and oblique planes) of each area. Therefore, localisation of the pain or neurolocalisation is crucial before using MRI as an investigating modality. MRI should not be used as hunt tool.

MRI is used mainly used to **investigate neurological conditions** (brain and spine) (Figure 180); however, other parts of the body are routinely scanned such as joints (shoulder, less commonly stifles, elbows, distal limbs) and nasal cavity. MRI is the best diagnostic method to evaluate tendons, which is more often used in large animals (equine).

MRI can be used to detect early stages of inflammatory/infectious diseases or neoplasia that cannot be detected with other diagnostic imaging modalities. **MRI is the gold standard modality for identification of migrating foreign bodies (grass seeds).**

MRI Safety

The MRI primary feature is a powerful magnet, which creates a static magnetic field which is measured in teslas. The magnetic field is weakest outside the room (Faraday cage), but strength increases rapidly in the immediate vicinity of the magnet.

The most significant known danger of the MRI is the risk associated with the attraction of ferromagnetic objects (i.e. iron, cobalt, nickel etc.) causing them to become projectiles which pose a great risk to the patient or anyone in their path.

The effect of the magnetic field within the magnet bore is a rotational force. **Nonspherical metallic objects inside or outside the body experience a torque.** The induced rotation of objects inside the body can cause the object to move or dislodge and tear the surrounding tissues. Microchips, vascular clamps, intravascular coils, or stents become stable once scarring has settled. Other implants, such as pacemakers may fail due to components being displaced inside the device. Iron aneurysmal clips have been reported to rotate and cause haemorrhage followed by death. Some of these devices are not common in veterinary patients, however this information is important to avoid anyone entering the MRI unit if they contain a pacemaker, defibrillator, aneurysmal clips, or other medical devices.

In addition, metallic implants or other objects may cause signal loss or alter MR images making it difficult for the radiologist to see the images correctly. This may be unavoidable, but if the radiologist knows about it, allowances can be made when obtaining and interpreting the MR images (i.e microchip) (Figure 181).

A knowledge of the entire clinical history of the patient is important to screen for previous surgeries that involved metal implants. Many orthopaedic implants are now made of titanium alloy and considered to be compatible with MRI at 1.5 T.

Items such as, cards with a magnetic strip (ID/work badges, credit cards, hotel keys), analogue and digital watches, hearing aids, cell phones and pagers, cameras, medical instruments (scissors, thermometers, stethoscopes etc.), keys, hair clips and bobby pins, clip boards, pens, paper clips, and noncompatible MRI medical devices (patient monitors, infusion pumps, ventilators etc.) should not be allowed in the MRI unit due to their ferromagnetic composition and high risk of projectile movement by the magnet.

Other hazards in the MRI include high level acoustic noise and systemic and localized heating.

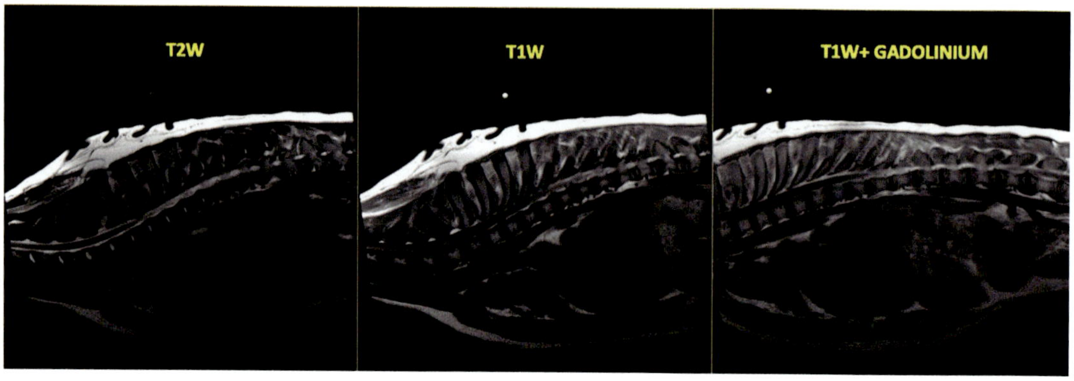

Figure 180. MRI of the thoracic spine (sagittal sequences) of a skeletally mature dog demonstrating T2W, T1W and postcontrast T1W sequences.

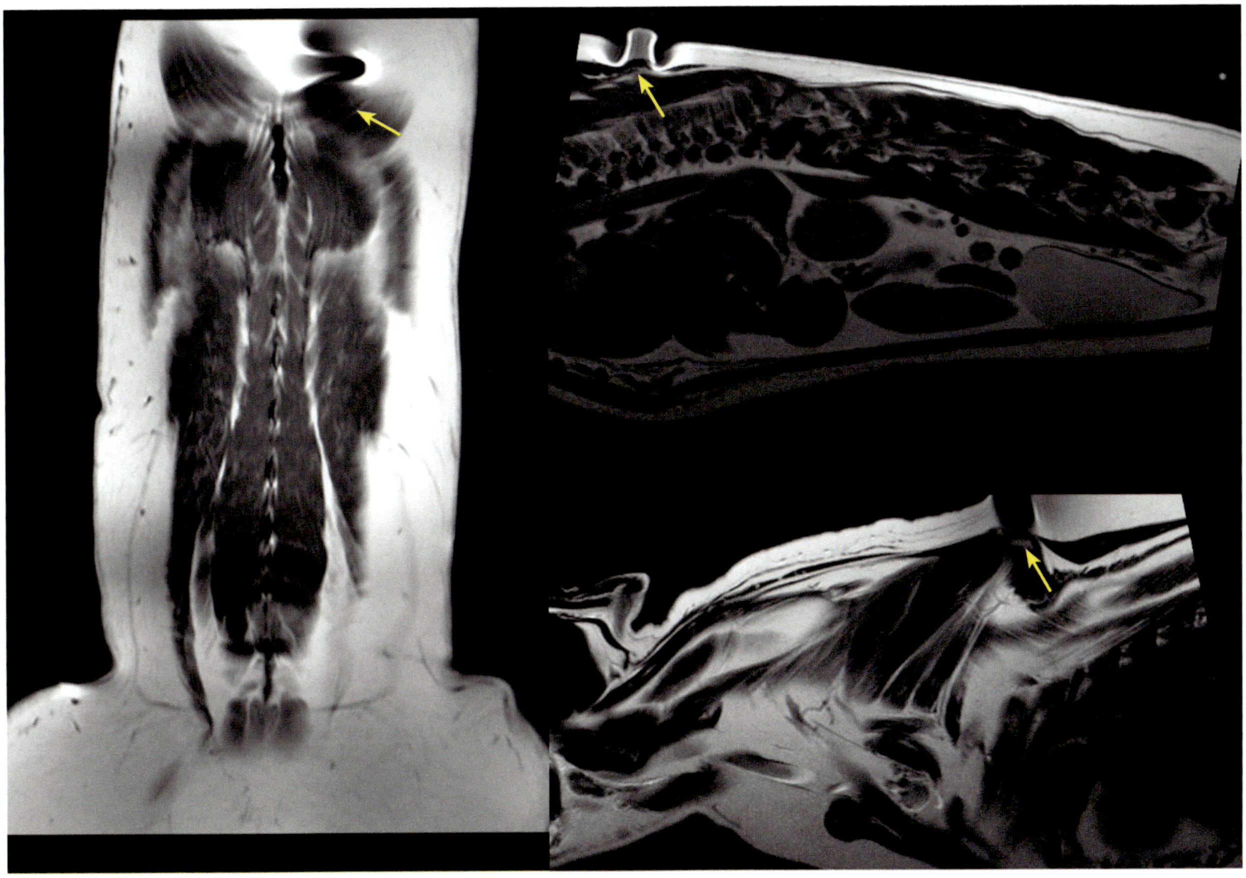

Figure 181. MRI images showing microchip artefact (yellow arrows).

Nuclear Medicine (Scintigraphy)

Scintigraphy is a branch of nuclear medicine routinely used in large animals (equine) but not so much in cat and dogs. The technique consists of the administration of a radionuclide which accumulates in the tissue of interest and is detected by a γ-ray camera. The γ-rays are converted into signals by the camera from which a computer produces a digital format that is used to construct an image.

Nuclear medicine images are described in terms of uptake of the radiopharmaceutical.

The primary limitation of scintigraphy is poor spatial resolution. Scintigraphy has a high sensitivity for detection of bone metabolism (bone destruction, remodelling, arthropathy), but is not specific to the changes. Hence, radiography is usually used alongside with scintigraphy, to obtain a more accurate diagnosis.

Scintigraphy in orthopaedic patients is used primarily to identify possible sites of occult fracture or bone lesions not detected by other imaging modalities or localisation of the site of lameness (single or multifocal).

Scintigraphy is very sensitive in the detection of stress fractures or occult fractures which have not been identified on X-rays. This technique is used more commonly in horses than cats or dogs. Scintigraphy can identify a stress fracture within 24–72 hours of injury. However, this can be correlated with clinical history, the degree of lameness, the degree of uptake and if there is any additional information from other diagnostic imaging modalities.

In dogs, bone scintigraphy has been used to identify primary neoplasm and/or metastases. In cats, it often used to identify ectopic thyroid/parathyroid tissue to plan surgery and prior to the start of radioactive iodine treatment. (Figure 182).

Nuclear scintigraphy can also provide physiological information about perfusion and ventilation of the lung, renal function, gastric emptying, and detection of gastrointestinal bleeding. However, it is rarely performed in small animals.

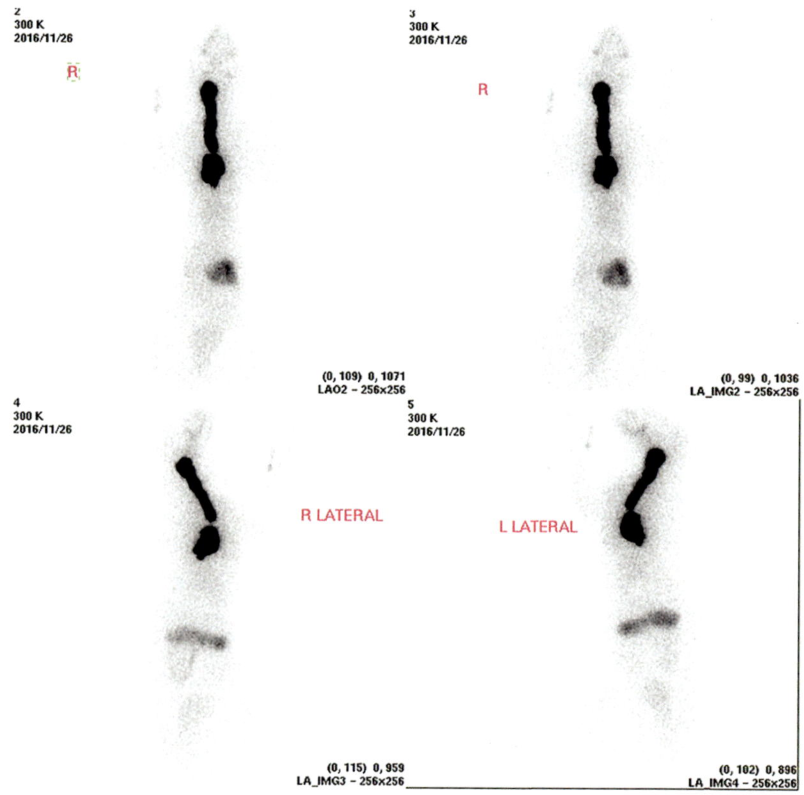

Figure 182. Scintigraphy images of a cat with marked radiopharmaceutical uptake demonstrating the localisation of ectopic thyroid tissue from the neck up to the mediastinum.

Bibliography

■ Ayers, S. (2012) *Small animal radiographic techniques and positioning*. West Sussex, Wiley-Blackwell.

■ Baines, E. & Holloway, A. (2019). Principles of radiological interpretation. *BSAVA Manual of Canine and Feline Radiography and Radiology*. Gloucester, BSAVA, pp.355–386.

■ Bansal, GJ. (2006) Digital radiography. A comparison with modern conventional imaging. *Postgraduate Medical Journal*. 82(969), 425–428.

■ Barr, F. & O'Brien, R. (2008) Approach to abdominal imaging. *BSAVA Manual of Canine and Feline Abdominal Imaging*. Gloucester, BSAVA, pp. 1–4.

■ Barrett, E. (2019) Radiology of the abdomen. *BSAVA Manual of Canine and Feline Radiography and Radiology*. Gloucester BSAVA, pp.176–239.

■ Beal, M.W. (2018) Interventional management of urethral obstructions. *The Veterinary Clinics of North America, Small Animal Practice*. 48(5), 863–874.

■ Beigel, R., Cercek, B., Arsanjani, R., & Siegel, R.J. (2014) Echocardiography in the use of non–invasive hemodynamic monitoring. *Journal of Critical Care*. 29(1), 184.e1–184.e8.

■ Berent, A.C. (2016) Interventional radiology of the urinary tract. *The Veterinary Clinics of North America. Small Animal Practice*. 46(3), 567–596.

■ Bochmann, M., Ludewig, E., Krautwald-Junhanns, M., & Pees, M. (2011) Comparison of the image quality of a high-resolution screen-film system and a digital flat panel detector system in avian radiography. *Veterinary Radiology & Ultrasound*. 52(3), 256–26.

■ Boysen, S.R., & Lisciandro, G.R. (2013) The use of ultrasound for dogs and cats in the emergency room: AFAST and TFAST. *The Veterinary Clinics of North America. Small Animal Practice*. 43(4), 773–797.

■ Boysen, S. (2014) Interventional Ultrasound-Guided Procedures. *Focused Ultrasound Techniques for the Small Animal Practitioner*. G.R. Lisciandro (Ed.)

■ Bradley, K. (2005) Practical contrast radiography 2 gastrointestinal studies. In Practice. 27(8), 412–41.

■ Bradley, K. (2008) The small intestine. *BSAVA Manual of the Canine and Feline Abdominal Imaging*. Gloucester, BSAVA, pp. 110–131.

■ Bradley, K. (2019) Radiology of the thorax. *BSAVA Manual of Canine and Feline Radiography and Radiology*. Gloucester, BSAVA, pp.109–175.

■ Brown, D., Gaillot, H., & Cunningham, S. (2015) Heart. *Atlas of small animal ultrasonography*. Iowa, Wiley Blackwell, pp. 111–181.

■ Caine, A., & Dennis, R. (2019) Principles of radiography. *BSAVA Manual of Canine and Feline Radiography and Radiology*. Gloucester, BSAVA, pp. 21–46.

■ Canty, D.J., Royse, C.F., Kilpatrick, D., Bowman, L., & Royse, A.G. (2012) The impact of focused transthoracic echocardiography in the pre operative clinic. *Anaesthesia*. 67(6), 618–625.

■ Cardoso, H.M., Tocheto, R., Padilha, V.S., Silva, G., Comassetto, F., Newton Bizetto Meira de Andrade, J., & Oleskovicz, N. (2018) Echocardiographic evaluation of dogs subjected to different protocols of anaesthetic induction. *Ciência Rural*. 48(8).

■ Clark, L., Kavanagh, J.A., Pang, D.S.J., Gurney, M.A., Bradbrook, CA., Gibson, S. M., & Oliveira, P. (2020) Impact of preanaesthetic echocardiography on the planned anaesthetic management of cats. *Veterinary Anaesthesia and Analgesia*. 47(5), 614–620.

■ Clarke, D.L. (2018) Interventional radiology management of tracheal and bronchial collapse. *The Veterinary Clinics of North America. Small Animal Practice*. 48(5), 765–779.

■ Cléroux, A., Hersh–Boyle, R., & Clarke, D.L. (2018) Interventional equipment and radiation safety. *The Veterinary Clinics of North America. Small Animal Practice*. 48(5), 751–763.

■ Cole, L., Pivetta, M., & Humm, K. (2021) Diagnostic accuracy of a lung ultrasound Protocol (vet BLUE) for detection of pleural fluid, pneumothorax and lung pathology in dogs and cats. *Journal of Small Animal Practice*. 62(3), 178–186.

■ Costello, M. (2008) The male reproductive system. *BSAVA Manual of the Canine and Feline Abdominal Imaging*. Gloucester, BSAVA, pp. 237–245.

■ Culp, W.T.N., & Griffin, M.A. (2018) Interventional radiology management of vascular malformations. *The Veterinary Clinics of North America. Small Animal Practice*. 48(5), 781–795.

■ Darnis, E., Boysen, S., Merveille, A., Desquilbet, L., Chalhoub, S., & Gommeren, K. (2018) Establishment of reference values of the caudal vena cava by fast-ultrasonography through different views in healthy dogs. *Journal of Veterinary Internal Medicine*. 32(4), 1308–1318.

■ Dennis, R. (2010) *Handbook of Small Animal Radiology and Ultrasound: Techniques and Differential Diagnoses* (2nd ed.). Churchill Livingstone/Elsevier.

■ Dennis, R. (2019) Physics and equipment. *BSAVA Manual of Canine and Feline Radiography and Radiology*. Gloucester, BSAVA, pp. 1–20.

■ Domenech O, Oliveira P. (2013) Transoesophageal echocardiography in the dog. *Vet J*. 198(2):329–38.

■ Drost, W.T., Reese, D. J., & Hornof, W.J. (2008) Digital radiography artifacts. *Veterinary Radiology & Ultrasound*. 49(s1), S48–S56.

■ Dunn, M., & Scansen, B. A. (2018) Interventional radiology management of vascular obstruction. *The Veterinary Clinics of North America. Small Animal Practice*. 48(5), 819–841.

■ Gallagher, A. (2018) Interventional radiology and interventional endoscopy in treatment of nephroureteral disease in the dog and cat. *The Veterinary Clinics of North America. Small Animal Practice*. 48(5), 843–862.

■ Gashen, L. (2008) The large intestine and perianal region. *BSAVA Manual of the Canine and Feline Abdominal Imaging*. Gloucester, BSAVA, pp. 132–143.

■ Hammond, G. (2008). The female reproductive system. *BSAVA Manual of the Canine and Feline Abdominal Imaging*. Gloucester, BSAVA, pp. 222–236.
■ Hammond, G. & McConnel, F. (2019) Radiology of the appendicular system. *BSAVA Manual of Canine and Feline Radiography and Radiology*. Gloucester, BSAVA, pp.240–301.
■ Hespel, A., & Cole, R.C. (2018) Advances in high-field MRI. *The Veterinary Clinics of North America. Small Animal Practice*. 48(1), 11–29.
■ Holloway, A. & Avner, A. (2019) Radiology of the head. *BSAVA Manual of Canine and Feline Radiography and Radiology*. Gloucester, BSAVA, pp.302–354.
■ Iwatsuki, K., Yoneda, H., Onishi, T., Ishii, H., Kurimoto, S., Yamamoto, M., Tatebe, M., & Hirata, H. (2020) Compatibility of magnetic resonance imaging in patients with orthopaedic implants: manufacturer questionnaires. *Nagoya Journal of Medical Science*. 82(1), 79–84.
■ John, M.S. and Durham, H.E., Jr. (2017) Echocardiography and Doppler Study. *Cardiology for Veterinary Technicians and Nurses*. H.E. Durham (Ed.).
■ Kealy, J.K., McAllister, H., & Graham, J.P. (2011) *Diagnostic radiology and ultrasonography of the dog and cat* (5th ed.). Saunders.
■ Kent, A. (2020) Guide to interventional radiology in cats and dogs. *In Practice*. 42: 476–487.
■ King, A. (2018) An insight into digital radiography use in small animal practice in the UK. *Veterinary Record*. 182(8), 222–224.
■ Larson, M.M. (2008) The kidneys and ureters. *BSAVA Manual of the Canine and Feline Abdominal Imaging*. Gloucester, BSAVA, pp. 185–204.
■ Liffman, R. and Courtman, N. (2017) Fine needle aspiration of abdominal organs: a review of current recommendations for achieving a diagnostic sample. *J Small Anim Pract*. 58: 599–609.
■ Lisciandro, G.R., & Wiley Online Library (Online service). (2020). *Point-of-care ultrasound techniques for the small animal practitioner* (2nd ed.). Wiley-Blackwell.
■ Lisciandro, G.R., & Fosgate, G.T. (2017) Use of urinary bladder measurements from a point-of-care cysto-colic ultrasonographic view to estimate urinary bladder volume in dogs and cats. Journal of Veterinary Emergency and Critical Care. 27(6), 713–717.
■ Lisciandro, G.R., Fulton, R.M., Fosgate, G.T., & Mann, K.A. (2017) Frequency and number of B-lines using a regionally based lung ultrasound examination in cats with radiographically normal lungs compared to cats with left-sided congestive heart failure. *Journal of Veterinary Emergency and Critical Care*. 27(5), 499–505.
■ Lisciandro, G.R. (2016) The use of the diaphragmatico hepatic (DH) views of the abdominal and thoracic focused assessment with sonography for triage (AFAST/TFAST) examinations for the detection of pericardial effusion in 24 dogs (2011–2012). *Journal of Veterinary Emergency and Critical Care*. 26(1), 125–131.
■ Lisciandro, G.R. (2014) *Focused ultrasound techniques for the small animal practitioner*. Wiley Blackwell.
■ Lisciandro, G.R., Fosgate, G.T., & Fulton, R.M. (2014) Frequency and number of ultrasound lung rockets (b-lines) using a regionally based ultrasound examination named vet blue (veterinary bedside lung ultrasound exam) in dogs with radiographically normal lung findings. *Veterinary Radiology & Ultrasound*. 55(3), 315–322.
■ Lisciandro, G.R. (2011) Abdominal and thoracic focused assessment with sonography for trauma, triage, and monitoring in small animals. *Journal of Veterinary Emergency and Critical Care*. 21(2), 104–122.
■ Lisciandro, G.R., Lagutchik, M.S., Mann, K.A., Fosgate, G.T., Tiller, E.g. Cabano, N.R., Bauer, L.D., Book, B.P., & Howard, P.K. (2009) Evaluation of an abdominal fluid scoring system determined using abdominal focused assessment with sonography for trauma in 101 dogs with motor vehicle trauma. *Journal of Veterinary Emergency and Critical Care*. 19(5), 426–437.
■ Lisciandro, G.R., Lagutchik, M.S., Mann, K.A., Voges, A.K., Fosgate, G.T., Tiller, E.g. Cabano, N. R., Bauer, L. D., & Book, B. P. (2008) Evaluation of a thoracic focused assessment with sonography for trauma (TFAST) protocol to detect pneumothorax and concurrent thoracic injury in 145 traumatized dogs. *Journal of Veterinary Emergency and Critical Care*. 18(3), 258–269.
■ MacDonald, M.R., Hawkins, N.M., Balmain, S., Dalzell, J., McMurray, J.J.V., & Petrie, M. C. (2008) Transthoracic echocardiography: A survey of current practice in the UK. QJM : *Monthly Journal of the Association of Physicians*. 101(5), 345–349.
■ Mcconnell, J.F. (2008) Abdominal radiography. In O'Brien, R., & Barr, F. (eds.) *BSAVA Manual of the Canine and Feline Abdominal Imaging*. Gloucester, BSAVA, pp. 5–17.
■ Menciotti, G., and Borgarelli, M. (2017) Review of Diagnostic and Therapeutic Approach to Canine Myxomatous Mitral Valve Disease. *Veterinary Sciences*. 4: 47.
■ Milley, E., Boysen, S., & Stillion, J. (2017) A general practitioner's guide to FAST cageside ultrasound techniques. *Companion Animal*. 22(7), 388–393.
■ Murphy, S.D., Ward, J.L., Viall, A.K., et al. (2021) Utility of point-of–care lung ultrasound for monitoring cardiogenic pulmonary edema in dogs. *J Vet Intern Med*. 35: 68 77.
■ Moore, A.H. (2008) The bladder and urethra. *BSAVA Manual of the Canine and Feline Abdominal Imaging*. Gloucester, BSAVA, pp. 205–221.
■ Oyama, M.A. (2004) Advances in echocardiography. *The Veterinary Clinics of North America. Small Animal Practice*. 34(5), 1083–1104.
■ Penninck, D., d'Anjou, M., & Mellor, B. (2015) *Atlas of small animal ultrasonography* (2nd ed.). John Wiley & Sons Incorporated.
■ Richmond, P. (2018). Canine pericardial effusion — a veterinary nurse's guide. *Veterinary Nurse*. 9(4), 208–214.
■ Robertson, I.D., & Thrall, D.E. (2018) Digital radiographic imaging. *Textbook of Veterinary Diagnostic Radiology*. Missouri, Elsevier, pp. 23–38.
■ Schwarz, T & Holloway, A. (2019) Radiology of the vertebral column. *BSAVA Manual of Canine and Feline Radiography and Radiology*. Gloucester, BSAVA, pp.355–386.
■ Royse, C.F., Seah, J.L., Donelan, L., & Royse, A.G. (2006) Point of care ultrasound for basic haemodynamic assessment: Novice compared with an expert operator. *Anaesthesia*. 61(9), 849–855.

■ Sage, J.E., & Gavin, P. (2016) Musculoskeletal MRI. *The Veterinary Clinics of North America. Small Animal Practice.* 46(3), 421–451.
■ Samoy, Y., Van Ryssen, B., Van Caelenberg, A., Gielen, I., Van Vynckt, D., Van Bree, H., De Bacquer, D., & Peremans, K. (2008) Single–phase bone scintigraphy in dogs with obscure lameness. *Journal of Small Animal Practice.* 49(9), 444–450.
■ Scansen, B.A. (2016) Interventional radiology: Equipment and techniques. *The Veterinary Clinics of North America. Small Animal Practice.* 46(3), 535–552.
■ Scansen, B.A. (2018) Cardiac interventions in small animals: Areas of uncertainty. *The Veterinary Clinics of North America. Small Animal Practice.* 48(5), 797–817.
■ Schwarz, T., Johnson, V.S., Voute, L., & Sullivan, M. (2004) Bone scintigraphy in the investigation of occult lameness in the dog. *Journal of Small Animal Practice.* 45(5), 232–237.
■ Seiler, G. (2008) The stomach. *BSAVA Manual of the Canine and Feline Abdominal Imaging.* Gloucester, BSAVA, pp. 87–109.
■ Seiler, G., Dukes-McEwan, J., & Gaschen, L. (2011) Basics of thoracic ultrasonography. Schwarz T., & Johnson, V. (eds) *BSAVA Manual of Canine and Feline Thoracic Imaging.* Gloucester, BSAVA, pp. 20–65.
■ Smith, J.A. (2010) Hazard safety and Anaesthetic consideration for Magnetic Resonance Imaging. *Companion Animal Medicine.* 25 (2), 98–106.
■ Thomas, W.P., Gaber, C.E., Jacobs, G.J., Kaplan, P.M., Lombard, C.W., Vet, M., Moise, N.S. and Moses, B.L. (1993) Recommendations for Standards in Transthoracic Two-Dimensional Echocardiography in the Dog and Cat. *Journal of Veterinary Internal Medicine,* 7: 247–252.
■ Thrall, D.E. (2018) *Textbook of Veterinary Diagnostic Radiology* (7th ed.). Saunders.
■ Thrall, D. E. (2013). *Textbook of Veterinary Diagnostic Radiology* (6th ed.). Elsevier Saunders.
■ Thrall, D. E., & Widmer, W. R. (2018) Radiation protection and physics of diagnostic radiology. *Textbook of Veterinary Diagnostic Radiology.* Missouri, Elsevier, pp. 2–22.
■ The Ionising Radiations Regulations 1999
■ The Ionising Radiation (Medical Exposure) Regulations 2017
■ The Ionising Radiations Regulations 2017
■ Vezzosi, T., Mannucci, T., Pistoresi, A., Toma, F., Tognetti, R., Zini, E., Domenech, O., Auriemma, E., & Citi, S. (2017) Assessment of lung ultrasound B-Lines in dogs with different stages of chronic valvular heart disease. *Journal of Veterinary Internal Medicine.* 1(3), 700–704.
■ Walters, A.M., O'Brien, M.A., Selmic, L.E., Hartman, S., McMichael, M., & O'Brien, R.T. (2018) Evaluation of the agreement between focused assessment with sonography for trauma (AFAST/TFAST) and computed tomography in dogs and cats with recent trauma. *Journal of Veterinary Emergency and Critical Care.* 28(5), 429–435

Test

1. **Why lower mAs and high KvP technique is used for thoracic radiographs?**
   a. To reduce motion artefact by the breathing.
   b. To increase contrast.
   c. To increase brightness.
   d. To decrease brightness.

2. **What does ALARA stand for?**
   a. As low as responsible as possible.
   b. As low as reasonably achievable.
   c. As low as responsible achievable.
   d. As low as reasonably as possible.

3. **Which positive contrast medium would be safest to use in a patient with suspected bladder rupture?**
   a. Barium.
   b. Ionic Iodinated contrast medium (i.e. Urografin®).
   c. Non-ionic iodinated contrast medium (i.e. Omnipaque®).
   d. Air.

4. **Identify the five radiographic opacities**
   a. Air, soft tissue, fat, bone, and metal.
   b. Air, fluid, soft tissue, bone, and mineral.
   c. Fluid, mineral, metal, air, and fat.
   d. Fluid, soft tissue, metal, and fluid.

5. **What are the sites examined on AFAST?**
   a. Diaphragmatico renal, splenorenal, hepatorenal, right renal.
   b. Hepatorenal, splenorenal, diafragmatico hepatic and cystocolic.
   c. Cystocolic, splenorenal, right renal and diaphragmatico hepatic.
   d. Hepatorenal, splenorenal cystouterus and diaphragmatico hepatic.

6. **Which view on AFAST is used to assess the cardiac silhouette for pericardial effusion?**
   a. Diaphragmatico hepatic.
   b. Splenorenal.
   c. Diaphragmatico renal.
   d. Hepatorenal.

7. **TFAST and VetBlue. Which ultrasonographic feature is identified in a patient with cardiogenic pulmonary oedema.**
   a. A-lines.
   b. B-lines.
   c. C-lines.
   d. D-lines.

Answers on page 302

8. **Which ultrasonographic feature is important for the exclusion of pneumothorax on TFAST and VetBlue?**
   a. B-lines.
   b. Rocket lines.
   c. Comet sign.
   d. Sliding sign.

9. **Right parasternal short axis view. What is the ratio that indicates left atrium enlargement?**
   a. LA: Ao <1.6.
   b. LA: PA <1.6.
   c. LA:Ao >1.6.
   d. RA: Ao <1.6.

10. **Which of the following can be used to measure high velocities in echocardiography without causing aliasing?**
   a. Colour Doppler.
   b. Continues wave Doppler.
   c. Pulse wave Doppler.
   d. B-Mode.

Clinical Case

Walter, a 5-year-old, male neutered Labrador with long intermittent history of lower urinary tract disease, pollakiuria, occasional stranguria and haematuria. The dog presented out-of-hours with stranguria, straining and haematuria. He has been treated for cystitis several times but never had a full workup of the urinary trat.

Walter was sedated and underwent an abdominal ultrasound which showed a markedly distended bladder with multiple cystoliths which was most likely causing an obstruction.

An attempt of placement of a urinary catheter was made but unsuccessful. The dog was then anaesthetised, and you were asked to prepare the X-ray room for abdominal radiographs, retrograde urethrocystogram and assist in the positioning of the patient.

1. **Where will be the centring for this radiograph?**
2. **Which views should be taken?**
3. **Why do you think a retrograde urethrocystogram should be performed?**
4. **Which type of contrast can be used?**
5. **What things should be considered when performing this type of procedures for patient and personnel safety?**

Notes

Correct answers:

Test

1. a
2. b
3. c
4. a
5. b
6. a
7. b
8. d
9. c
10. b

Clinical Case

1. **Where will be the centring for this radiograph?**
Caudal abdomen including the perineum and the entire trajectory of the urethra.

2. **Which views should be taken?**
Right lateral views with hind limbs in neutral position and pulled forwards.

3. **Why do you think a retrograde urethrocystogram should be performed?**
To evaluate the urethra and identify the uroliths that could be the cause of the obstruction in the urethra or bladder.

4. **Which type of contrast can be used?**
Ionic iodinated or non-ionic iodinated contrast medium.

5. **What things should be considered when performing this type of procedures for patient and personnel safety?**
    - These procedures should be performed in a controlled area. The staff allowed in the room should have been trained to use the X-ray unit and understand the local rules. Only essential staff should be allowed in the room.
    - Everyone should where a dosimeter badge.
    - Always communicate with the anaesthetist or nurse performing the anaesthesia to make sure patient is stable.
    - Do not allow any pregnant staff to partake on the procedure or be in the room.
    - Personnel closer to the primary beam during contrast administration should wear appropriate PPE (lead gown, gloves, and thyroid shield).

Notes

Preparation for Surgery

Darren Barnes

Chapter Summary:

- **The principles of surgical technique.**
- **Suture materials and suture principles. Suture patterns and techniques.**
- **Main pathways of haemostasis and control of haemorrhage at surgery.**
- **Surgical instrumentation – nomenclature and instrument handling.**
- **Pathophysiology of gastric dilation/volvulus (GDV).**
- **Pathophysiology of a variety of surgical conditions of the gastrointestinal tract, options for treatment and complications such as peritonitis.**
- **Surgery of the head and neck (BOAS, maxillectomy/ mandibulectomy, TECA-LBO and ophthalmic surgery.**
- **Pathophysiology of pyometra and treatment.**
- **Endoscopic surgical equipment for laparoscopy/ thoracoscopy.**

Surgical Planning

Planning a surgery requires a thorough appraisal of a patient's condition using preoperative investigations such as a clinical examination, laboratory tests, and diagnostic imaging. With these evaluations complete in preparation for surgery, this allows for informed discussions between the care team and surgeon, maximises preparedness, and increases the likelihood of a successful outcome. Key to bringing this about is good team communication.

Communication between the surgical team, anaesthetists, and theatre staff is vital to ensure the patient is prepared optimally and all necessary equipment is available. **To achieve this, surgical request forms** (Figure 1) are a useful way for the surgeon to appraise the procedure with respect to patient clipping, skin sterilisation, positioning for optimal surgical access. In turn this facilitates appropriate preoperative medication and availability of necessary equipment, in order to maximise the efficiency of the surgical procedure (i.e. the appropriate electrosurgical equipment, retraction, and implants are available and ready for use). Anaesthetists also want to plan the appropriate analgesia for optimal safety and to minimise morbidity.

Surgical Safety Checklists

Safety checklists are common in other high-risk occupations such as in aviation and construction. The surgical safety checklist is a simple tool designed to improve communication and teamwork by bringing together the surgeons, anaesthetist, and nurses involved to confirm that critical safety measures are undertaken before, during and after an operation. (Figure 2).

The **World Health Organisation developed a template surgical safety checklist,** which is used widely in human surgery, and is also applicable to veterinary patients. The checklist introduces **three focussed periods of pausing** to check patient details before proceeding to the next stage of the procedure.

- A **sign-in** is performed prior to anaesthetic induction with the priority being to check the patient's identity and procedure, and the preparedness of the anaesthetic equipment. At this stage any patient allergies should be documented and if haemorrhage is considered a high risk, then a strategy prepared to manage it.
- In theatre, prior to the first incision, a **time-out** should be undertaken. The idea is that with all members of the surgical team present, this ensures that everyone is known to their colleagues and their roles clearly defined. Also, it is confirmed that all the necessary equipment and diagnostic imaging that may need to be referred to is prepared. Then the surgeon and anaesthetist should reiterate any specific patient concerns so that the whole team is aware of any critical issues.
- At the end of the procedure, a **sign-out** should be undertaken before any team member leaves theatre. This should review the procedure and that all planned steps have been completed, check the swab and sharp count, review postoperative care plans, along with specimen labelling and handling.

As stated at the bottom of this sample WHO checklist this is not intended to be comprehensive, with additions and modifications to fit local practice encouraged. Figure 3 shows an adaptation of this checklist used in a veterinary referral clinic, to optimise for the specific caseload and team's protocols.

PATIENT DETAILS	
Last name:	
First name:	
Breed/Age:	
Patient Number:	

Pre-op imaging:	
Post-op imaging:	
Display imaging:	

Bloods pending:	CBC MBC Coag Type
Feeding tube:	O G J→G PEG

Urinary catheter	Throat pack
Purse string	Hanging limb
Positioning:	

Antibiotics:	None Zinacef Other: Pre-op / Post sampling
Anti-inflammatory:	
Gastroprotectants:	
Tranexamic Acid:	

INSTRUMENT REQUESTS			
Basic kit			
Ligasure	Precise		
	5mm		Short
	10mm		Long
Harmonic Scalpel			Mono
			Bipolar
			Shears
Cautery	Mono		Bipolar
Gelpi	Mini	Med	Large
Gosset	Small		Large
Finochietto	Small		Large
Drill / Saw	Arthrex		
	Minidriver		
	Colibri		
Stapler (Size)	TA GIA Endo GIA		
	30 60 90		
Suction	Poole Frazier Yankauer		
Scope	2.7mm Cysto		
	5mm Lap 30°		
	10mm Lap 0°		
Caesarian Drape	Laparoscopy Kit		
4 Quarter Drapes	Pin & Wire Kit		
Bowl	Ophthalmic Kit		
Lap Sponges	Biopsy Kit		
Syringes	2.3 5 10 20 50		
Saline	100 500 1000		

PROCEDURE DETAILS				
Procedure name:				
Procedure date:		Surgeons:		
Consent status:	To Be Confirmed	Signed Consent	RX log Verbal Consent	Consent for Study

CLIPPING & POSITIONING INSTRUCTIONS

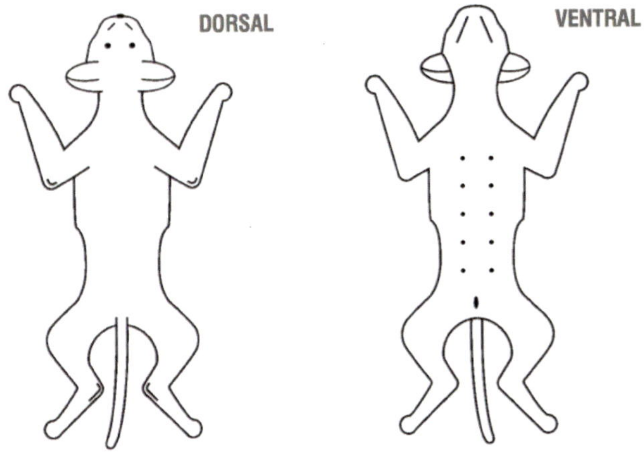

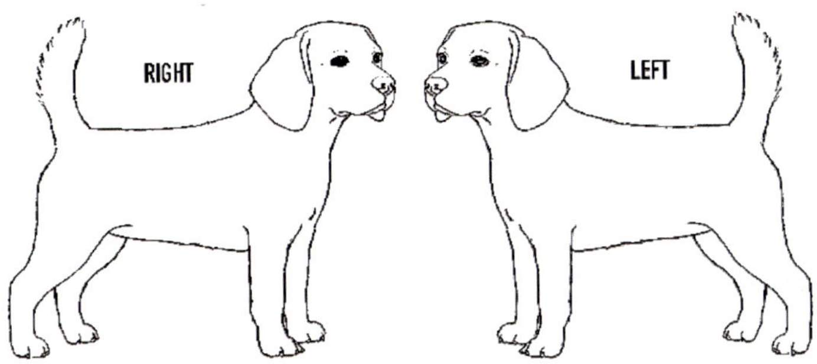

MARK POSITION OF KIT TROLLEY/SCOPE TOWER/ANAESTESTIC MACHINE

☐ NO CLIPPING

Requests for epidural / loco-regional analgesia?

What is the anticipated blood loss risk?
☐ Minimal ☐ >10% blood volume ☐ Life threatening

Is an internal referral request form required? ☐ No ☐ Yes; from whom?: **Do we need to charge an internal referral fee?** ☐ No ☐ Yes **Do we need to add to the soft tissue reports list?** ☐ No ☐ Yes: please tick when actioned: ☐	**Procedure charging?** ☐ 1st Surgery (default) ☐ 2nd Surgery ☐ Vet's time **Nurse text owner post op?** ☐ Yes

OTHER NOTES / KIT REQUIREMENTS		
	Scrubbed assistant needed?	Yes

Figure 1. Surgical request form.

Surgical Safety Checklist

World Health Organization | Patient Safety
A World Alliance for Safer Health Care

Before induction of anaesthesia → **Before skin incision** → **Before patient leaves operating room**

Before induction of anaesthesia

(with at least nurse and anaesthetist)

Has the patient confirmed his/her identity, site, procedure, and consent?
- ☐ Yes

Is the site marked?
- ☐ Yes
- ☐ Not applicable

Is the anaesthesia machine and medication check complete?
- ☐ Yes

Is the pulse oximeter on the patient and functioning?
- ☐ Yes

Does the patient have a:

Known allergy?
- ☐ No
- ☐ Yes

Difficult airway or aspiration risk?
- ☐ No
- ☐ Yes, and equipment/assistance available

Risk of >500ml blood loss (7ml/kg in children)?
- ☐ No
- ☐ Yes, and two IVs/central access and fluids planned

Before skin incision

(with nurse, anaesthetist and surgeon)

- ☐ **Confirm all team members have introduced themselves by name and role.**
- ☐ **Confirm the patient's name, procedure, and where the incision will be made.**

Has antibiotic prophylaxis been given within the last 60 minutes?
- ☐ Yes
- ☐ Not applicable

Anticipated Critical Events

To Surgeon:
- ☐ What are the critical or non-routine steps?
- ☐ How long will the case take?
- ☐ What is the anticipated blood loss?

To Anaesthetist:
- ☐ Are there any patient-specific concerns?

To Nursing Team:
- ☐ Has sterility (including indicator results) been confirmed?
- ☐ Are there equipment issues or any concerns?

Is essential imaging displayed?
- ☐ Yes
- ☐ Not applicable

Before patient leaves operating room

(with nurse, anaesthetist and surgeon)

Nurse Verbally Confirms:
- ☐ The name of the procedure
- ☐ Completion of instrument, sponge and needle counts
- ☐ Specimen labelling (read specimen labels aloud, including patient name)
- ☐ Whether there are any equipment problems to be addressed

To Surgeon, Anaesthetist and Nurse:
- ☐ What are the key concerns for recovery and management of this patient?

This checklist is not intended to be comprehensive. Additions and modifications to fit local practice are encouraged.

Revised 1 / 2009

© WHO, 2009

Figure 2. WHO surgical safety checklist.

Patient Preparation

Preemptive analgesia should be considered where possible, including epidural analgesia or peripheral nerve blocking techniques. The specifics of analgesic techniques are covered in Chapter 4.

Before moving the anaesthetised patient to the operating room, the surgeon should check the extent of the clipping and that it is adequate for the procedure. The patient is then positioned for optimal surgical access and the comfort of the surgical team.

Preparation of the Surgical Team

Gowning and Gloving

The surgeon disinfects their skin by scrubbing with skin disinfectant or alcohol skin-rub solutions. To further reduce the risk of contaminating the surgical site, surgical staff should wear sterile gowns and gloves.

Gowns should be made of a material which is impenetrable to fluids, free from linting, and provides a barrier to the passage of airborne particles and microbes between the surgeon and the patient. The ideal gowns are **single use, disposable gowns.** These are manufactured to meet quality control standards for surgical use, prefolded for ease of donning and sterilised using ionising radiation. Gowns should be donned in a low traffic area, specified for this purpose to minimise the risk of contamination of the gown.

Surgical gloves are ideally donned using a closed gloving technique to minimise contamination. Glove perforations are reported in around a quarter of surgical procedures. Risk factors for glove perforation included:

- the duration of surgery being longer than one hour
- performing orthopaedic procedures
- any procedure using powered instruments or orthopaedic wire.

SIGN IN (to be read out loud)
Before induction of anaesthesia

Has the patient identity been confirmed?
□ Yes
Has a surgical request form been completed?
□ Yes
What is the procedure to be undertaken?

Do we have consent for the procedure?
□ Yes: Written / Verbal

Have the anaesthetic machine and monitor checks been completed?
□ Yes
Has a patient warming device been prepared?
□ Yes □ No, not required for this patient
Have CBC, MBC, coagulation times been checked?
□ Yes □ Not required

What is the ASA Status of the patient?
□I □II □III □IV □V □E
Is the patient currently receiving any medications?
□ No □ Yes:

Antibiotics to be administered after induction?
□ No □ Yes:

Does the patient have any known allergies?
□ No □ Yes:
Difficult airway/aspiration risk?
□ No □ Yes, and equipment/assistance available
Risk of >10% blood loss?
□ No □ Yes: transfusion planned?
Blood type? ____________
Previous transfusions? □ Yes □ No
Are blood products available?

Has an internal referral request form been completed?
□ Yes / Surgeon confirmed not required

PATIENT DETAILS	
Last name:	
First name:	
Breed/Age:	
Patient Number:	

⇨

TIME OUT (to be read out loud)
Before start of surgical intervention

Have all team members introduced themselves by name and role?
□ Yes

Confirm the procedure and feeding tube requirement:
□ Checked as planned / Noted changes to plan:

Are there any critical or unexpected steps you want the team to know about?

Are there any patient specific concerns?
□ No □ Yes:

Do we need to notify ICU to prepare for recovery?
□ No □ Yes

Has the sterility of the instruments been confirmed?
□ Yes
Have electrosurgical devices been connected and turned on?
□ Yes
Have instruments and swabs been counted?
□ Yes (Tally swabs below)
Are there any equipment issues or concerns?
□ No □ Yes:

Have pre-operative antibiotics been administered?
□ Not requested □ No □ Yes:
Has pre-surgical imaging been reported?
□ Yes / not applicable
Is essential imaging displayed?
□ Yes / not applicable
Has the air conditioning been set to 21°C?
□ Yes

SWAB & SHARP TALLY					
		Counted In		Counted Out	
10x10	**20x20**				
Cotton tips					
Needles					
Blades					

⇨

END OF SURGERY (to be read out loud)
Before any team member leaves theatre

Name of procedure undertaken?

What are the key concerns for recovery and management of this patient?

Post-operative requirements:
□ **Medications:**

□ **Checks:**

□ **Feeding:**

Is a buster collar required?
□ Hard □ Soft □ None
Is a bandage or dressing required?
□ No □ Primapore □ Other:
Are instrument, swabs and sharp counts complete?
□ Yes
Are throat packs, rectal swabs and purse strings removed?
□ Yes
Have the specimens been labelled & preserved?
□ Yes
Nominee to sign out & submit specimens?

Have any equipment problems been identified?
□ No □ Yes:

SIGN OUT
Before nominee leaves the prep room
Have the laboratory request forms been completed and specimens collected?
□ **Yes. Signed:**

ACCOUNT COMPLETION	
Before scanning records	**Y**
Post-op medications been dispensed?	
Has the procedure been priced & logged? (correct date/surgeon/cost centre)	
Internal Referral Fee / Soft Tissue Reports List	

Figure 3. Surgical safety checklist.

Data shows **wearers are poor at detecting perforations,** with a sensitivity of 30.8% (Hayes et al., 2014). Therefore, the use of thicker gloves and double gloving are advocated for orthopaedic surgery. The use of colour-indicator under-gloves is shown to aid in the swift identification of outer glove perforations (Meakin et al., 2016). Regular changing of gloves (every hour) during longer surgeries, particularly those involving implants, helps reduce the risk of contamination of the surgical site. When changing gloves, the damaged gloves should be removed and then replaced using an open-gloving technique to prevent contamination of the hands from further up the arms.

Surgical Exposure

Surgical Access

Various factors determine the best site for surgical access; these include:

- the nature of the procedure
- the organ or tissue requiring exposure
- the position of a lump to be removed
- required access: keyhole approach vs extensive opening for hand access
- surgeon preference
- availability of equipment
- cost
- patient benefit vs risk.

Take the example of an intrathoracic mass. Depending on the size, location, and attachments the mass may be considered for removed via an intercostal thoracotomy, median sternotomy, or minimally invasive thoracoscopy (Figures 4, 5, 6). Each approach has advantages and disadvantages, such as intercostal thoracotomy allowing access to a limited region of the thorax on one side, whereas a median sternotomy allows more thorough exploration of the thorax but is a more invasive procedure, whilst thoracoscopy is certainly less invasive but allows only a limited, but magnified field of view and working space within the thorax.

As a general rule **access to abdominal structures is via a ventral midline approach,** dissecting between the abdominal musculature and gaining access via the linea alba. Occasionally, other approaches are made to the abdomen e.g. a limited inguinal approach for cystostomy tube placement or a paracostal incision in addition to a midline incision to increase access to the right side of the liver and right adrenal gland.

Positioning for Surgery

Optimal patient positioning on the operating table is an essential part of presurgical planning. This ensures the surgeon has the best access to the surgical site to maximise the efficiency of the surgery, hence reducing surgical trauma.

Points for Consideration

- **Patient positioning on the operating table:** the patient needs to be orientated appropriately to allow ease of access to the surgical site (Figure 7). Typically, the area to be incised is uppermost, except in the case of perineal or oral surgery where the region is positioned at the end of the operating table on an incline towards the surgeon.
- **Operating table position within the operating room:** whilst the surgical lights are moveable and orientated towards the surgical site, optimisation may require specific positioning of the operating table and other equipment.
- **Surgical site exposure:** may require tying the limbs and tail in one direction or another to keep them out of the surgical field, or indeed, hanging them for clipping and preparation. Often sandbags, foam wedges, packs of swabs, or beanbags are required to support, stabilise and elevate the surgical site, e.g. for surgery on the neck (Figure 8).

The use of a **surgical request form** prompts the surgeon to consider patient surgical positioning and required equipment ahead of surgery. This allows the theatre team to prepare the operating room in advance and have the appropriate equipment available, along with that required in the event of intraoperative surgical complications. This minimises traffic in the operating room during the procedure, which helps maintain a sterile field.

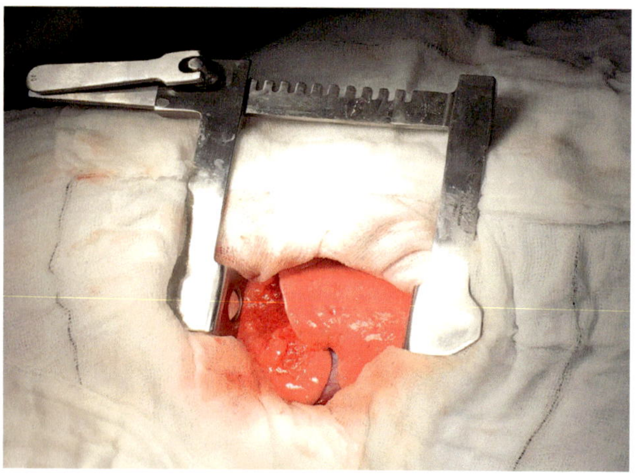

Figure 4. Intercostal thoracotomy.

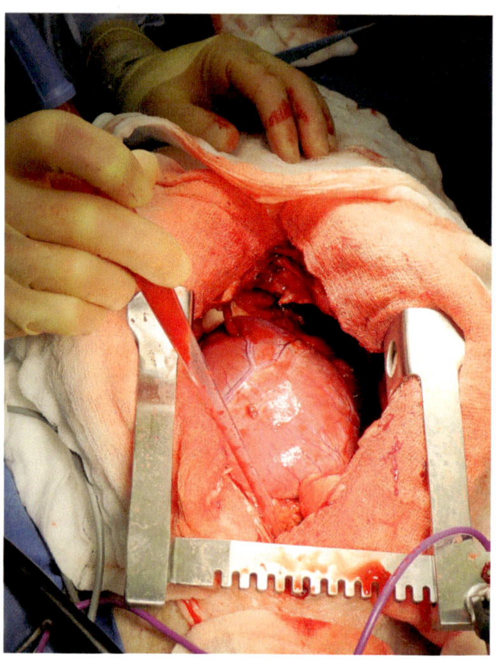

Figure 5. Median sternotomy.

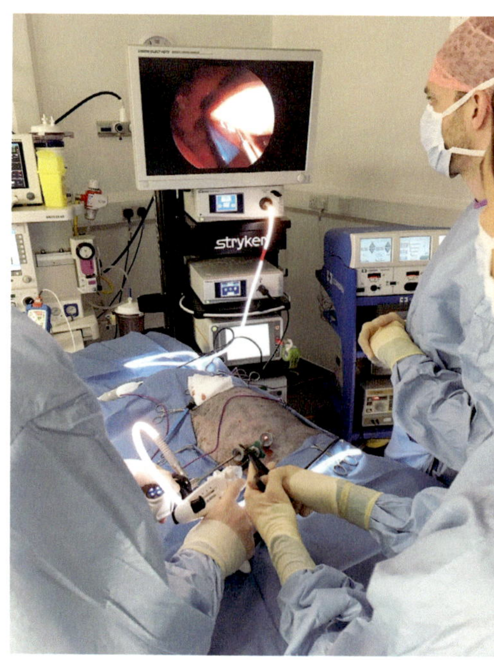

Figure 6. Thoracoscopy.

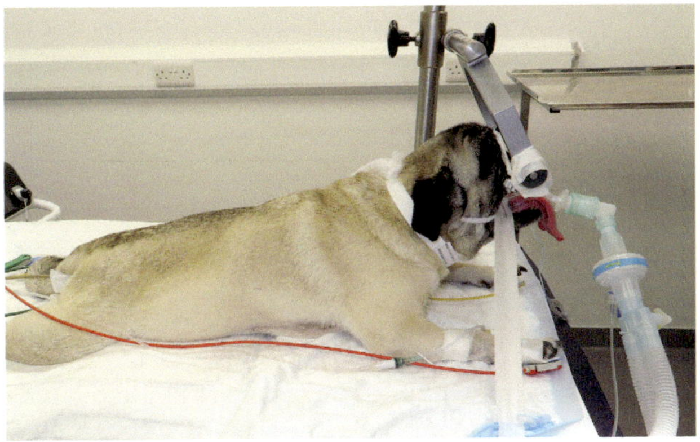

Figure 7. BOAS (Brachycephalic obstructive airway syndrome) positioning for surgery in a custom made stand.

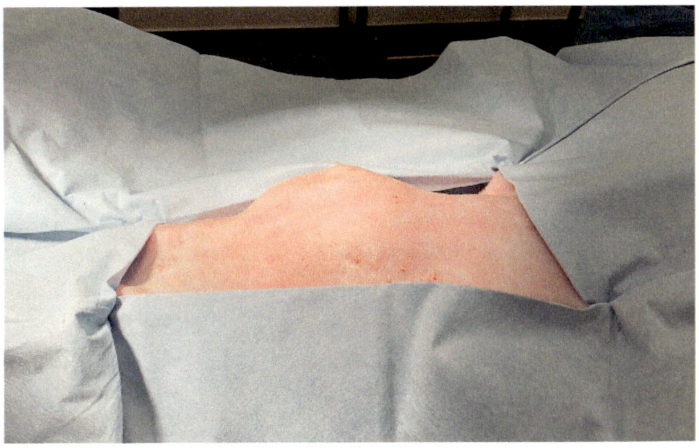

Figure 9. Four-quarter draping.

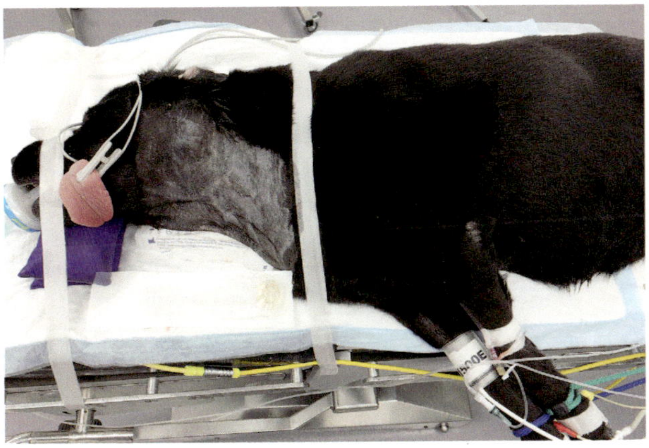

Figure 8. Tie-back positioning.

Draping for Surgery

The patient and entire operating table should be covered with surgical drapes to create a sterile operating field, which is then continuous with the surgical team and the kit trolley. The surgeon may choose to drape with a single or double layer of drapes depending on the nature of the surgery. With double layer draping it is common to employ four-quarter draping for the base layer (Figure 9).

Incision drapes (e.g. OpSite®), including those impregnated with iodine (e.g. Ioban®) are not proven to significantly reduce surgical site infection rates, however these are often chosen to minimise skin contact, particularly for orthopaedic surgery and other procedures involving surgical implants, and avoid the use of towel clamps where this is advantageous, i.e. when intraoperative imaging is performed, as well as having potential benefits in keeping the patient dry. For this latter purpose, pouch drapes designed for human caesarean surgery are useful when performing coeliotomy and large volume abdominal lavage, e.g. in cases of septic peritonitis. (Figure 10).

A

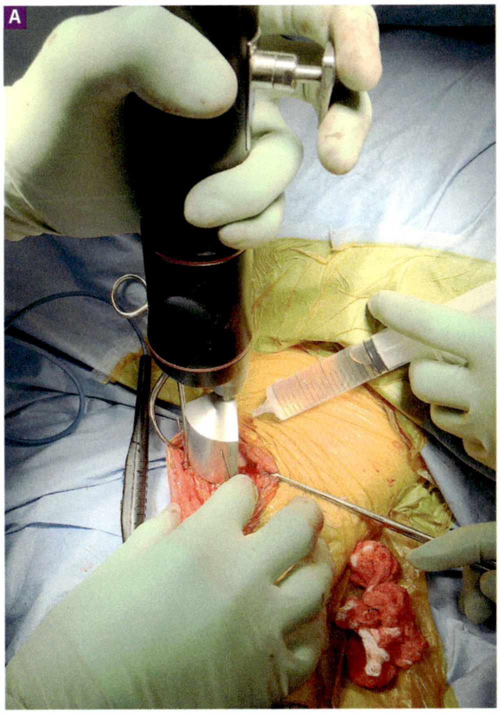

B

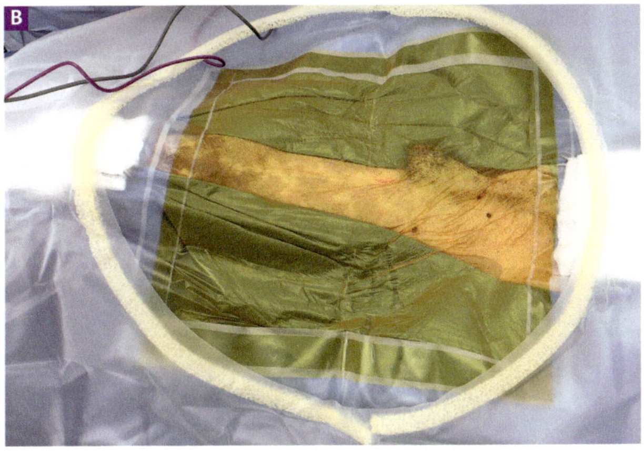

Figure 10. A. Iodine impregnated incise drape;
B. Iodine impregnated caesarean drape.

Halsted's Principles

William Stuart Halsted (1852–1922) (Figure 11) was a revolutionary American surgeon who advocated **strict aseptic technique during surgical procedures.** He was an early champion of newly discovered anaesthetics (which he tested on himself), and introduced several surgical procedures, as well as designing surgical instruments. Halsted operated on patients with great confidence and had excellent surgical outcomes, ahead of his time. He was later proclaimed as the Father of Modern Surgery.

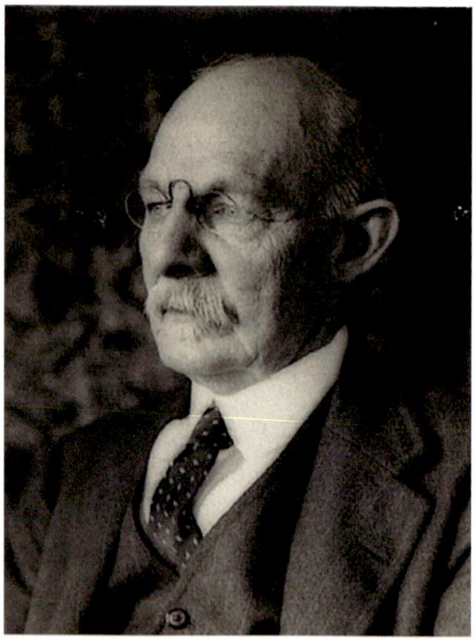

Figure 11. William Stuart Halsted.

Halsted's principles are the basis of soft tissue handling which surgeons strive for to this day:

- Gentle tissue handling.
- Meticulous haemostasis.
- Strict asepsis.
- Preservation of blood supply.
- Elimination of dead space.
- Accurate tissue apposition with minimal tension.

Gentle Tissue Handling

Body tissues are fragile, especially when inflamed, and require **delicate handling** to minimise additional trauma, which is associated with delayed healing, pain, increased infection risk, and hence morbidity and mortality. It is important to select the **appropriate instruments** for the surgery, to minimise trauma due to surgical manipulation and to increase surgical efficiency. **Surgical time is correlated with infection risk and morbidity.**

Other considerations for tissue handling are:

- Can the tissue be **handled more delicately manually** rather than with surgical instruments? (e.g. using an assistant's fingers to gently occlude bowel during an enterectomy procedure, rather than Doyen bowel clamps). (Figure 12).
- Can **stay sutures be used rather than clamps** to support delicate tissues? (e.g. for retracting the bladder during cystotomy). (Figure 13).
- **Tissue should be kept moist** and covered to protect it from desiccation under hot theatre lights.

Meticulous Haemostasis

The **avoidance of major haemorrhage** is always at the forefront of the surgeon's mind. It's also important to appreciate that **cumulative oozing from multiple smaller vessels can also cause significant blood loss,** especially in anaemic patients,

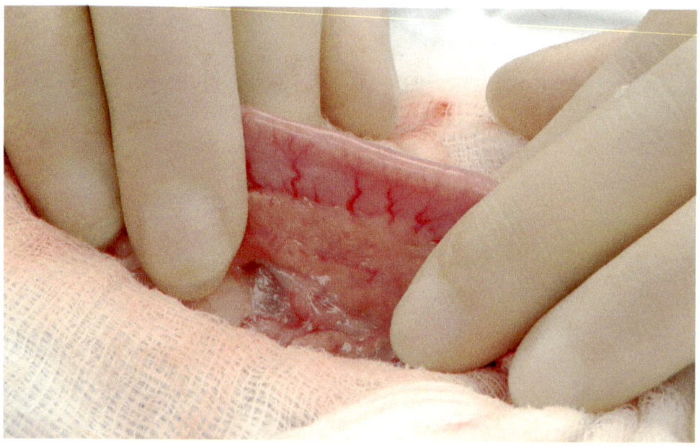

Figure 12. Finger bowel occlusion.

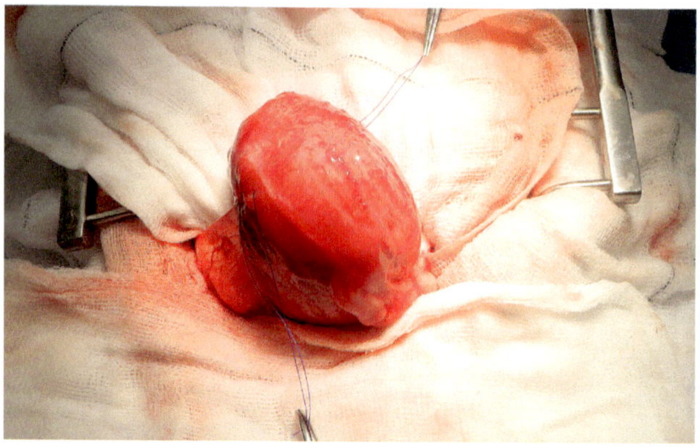

Figure 13. Bladder being manipulated with stay sutures.

those with coagulopathies, or where haematoma formation may cause unwanted compression and dysfunction (e.g. adjacent to the central nervous system) or may predispose a risk of surgical site infection (as a haematoma is an ideal breeding ground for many bacteria).

Haemostasis may be achieved by several means:
- **Direct application of pressure** using a digit or pair of haemostatic forceps, or indirectly by packing an area with a sterile surgical swab. Application of pressure to a vessel or bleeding surface of a tissue is required for a period of time (often five minutes is used as a rule of thumb) to allow coagulation of the vessel.
- **Ligation of a vessel with suture** is appropriate for managing discrete bleeding from an isolated vessel of any size. Different knots and numbers of ligatures are used for different clinical situations; for example, a small cutaneous vessel may require a simple encircling ligature, whereas a major artery such as a renal artery requires placement of a transfixing ligature (one which passes through the tissue or vessel being ligated to anchor it to that tissue) and secondary encircling ligature to prevent slippage. Ligation may also include the use of metal staples/vascular clips.
- **Indirect reduction in blood flow to a bleeding tissue by the application of a tourniquet** (e.g. high up a limb to control bleeding from a foot) or ligation of a major artery supplying an area of significant bleeding (e.g. carotid artery ligation for management of severe epistaxis or bleeding following a maxillectomy surgery), where the bleeding cannot be managed directly.
- **Application of topical haemostatic agents** to the bleeding surfaces either to plug the blood flow or to act as a scaffold on which a clot can preferentially form. Examples are listed below:
  - **Omentum:** a native tissue which provides vascular supply and hence clotting factors, as well as acting as a scaffold and providing surgical drainage.
  - **Cellulose:** Surgicel® which is acidic and reacts with blood to form a clot-like substance.
  - **Gelatin:** Gelfoam® which absorbs blood and acts as a scaffold for clotting.
  - **Collagen:** Lyostypt® which activates factor XII and causes platelet adhesion. This product is rapidly absorbed thereafter.
  - **Bone wax:** made from beeswax and used to plug bones, physically preventing bleeding.
  - **Fibrin sealants:** are combinations of thrombin and fibrinogen, which are part of the clotting cascade and actively facilitate clot formation.
- **Electrosurgical devices** to perform electrocautery or vessel sealing using a variety of radiofrequency devices.

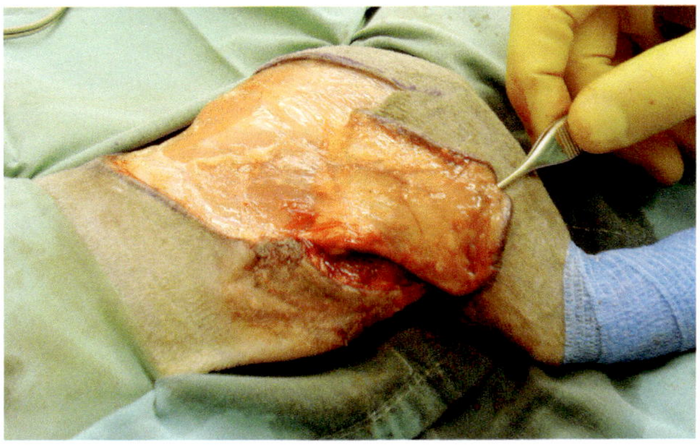

Figure 14. Skin flap preparation, to ensure maintenance of its blood supply.

Strict Asepsis

Aseptic technique is paramount to prevention of surgical site infection. Surgical contamination classification and rational use of antibiotics as well as preparation of the patient, theatre environment, surgical team, and equipment are covered elsewhere. Additional factors important for surgical asepsis are **minimising surgical and anaesthesia times** and **minimising hypotension** by appropriate surgical preparation, knowledge of anatomy, and appropriate anaesthetic and surgical techniques.

Preservation of Blood Supply

Maintenance of tissue blood supply is essential for tissue viability and wound healing. Hence knowledge of the vascular anatomy to the tissues undergoing surgery is essential to maintain blood supply following surgery. An example of this is skin flaps. Skin flaps and reconstructive surgery are discussed later in this chapter, but where skin is moved as a flap, it is essential that the surgeon understands the blood supply to the skin, to give that flap the best chance of surviving the transfer. (Figure 14).

Elimination of Dead Space

Dead space is the term applied to the space, or potential for space between tissues following a surgical procedure, for example removal of a tumour. This empty cavity, or dead space, has the potential to fill with fluid postoperatively, resulting in seroma formation. Seroma might delay wound healing and mean a protracted period of exercise restriction and rest for the patient following surgery, but also the nutrient rich fluid is a potential breeding ground for bacteria which evade the immune system and may cause a surgical site infection. Hence, wherever possible, action should be taken at the time of surgery to prevent leaving dead space:

- **Minimise unnecessary dissection:** whilst it is essential the surgeon has adequate surgical exposure, ensuring that dissection does not extend beyond the necessary extent is helpful in minimising dead space following surgery.
- **Walking sutures:** when dead space is created under the skin by a dissection, closing this space as part of the closure helps to prevent large fluid pockets collecting. This is achieved by placing interrupted sutures to reattach the skin and subcutis to the underlying tissue. (Figure 15).
- **Surgical drainage:** when suturing closed a dead space is not achievable (due to the size of the cavity, expected volume of fluid ooze from the cut surface, or risk of entrapment of vital structures preventing suture placement), then the surgeon should consider surgical drainage. In the simplest form this means leaving part of the incision open to allow fluid to drain passively. A surgical drain is the name given to any temporary implant which when placed within the surgical site, allows fluid to be removed following surgery.

- **Types of drain:**
  - **Omentum:** the omentum has many functions but can be used as a biological drain, by nature of its immense vasculature supply.
  - **Penrose drains:** these are passive drains, made of soft latex tubing, made in a variety of sizes, which allow fluid to pass by gravity flow and capillary action over the surface of the drain. These drains are anchored deep in the surgical site and at the point of exit through the skin, separate from the main surgical incision. The exposed portion of the drain requires covering with a sterile dressing or swabs, which are changed as often as needed when they become saturated to prevent ascending infection. (Figure 16).
  - **Closed suction drains:** these are cylindrical tubes made of silicone, polyurethane, or polyethylene, which connect to an external container, which can be emptied to generate negative pressure, which draws fluid out from the surgical site. Similar to Penrose drains these exit through a separate stab incision. (Figure 17).
- **Bandages:** bandages may be used either in isolation or in combination with drains. They provide external compression of the tissues to minimise dead space capacity (Figure 18). They may be very effective if well placed over the limbs but are more limited when the pressure under the dressing is limited, i.e. over the thorax/cervical region.

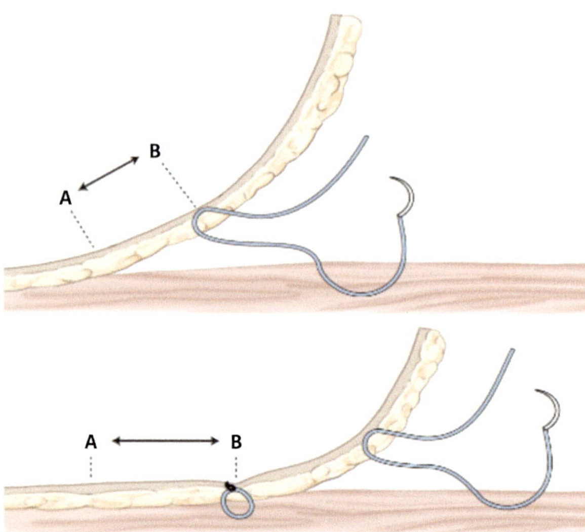

Figure 15. Walking sutures.

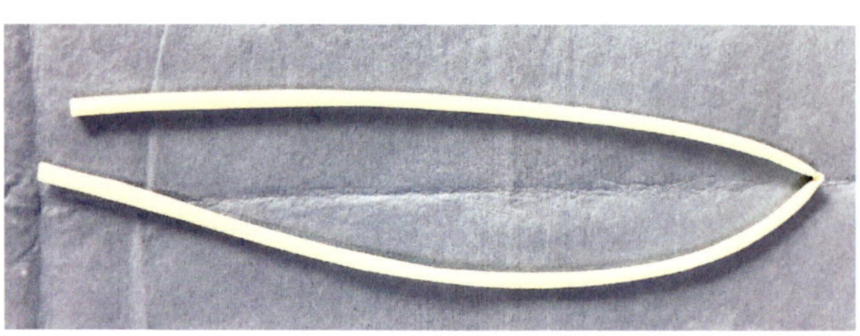

Figure 16. Penrose drain.

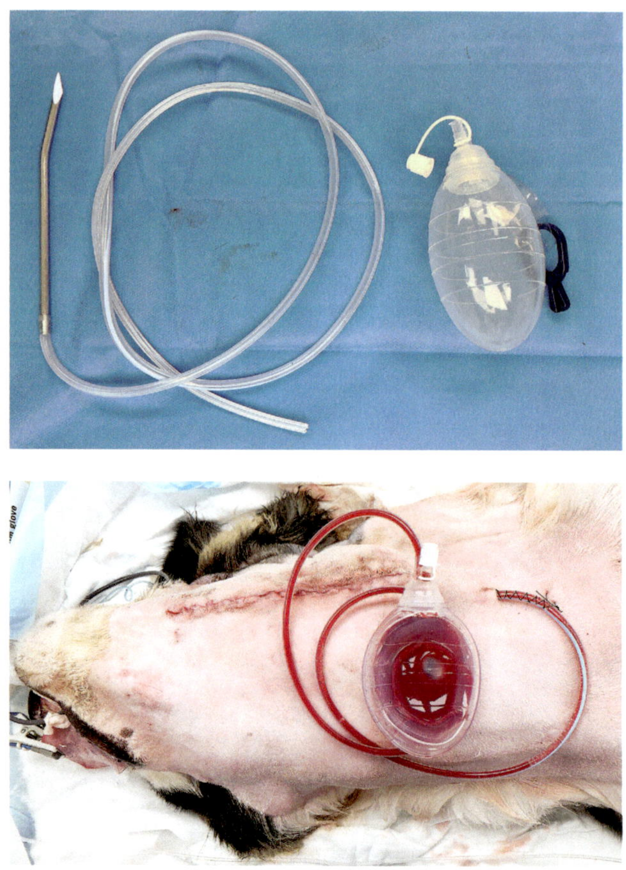

Figure 17. Closed suction drain.

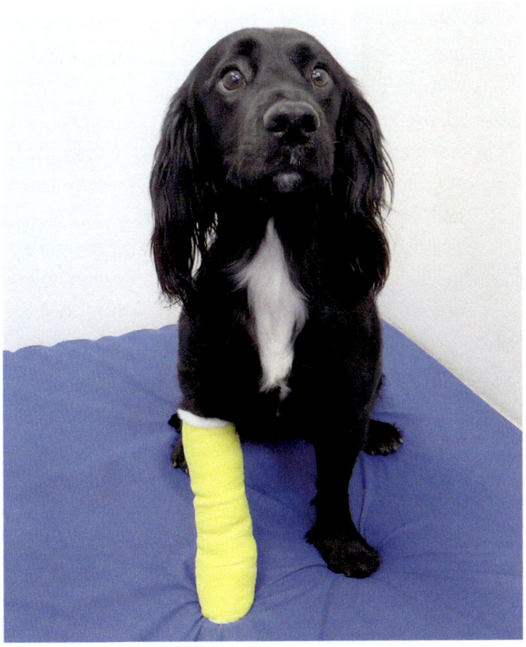

Figure 18. Bandage.

Accurate Tissue Apposition with Minimal Tension

Appropriate tissue tension is important for healing. Leaving tissues very loosely apposed predisposes to dead space and seroma formation, however if tissues are closed too tightly this compresses the blood supply and reduces tissue viability; so **minimising tension is also an essential of surgical site closure.**

Suture Materials

Properties of Suture Materials

Many suture materials are available, many of which are appropriate for specific uses. These properties can be classified in different ways:

- **Manufacturing properties**
  - Naturally occurring or synthetic: some naturally occurring materials are processed into manufactured suture materials, whereas other materials and polymers are generated in the laboratory and extruded into uniform fibres.
- **Persistence**
  - Sutures may be absorbable or non-absorbable. Those that are absorbable vary in their rate of absorption and hence, how long they persist in the surgical site. Non-absorbable sutures become walled off in fibrous tissue and generally their use is restricted to temporary use in the skin. Chronic infections and drain tracts can be seen where non-absorbable sutures are used and not removed.
- **Monofilament vs multifilament/braided**
  - Monofilament sutures are a single, smooth, uniform strand of extruded material; whereas braided materials are made of multiple filaments interwoven to create a rope-like fibre. Braided materials usually have higher relative tensile strength and knot security, but also a higher capillarity and hence risk of infection (bacteria can hide out between the fibres and evade the immune system).
- **Coating**
  - Some braided sutures are coated to smooth their surface, giving them some of the benefits of both monofilament and braided materials.
- **Dying/colouring**
  - Many suture materials are colourless, whilst others are dyed to enhance their surgical visualisation. Coloured sutures used intradermally may be visible through non-pigmented skin and not be ideal for cosmetic reasons.
- **Sterility/packaging**
  - Modern suture materials are coiled onto card or plastic cassettes and sealed in foil packets, which are sterilised by γ-irradiation or ethylene oxide. Older sutures may be coiled on reels for multi-patient use. The latter should be considered as surgically clean, not sterile.
- **Size**
  - Two classification systems are commonly used, and both are usually displayed on the packet, although the first is usually more prominent:
    - **United States Pharmacopoeia (USP)**/European Pharmacopoeia (PhEur): this system varies with suture diameter, strength, and knot security. In general, large integers represent larger sutures, and the larger integers followed by a backslash zero (/0) are decreasing size. (Note two different materials with the same USP may be different diameters if one is synthetic and one is naturally occurring).
    - **Metric system:** this system is based solely on suture size and suture diameter is measured in units of tenths of a millimetre.

For commonly used synthetic sutures this conversion chart shown in Table 1 applies.

- **Mechanical properties**
  - **Tensile strength:** the ability of the suture to resist failure under load per unit area. Strength varies with linear tensile (stretching) strength and knot strength.
  - **Elasticity:** the degree of lengthening and recoil when loaded.

- **Plasticity:** the ability of the suture material to have its shape distorted. This is beneficial with respect to knot security; however, it can make materials more challenging to handle due to their propensity to kink.

- **Rate of loss of strength**
  - The absorption profile of the suture affects its strength through the healing process. The rate of loss of strength varies with the environment of the suture, e.g. in stomach acid or in alkali urine within the bladder.
- **Mechanism of absorption**
  - Synthetic sutures are generally absorbed by hydrolysis, which occurs at a linear and predictable rate. Natural sutures, such as catgut, incite an inflammatory response and are absorbed by phagocytosis and proteolysis; but the rate of this absorption varies depending on patient and local wound factors, which may supress or accelerate the inflammatory response.
- **Handling properties**
  - **Knot security:** knot security is dependent on a number of other factors, including plasticity, pliability, memory, and friction; but also, may vary with absorption and the inflammatory response incited by the suture material. This is of particular concern with catgut sutures which are known to rapidly loosen following placement.
- **Pliability**
  - The tendency for a suture to change shape in response to forces acting on the suture. Sutures range from limp e.g. silk, which flows freely smoothly, to stiff, e.g. stainless steel, which requires significant forces to be applied to deform a strand. These properties are used to the surgeon's advantage in different clinical scenarios.
- **Memory**
  - The tendency for a suture to retain its original shape, e.g. that in which it comes in the suture packet. Generally, memory is an undesirable trait in a suture material as it makes its manipulation more challenging for the surgeon.
- **Tissue drag/friction**
  - Knot security relies on friction of the suture material against itself, however excess drag when passing through tissues is undesirable as this causes additional tissue trauma. Some sutures are coated to reduce their friction. Silk may be moistened when used to reduce its drag.
- **Tissue interaction**
  - **Inflammatory response:** natural sutures stimulate a greater inflammatory response, which affects their strength and rate of absorption. Synthetic materials generate less inflammatory response and hence their absorption characteristics are more predictable.
- **Potentiation for infection**
  - Triclosan coating of some modern sutures is suggested to provide some increased resistance to infection and reduce the risk of surgical site infection.
- **Capillarity/wicking**
  - The propensity for a suture to allow fluids and bacteria to travel along and within its fibres. This is of particular concern with braided materials, and generally these are not recommended for use in contaminated surgical sites such as in surgery of the skin, gastrointestinal or urogenital tracts.

Table 1. Conversion chart for synthetic sutures.

Diameter	Metric size	USP/PhEur size
0.02 mm	0.2	10/0
0.04 mm	0.4	8/0
0.07 mm	0.7	6/0
0.15 mm	1.5	4/0
0.2 mm	2	3/0
0.3 mm	3	2/0
0.35 mm	3.5	0
0.4 mm	4	1

Types of Suture Material

Rapidly Absorbable Sutures

Multifilament Sutures

- **Catgut**
  - multifilament made from the collagenous submucosa of sheep intestine
  - often treated with chromium salts which slow its degradation by macrophages
  - produces an intense tissue reaction and shows a rapid loss in strength and knot security
  - retains its strength for 7–10 days (10–14 days for chromic gut)
  - complete absorption in 70 days (90 days for chromic gut)
  - suitable only for superficial blood vessel ligation and opposing subcutaneous tissue
- Polyglycolic acid (e.g. **Dexon®**)
  - synthetic, braided multifilament, absorbable
  - absorption by hydrolysis occurs more rapidly in alkaline environments and so is not recommended for use in the bladder
  - loses 33% strength in 7 days and 80% in 14 days

- high tissue drag, can be reduced by wetting the suture before use

– Polyglactin 910 (e.g. **Vicryl®**) (Figure 19 A)
- synthetic, braided multifilament, absorbable
- coated to reduce tissue drag
- loses all strength by 21 days
- complete absorption by 56–90 days

Vicryl Rapide® is manufactured to be more quickly absorbed, losing half of its strength in 5–6 days and all strength in 10–14 days. Completely absorbed in 42 days. **Vicryl Plus®** is coated with triclosan, an antibacterial agent, which has been shown to reduce surgical site infection risk in some instances in humans.

– Lactomer 9-1 (e.g. **Polysorb®**)
- synthetic, braided multifilament, absorbable
- similar to polyglactin 910 but a finer filament, makes this softer and more pliable, with better knot security
- the strongest braided suture material available
- loses 70% of its strength in 21 days.

Monofilament Sutures

– Polyglytone 6211 (e.g. **Caprosyn®**)

synthetic, monofilament, absorbable
loses all strength by 21 days

– Poliglecaprone 25 (e.g. **Monocryl®**) (Figure 19 B)
- synthetic, monofilament, absorbable
- loses 50% strength by 7 days, which is slower than polyglytone 6211
- loses all strength by 21 days
- complete absorption 120 days
- high tensile strength

Monocryl Plus® is coated with triclosan, an antibacterial agent, which has been shown to reduce surgical site infection risk in some instances in humans.

Slowly Absorbable Sutures

Multifilament Sutures

– Poly L-lactide/glycolide (e.g. **Panacryl®**)
- synthetic, braided, absorbable
- the only braided, absorbable suture, which provides long term support
- only available in large sizes for orthopaedic joint stabilisation/ligament reconstruction.

Monofilament Sutures

– Glycomer 631 (e.g. **Biosyn®**)
- synthetic, monofilament, absorbable
- the strongest monofilament suture second only to steel
- but it is brittle
- complete absorption in 90–110 days

– Polydioxanone (e.g. **PDS®**) (Figure 19 C)
- synthetic, monofilament, absorbable
- knot security is poor – so extra throws are recommended
- loses 50% strength in 6 weeks
- minimal absorption in first 90 days, provides prolonged wound support

– Polyglyconate (e.g. **Maxon®**) (Figure 19 D)
- synthetic, monofilament, absorbable
- loses 50% strength in 3 weeks
- complete absorption in 180 days
- maintains strength and wound support in an acid environment.

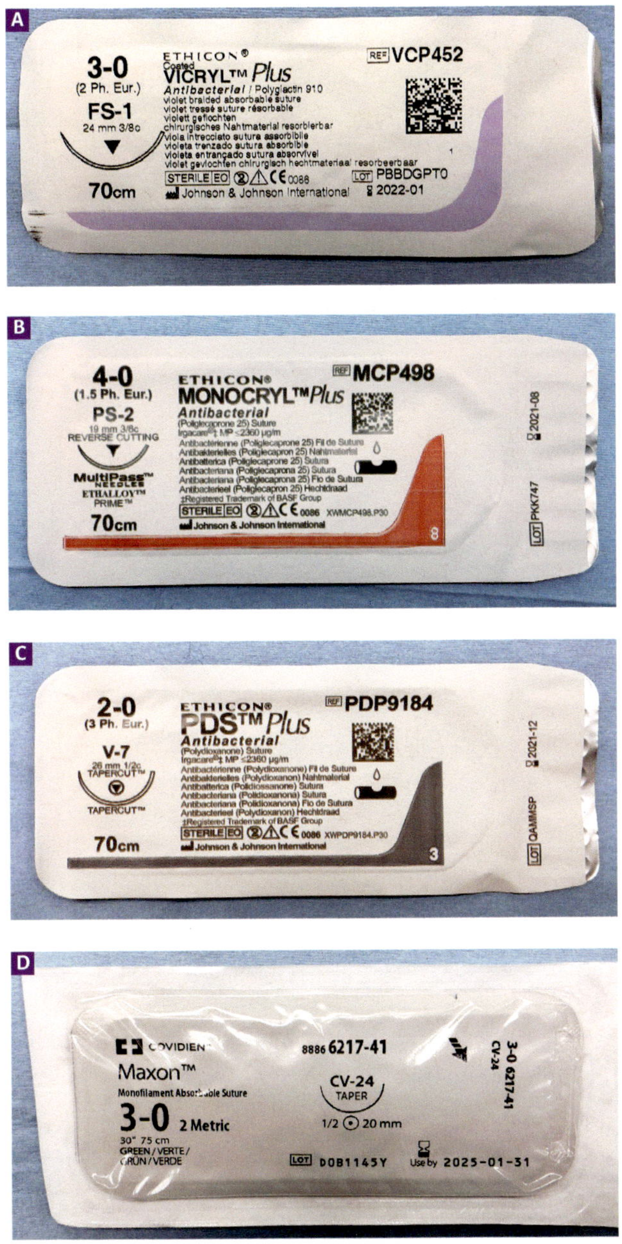

Figure 19. A. Vicryl®. **B.** Monocryl®. **C.** PDS®. **D.** Maxon®.

Non-absorbable Sutures

Silk (e.g. Mersilk®) (Figure 19 E)

- natural fibre made from the cocoon of the silkworm, which initiates a stronger inflammatory reaction than other non-absorbable sutures
- twisted or braided multifilament, sometimes coated in beeswax to reduce tissue drag and capillarity, otherwise, it may be moistened in saline to reduce drag
- although classified as non-absorbable, it is slowly absorbed over 2 years
- excellent handling, pliability and knot security historically make it many surgeons preference for ligation of larger blood vessels.

Stainless Steel (e.g. Flexon®)

- available as monofilament or twisted multifilament, non-absorbable
- biologically inert
- difficult to handle due to plasticity
- repeat bending leads to fracture and failure.

Polyamide (e.g. Nylon®) (Figures 19 F and 19 G)

- available as a monofilament e.g. **Monosof®, Ethilon®, Dermalon®;** or a multifilament e.g. **Nurulon®, Surgilon®, Bralon®**
- used for skin suturing due to its pliability and elasticity
- sharp, irritating ends are also not suitable for burying due to tissue irritation.

Monosof® is more plastic than other forms resulting in better handling characteristics and knot security. Hence, Monosof® sutures are secure with three throws, but other nylons require four or five tightly placed throws for a secure and stable knot. Nylon® is hydrolysed very slowly but retains 72% of its tensile strength after two years.

Polypropylene (e.g. Prolene®, Surgipro®, Surgilene®) (Figure 19 H)

- low tissue adherence makes this suture easily removeable
- maintains its tensile strength and not degraded by tissues, hence polypropylene is often used for tendon repair
- low thrombogenicity makes it ideal for vascular surgery.

Polymerised Caprolactam (e.g. Supramid®, Vetafil®)

- twisted multifilament polyamide wrapped in a sheath of proteinaceous material
- cheaply produced on a reel, in a cassette in a chemical disinfectant but is not sterile and so not suitable for safe implantation within tissues
- skin wounds closed with this material show greater inflammation and suture tracts than those closed with monofilament Nylon®.

Polyester (e.g. Surgicac®, Mersilene®, Dacron®, Ethibond®, Ethiflex®, Ticron®, Tevdek®)

- braided non-absorbable, synthetic suture
- may be uncoated; or with a variety of coatings which reduce tissue drag and improve knot security
- high tensile strength
- elicits a marked tissue reaction which may potentiate wound infection and inflammation.

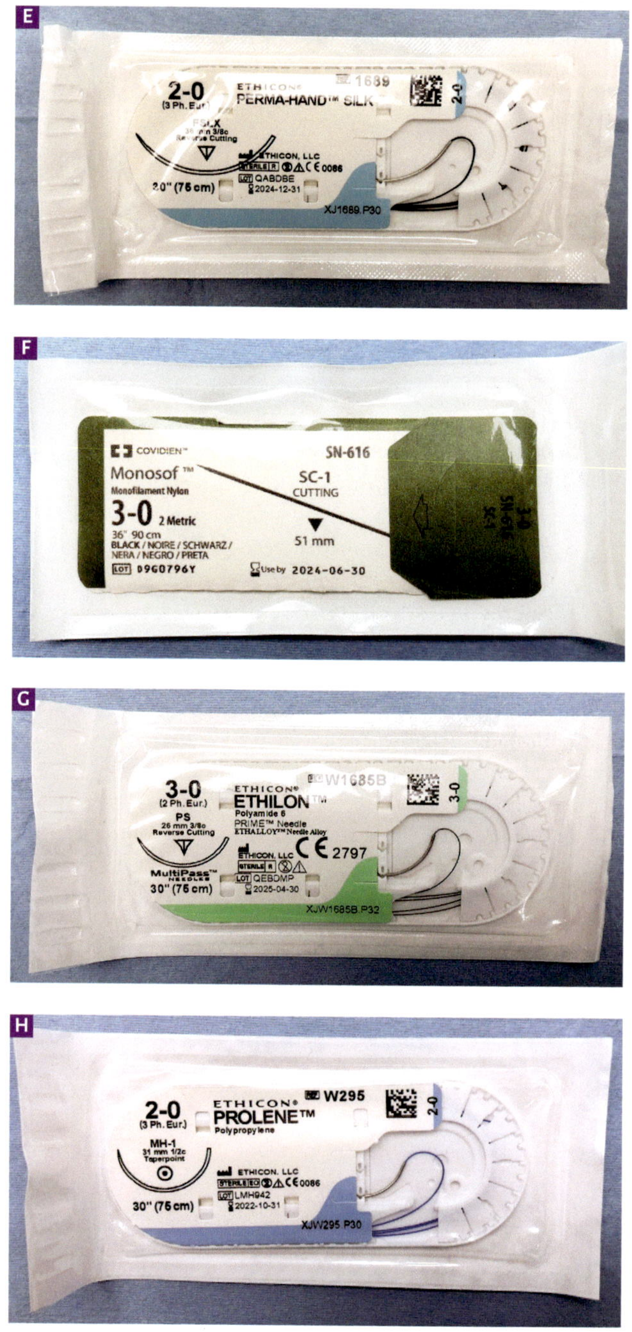

Figure 19. E. Silk. **F.** Monosof®. **G.** Ethilon®. **H.** Prolene®.

Selection of Suture Material

Suture selection varies with surgeon preference and training, but there are some principles to consider when choosing a suture for a specific purpose:

- **Duration of support:** the suture only needs to provide wound support until the wound has adequately healed. Visceral incisions and skin heal quickly and may only need support for 2–3 weeks, whereas fascial tissue and tendons take months to years to heal and may never return to their former strength and so prolonged wound support is warranted.
- **Multifilament sutures** cause wicking which allows bacterial seeding and protection from the immune system, so they are poorer choices in infected or contaminated wound environments. Surgeons may prefer the increased knot security and the soft, less irritating suture ends, which are especially important for ophthalmic use.

Box 1 shows several examples of suitable suture material for different clinical applications.

Box 1. Suitable Suture Material for Different Clinical Applications:

- **Monofilament, non-absorbable: polyamide.** Suturing of the skin with simple interrupted skin sutures following a routine spay in a healthy Labrador.
- **Monofilament non-absorbable: polypropylene.** Repair of a ruptured Achilles tendon in a cat.
- **Braided, non-absorbable: silk.** Ligating a patent ductus arteriosus in a West Highland White Terrier puppy with a continuous heart murmur.
- **Monofilament absorbable: poliglecaprone 25.** Suturing a palatoplasty incision in a Bulldog having airway surgery.

Suture Needles

Suture needles are made of **high-grade stainless steel,** strong enough to maintain their form with normal handling. They should be **small but strong and sharp** enough to penetrate the tissue with minimal trauma. They should be **sterile** and corrosion free.

Suture needles may be eyed to allow attachment of a free piece of suture material or manufactured with **suture material swaged on.** Swaged on needles are crimped on to the suture material during manufacturing. Swaged on needles allow for ease of use, but also cause **less tissue trauma** as the needle diameter is minimised and are sterilised with the suture material.

Suture packets are labelled with the suture material type, coating information, suture size, colour, length, needle type, needle shape, needle size, curvature, and number of needles: (some sutures have swaged on needles at both ends). This is of particular importance to note during sharps counts at the end of surgery on the surgical safety checklist.

Suture needles may be **curved or straight.** Straight needles are most frequently used for hand suturing of the skin or for anchoring of feeding tubes and drains. **Simple curved needles are classified by the proportion of the diameter of a circle** along which their curve extends (e.g. ½), as well as their curved length. Half-curved needles have a straight shaft, with a curved portion nearest to the tip, e.g. J-shaped needles commonly used for fabello tibial leader line Nylon® suture placement for cruciate ligament disease. Compound curved needles may have different radii of curvature along their length. (Figure 20).

Needle tips and shafts are designed to allow ease of passage through different types of tissue, whilst minimising trauma.

Round Bodied Needles

These needles have a **smooth conical tip and cylindrical body and are minimally traumatic to tissue.** They are difficult to pass through tougher types of tissue such as skin and **blunt quickly.** They are most useful for **parenchymatous tissues** with a low collagen content, e.g. fat, liver, muscle.

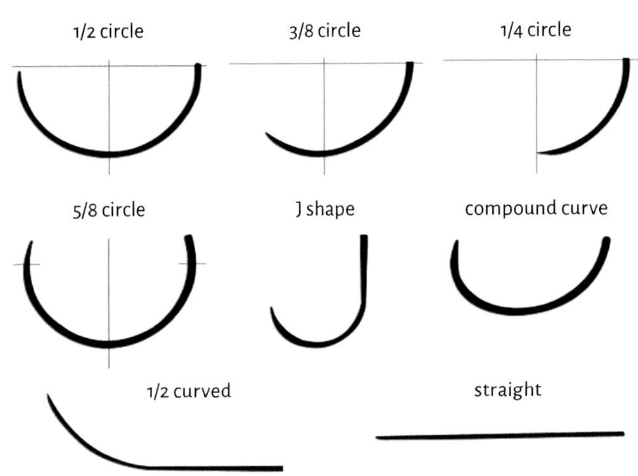

Figure 20. Needle shapes.

They are also used for vascular, urinary tract and intestinal surgery to minimise the risk of tissue tearing and leakage following suturing.

Cutting Needles

These needles have a **pyramidal tip with sharp edges,** which help them to cut and divide tissue, making them **suitable for tougher, more fibrous tissue.** Taper cut needles have a smooth round shaft and have a cutting portion only at the tip.

Conventional cutting needles have a sharp cutting edge along the concave, inner aspect of the curve of the needle. Reverse cutting needles have the sharp cutting edge on the outer, convex aspect of the curve of the needle, designed so that subsequent tightening of the suture is less likely to propagate in the direction of the cut of the needle and tear through the tissue. **Spatula tip needles** have a flatter profile with a cutting tip and are most commonly used for ophthalmic surgery. (Figure 21).

Suturing Principles

Surgical Knots

The surgical knot secures the suture material within tissue, but due to acute kinking of the suture at this point, this is mechanically **the weakest point** and frequently the source of failure. Whilst knots are a weak point, tying secure knots reduces the risk of suture loosening. Knots work by creating friction between the strands of suture. Maximising contact and hence friction, coupled with tight bending of the suture prevents suture ends slipping.

The key surgical knot is the square knot (also known as **a reef knot).** This is a simple twist of the two strands in one direction (one throw) followed by a twist back on itself and a second twist in the opposite direction (second throw). (Figure 22).

A square knot is secure in itself but due to the nature of different suture materials, including their plasticity, memory, and

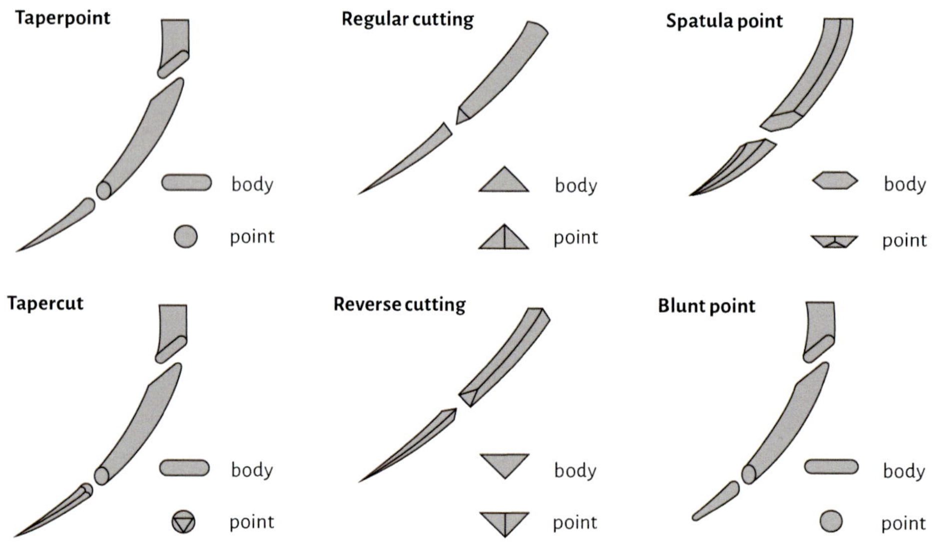

Figure 21. Needle profiles.

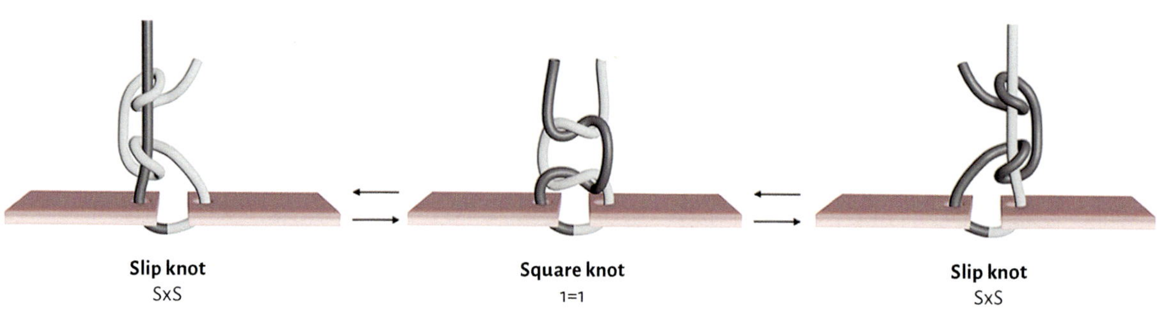

Figure 22. Slip and square knots.

stiffness; additional throws are required for knot security. Typically for a simple knot four throws are required for monofilament sutures or three for multifilament sutures. When tying continuous suture patterns, an additional throw is recommended at the start of the suture line (when started with a square knot) and two additional throws at completion with a square knot, at this point a loop is tied to a strand rather than tying two strands. (Table 2).

Table 2. Throws per knot.

Suture material	Interrupted pattern	Continuous pattern	
		Start	End
Polydioxanone	4	5	7
Polyglactin 910	3	3	6
Polyglycolic acid	3	3	5
Polyamide	4	5	6
Polypropylene	3	3	3

Cutting Suture Ends

Suture ends should be cut with dedicated suture scissors, which have a serrated edge. The suture ends (tags) are typically 3–5 mm for buried sutures (which can typically be judged against the width of the scissor blade as demonstrated). **Leaving long enough ends is important to prevent the knot unravelling** with any slippage or loosening. Cutting using the width of the scissor blade as a guide can be achieved by rotating the suture scissors 90° and sitting the back edge of the blade on the knot. **Skin sutures that require removal are left longer (10–15 mm)** to facilitate their removal.

Suture Patterns

Interrupted Suture Patterns

Interrupted suture patterns refer to individual sutures placed, each with their own knot.

- **Simple interrupted sutures** are the most commonly used interrupted suture pattern (Figure 23). These are single suture loops placed along the incision, each secured with an individual knot. Simple interrupted sutures may be slid into position and tightened by adjusting tension on the suture ends. All the tension on one suture end causes the suture to slide, but sharing the tension evenly tightens the knot and the suture loop. Tensioning the suture flat to the tissue tightens the suture loop. Tensioning the suture ends away from the

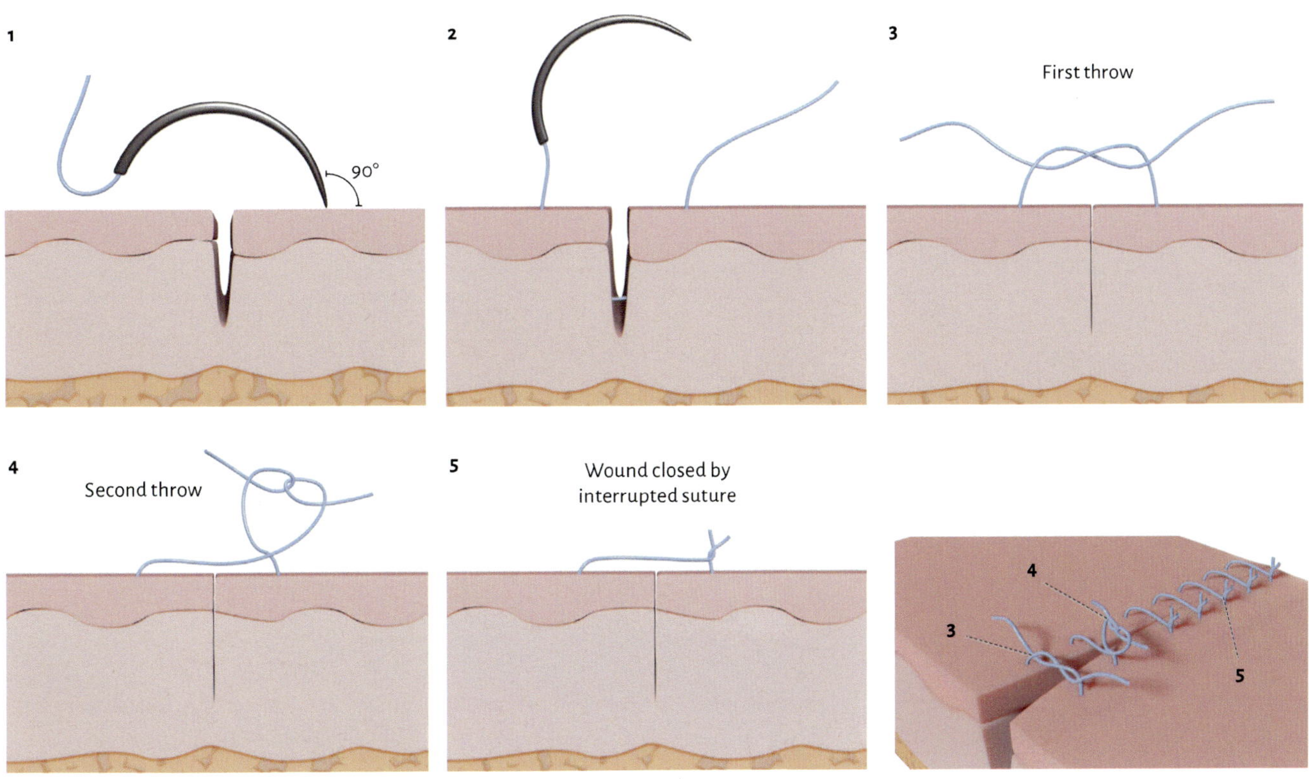

Figure 23. Simple interrupted suture.

tissue surface tightens the knot without tightening the suture loop.

- **Mattress sutures** are double-bite, interrupted sutures which share the load across each side of the incision and hence are sometimes used to **manage tissue tension, but may also invert or evert the tissue edges** rather than perfectly opposing them. They are used on their own or placed as every other suture, alternating with simple interrupted sutures, along the length of the wound, to maintain tissue apposition. (Figure 24).
- **Cruciate sutures** are double-bite sutures which cross over externally and are an efficient way of placing a reduced number of interrupted sutures without creating a continuous suture line. (Figure 25).
- **Transfixing sutures** are sutures typically used to ligate the lumen of a tube, (e.g. a larger blood vessel, bile duct, or the uterus), by passing through the tissue they are secured around in order to prevent slippage. (Figure 26).

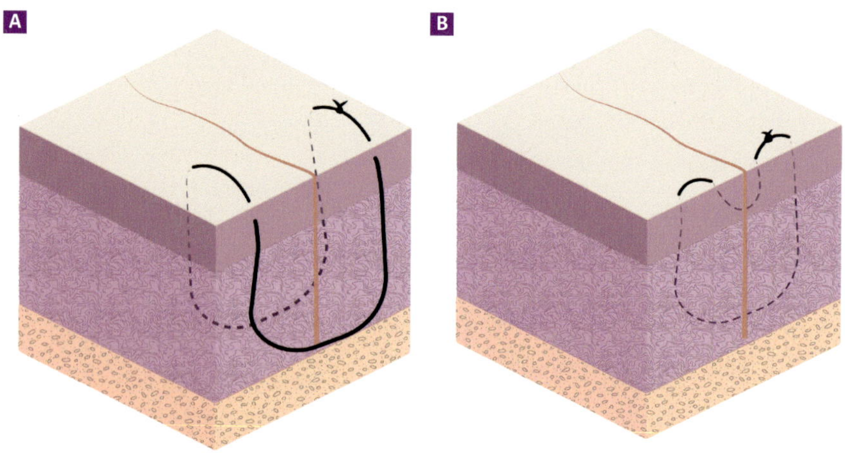

Figure 24. A. Horizontal mattress; **B.** Vertical mattress sutures.

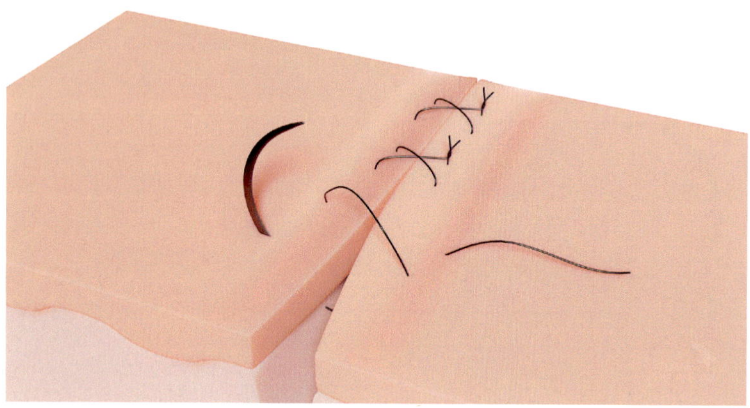

Figure 25. Cruciate interrupted suture.

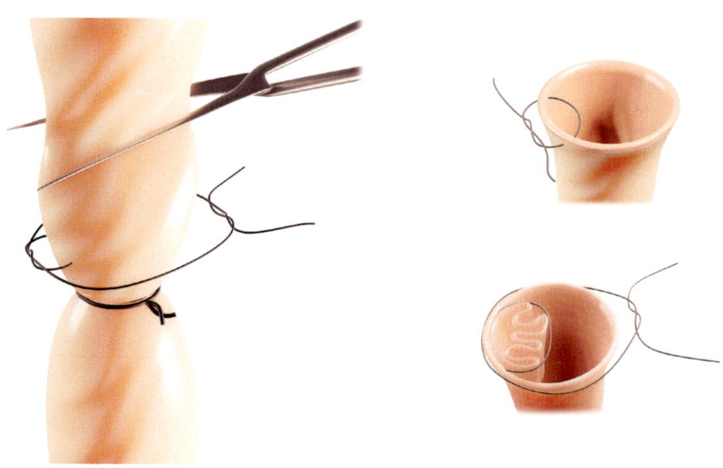

Figure 26. Transfixing suture.

Continuous Suture Patterns

Continuous suture patterns have one knot at the beginning and one knot at the end of a long suture line with multiple bites along its length. This helps evenly distribute tension along the length of the wound, which is advantageous for a linear wound, but is **not appropriate for irregularly shaped wounds** where tension is uneven. Continuous sutures are **quicker to place** and, as the knot is the weakest part of a suture, avoids multiple weak points along the closure. But if suture failure does occur the consequences are potentially more serious as the entire suture may unravel and wound dehisce.

Continuous suture patterns may be initiated and completed with square knots (Figure 22), but other knots may also be considered. **Aberdeen knots** are a common means of completing a continuous suture line. (Figure 27).

- **Simple continuous sutures** are a simple run of bites along the suture line, opposing the wound edges. (Figure 28).
- **Ford interlocking sutures** are a continuous running suture, most commonly used for suturing skin, whereby each opposing suture bite passes through the previous suture loop to align the suture loops across the incision edge, whilst leaving suture loops accessible for removal in due course. (Figure 29).
- **Everting or inverting suture patterns** have been described for sealing visceral organs in certain circumstances, or as reinforcing layers following an appositional suture pattern. However, in modern surgery they are infrequently used as most surgeons adhere to appositional suture patterns which achieve more rapid tissue healing.

Knotless Suture

Recently suture materials which do not require knot tying have been developed. These are quick to place and useful for minimally invasive surgery, **where knot tying is particularly**

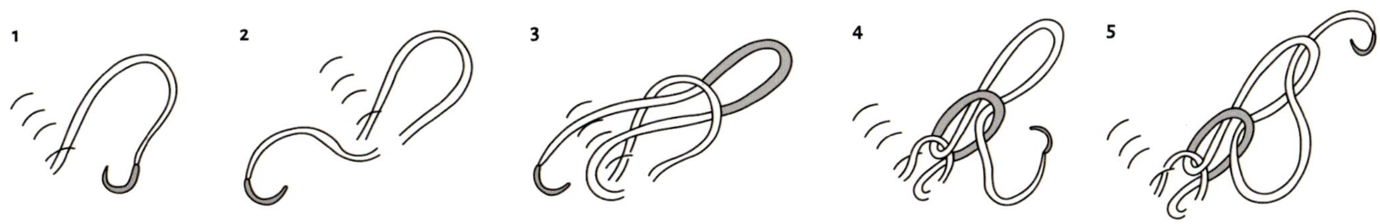

Figure 27. Aberdeen knot.

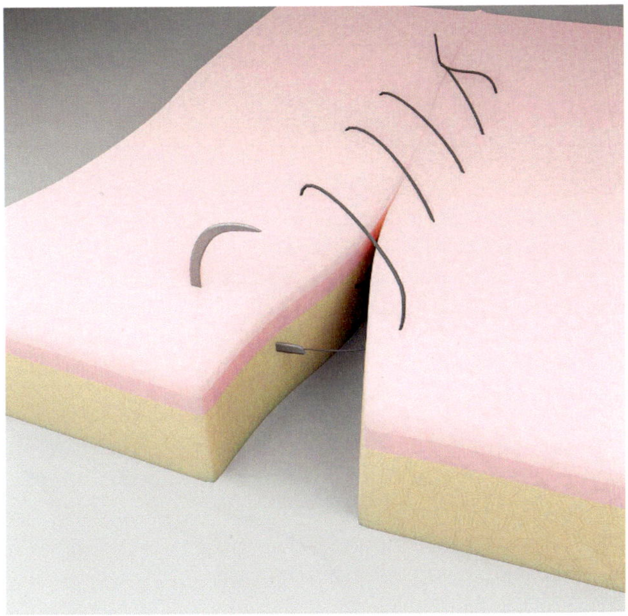

Figure 28. Simple continuous suture.

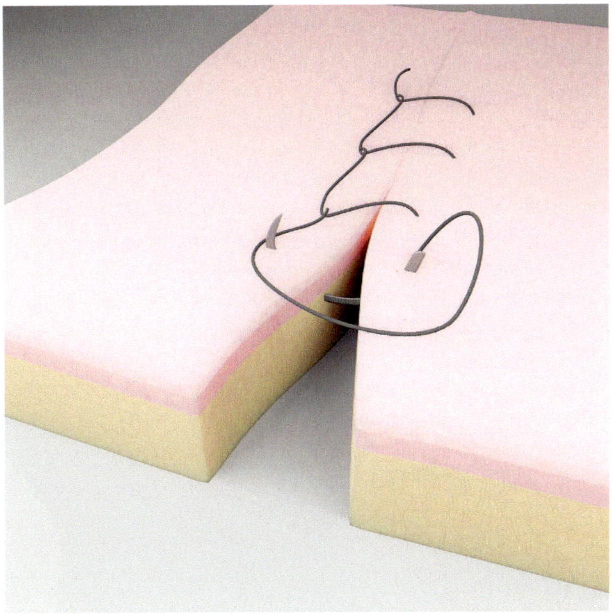

Figure 29. Ford interlocking suture.

challenging using long instruments hidden from view inside a body cavity. The sutures are designed with barbs along their length which allow them only to pass one way through tissue and therefore **cannot be retracted.** A suture size one larger than would otherwise be selected for non-barbed suture is advised as the barbs are cut into the suture strand, making the suture only of equivalent strength to a size smaller of the suture material. (Figure 30).

Knotless sutures are unidirectional, with a loop at one end and a needle at the other. The suture is anchored in tissue and then the needle passed through the loop to anchor the start of the suture line. **Bidirectional sutures** have needles at each end and barbs running in opposing directions from the midpoint of the suture strand outwards. **The first bite must be taken at the midpoint of the surgical incision.** In either case the suture line is ended by taking one bite of tissue forwards and then making a tight 180 degree turn and a second bite back through the same tissue to anchor the barbs at the end of the suture before cutting, without the need for a knot.

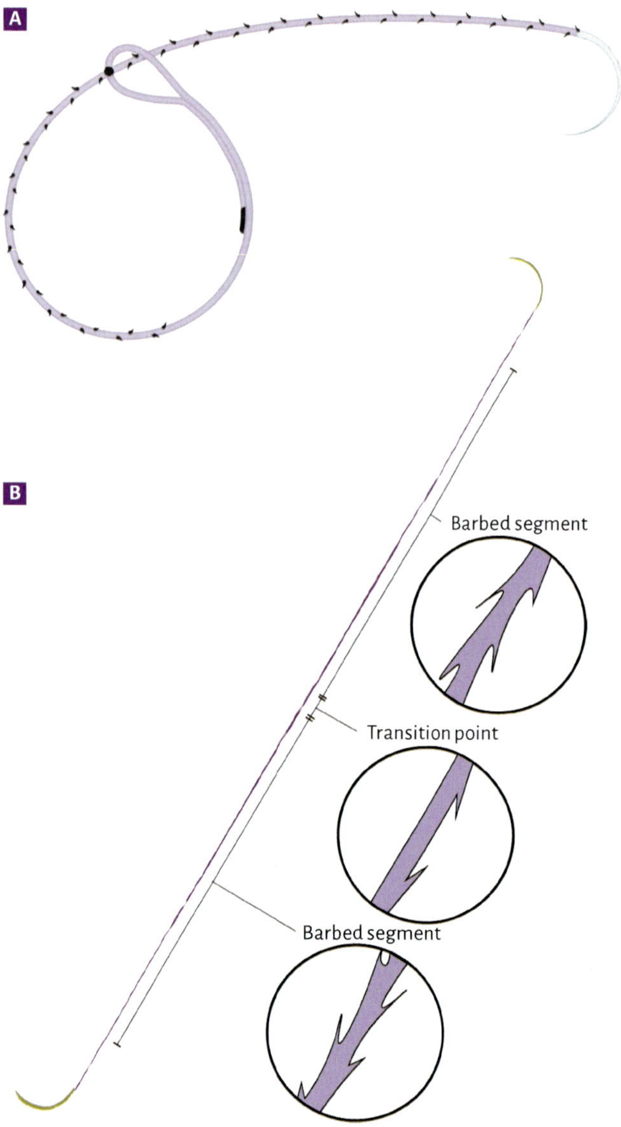

Figure 30. A. Unidirectional knotless suture; **B.** Bidirectional knotless suture.

Skin Staplers

Surgical staples are made of medical grade stainless steel. Surgical staplers are rapid to use and produce highly reproduceable results when used correctly and in the right clinical setting. They are not however a replacement for meticulous surgical technique. There are a variety of staplers designed for specific clinical scenarios. The big drawbacks of the use of some surgical staplers is familiarity with their use, which is needed for consistent results, and the cost.

Skin staplers are the most commonly used surgical staplers. They fire a rectangular shaped loop conformation of staple, which holds apposed the tissue to which they are applied but should not compress or constrict the tissue. They can, however, rotate in the tissue and sometimes release from the tissue and migrate. They are **removed with a dedicated staple removing device,** which bends the staples along the exposed long edge to release them from the tissue. (Figure 31).

Skin staplers are designed for application to the skin; however, some surgeons have also demonstrated their safe application for enterotomy and enterectomy in both dogs and cats (Rosenbaum et al., 2016; Schwartz and Coolman, 2017; Schwartz and Coolman, 2018).

Thoracoabdominal Staplers

Thoracoabdominal or TA staplers (Figure 32) have a long hand piece with a pistol-style grip and load a staple cartridge, which fires staples in a line perpendicular to the shaft of the stapler. The **open staples are U-shaped, but close to become B-shaped** when secured within the tissue.

The stapler can be closed to secure the tissue to be stapled within the jaws, but at this stage can be released and repositioned if needed. Once appropriate positioning is confirmed, the staples are fired. Before releasing the cartridge, the tissue can be cut along the edge of the cartridge without damaging the staple line, but maximising the amount of tissue which is removed, which may be important when achieving surgical margins for tumour removal.

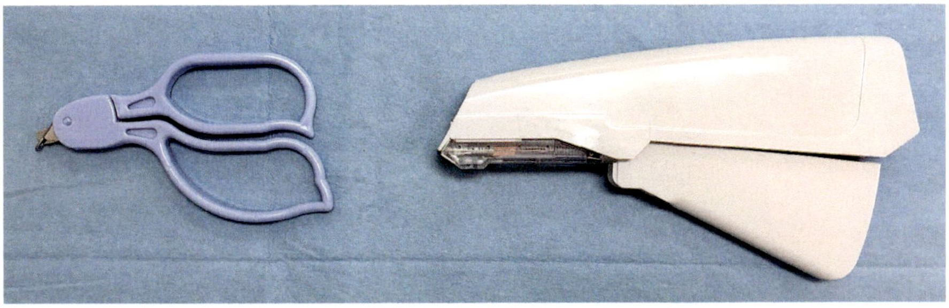

Figure 31. Skin staple remover and skin stapler.

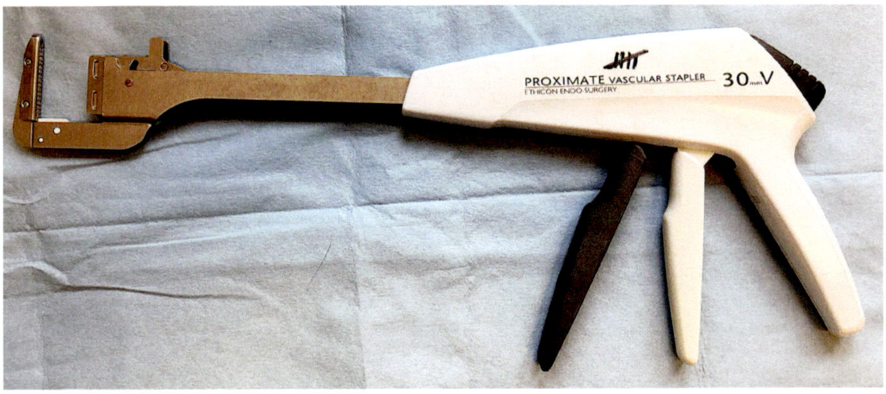

Figure 32. TA stapler.

Staplers and staple cartridges vary in length, the number of rows of staples, and the size of the staples. Cartridges either contain two or three (vascular) rows of staples, which are staggered and overlap with one another, in order to form an airtight seal on the tissue they are applied to. **It is essential to use an appropriate size of staple** (Table 3), as small staples applied to thick tissue will crush the tissue, whereas large staples in thin tissue will be loose and not prevent bleeding and leakage.

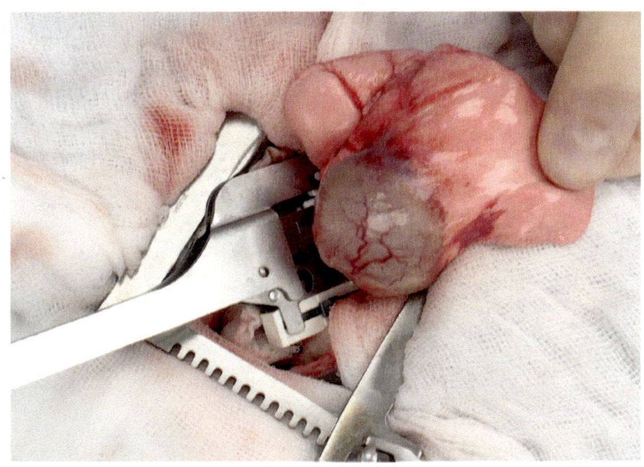

Figure 33. A TA stapler being used to perform a lung lobectomy to remove a primary lung tumour.

Table 3. TA staple sizes.

Staple* dimensions (mm)	Closed height (mm)	Wire diameter (mm)	Number of rows	Cartridge colour	Available cartridge widths (mm)
3.0 x 2.5	1.0	0.21	3	White	30
4.0 x 3.5	1.5	0.23	2	Blue	30, 55, 90
4.0 x 4.8	2.0	0.28	2	Green	30, 55, 90

*Crown width x leg length

TA staplers are most frequently **used for lung lobectomy, liver lobectomy,** and (in combination with a linear cutter stapler) for **performing a functional end-to-end anastomosis of the intestine.** (Figure 33).

Linear Cutter Staplers

Linear stapler cutters (Figure 34) do as their name suggests and both seal tissue with staples and then cut the tissue in line with the staples. They are also referred to as **gastrointestinal anastomosis (GIA) staplers,** which refers to one of their more frequent applications. As opposed to the TA staplers, they **fire staples in the same axis as the handle,** in rows (typically six rows) and then cut the tissue between the third and fourth rows of staples, leaving a seal in the tissue on either side of the incision.

There are handpieces designed for use in open surgery, as well as longer devices intended for use in minimally invasive surgery (e.g. the EndoGIA®). (Figure 35).

Linear stapler cutters are most frequently used in intestinal surgery to perform an end-to-end anastomosis following enterectomy. They are placed into the two cut ends of the bowel, intended to be joined and then fired to join and cut a connection between the two loops, like a pair of trousers. The open end (waistband of the trousers) is then sealed with a second firing of the linear cutter stapler or more frequently a TA stapler. (Figure 36).

Linear cutter staplers are used for **partial liver lobectomy, partial lung lobectomy and partial gastrectomy procedures.**

Vascular Clips

Vascular clips place V-shaped staples, which are compressed to seal smaller vessels and ducts. They also come in a variety of sizes but are designed so that the ends of the staple should overhang the tissue by at least a third of the length of the staple. Some clips have a locking mechanism to increase security, whilst others may be prone to slippage.

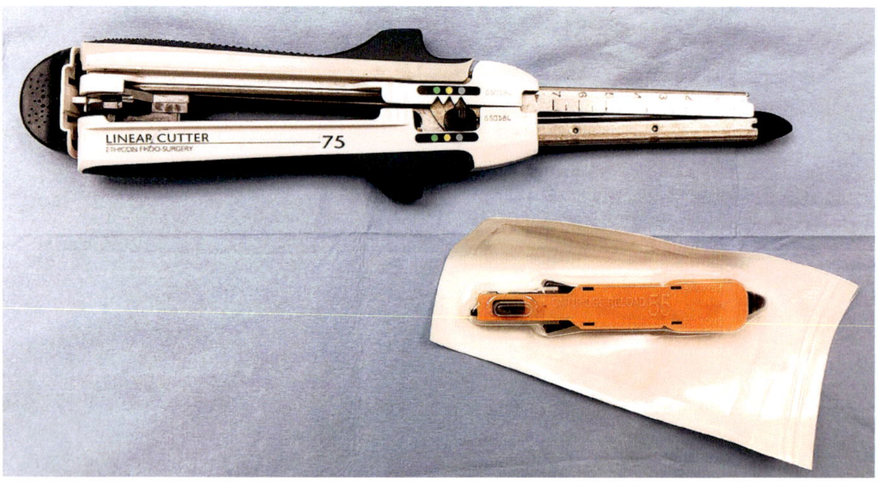

Figure 34. Linear cutter.

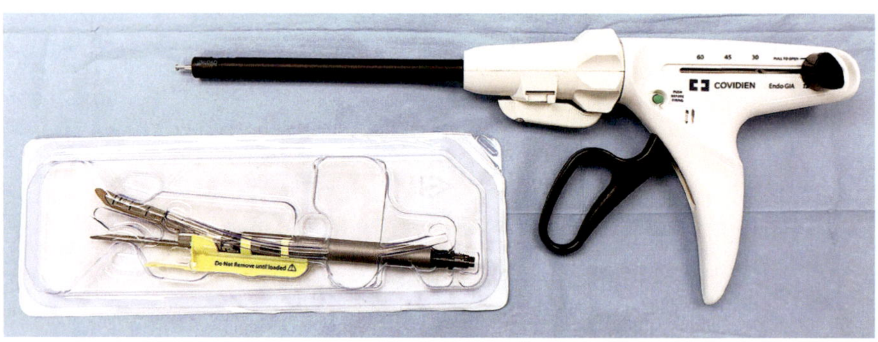

Figure 35. EndoGIA®.

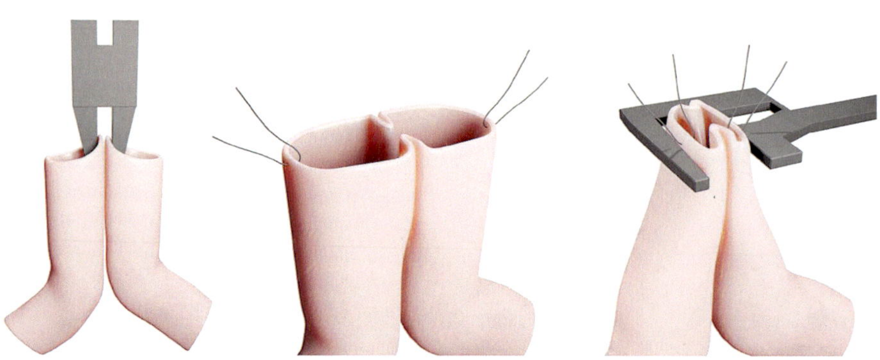

Figure 36. FEEA (Functional End-to-End Anastomosis) performed using a linear cutter followed by a TA stapler.

Vascular clips can also be made of absorbable materials, as well as stainless steel. (Figure 37).

As well as sealing small vessels, they are used to **seal the cystic duct during cholecystectomy** and to **secure cellophane bands to attenuate portosystemic shunts.**

Ligate and Divide Staplers (LDS)

Ligate and divide staplers (LDS) have a pistol-grip and apply C-shaped staples to bunch and ligate the tissue placed within their jaws, placing one staple either side of the tissue which is then cut between. These are frequently used for **surgeries requiring ligation of multiple branch vessels, e.g. splenectomy.**

Circular Staplers

Circular staplers are a special design of stapler for performing end to end intestinal anastomosis. They are of **limited use** as they require access either being passed through the anus for use in the colon and rectum or requiring a separate incision for placement elsewhere along the small intestine.

Stages of Haemostasis

Primary Haemostasis

The first stage of haemostasis is the body's initial response to vascular injury, which involves **vasoconstriction and formation of the primary platelet plug.** (Figure 38).

Vessels are lined by a single layer of endothelial cells, which act as a semipermeable membrane, allowing transfer of nutrients and waste products into and out of the bloodstream. These cells **normally have an inhibitory role in clot formation** to prevent thrombosis within a vessel. **When the endothelium is damaged and disrupted, platelets are able to adhere** to the damaged surface binding to cell surface receptors called **tissue factor** (also known as factor III). The damaged, activated cells release locally active chemicals, which cause temporary vasoconstriction to slow the blood flow, reducing blood loss to allow platelet clot formation with minimal mechanical disruption.

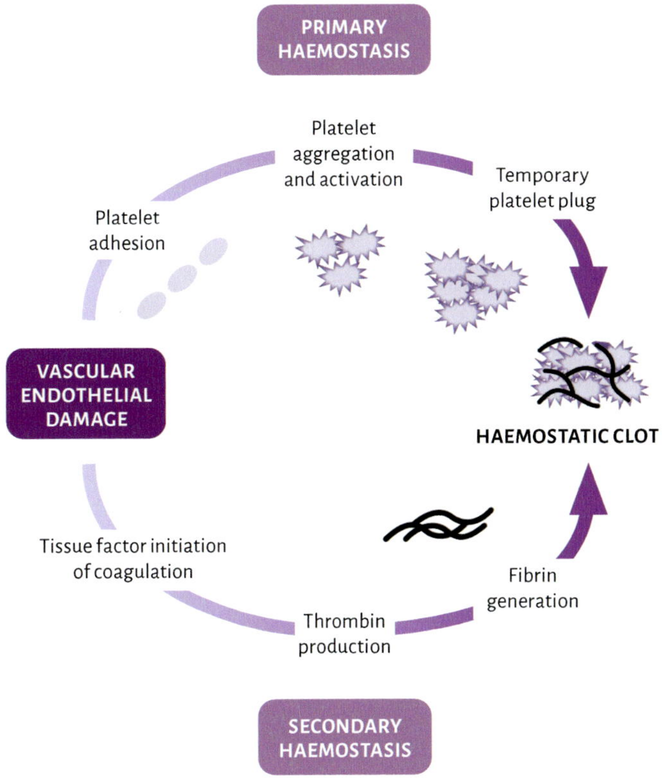

Figure 38. Primary and secondary haemostasis working in parallel to result in formation of a stable blood clot.

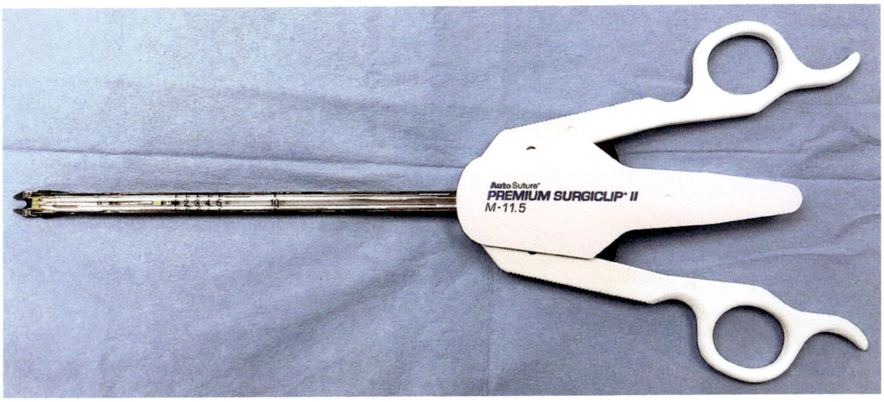

Figure 37. Vascular clip.

Platelets are tiny cell fragments containing cytoplasm but no nucleus or organelles. They are formed from giant cells called megakaryocytes in the bone marrow. Platelets stick to the damaged vessel wall, binding to exposed collagen. Binding activates the platelets, which leads to a change of shape from their smooth disc shape (ideal for flow through the bloodstream), to become a sticky, spikey shape which further binds to platelets to form a network, which acts as a primary plug of the damaged blood vessel. This activation of the platelets also releases local chemicals which recruits the adhesion of other passing platelets to join the plug. Platelets express an enzyme called **cyclooxygenase 1 (COX-1)** which is essential for their activation for aggregation and adhesion. COX-1 inhibitors such as aspirin and non-steroidal anti-inflammatory medications (NSAIDs) which are not designed to be selective only for **COX-2** (which is part of the inflammatory pain pathway), may reduce platelet activity. Calcium is also required for platelet activation and adhesion, and so calcium-channel blocker medication such as the antiarrhythmic medication diltiazem can affect platelet plug formation. On the other hand, calcium containing products can be used to aid haemostasis.

Von Willebrand factor (vWf) is released from the damaged endothelial layer of the vessel wall. This long chain glycoprotein molecule acts as a linking scaffold between activated platelets, contributing to the stability of the platelet plug. vWf also carries factor VIII, which is an important protein involved in secondary haemostasis.

Disorders of Primary Haemostasis

Disorders of primary haemostasis result in spontaneous bleeding, which might be observed as pinpoint petechiae or larger ecchymoses within the mucosa, or as bleeding from bodily orifices, neurological signs with intracranial bleeding, or weakness/collapse associated with third space loss of blood into a body cavity.

Disorders may result from low platelet number due to reduced production in the bone marrow or the increased use of consumption of loss. These may result due to infectious diseases, toxin exposure, primary bone marrow disorders, platelet destruction due to immune-mediated thrombocytopaenia (ITP), or consumption with disseminated intravascular coagulation (DIC). Patients with normal platelet numbers may suffer spontaneous bleeding in the event of abnormalities of platelet function. One example is in patients with von Willebrand's disease, which is a common congenital condition of the Dobermann but is also seen in some other breeds that lack vWf.

Secondary Haemostasis

Secondary haemostasis is the activation and amplification of the clotting cascade (a series of progressive reactions within the bloodstream), **which results in the formation of fibrin, which acts as a scaffold for stabilisation of a blood clot.** (Figure 38).

The clotting cascade (Figure 39) **is a sequence of enzymatic reactions, which result in the production of fibrin from its precursor fibrinogen.** There are **12 clotting factors** that are involved in the pathways, and these are usually referred to by their numbers in Roman numerals. The simplified coagulation cascade in the diagram, shows an oversimplified model of the process, with the extrinsic pathway stimulated by vessel damage and the exposure/expression of tissue factor (III) which initiated and drives the clotting process extrinsically. Once initiated, the intrinsic pathway amplifies the process, with both pathways resulting in activation of a common pathway, which leads to the formation of fibrin to stabilise the clot. The importance of the intrinsic and extrinsic pathways is that **deficiency of a single factor in either pathway, may result in spontaneous bleeding,** and hence testing of the pathways is important for diagnosis of a specific deficiency.

Clotting factors are proteins, largely synthesised in the liver. Some of the clotting factors (II, VII, IX and X) are **dependent on the presence of vitamin K for their production** (Figure 40). Liver disease is a common cause of disorders of secondary haemostasis; although the risk of spontaneous bleeding is rare,

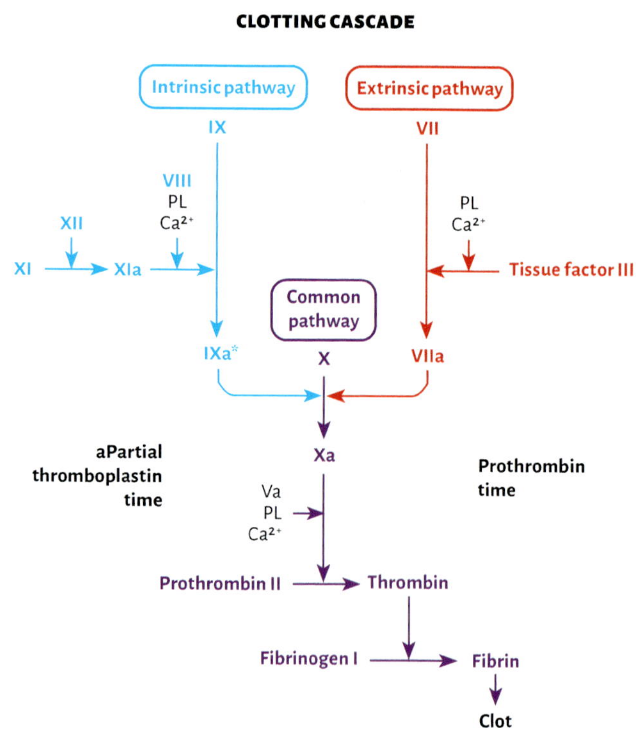

Figure 39. Clotting cascade. Roman numerals represent the clotting factors, those annotated with an 'a' are the activated version which propagates the next stage of the cascade. PL represents platelets.

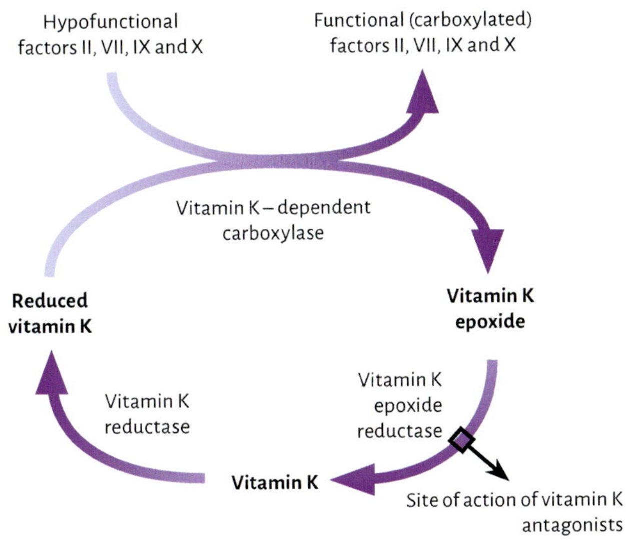

Figure 40. Vitamin K recycling within the liver.

these patients are at risk of bleeding at the time of surgery or biopsy and so coagulation testing should be performed prior to these procedures. Disorders of secondary haemostasis may also occur with vitamin K deficiency, which most commonly results from impaired intestinal absorption or due to rodenticide poisoning. ***Angiostrongylus vasorum* (lungworm) infection also causes coagulopathy,** however the exact mechanism is poorly understood. Disseminated intravascular coagulation (DIC) may result in the consumption of clotting factors and hence eventually result in spontaneous bleeding.

Tertiary Haemostasis

The final stage of haemostasis is the remodelling and eventual dissolution of the formed clot with repair of the vascular wall.

Degradation of the fibrin clot is referred to as fibrinolysis, and performed by fibrinolytic enzymes, primarily plasmin. Plasmin is released in response to the activation of endothelial cells, which are dividing and growing to repair the vessel, forming a seal to the damaged vessel lining, hence indicating that the clot is no longer required. Fibrinolysis results in the release of fibrin degradation products (FDPs) and D-dimers.

The clotting cascade and fibrinolysis processes are both kept in balance by inhibitory enzymes to ensure clots do not form inappropriately. **When the balance of these processes is lost, disseminated intravascular coagulation (DIC) may occur,** with clots forming inappropriately, but then also being broken down and this may be detected by the consumption of platelets and clotting factors, as well as by measuring elevations in FDPs and D-dimers in the blood, and possibly by spontaneous bleeding.

Haemostatic Testing

Surgical patients should have a full clinical history taken (including any previous episodes of spontaneous bleeding) and be thoroughly examined prior to surgery (including assessment for evidence of spontaneous bleeding, which may be noted as petechiae, ecchymoses or pallor associated with third space blood loss into a body cavity). **Patients with a history of previous bleeding or liver disease should undergo further haemostatic testing prior to surgical treatment.**

Tests of Primary Haemostasis

Platelet Count

A normal platelet count in dogs and cats is approximately 150–450 × 10^9/l. Spontaneous bleeding is not usually observed until platelet numbers drop below 30–50 × 10^9/l.
Spurious low platelet counts can occur:

- **due to platelet clumping:** these can usually be seen at the feathered edge of a blood film hence, alongside use of an automated analyser counter smears should be visually examined. Clumping can occur due to traumatic sampling, leading to activation of coagulation, or due to the anticoagulant used;
- **large platelet size:** common in certain breeds, more frequently seen in Cavalier King Charles Spaniels. These larger platelets function similarly to many smaller platelets and are considered a normal variant; and
- **ageing of the sample.**

A manual estimate of the platelet count is obtained by examining a red cell monolayer under high power on a microscope, with an **expectation of 8–12 platelets per high power field.** The average number over 5–10 high power fields can be multiplied by 20 × 10^9/l to give an estimate of platelet count.

Buccal Mucosal Bleeding Time (BMBT)

This is an in vivo test of primary haemostasis in patients with normal platelet counts. It is not necessary in patients with low platelet counts but can be used as a test of platelet function, for von Willebrand's disease screening prior to surgery in at risk breeds, and dogs with *Angiostrongylus vasorum* (lungworm) infections.

A spring-loaded automated device is used to make a **standardised superficial cut in the mucosa of the inside of the upper lip.** The blood is blotted away with blotting paper from adjacent to the incision but taking care not to disrupt the clot formation on the incision itself. **Normal clotting times should be <4 minutes in dogs, and <2.5 minutes in cats.**

Von Willebrand Factor (vWf)

Following an abnormal BMBT in an at-risk breed of dog, a quantitative assessment of vWf levels should be performed, as well as genetic testing in some breeds such as the Dobermann Pinscher.

Tests of Secondary Haemostasis

Clotting tests are relatively insensitive, only becoming abnormal when there is a reduction of a clotting factor to less than 30% of its normal value. These tests have been designed for use in humans for monitoring response to treatment with anticoagulant medications rather than as screening tests for disease in animals and so their results should be interpreted with caution. (See Figure 39).

Activated Clotting Time (ACT)

This is a test of the intrinsic and common pathways. This test **provides similar information to the APTT but is less sensitive.**

Activated Partial Thromboplastin Time (APTT)

This is also a test of the intrinsic and common pathways. Prolongation of APTT in isolation may represent an intrinsic pathway disorder such as haemophilia A (factor VIII deficiency), haemophilia B (factor IX deficiency), or deficiencies of factors XI or XII.

Prothrombin Time (PT)

This is a test of the extrinsic and common pathways. Prolongation of PT in isolation may represent factor VII deficiency, early rodenticide poisoning, or vitamin K deficiency (as factor VII has the shortest half-life of the vitamin K dependent factors). Prolongation of both APTT and PT may represent a common pathway deficiency or deficiency of multiple factors which result from rodenticide poisoning, vitamin K deficiency, or liver disease. Prolongation of APTT, PT, BMBT and a reduction in platelet numbers is indicative of DIC or hepatic failure, although the patterns may be variable with these conditions.

Thromboelastography (TEG)

TEG is a global test of coagulation. It requires specialised, highly sensitive equipment and so is not widely available. The test uses a wire moving within a sample, to assess the rate of clot formation, clot strength, and subsequent degradation of the clot. (Figure 41).

Haemostatic Aids

Blood Flow Reduction

- **Tourniquets/vascular occlusion:** placing a tourniquet proximally on a limb prior to surgery on the extremity helps limit flow during the procedure. This is not at the expense of surgical haemostasis but may allow for a clear field of view and reduce surgical time. **The duration of tourniquet placement should be limited** to prevent ischaemic injury to the affected tissue. Similarly, temporary ligation, clamping, or use of Rumel tourniquets is helpful to limit bleeding during other surgeries, e.g. the carotid arteries for maxillofacial surgery, or the Pringle manoeuvre to limit blood flow to the liver for major liver resections.

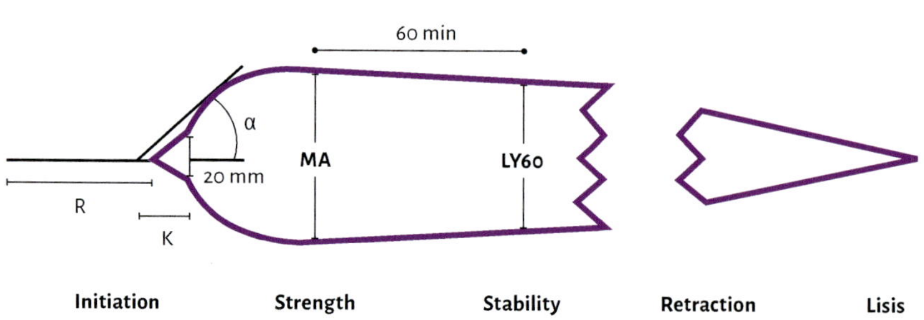

Figure 41. TEG trace showing the production and degradation of a clot over time (from left to right), with height of the graph representing clot strength. Reaction time (R) is a measure of the speed of activation of the clotting cascade, clotting time (K) is an assessment of the speed of initial clot formation, alpha angle (α) is an assessment of the speed of fibrin clot stabilisation, maximum amplitude (MA) is a measure of strength of the fibrin clot, LY60 is a measure of the retraction and breakdown (lysis) of the clot over 60 min.

- **Pressure/tamponade:** applying pressure to a bleeding vessel slows blood flow and allows time for a platelet plug to form and stabilise, to prevent ongoing bleeding. Pressure should be maintained for up to five minutes. Thereafter, the pressure can be released, taking care not to disrupt the clot. For severe bleeds this may be a temporary measure which stems the flow and allows for identification and sealing of the source of the bleeding.
- **Topical vasoconstrictors:** adrenaline or ephedrine may be administered topically and cause local vasoconstriction. They are however systemically absorbed and may result in systemic cardiovascular effects. Ice cold saline, similarly, can be used to cause temporary local vasoconstriction. Any topical vasoconstrictor should be used with care to reduce the risk of local ischaemic necrosis.

Topical Haemostatic Agents

- **Mechanical agents:** these products absorb blood and provide a matrix for clot formation and stabilisation. They are absorbable and so can be left in place so as not to disrupt the clot that forms at the end of surgery. Commonly used products are gelatins, collagens, and cellulose. Bone wax is also a mechanical agent, a sterile purified form of beeswax, which can be used to physically plug and seal openings in bone to occlude bleeding.
- **Active haemostatic agents:** thrombin (factor II), is available in bovine, human and recombinant formulations, and contributes to the normal coagulation cascade, directly promoting the formation of fibrin from its precursor fibrinogen (the last step of the clotting cascade). See Figure 39.
  - **Alginates** are commonly used as wound dressings (discussed in Chapter 8). They are derived from seaweed and are a rich source of calcium, which helps to activate the clotting cascade. They are not suitable for intracavitary use due to the foreign body reaction they cause and must be removed with saline irrigation.
- **Sealants:** these are the equivalent of biological glues and work independently of the patient's clotting mechanism. The most common of these is fibrin, the end product of coagulation, used pre-prepared in its own right. These products are prepared from human plasma.

Antifibrinolytics

Fibrinolysis is normal following coagulation, to allow remodelling and clot resolution of the sealed vessel. In some circumstances, delaying this process is beneficial to the patient, most notably, when fibrinolysis proceeds more quickly than is ideal. This is frequently observed in sighthounds, who are at risk of delayed postoperative bleeding and severe bruising following surgery. **Hence treatment with antifibrinolytics such as tranexamic acid is common in sighthounds undergoing surgery, and for 3–5 days following surgery.**

Instrument Manufacture and Care

Kit Organisation

It is the role of scrubbed surgical assistants to open and lay out the surgical kit prior to a procedure. Knowledge of the procedure and the surgeons preferred equipment choices, plus the surgical request form helps ensure the correct equipment is available.

It is important to **use a routine layout** when organising the kit on the trolley so that under pressure the correct instrument is obtained rapidly. **Grouping instruments by type should be considered,** with the handles nearest to the person responsible for speed of access or arranging the instruments in order of requirement. Special attention should be paid to keeping sharps in a dish or swab (to prevent perforating the drapes) in one area of the trolley, to protect the team from injury. Contaminated instruments (e.g. by gastrointestinal content or following neoplastic resection) should always be kept in a designated and clearly identifiable region of the trolley. (Figure 42)

It is essential the scrubbed assistant has a **good knowledge of the names of surgical instruments.** They must pass instruments positively to the surgeon, with the handles placed firmly into the surgeon's open hand to ensure they are not dropped, as the surgeon may be focussed on the surgical field and not be looking at the instrument. (Figure 43).

Instrument Manufacture

Most surgical instruments are manufactured from **high-grade stainless steel.** Stainless steels are a group of iron-based metal alloys, which are corrosion resistant due to the addition of chromium. They are not truly stainless and will corrode if not cared for appropriately i.e. storing instruments in a moist environment, in contact with reducing agents (inorganic tissue or cleaning product residues), or by storing different metals in contact with one another.

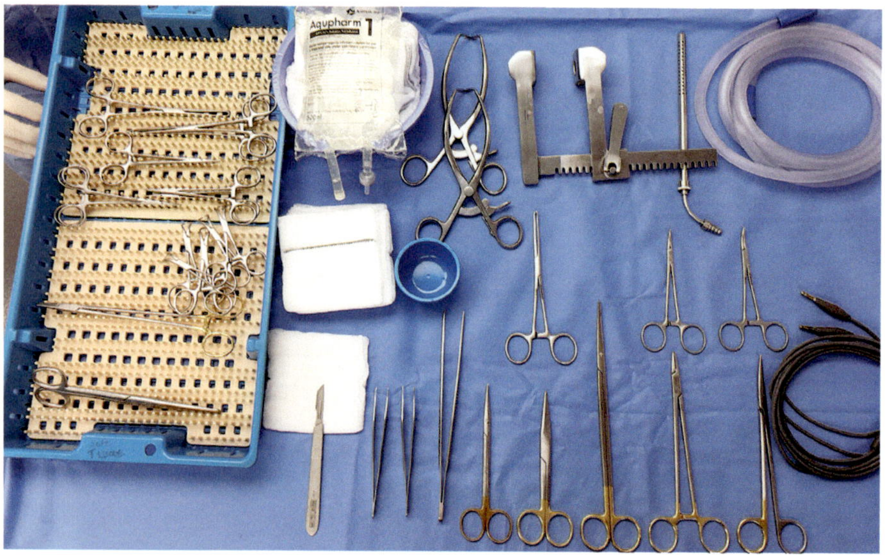

Figure 42. A Kit trolley laid out ready to start surgery.

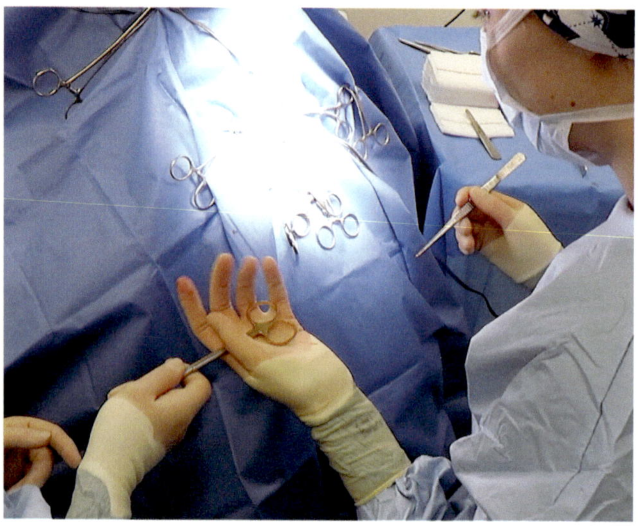

Figure 43. Positive passing. Instruments should be passed firmly into the hand of the surgeon in the correct orientation for use, so that the surgeon can maintain focus on the surgical field without dropping the instrument.

A high carbon content in stainless steel is critical to improve the hardness of instruments. This is ideal for manufacture of sharp instruments e.g. scissors, however a high carbon content also increases the brittleness of instruments, making them more prone to breakage and corrosion. When even harder materials are needed, such as the tip of needle holders, some scissors and pin and wire cutters, instruments may have inserts of tungsten carbide at the tips. This layer is very hard but also brittle and so is reinforced by stainless steel. **Scissors with tungsten carbide cutting edges are identified by having their handles electroplated with gold.** Formation of chromium oxide is encouraged on the surface of the instrument during a process of passivation in nitric acid which prevents exposure of the iron content, which might otherwise corrode causing staining.

Instrument Care

Instruments should be appropriately **cleaned, dried, and lubricated** (if appropriate) soon after each use to maintain them in the best condition. Immediately following use gross contamination should be removed using warm water and detergent. Where possible **the instruments should be opened** and/or dismantled to allow thorough cleaning of each constituent part including the joins, ratchets, and box-junctions. Once grossly clean, **the use of enzymatic cleaners and ultrasonic cleaning baths help remove smaller particulate debris.** This should be done with all box/hinge joints open to allow penetration and complete cleaning. Instruments may be immersed in instrument milk (an emulsion of oil and water) at this stage or oiled after drying.

Each instrument should be inspected to ensure thorough cleaning, and also faults and damage identified. The ratchets should also be checked to ensure they engage and release appropriately. Hinges of hinged instruments, such as scissors should be checked to ensure they are appropriately tight; when scissors are held fully open and with the handles one above the other vertically, if the top handle is released the jaws should come naturally to a close with roughly one-third of the tips still open. Scissors should open with a smooth action along the full length of the blades and be able to cut along their length, being particularly effective towards the tip. When blunt, scissors should be sent to an instrument specialist for sharpening. The tips of needle-holders and haemostatic forceps should meet perfectly and completely and be secure even when tightened on only the first notch of the ratchet. Cutting surfaces should be inspected for areas of damage. As noted previously, tungsten carbide inserts of such instruments, whilst being hard are brittle.

Instrument Marking

Instruments may be marked during manufacturing by etching or engraving prior to the passivation process to seal and protect the outer coating and prevent staining of the instrument. Subsequent engraving should be discouraged as this leaves the uncoated stainless seal exposed and allows corrosion. (Figure 44)

Autoclave resistant coloured tape or silicone rings are often used to colour code instruments, e.g. for a specific kit (Figure 45). However, these can create crevices which are challenging to clean and may harbour infection.

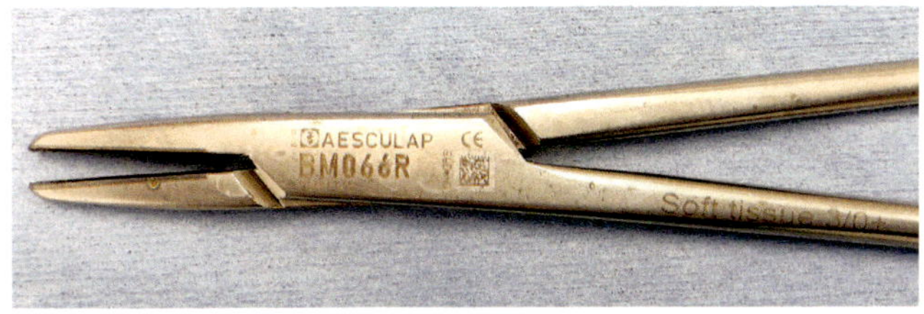

Figure 44. This pair of Mayo-Hegar needle holders are engraved with the manufacturer and product code, plus the users "soft tissue" kit designation and the suture size they are designed to use, i.e. 3/0 and larger.

General Surgical Instruments

Scalpels

The scalpel is the basic cutting instrument for surgery. The handle most widely used for small animal surgery is the #3 design. **Blades frequently used are the #10, smaller #15 and pointed #11. #12 has a curved blade and is used for skin suture removal.** (Figure 46).

Holding the scalpel in **pencil-grip** (Figure 47 A) uses the tip of the blade and is used for making stab incisions. Holding the

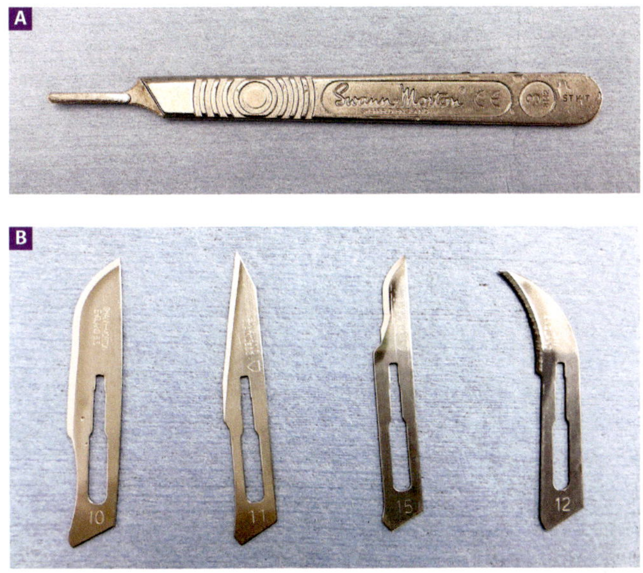

Figure 46. A. Scalpel handle #3; **B.** Scalpel blades: #10, #11, #15 and #12.

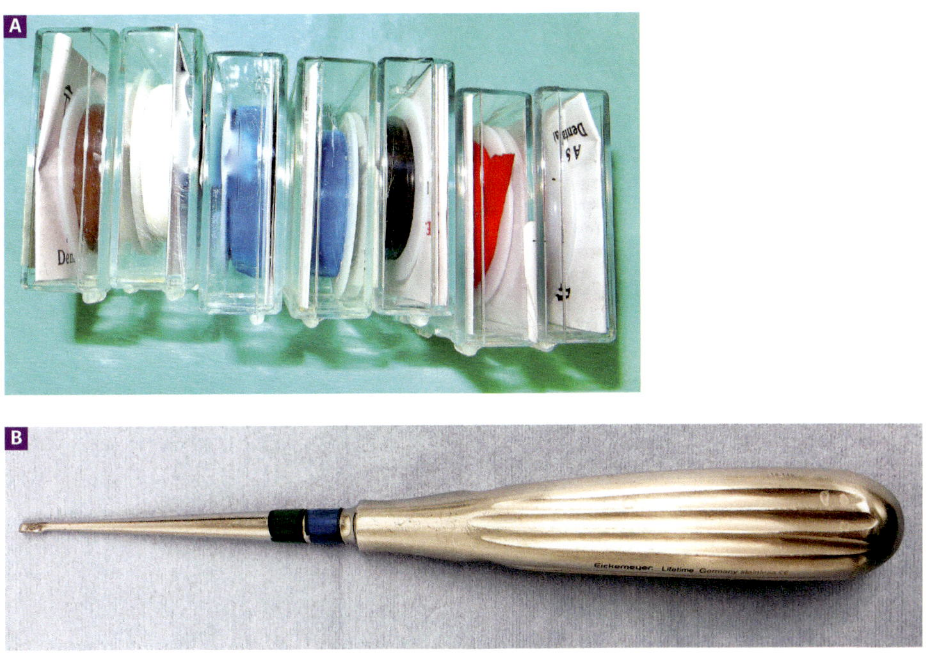

Figure 45. A. Coloured tape; **B.** Tape marked.

scalpel in **finger-grip** (Figure 47 B) brings the curve of the blade into contact with the tissue surface and is commonly used for longer incisions. **Palm-grip** (Figure 47 C) gives a sturdier grip, which allows more force, but with less precise control.

Scissors

Metzenbaum scissors (Figure 48) **are a delicate, lightweight design for fine tissue dissection.** Longer versions are useful for deep cavity surgery and use at the back of the pharynx and larynx via an intraoral approach.

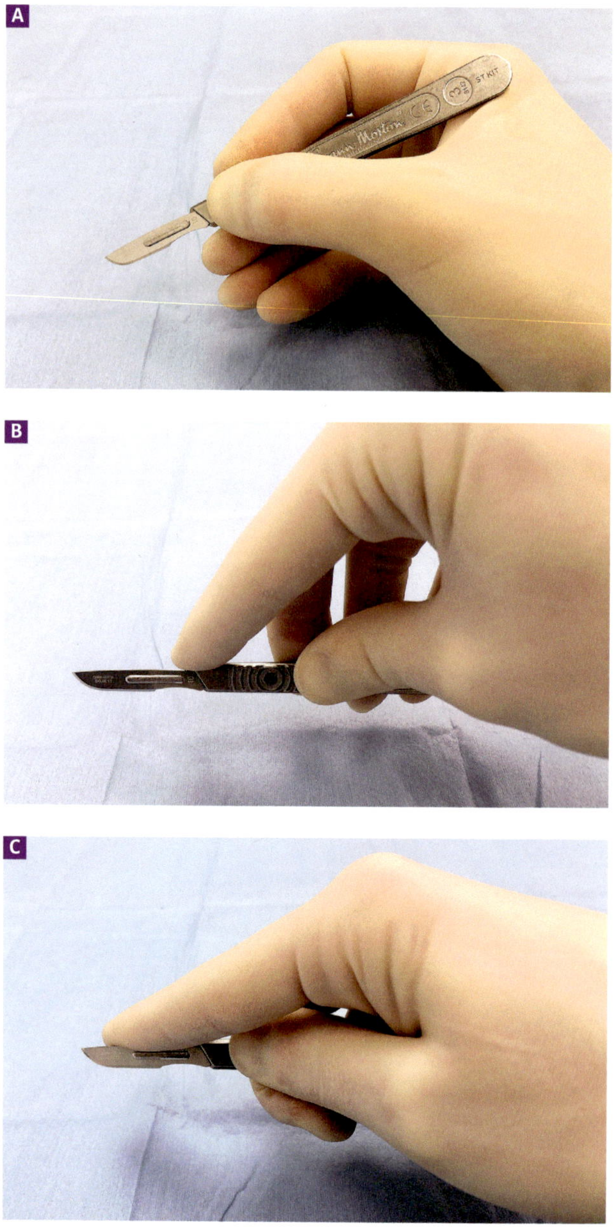

Figure 47. A. Pencil-grip; **B.** Finger-grip; **C.** Palm-grip.

Mayo scissors are a heavier, more robust design for cutting though tougher tissues, e.g. fibrous tissue and cartilage. Carless suture scissors differ as they have a serrated blade. Drape scissors are specific, heavier scissors for cutting drape material and should not be used for incising tissue or sutures. There are also a variety of smaller, more delicate specialist ophthalmic scissors (e.g. iris scissors and tenotomy scissors), which are also useful for ureteral and urethral surgery and vascular surgery.

Scissors (Figure 49) are usually grasped in a conventional tripod grip, with the thumb and fourth finger, with the index finger directed along the shaft to control the tip of the instrument precisely. Scissors can be used to **scissor-cut** by opening and closing, or to **push-cut** holding the blades half open and sliding along to separate a tissue plain; this latter technique is often used to separate the linear alba.

Thumb Forceps

Thumbs forceps are used for grasping tissue and vary most with respect to the size and number of teeth at their tips. Generally, the larger and more numerous the teeth, the more traumatic the forceps. More delicately toothed forceps are intended for use with more delicate tissues. Commonly used designs are the fine rat-toothed Adson forceps, Brown-Adson forceps with a short row of fine interlocking teeth, and the longer DeBakey serrated and ridged forceps. There are also heavier Treves forceps for tougher tissues. These are all designed to be held with a pencil grip and used as gently as possible to grasp the tissue. (Figure 50).

Needle Holders

A variety of designs of needle holder are available. The most appropriate design for general surgery is the **Mayo-Hegar**

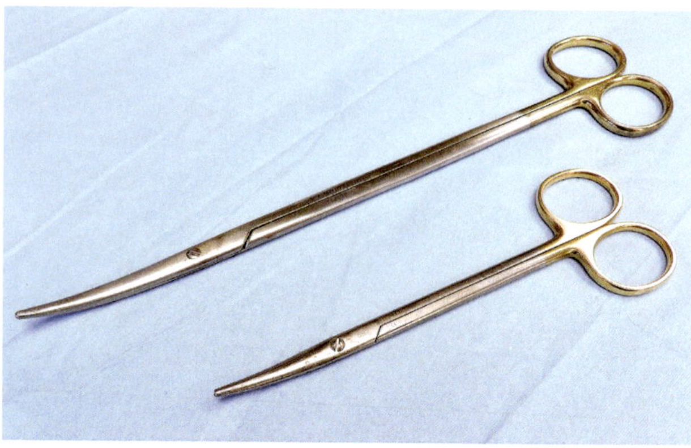

Figure 48. Metzenbaum scissors.

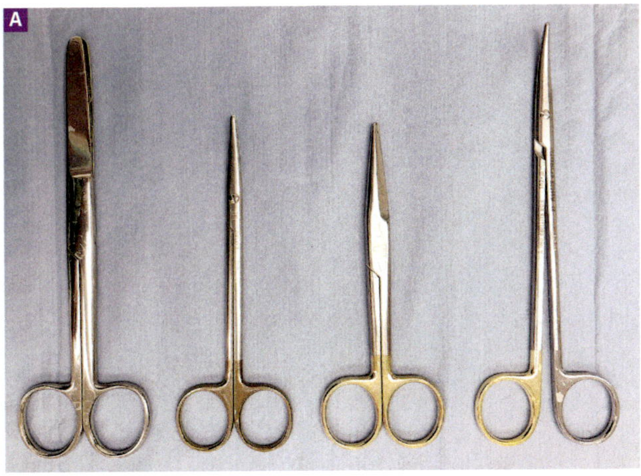

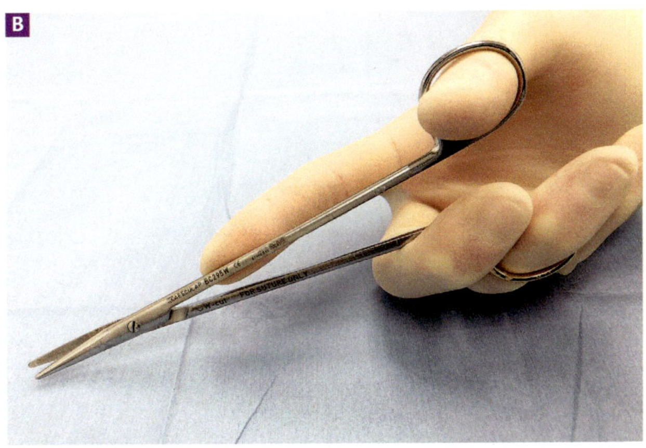

(Figure 51), which is a long, straight handled, ringed, single function instrument. **Olsen-Hegar** needle holders incorporate suture scissors. Both designs are held with the conventional tripod grip, as previously described for scissors. The Thenar grip is an alternative palm grip sometimes used, closing the ratchet with the base of the thumb, to aid control for continuous sutures, and to improve the force able to be generated to pass the needle through tougher tissue. (Figure 52).

Gillies have a distinctive, unique, asymmetric design. They are not suitable for deep suturing due to their short design.

Figure 49. A. Selection of scissors: drape, Metzenbaum, Mayo, suture scissors from left to right; **B.** Scissors grip.

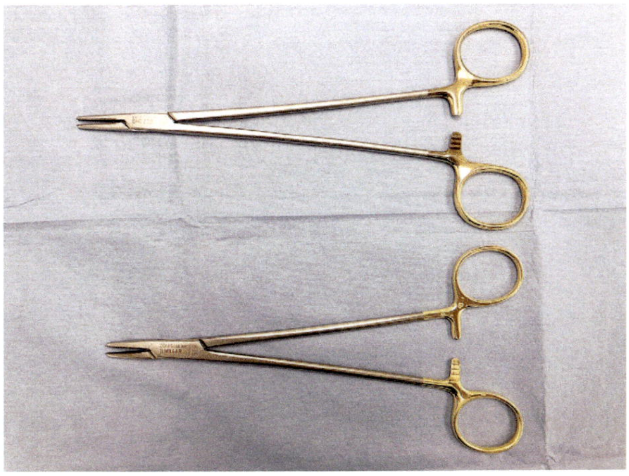

Figure 51. Mayo-Hegar needle holder.

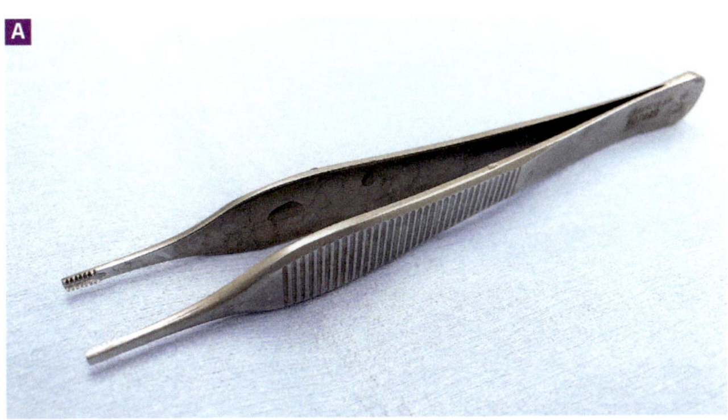

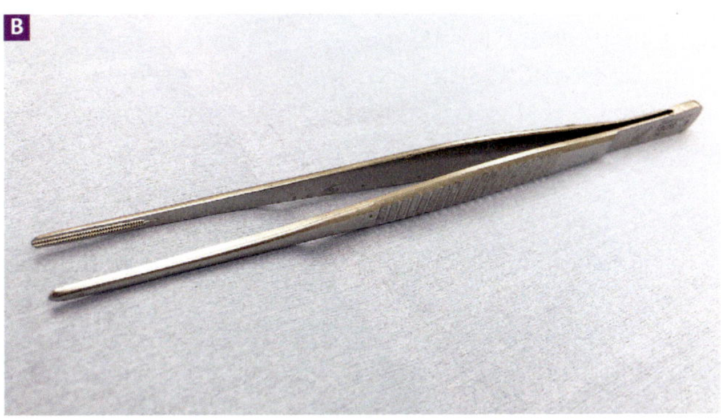

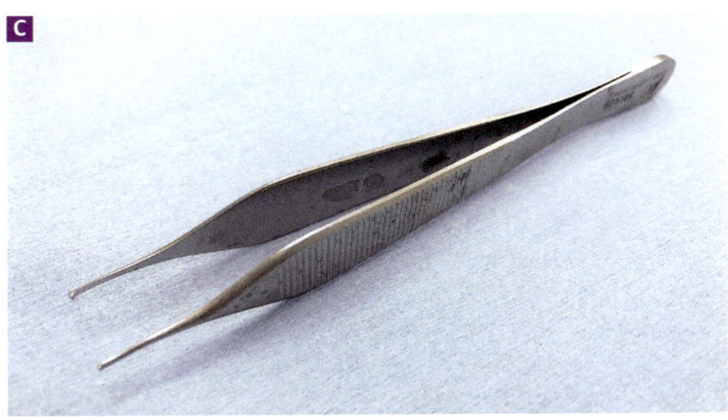

Figure 50. A. Brown-Adson; **B.** DeBakey; **C.** Adson.

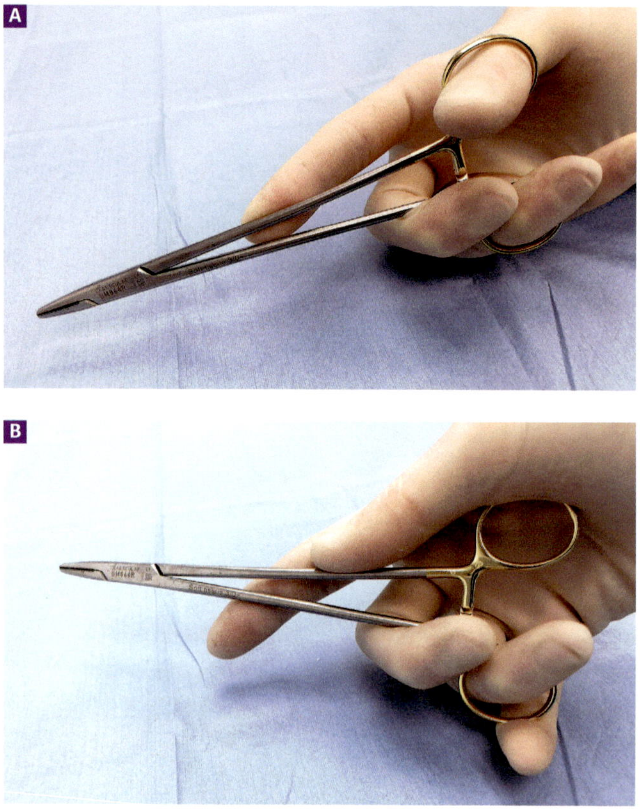

Figure 52. A. Tripod grip; **B.** Thenar grip.

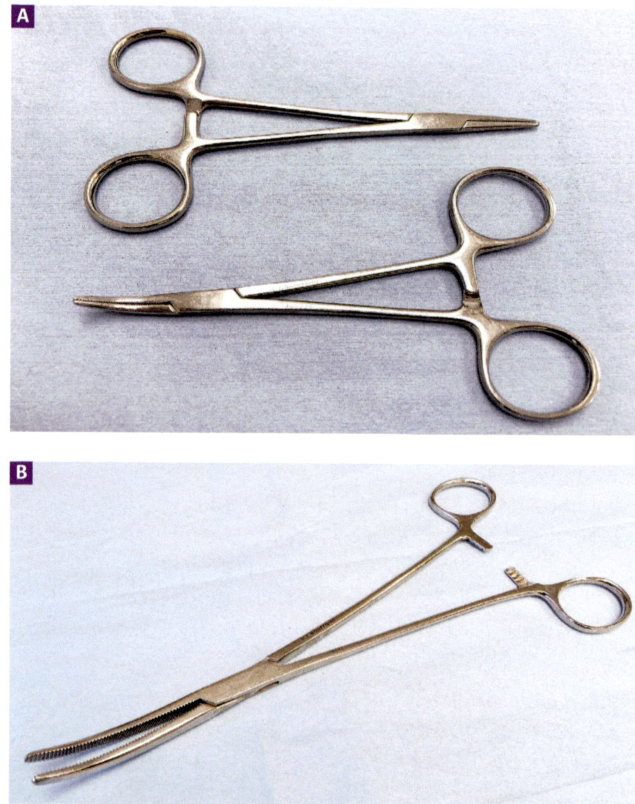

Figure 53. A. Halsted mosquito forceps (straight and curved varieties); **B.** Kelly forceps.

They encourage a different wrist movement due to their asymmetry, which is not favoured by most surgeons and lack a ratchet to grasp and hold the needle. These also incorporate a suture scissor. As with other multifunction instruments neither function is optimised, and cutting is only possible deep within the jaws of the instruments which is not ideal for delicate suture cutting deep in body cavities. **Castroviejo needle holders** are a more delicate, spring-loaded design, suited to ophthalmic use.

The needle should be held in the tips of the needle holders by pyramid shaped teeth designed for this purpose; these should be an **appropriate size for the needle:** too small and the needle twists, rocks or jumps; too large and the jaws bend the needle, increasing tissue trauma. Hence, it may be necessary to have needle holders of different sizes within a basic surgical pack.

The needle should be gripped roughly one third of its length from the base. Suture packs are usually constructed to facilitate picking up the needle from the pack in this position for the right-handed surgeon. **The needle should be driven along its long axis,** which for a curved needle requires supination (rotation) of the wrist.

Haemostatic Forceps

There are a variety of haemostatic forceps, including Halsted, Dunhill, and Kelly; which usually feature transverse grooves. These are available in different sizes, with the smallest size commonly around 3.5-inches in length, referred to as **mosquito forceps.** They are also available in straight and curved varieties. Curved instruments are designed to allow placement without impeding the surgeons view of the tips. (Figure 53).

Rochester-Carmalt forceps have a longer blade, with longitudinal grooves, which crush through fatty tissue and are preferred by some surgeons for procedures, such as ovariohysterectomy, where sutures may be placed in precrushed tissue.

Right-angled designs of haemostatic forceps are particularly useful for dissecting around vessels and ducts, e.g. for cardiovascular procedures, cholecystectomy and portosystemic shunt surgeries. The image shows designs with and without ratchets which can clamp tissue as well as being used for dissection and suture passing (Figure 54).

There are a range of specific, atraumatic vascular clamps used for cardiovascular surgery such as **Satinsky clamps** (Figure 55),

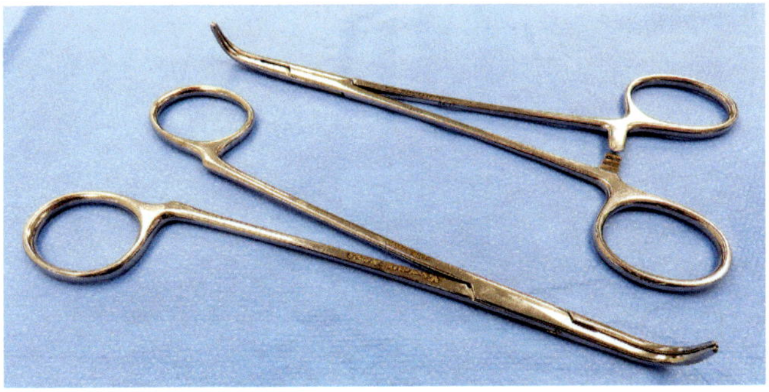

Figure 54. Right-angled forceps.

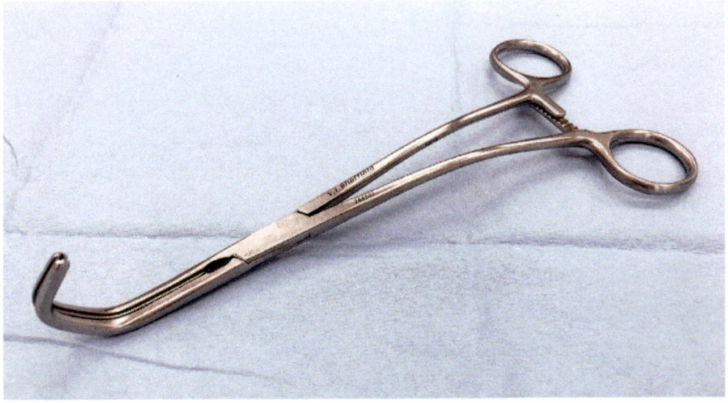

Figure 55. Satinsky vascular clamp.

designed to be applied longitudinally to vessels to allow incision of the vessel within the portion sealed by the clamp, whilst allowing flow past the clamped off portion of the vessel. These are also designed to be atraumatic as the vessel will be released and blood flow restored following repair of the incision.

Tissue Forceps

Tissue forceps are used to grasp tissue directly and should be appropriate for the tissue being grasped. Ideally, tissues should be handled remaining in the patient as little and atraumatically as possible. (Figure 56).

Allis tissue forceps have traumatic serrated jaws with interdigitating teeth. They should only be used on relatively tough, avascular, connective tissues, and are commonly used to secure suction tubing and electrical cables to drapes.

Babcock's have smooth jaws and may be used on more delicate tissues more gently if needed, but even these are not atraumatic and leave a crush line on tissue.

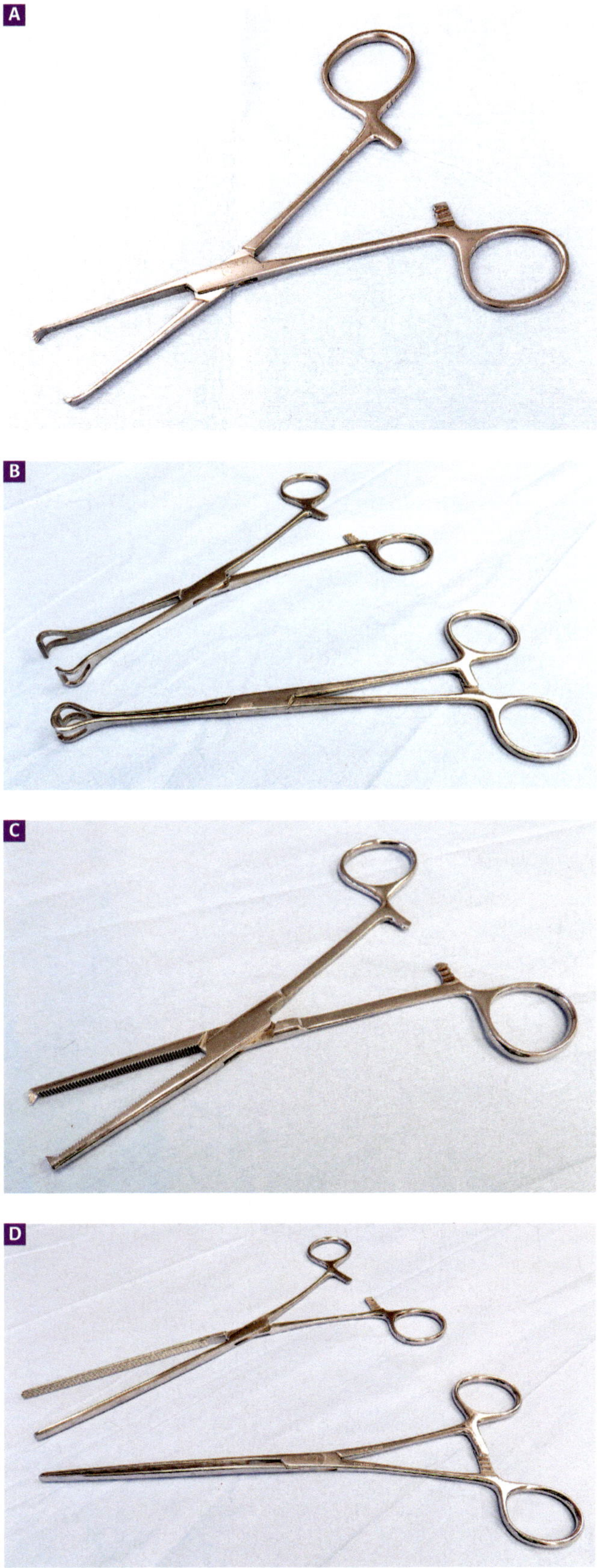

Figure 56. A. Allis; **B.** Babcock; **C.** Cocker; **D.** Doyen forceps.

Cocker forceps are rat-toothed and very traumatic but grip tissue securely. They may be used to grasp the cartilage of an ear canal as a handle, when being removed during a total ear canal ablation procedure.

Doyen forceps are designed for occluding the bowel with their long, flexible, relatively atraumatic blades. The bowel should be placed in the widest part of the jaws and grasped as gently as possible, ideally with only one click on the ratchet.

Retractors

Tissue retractors are used to **improve the surgeon's view and access** and may be self-retaining by means of a ratchet or handheld.

Gelpi retractors are the most widely used self-retaining retractors, with ringed handles, which take some experience to become familiar with as the hinged mechanism is counterintuitive (the tips open as the handles close), contrary to other ringed instruments. Gelpi's have a single hooked tip at the end of each leg and come in a variety of sizes, with legs of different lengths appropriate for use at different depths within tissue. (Figure 57).

West, Weitlander, and Sternomastoid retractors are similar in design to Gelpi's but have multiple prongs on the end of each limb, hence retracting a broader surround of tissue, making them less prone to rotating out of position and particularly useful for perianal surgery where multiple points of contact reduce the risk of instruments misplacing and falling to the floor.

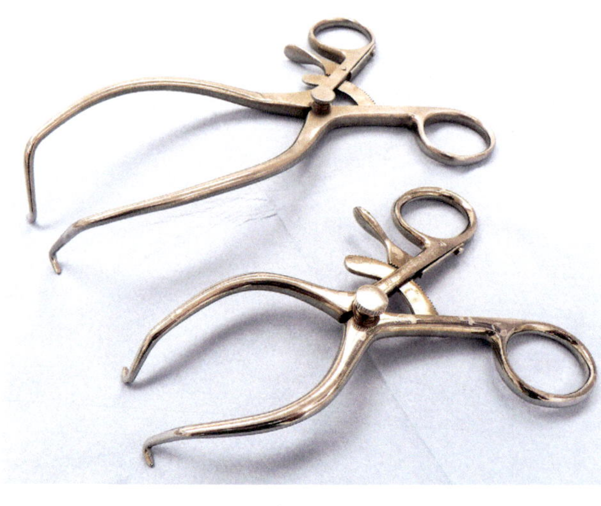

Figure 57. Gelpi retractor.

Gosset and Balfour retractors are specifically designed for abdominal wall retraction for coeliotomy procedures, the latter with a third blade (or spoon) which can be attached under the xyphoid cranially.

Finochietto rib spreaders have a rotary crank and are used to retract ribs and median sternotomy incisions for thoracic surgery, although Gelpi's may suffice for this purpose in smaller patients. (Figure 58).

Army and Navy, Green, and Morris & Langenbeck are different designs of handheld retractors, which have a basic flat blade design, perpendicular to the axis of the handle. The **Senn retractor** is a smaller, lighter design, which also has a row of sharp, hooks at the other end, which gives it its alternative name of the cat's paw retractor; which when held should be wrapped in a surgical swab to prevent glove perforation. **Mergerding retractors** are similar to Langenbeck but with a single ring for retraction. **Malleable (or ribbon) retractors** are smooth, flat paddles, which are indeed malleable and can be bent into the desired shape to provide gentle retraction from a distance, which is particularly useful for retracting delicate tissues deep within body cavities (e.g. the liver or lung) and are commonly used indirectly over a moist laparotomy sponge to prevent trauma to those delicate tissues. (Figure 59).

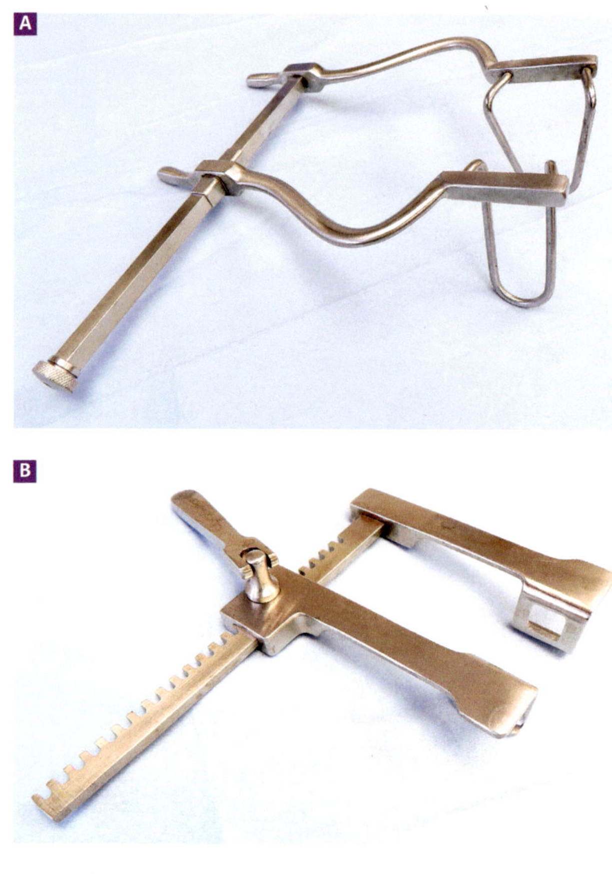

Figure 58. A. Gosset retractor; **B.** Finochietto rib spreader.

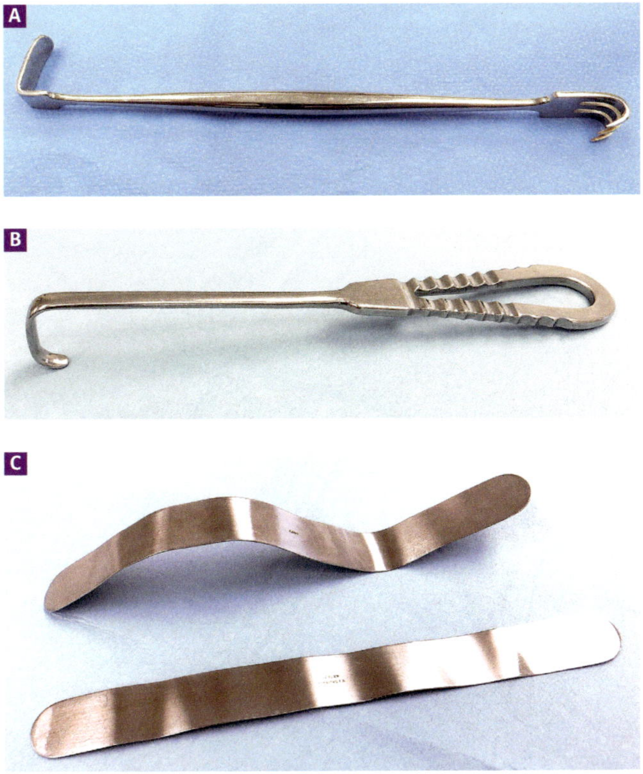

Figure 59. A. Senn; **B.** Langenbeck; **C.** Malleable retractors.

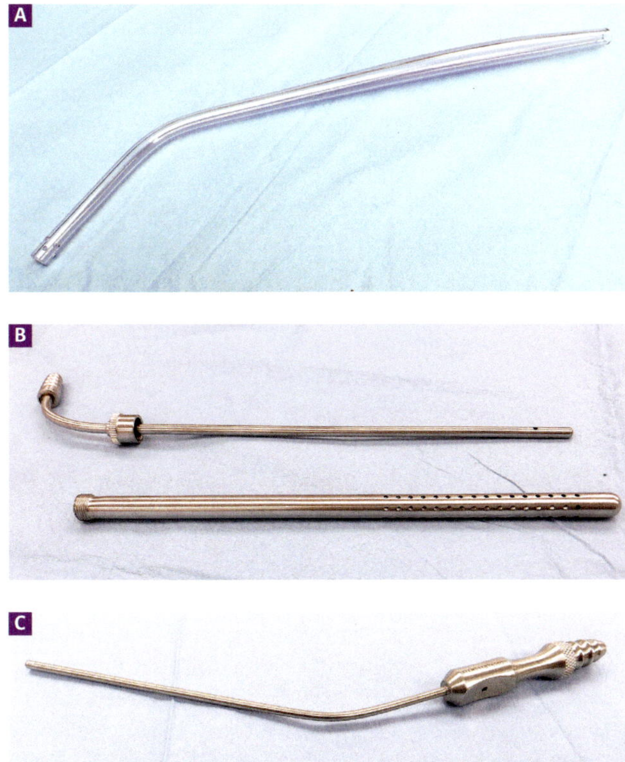

Figure 60. A. Yankauer; **B.** Poole; **C.** Frazier suction tips.

Suction Tips

The **Yankauer tip** is a large bore, blunt ended design with fenestrations on each side at the tip and at the end of the tip, designed for rapid suction of larger fluid volumes. Care is required at higher pressures, to avoid traumatising tissue which contacts the tip.

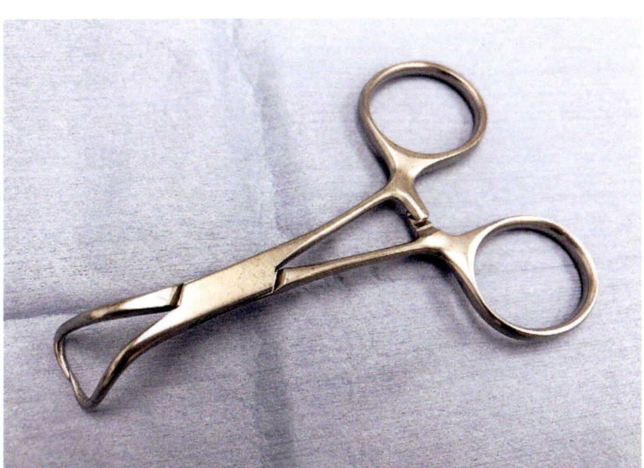

Figure 61. Backhaus towel clamp.

The Poole design has an inner narrow cannula with single aperture at its tip, which may be used independently, or with an outer sheath with many fenestrations along its length. It is designed to prevent obstruction by tissue, (e.g. omentum) when draining the abdominal cavity.

Frasier tips come in different sizes and are a fine cannula with a single aperture at the tip and a bent shaft for focussed suctioning, with a valve at the base of the handle which is occluded by the surgeon when suction is desired. The narrow bore capacity of these tips means they frequently block and often have an accompanying stylet or can be reverse flushed with saline applied with a syringe from the handle towards the tip with the valve covered. (Figure 60).

Miscellaneous Surgical Instruments

Towel Clamps

As the name suggests, these are used to secure drapes to the patient. **Backhaus** are the common ringed design with a ratchet lock (Figure 61). A cross-sprung, **Jones design** is also available. In the era of increasing frequency of minimally invasive surgery and more frequent intraoperative imaging modalities, often it is ideal to avoid the use of towel clamps altogether as they are universally radiopaque and therefore adhesive drapes may be preferred.

Galliban Forceps

These are a little used instrument, which **resemble a bent-tipped haemostat with no ratchet and completely smooth blades at the tip** (Figure 62). They are specifically designed to apply pressure to stabilise the first throw of a suture, maintaining tension whilst the second throw is applied, whilst causing minimal trauma to the suture material. These are commonly used for arytenoid lateralisation procedures in cases of laryngeal paralysis.

Rongeurs

Rongeurs are used to remove bone fragments and cartilage, most commonly in maxillofacial surgery and bulla osteotomy techniques. They are spring loaded instruments, come in an array of sizes and may be single or double action; the latter increasing the mechanical advantage and hence the force applied to the tissue. The standard **Lempert** design has jaws pointing in line with the handles at the tip of the instrument. **Kerrison** rongeurs have a footplate at the end, which is cut down onto by a sliding blade, and removes bone edges at an angle perpendicular to the shaft of the instrument. This design is most useful for spinal surgery but is also useful for bulla osteotomies and rhinotomy procedures. (Figure 63).

Curettes

Curettes are sharp-edged stainless-steel scoops, used to scrape soft tissue from bone. These come in a variety of shapes and handle styles. The **Volkmann spoon** is a double-ended curette with different sizes at either end. The **Spratt curette** has a single scoop with a broader handle allowing more forceful scraping of tissue. Within soft tissue surgery, curettes are most frequently used to assist bulla osteotomy procedures and to curette necrotic tissue from abscesses. (Figure 64).

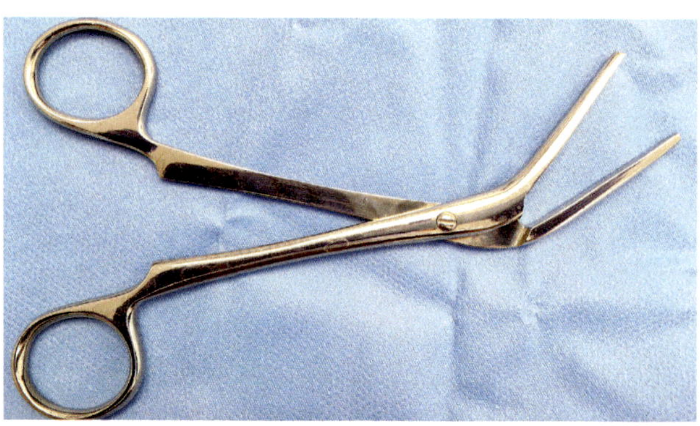

Figure 62. Galliban forceps.

A variety of other orthopaedic instruments including saws, osteotomes, mallets, bone cutters, orthopaedic wire and other powered instruments are sometimes used for soft tissue surgery, but more frequently used for orthopaedics and reviewed in the orthopaedic chapter.

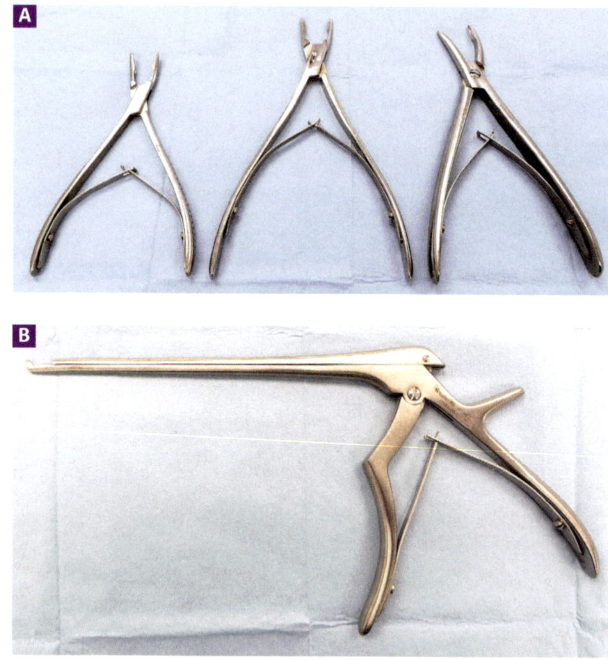

Figure 63. A. Lempert rongeurs; **B.** Kerrison rongeurs.

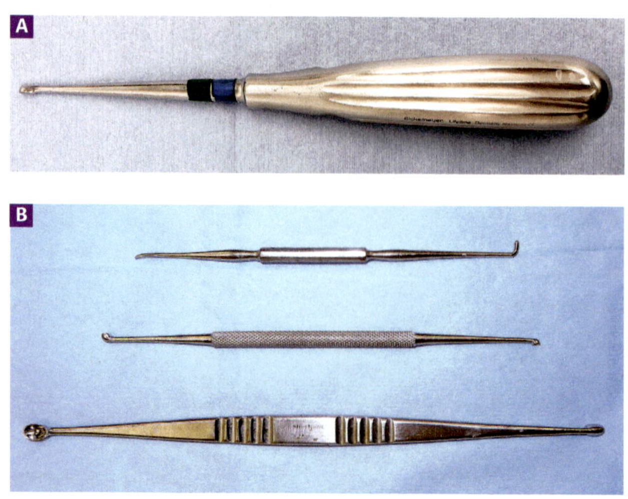

Figure 64. A. Spratt curette; **B.** Varieties of Volkmann spoon curette.

Electrosurgical Devices

- **Monopolar cautery** travels from the tip of the hand-piece through the patient to the earth plate, which must be placed in good contact with the skin over the chest or abdominal wall at the start of the procedure. Failure to have a good contact may result in the current being focussed in a smaller area and lead to an electrical burn. Different forms of monopolar cautery can be used to produce either just coagulation or both cutting and coagulation at the same time. When using monopolar cautery for tissue dissection, suction should also be used to prevent inhalation of the smoke created wherever possible. Diathermic cautery uses radiofrequency to **coagulate vessels of up to 2 mm diameter.** (Figure 65).
- **Bipolar cautery** uses electrified tissue forceps, with the current running between the tips and therefore a grounding plate is not required. Less current is required with bipolar cautery and this is effective in a wet tissue field. More advanced electrosurgical devices are also available for tissue dissection and sealing of large vessels. Bipolar vessel sealing devices such as Ligasure® (Figure 66) are applied to tissue like haemostatic forceps, but the electrical feedback within the generator measures tissue impedance to judge when the tissue is adequately coagulated, and a sound alerts the surgeon to discontinue application. The instrument then allows the tissue to be cut along the sealed area. Bipolar vessel sealing devices may be used to seal some vessels up to 7 mm in diameter.
- **Harmonic ultrasonic dissectors** use high frequency sound waves to coagulate and divide tissue. These produce minimal thermal injury to the surrounding tissue and may seal some vessels up to 5 mm in diameter. (Figure 67).
- **Ultrasonic surgical aspirators** such as CUSA® combine an ultrasonic dissector and suction, to dissect soft parenchymatous tissue whilst maintaining an excellent view for the surgeon and minimising trauma to the surrounding tissue and vascular structures, having advantages for brain and liver dissection. (Figure 68).

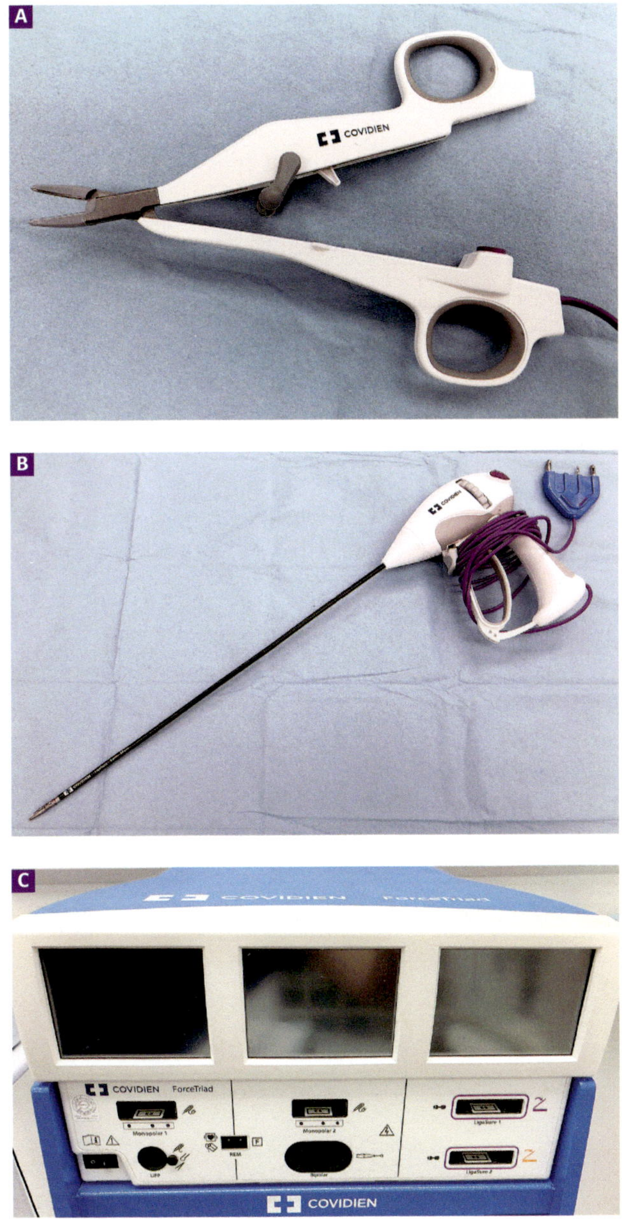

Figure 66. A and **B.** Variations of Ligasure® bipolar vessel sealing device hand-pieces; **C.** Force Triad generator.

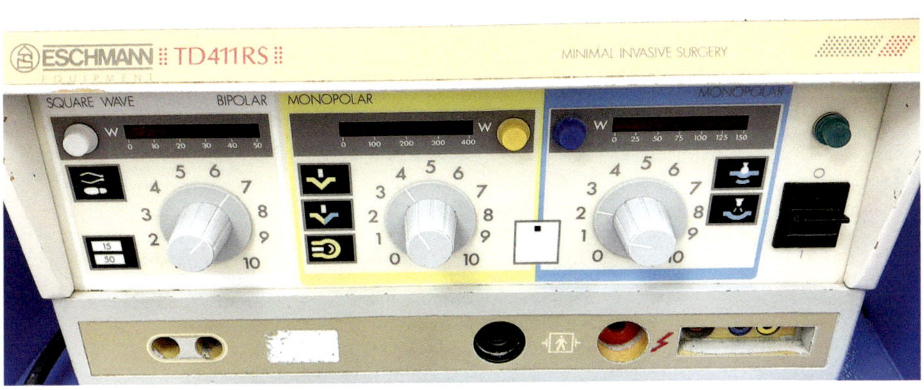

Figure 65. Electrocautery generator.

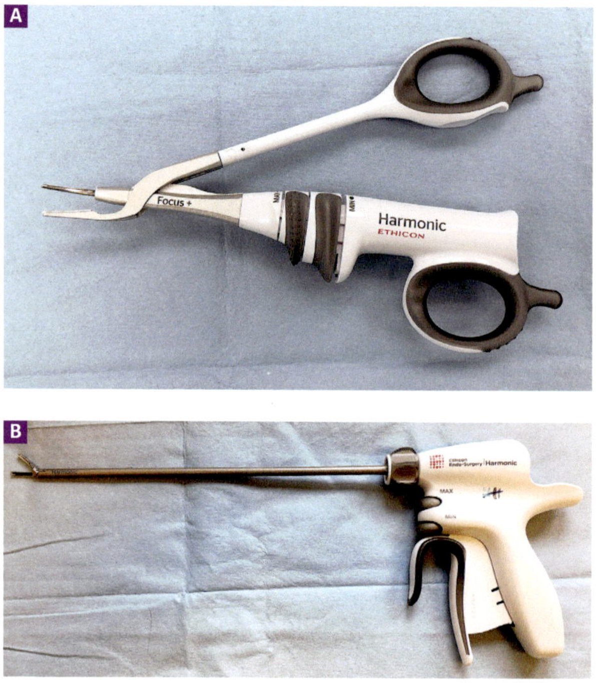

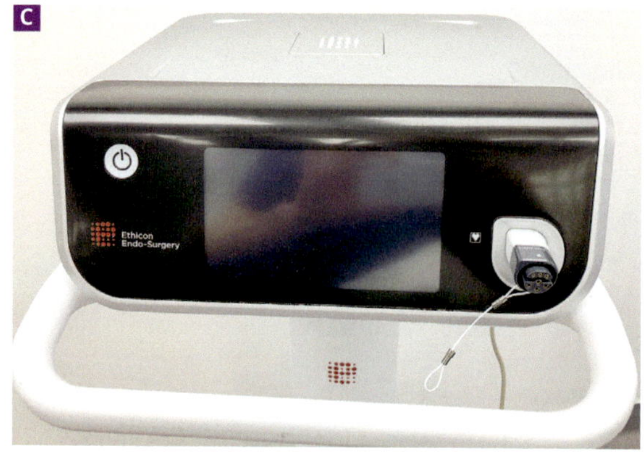

Figure 67. A and **B.** Harmonic ultrasonic dissector; **C.** Ethicon generator.

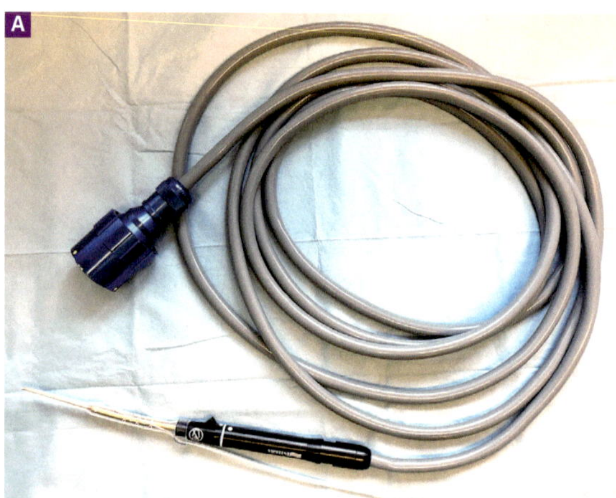

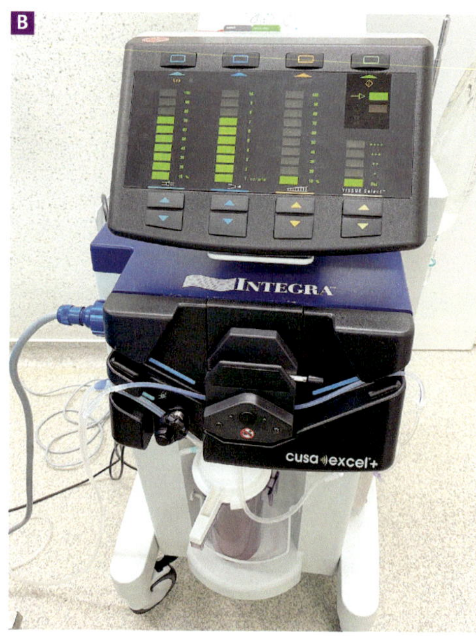

Figure 68. Cavitron Ultrasonic Surgical Aspirator (CUSA®) handpiece (**A**) and control unit (**B**).

Lasers

Surgical lasers vary in wavelength, which affects the depth of tissue penetration and hence the surgical application (Figure 69). Each laser type comes with its own safety protocols, including the use of protective eyewear and safety notices which should be displayed around the room where the laser is used. The most common use of lasers in modern soft tissue surgery is via cystoscopy for management of intramural ectopic ureters in young dogs with urinary incontinence.

Surgical Staplers

There are different surgical stapling devices available, each with different conformations, and varieties of staple number

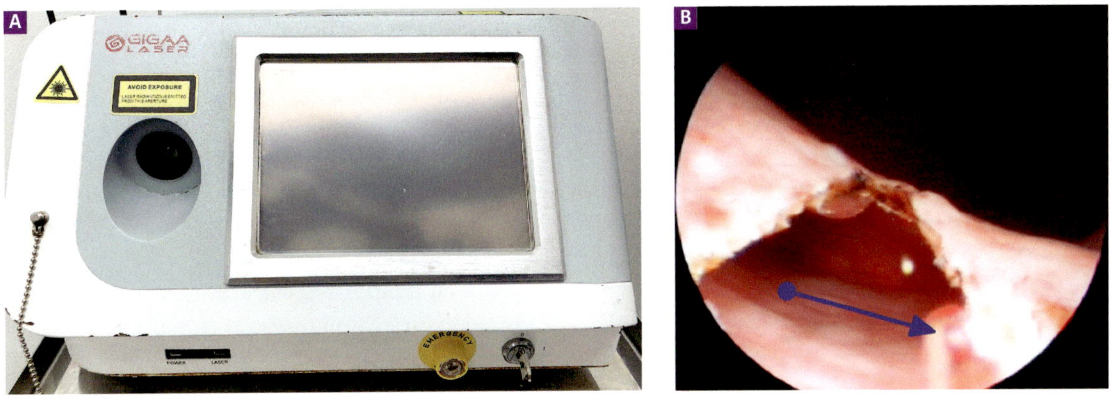

Figure 69. A. Laser generator; **B.** Laser ablation of an ectopic ureter being performed under cystoscopic guidance.

and sizes for specific applications. The most common applications for stapling are lung lobectomy, liver lobectomy, intestinal anastomosis, and closing skin incisions. These were covered in more detail earlier in this chapter alongside suture materials.

Endoscopic Surgical Equipment

Instrumentation and Handling

Minimally invasive surgery is increasing in popularity, largely arising from a demand for smaller scars, reduced hospitalisation times, and quicker return to function as seen with minimally invasive surgery in man. These advantages are not always so clearly apparent as our veterinary patients appear to return to function more rapidly than their human counterparts undergoing similar procedures. That said, there are clear advantages to performing some routine surgeries in a minimally invasive manner such as liver biopsy, gastropexy, and ovariectomy. For the surgeon, some of the advantages are an improved and magnified surgical view.

Endoscopic surgery of the abdominal cavity is referred to as laparoscopy and thoracic cavity as thoracoscopy or video-assisted thoracic surgery (VATS). Some surgical procedures may be performed by placing endoscopes through other orifices, e.g. urethroscopy, cystoscopy, tracheobronchoscopy, gastroscopy. This section focuses on rigid endoscopy, most frequently utilised for laparoscopy and thoracoscopy.

Endoscopic surgery requires several elements of instrumentation:

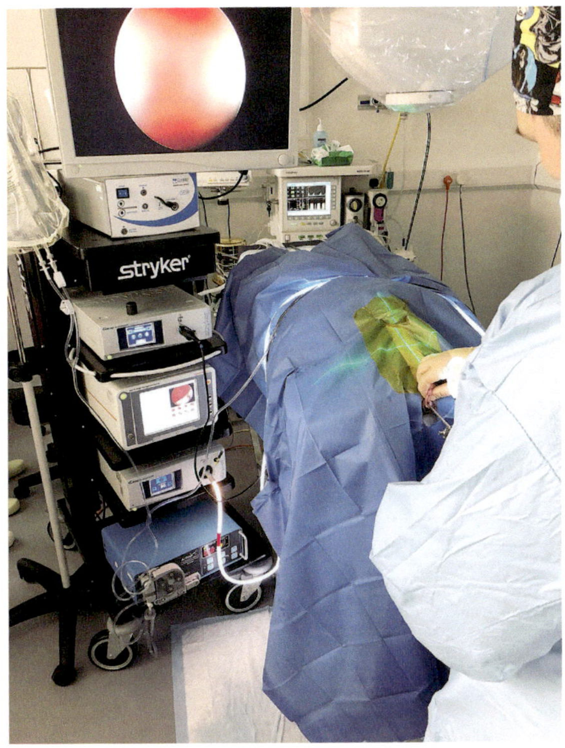

Figure 70. Scope tower.

- rigid endoscope
- light source and light cable
- camera, monitor and image capture device
- cannula(s)
- insufflator and source of carbon dioxide
- endoscopic surgical instruments.

For ease of use the **light source, monitor, insufflator, and image capture** devices are usually combined into a **multi-platform tower** (Figure 70).

Rigid Endoscopes

Rigid endoscopes are a series of delicate glass lenses, arranged and supported within a metal tube, with attachment points for a light source and camera. (Figure 71).

Rigid endoscopes vary in length, diameter, and the angle of their tip, which standardly may be 0° to allow vision straight in line with the endoscope, or 30° to allow a slight angle to the view. This angle of view can be rotated by turning the endoscope, which allows for a greater field of view, and creates some ability to see around corners.

- **5 mm and 10 mm diameter,** 29 cm long endoscopes are commonly used for laparoscopy and thoracoscopy in dogs and cats.
- **Smaller 3 mm,** 14 cm long endoscopy systems are suitable for laparoscopy in smaller patients.
- **2.7 mm endoscopes** are commonly used for urethrocystoscopy.
- **Smaller 2.4 mm and 1.9 mm** endoscopes are used for arthroscopy.

Light Source

Endoscopes are usually used to visualise dark body cavities and additional illumination is essential via an external light source and cable. The light is accompanied by heat and so care should be taken not leave the end of a light cable or connected endoscope in contact with the patient or combustible surgical drapes. When not in use turn the light source should be turned off. Light sources usually use halogen or xenon bulbs. Xenon is preferred as the high intensity light emitted is similar in wavelength and colour to that of natural daylight. Light cables are fibre optic and should be handled with care to prevent damage to the delicate fibres.

Camera

An endoscopic camera attaches to the endoscope, to avoid having to directly peer down through the lens. This usually requires a separate monitor and cable, which allows visualisation of the magnified image on the screen. When positioning the screen, where possible the screen should be aligned with the surgeon and patient, so the surgical field is between the surgeon and the display, to facilitate the surgeon's orientation. An image capture device attached to the camera system is also useful for storage of images and videos.

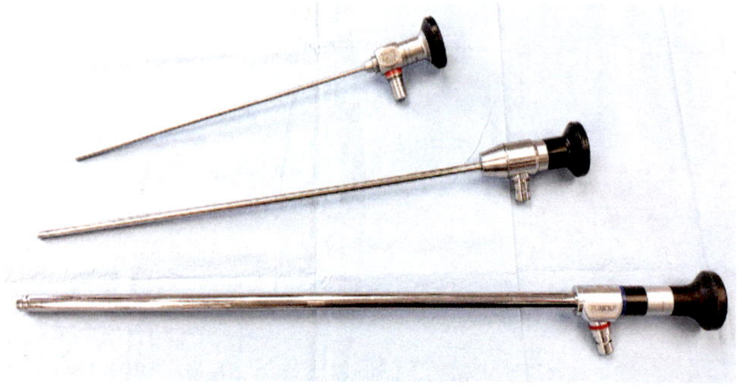

Figure 71. Rigid endoscopes.

Cannulas

Cannulas are portals, via which the endoscope and endosurgical instruments are placed and introduced into the body cavity, maintaining the opening for the interchange of instruments. They come in a variety of sizes, specific to the instruments that pass through them; commonly 12 mm to allow passage of 10 mm diameter instruments and 6 mm to allow use of 5 mm diameter instruments. There are also multiport cannulas which are larger but allow passage of several instruments through a single port, for example the single incision laparoscopic surgery (SILS®) port (Figure 72).

Cannulas usually have blunt trocars to facilitate placement with minimal risk to the underlying body tissues. Those used for thoracic surgery often have an external thread, which allows them to be slowly screwed through the thoracic wall, to a controlled depth of entry into the thoracic cavity (Figure 73). Some cannulas also incorporate a channel for attachment of the insufflation tubing.

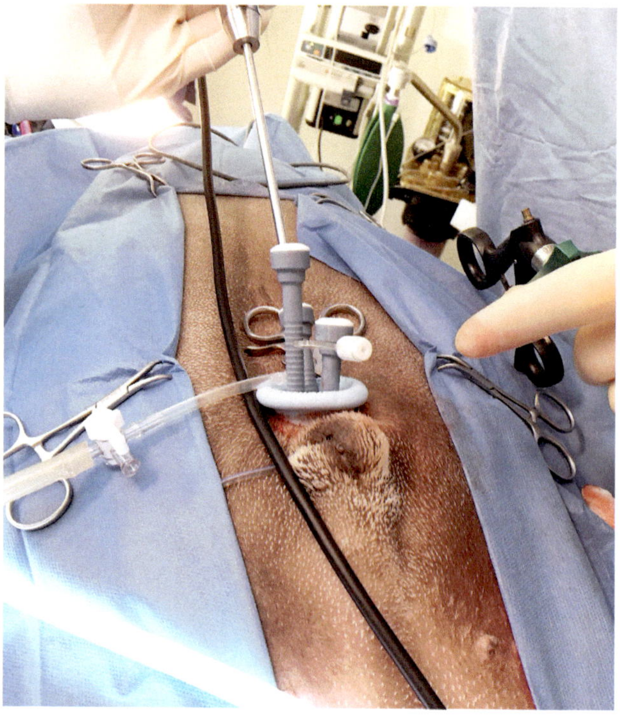

Figure 72. SILS® laparoscopy port.

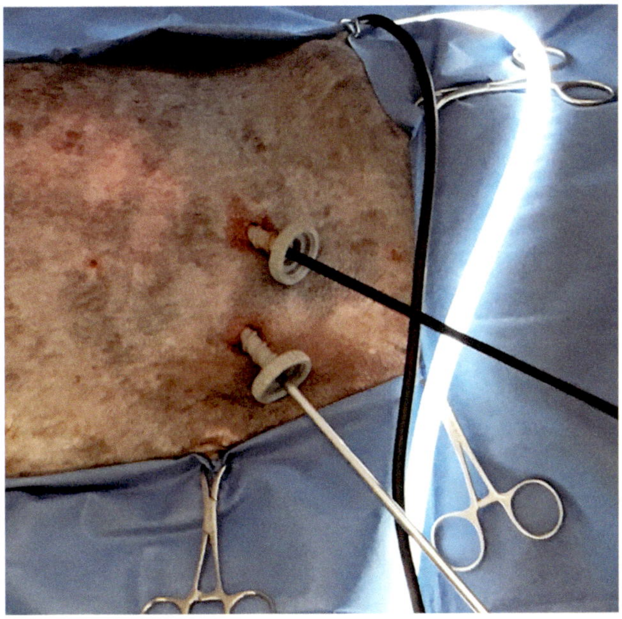

Figure 73. Threaded cannulas.

When performing cystoscopy, the 2.7 mm rigid cystoscope uses its own sheath, with ports to attach fluids for insufflation and an instrument channel through which to pass biopsy forceps, graspers, or a laser. (Figure 74).

Insufflator

The insufflator is a pump, with a source of carbon dioxide, which is used to distend the abdomen or partly suppress lung inflation in the thorax, to create space between the organs, such that the surgeon has room to work and can see the organs. **Carbon dioxide** is used as it is relatively inert inside the body and prevents fire from electrosurgical instruments, which might occur in an oxygen rich environment. The insufflator is usually pressure limited. Typical pressure settings used for laparoscopy in large dogs would be 10 cm H_2O, and 6 cm H_2O for cats and toy breed dogs.

When performing cystoscopy or endoscopy of some other bodily spaces (e.g. tracts in the neck created by stick injuries), then saline and an infusion pump or pressurised fluid bag and giving set are used to distend the tissue in a similar way.

Endoscopic Surgical Instruments

There are a variety of fine, extra-long surgical instruments designed for endoscopic use, which are based on common surgical instruments used for open surgery. These include **Metzenbaum scissors, Babcock tissue forceps, needle holders** (typically two pairs are needed to allow the needle to be passed from one hand to the other), **haemostatic forceps** including right-angled forceps and tissue graspers (which mimic the function of thumb forceps). There are also novel surgical instruments which are designed specifically for endoscopic use.

A

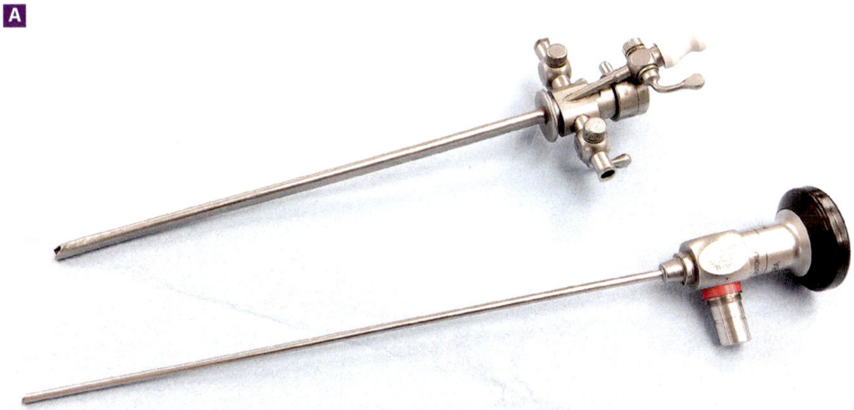

B

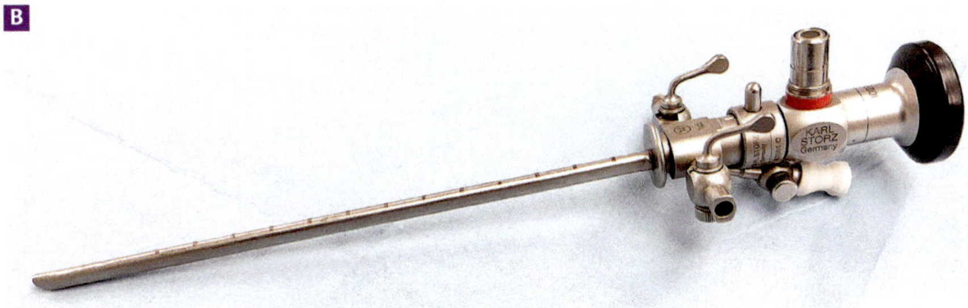

Figure 74. A. Cystoscope with sheath;
B. Cystoscope assembled.

These include:

- **Fan retractor:** has an array of flat, relatively atraumatic paddles, which fan out on activation of the hand-piece to create a larger surface. May be used to gently hold tissue back to improve a surgeon's view.
- **Articulated forceps:** which allow the tips to be angled once introduced through the trocar, to allow dissection in a different plane to the direction of the introduced instrument.
- **Specimen retrieval bags:** once tissue sample is freed within a body cavity, the next challenge is to retrieve it in one piece through a portal. Specimen retrieval bags facilitate this, containing the tissue, preventing leakage, or contamination with cancerous cells as the sample is manipulated through the port and out of the body cavity.

Many electrosurgical tools, such as monopolar cauterising probes, bipolar vessel sealing devices, and harmonic scalpels also have handpieces designed specifically for endoscopic use, such as the articulating EndoGIA® staplers in a range of sizes. (See Figure 35).

Other innovations useful for endoscopy are **pretied suture loops and barbed knotless sutures,** as intracorporeal (inside the body) knot tying is challenging. These are also useful during open surgery for stress free ligation of large vascular pedicles, e.g. for partial or complete liver lobectomy or lung lobectomy.

Endoscope Maintenance and Storage

Rigid endoscopes are delicate instruments which require handling, cleaning, and storing with the utmost care to avoid bending, dropping, or scratching the lenses. **The endoscope should be dismantled straight after use** to allow thorough cleaning, to prevent residues drying on and facilitate atraumatic cleaning. Endoscopes are usually hand-washed, with the light cables and cameras wiped with a soft cloth soaked in enzymatic cleaning solution, although metallic accessories and attachments may undergo ultrasonic cleaning as per other instruments. A soft brush may be used to clean the lens, to avoid scratching. **Leaving endoscopes in contact with cleaning solutions for longer than recommended should be avoided** and they should be rinsed with demineralised water where practical.

Endoscopes may be autoclaved carefully in purpose designed cases, sterilised in ethylene oxide, or cleaned in high-level disinfectant immediately prior to use. Camera and light cables may be sterilised in ethylene oxide or cleaned in high-level disinfectants prior to use.

Rigid endoscopes should be stored in purpose made boxes, cushioned in rubberised plastic or foam. (Figure 75).

During the preparation for surgery, the components of the endoscopy system should be carefully opened and **those being prepared rinsed in high-level disinfectant with sterile saline** and then dried carefully before use. The light post and camera should be fitted securely to the endoscope. Then, prior to the start of surgery, **white balancing** should be performed to adjust the colour appropriately. When in use **the camera should always be supported in an upright position** to ensure the surgeon does not become disorientated. It is essential not to bend the endoscope by forcing it in one direction or another. If it starts to bend, a grey crescent is often observed at the edge of the field of view and the pressure should be released. With a 30° angled telescope, the field of view is directed opposite to the attachment point of the light post, and so to alter the viewing angle, the camera is kept still, and the light post is rotated around the long axis of the telescope. (Figure 76).

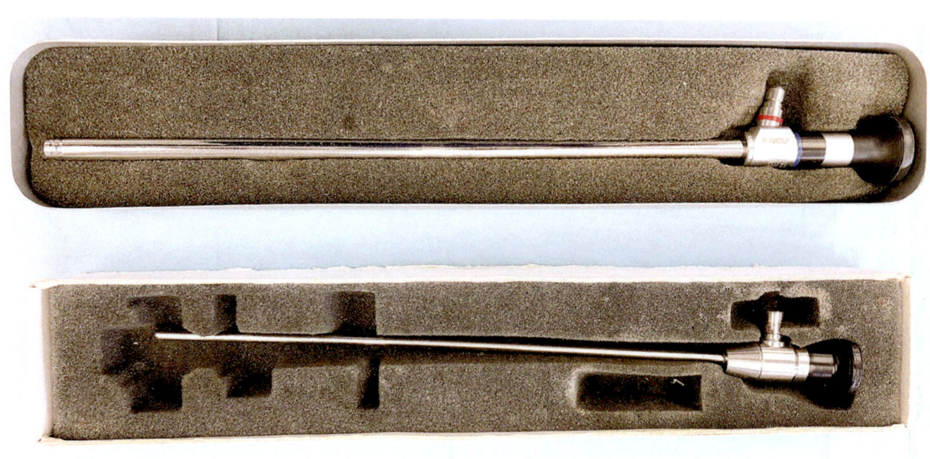

Figure 75. Endoscope storage.

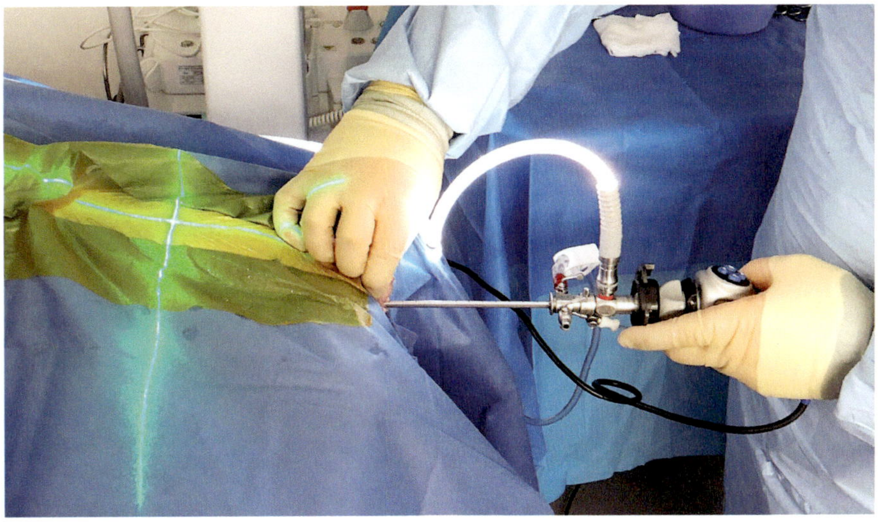

Figure 76. Endoscope assembly and handling.

Anatomy of the Skin

Functions of the Skin

The skin is a large, multifunctional organ, comprising on average 24% of the mass of a puppy, and 12% of the mass of an adult dog. However, there is significant breed variation, for example in the quantity and functionality of the skin of a Greyhound compared to that of Shar Pei. Puppies grow into their skin and so skin elasticity and mobility both reduce with age.

Functions of the skin:
- sensation allowing interaction with the environment and assessment of heat/cold, touch
- production of vitamin D through exposure to light
- thermoregulation and insulation
- storage of water, fat, carbohydrate, and protein
- defensive barrier to chemicals, desiccation, UV radiation.

Skin Structure

The skin (Figure 77) comprises **three basic layers:**
- epidermis
- dermis
- hypodermis or subcutis.

The thickness and structure of the layers varies widely with species, breed, and body location, with certain areas specifically adapted for different functions.

Where **skin is most mobile,** it has more elastic properties and less tough, fibrous tissue and more subcutaneous tissue, e.g. around the neck of most dogs and cats. Where the skin is less mobile, it has a greater fibrous component, with less elastic tissue and less underlying subcutaneous tissue, e.g. over the inside of the pinnae.

The **epidermis is thickest** where there is an absence of hair, as this provides an alternative protective barrier.

The dermis contains hair follicles and adnexal structures, including pressure and temperature sensory organelles and is thickest where the coat is thickest, e.g. along the dorsum and thinnest in non-haired areas such as the axilla and groin. The density of pressure sensory organelles is greater in the digits and face than on the trunk of the body.

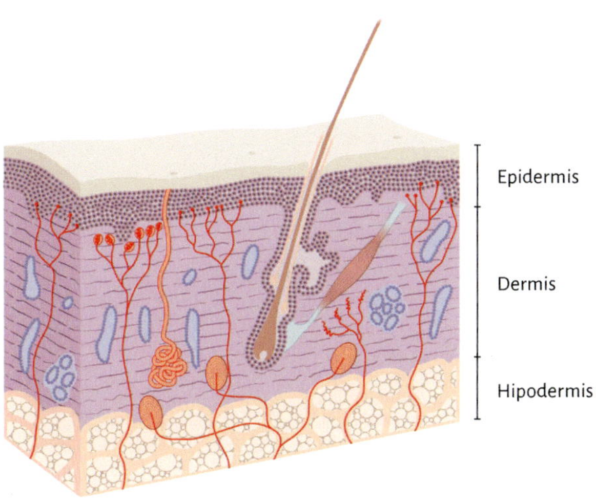

Figure 77. Skin anatomy.

The subcutis is a loose network of elastin, collagen and fat. There are two layers, the stratum adiposum, which consists mostly of fat, and the stratum fibrosum, which is more fibrous and contains the panniculus muscle which has a function in skin movement, but also an important role in reconstructive surgery.

The vascular supply to the skin (Figure 78) has two main components:

- **Musculocutaneous arteries,** which supply muscles and the area of skin overlying that muscle. This is the most common form in humans.
- **Direct cutaneous arteries,** which run straight to the superficial, panniculus muscle layer, the stratum fibrosum in the subcutis and then run parallel to the skin and fan out to supply nutrients over a wider area. As such, one direct cutaneous artery supplies a large area of skin via a subcutaneous plexus of branching and interconnecting vessels. This type of blood supply predominates in the dog and cat.

The elasticity, abundance, type of blood supply, and mobility of canine and feline skin make reconstructive surgery in small animal species very different from in other species, i.e. humans and horses. Skin flaps are only feasible due to the direct cutaneous arterial vascular supply to the skin in dogs and cats and the elasticity of the skin in our small animal veterinary patients.

Skin Tension Lines (Figure 79)

The tension in the skin has a directional bias which influences how surgery can be performed. The picture depicts the lines of skin tension in dogs and cats. A general rule is to **make an incision parallel with these tension lines to minimise tension**

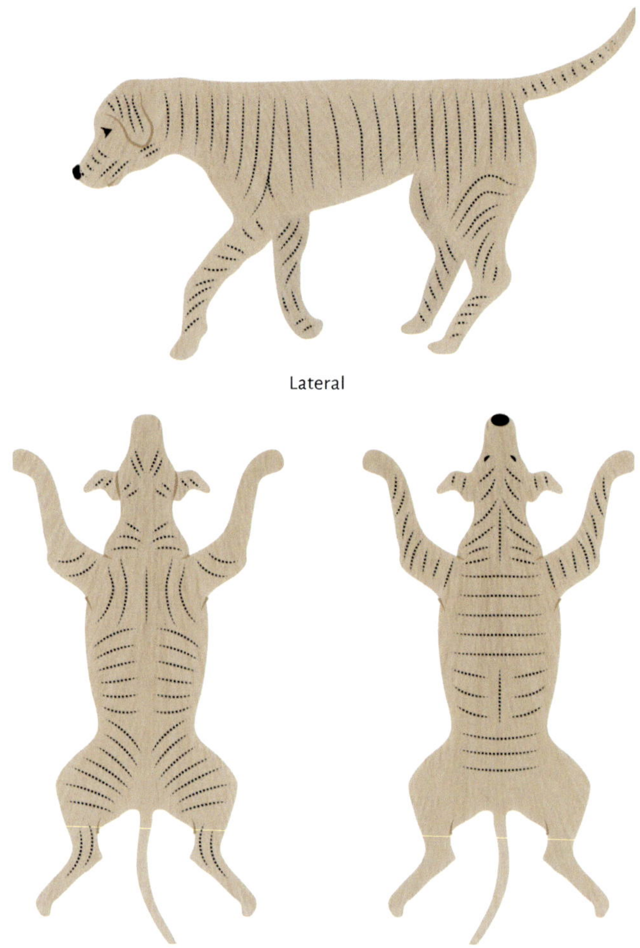

Figure 79. Skin tension lines.

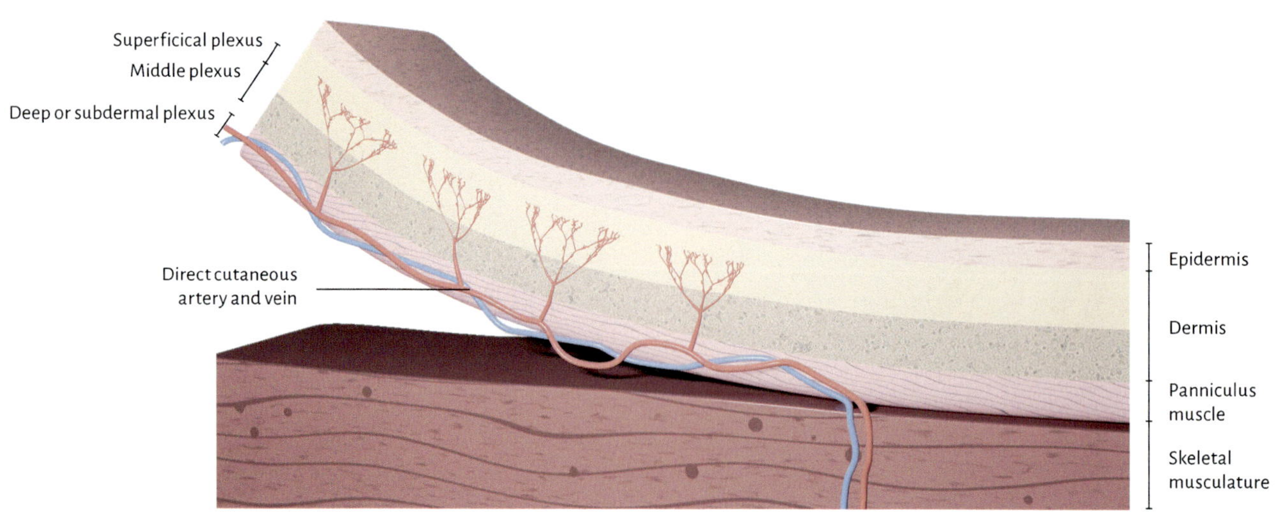

Figure 78. Skin vascular supply.

on the closure of the incision (remember Halsted's principles). In practice when removing an area of skin, and closing a wound, the surgeon should inspect the site and attempt to mobilise the skin with the patient asleep prior to surgery to finalise a surgical plan, so tension is minimised and hence the likelihood of uneventful wound healing is increased.

Wound Healing

Understanding how wounds naturally heal is essential for the management of open wounds. Wound management aims to promote tissue healing as efficiently as possible and negate factors which might compromise normal healing, hence directing and assisting the natural healing process. This applies both to surgical incisions and to traumatic open wounds, however the timelines for the healing processes vary depending on the location, depth, width, and nature of the wound. A specific discussion of wound types, open wound management, and dressings follows in Chapter 8.

Phases in wound healing (Figures 80 and 81):

- the **inflammatory phase:** occurs immediately and for up to a week postinjury
- the **proliferative phase:** begins around day 3 following injury
- the **remodelling phase:** begins around days 5–7 following injury.

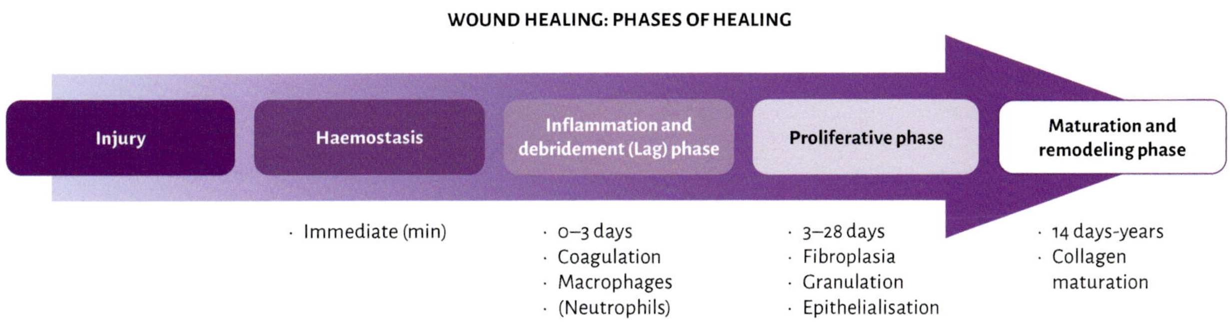

Figure 80. Phases of wound healing.

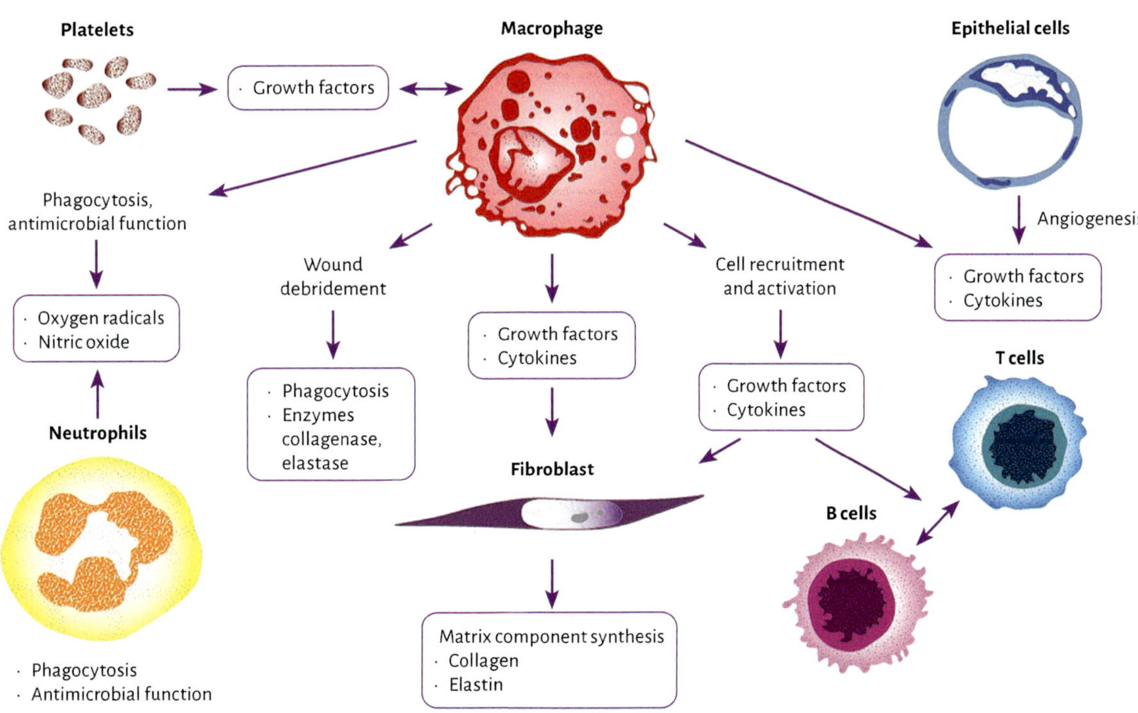

Figure 81. Wound healing.

The durations of each phase vary with the nature of the wound and the healing environment; these phases overlap and occur simultaneously in different regions within the same wound.

The inflammatory phase has early and late stages.

Early Inflammatory Phase

The first essential step in wound healing is haemostasis. In brief, platelet adherence within the wound culminates in coagulation, release of inflammatory mediators, and the activation of complement. Neutrophils are the first inflammatory cells present in the wound and initially begin to debride the wound and neutralise bacteria.

Late Inflammatory Phase

Under the influence of inflammatory mediators further neutrophils and importantly macrophages are recruited to the wound site by a process known as chemotaxis (chemical signalling). **Macrophages are the key cell for wound healing in the inflammatory phase and healing cannot progress without them.**

The role of macrophage includes:

- **Debridement:** macrophages debride and ingest foreign material, bacteria, injured host cells, and platelet clots.
- **Fibroblast proliferation and fibrosis:** activated macrophages release growth factors which stimulate fibroblasts to form and build a collagen scaffold within the wound. This scaffold allows the ingrowth of other tissues such as blood vessels as well as allowing contraction of the scar later in the remodelling phase.
- **Angiogenesis:** also stimulated by growth factors from activated macrophages, new capillaries grow into the wound along the collagen scaffold.
- **Stimulation of epithelialisation:** growth factors encourage epithelial cells at the margins of the wound to replicate and migrate under the clot, over the collagen scaffold and towards the centre of the wound, lifting the clot away as a scab.

The proliferative phase is marked by the development of granulation tissue under the influence and direction of macrophages. **Granulation tissue is a network of collagen which is produced and remodelled by fibroblasts and the new capillaries which grow into the collagen scaffold** (Figure 82). This process is reliant on a well oxygenated environment and good nutrition. Granulation tissue has a rich pink/red colour and is delicate to the touch due to the vascular proliferation. Granulation tissue formation occurs more rapidly in dogs than in cats. **Once a wound is sealed with a bed of granulation tissue, it has its own natural resistance** to infection due to the excellent vascular supply and the presence of inflammatory cells. **Hence antibiotics are not usually needed when a wound is covered by a granulation bed.** Even though the surface is commonly contaminated by bacteria, these are unable to colonise and cause infection.

Over the granulation bed, epithelial cells continue to proliferate, covering the wound from the edges inwards with new epithelium, at a maximal rate of around 1 mm per day given an ideal, moist wound healing environment. Wound contraction also begins by reorganisation of the initial haphazard collagen scaffold which is dismantled and shortened pulling the wound edges closer together. (Figure 83).

The remodelling phase sees a continuation of collagen scaffold reorganisation, with randomly produced type III collagen progressively replaced by more orderly and mechanically stronger type II and then type I collagen to restore the structure of normal skin. The direction of orientation of these collagen fibres becomes organised along lines of tension. As with most damaged tissue the healed skin never returns completely to full preinjury strength and extensive scars continue to remodel, contract, and strengthen for years after injury. But they remain weaker than the surrounding tissue, **reaching only 80% of preinjury strength in the long term.** Scarred skin tissue also lacks the adnexal structures (sensory organs and hair follicles).

Surgical Incision Strength and Suture Removal

With regards to wound strength, initially a perfectly apposed, sutured surgical incision relies on the sutures, fibrin clot (which seals the wound in 6–10 hours), and epithelial cells, (which seal the wound within the first 24–48 hours).

Thereafter granulation tissue within the incision adds some minor additional strength.

For dogs, in the absence of infection or poor wound healing for other reasons, **suture removal should be possible around 7–10 days following incision** when collagen is forming across and bridging the incision, although wound strength will

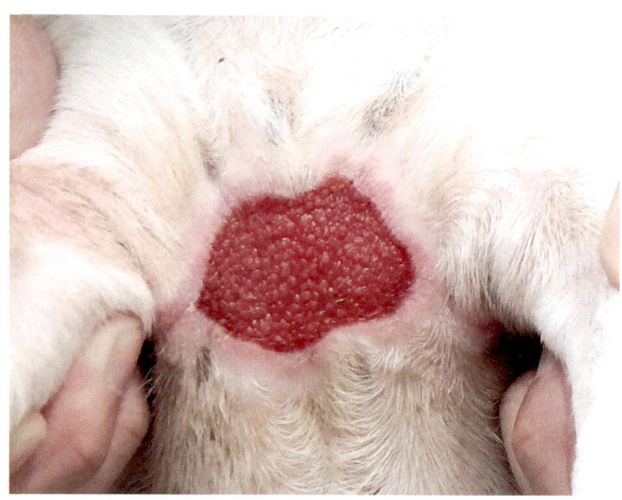

Figure 82. Granulation tissue.

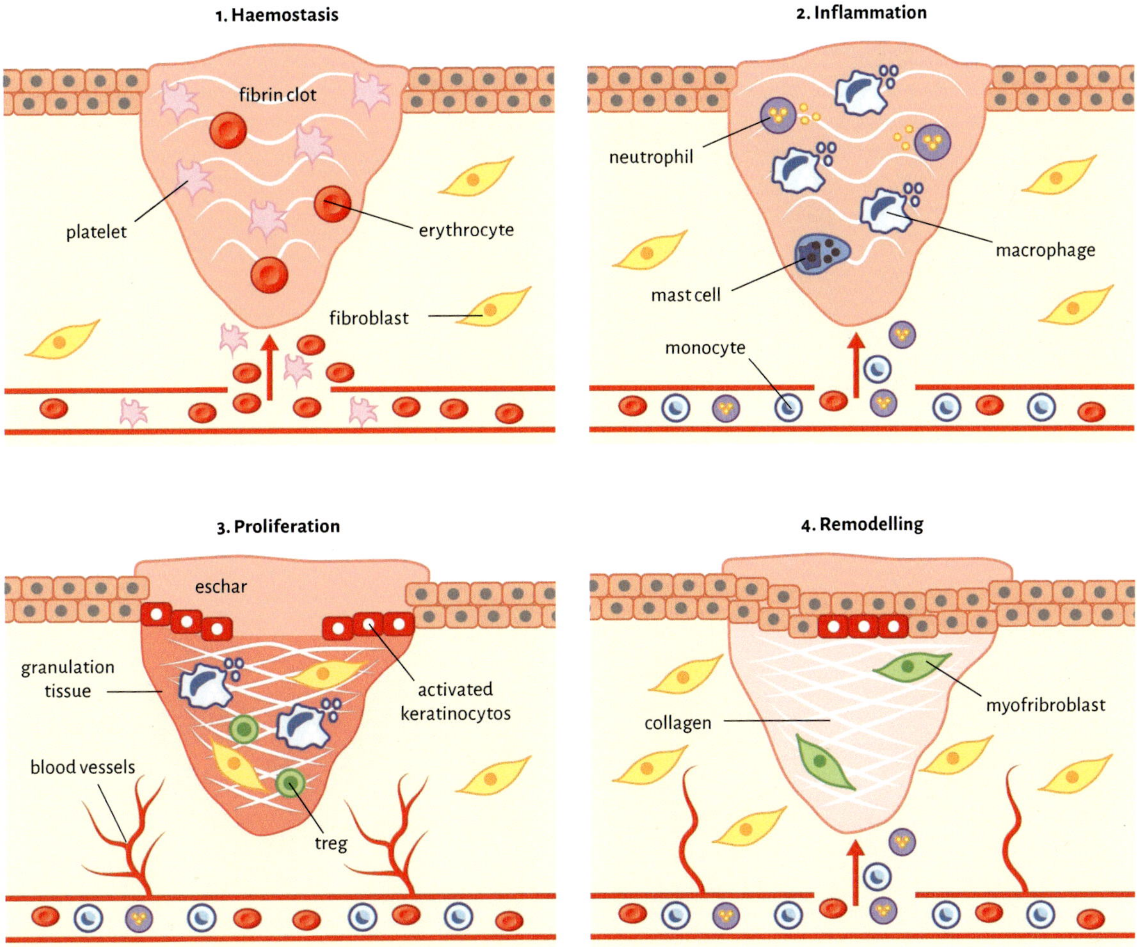

Figure 83. Phases of wound healing.

be only 50% of preincision levels at this time. **For cats, sutures should be left for 14 days** due to slower wound healing. In dogs with delayed wound healing e.g. due to steroid treatment, endocrinopathy, or other chronic disease states, sutures should also be left in place longer.

Wound Closure

Appositional Closure

Appositional closure is the term used to refer to direct closure of the edges of a wound (whenever this takes place with regards to the creation of the wound). With direct apposition, the edges are drawn together like curtains. To achieve this and respect Halsted's principles, tension must be minimised. Whilst this might not be a concern with a linear incision made to access deeper tissues, e.g. for abdominal surgery, when removing skin tumours or areas of wounded skin and closing a defect, to achieve appositional closure where the skin does not easily close, additional measures may be taken to advance the skin edges to allow appositional closure:

- **Undermining:** blunt dissection under the hypodermis layer and the dermal plexus of interconnecting blood vessels supplying the skin helps to release the skin from the underlying tissue, and the wound edges are then advanced towards each other with reduced tension using the skin's natural elasticity. The amount to which the skin can be advanced to close a wound depends on direction of tension lines and bodily location and can be assessed preoperatively.
- **Walking sutures:** these are sutures used to close dead space but also following undermining, to advance the skin and tether it to the underlying tissue away from the cut edge, but closer than its origin, which helps relieve tension on the incision edges. (Figure 84).
- **Relaxing incisions:** are incisions made away from the primary incision, which release the skin and increase the length of the skin (in combination with undermining).

This additional skin stretch allows closure of the primary incision, whilst leaving a defect elsewhere. This secondary incision is chosen to be somewhat more amenable to management as an open wound or allow preferential closure over a joint or a surgical implant, which might not otherwise be possible. Often the surgeon might use a **number of small releasing incisions** (Figure 85) rather than one large incision as this may speed the process of healing as each smaller wound heals quicker than one bigger wound. Relaxing incisions are made in parallel with the main wound closure.

– **Plasties:** where there is adjacent free skin running parallel to an incision but the tension is perpendicular to the incision, then an alternative to releasing incisions (which leave an open wound) are local plastic surgical procedures. These change the direction of tension to help the surgeon close a wound. Examples are the V-to-Y-plasty, and Z-plasty (Figure 86). When considering these procedures, it is helpful to plan ahead and draw the incisions on the skin with a sterile surgical marker pen prior to surgery.

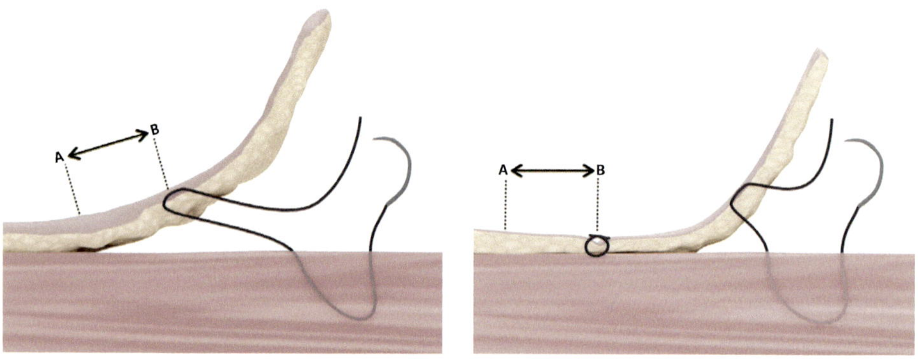

Figure 84. Walking sutures.

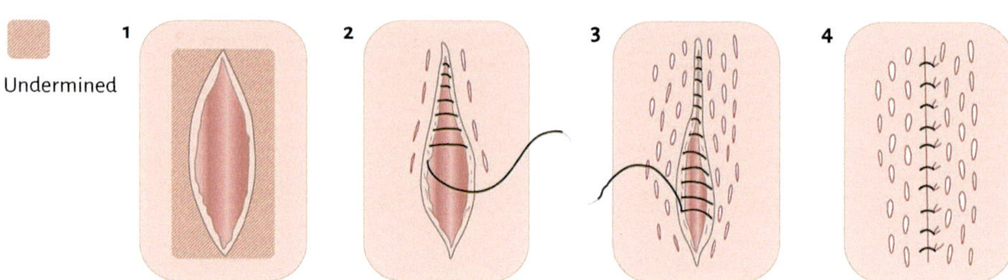

Figure 85. Releasing incisions.

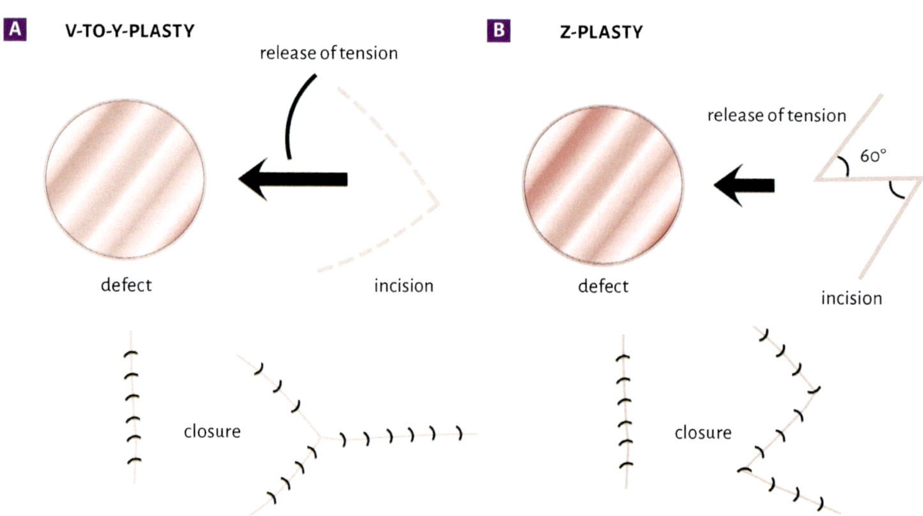

Figure 86. A. V-to-Y-plasty; **B.** Z-plasty.

Skin Flaps

Where regular techniques to mobilise the skin edges are insufficient to close a wound, it may be possible to **utilise nearby areas of loose skin by means of a local skin flap.** These rely on maintaining the **subdermal plexus of blood vessels** and gentle handling to allow tissue transfer without compromising the blood supply. There are two major classifications of local skin flaps:

- random flaps
- axial pattern flaps.

Random Flaps (or subdermal plexus flaps)

These are skin flaps that **rely on maintaining sufficient local blood flow** via the subdermal plexus from at least one end of the skin flap. They may be performed anywhere on the body with sufficient local free skin. They mobilise skin and move it to the area of requirement by means of either:

- **Advancement flap** (Figure 87): parallel skin incisions are made away from the main incision until sufficient skin is freed as a long rectangle to slide forwards and achieve closure with minimal tension.
- **Rotational flap** (Figure 88): where free skin is rotated from the adjacent tissue on a curve to fill a defect.
- **Transposition flap** (Figure 89): a flap is lifted from tissue in a line connecting with one end of the original incision and again rotated into position but extending beyond the margins of that original incision.
- **Interpolation flap** (Figure 90): a flap is lifted from tissue in a line not connecting with one end of the original incision and again rotated into position, with a bridging incision to allow the skin to be brought into the original incision.

ADVANCEMENT FLAP

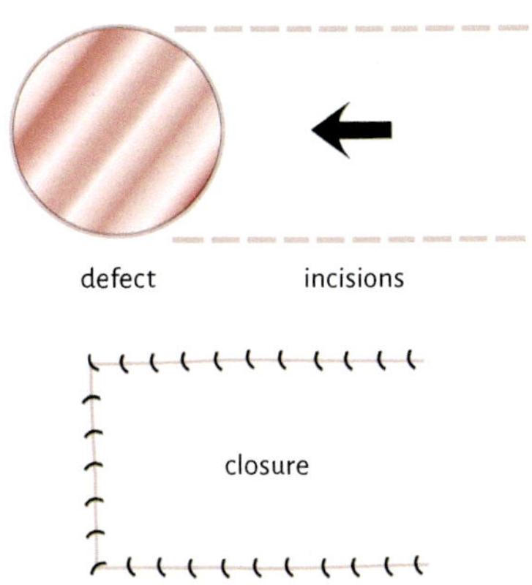

Figure 87. Advancement flap.

ROTATIONAL FLAP

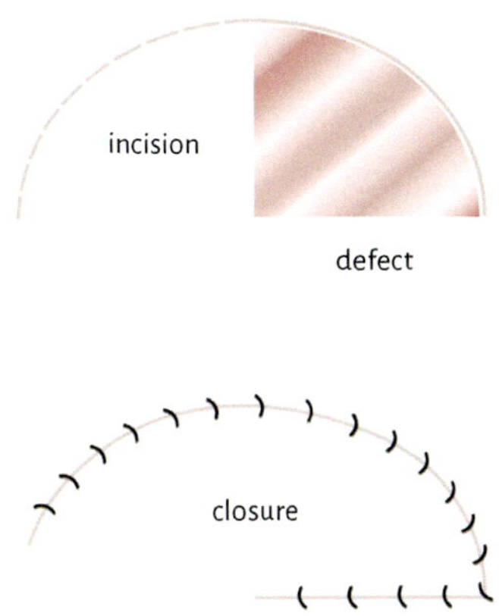

Figure 88. Rotational flap.

TRANSPOSITION FLAP

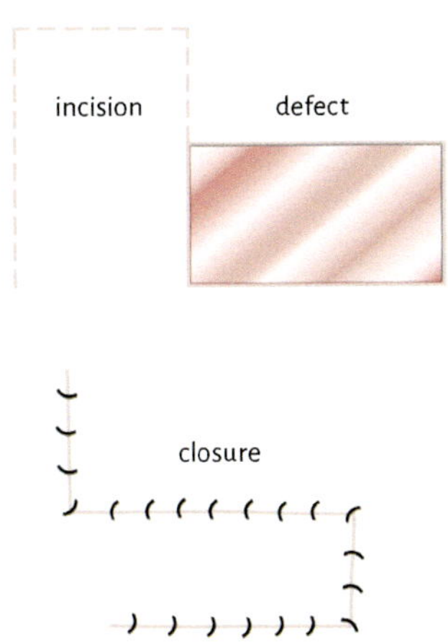

Figure 89. Transposition flap.

INTERPOLATION FLAP

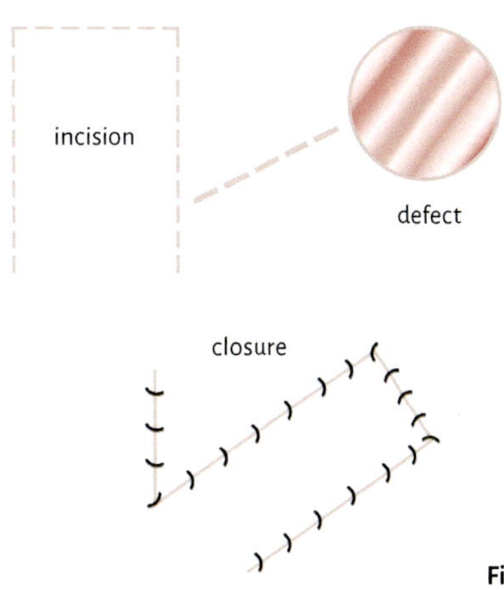

Figure 90. Interpolation flap.

Based on these principles, in addition to the use of random flaps, the same rationale can be used to mobilise the free baggy skin folds often present in the axilla and inguinal region as rotational flaps to mobilise skin to any of the adjoining regions over the trunk or proximal limbs. (Figure 91).

Axial Pattern Flaps

These flaps are specifically planned to maintain a main trunk direct cutaneous artery within the flap to maximise the blood supply and hence survival potential of the flap.

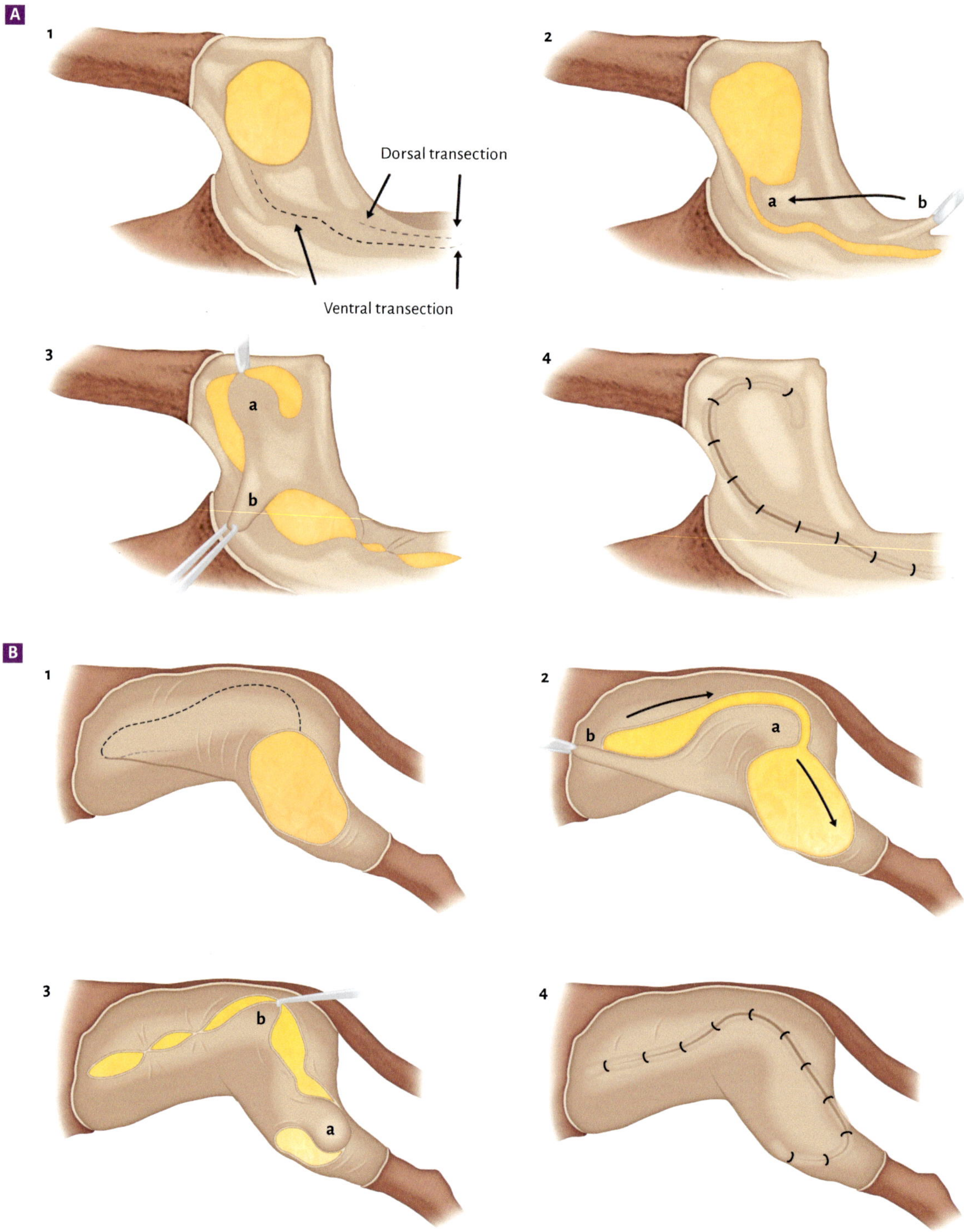

Figure 91. Skin fold flap (Hunt et al., 2001). **A.** Rotational flap from the axilla to the proximal limb; **B.** Rotational flap from the inguinal region to the hind limb.

Hence there are several specific, named vessels on which these flaps are based. Below are a few of the most used examples:

- **Caudal superficial epigastric:** utilises the main artery which feeds the caudal part of the mammary chain, based on its exit through the inguinal canal, and rotated to cover deficits of skin in the perineum and around the thigh and caudal body wall.
- **Thoracodorsal:** utilises the thoracodorsal artery which supplies the skin below the scapula spine over the side of the chest, based on the start of the vessel in the caudal axillary region, and used to cover defects in the axilla and proximal forelimb. (Figure 92).

There are numerous examples, which are used less frequently, but have specific uses for reconstruction of wounds in otherwise hard to close locations.

By their nature, skin flaps often entail quite large dissections and so require advanced planning to allow adequate skin clipping and aseptic preparation, appropriate positioning (as the skin may be moved from an area less accessible than the main incision), adequate analgesia, and placement of a closed suction drain to manage the dead space created.

Free Skin Grafts

When wound closure fails by the use of local tissue or the skin cannot be mobilised sufficiently, most commonly affecting deficits distal to the elbow and stifle, then free skin grafting should be considered. As the name suggests, skin is harvested from an area where it is plentiful, (often the side of the thorax or abdominal wall), separated completely from its blood supply and transferred to fill a defect. **The skin is then reliant on reestablishing new blood supply from the wound bed.**

Skin may be transferred as:

- **unmeshed sheets:** sheets of skin without openings
- **meshed sheets (pie crust):** sheets of skin with openings to allow greater wound coverage and drainage. These often conform well to the shape of the recipient wound bed
- **pinch or punch grafts:** small islands of skin, which are often harvested with a skin punch biopsy
- **strip grafts:** narrow strips of skin.

The transferred skin must be prepared by removal of the subcutaneous tissue as this is a barrier to nutrition and vascular ingrowth, and hence graft survival. (Figure 93).

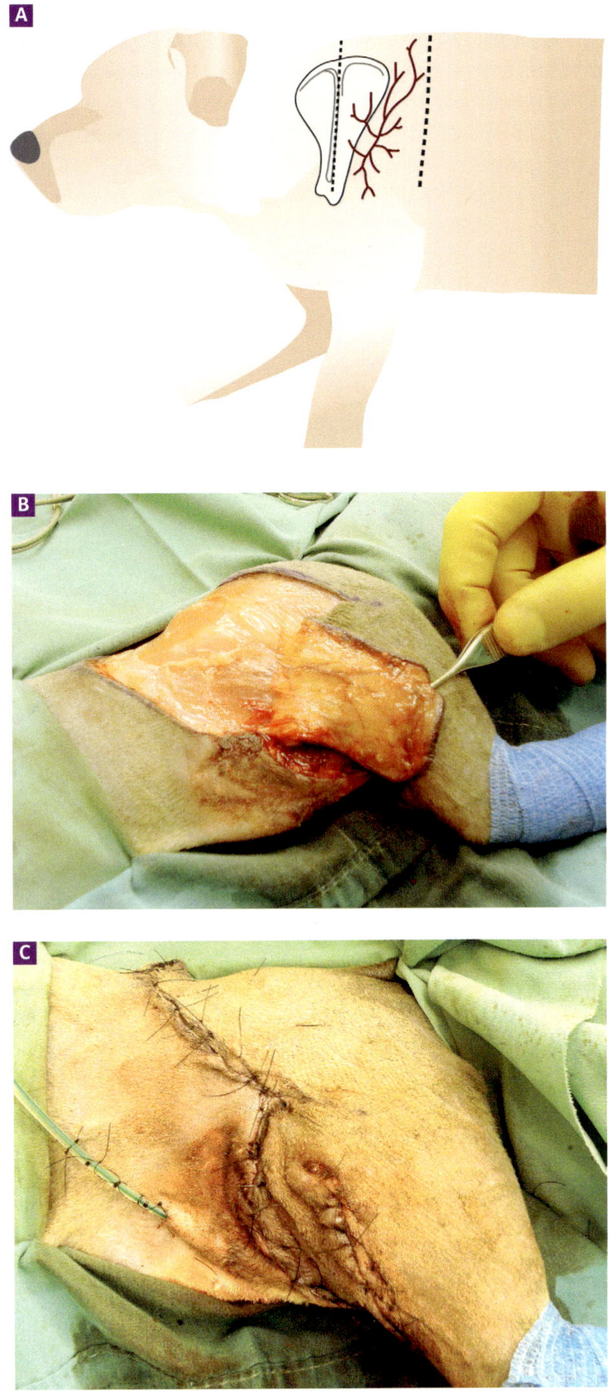

Figure 92. Thoracodorsal axial pattern flap. **A.** Anatomy of the thoracodorsal artery running up the caudal edge of the scapula. **B.** The vessel during flap creation in a cat. **C.** Flap used to close a wound in the axilla, caused by the cat trapping his leg through a collar.

Free skin grafting relies on the grafted skin acquiring nutrients from the wound bed and being revascularized. For this to happen **the graft must be immobilised** in contact with a well vascularised, aseptic, fresh surgical wound bed or a healthy bed of fresh granulation tissue. Graft take (Figure 94) is a complex process with a few key stages which should be considered when placing and then managing the graft postoperatively:

- **Adherence:** over the first 24 hours following graft placement, fibrin exuded from the wound surface acts as a sealant to loosely stick the graft to the wound bed. This adherence is initially weak and easily disrupted and so the recipient site must be immobilised and protected.
- **Plasmatic imbibition:** for the first 2–3 days following graft placement, the transferred skin is reliant on absorption of protein, blood, and fluid from the recipient bed. This causes some swelling and discolouration of the graft at this stage.
- **Inosculation:** by days 2–3 after graft placement, as long as movement between the graft and recipient bed has been prevented then capillary buds from the bed start to connect to the old vessels within the graft and re-establish a rudimentary form of circulation to nourish the graft.
- **Revascularisation:** finally, 1–2 weeks following graft placement new vessels grow into the graft and establish a more organised and complete circulatory pattern which allows the graft tissue to continue to heal and function as normal.

Graft take is reliant on several factors:

- **Graft contact and adequate drainage:** hence grafts are often meshed to allow drainage and held in place with non-adherent dressings. These dressings may be left in place for 3–4 days at a time to minimise interference with the graft. Dressings are changed under heavy sedation/anaesthesia to prevent removal or movement of the graft with the dressing, which should be moistened to facilitate removal.
- **Immobilisation:** when grafts are placed close to joints, they are often placed in combination with external skeletal fixators to prevent movement of the recipient bed and displacement of the graft.
- **Absence of infection:** cultures are usually taken prior to skin grafting and often grafts are treated topically with antibacterial agents.

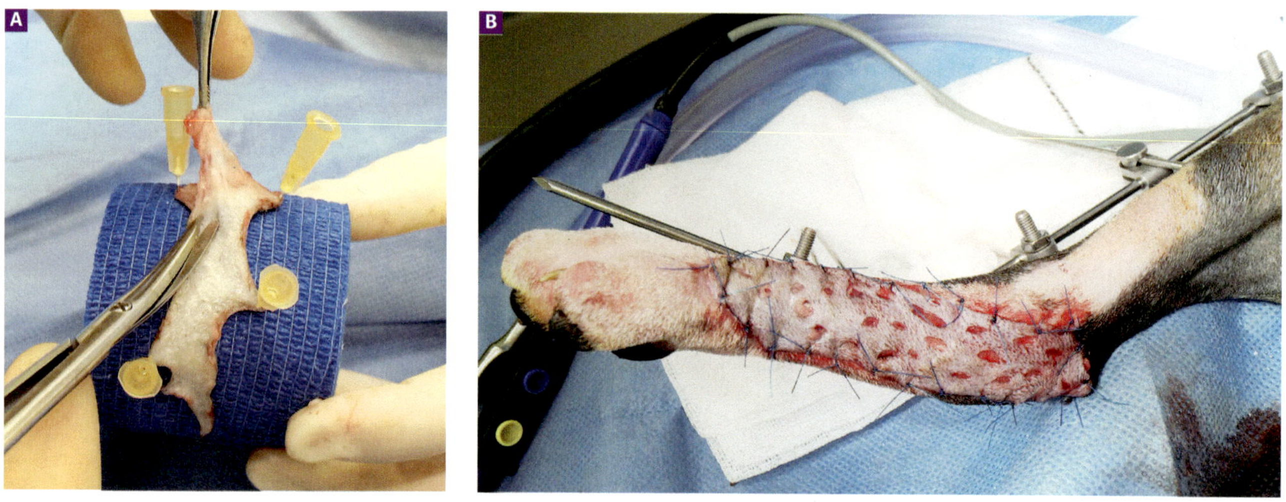

Figure 93. A. Graft preparation; **B.** A meshed skin graft sutured in place.

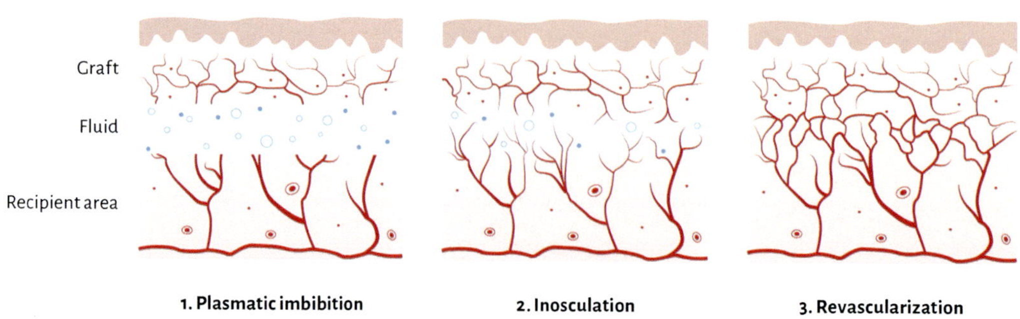

Figure 94. Phases of graft take.

– **Adequate vascularisation of the recipient bed:** hence the need for a healthy granulation bed or well vascularised surgical wound.

Gastric Surgery

Anatomy of the Stomach

The stomach (Figure 95) functions to store, begin the digestive process, mix, and then pass food on into the small intestine for absorption and further digestion. The stomach is lined by a mucosa which secretes a layer of protective mucus and secretes digestive enzymes and acid to initiate the digestive process. The mucus protects the stomach wall itself from these digestive enzymes and acid.

The stomach sits in the cranioventral abdomen, with the fundus sitting to the left side, the body crossing the midline and pylorus on the right side. The stomach wall comprises five layers:

- inner mucosa backed by a submucosa, the supporting layer
- two muscular layers
- an inner concentric layer
- outer longitudinal layer
- a covering film of serosa.

Gastrotomy

Gastrotomy (Figure 96) **refers to a surgical incision into the stomach,** often performed for removal of obstructive gastric foreign bodies, but also for removal of tumours, biopsy procedures, and placement of gastrostomy feeding tubes. **Compared to surgery on other parts of the gastrointestinal tract the risk of complications from healing of the stomach wall**

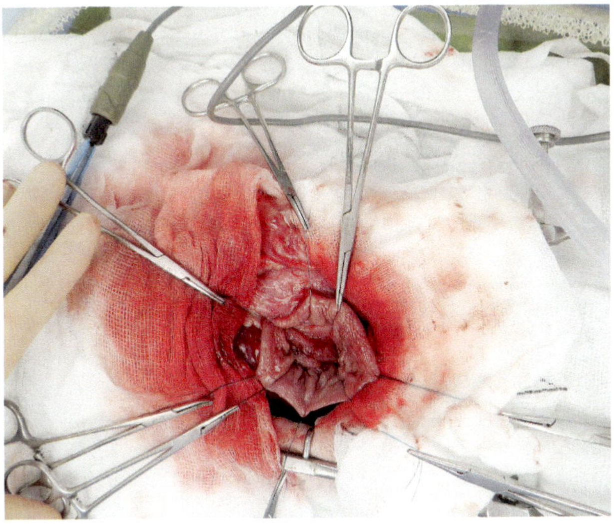

Figure 96. Gastrotomy.

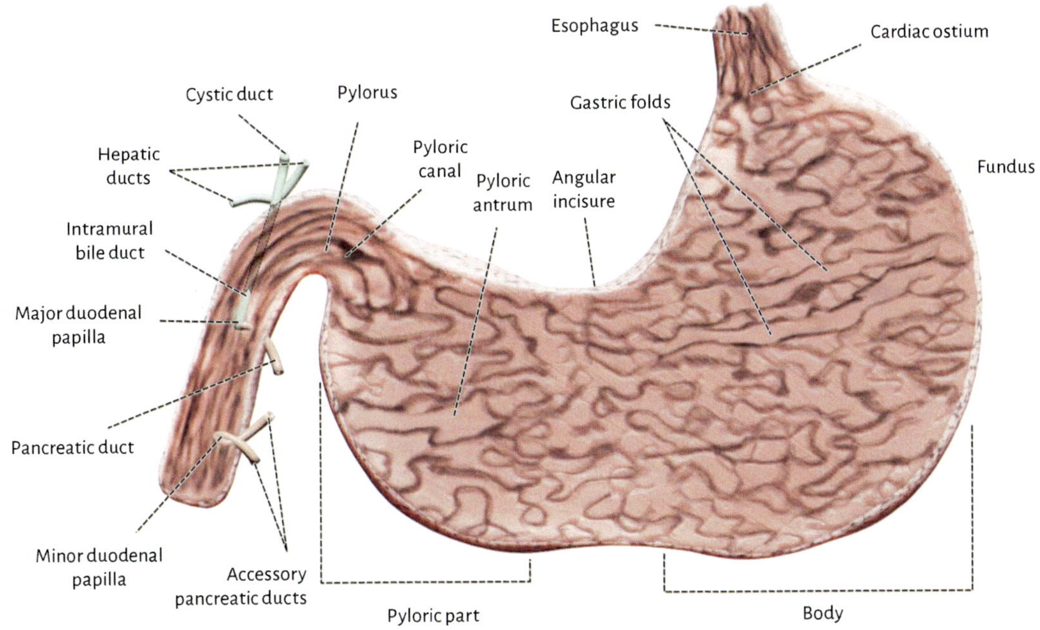

Figure 95. Stomach anatomy.

are low and so gastrotomy may be the approach of choice to remove distal oesophageal foreign bodies, and those from the small intestine, which can we successfully manipulated back into the stomach. Reasons for this reduced complication risk may be in part due to the thickness of the gastric wall, the blood supply with vessels running along both the greater and lesser curvatures and branching across the gastric wall, and the great capacity of the stomach, which with appropriate small regular meals following surgery is less likely to be under strain and therefore the suture line under less pressure during healing.

When gastrotomy is planned, perioperative antibiotics are indicated as this is classified as clean-contaminated surgery. During surgery, **the entire abdomen should be thoroughly explored** to ensure additional foreign bodies or disease are not missed. **The stomach should then be isolated with moist laparotomy sponges,** so that any minor spillage is contained and does not cause global abdominal contamination. An assistant supports the gastric wall, using fingers or stay sutures. An incision should be made on the underside of the stomach, midway between the greater and lesser curvatures to avoid the vessels on the gastric surface. When the stomach is fluid filled, passing a stomach tube through the mouth may also be indicated to decompress the stomach and reduce the chance of abdominal contamination. Suction should also be available to evacuate residual fluid directly from the stomach.

Instruments entering the gastric lumen are contaminated and should not be returned to the sterile field on the instrument trolley. Contaminated instruments may either be discarded (if they have been used for foreign body retrieval from the stomach and are no longer needed) or kept in a separate, well demarcated area of the kit trolley, to prevent cross contamination.

Closure of the stomach wall is usually performed in two layers as the stomach wall separates with incision. **Polyglyconate (Maxon®) is the ideal suture for gastric wall closure as unlike PDS®, it does not loose strength more rapidly in an acidic environment, should the sutures penetrate the gastric lumen.**

Gastric Dilation/Volvulus

Aetiology

Gastric dilation/volvulus (GDV) is an infrequent condition, usually **of older, deep-chested large and giant breed dogs, more commonly affecting males than females.** Although the exact circumstances which lead to the condition are poorly understood, increased mobility of the pylorus allows displacement from its usual location on the right side of the abdomen, across to the left, in combination with gas filling the stomach. It is unclear if the gas filling is primary or secondarily to obstruction and fermentation of gastric contents or a combination of the two. Displacement of the stomach is shown in Figure 97.

This displacement obstructs the outflow of the stomach in both directions (orad and aborad) and so bloating progresses. As the stomach becomes more distended, this increased intra-abdominal pressure compresses the caudal vena cava, restricting return of blood from the caudal half of the dog to the heart, leading to **cardiorespiratory compromise and distributive shock.** Hence rapid diagnosis and presurgical management of GDV is an **acute emergency.**

Multiple factors are implicated as the cause of GDV, from frequency of feeding, type of diet (wet or dry, biscuit size), speed of eating, elevation of food bowls, and timings of feeding and exercise. But in the largest studies, the only risk factors which were shown to be associated with increased risk of GDV were feeding **one large meal a day, feeding from a raised food bowl (thought to be due to a greater air intake with the food in this position) and having a fearful temperament** (Glickman et al., 2000; Raghavan et al., 2004).

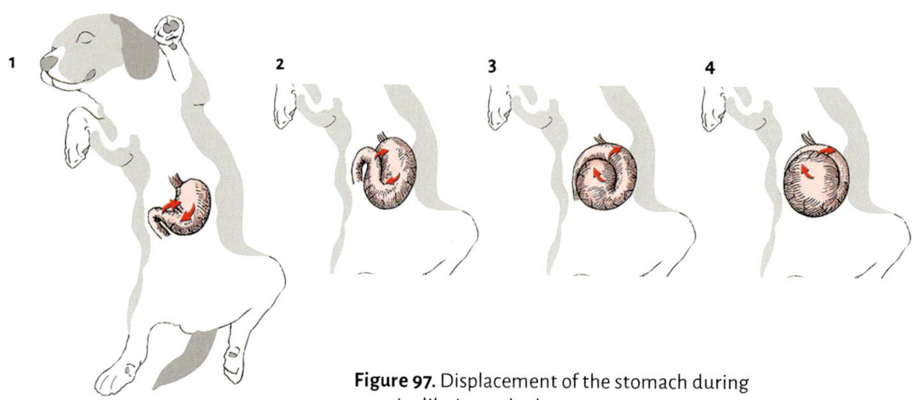

Figure 97. Displacement of the stomach during gastric-dilation-volvulus.

Diagnosis

Diagnosis is usually made over the telephone, with a classic history of an at-risk breed, older dog reporting acute onset abdominal distension, and unsuccessful attempts to vomit, usually within hours of the last feed. Typically, these cases present more frequently in the evening.

On presentation, clinically patients have a **distended, drum like abdomen,** which can be balloted to confirm the presence of air. Patients may be in variable stages of **shock, with weak pulses and tachycardia.** If necessary, radiographs can confirm the diagnosis by observing a classic double-bubble or inverse-C created by the silhouette of the gas filled stomach on a right lateral abdominal radiograph. Radiography should not be prioritised however over immediate presurgical stabilisation and management. (Figure 98).

Presurgical Stabilisation

Emergency stabilisation treatment is the priority for a patient presenting with suspected GDV. Expecting a patient to arrive with this condition should prompt preparation of essential equipment before the patient arrives at the practice.

The initial treatment goals are:
- achieve gastric decompression
- volume resuscitation of the patient.

Both goals are best served by addressing decompression first, as this allows return of the venous blood in the caudal half of the patient to the circulation. **Decompression is rapidly achieved by passing an orogastric tube,** which is usually achievable in most patients, by placing a large new VetWrap® or equivalent in the patient's mouth whilst an assistant holds the mouth closed around it, and a well-lubricated feeding tube is fed into the mouth with the head lowered. **The length of tube should be premeasured from the last rib to the tip of the nose** and the tubing marked with a marker pen or a piece of sticky tape. There is likely be resistance to passage of the tube at the lower oesophageal sphincter due to the twisting of the stomach, but this is often overcome by maintaining gentle pressure, and sometimes by changing the recumbency of the patient. Once passed the tube should allow rapid decompression.

If this is not achievable, then the next option is to quickly clip and prepare a small square of skin over the area of most obvious distension and gas filling on ballottement, and then **pass a large bore intravenous catheter into the stomach directly** as a trocar to allow decompression; partial decompression by this means often then allows easier passage of an orogastric tube.

Intravenous fluid therapy should be via **cephalic catheters placed in both forelimbs,** as the venous return from the caudal half of the patient may still be impaired. Aggressive fluid therapy is required, but should be appropriate and targeted, based on the patient's cardiovascular parameters as well as electrolyte and lactate assessments. (Figure 99).

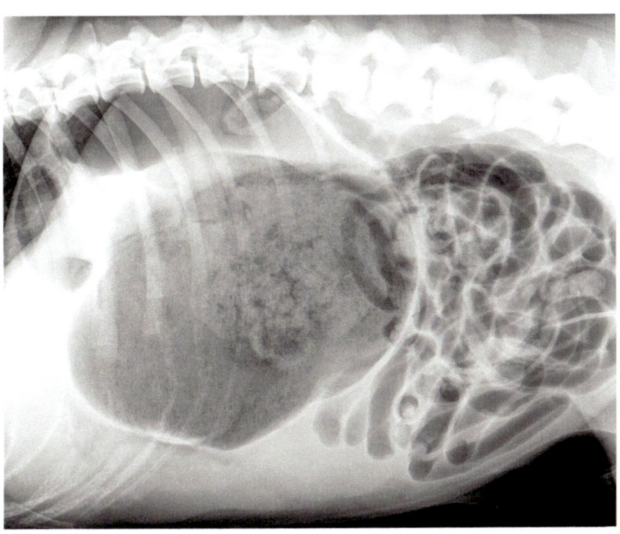

Figure 98. Radiograph of a patient suffering with GDV.

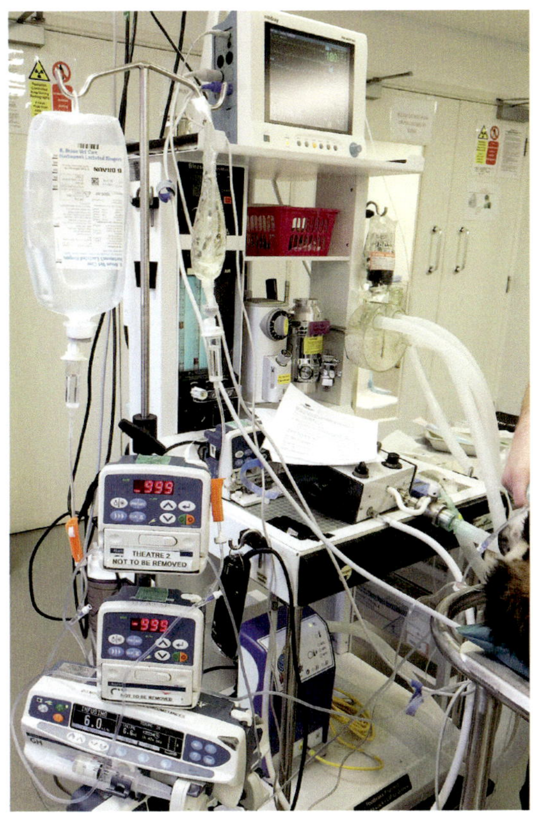

Figure 99. Fluid bolus administration using multiple drip pumps.

Surgical Treatment

Surgical treatment of GDV (Figure 100) is not in itself an emergency and should be delayed until the patient is sufficiently volume resuscitated to allow a safer general anaesthesia. That said, prolonged delay to surgery may necessitate repeat orogastric intubation as the stomach continues to bloat. Also, prolonged severe gastric rotation does lead to reduced blood flow to the gastric wall which may be more likely to result in necrosis requiring surgical resection or invagination into the stomach.

The aim of surgery is to derotate the stomach, assess the integrity of the stomach wall (and the spleen) and perform a full abdominal exploration for additional pathology or inciting causes.

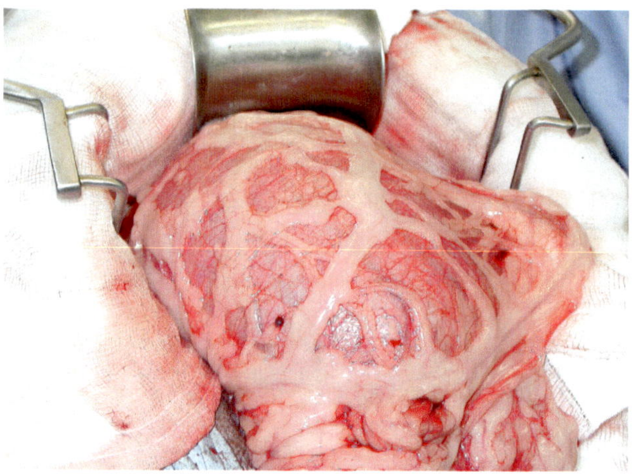

Figure 100. GDV exploratory laparotomy.

The final stage of surgery is then **to anchor the stomach** to prevent repeat rotation in the future. This has been described by several techniques, but the simplest method is the **incisional gastropexy,** whereby a partial thickness incision is made into the stomach at the body near to the pylorus and a matching incision in the body wall behind the last rib on the right side and then these incisions are sutured together with a continuous suture.

A right sided, tube gastrostomy (Figure 101), in the same location, allows for the provision of early enteral nutrition, as well as allowing ongoing gastric decompression and administration of medication should the patient not be amenable to oral administration.

Aftercare

Following surgery, analgesia and fluid therapy should be continued as required and until nutritional demands are managed enterally. If a feeding tube is in place, low volume tube feeding should be initiated following anaesthetic recovery, however gastric motility and emptying should be assessed by draining the gastric contents before the next feed, and the process repeated every few hours. De-rotation of the stomach can release inflammatory mediators which have prolonged effects on cardiac output and cause ventricular premature contractions (VPCs). **This should be monitored with an ECG** and may require treatment with a lidocaine infusion if there are prolonged periods of arrhythmia associated with loss of blood pressure.

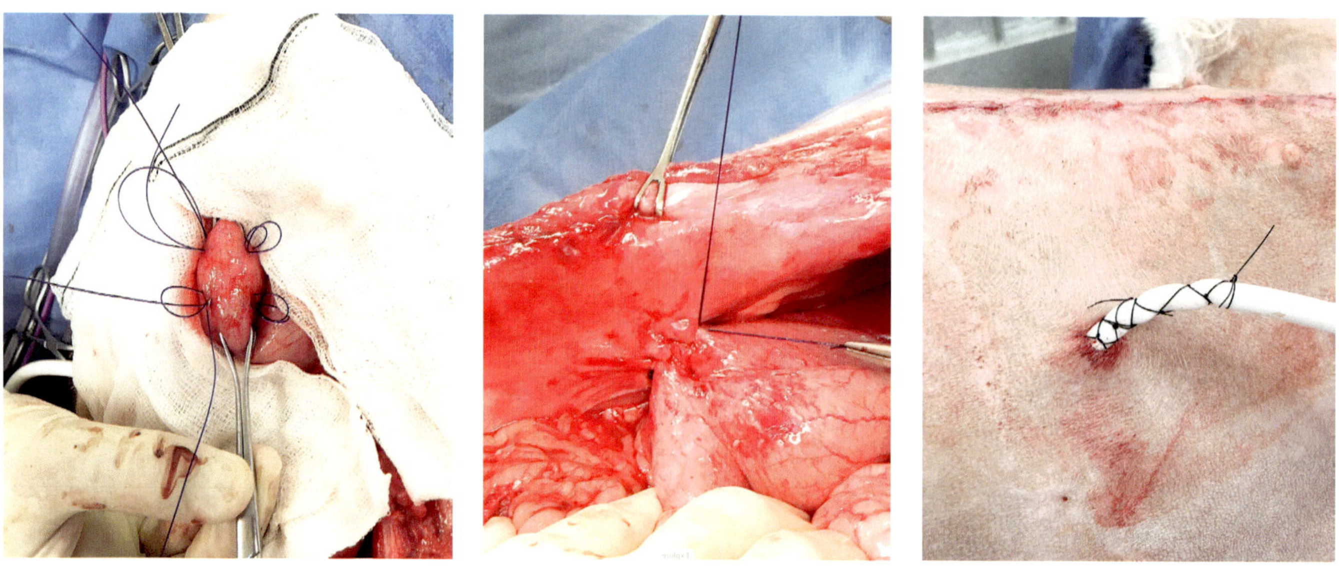

Figure 101. Gastrostomy tube placement.

Prevention

Prophylactic gastropexy at the time of routine neutering, other abdominal surgery (e.g. foreign body removal), or planned independent surgery is gaining popularity in at-risk breeds. This may even be performed laparoscopically, with minimal risk of negative consequences, except in one report in military working German Shepherd dogs, which subsequently appeared at increased risk of intestinal torsion (a rare condition, more frequently seen in German Shepherd dogs, with a very high mortality rate) and so perhaps this group should be excluded from this preventative treatment in the future (Ward et al., 2003; Deroy et al., 2019; Andrews et al., 2018).

Intestinal Surgery

Anatomy of the Intestine

The intestine of carnivores is roughly five times the length of their trunk, with the small intestine predominating. The intestine is a tube with different subdivisions, but with the same basic anatomy, like the stomach, with an inner mucosal layer, submucosa, muscularis (composed of an inner circular muscle layer and outer longitudinal layer) and covering film of serosa (Figure 102). The thickness and function of these layers, particularly the mucosa varies along the length of the intestine.

The small intestine stems from the pylorus as the duodenum and is joined by the pancreatic and bile ducts at the major and minor papillae. The duodenum descends the abdomen as the furthest lateral loop of intestine on the right side, and then turns at the pelvic canal with an attachment of its mesentery to that of the colon (the duodeno-colic ligament). **The duodenum** then ascends and becomes the **jejunum,** which is more free-form with mobile loops of bowel which are apparent when entering the abdomen via coeliotomy. These loops hang from the mesentery, which is rooted craniodorsally around the cranial mesenteric artery. **The terminal jejunum becomes the ileum,** which is notable for having a vessel running along its antimesenteric border, which stems from the attachment with the caecum. At the **ileocaecocolic junction** the ileum connects to the caecum and ascending colon, in the right cranial abdomen. From there the colon traverses to the left and then descends to and through the pelvis as the most lateral loop of intestine on the left side of the abdomen. (Figure 103).

Intestinal Biopsy

Full thickness, surgical, intestinal biopsy is a procedure which is not without risk as the bowel wall is perforated and hence there is a small (1.0–2.3%) risk of poor healing, leakage, and peritonitis; but is indicated where mucosal biopsy (achieved endoscopically) provides insufficient information for diagnosis of intestinal disease (most commonly to differentiate inflammatory bowel disease from intestinal lymphoma) (Swinbourne et al., 2017).

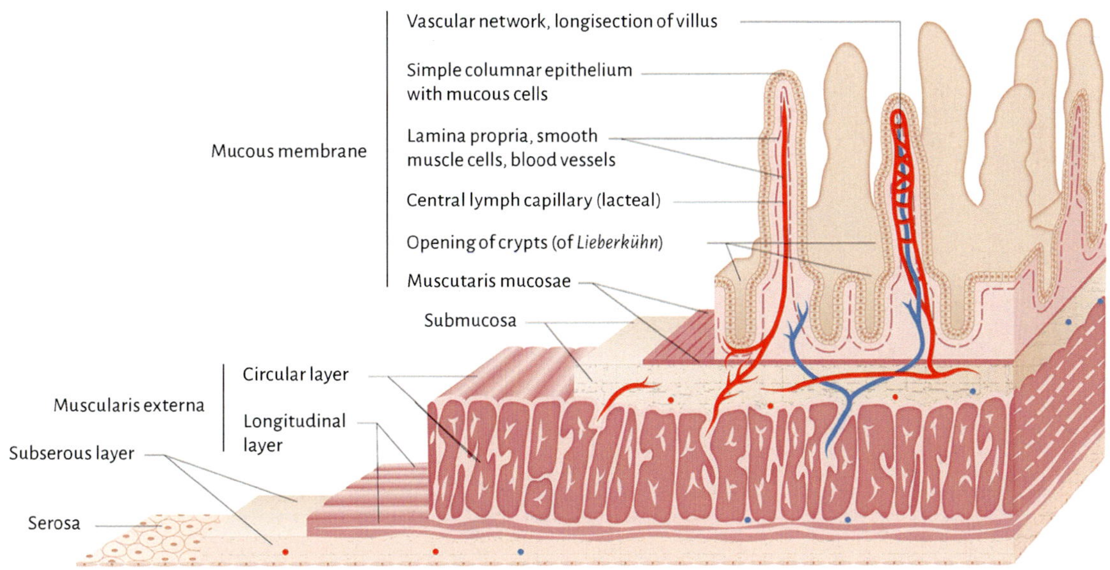

Figure 102. Intestinal wall.

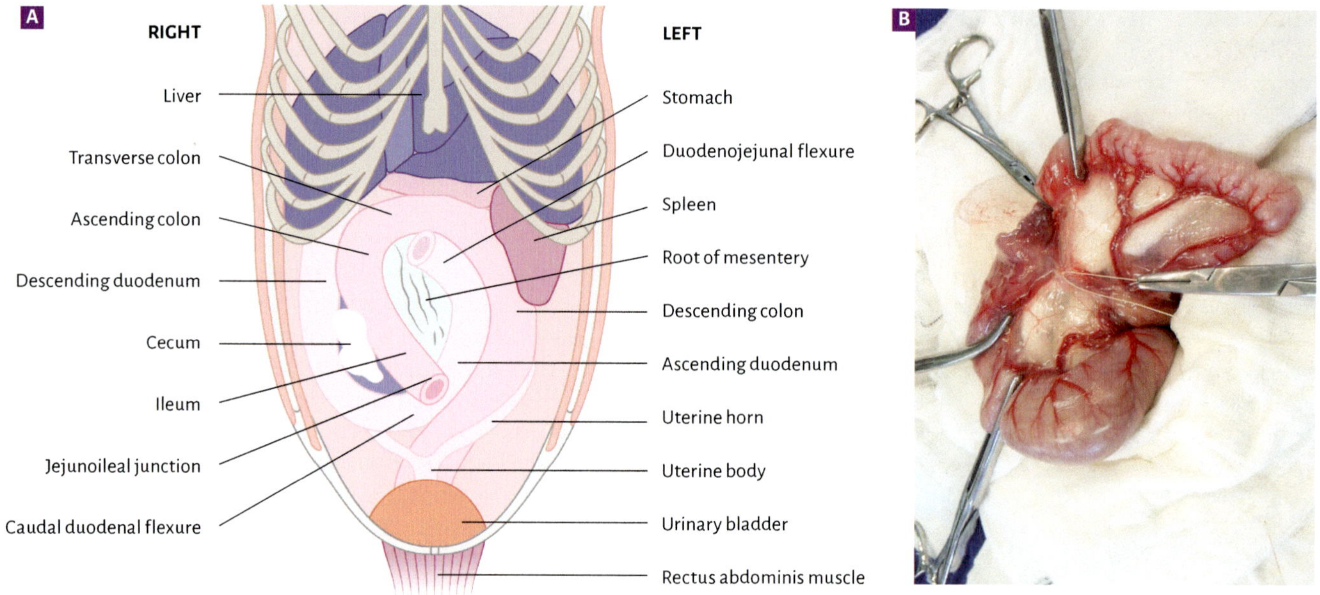

Figure 103. A. Intestinal position; **B.** Mesenteric vasculature.

Intestinal biopsy (Figure 104) **is a clean-contaminated procedure and so perioperative antibiotics are indicated.** An intestinal loop is isolated with moist laparotomy sponges to prevent contamination of the abdomen. The surgical assistant milks the intestinal contents to either side and then uses their fingers to gently occlude the bowl. The surgeon then cuts a sample of the bowel wall using a number 11 scalpel blade or a skin punch biopsy. The instruments should be discarded or isolated in a designated contaminated kit area. Small samples may be collected on the card insert from a suture packet for ease of transfer into formalin for submission for histopathology. The intestinal incision is then **sutured closed, usually with simple interrupted, appositional sutures, using monofilament, absorbable suture material,** and a non-cutting needle. Leak testing is performed by injecting sterile saline into the isolated bowel loop, using a 20 ml syringe and 25G needle.

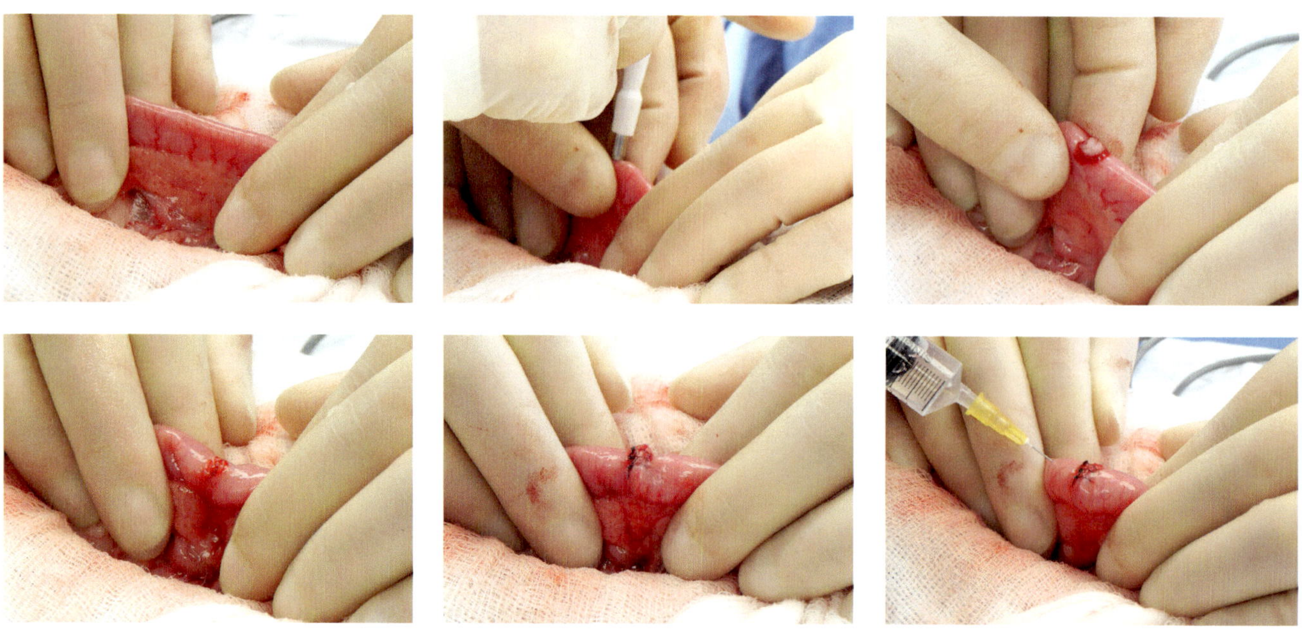

Figure 104. Intestinal biopsy: the bowel loop is isolated, a punch biopsy is taken from the antimesenteric border. Then the defected is sutured closed and the repair leak tested.

Enterotomy

Enterotomy is a surgical incision into the small intestine, most commonly performed for foreign body removal. The procedure is as for intestinal biopsy, with the incision made at the antimesenteric border. To allow visualisation within the lumen of the bowel (e.g. to cannulate the bile duct), placing temporary stay sutures in the incisional edges is helpful, along with lavage and suction of the intestinal contents.

The incision should be closed along its length, usually with a simple appositional suture pattern, either with interrupted or continuous sutures, using monofilament, absorbable suture material, and a non-cutting needle, to prevent tearing of the delicate bowel wall.

Enterectomy

Enterectomy (Figure 105) **is the surgical removal of a loop of intestine,** which may be performed to excise a tumour or remove a portion of damaged bowel following obstruction with a foreign body, an intussusception, abdominal trauma, or other injury. As with other abdominal surgeries, the entire abdomen should be explored for additional findings and the area of interest isolated with moist laparotomy sponges. The margins for intestinal removal should be assessed, with damaged bowel, the surgeon would remove only the damaged portion trying to spare as much healthy tissue as possible, whilst for a tumour, commonly 4 cm margins orad and aborad to the tumour are taken to achieve clean removal of the tumour based on common intestinal tumour types and degree of expected

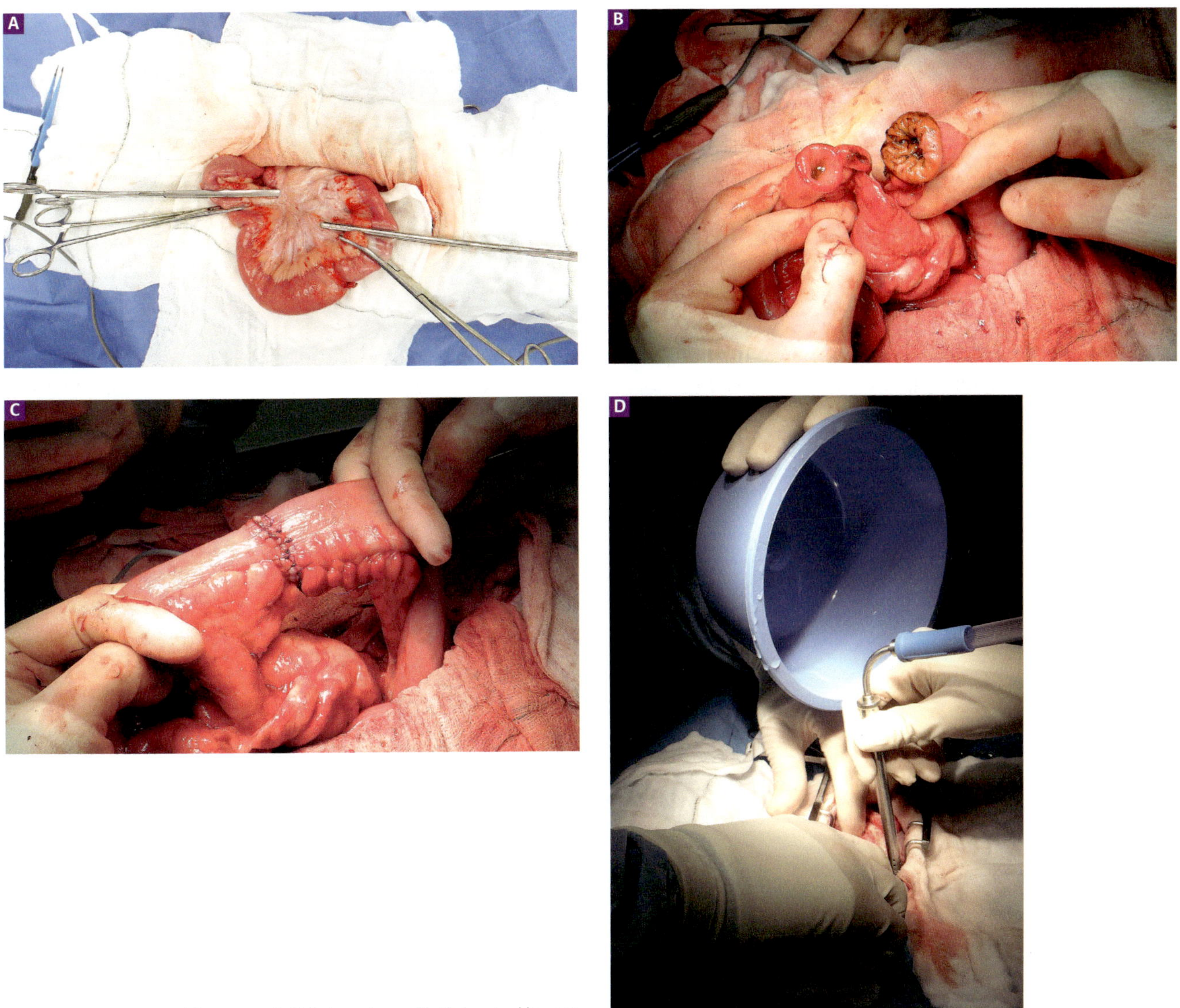

Figure 105. A-C. Enterectomy; **D.** Abdominal lavage.

infiltration. When excising the bowel, it is important to inspect and maintain the blood supply to the bowel which remains to ensure the sutured tissue is viable and heals with the lowest possible risk of complications (Morrice et al., 2019).

Instruments used for enterectomy are considered contaminated. A new, sharp scalpel blade should be used to excise the isolated bowel loop. The bowl either side is ideally clamped in the fingers of a surgical assistant, although if not available then Doyen bowel clamps placed as atraumatically as possible on the bowel ends can be used, using the widest part of the jaws and the minimal tension on the ratchet to occlude but not crush the bowel. The ends of the bowel loop which are being removed may be clamped with artery forceps to seal the excised loop, as this tissue is removed from the body.

The affected bowel loop should be removed and the free ends of the bowel brought together and sutured in apposition, using absorbable monofilament suture material on a non-cutting needle. Most frequently, bowel is sutured with simple interrupted or simple continuous sutures and then a **leak test** (Figure 106) **performed (using a 20 ml syringe and 25G needle)** to ensure adequate sealing of the bowel. An alternative to hand suturing of the anastomosis is to use surgical stapling equipment. (See Figure 36).

The operated loop is then lavaged (Figure 105 D), before more thorough abdominal lavage and closure.

Intussusception

Intussusception is the telescoping of one loop of intestine into an adjacent loop. This most commonly occurs in puppies, associated with intestinal hypermotility, which may accompany other gastrointestinal disease including parasitic and viral diseases. Intussusception less commonly occurs in adult patients but may occur secondarily to tumours or foreign bodies.

Intussusception (Figure 107) **most commonly occurs at the ileocolic junction** with the ileum passing into the colon. The effect of an intussusception is similar to a foreign body obstruction, causing vomiting, diarrhoea, and abdominal pain, but the internal loop of intestine, **(interssusceptum)** may also

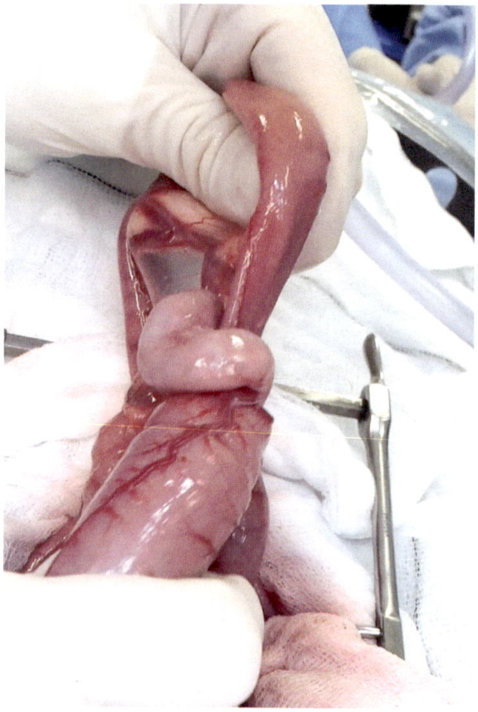

Figure 107. Intussusception of the ileum into the colon.

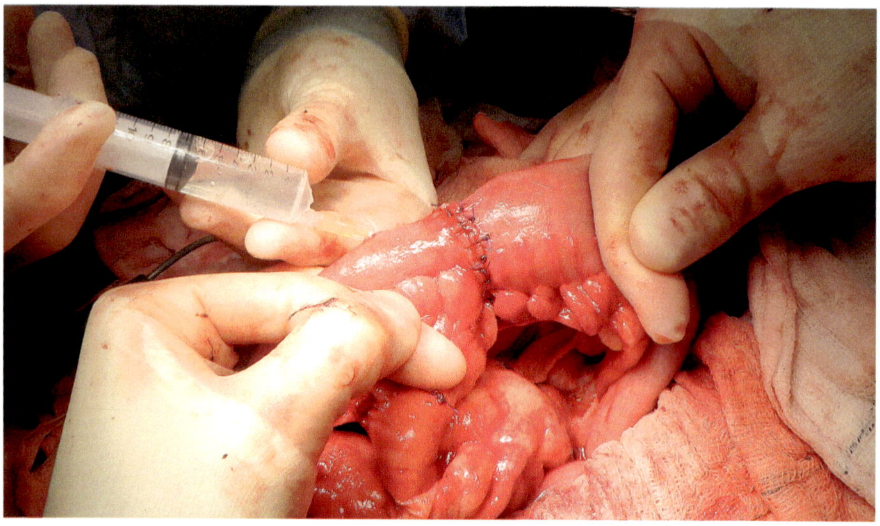

Figure 106. Leak testing of a hand sutured intestinal anastomosis.

have compromised blood flow and with time, adhesions form which make reduction from the outer loop **(intussuscentiens)** more challenging, at least without causing damage.

Diagnosis is made based on patient signalment, palpation of a sausage-like firm loop of intestine in the mid abdomen and confirmed **with ultrasound which shows concentric rings of intestinal wall** inside each other and obstruction to flow with fluid accumulation orad to the obstruction.

At surgery the affected loop of bowel is isolated. When possible, the intussusception should be gently reduced. If this is challenging it may still be worth persisting as small tears in the bowel may require removal of the damaged portion, but often a smaller section of bowel might require resection following reduction of the intussusception than would be needed to remove it completely. Thereafter an enterectomy of the non-reducible portion and damaged portion is performed.

Enterectomy may not be required when an intussusception is identified early, reduced, and the bowel wall appears viable. Following reduction, some surgeons consider performing **enteroplication** (tacking of adjacent bowel loops with simple interrupted sutures) to try to reduce the risk of repeat events following surgery. (Figure 108).

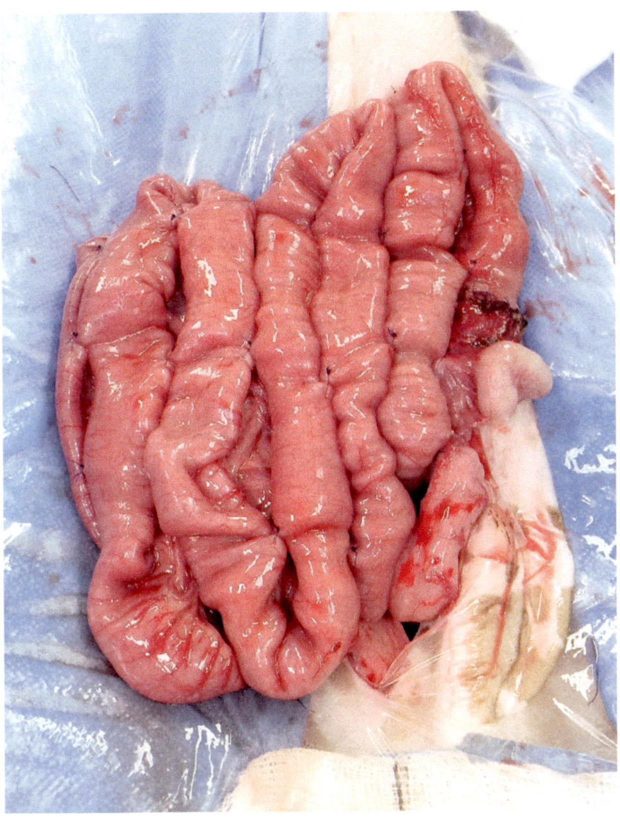

Figure 108. Enteroplication of the small intestine.

It is essential to investigate and treat for underlying gastrointestinal disorders, including administration of parasite control to patients suffering intussusception to try to prevent recurrence.

Linear Foreign Bodies

Intestinal obstruction with linear foreign bodies, often caused obstruction and damage to the intestine at multiple levels. Cats eating string or cotton thread or dogs chewing strips off towels or eating undergarments are common scenarios. With cats, the foreign body is often anchored around the base of the tongue, but more commonly in dogs a portion of the foreign body becomes wedged in the stomach, whilst a free strand of the foreign body then passes through the intestine causing corrugation of the intestine. This leads to cheese-wiring through the intestinal wall if left.

Radiographically and on ultrasound examination **the intestine appears bunched and corrugated.** Surgery requires release of the anchoring point of the foreign body and then milking the foreign body through the intestine to allow its complete removal through as few incisions as possible. The hub and bung from an intravenous cannula may be attached to the end of a foreign body to facilitate milking through the intestine. Following removal of the foreign body by enterotomy/enterotomies, the entire bowel wall is inspected for evidence of perforations and if necessary, enterectomy performed to remove a damaged portion.

Septic Peritonitis

Septic peritonitis is the presence of, and inflammatory process associated with, bacterial proliferation within the peritoneum, outside of the abdominal visceral organs. In dogs this is usually secondary to intestinal perforation, leakage following surgery, foreign body (Figure 109 A, B) penetration, or neoplastic infiltration and compromise of the intestinal wall. But it may also occur due to rupture of the biliary or urinary systems when bacteria are present (e.g. with urinary tract trauma or obstruction in a patient with cystitis, rupture of a pyometra, or rupture of an infected gallbladder mucocoele), or due to penetrating injury to the abdomen.

In cats, the cause of peritonitis is not always clear and bacterial translocation across the bowel wall or seeding from the blood stream may be suggested in cases without previous trauma or inciting cause. **Septic peritonitis is usually generalised in cats and dogs** (Figure 109 C, D), but occasionally can be focal associated with an abscess which is isolated by the omentum. Septic peritonitis is the most serious complication of intestinal surgery. Diagnosis and treatment are challenging and discussed at length in Chapter 8.

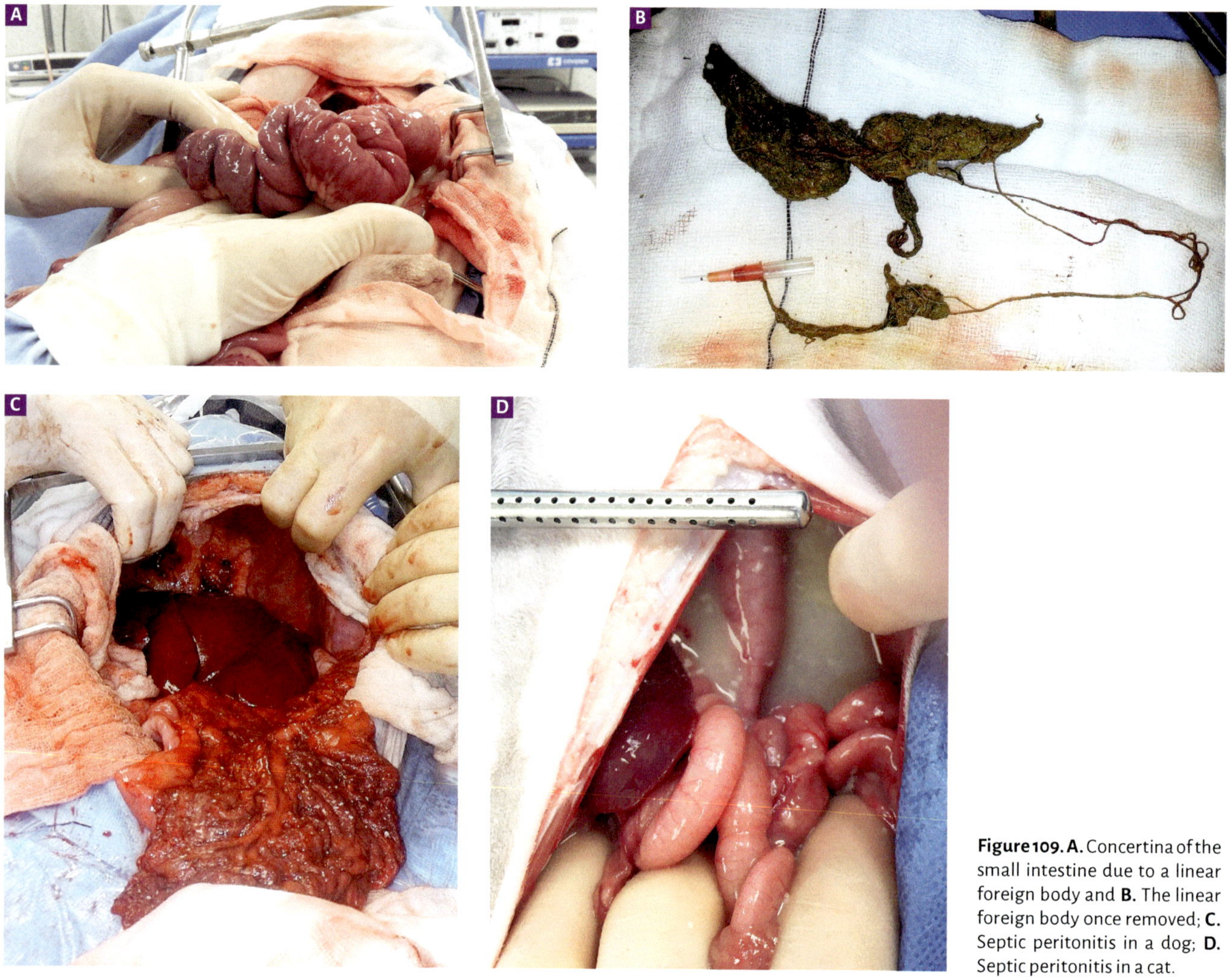

Figure 109. A. Concertina of the small intestine due to a linear foreign body and **B.** The linear foreign body once removed; **C.** Septic peritonitis in a dog; **D.** Septic peritonitis in a cat.

Spleen

Anatomy of the Spleen

The spleen is a strap-like, delicate, parenchymatous organ which sits along the left side of the abdominal wall, just behind the last rib along the greater curvature of the stomach, sharing the blood supply to the stomach via the short gastric arteries and veins. (Figure 110 A).

The spleen has **three primary functions:**

- **Reservoir:** 10–20% of a dog's red blood cells and 30% of the platelets are stored in the spleen. These can be mobilised into the circulation at times of increased requirement or after blood loss, by the contraction of smooth muscle tissue within the spleen. This muscle is under the influence of vasodilatory and vasopressor medications.
- **Haematopoiesis:** the red pulp tissue of the spleen is responsible for final maturation of blood cells which originate in the bone marrow, prior to release into the circulation.
- **Immunological function:** the white pulp tissue of the spleen consists of diffuse and nodule regions of lymphoid tissue, which filter the blood and stimulate the production of B-cells and T-cells, and subsequently secretion of antibodies.

Diseases of the Spleen

Generalised Splenomegaly

The spleen may become generally enlarged for several reasons:

- inflammation with splenitis

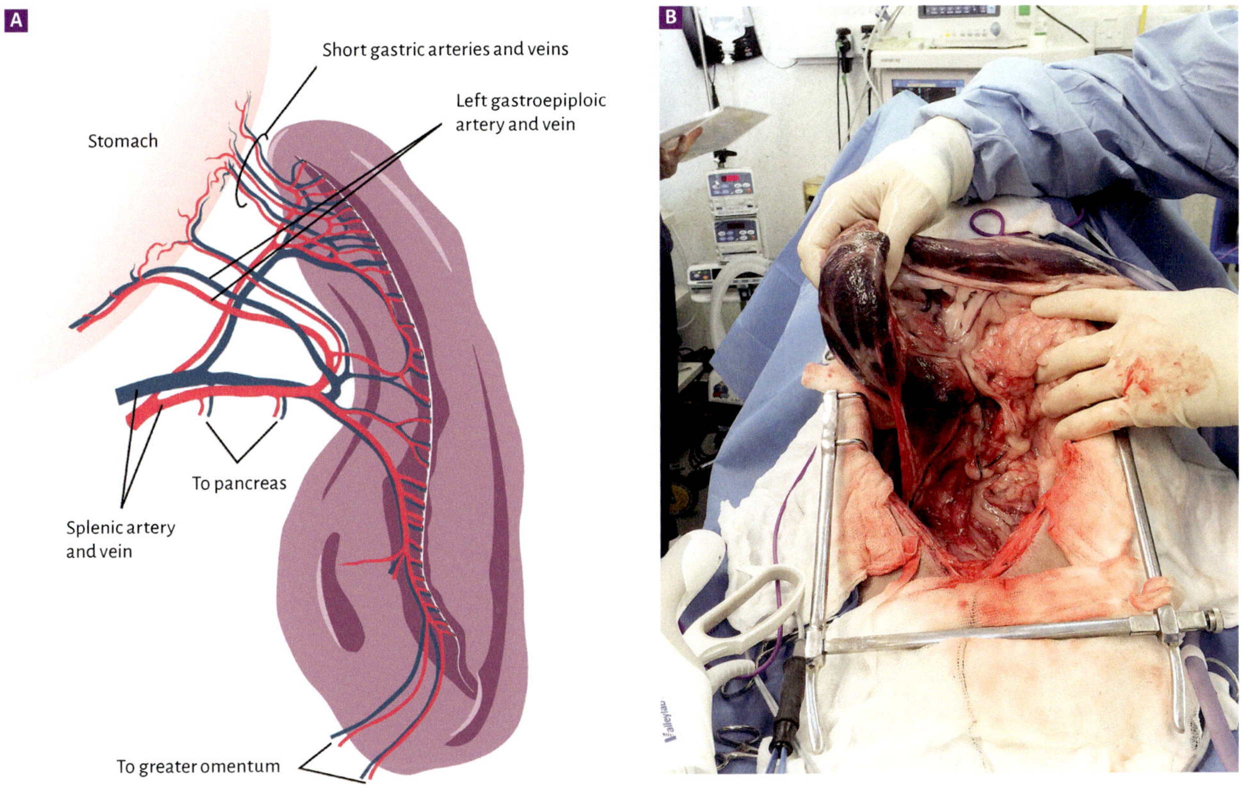

Figure 110. A. Spleen anatomy; **B.** Splenic torsion.

- cellular hyperplasia as the result of immune stimulation
- congestion due to:
  - congestive heart failure
  - vascular outflow obstruction secondary to:
    - splenic vein restriction (e.g. due to splenic torsion (Figure 110 B); or
    - portal hypertension due to liver disease (see notes on the liver in the next section)
- capsular relaxation under the influence of barbiturates (e.g. phenobarbital) or phenothiazines (e.g. acepromazine)
- infiltration as seen with some neoplastic diseases (e.g. lymphoma, histiocytic sarcoma, or mast cell tumour).

Localised Splenomegaly

The spleen may also become focally or multifocally enlarged with nodules for several reasons:

- nodular hyperplasia: a common age-related change in dogs, with multiple benign lumps of the surface of the spleen
- benign hamartoma or haemangioma
- haematoma, which may result from splenic trauma
- abscesses (rare)
- neoplasia: haemangiosarcoma (the most common), sarcoma, lymphoma, mast cell tumour, histiocytic sarcoma, plasma cell tumours.

Diagnosis

Splenic enlargement may be noted during abdominal palpation or abdominal imaging investigations. Splenic tissue is ultrasonographically compared to that of the liver, with **normal spleen tissue being more echogenic and with a finer echotexture than the liver. The texture of the spleen is normally smooth,** and areas of different echotexture may be investigated by fine needle aspiration for cytology in patients with adequate haematocrit, platelet numbers, and coagulation profiles (due to the risk of intra-abdominal haemorrhage).

With larger splenic lesions most surgeons prefer not to risk bleeding from aspiration of the spleen, and instead elect to remove the spleen for diagnostic testing, without the risk of spontaneous internal bleeding from rupture of a fragile mass.

Roughly two-thirds of splenic masses are malignancies, with two-thirds of those having metastasised at the time of diagnosis. Therefore, **staging should be performed prior to surgical intervention** by full assessment of the abdomen by ultrasonography and three view inflated thoracic radiography or CT scanning both the thorax and abdomen. **Haemangiosarcoma may also metastasise to the heart base and right side of the heart** and so structural echocardiography and assessment for associated pericardial effusion should be performed as part of staging prior to surgery.

Haemoabdomen

Rupture of a splenic mass is the most common cause of non-traumatic haemoabdomen. Patient's with haemoabdomen present with weakness, lethargy, collapse, and varying degrees of pallor of the mucous membranes, and circulatory collapse.

Diagnosis is by sampling of the abdominal fluid following abdominal imaging, and comparison of the PCV of the fluid to that of the patient's general circulation – similar PCV values confirm acute bleeding.

Targeted intravenous fluids should be administered, assessing the response to fluid bolus administration, whilst being aware there is almost certainly ongoing bleeding, so at the same time the patient should be prepared for surgical intervention to limit ongoing bleeding. Assessment of the patient's blood type should be performed in preparation for transfusion if needed.

Splenectomy

Splenectomy is performed by ventral midline coeliotomy. The patient should be prepared for full exploration of the entire abdominal cavity as with haemangiosarcoma, additional metastatic lesions may be present, commonly associated with the liver and diaphragm.

In the case of haemoabdomen, preparations should be made for the large volume of free abdominal blood, with **adhesive caesarean drapes ideal for preventing spillage** and soaking of the patient; these also maintaining sterility should it be necessary to suction the blood into a cell-saver device, mixed with citrate anticoagulant, filtered, and autotransfused.

Splenic masses (Figure 111) **are fragile and so should be handled with care.** Removing the spleen requires ligation and sectioning of the vessels supplying the spleen. This may be performed along the splenic margin, or by ligation of the trunk vessels supplying the branches which join the spleen but **taking care not to disrupt the blood supply to the pancreas and stomach.** Splenic vessel ligation may be performed by hand suturing, surgical stapling using vascular staples or a ligate and divide stapler or using a bipolar vessel sealing device. (Figure 112).

Following surgery, **multimodal analgesia** should be administered, and the patient monitored for ongoing bleeding: this is done by **regular documenting of heart rate, respiration rate, pulse rate, and quality, mucous membrane colour and blood pressure.** Up to half of patients undergoing splenectomy suffer periods of ventricular tachycardia for 1–5 days following surgery, which may be monitored by electrocardiography during surgical recovery, and may require treatment with **lidocaine infusion** if prolonged and associated with hypotensive episodes. Hypoxia may be associated with acute blood loss in cases of haemoabdomen and may require oxygen therapy and blood product administration perioperatively.

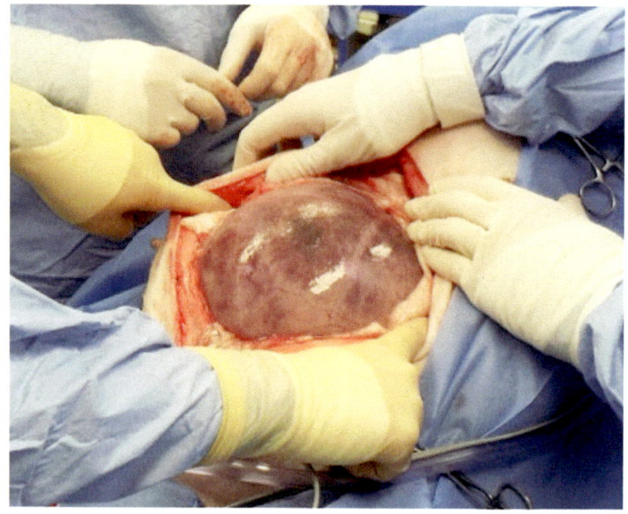

Figure 111. Splenic mass.

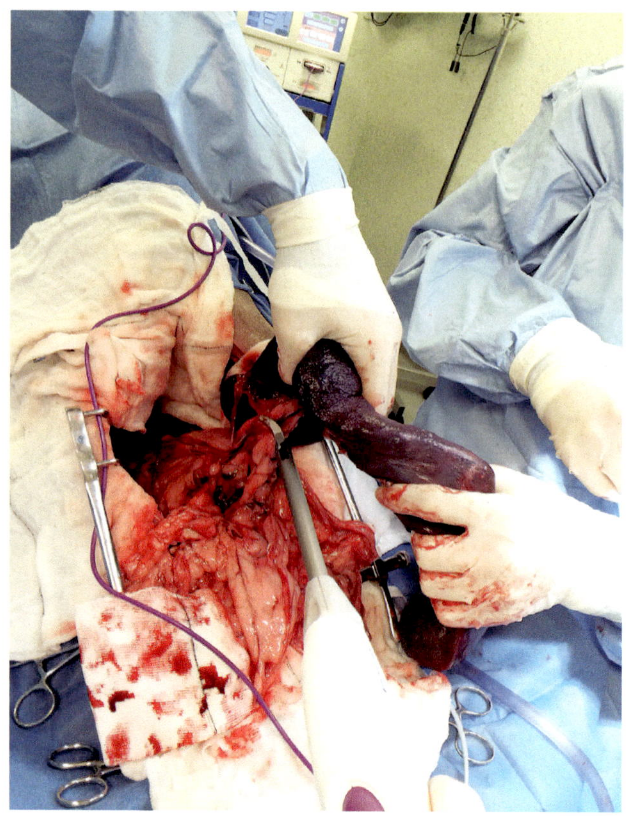

Figure 112. Splenectomy being performed using a bipolar vessel sealing device.

LIVER

Anatomy of the Liver

The liver (Figure 113) **is a fragile parenchymatous organ which sits in the cranial abdomen in contact with the diaphragm.** It is divided into several lobes as shown in the figure. The liver has many functions including:

- protein synthesis, including albumin and coagulation factors
- carbohydrate metabolism, maintaining blood glucose levels by glycogenolysis and gluconeogenesis
- storage of fat, glycogen, vitamins, and trace elements
- heat generation
- bile production and bile sale circulation
- degradation of ammonia, excess protein, drugs, and toxins
- immune regulation.

The liver receives 20% of its blood supply and 50% of its oxygenation directly from the hepatic artery, and a further 80% of its blood supply and the other 50% of its oxygenation via the portal vein, which collects blood returning from the gastrointestinal tract, spleen and pancreas for filtration and extraction of nutrients prior to return to the general circulation. The liver lobes each stem from the hilus in the middle of the liver, centred around the caudal vena cava, into which the blood from the liver drains, following filtration through the sinusoids (capillaries of the liver tissue). (Figure 114).

The gallbladder stores bile, which is produced in the liver. Following feeding, contraction secretes bile into the duodenum via the common bile duct, in association with gastric emptying. The common bile duct remains separate from the pancreatic ducts in the dog but joins with the major pancreatic duct before entering the duodenum in the cat, which makes it more prone to obstruction and inflammation as the result of triaditis (inflammation of the bowel, pancreas, and hepatobiliary system).

Liver Biopsy and Liver Lobectomy

Liver biopsy is performed as a diagnostic procedure for investigation of generalised liver disease, or for sampling of a focal nodular lesion within the liver at the time of abdominal exploration for other purposes. Liver lobectomy is most frequently performed as a treatment for tumours or abscesses of the liver.

Before performing surgery for liver biopsy or liver lobectomy, it is advisable to **check platelet counts and coagulation times** to reduce the risk of intraoperative or postoperative bleeding, especially as liver disease may result in reduced protein synthesis, including that of the coagulation factors.

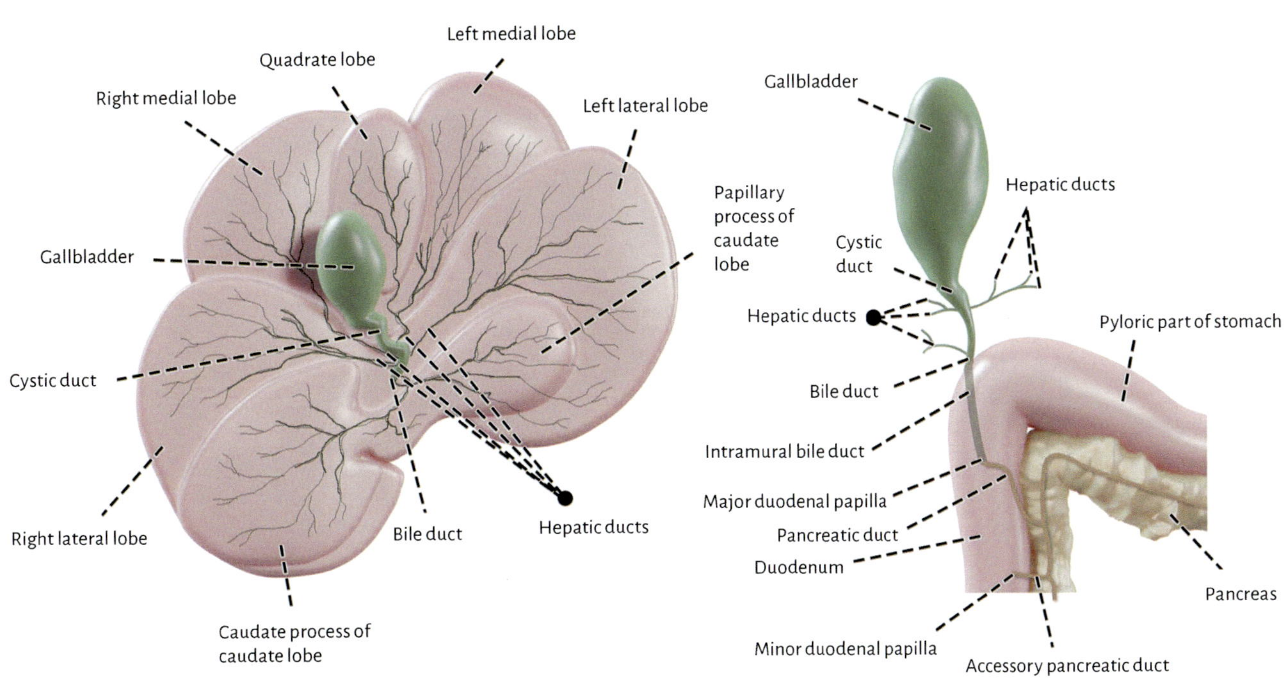

Figure 113. Liver anatomy.

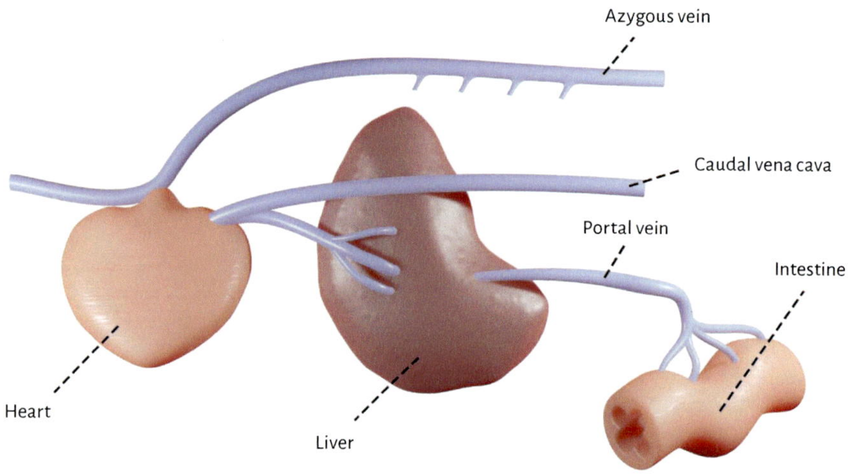

Figure 114. Normal liver vasculature.

Biopsy Techniques

- **Guillotine/suture fracture technique:** removing a small biopsy from the margin of the liver can be performed simply by crushing the tissue near to the margin with a suture or a pair of haemostats, and then cutting away the margin of tissue beyond the crush site. This technique is also used to grab biopsies from the margin of the liver, using a laparoscopic technique.
- **Punch biopsy:** using a skin punch, a core of tissue is taken from the flat surface of a liver lobe. Care should be taken to avoid taking biopsies directly over larger concealed vessels, which are more likely to be present near to the hilus of the liver. Following removal of the liver tissue from the core, the hole left behind is often packed with a haemostatic agent such as a gelatine or cellulose sponge to limit bleeding.
- **Tru-Cut® biopsy:** a Tru-Cut® needle is a spring-loaded device which cuts a narrow core of tissue but can reach deep into the substance of a liver lobe. This technique can be used in open surgery, but more frequently may be performed under ultrasound guidance as an alternative to open surgery. The samples taken are slender and there is moderate risk of haemorrhage with this technique, and so it is used with caution in many veterinary surgeons' hands.

Lobectomy/Partial Lobectomy Techniques

- **Finger fracture:** this technique involves gently breaking down the liver tissue with fingers or a suction tip, to expose the individual vessels and ducts which are ligated individually.
- **Stapling:** a thoracoabdominal stapler (TA) is used to place overlapping rows of staples across the hilus of the liver lobe. Their use is rapid, however limited by their size (length of the staple line and width of the jaws) and challenges placing them appropriately without damaging the surrounding tissues, and so may not be appropriate for every case.
- **Bipolar vessel sealing device:** used to dissect the liver tissue and seal vessels of up to 7 mm in diameter.
- **Encircling suture:** this technique uses a pretied loop of suture to place a noose around the liver lobe and is gradually tightened, dissecting its way through the liver tissue, and bunch ligating the vessels and duct. This is demonstrated for a partial liver lobectomy in the video below. Sufficient tissue must remain beyond the suture to prevent slippage, and so again this may not be appropriate for every application (Risselada et al., 2010).

Cholecystectomy

Cholecystectomy is the removal of the gallbladder. This is feasible as it sits on a side branch of the connection of the intrahepatic bile ducts and the common bile duct which enters the duodenum. **Removal merely results in a loss of the storage function.**

Cholecystectomy is most commonly performed in humans due to obstruction with gallstones. Whilst these do occur in cats and dogs, they are rare. Far more commonly the gallbladder may require removal due to biliary mucocoele, or occasionally due to traumatic rupture of the gallbladder, which results in bile peritonitis.

A gallbladder mucocoele (Figures 115, 116) **is overproduction and filling of the gallbladder with thick jelly-like material.** This is produced by the gallbladder wall and removal of the gallbladder resolves the issue, although some cases also require flushing of the common bile duct due to overflow of mucus causing obstruction and jaundice/icterus. This disease is more frequently observed in Border Terriers in the UK, and in Shetland Sheepdogs in the USA, although other breeds may be affected. Dogs present with abdominal pain, lethargy, inappetence, vomiting, and sometimes with jaundice.

Ultrasonography of the abdomen reveals a distended gallbladder filled with echogenic material (the normal appearance is anechoic (black) liquid content), which is said to have the **appearance of a kiwi fruit.** At surgery, via ventral midline coeliotomy, the gallbladder is dissected free from the liver, where it is nestled between and attached to the right medial and quadrate lobes. The surgeon should prepare to manage bleeding from the liver surface with electrocautery and topical haemostatic agents.

The bile ducts should be inspected for signs of obstruction and if necessary (Figure 117), the gallbladder opened to suction the contents and allow flushing of the bile ducts until patent. Alternatively, an incision can be made into the duodenum to allow retrograde flushing back from the common bile duct opening. The gallbladder is then removed, and the stump of the cystic duct ligated. The abdomen is then lavaged and closed.

Following hepatobiliary surgery some patients can be extremely painful and show signs of systemic inflammatory

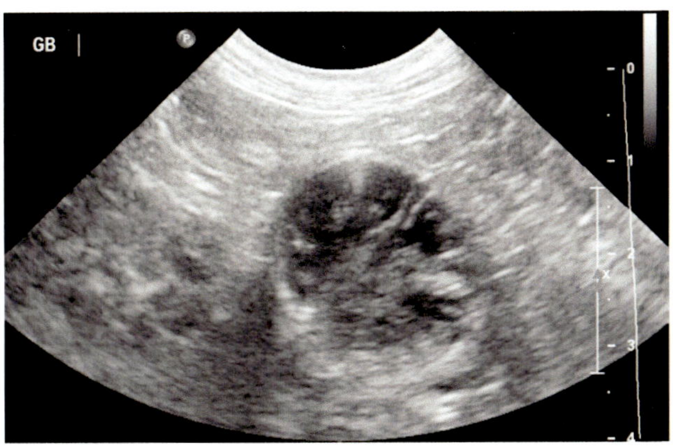

Figure 115. Gallbladder mucocoele appearance using ultrasound.

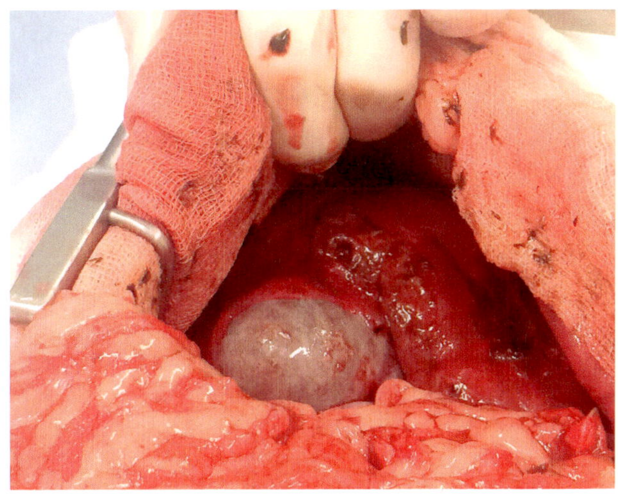

Figure 116. Gallbladder mucocoele appearance at surgery.

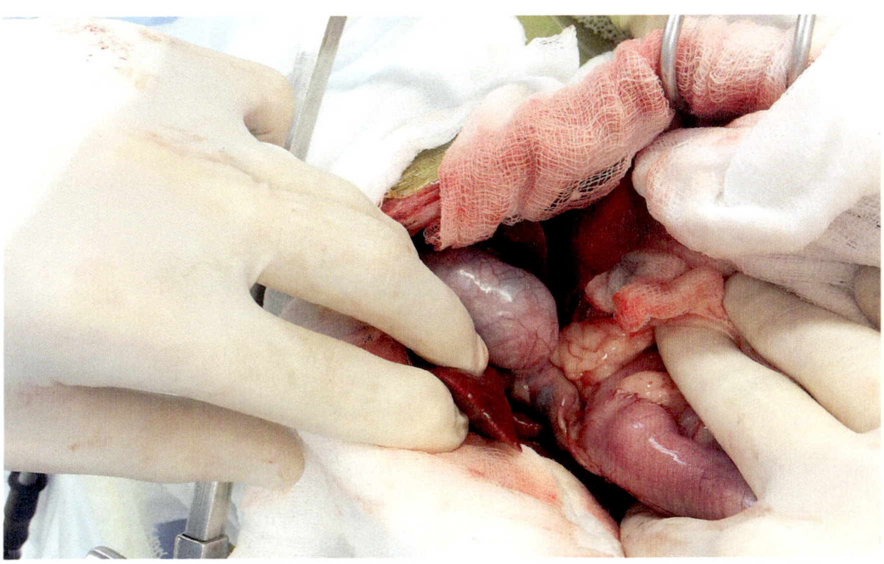

Figure 117. Obstruction of the common bile duct causing distension.

response syndrome (SIRS). Multimodal analgesia is required, best provided by an epidural catheter to reduce the systemic side effects of the high doses of opioids and lidocaine infusions which are frequently needed. Patients may also require nutritional support following surgery and placing a gastrostomy tube following cholecystectomy should be considered.

Portosystemic Shunts

Portosystemic shunts are abnormal vessels which allow blood to bypass the liver; hence evading the filtration system and immunological function of the liver, and exposing the rest of the body to toxins, bacteria, and metabolites which are normally removed. The reduction in blood flow to the liver also impairs development of the liver both with respect to its size and ability to perform protein synthesis and carbohydrate metabolism to maintain blood glucose levels. **Portosystemic shunts may be congenital or acquired.** The figures 114, 118, 119 and 120 show the normal portal vascular drainage to the liver from the digestive tract, as well as common conformations of congenital portosystemic shunts, which may occur within the liver, or outside of the liver between the portal vein and the caudal vena cava, or between the portal vein and the azygous vein. The larger the shunting vessel the greater the increase in preferential flow through the shunt, rather than the liver.

Acquired shunts typically occur in older animals as **the result of end stage liver disease or cirrhosis.** In this setting the liver function is reduced, and the liver is no longer able to accommodate the blood flow it receives, so multiple small vessels develop to allow drainage back into the circulation, usually around the left kidney. (Figure 121).

Young animals with congenital portosystemic shunts may **present with neurological signs or seizures** from the toxic effects of metabolites on the brain, due stunted growth, which is associated with polyuria/polydipsia and

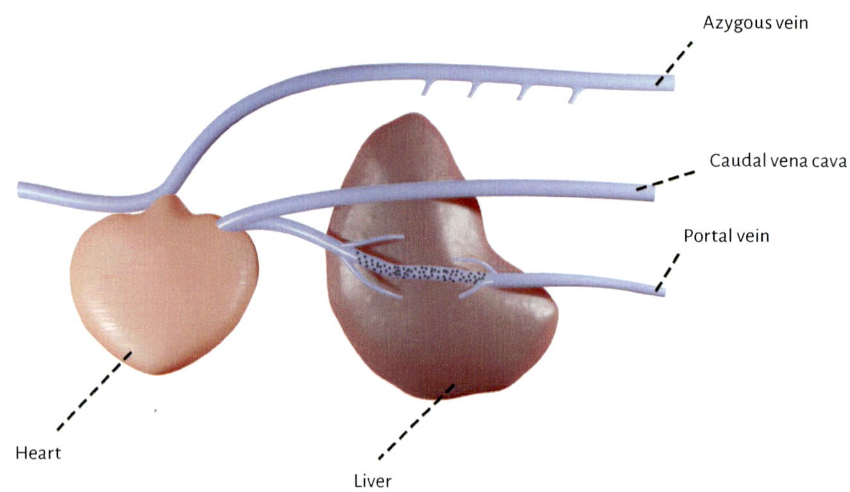

Figure 118. Intrahepatic shunt.

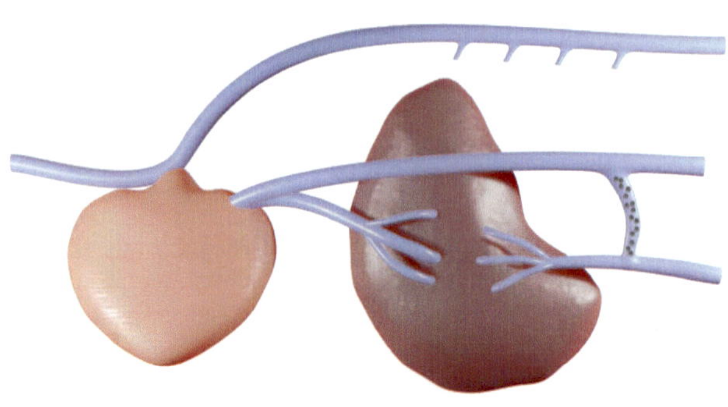

Figure 119. Portocaval shunt.

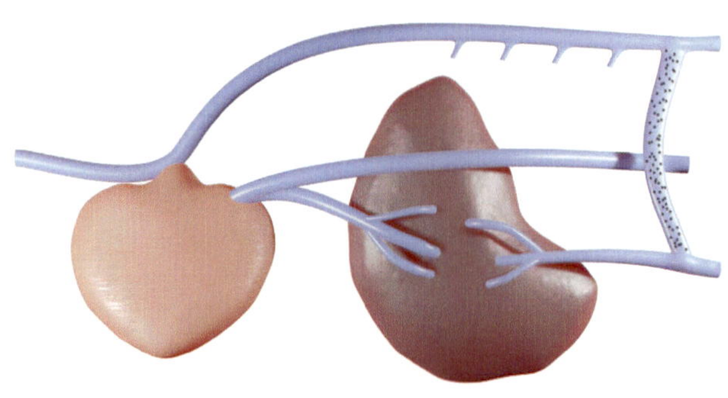

Figure 120. Portazygous shunt.

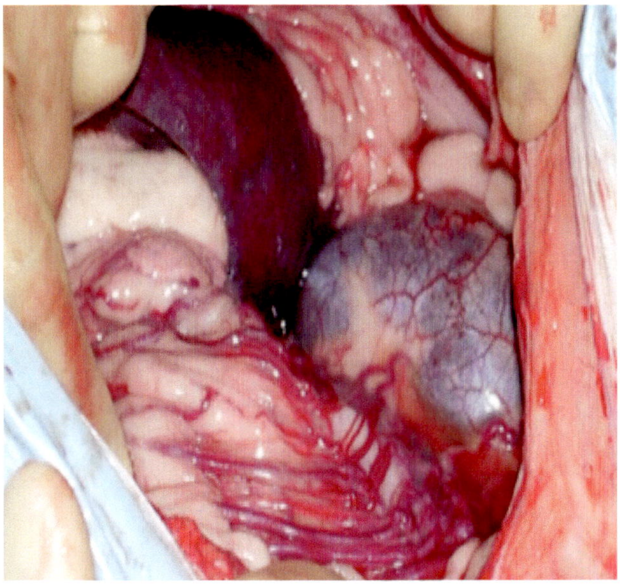

Figure 121. Multiple acquired shunts draining towards the left kidney.

gastrointestinal signs, or due to urinary tract obstruction with urolithiasis due to the propensity to form urate calculi.

Laboratory testing reveals mild elevation of liver enzymes (ALT, AST) with low BUN, cholesterol, and albumin. Bile acids are elevated, even more so following feeding in a bile acid stimulation test, as the bile acids are normally cycled between the intestine and the liver via the portal vasculature and the biliary system, but with a shunt they make their way into the general circulation bypassing the liver.

Patients are initially managed medically, with lactulose (orally, or by enema in acute emergency situations) to reduce intestinal transit time and reduce the accumulation of bacteria and their metabolites and trap ammonia within the gastrointestinal tract, antibiotics to limit intestinal flora and a restricted-protein diet. **Long term survival is better for patients undergoing surgical management** than those maintained medically and so surgery is recommended after a month of medical stabilisation (Greenhalgh et al., 2014).

Diagnostic imaging by means of ultrasound or computed tomography angiography (CTA) is performed to identify the location of the shunt vessel, and most importantly its point of entry into the normal circulation. The aim of surgery is to locate this point of communication within the general circulation and either acutely ligate or slowly attenuate the shunt vessel at this level, depending on the size of the vessel, the development of the liver and its internal vascular structure and the ability of the liver to cope with redirection of blood flow.

Gradual attenuation of the shunt vessel is achieved by placing of an ameroid constrictor (a metal ring lined with a hygroscopic material which, slowly absorbs water from the body, closing the space at its centre around the vessel) or cellophane band (secured with vascular staples). **Intrahepatic shunts,** which are more common in larger breeds of dog, may be managed by interventional procedures using coils and stents to close the shunt vessel off from the inside to avoid significant surgical risk.

Following surgery patients must be monitored for postattenuation neurological syndrome (PANS) including seizures (due to the change in exposure of the brain to toxins). Also, there are risks of increased pressure in the portal vein, which can cause abdominal pain, ileus, and diarrhoea, as well as ascites and abdominal distention. Most complications occur in the first 72-hours following surgery.

Long-term, following complete shunt occlusion the liver develops to a normal size and the patient may gradually have medication discontinued and return to a normal diet.

Urogenital System

Anatomy of the Urogenital System

The kidneys receive 25% of cardiac output via the paired renal arteries. The blood is filtered, and urine produced, which flows from the renal pelvis down the ureters to the bladder, where urine is stored prior to micturition. Urine then passes via the urethra, which varies in both length and diameter significantly between sexes. The shorter wider urethra in females (Figure 122), leaves them at increased risk of ascending urinary tract infection and incontinence associated with either ectopic ureters or urethral sphincter mechanism incompetence. Whilst males are at lower risk of these clinical problems, their longer, narrower urethras are more prone to obstruction by either urethral spasm or due to urolithiasis.

The female reproductive tract consists of **paired ovaries,** suspended caudal to the kidneys on each side from the dorsal body wall by the suspensory ligaments. They receive their blood supply from the ovarian arteries through a fatty, vascular pedicle. **The ovary then attaches to the uterine horn by the proper ligament.** The uterine horns come together in the caudal abdomen to form the uterine body and then the cervix, which sits sandwiched between the bladder neck ventrally and the rectum dorsally. The vagina then extends through the pelvis, with the urethra entering the floor of the vestibule.

The male testes descend from a location similar to that of the ovary during development and pass through the inguinal canal and into the scrotum. Hence the vas deferens traces this

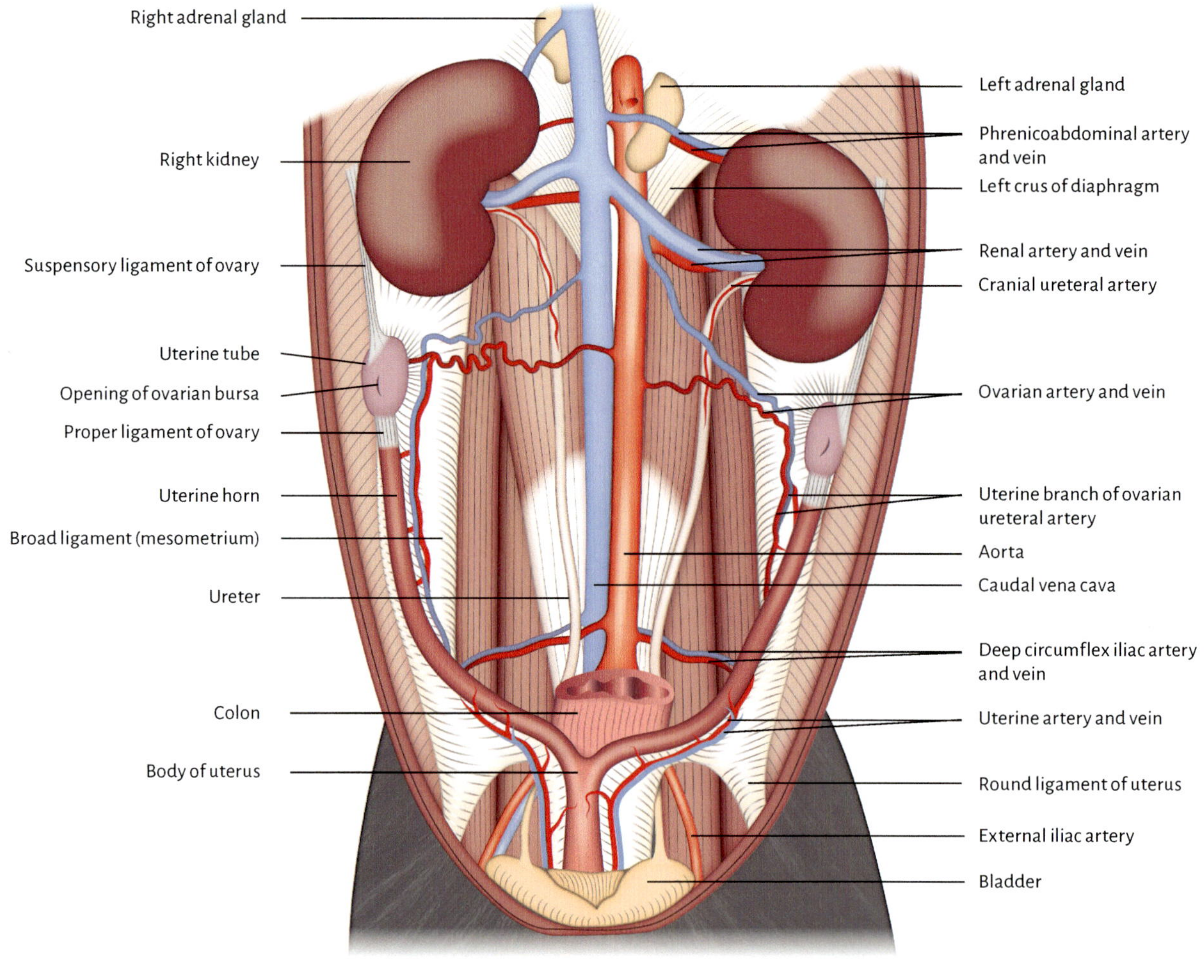

Figure 122. Female urogenital system.

course back through the inguinal canal and loops around to meet the prostate gland dorsally, caudal to the bladder neck. The male urethra runs a similar course to that of the female along the floor of the pelvis, but then continues in the male dog around the ischial arch and along the ventral aspect external to the pelvis and along the length of the penis. **The narrowest point, which is frequently a site of obstruction with uroliths,** is where the urethra enters the os penis. In cats the course is less tortuous, ending in the perineal region, but still longer and markedly tapered through the feline penis.

Pyometra

Aetiology

Pyometra (Figure 123) **is common in middle-aged entire bitches,** with around 25% of non-neutered female dogs being affected by the age of 10 years (it is much less common in cats). Uterine infection results secondarily due to cystic endometrial hyperplasia (CEH) **under the influence of the hormone progesterone.** Progesterone promotes the development of endometrial glandular tissue, which produces secretions, as well as reducing uterine contractility, allowing secretions to accumulate, providing an ideal environment for bacterial growth. Added to this the local immunity is also compromised under the influence of progesterone. *E. coli* are the most commonly identified bacteria associated with pyometra.

Presentation

Dogs most frequently present with pyometra around 6–8 weeks following a season, and typically show lethargy, inappetence, abdominal discomfort, and polyuria/polydipsia, with vaginal discharge present in more than 50% of cases (open pyometra). Hyperthermia, tachypnoea, and tachycardia are frequently noted on physical examination, with more than half of cases showing systemic inflammatory response syndrome (SIRS).

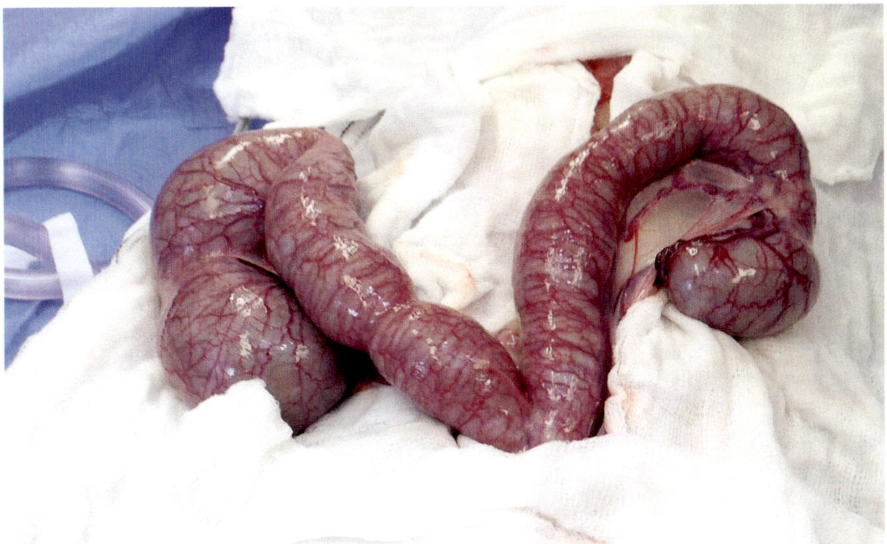

Figure 123. Appaearance of the uterus with pyometra at surgery.

Diagnosis

Blood work reveals elevated neutrophil numbers, with a degenerative left shirt and toxic change often with normocytic, normochromic anaemia, due to loss into the uterus and reduced production due to bone marrow suppression. Polyuria/polydipsia is proposed to be the result of an *E. coli* toxin induced effect, or as the result of glomerulonephritis and may be associated with azotaemia.

Abdominal imaging reveals a fluid filled and distended uterus. Infrequently, uterine rupture may be associated with abdominal effusion and septic peritonitis.

Treatment

Without doubt the treatment of choice is ovariohysterectomy, which generally results in a rapid recovery and performed appropriately prevents recurrence. Preoperative stabilisation however is key, with administration of **intravenous fluids** to restore circulating volume and broad-spectrum **perioperative antibiotics.** Standard ovariohysterectomy is performed by releasing the suspensory ligaments of the ovaries, ligating the ovarian and uterine arteries and veins, as well as larger branching vessels in the broad ligaments which support the uterine horns. The vessels are typically much more developed and engorged during pyometra than during routine ovariohysterectomy in a healthy bitch. The uterine body is itself clamped to prevent spillage and then ligated, often with a transfixing suture to prevent slippage, as close to the cervix as possible. The stump is then lavaged before abdominal closure.

Following surgery, patients should remain on intravenous fluid therapy until adequate oral intake is achieved and receive appropriate multimodal analgesia. Antibiotics are continued postoperatively in patients who are systemically unwell with sepsis, urinary tract infection, or in those with surgical contamination. The mortality rate with surgery is reported to be less than 5%, with risk of mortality higher in those who are systemically unwell at the time of assessment and treatment.

Medical management may be considered in bitches who are not systemically unwell with SIRS, if the bitch is intended for future breeding, or has co-morbidities which otherwise complicate surgical treatment. Treatments consists of at least 14 days of appropriate antibiotic therapy, to prevent bacteraemia and sepsis, as well as medication to stimulate cervical relaxation and uterine contraction to eliminate the infection. Treatment has been reported to be effective in 75% of cases and should be monitored by documenting vaginal discharge with repeat assessment of uterine emptying on ultrasonography. With successful medical treatment there **remains a similar risk of recurrent disease** in the future of between 30 and 50%. In cases which do not respond to medical management, transcervical catheter placement for uterine lavage and drainage has been reported with a good outcome in 75% of cases (Gobello et al., 2003).

Urolithiasis

There are a variety of uroliths which may form at any level within the urinary tract. Generally, **uroliths form more frequently in concentrated urine,** and often as the result of a **metabolic or nutritional abnormality** which results in a saturated solution of precursors for the uroliths. Discussion of all the metabolic causes and management advice is beyond the scope of this text, but further information is available on the urolith centre website: www.urolithcenter.org.

The most commonly identified uroliths are:

- **Oxalate:** these are common, calcium based radiopaque uroliths.
- **Struvite:** these common uroliths are less radiopaque. They form as a consequence of urinary tract infection due to bacterial production of the enzyme urease. They may often be dissolved if not causing an acute obstruction, by treating the underlying infection, and acidifying the urine by dietary modification.
- **Urate:** these stones are most commonly identified in Dalmatians, (who lack a transporter responsible for the degradation of uric acid) and patients with portosystemic shunts.
- **Cystine:** these stones are most common in entire male dogs due to an androgen responsive defect in transporters of cystine in the renal tubules. Treatment includes castration to manage the condition and prevent genetic transmission.

Urethral Obstruction and Bladder Stones

Uroliths form within the bladder and irritate the lining, causing **signs of cystitis** such as haematuria, pollakiuria, and stranguria. The uroliths may move and if too large to be voided lead to **acute obstruction of the urethra,** causing stranguria and anuria. In turn this causes **postrenal obstruction,** with azotaemia, lethargy, vomiting and even bladder rupture.

Patients with urinary tract obstruction **develop hyperkalaemia,** which progressively causes bradycardia and cardiac dysfunction. Emergency treatment requires establishment of urine drainage by urethral catheterisation past the obstruction or urinary diversion by cystostomy tube placement across the abdominal wall. Fluid therapy is essential to correct electrolyte disturbances. In extreme cases, this may be aided by the administration of glucose and insulin to cause potassium to be taken up into cells along with the glucose under the influence of the potassium. Calcium may have a cardioprotective effect.

Radiopaque uroliths may be observed on abdominal radiographs (Figure 124). If uroliths are radiolucent, they may be highlighted by performing a retrograde urethrogram with iodinated contrast to outline the uroliths. Ultrasonography reveals shadowing due to the presence of uroliths within the bladder and urethra but cannot assess the intrapelvic portion of the urethra.

Following emergency stabilisation, the patient most frequently requires surgery to remove the uroliths by cystotomy, although endoscopy and laser lithotripsy may be possible at centres with appropriate equipment.

Cystotomy (Figure 125) is performed by caudal midline coeliotomy, the bladder is handled gently with stay sutures, and isolated with moist laparotomy sponges. An incision is made into the bladder with a fresh number 11 scalpel blade and enlarged to allow removal of the uroliths with a surgeon's finger, sterile teaspoon, or curette. The largest rigid urinary catheter possible should be passed and repeatedly flushed through with warm sterile saline, along the length of the urethra, to hydropulse any urethral uroliths back into the bladder for removal until the surgeon is satisfied the catheter passes easily without any ongoing resistance. Following surgical closure, radiography should be repeated to ensure all the uroliths were removed.

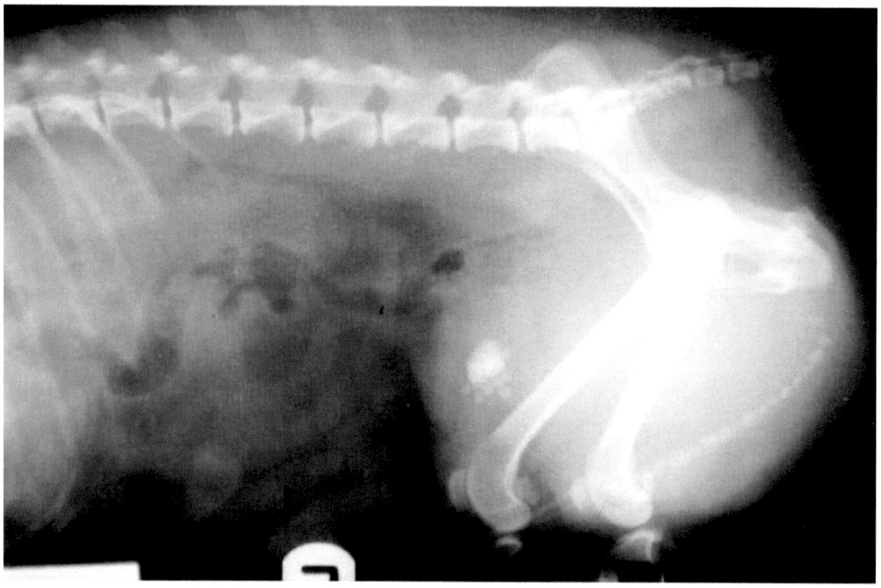

Figure 124. Abdominal radiograph showing urolithiasis within the bladder and extending along the length of the urethra.

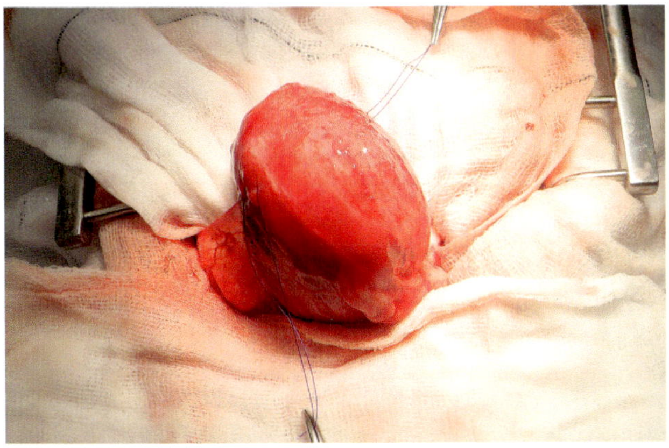

Figure 125. The bladder exposed and isolated at surgery for open cystotomy.

Alternatively, **laparoscopic assisted cystotomy minimises the incision size** into the abdominal wall and bladder and provides a magnified view inside the bladder and proximal urethra to aid in the detection and removal of uroliths. (Figure 126).

Ureteral Obstruction

Uroliths may also form in the kidneys (nephroliths), which then fragment and pass into the ureters. Signs of ureteral obstruction are similar to those of urethral obstruction but without straining to void urine, and are most commonly seen in **middle-aged to older cats due to calcium oxalate stone formation.** Ureteral obstruction in dogs and cats may also occur due to inadvertent entrapment of the ureters during suture placement for ovariohysterectomy.

Following initial medical stabilisation surgery is usually required to alleviate the obstruction. Obstruction is alleviated by **ureterotomy for stone removal,** which requires the use of an operating microscope due to the small size of the ureter. Alternatively, the obstruction is bypassed by the passage of a ureteral stent to allow flow through the ureter past the urolith. **Ureteral stents** (Figure 127) are placed over a guidewire, passed from the kidney or the bladder, along the length of the ureter and require the use of fluoroscopy or intraoperative radiography to assess correct placement. The stent is then retained in place by the pigtail shape at either end.

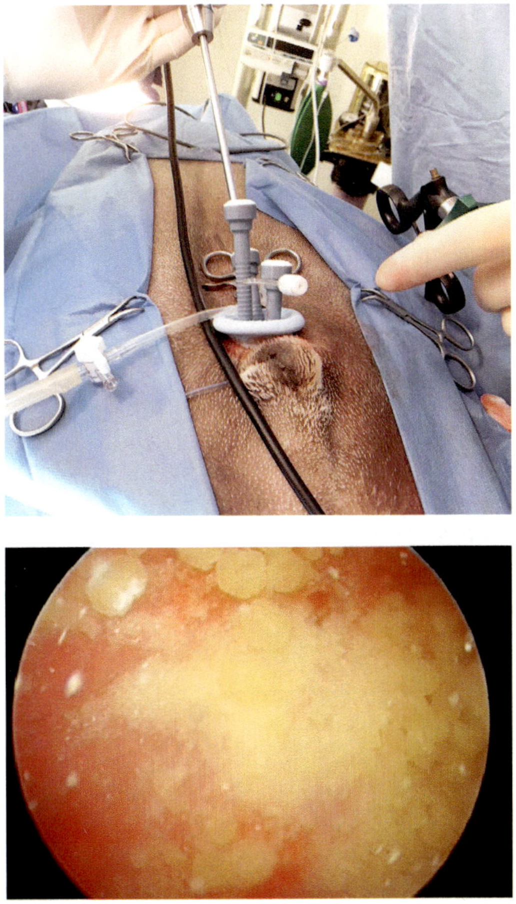

Figure 126. Laparoscopic-assisted cystotomy performed in a dog to remove uroliths.

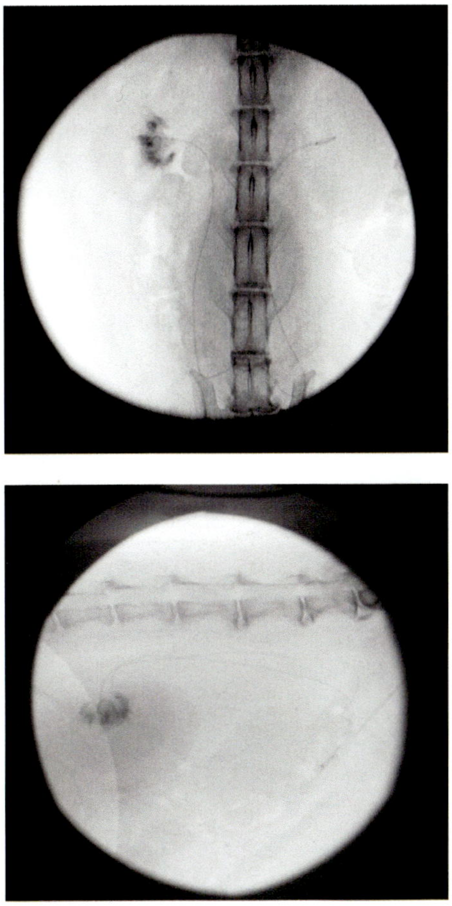

Figure 127. Ureteral stent placement at surgery visualised with fluoroscopy.

An alternative is placement of a **subcutaneous ureteral bypass (SUB) device** (Figure 128). This consists of pigtailed catheters being placed through the walls of the kidney and bladder and sealed in position with sutures and glue to hold a Dacron patch seal around the connection. The tubes are then linked by a port which sits under the skin over the abdominal wall. The port allows for sampling and flushing of the SUB device to check its patency and assess for evidence of infection.

Following surgical treatment, the patient should continue on **intravenous fluid therapy** with close attention to electrolyte balance and resolution of azotaemia during recovery. **The use of non-steroidal anti-inflammatory medications should be avoided,** so analgesia may be largely opioid based. The patient should be monitored for sufficient urine production, evidence of urinary tract leakage, and uroabdomen. Following alleviation of an obstruction the kidneys often show a **rebound postobstructive diuresis,** over-producing dilute urine, and therefore fluid therapy should be adjusted to match urine output until normalisation and adequate oral intake of fluid. This requires diligent record keeping and weighing of litter trays and bedding if urinary catheters are not in place.

Ectopic Ureters

Ectopic ureters are a common cause of **continuous urine leakage incontinence** in young puppies. During development the connection of the ureters to the bladder does not form appropriately, with the ureters bypassing the bladder neck and entering the urethra more caudally, either passing within the wall of the bladder and urethra (intramural) or independently (extramural). Urine from the affected ureter(s) is not stored and leaks constantly via the urethra.

Diagnosis

Diagnosis is confirmed by ultrasonographic or intravenous urography (IVU), and ideally imaged by CT for assessment of the location of the ureters and their openings with respect to the bladder neck. The openings can be observed directly by urethrocystoscopy.

Treatment

Intramural ectopic ureters (Figure 129) can be treated **by laser ablation of the partition** in the wall of the urethra and bladder neck which prevents urine from entering the bladder. This requires the use of a cystoscope, surgical diode laser and fluoroscopy or intraoperative radiography to check positioning and to assess for urinary tract integrity at the end of the procedure. (Figure 130).

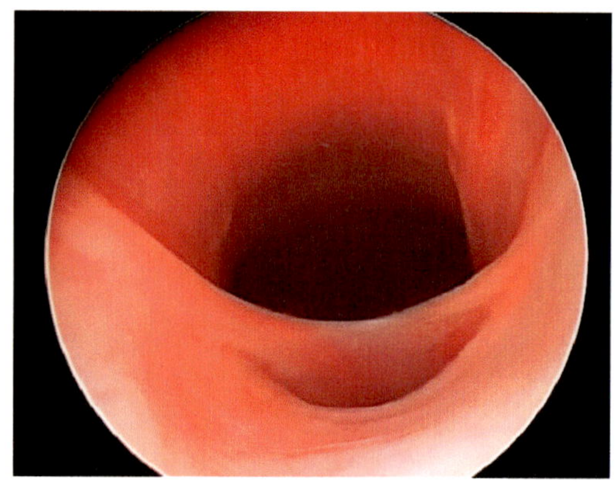

Figure 129. An Intramural ectopic ureter seen opening into the urethra of a puppy on cystoscopy.

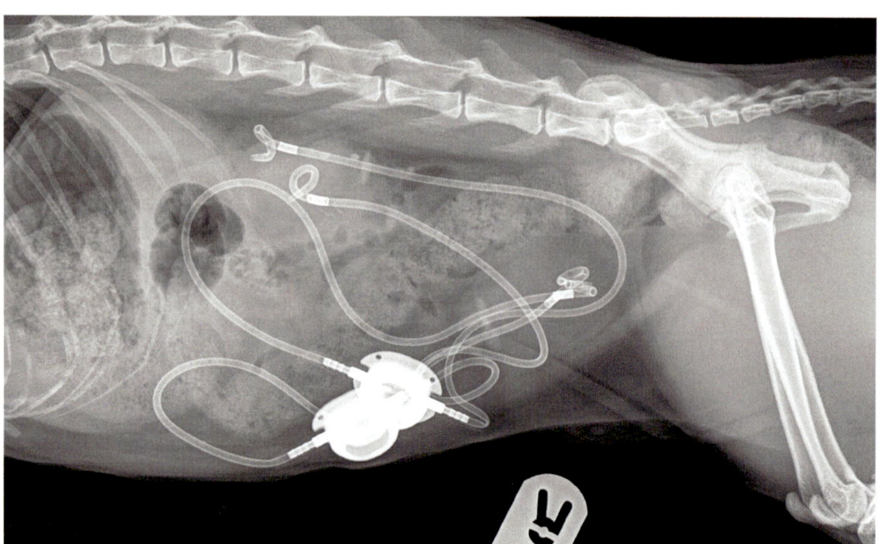

Figure 128. Subcutaneous ureteral bypass (SUB) devices placed bilaterally in a cat.

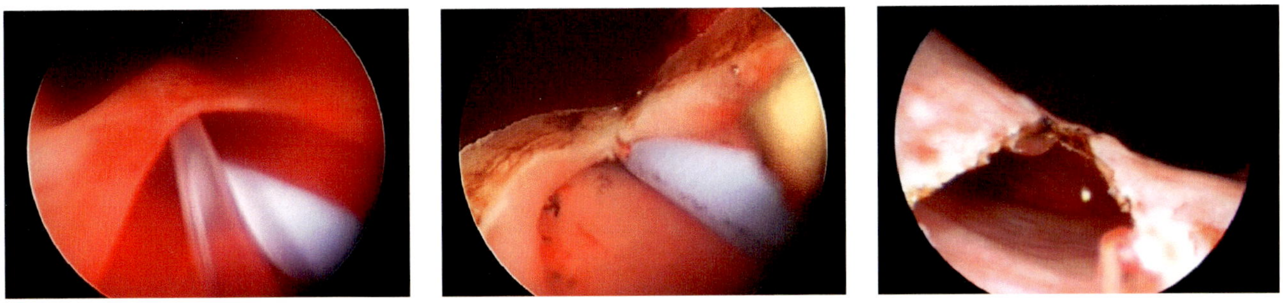

Figure 130. Laser ablation of the partition separating the intramural ectopic ureter from the urethra and bladder under cystoscopic guidance.

Extramural ectopic ureters require surgical resection and reimplantation into the bladder, which in smaller patients may require magnification with surgical loupes or an operating microscope.

Thoracic Anatomy and Surgical Access

Anatomy

The thoracic organs of dogs and cats are protected within the **cage formed by the spine, 13 pairs of ribs, and the sternum.** The thoracic wall enables breathing by expanding outwards to generate a negative intrathoracic pressure, causing expansion of the lungs, drawing air into the lungs. Both features create challenges for surgery. Firstly, **access is limited** to incisions between the ribs (intercostal thoracotomy), splitting the sternum (median sternotomy), or removal of diseased portions of the thoracic wall. Intercostal thoracotomy allows access through a narrow surgical window to the thorax. Secondly, **opening the thoracic cavity immediately eliminates the negative pressure needed to drive ventilation,** and so positive pressure ventilation must be performed by the anaesthetist, either manually or using a mechanical ventilator for the duration of the surgical procedure. Further complicating access into the thorax are the muscles of the thoracic wall. There are the muscles which attach the forelimb to the trunk, muscles which support and move the cervical spine, muscles of the abdominal wall and the intercostal muscles themselves. Figure 131 shows those muscles, with the forelimb removed.

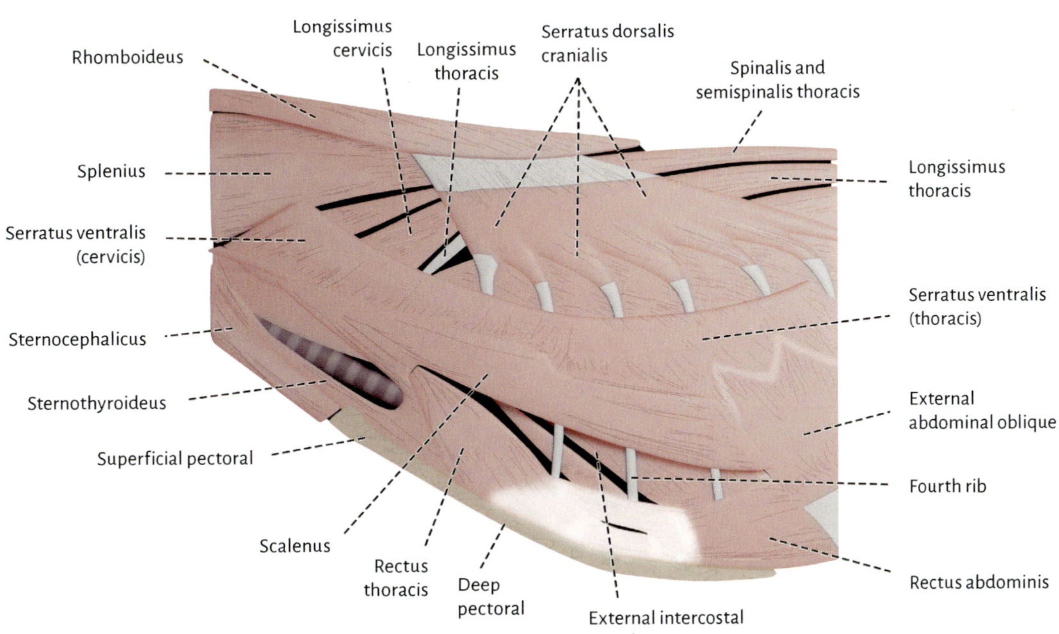

Figure 131. Thoracic wall anatomy.

Access via the sternum (Figure 132 and 133) **requires** less muscular dissection, as only the pectoral muscles attach to the sternebrae, however access requires orthopaedic instruments for access and closure.

The major vessels and nerves to the thoracic wall run immediately behind each rib (intercostal vessels and nerves). The internal thoracic vessels also run parallel to the sternum.

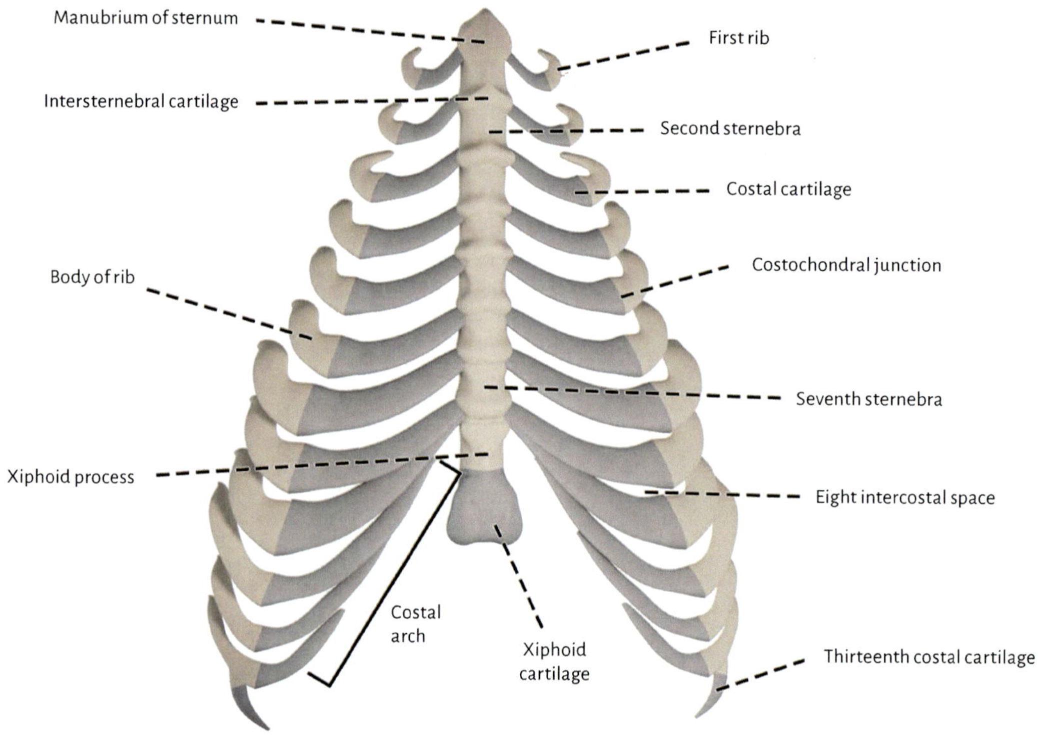

Figure 132. Sternum.

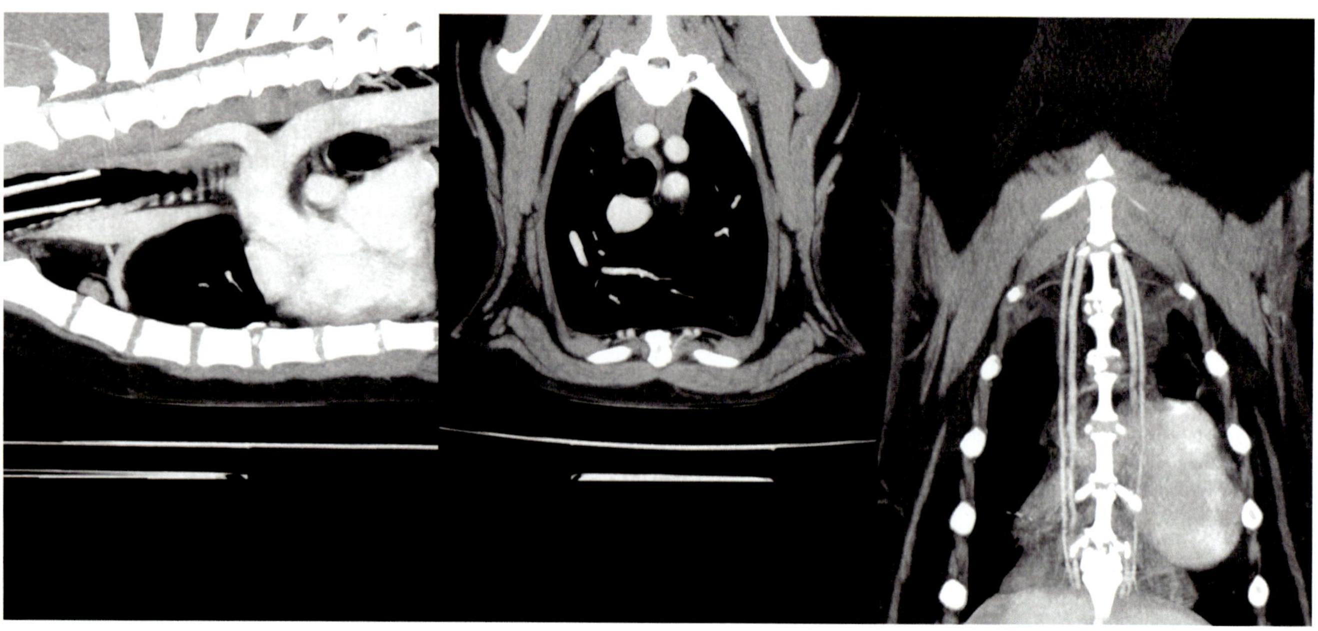

Figure 133. Appearance of the sternum on a CT scan.

The lungs (Figure 134) **of the dog and cat are subdivided into seven lobes.** On the left the cranial and caudal parts of the left cranial lung lobe are incompletely divided; meaning they are frequently removed as one when lung lobectomy is required. There is a large left caudal lobe. On the right side there are cranial, middle, and caudal lobes, with an accessory lobe, arising from the right caudal bronchus, with the accessory lung lobe sitting caudal to the heart in the midline within a reflection of the mediastinum, with the caudal vena cava on one side and the aorta and oesophagus on the other.

Surgical Access

Intercostal Thoracotomy

Intercostal thoracotomy (Figures 135, 136, 137) allows **access to a limited area** of the thoracic cavity on one side of the thoracic cavity. This technique is most useful for **accessing the lungs and the heart base.** The surgeon must consider the surgery to be performed inside the thorax when considering where to make the intercostal thoracotomy due to the limited access. Note that although the lungs may inflate and fill the thorax, generally, removal of a lung lobe requires access to the hilus of the lungs at the heart base, and so most lung lobectomies can be performed by a fifth intercostal thoracotomy. (See Table 4).

When preparing for thoracic surgery, it is important to consider the surgery to be performed, and also drain placement at the end of surgery to allow restoration of the intrathoracic negative pressure (needed for ventilation), so **the entire thoracic wall must be clipped, prepared, and draped out for surgery.** This also assists the surgeon in counting the ribs to ensure the incision is made at the appropriate intercostal space.

A linear incision is made dorsoventrally at the appropriate intercostal space. Dissection continues through the thin

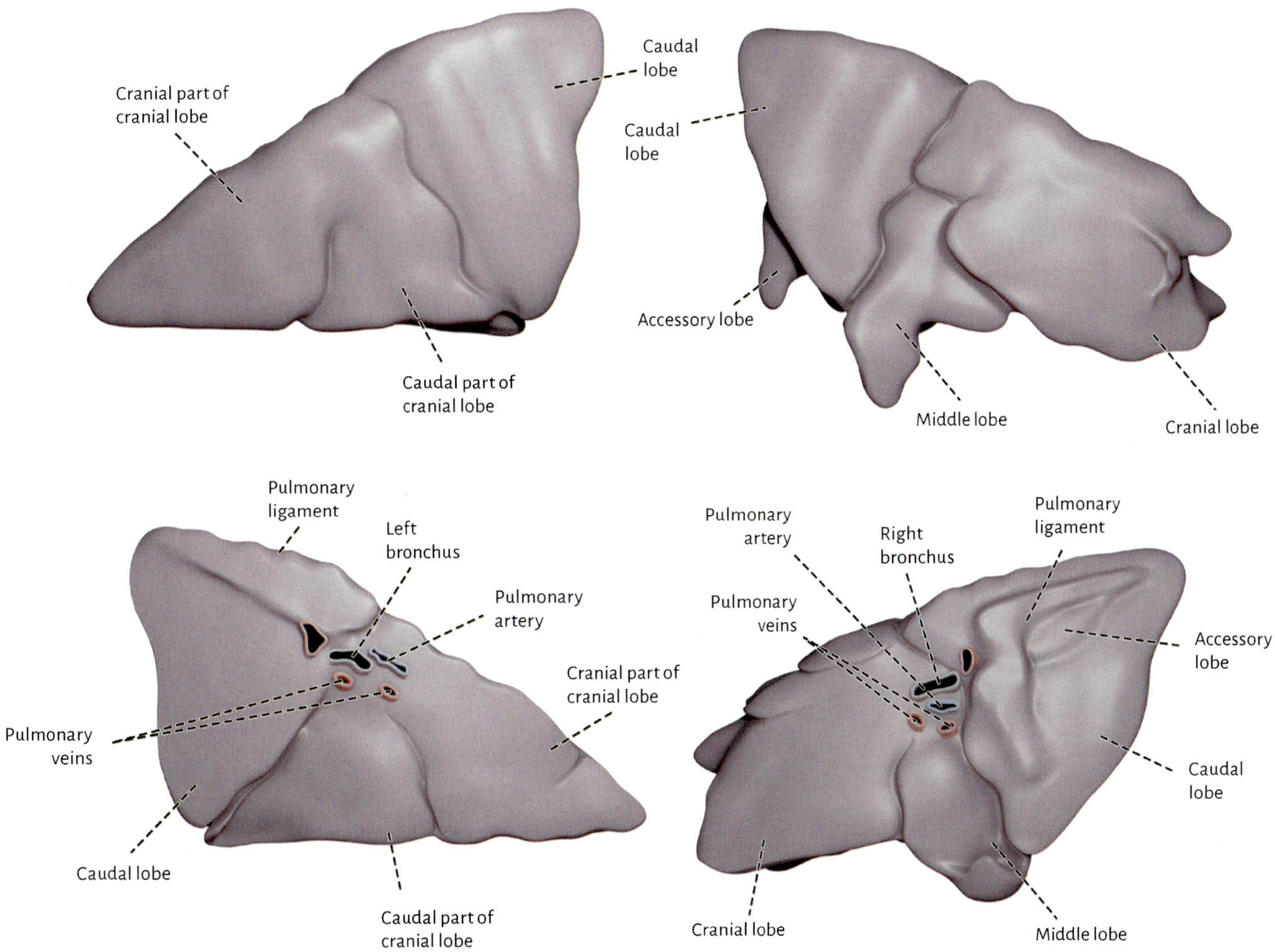

Figure 134. Lung anatomy.

cutaneous trunci muscle and subcutaneous tissue and then the latissimus dorsi is retracted dorsally by a surgical assistant using a Langenbeck retractor.

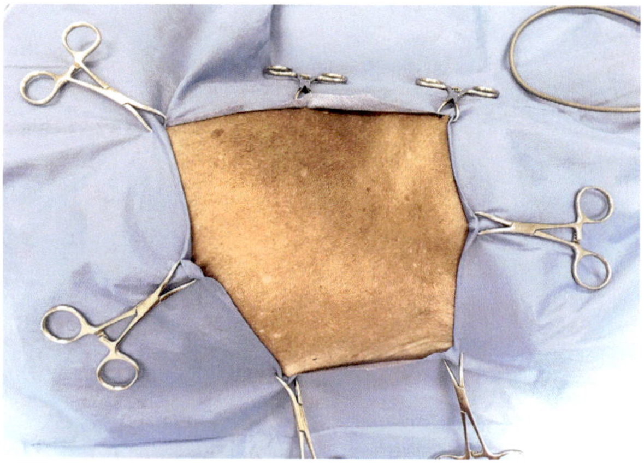

Figure 135. Intercostal thoracotomy draping.

Table 4. Intercostal location.

Thoracic structure		Intercostal space	
		Left	Right
Heart		4–5	
Right atrium			4–5
PDA		4	
Pulmonic stenosis		4	
Pericardiectomy		5	
Lung		4–6	
Cranial lobe		4/5	4/5
Middle lobe			5
Caudal lobe		5/6	5/6
Diaphragm		7–10	7–10
Thoracic duct	Dog		8–10
	Cat	8–10	
Oesophagus	Cranial/mid	4–6	
	Mid/caudal	7–9	7–9

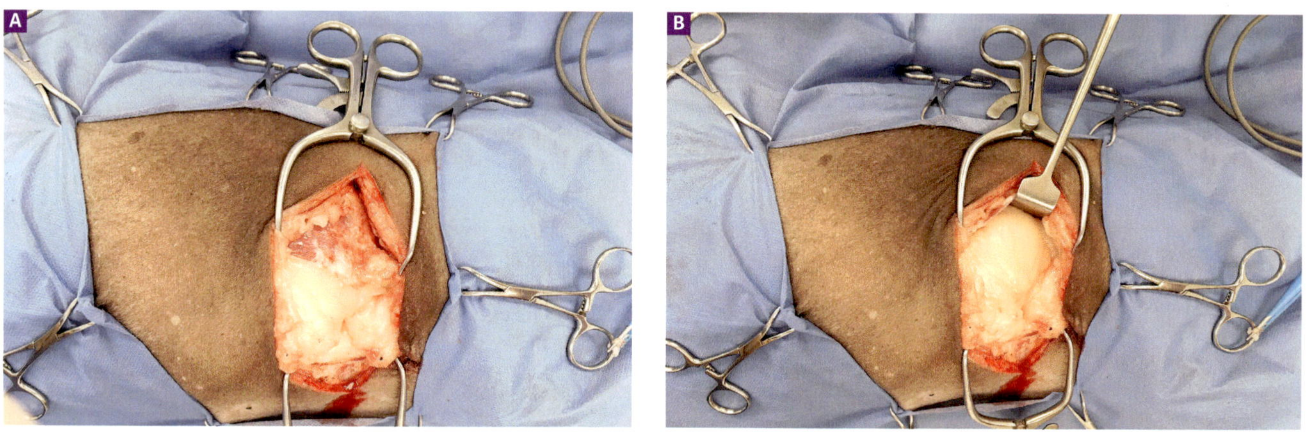

Figure 136. A. Intercostal thoracotomy incision; **B.** Intercostal thoracotomy with latissimus dorsi retracted using a Langenbeck.

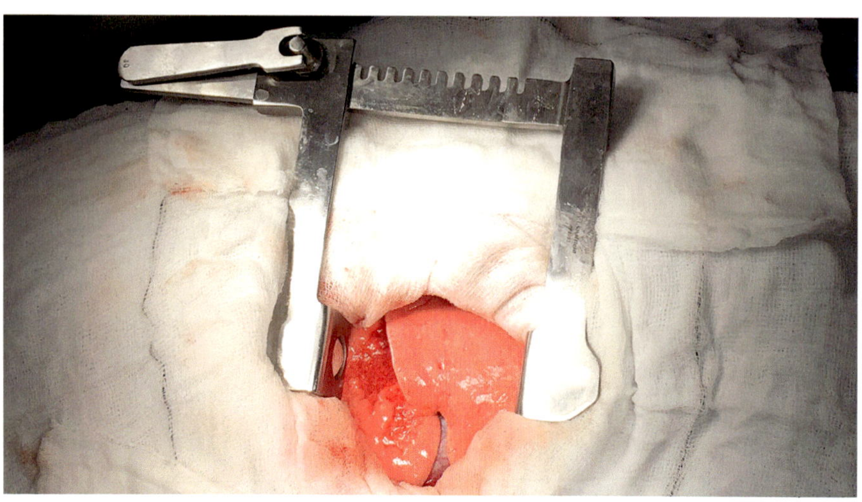

Figure 137. Finochietto placement to retract the ribs.

Dissection continues between the muscles to expose the intercostal space. The intercostal muscles are split to open the thorax, remembering that the vessels and nerves are just behind each rib, so **the incision is made slightly more caudal than halfway between the ribs.** The anaesthetist should prepare to ventilate the patient. Moist laparotomy sponges are used to pack off the chest wall and protect the ribs and Finochietto rib spreaders used to open the thoracic access. In very small patients, Gelpi's may suffice (Figure 137).

Prior to closure of the thoracic wall, it is **essential to place a thoracic drain.** The ribs are reapposed by placing interrupted sutures around the ribs immediately in front of and behind the intercostal incision. This must be performed delicately to avoid perforating the intercostal vessels behind those ribs or the lungs which continue to inflate and move inside the thorax during the procedure. Hence the surgeon passes the blunt end of the needle around the rib to reduce the risk of injury as the needle bluntly dissects its path through the chest wall. Therefore, the needle should be loaded in reverse as shown in Figure 138.

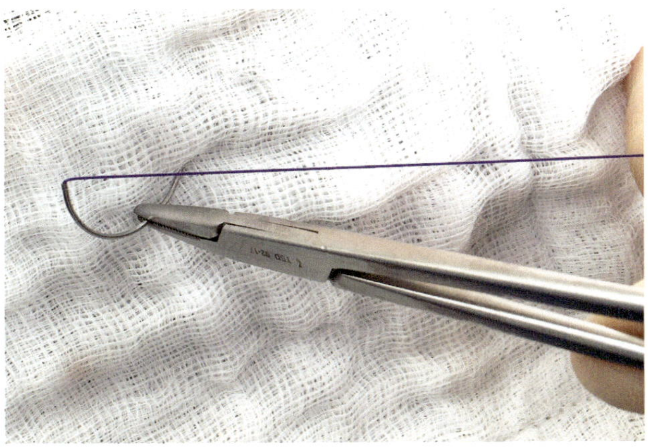

Figure 138. Reverse needle grip for passage around the ribs.

Each interrupted suture is **preplaced as a stay suture** as tightening one prohibits safe placement of the next. All the sutures are closed in turn once all are in place. Each one is tightened sufficiently to reappose the ribs but not to overlap them and deform the chest wall. As a result the chest wall is not air-tight until the muscles and subcutaneous tissue are reconstructed over the ribs. During this time the chest drain should be left open to allow the pressure to equalise and prevent a tension pneumothorax which would prevent ventilation. The chest drain is only drained and sealed at the end of surgery. (Figure 139).

Median Sternotomy

Median sternotomy, splitting part or all the sternum, gives **access to both sides of the thorax** which may be required for full exploration of the thorax to treat more diffuse disease affecting the mediastinum and pleura. Surgical access is less restricted and so this method is preferred for removal of larger lung masses, which may not be possible through a smaller intercostal incision. However, access to the lung hilus is more challenging due to the depth of the chest with the ventral incision. In preparation, **the entire thoracic wall should be clipped and prepared.** Draping should allow exposure of the sternum but also allow for thoracic drain placement. (Figure 140).

Median sternotomy (Figure 141) **requires a skin incision along the ventral midline.** The pectoral muscles are elevated off the midline to allow access to the bone; this is achieved with a **periosteal elevator or monopolar diathermy.** Once prepared the sternebrae are cut one by one with an **oscillating saw,** whilst under constant irrigation and suction to cool the saw blade. Once open the incised edges are protected with moist laparotomy sponges and the sternebrae retracted using Finochietto rib spreaders. The sternal incision may be the entire length of the sternum, but commonly surgeons **maintain the**

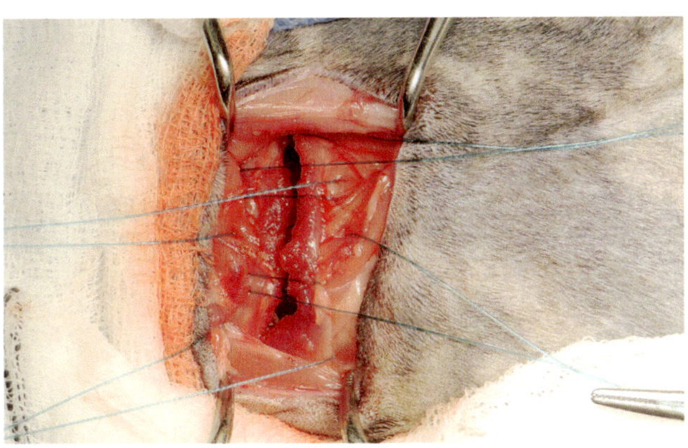

Figure 139. Intercostal closure.

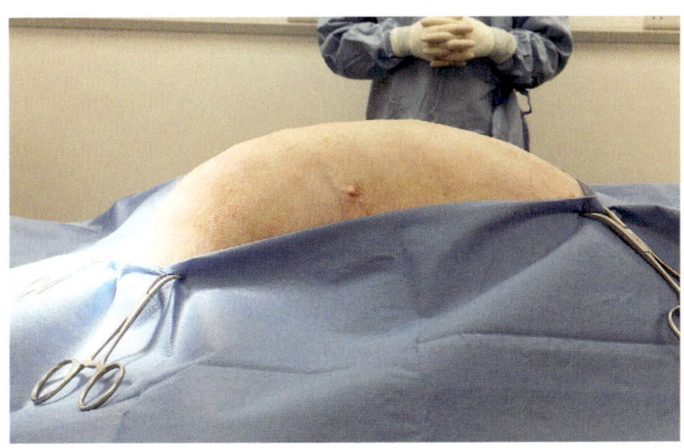

Figure 140. Sternotomy draping.

integrity of either the manubrium or the xyphoid at one end, to provide some inherent stability following closure.

When closing the sternum (Figure 142, 143, 144), at least for larger patients, the sternebrae are secured with orthopaedic wire. This requires not only the wire, but a graft passer to allow the wire to be atraumatically passed around the sternebrae, avoiding puncture of the internal thoracic vessels. The wire is then secured by twisting using snub-nosed wire twisters and the ends cut with pin and wire cutters. Wires are then sequentially tightened and cut short to leave two or three twists. The wire ends are flattened to the chest wall and covered by the pectoral muscles during closure of the incision.

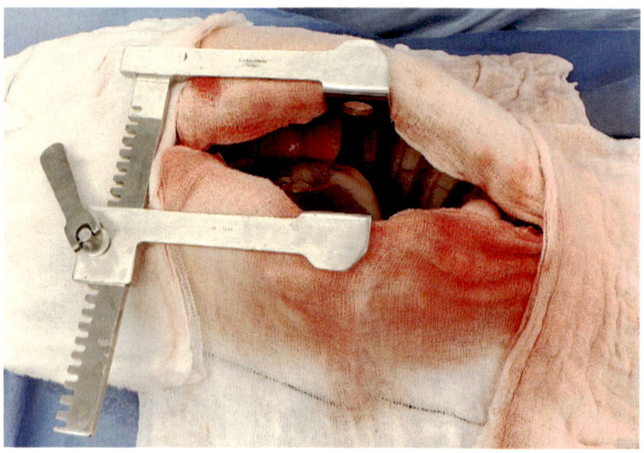

Figure 141. Median sternotomy.

Thoracoscopy

Thoracoscopy is performed with the patient in lateral recumbency or dorsal recumbency with ports placed intercostally, and/or under the xyphoid. (Figure 145).

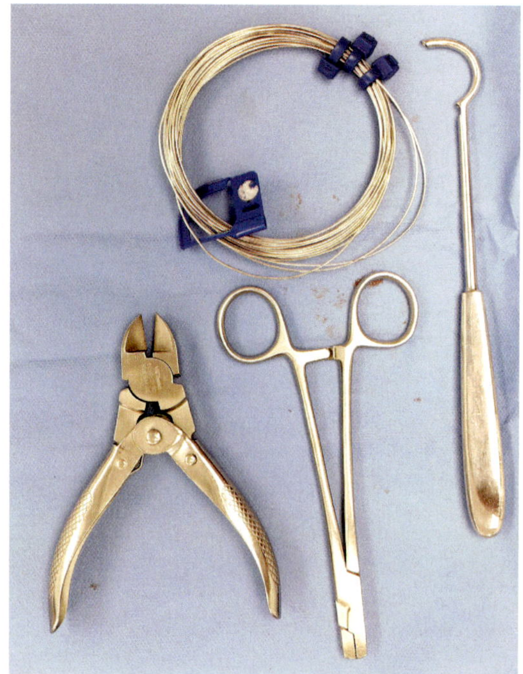

Figure 142. Sternal closure kit.

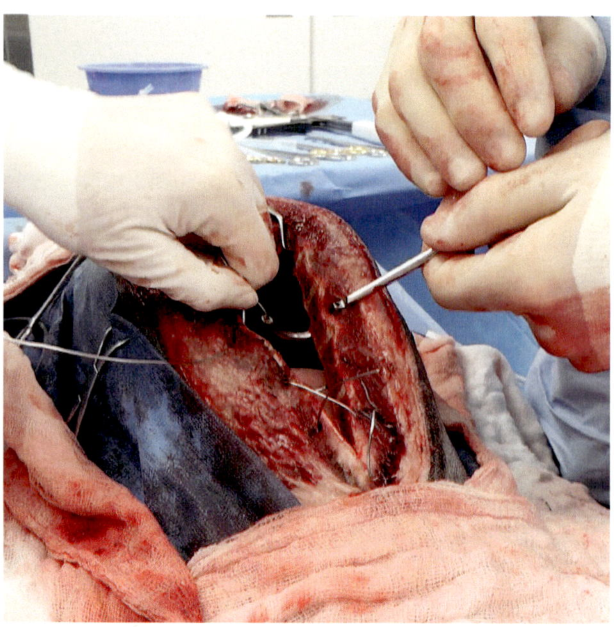

Figure 143. Sternal wire placement.

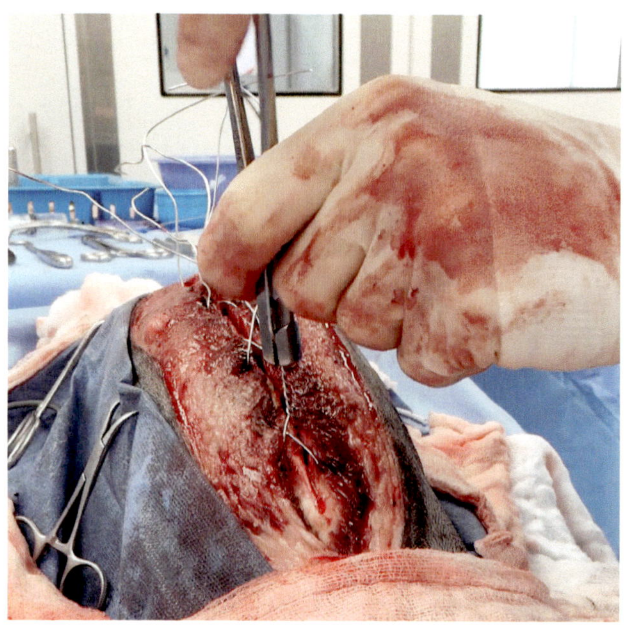

Figure 144. Sternal wire tightening.

When performing thoracoscopy there is a limited space inside the thorax for the surgeon to work, and so often one lung ventilation (Figure 146) is performed in the opposite side of the chest so that the operated lung collapses to create space for surgery. This **requires placement of a long endotracheal tube into a single bronchus,** or placement of an endobronchial blocker into the bronchus of the lung not to be inflated, using endoscopic guidance prior to surgery.

The operating room equipment must be arranged so the patient is in a line between the surgeon and the endoscope tower, to allow ergonomic use of the equipment. During thoracoscopy (Figures 6, 147 B, 148) with the patient in dorsal recumbency, e.g for thymoma removal or pericardiectomy, both lungs are only partially inflated to give room for surgical access.

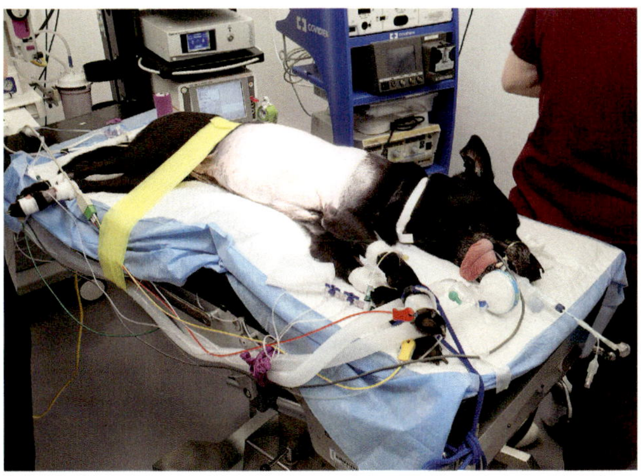

Figure 145. Thoracoscopy positioning (a patient being prepared for lateral thoracoscopy for removal of a lung lobe tumour).

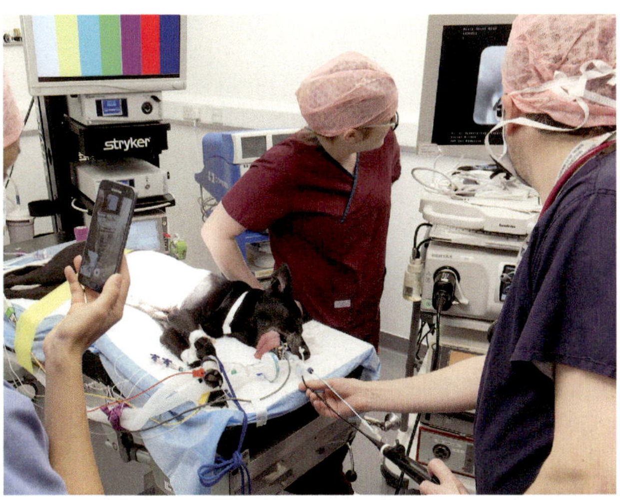

Figure 146. One lung ventilation being achieved by placement of an end-bronchial blocker in the upper most bronchus under endoscopic guidance.

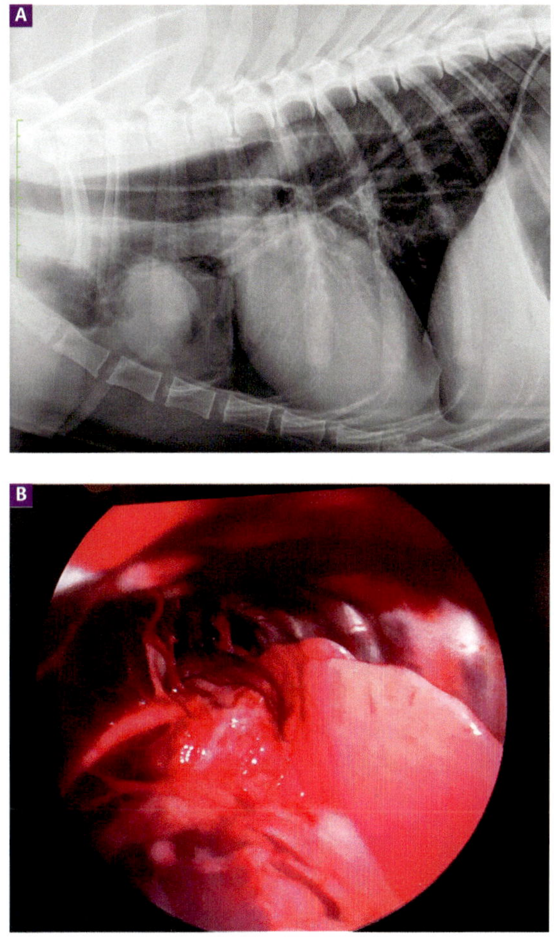

Figure 147. A. Radiograph of a patient with a thymoma; **B.** Thoracoscopic view of the same thymoma. The lungs can be seen on either side of the image. The tumour is in the centre of view just in front of the heart. Dissection of the mass requires the use of endoscopic vessel sealing devices and surgical staplers. Following freeing of the mass, the mass is placed into an endoscopic specimen retrieval bag to aid extraction, or as shown in Figure 148, one of the instrument ports is expanded and held wide open using an Alexis® wound retraction device to both protect the tissues and provide 360° retraction).

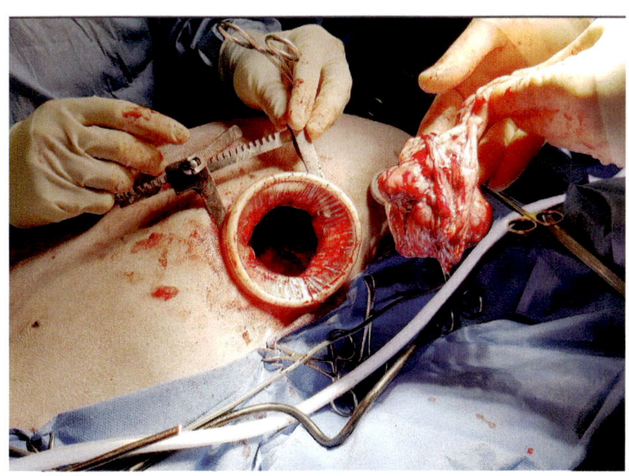

Figure 148. Alexis® wound retraction device.

Surgical Thoracic Pathology

Lung Tumours

Primary tumours (Figure 149) **of the lungs are uncommon in dogs and cats** accounting for 1% of tumours, most frequently affecting older patients. Almost all tumours of the lungs are **carcinomas,** derived from the epithelial tissue. Patients with lung tumours usually present with a cough, but may also suffer dyspnoea, haemoptysis, pyrexia, and exercise intolerance.

Diagnosis is by radiography or CT of the thorax (Figure 149). Sampling by ultrasound-guided fine needle aspiration might be possible for peripheral lesions, or by bronchoalveolar lavage or grab biopsy for lesions accessible by bronchoscopy.

Prognosis is more guarded for larger tumours, those with lymph node involvement, or not amenable to surgical removal. **CT provides the best preoperative assessment** of feasibility of removal and size of the tracheobronchial lymph nodes. At surgery the mass may be removed by lung lobectomy (Figure 150), or possibly by pneumonectomy (removal of an entire lung) for larger lesions close to the hilus or affecting more than one lobe. When possible, the draining lymph nodes are also removed to aid clinical staging.

Pneumothorax

Pneumothorax may result from blunt trauma to the thorax, penetrating injury to the chest wall, migrating foreign body penetration of the lung internally, neoplastic erosion of the lung, or due to spontaneous rupture of pulmonary bullae (air-filled pockets, commonly of unknown aetiology) (Figure 151) which rupture and create an air leak and a one-way valve in the affected lung, leading to tension pneumothorax.

In the acute setting, the pneumothorax must be managed by thoracic drain placement. It is essential that drain placement and investigation are performed to **maintain negative pressure and spontaneous ventilation,** because if the patient is anaesthetised and positive pressure ventilation performed this could rapidly worsen the pneumothorax (by pushing air through the one-way valve of the ruptured pulmonary bulla).

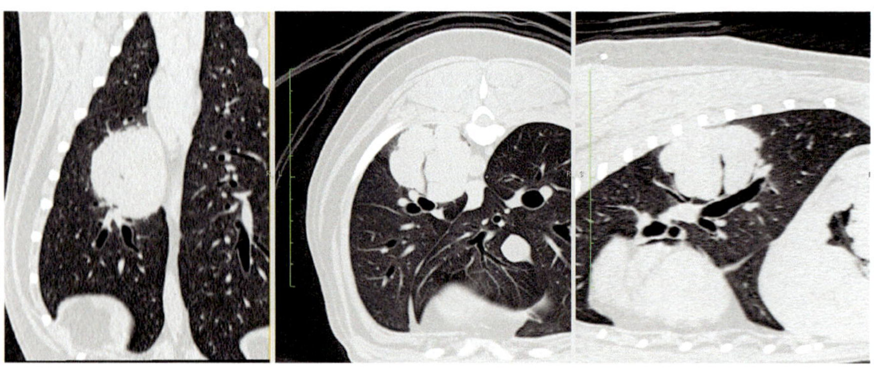

Figure 149. Lung mass diagnosed on CT.

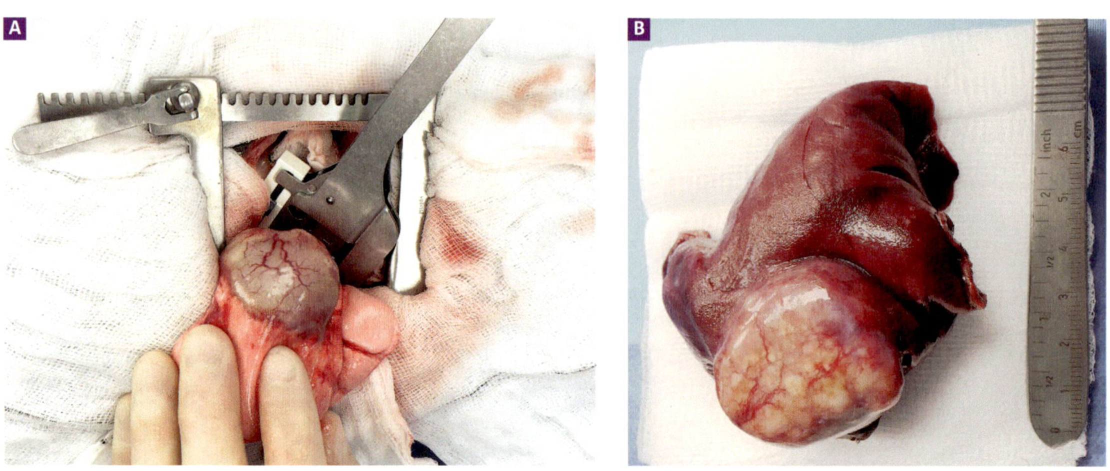

Figure 150. A. Lung lobectomy being performed using a TA stapler;
B. Lung mass following surgical removal.

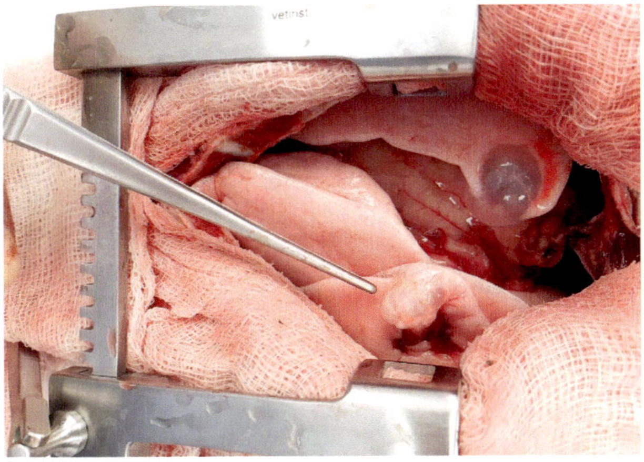

Figure 151. Bullae seen at the periphery of the lung lobes.

Continued thoracic drainage may lead to a natural sealing of the damaged pulmonary tissue, but relapses are common and so surgical removal of the damaged lung is usually considered. The location of the air leak, as well as secondary lesions cannot be guaranteed preoperatively even when CT is performed, and so median sternotomy and thorough inspection of each lung lobe is essential. **Each lung lobe is leak tested** by submerging in warm saline and manually inflating the lung tissue to a maximal physiological pressure: usually 20 cm H_2O. The damaged lung lobes or damaged portions of the lung lobes and those with other intact bullae are removed.

Lung Lobe Torsion

This is **an uncommon condition** whereby a lung lobe spontaneous twists and becomes engorged with blood (Figure 152). Patients present with acute onset dyspnoea or more chronic progressive coughing and tachypnoea. The condition most frequently affects the **left cranial lung lobe in young male Pugs,** and the left cranial and right middle lung lobes of large deep chested dogs, such as sighthounds and Afghan Hounds.

The condition is diagnosed on thoracic radiography or CT, sometimes complemented by thoracic ultrasound. **Treatment is removal of the affected lobe by intercostal thoracotomy,** taking care not to de-rotate the affected lobe as this is associated with release of potassium and toxins (reperfusion injury) which can be fatal.

Lung Lobectomy

This may be performed by hand suturing of the vessels and bronchi of the lobe to be removed, but more commonly, using TA surgical staplers or pretied ligatures Endoloop™. Following any lung lobectomy, the **closure site is submerged in warm saline and leak tested at 20 cm H_2O of inflation**

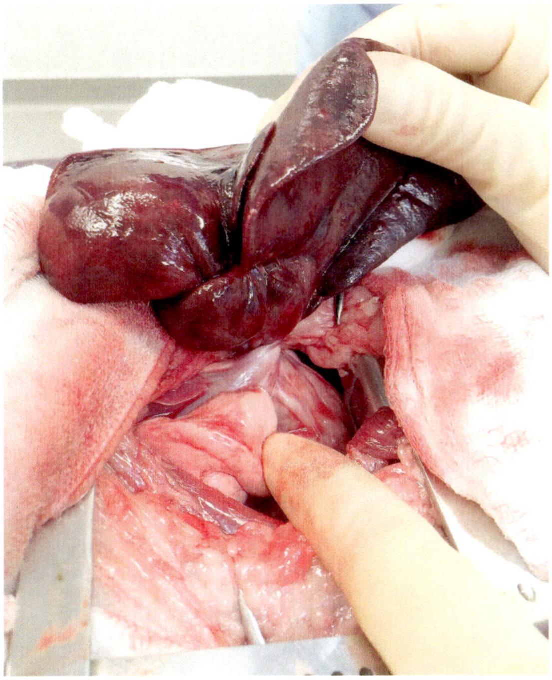

Figure 152. Lung lobe torsion.

pressure as discussed above for spontaneous pneumothorax assessment (Cronin et al., 2018).

Thoracic Cavity Disease

Pyothorax

Pyothorax is the development of severe infection and inflammation in the pleural cavity (Figure 153). This is usually a process which affects the entire thoracic cavity and may be caused by penetration of the thoracic wall or rupture of a pulmonary abscess (formed due to a tumour or more commonly migration of an inhaled foreign body such as a grass seed); Springer spaniels are over-represented in the latter group.

Patients present with progressive lethargy, pyrexia, tachypnoea, and dyspnoea. Thoracic imaging reveals **free fluid** with marked thickening of the mediastinal tissues including the pericardium. Rarely a foreign body is identified on diagnostic imaging, but in the absence of other causes, foreign body migration is assumed. Clinicians debate managing pyothorax cases medically by drain placement, daily thoracic lavage and prolonged antibiotics, versus surgical debridement of the thoracic cavity in the hope of removal of the inciting cause and removing as much inflammatory tissue as possible. **Surgery is typically indicated in the presence of a foreign body, abscess, or with failing medical management.** If surgery is performed this should be by median sternotomy.

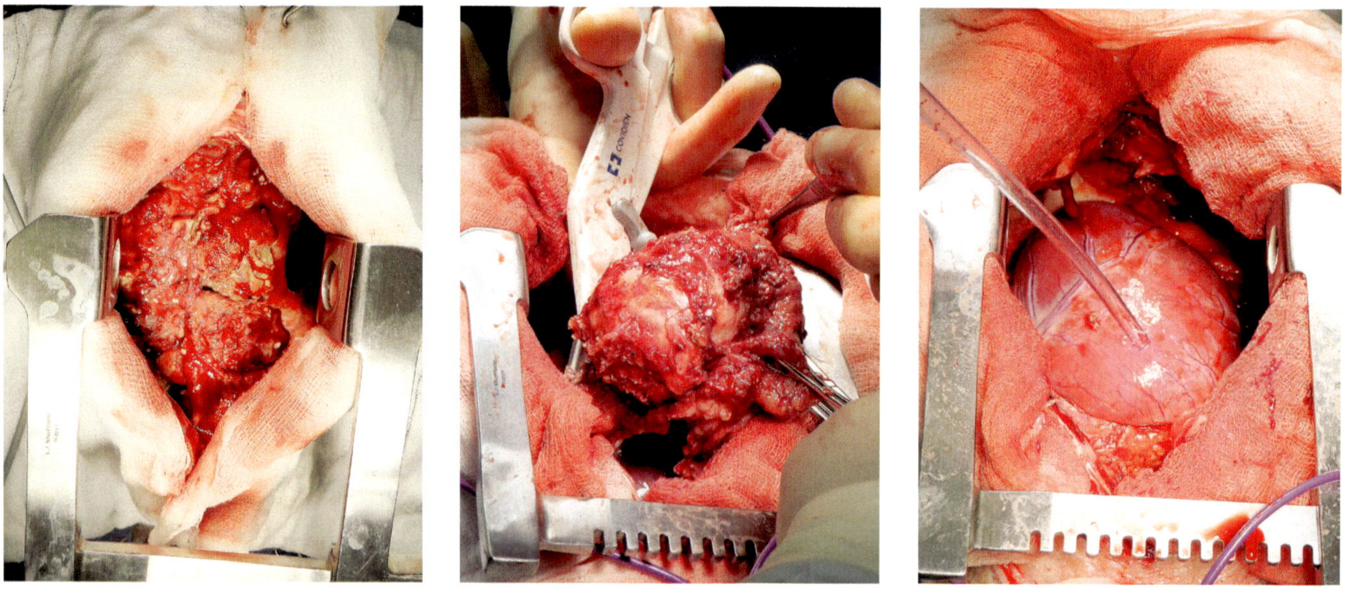

Figure 153. A case of pyothorax. The thickened and inflamed mediastinal tissues and pericardium are removed.

The mediastinum and pericardium are massively thickened and removed as extensively as possible, below the level of the phrenic nerves on each side which run the length of the chest cavity to control movement of the diaphragm. Samples are submitted for histopathology and for culture and sensitivity testing. Lung abscesses may also be removed by lung lobectomy (Stillion, Letendre, 2015).

Thymoma

Thymoma is a benign tumour of the remnant of the thymus gland, which in the growing animal is responsible for T-cell development and immunological function. The gland usually regresses at skeletal maturity. Older Labradors and Golden Retrievers are most frequently affected. Thymomas may cause clinical signs as the result of their physical presence causing **coughing or dyspnoea,** but may also cause:

- **hypercalcaemia:** which presents as polydipsia and polyuria; or due to
- **neurological changes:** including regurgitation due to megaoesophagus as a result of myasthenia gravis; and
- **head swelling:** due compression of the cranial vena cava, restricting venous return from the head.

Diagnosis is by diagnostic imaging of the thorax and fine needle aspiration of the cranial mediastinal mass for cytology and flow cytometry. Achieving a cytological diagnosis is important as the **major differential diagnosis for thymoma is mediastinal lymphoma,** for which surgery is not indicated, as this condition is managed by chemotherapy and/or radiotherapy. See Figures 147 A and 154.

Surgery may be performed to remove the thymoma, with the surgical approach depending on the patient size and extent of the mass. Smaller masses might be amenable to removal by

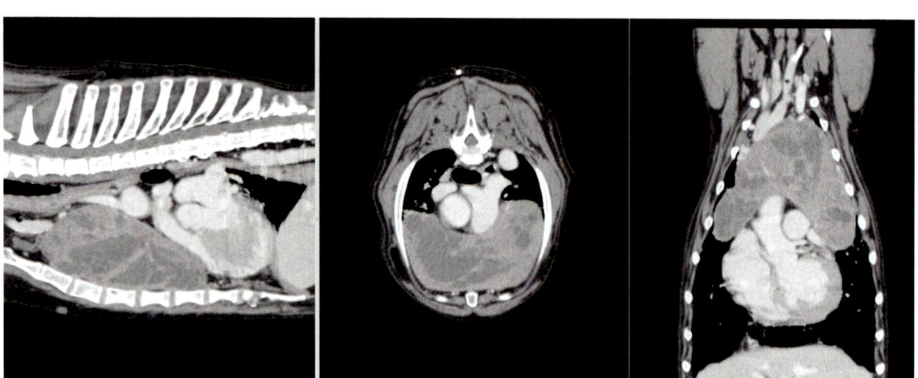

Figure 154. Thymoma CT.

intercostal thoracotomy or even thoracoscopy (see later), but larger masses require median sternotomy for full assessment and safe dissection from the neurovascular structures of the cranial thorax. (See Figures 155 and 156).

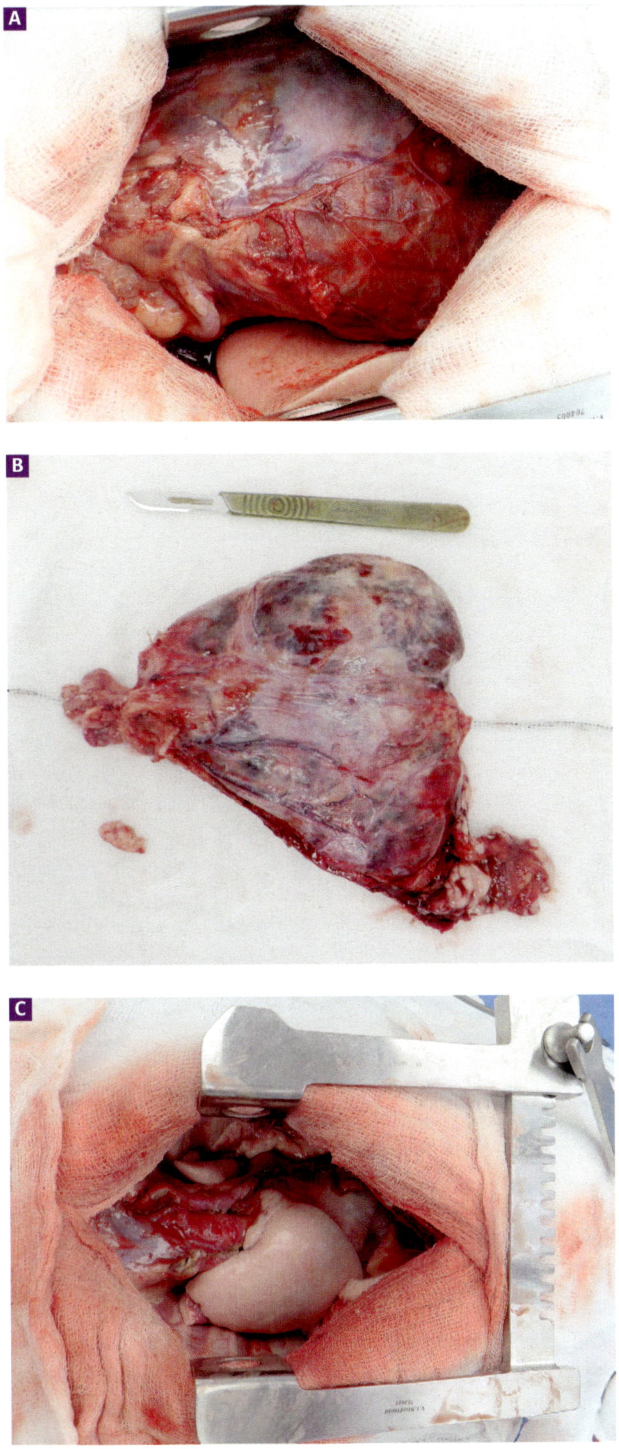

Figure 155. A. Intraoperative view of a thymoma via median sternotomy; **B.** Thymoma removed; **C.** View inside the thorax following thymoma removal.

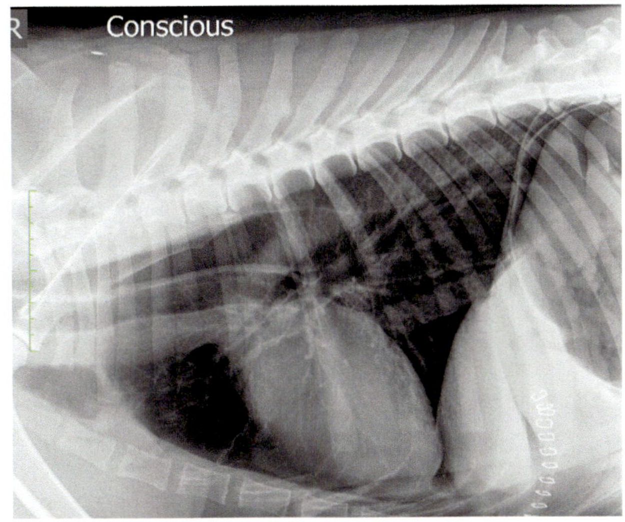

Figure 156. Radiograph of a thorax following thymoma removal.

Complications of surgery include:
- major haemorrhage
- pneumothorax
- regurgitation and aspiration pneumonia
- intraoperative cardiac arrest
- nerve injury to the recurrent laryngeal nerves causing laryngeal paralysis or phrenic nerves causing paralysis of the diaphragm
- postoperative development of myasthenia gravis.

However, patients that do recover from surgery have a good prognosis.

Thoracic Wall Disease

Chest Wall Tumours

Tumours arising from the ribs are usually firm and immobile. Sarcomas are the most common tumours of the thoracic wall, including chondrosarcoma, osteosarcoma, and fibrosarcoma. Diagnosis is by thoracic radiography or CT (Figure 157), to assess the lesion and the presence of pulmonary metastases. Histological diagnosis is made by biopsy of the mass.

Surgical treatment of the mass is removal with wide surgical margins, usually considering 2–3 cm margins of unaffected surrounding tissue, including one affected rib in front of and behind the tumour. This leaves a defect in the thoracic wall which requires reconstruction, either using local muscle flaps, a combination of omentum and fascia graft, or surgical mesh implants.

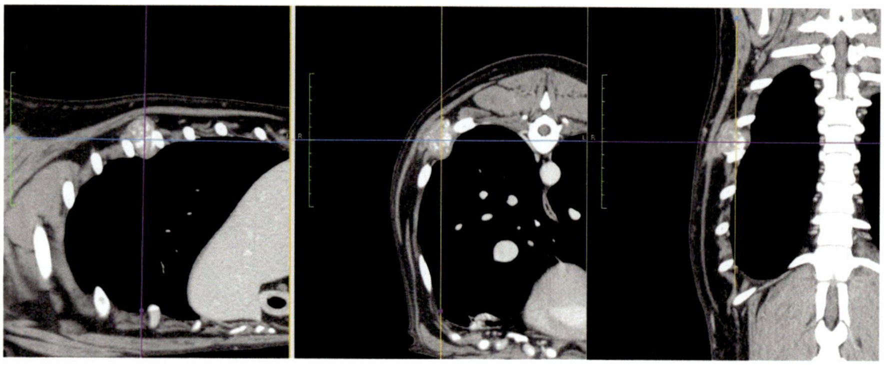

Figure 157. Chest wall mass CT.

Penetrating Injury

Penetrating injuries to the thoracic wall commonly occur as the result of bite wounds, usually larger dogs attacking smaller dogs or cats, or impalement injuries due to chasing and/or jumping on sticks. (Figure 158).

Both bite wounds and impalement injuries may leave only small entry wounds, but these can frequently be the tip of the iceberg with far more extensive internal injury, either due to impalement with or without retention of a foreign body, or due to bite wounds causing crushing injury and devascularisation of deeper structures. Hence penetrating injuries to the body wall should undergo extensive diagnostic imaging investigation and then surgical exploration and debridement of the affected region (Matiasovic et al., 2017; Frykfors et al., 2020).

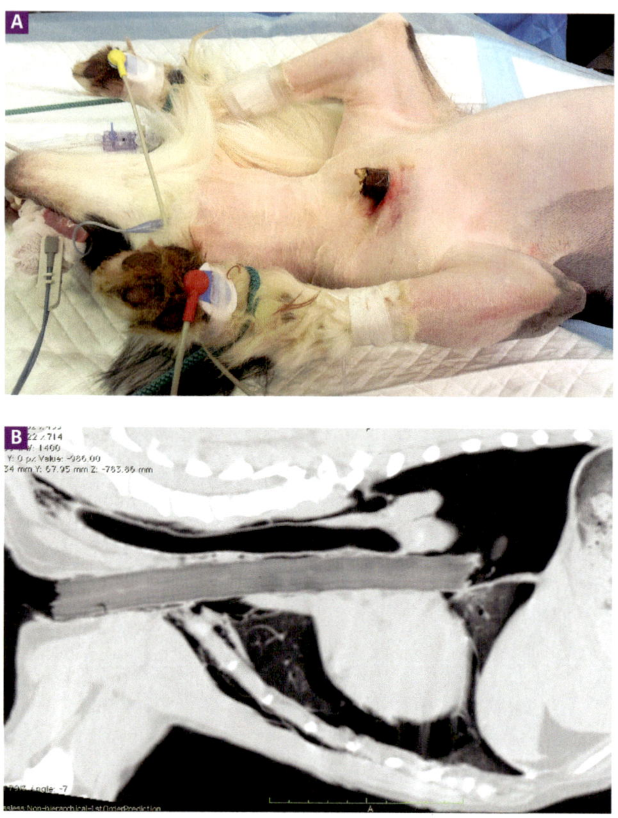

Figure 158. A. Photograph of a patient suffering an impalement; **B.** CT scan of the same patient showing the extent of the penetrating injury internally.

Cardiovascular Disease

Pericardial Effusion

Pericardial effusion is the accumulation of fluid in the pericardial sac around the heart. As this accumulates it may restrict cardiac filling and therefore cause a reduction in cardiac output. This causes the patient to suffer weakness, lethargy, and exercise intolerance. Diagnosis is confirmed by echocardiography, and the fluid drained. The condition can be caused by mass lesions at the heart base or as an idiopathic condition without known cause. For idiopathic cases, in the event of recurrence following drainage, **surgery is often considered to remove the pericardium** to prevent the tamponade of the heart and hopefully reduce the production of fluid. Subtotal pericardiectomy is performed, as the most dorsal portion is not removed due to the presence of the phrenic nerves running to the diaphragm on both sides. Subtotal pericardiectomy is commonly performed by intercostal thoracotomy (from either side) but may also be performed thoracoscopically.

Patent Ductus Arteriosus (PDA)

During foetal development blood vessels bypass the lungs and liver, which are not used until after birth. These bypass vessels usually close completely in the first few days after birth under the influence of prostaglandins. The ductus arteriosus (Figure 159) is a communication between the aorta and the pulmonary artery, which allows blood from both sides of the heart to be pumped around the body but following birth if this communication persists, this causes an overload of pressure in the pulmonary vasculature and **a continuous machinery type murmur on thoracic auscultation.** Diagnosis is confirmed by echocardiography.

Treatment may then be interventional by placement of an Amplatzer occluder inside the affected vessel to block the vessel, or by surgical dissection and ligation of the vessel. Surgery is performed via a left 4th or 5th intercostal thoracotomy. The vagus nerve is retracted dorsally and the abnormal vessel identified, dissected free, and then tied at both the connection with the aorta and pulmonary artery, traditionally with silk. The murmur should resolve immediately following ligation. The anaesthetist may see temporary postligation bradycardia due to the Branham Reflex.

Vascular Ring Anomalies

Vascular ring anomalies are abnormalities of development of the heart and major vessels, which form in the embryo from a complex system of vessels. Various abnormalities can develop and are only significant if the abnormality forms a restriction around the oesophagus, preventing passage of solid food, usually noted at the time of weaning, causing regurgitation and risking aspiration pneumonia.

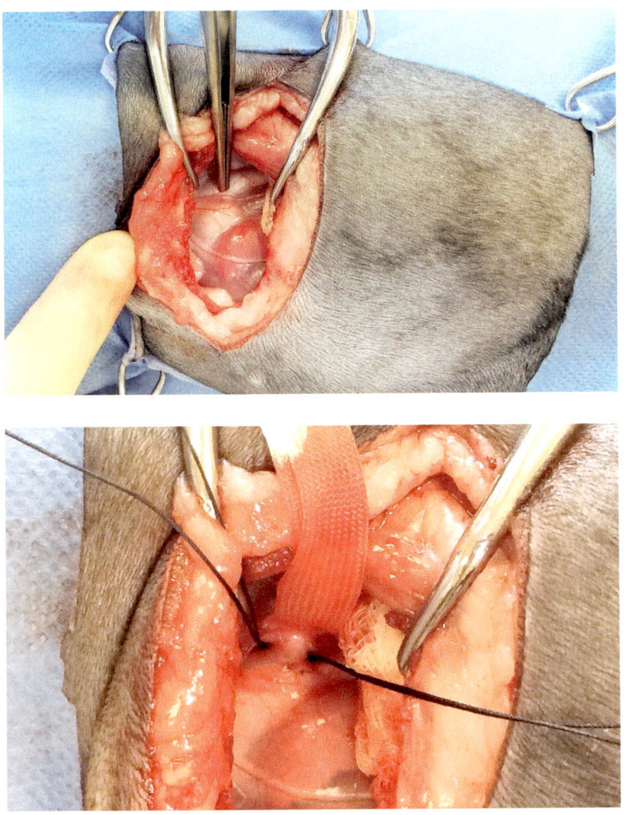

Figure 159. A patent Ductus Arteriosus (PDA) is identified, isolated and ligated at surgery.

Plain radiography can be suggestive of the anomaly, which is highlighted using barium swallowed as a contrast agent. CT is used to further investigate the specific abnormality present. The most frequent anatomic variation is development of the aorta on the right side instead of the left, otherwise known as Persistent Right Aortic Arch (PRAA). The PRAA is associated with a residual ligament from the ductus arteriosus. This ligament on the left side (left ligamentum arteriosum: LLA), encircles the oesophagus. Surgery therefore is a left 4th or 5th intercostal thoracotomy to dissect the ligamentum arteriosum, ligate (in case any flow remains) and divide the ligament to release the oesophagus. (Figure 160).

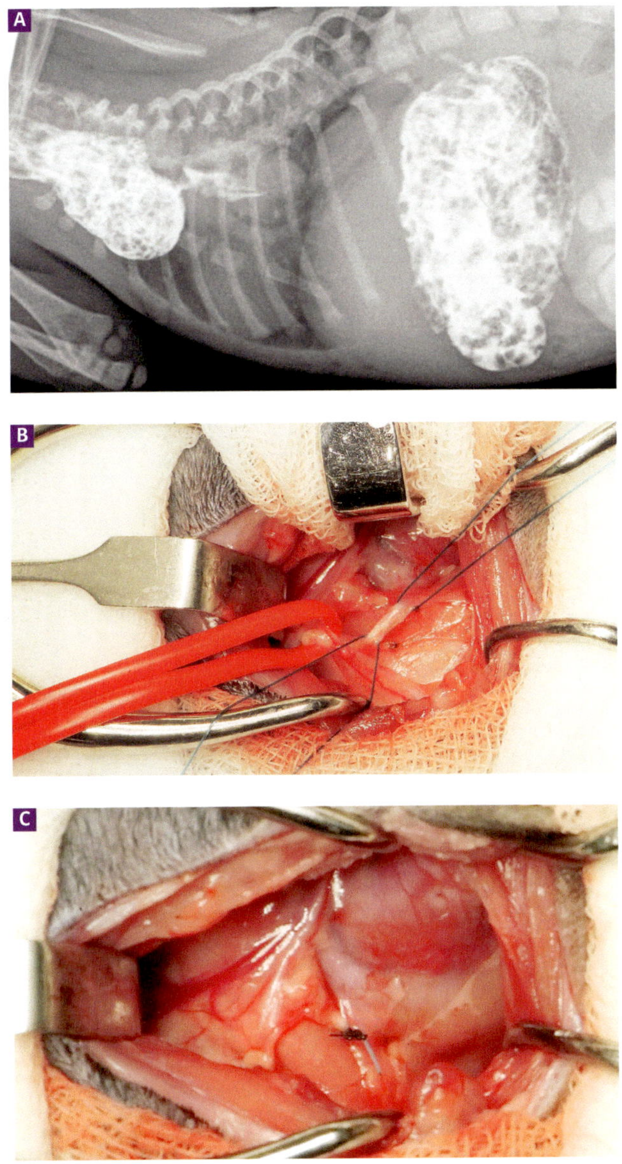

Figure 160. A. Radiographic barium study of a patient with a Persistent Right Aortic Arch (PRAA); **B.** The left ligament arteriosum (LLA) is identified and isolated at surgery; **C.** Intraoperative appearance following LLA ligation and division.

Postoperative Care

Thoracic Drainage

An essential part of any thoracic surgery is the drainage of air from the thorax to allow reinflation of the lungs, and in most cases to allow removal of further fluid (air, blood, inflammatory fluid, chyle) which may accumulate within the thorax following surgery. For surgeries where no ongoing fluid accumulation is anticipated, (e.g. after repair of a ruptured diaphragm when there is no injury to the intrathoracic tissues) following placement of the final suture, which creates an air tight seal, the thorax may undergo one-off needle drainage through the diaphragm or the chest wall.

When further fluid accumulation is anticipated and is a risk which needs to be mitigated, (i.e. the risk of air leakage following a routine lung lobectomy), then a thoracic drain should be placed prior to closure of the thoracic cavity. Some patients may have had drains placed prior to surgery as part of their investigations or stabilisation before anaesthesia and often these drains are maintained following surgery if adequately placed and secured.

Drain placement requires consideration preoperatively, with adequate clipping and skin preparation and placement of the drapes to enable placement. Typically, a drain is placed into the thorax through the 7th or 8th intercostal space (on one or both sides depending on the nature of the disease process, the volume of ongoing fluid accumulation anticipated, and the surgery performed). **The drain is tunnelled under the skin** from the caudal skin incision to the desired penetration point through the thoracic wall. **This position is appropriate for drains placed following sternotomies and the most common 4th/5th intercostal thoracotomies,** as drain placement should not be through the main surgical incision. Where the 7th/8th intercostal spaces are within the surgical exposure, e.g. for chest wall tumour resections, then drain placement should be adjusted to avoid this region. The specific entry point is not critical, with the priority being the placement such that the drain runs the length of the thoracic cavity to provide adequate drainage.

The fluids most commonly drained from the thorax following surgery are not overly viscous and so narrow-gauge drains are preferred to reduce postoperative morbidity. Most surgeons **use 12 to 14-gauge drains** (placed by the Seldinger technique),

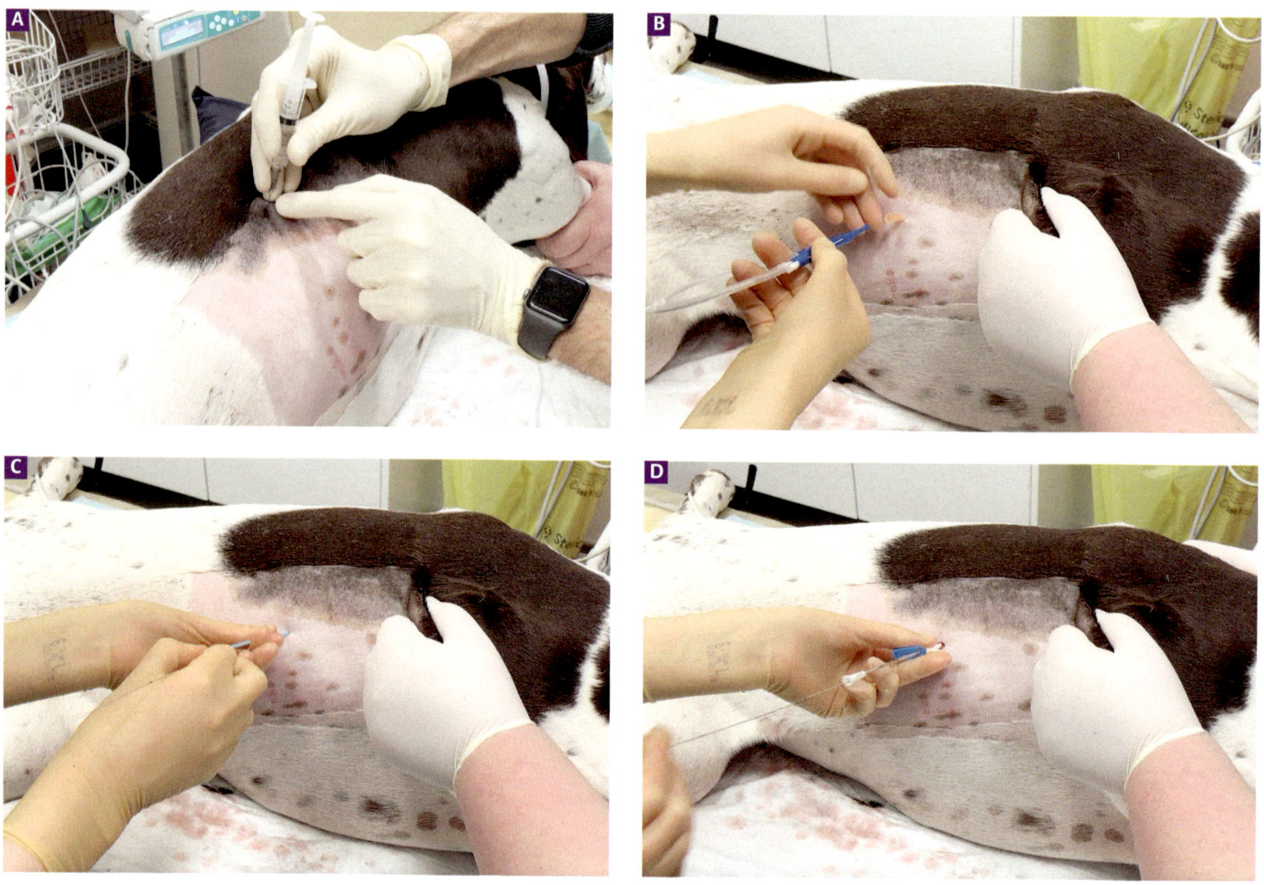

Figure 161. A. Intercostal nerve block; **B, C, D.** Over the wire chest drain placement (Seldinger technique).

although larger bore trocar drains are also available. An intercostal nerve block is commonly performed for analgesia prior to drain placement.

Once placed, **initially the thoracic drain is left open while the thoracic wall incision is closed,** in order to prevent a tension pneumothorax. Once the thoracic wall is sealed the drain is then closed and promptly emptied appropriately.

The drain is anchored to the skin at the point of entry by sutures through eyelets on the drain or by a finger-trap suture (Figure 162). The entry point of the drain into the skin should be treated aseptically as a surgical incision; it is a potential point of entry for nosocomial infection and so should be appropriately covered and regularly cleaned, inspected, and recovered.

A drain, whilst essential for removing fluids from the thorax, is also a risk for allowing air entry into the thorax if not kept well closed and sealed. Hence, **at least two methods should be used to close off the drain,** i.e. a clamp on the drain itself, 3-way tap in the off position with bungs on the outlet ports. **Staff should be trained in how to use a 3-way tap** as failure to appreciate the mechanism is a common cause of problems associated with thoracic drainage.

It is paramount the drain is protected from interference by the patient, using a hard, Elizabethan collar, often plus a body suit to prevent removal by a cat's rear paws.

Ongoing Thoracic Drainage

Thorax drainage may be performed intermittently or continuously. Intermittent drainage is usually performed by a trained nurse or veterinarian using a syringe, with an aseptic technique and ensuring the chest drain always remains sealed closed to prevent air entry. Continuous drainage in less frequently used and requires connection to a dedicated pump; it may be considered for cases where high volumes of air are leaking inside the thorax to prevent a tension pneumothorax.

An advantage of continuous drainage systems is that they can be calibrated to perform drainage at a specific negative pressure, which is beneficial to allow a slow controlled re-expansion of the lungs following previous trauma or following more major resections (such as pneumonectomy, the removal of one entire lung) to gradually allow expansion of the remaining lung tissue to fill the thorax without overstretching and traumatising the lung.

Following surgery, the surgeon will decide on the frequency of thoracic drainage. The initial frequency depends on **the anticipated rate of fluid accumulation and the risks associated with that fluid accumulation.** Generally, the drainage frequency reduces over time as the production of fluid diminishes. **The presence of a drain itself in the thorax causes the production of a small volume of inflammatory fluid** (often suggested to be up to 2 ml/kg/day). Drainage may need to be performed with the patient in different recumbencies to allow the fluid within the thorax to be in contact with the drain, (depending on the position of the drain and the volume of fluid present). It is important to remember, **air rises within the thorax and liquid falls under gravity,** so the position of the drain (from knowledge of its position at surgery or based on postoperative thoracic radiographs) and the expected location of the fluid should be considered.

Drainage Records

The volumes and nature of fluid removed from the thorax should be documented so as to allow the veterinary surgeon to adjust the frequency of drainage and decide when to remove the drain.

Removal of substantial volumes of blood from the thorax should prompt investigation. The fluid's PCV should be

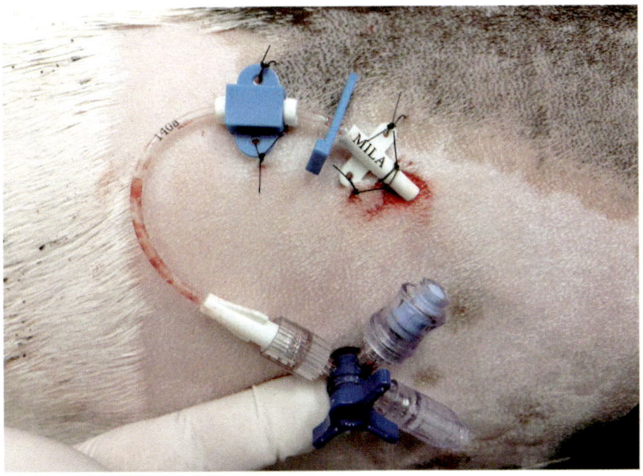

Figure 162. The chest drain is sutured to secure it to the body wall and sealed with a closed three-way tap and injection port bungs.

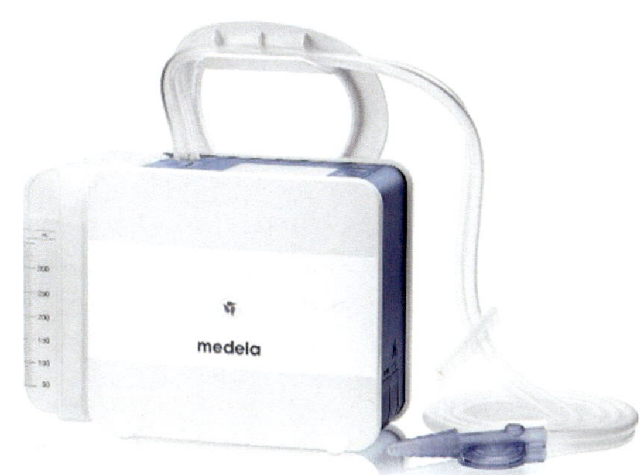

Figure 163. Continuous thoracic drainage device.

compared to that in the patient's circulation to help **assess for active intrathoracic haemorrhage.** If a large volume of frank blood is drained, it is advisable to aseptically collect the blood into syringes or a blood collection bag which is preloaded with citrate anticoagulant for autotransfusion if required.

Turbid, cloudy liquid, especially if it progressively increases in volume, may indicate surgical site infection and fluid analysis (cytology and white blood cell counts) are advisable, to compare with previous samples.

Drain Removal

Thoracic drains should be removed aseptically. The sutures that anchor the drain should be cut, which should allow the drain to be gently withdrawn without resistance in an unsedated patient. The tip of the drain should be kept and if desired submitted for bacteriology testing, for hospital infection monitoring or as indicated by the patient's status.

Analgesia

Intrathoracic surgery is generally well tolerated in dogs and cats, with most regaining mobility rapidly after surgery. That said, it should be anticipated that thoracic surgery may be a cause of significant pain and morbidity and **adequate analgesia provided.** Surgeries which require thoracic wall resections e.g. to remove tumours or dissect drain tracts due to penetrating injury or migrating foreign bodies, are more painful than surgeries which preserve normal anatomy.

The surgical team can influence the patient's comfort postoperatively by:

- respecting anatomy
- meticulous technique
- retracting rather than transecting muscle layers
- using smaller thoracic drains where possible
- not incising the full length of the sternum if avoidable, so as to improve sternotomy stability postoperatively
- placing secure implants to close the sternum
- rigidly immobilising bone fragments for healing.

As part of a multimodal analgesia protocol **intermittent, intrapleural administration of local anaesthetics (e.g. levobupivicaine) postoperatively** provides improved analgesia for the patient. Administration should be timed immediately following pleural drainage, so as not to add the medication to a soup of fluid in the thorax, which then dilutes its benefit. Intrapleural analgesia is of particular benefit for patients undergoing median sternotomy, due to the dependent position of the incision in a sitting or standing patient.

Airway Surgery

Brachycephalic Obstructive Airway Syndrome (BOAS)

Aetiopathogenesis

Brachycephalic obstructive airway syndrome (BOAS) refers to the combination of an **overlong soft palate and stenotic nares** (Figure 164), commonly seen in brachycephalic (short-nosed) breeds. Additionally, most dogs with BOAS also have **congenital trachea hypoplasia.** These anatomic abnormalities can subsequently lead to secondary changes within the airway:

- stenotic nares greatly reduce airflow through the nose
- an overlong soft palate fills the pharynx and blocks airflow through the larynx.

Struggling to breath leads to inflammation, swelling, and further thickening of the palate due to the negative airway pressure created. Negative airway pressure frequently leads to progressive collapse of the larynx. Commonly the **laryngeal saccules (tissue pockets just in front of the vocal cords) turn inside out becoming balloons,** which further obstruct airflow. This may also progress to weakening and **inward collapse of the arytenoid cartilages,** which support the vocal cords, increasing the degree of airway obstruction. **Tonsillar enlargement** occurs secondary to airway inflammation causing activation of the immune system as well as the result of suction on these delicate structures. **Regurgitation is also common** in affected dogs due to negative airway pressures promoting stomach acid reflux as well as a common association with **hiatal hernia** (a congenital weakness of the diaphragm through which the stomach slides back and forth) in addition to reducing tone of the lower oesophageal sphincter.

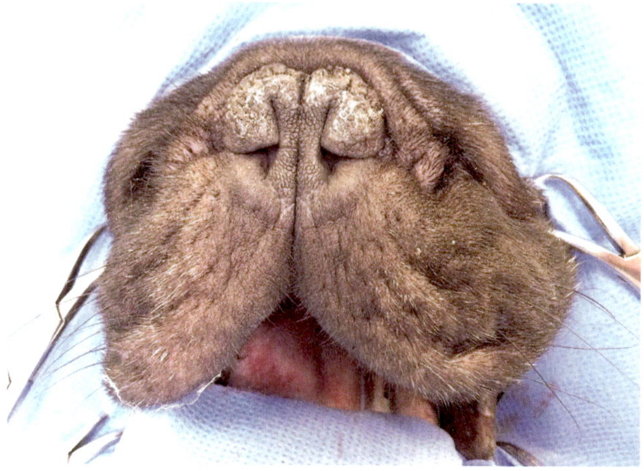

Figure 164. Stenotic nares.

Symptoms

Dogs with elongated soft palates generally have a history of **stertorous breathing and snoring,** especially upon inspiration. Some dogs will retch, gag or reverse sneeze due to choking on their overlong palate or catching of the epiglottis behind the soft palate. **Exercise intolerance, cyanosis and collapse** are common, especially following over-activity, excitement, or excessive heat/humidity. **Obesity** accentuates the problem by causing further airway narrowing and increasing the risk of overheating. Many dogs also regurgitate food, white frothy gastric mucus, or bile on a regular basis. In some dogs this is the primary clinical problem noted by the owner.

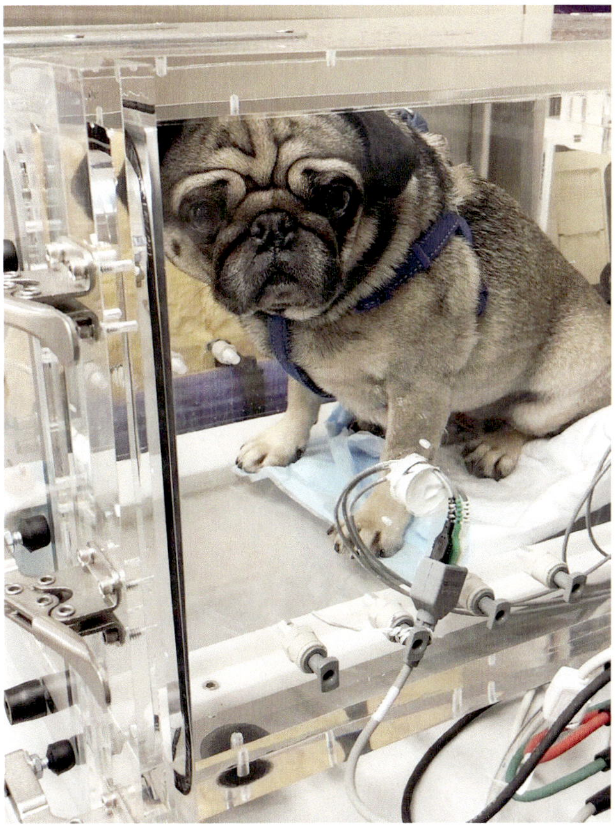

Figure 165. A pug undergoing plethysmography assessment of its breathing.

Diagnostics

On physical examination, stenotic nares are easy to spot. At this point the patient's body condition score (BCS) should also be assessed.

The functional grade of the condition is assessed based on the degree of respiratory noise, inspiratory effort, and if the patient presents dyspnoeic, cyanotic, or collapsed (Table 5). Mild or moderately affected dogs may undergo a three-minute exercise test at a moderate trot to assess changes in their breathing and clinical status. Functional grade can then be used to advise as to whether patients should be managed by weight loss and ongoing monitoring or surgical intervention.

Whole body plethysmography (Figure 165) **is a non-invasive means of assessing respiratory function.** The patient is positioned in a chamber and pressure changes in the box are used to infer the airway resistance and peak airflow pressures.

Definitive diagnosis of an elongated soft palate, tonsil enlargement, and laryngeal collapse are made under carefully monitored anaesthesia, using a laryngoscope and a blunt probe to retract the soft palate to allow laryngeal examination. The airway is also assessed for additional mass lesions,

Table 5. BOAS functional grades. (Ladlow, 2018).

		Respiratory noise	Inspiratory effort	Dyspnoea/Cyanosis/Syncope
Grade 0	Pre-ETT	Not audible	Not present	Not present
	Post-ETT	Not audible	Not present	Not present
Grade 1	Pre-ETT	Not audible to mild, or moderate intermittent nasal stertor when sniffing	Not present	Not present
	Post-ETT	Mild or moderate intermittent nasal stertor when sniffing	Not present to mild	Not present
Grade 2	Pre-ETT	Mild to moderate	Mild to moderate	Not present
	Post-ETT	Moderate to severe	Moderate to severe	Mild dyspnoea; cyanosis or syncope not present
Grade 3	Pre-ETT	Moderate to severe	Moderate to severe	Moderate to severe dyspnoea; may or may not present cyanosis. Inability to exercise
	Post-ETT	Severe	Severe	Severe dyspnoea; may or may not present cyanosis or syncope

or swellings which may exacerbate respiratory dysfunction. The airway should be secured promptly following airway evaluation. (Figures 166, 167).

Thoracic radiographs help evaluate the trachea, lower airways, and lungs for evidence of concurrent problems, especially aspiration pneumonia (Figures 168, 169). It is common to note **multiple spinal abnormalities** on radiographs of brachycephalic breeds (although these do not cause a clinical problem in most dogs). Skull radiographs may help assess the length and thickness of the soft palate prior to surgery. CT scans are sometimes performed and give a more thorough assessment of the palate dimensions as well as demonstrating aberrant, additional turbinate bone folds which contribute to airflow obstructions within the nasal passages.

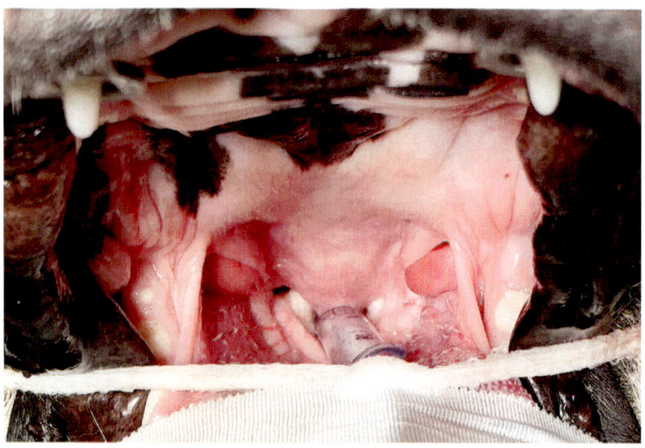

Figure 166. This image is a view of a patient positioned for surgery, demonstrating an overlong soft palate which extends all the way down into the larynx, and was obstructing the larynx during inspiration when the patient was awake. The tonsils to the sides of the soft palate are hypertrophied and bulging out from their crypts (pouches), further increasing airway resistance.

Additionally, dogs presenting primarily with regurgitation rather than respiratory compromise may undergo endoscopy of the stomach and small intestine to assess for hiatal hernia and biopsy to exclude other causes of intestinal disease, which contribute to the clinical problem.

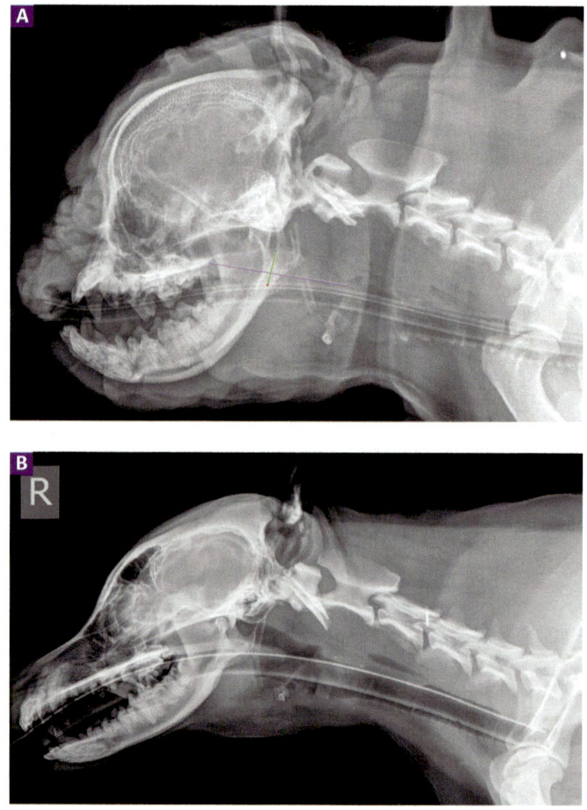

Figure 168. A. Radiograph of the head and neck of a BOAS patient taken for preoperative assessment; **B.** Comparative radiograph of a patient not suffering from BOAS. Note the difference in soft palate thickness and space of air passage above and below the soft palate.

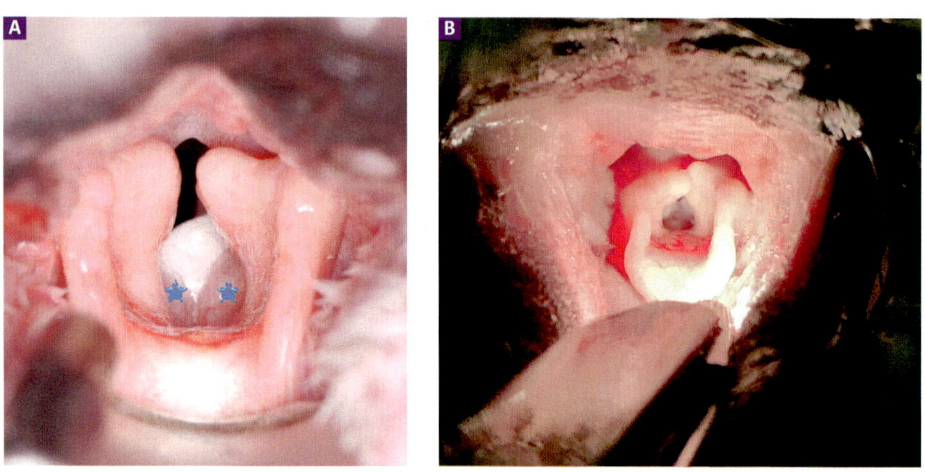

Figure 167. A. Stage 1 laryngeal collapse: elevating the soft palate with a probe is necessary to inspect the larynx itself. This image shows the larynx partially obstructed by the laryngeal saccules at the base of the larynx (blue stars), plus a mucus plug just above. **B.** Stage 2: this image shows folding in of the arytenoid cartilages with stage 3 laryngeal collapse.

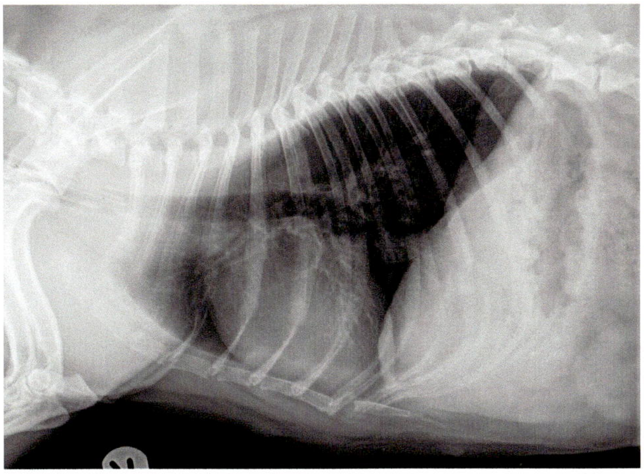

Figure 169. Thoracic radiograph of a BOAS patient taken for preoperative assessment.

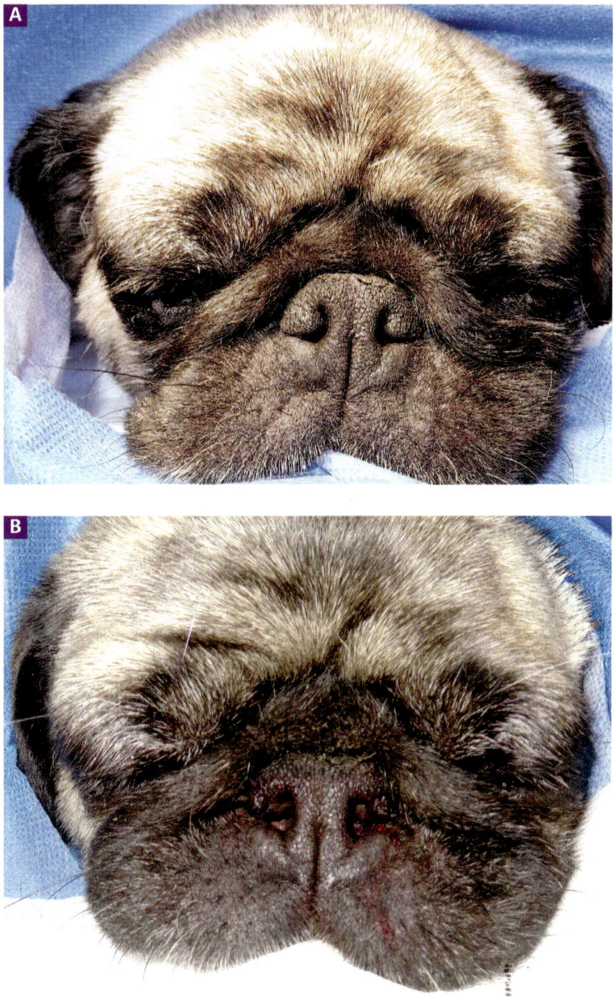

Figure 171. A. Pre-rhinoplasty; B. Post-rhinoplasty.

Treatment

In overweight patients with mild clinical signs, dietary changes alone may be advised initially. When patients are showing respiratory distress, exercise intolerance or frequent regurgitation then surgical management should be considered. Surgical treatment is not without risk, but this risk may increase if the patient is left longer, and clinical signs and stage of laryngeal collapse become more advanced. Surgical patients must be securely positioned to allow visualisation and access to the back of the mouth and the larynx for surgery. This may be achieved with a mouth gag, hanging the patient with gauze to support the upper jaw, or in a custom-made jig. (Figure 170).

Routine Surgical Treatment of BOAS

- **Rhinoplasty/alarplasty:** surgical widening of stenotic nares (Figure 171), by removing part of the alar cartilages, helps to improve nasal airflow.
- **Staphylectomy** (soft palate shortening) or **folded flap palatoplasty** (shortening combined with thinning of the palate) is performed to remove excess tissue and create space in the pharynx, relieving obstruction of the larynx.

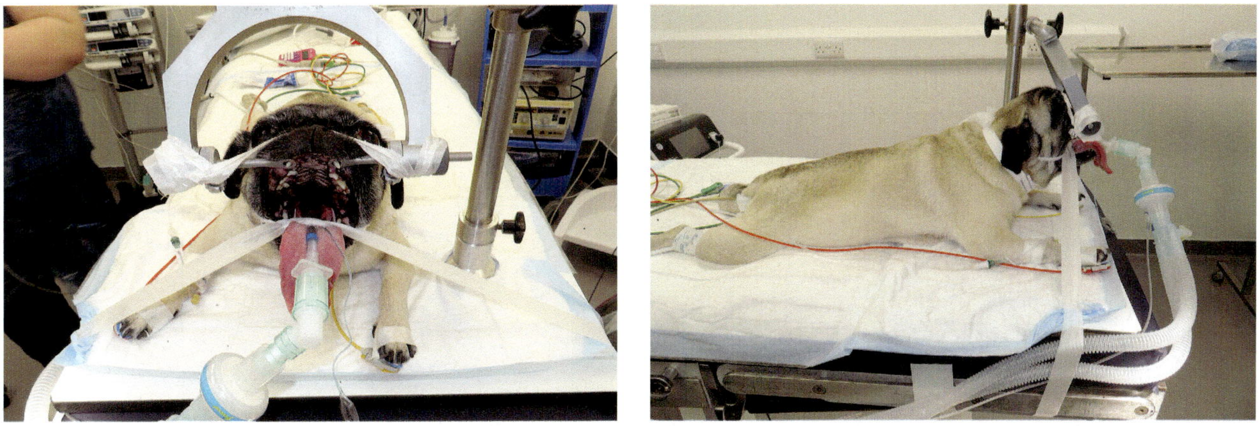

Figure 170. Positioning of a patient for BOAS surgery in a custom frame.

– **Tonsillectomy:** if the tonsils are enlarged and contributing to airway narrowing, they may be removed. They are clamped at their base and cut free, suturing over the clamp, or removed using a vessel sealing or electrosurgical device. Figure 172 demonstrates the appearance following tonsillectomy and folded flap palatoplasty. Note the larynx is clearly visible and no longer obstructed.
– **Sacculectomy:** removal of the everted laryngeal saccules, which obstruct the larynx. These are grasped with Allis tissue forceps and cut free with long Metzenbaum scissors.
(See Figure 167. Stage 1 laryngeal collapse).

Aftercare

Immediately after surgery and overnight thereafter, the patient **is monitored continuously in intensive care.** Significant inflammation or bleeding can obstruct the airway, making breathing difficult or impossible. Following surgery patients are usually medicated with steroids to help reduce airway swelling, and gastroprotectant medications (metoclopramide and omeprazole) to help reduce the risk of regurgitation. **Patients frequently require sedation,** often with CRIs of dexmedetomidine or butorphanol to keep them calm during surgical recovery. Occasionally (around 5% of cases) a temporary tube must be placed and maintained until the swelling in the throat subsides enough for the pet to breathe normally (usually 36–48 hours).

Outcome

The prognosis is good for young animals that are only moderately affected at the time of diagnosis. They generally breathe more easily and are more tolerant of exercise after resolution of the postoperative swelling a few weeks following surgery. **Regurgitation episodes are usually greatly reduced** in the longer-term following surgery; however, they can be aggravated immediately following anaesthesia and surgery and with the stress of hospitalisation. **The prognosis is less favourable for cases with advanced stage laryngeal collapse.**

For dogs with ongoing respiratory problems despite the treatment, computed tomography (CT) of the head and/or endoscopy of the nasal cavity can be used to **assess aberrant turbinates (additional bone folds)** which add to airflow obstruction. If found these may be amenable to removal with a surgical laser. In cases with severe laryngeal collapse it is sometimes recommended to perform an **arytenoid lateralisation** (tie-back) procedure on the larynx to help open the airway. Another alternative is to remove part of the larynx to create a wider opening. Permanent tracheostomy may be the only solution for cases with advanced stages of laryngeal collapse, although there are complications associated with this procedure.

Tracheostomy

Temporary tracheostomy is performed as an emergency procedure to bypass laryngeal or oronasal obstructions to airflow. Common causes of airway obstruction requiring tracheotomy include:
– laryngeal collapse
– laryngeal swelling and inflammation e.g. due to stick injuries/infection
– laryngeal tumours
– pharyngeal foreign bodies (choking)
– laryngeal paralysis.

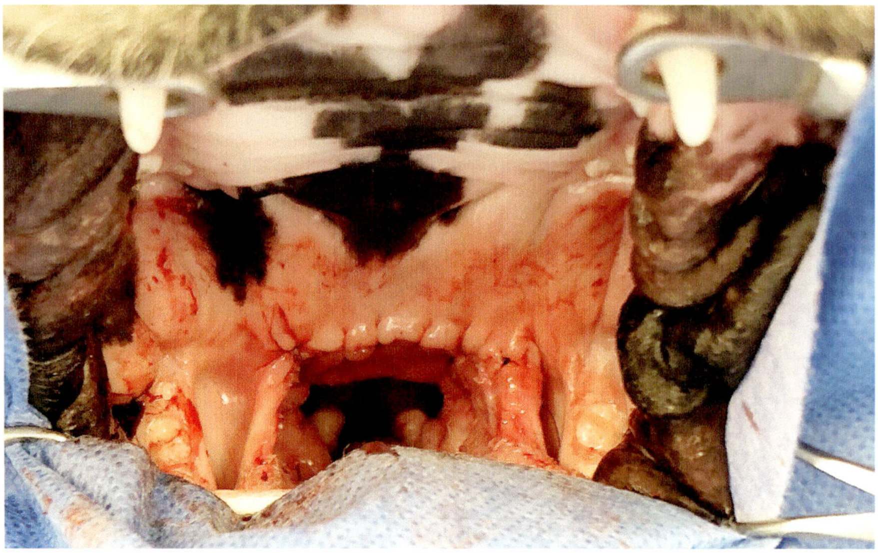

Figure 172. Postoperative appearance following folded flap palatoplasty.

The priority with airway obstruction is to act promptly but to secure an airway as best possible to stabilise a patient prior to surgical intervention.

Once the patient is anaesthetised, the **ventral cervical region is clipped and prepared** for a ventral midline approach to the trachea. (Figure 173).

Long Nylon® sutures are placed around the tracheal rings above and below the tracheostomy site and maintained as stay sutures. These sutures are lifted to elevate the trachea and widen the opening. (Figure 174).

The trachea should be opened circumferentially (up to 50% around the circumference) between two rings. The incision should not be too close to the thoracic inlet as this may risk air tracking between the cervical tissues, leading to pneumomediastinum. A sterile tracheostomy tube should be inserted through the incision. (Figure 175).

The stay sutures should be retained, and may be labelled, for ease of opening the trachea to replace the tube in an emergency should it become displaced or plugged with mucus. The surgical incision should be partially closed, but not so much as to interfere with tube removal and replacement. The tracheostomy site should be dressed around the tracheostomy tube, to secure the tube around the patient's neck (Figure 176). On recovery from anaesthesia, **the tube is maintained by regular nebulisation** (every four hours) and suction to remove the thick mucus which forms due to dry air and the tube irritating the airways.

Obstructed tubes often need to be changed and so **a sterile replacement tube should be kept on standby** along with a light source, suction machine, oxygen supply, appropriate induction agent, and cotton tipped applicators: this is to help clean, clear the airway or allow ease of reintubation in an emergency.

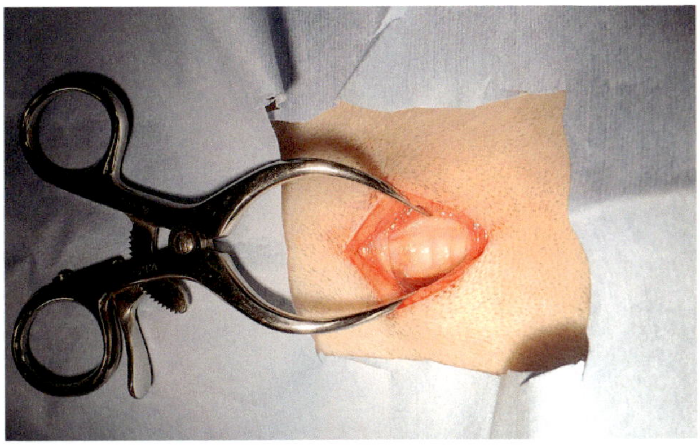

Figure 173. Ventral midline approach to the trachea.

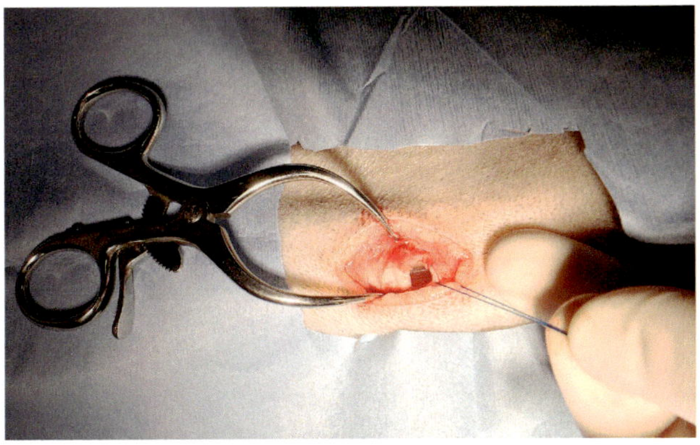

Figure 174. Placement of stay sutures around the tracheal rings.

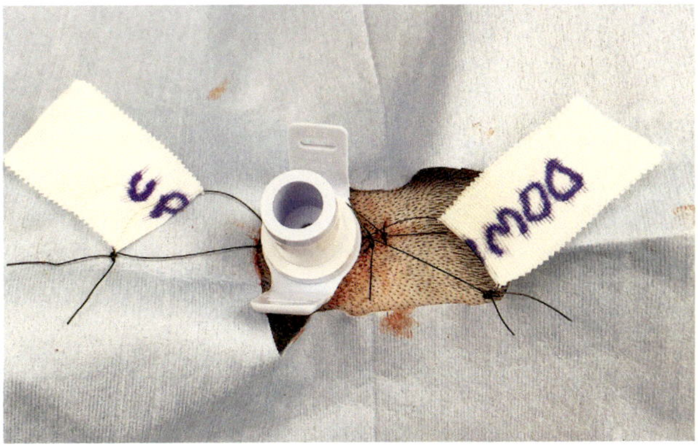

Figure 175. Tracheostomy tube placement at surgery.

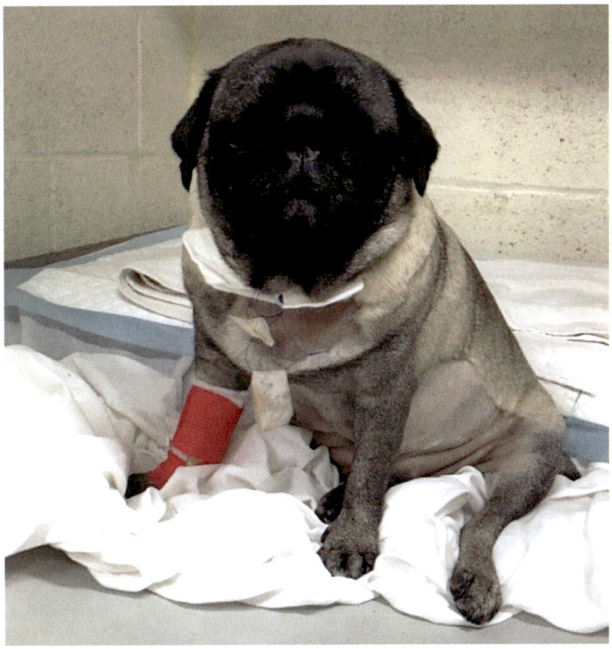

Figure 176. Postoperative appearance of a patient with a tracheostomy tube in place, with a dressing around the tracheostomy site.

Permanent tracheostomy, as the name suggests, is reserved for airway compromise which is refractory to other treatment options. This surgery is most commonly performed for cases of **severe laryngeal collapse,** where other options have failed or are not appropriate, or as a palliative option for laryngeal neoplasia.

The surgery requires a more extensive surgical preparation as a large skin fold may need to be removed to prevent obstruction of the stoma following surgery. This is best assessed in the conscious patient, prior to anaesthesia.

Usually, the ventral half of three to four adjacent tracheal rings are removed. The sternohyoideus muscles, which on the surgical approach covers the trachea, is tucked dorsal to the trachea with mattress sutures, hence elevating the trachea, making it more superficial in relation to the incision. The skin edges should be carefully opposed to the tracheal mucosa.

As for temporary tracheostomy, preventing obstruction of the stoma with mucus is key following surgery. **The stoma requires delicate cleaning,** with cotton-tipped applicators and suction, plus **frequent nebulisation** to loosen secretions and prevent desiccation of the lower airways. Over time, the airways remodel and become more resilient and require reduced frequency of care.

The main complications following surgery are stoma narrowing, skin fold obstruction, and aspiration pneumonia. For these reasons the stoma is made as large as reasonably feasible, with attention to the skin folds at the time of surgery. The patient should be maintained in slim body condition to minimise the risk of further skin fold formation. **It is essential the patient does not go swimming, as this would result in immediate drowning.**

Laryngeal Paralysis

Aetiology

Laryngeal paralysis results from loss of innervation of intrinsic muscles of the larynx, which move the arytenoid cartilages and hence the vocal folds, to open the airway to allow increased airflow. This loss of innervation most commonly occurs in large breed dogs in old age, for unknown reasons, and is referred to as **geriatric onset laryngeal paralysis (GOLP).** The condition may also arise as a congenital disease and is described in the Siberian Husky and Bouvier des Flandres. Additionally, laryngeal paralysis may occur as part of a wider polyneuropathy syndrome in older patients, coupled with loss of other functions, including hind limb weakness, and oesophageal dysfunction with megaoesophagus. The condition can also occur as a complication of trauma (including surgery) to the cervical region.

Clinical Presentation

Laryngeal paralysis is often insidious in onset with a change or loss of bark, reduced exercise tolerance (especially in warmer weather), gagging, retching, and an increasing respiratory noise known as stridor (a high-pitched noise over the larynx) commonly with a pathopneumonic reverberating noise (Figure 177). Due to the exacerbation with warm weather the disease more commonly presents in patients in the spring. Patients may arrive in acute respiratory distress due to the anxiety of being transported and frequently require **sedation to relieve anxiety, cooling to alleviate panting, and oxygen therapy.**

Anatomy

The larynx (Figure 178) is constructed of cartilage structures.

- Caudally, the **cricoid cartilage** is a ring-shaped extension of the trachea.
- The **thyroid cartilage** is U-shaped and cups the front of the cricoid cartilage on the outside ventrally, attaching to the cricoid by ligaments at its caudodorsal corners on each side.
- The **arytenoids** are two irregularly shaped paired

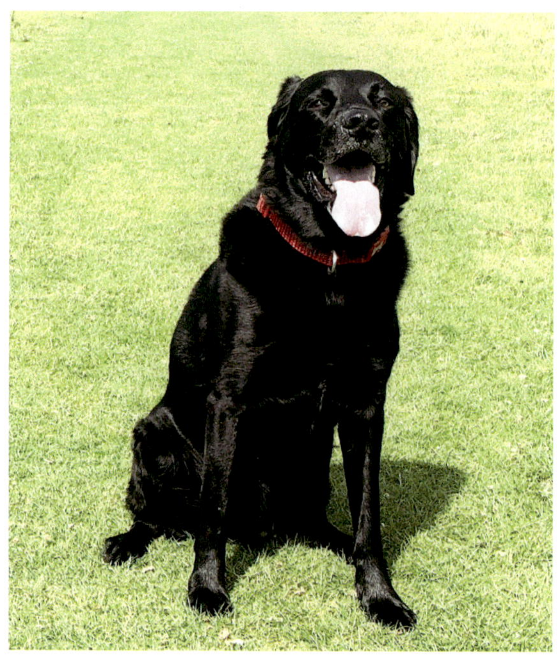

Figure 177. A dyspnoeic labrador, who has sat down and has stridorous breathing whilst on a walk on a warm sunny day. He was later confirmed to be suffering from laryngeal paralysis.

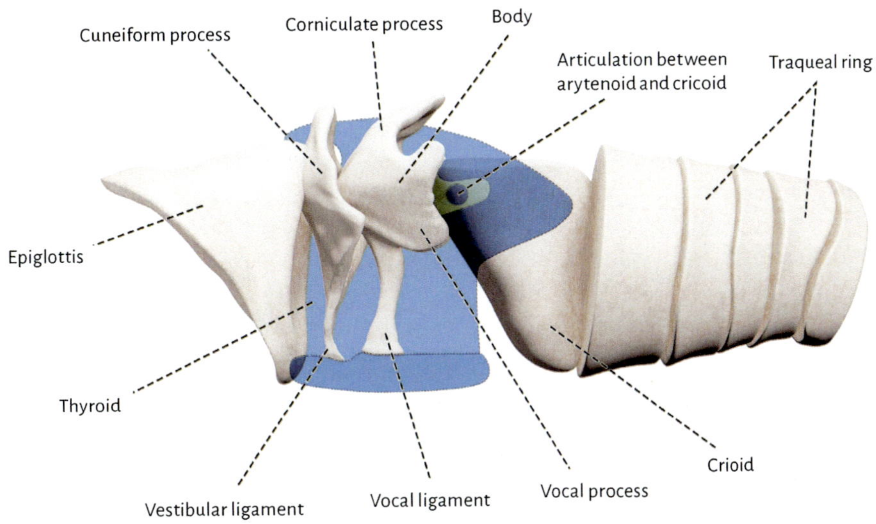

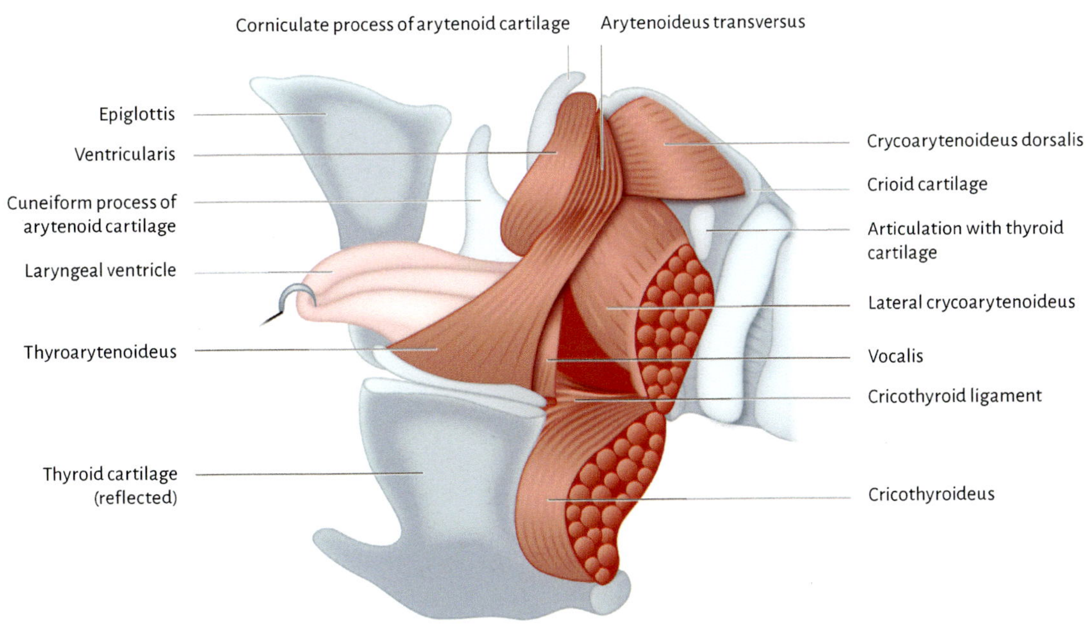

Figure 178. Larynx anatomy.

cartilages which hang over the front edge of the cricoid on the dorsolateral sides, supporting the **vocal cords** within the larynx and **mobilised by muscles** which lie sandwiched between the cricoid and thyroid cartilages.

- The **recurrent laryngeal nerves** mobilise the muscles, which have a long and tortuous course down through the neck, around the heart base and back up to the larynx. It is suggested their length and this course predispose to degeneration and dysfunction.
- The last of the cartilages is the **epiglottis**, which acts as a hood to cover the front of the larynx to provide additional protection to aspiration during swallowing.

Preoperative Assessment

Dogs presenting with laryngeal paralysis are **typically geriatric** and so a full general physical examination and routine health screening (with complete blood count (CBC) and serum biochemistry) is essential to screen for concurrent illness. **Neurological dysfunction** is common with hypothyroidism and so measuring T4 and TSH levels is advisable. Neurological assessment is also advocated to assess for evidence of concurrent polyneuropathy. The presence of additional neurological dysfunction may not change the urgent requirement for surgical treatment to improve the patient's ventilation but may affect the patient's long-term prognosis and the risk of postsurgical complications; so clinical findings should be documented and ensured the owner is adequately informed before surgery.

To assess the likelihood of megaoesophagus, it is helpful to question the owner about any history of regurgitation. Prior to surgery, where possible, the thoracic and cervical areas should be radiographed, and conscious lateral thoracic film taken to assess for megaoesophagus (as air distention of the oesophagus is a normal change following sedation or anaesthesia). Figure 179 demonstrates a distended, air-filled oesophagus due to megaoesophagus. Radiography also allows for assessment of presurgical aspiration pneumonia as well as possible cervical or thoracic lesions which might have compromised the course of the recurrent laryngeal nerves.

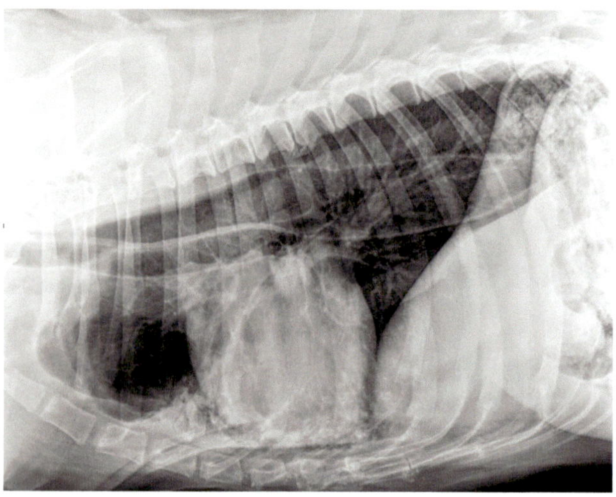

Figure 179. Megaoesophagus X-ray.

Patients are premedicated and a **light plane of anaesthesia induced to allow assessment of laryngeal function** (Figure 180). This requires the patient's gag and blink reflexes to just be intact, as deep anaesthesia paralyses the larynx, and it is essential an accurate diagnosis is achieved if surgery is to be performed. This also requires an assistant to inform the assessor when the patient is breathing inwards to ensure that the laryngeal movement is coordinated with inspiration.

It is most common for progressive paralysis to affect the left side of the larynx first and then progress to the right side. This is thought to be due to anatomic differences in the length and course of the nerves on each side. It is also for this reason that surgery is most commonly performed on the left side. Surgeon familiarity also then dictates that the left side is usually chosen for surgery in cases with bilateral paralysis.

Surgery

The patient is positioned in right lateral recumbency with the forelimbs withdrawn for a left arytenoid lateralisation surgery (tie-back). **The neck is supported, clipped, and prepared so as to expose the jugular groove.** The incision is made just ventral to the jugular at the bifurcation into the linguofacial and maxillary veins. (See Figure 8 for tie-back positioning).

The surgeon dissects down to the larynx and peels open the thyroid cartilage to expose the cricoid and left arytenoid. The aim of surgery is to place sutures to re-enact the dysfunctional muscles which move the arytenoid and hence the vocal cord to the side. This is commonly achieved by placing sutures from the back edge of the cricoid and thyroid cartilages through the muscular process of the arytenoid. (Figure 181).

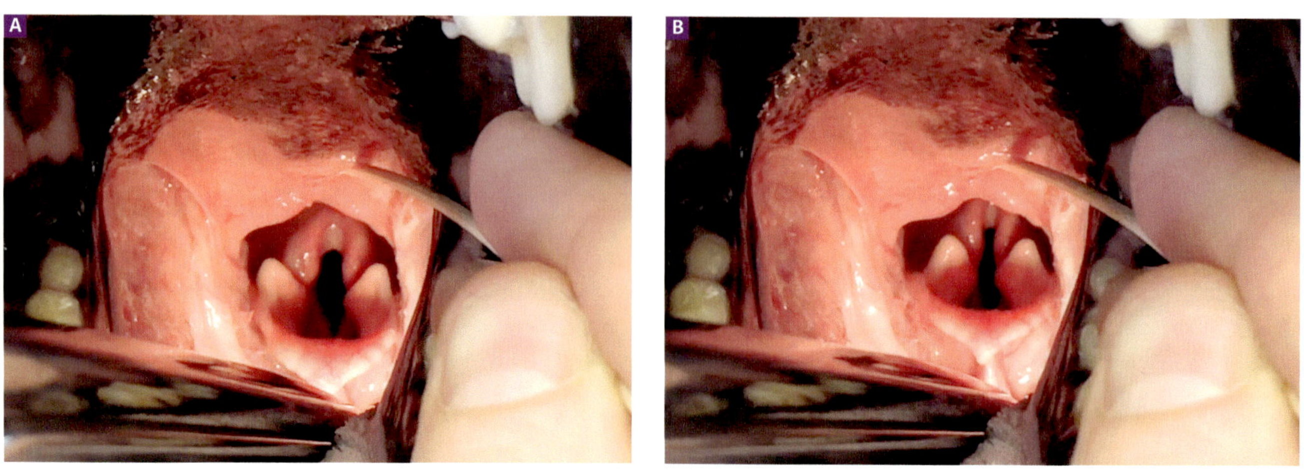

Figure 180. A. Larynx open; **B.** Larynx closed. These images show assessment of laryngeal movement. This dog has good movement on the right side (left of the picture) but weak movement on the left side.

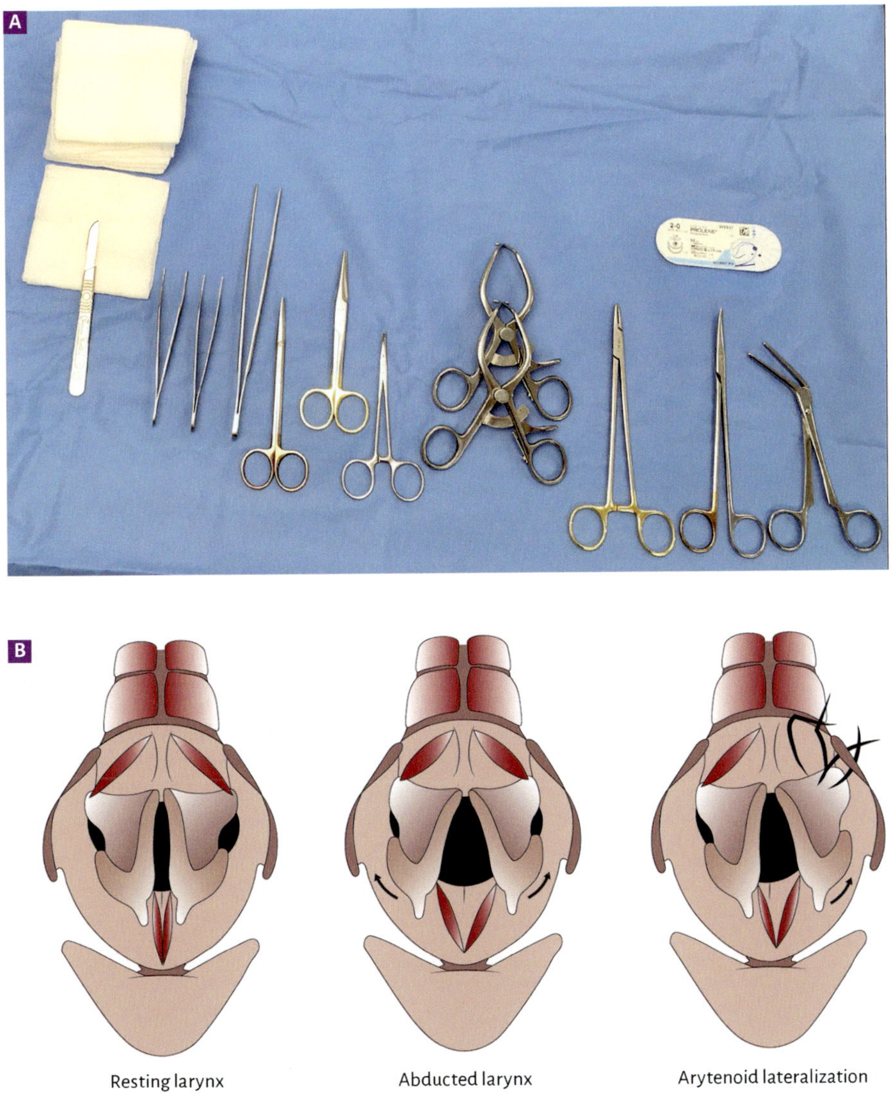

Figure 181. A. Kit trolley prepared to perform an arytenoid lateralisation (tie-back) surgery; **B.** Arytenoid lateralisation suture placement demonstrating the effect of suture placement.

Adequate tension must be maintained on the suture whilst the knot is secured, whilst taking care not to cheese wire through the fragile cartilage tissue. This is where Galliban forceps are used to hold the first throw of the knot whilst a second is placed. Their smooth jaws are designed to minimise damage to the suture which might risk suture failure.

Following surgery repeat airway assessment is made to ensure adequate opening of the larynx. The aim is to improve airflow sufficiently, without being overzealous and reducing airway defences which would result in increased risk of aspiration following surgery.

Aftercare

Following surgery patients are maintained on intravenous fluid therapy and the oral intake of food and fluids is withheld until the surgeon is happy the patient has fully recovered from anaesthesia, usually 24-hours following surgery. At that stage the patient should be hand fed, with balls of soft food to control the speed of eating and monitor that each mouthful is swallowed without choking. Long-term some surgeons recommend continuing to feed a soft food diet, as there is a perceived increased risk of aspiration pneumonia with dry, dusty foods or runny, liquid foods/drinks other than water.

Analgesia may be provided by means of local anaesthetic infiltration at surgery, and non-steroidal anti-inflammatories and/or paracetamol postoperatively. If possible, opioids should be avoided due to a reported increased incidence of aspiration pneumonia following this surgery (Wilson, Monnet, 2016).

Patients are lightly sedated to keep them calm and to prevent barking which might put undue strain on the sutures placed at surgery. When safe to do so, the patient should be discharged to prevent stress and barking in the hospital environment.

Complications

The main complications seen with this procedure are aspiration pneumonia due to impaired airway protection following surgery. This may manifest during surgical recovery or at any time in the future. Aspiration pneumonia is treated supportively with oxygen therapy and antibiotic administration.

Recurrent clinical signs may occur due to suture failure, which might require repeat surgery on the other side. As noted earlier, the patient may also suffer progressive neurological dysfunction affecting other body systems due to further nerve degeneration in polyneuropathy cases.

Mandibulectomy/Maxillectomy

Tumours of the Jaw

There are a variety of tumours which can arise in the mouths of dogs and cats. These may be noted during routine inspection of the mouth or cause as a of oral pain, reduced appetite, oral bleeding, or halitosis.

Investigation of oral tumours includes sampling the **primary tumour by fine needle aspiration** for cytology or incisional biopsy as well as assessing the jaw for evidence of invasion. It is also essential to **assess the draining lymph nodes** (mandibular, parotid, and retropharyngeal on both sides) by palpation of size, sampling and/or imaging. Finally, **thoracic imaging** to detect gross evidence of distant metastasis is essential prior to surgical intervention. This staging of the tumour is best performed by computed tomography (CT) of the head, neck, and thorax, or radiographs when this is not available. Radiography of the skull requires multiple projections and accurate positioning to obtain the most thorough assessment of the 3-dimensional structure of superimposed and overlapping bones of the skull. Thorough assessment of the extent of the lesion is essential for surgical planning. As with most cancer surgery the best prognosis is afforded to the patient by performing adequate surgery and achieving clean margins in the first instance.

Common **benign oral tumours include:**

- **Gingival hyperplasia/epulis** (Figure 182): a non-neoplastic overgrowth of the gums, resultant from poor dental hygiene, most commonly seen in the Boxer. These are firm proliferations around the base of the teeth. They can cause significant halitosis and dysphagia. They may be debulked surgically using electrocautery or a surgical laser.
- **Peripheral odontogenic fibroma** (fibromatous or ossifying epulis): a smooth, shiny, non-ulcerated, firmly attached proliferation from the gum which is frequently mineralised. They do not invade the bone, but complete removal requires surface removal of the bone to which they attach.
- **Basal cell carcinoma** (acanthomatous epulis): is a benign tumour, which acts locally aggressively by invading the surrounding bone. It often appears irregular and ulcerated. This tumour may be managed successfully by radiotherapy or by surgery to remove the mass with 1 cm of surrounding bone by partial mandibulectomy or maxillectomy.
- **Ameloblastoma:** a cystic, benign, expansile lesion, often with multiple lobes, which invades the mandible. This tumour is managed by removal with a 1cm margin, or by marginal excision and aggressive curettage or burring of the surrounding bone.

Common **malignant oral tumours** include:

- **Squamous cell carcinoma (SCC)** (Figure 183): this is the most common malignant tumour in the mouth of the dog and the cat. One form is an ulcerated, invasive mass, which displaces teeth and erodes the jaw; which is slow to metastasise and managed by wide local removal by mandibulectomy or maxillectomy with 1cm margins following staging of the lymph nodes and thorax. A second more aggressive form affects the frenulum on the underside of the tongue (commonly in the cat) and/or the tonsils, which has metastasised in 99% of cases at

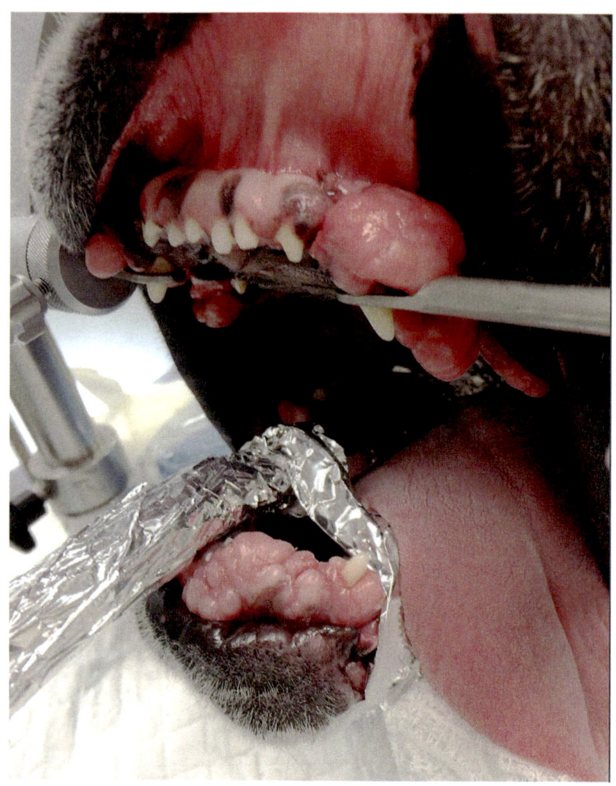

Figure 182. Epulis.

the time of diagnosis and so removal is only palliative.

- **Sarcomas (fibrosarcoma/osteosarcoma or OSA)** (Figure 184): these tumours are highly invasive locally and require wide local removal, with 2–3 cm lateral margins, and/or with adjunctive radiotherapy where it is not possible to achieve these margins. If radiotherapy may be required following surgery and the planned radiotherapy field includes the eye, enucleation may be required at the time of tumour removal due to the high risk of ocular ulceration, pain, and cataract formation as a side effect of the radiotherapy.
- **Malignant melanoma** (Figure 185): may present as a pigmented (black) or non-pigmented (amelanotic), ulcerated, necrotic mass which frequently invades surrounding bones and commonly metastasises to local lymph nodes and the lungs. Surgical removal with 1cm margins may achieve local control, but chemotherapy and/or the melanoma vaccine are often advocated by oncologists to help control the spread of disease.

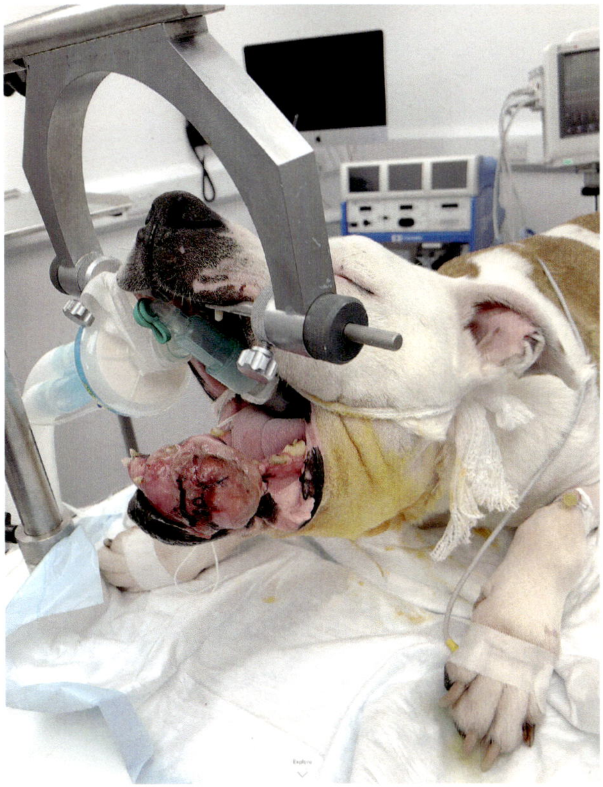

Figure 184. Oral osteosarcoma.

Anatomy of the Skull

The skull is a complex structure of multiple fused bones (Figure 186). Generally, **the term maxillectomy is used for surgical removal of tumours with portions of the upper jaw and mandibulectomy for removal of portions of the lower jaw.**

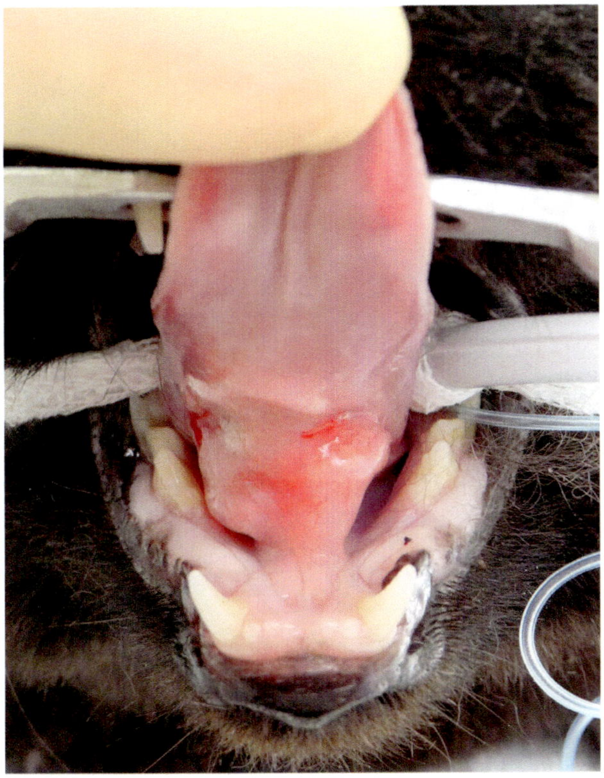

Figure 183. Sublingual squamous cell carcinoma.

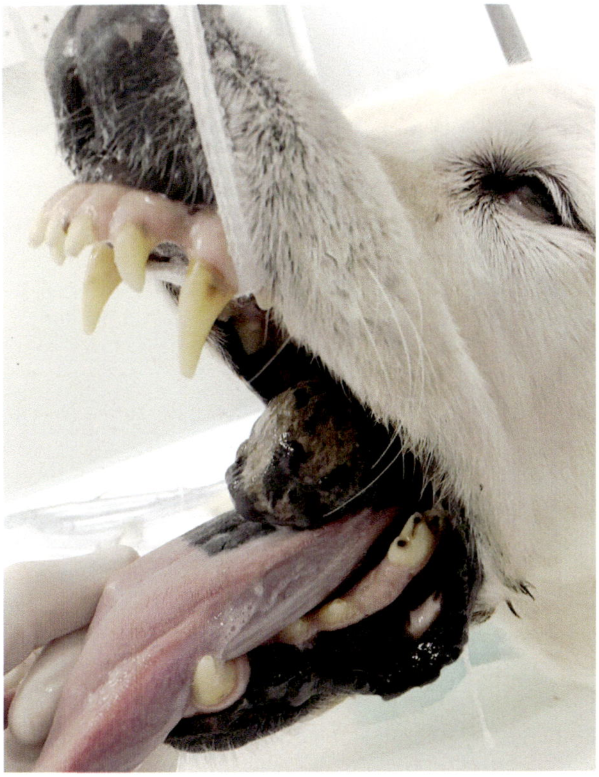

Figure 185. Oral melanoma.

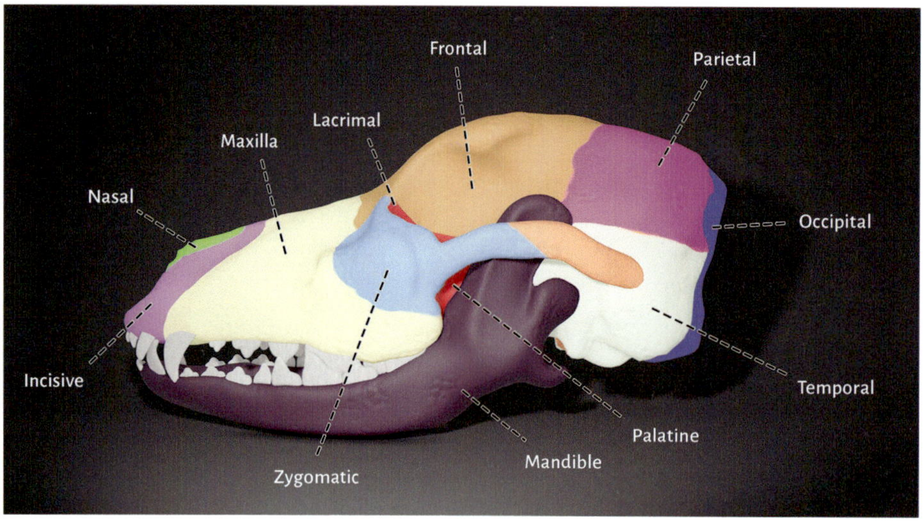

Figure 186. Skull anatomy.

Some procedures requiring access behind the eye necessitate removal of the zygomatic arch.

The blood supply to the maxilla and mandible is by the maxillary and mandibular arteries on each side, which branch from the carotid arteries. The maxillary artery has numerous branches to supply the skull. **The vessels are largely concealed within the bone, making access for ligation during surgery challenging,** hence the surgical team should have an appreciation of the surgical anatomy, and be prepared for significant blood loss by:

- blood typing the patient
- having type compatible blood available during more extensive surgeries
- managing bleeding from within the bone with appropriate electrosurgical devices, bone wax, and haemostatic agents
- bleeding may also be limited by ligation of the carotid artery on the ipsilateral side.

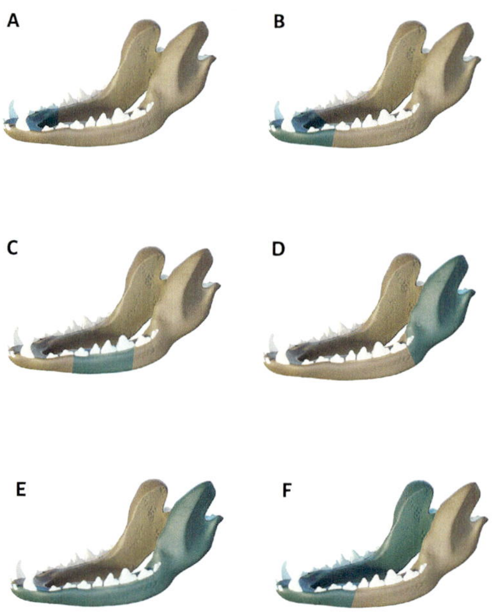

Figure 187. Types of mandibulectomy. **A.** Rostral hemimandibulectomy (unilateral rostral mandibulectomy); **B.** Rostral mandibulectomy (bilateral rostral hemimandibulectomy); **C.** Central hemimandibulectomy; **D.** Caudal hemimandibulectomy; **E.** Total hemimandibulectomy; **F.** Three-quarter mandibulectomy. (Adapted from Fossum T.W., 2007. Small animal surgery, 3rd ed, St Louis, Mosby/Elsevier).

Mandibulectomy/Maxillectomy

The specific names for procedures for removal of different segments and extents of the jaws are detailed in Figures 187 and 188.

Mandibulectomy and maxillectomy procedures (Figure 189), following dissection of the overlying soft tissues, require cutting of the bone using surgical saws and/or osteotomes and mallets. The soft tissues are also highly vascular and so electrosurgical devices are advisable for extensive oral dissections. Surgical positioning is challenging due to the 3-dimensional shape of the skull and requirement to access from multiple angles. The use of a head stand is helpful in some circumstances.

Following removal of the tumour, the soft tissues are sutured to cover the exposed cut surfaces of the bone. This is achieved

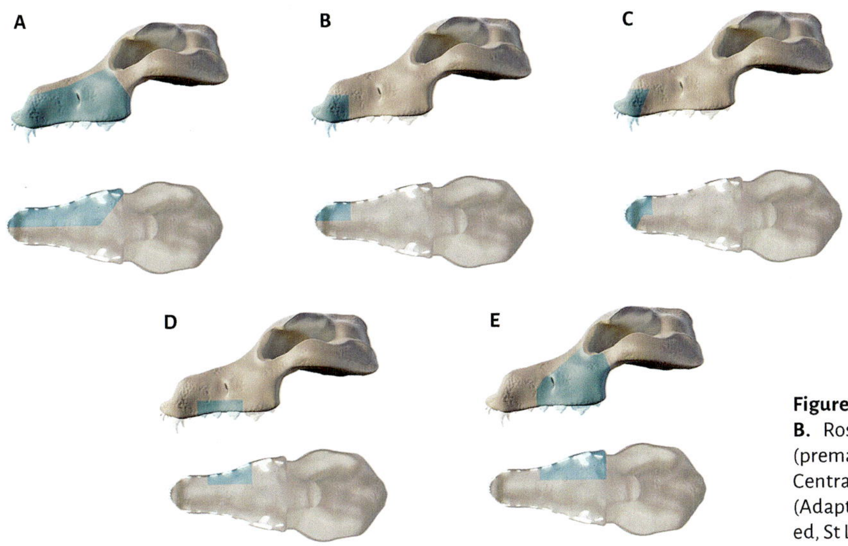

Figure 188. Types of maxillectomy. **A.** Hemimaxillectomy; **B.** Rostral hemimaxillectomy; **C.** Rostral maxillectomy (premaxillectomy or bilateral rostral hemimaxillectomy; **D.** Central hemimaxillectomy; **E.** Caudal hemimaxillectomy. (Adapted from Fossum T.W., 2007 Small animal surgery, 3rd ed, St Louis, Mosby/Elsevier).

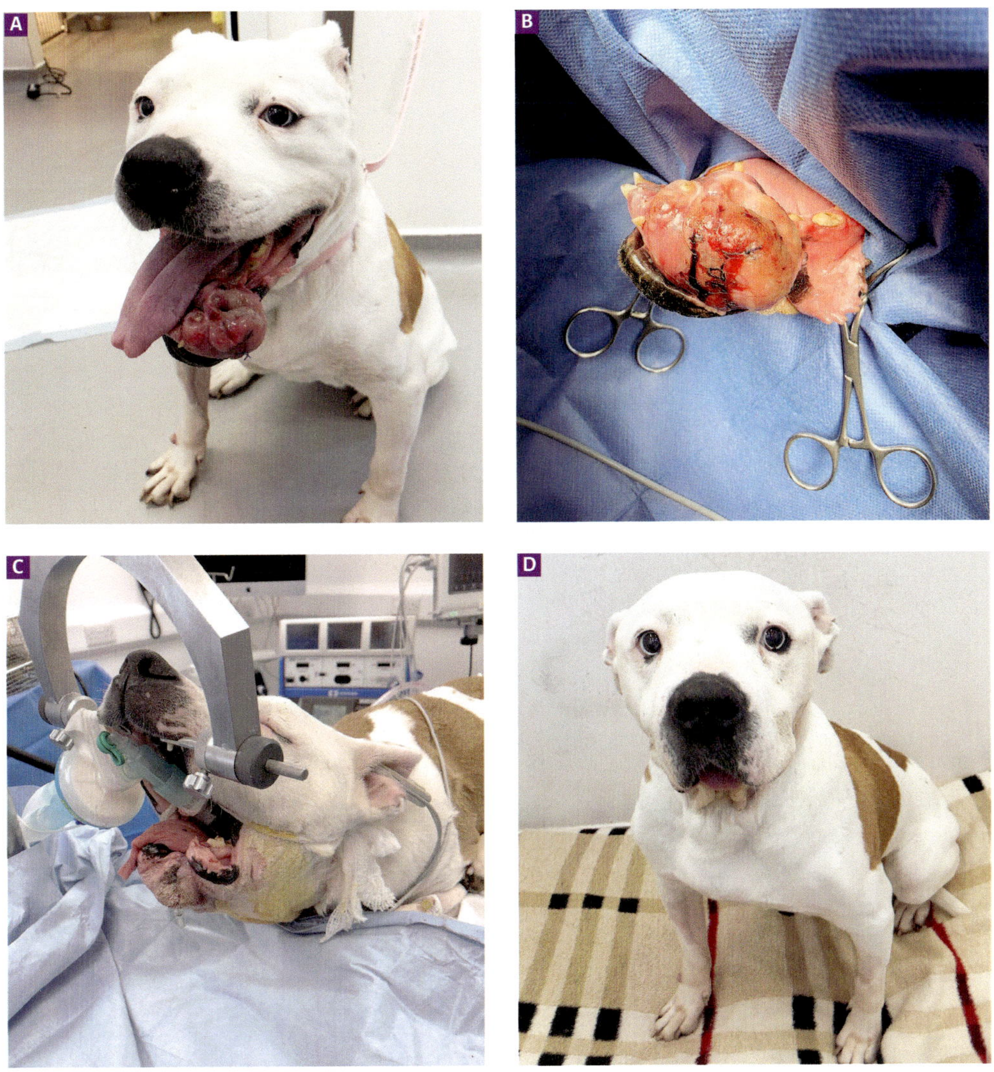

Figure 189. A. Mandibular osteosarcoma (OSA) preoperatively; **B.** Intraoperative appearance of the mandibular OSA; **C.** Intraoperative appearance following rostral mandibulectomy.; **D.** Appearance of the patient following recovery from anaesthesia.

by suturing the tissues to anchor points through bone tunnels drilled in the remaining bone, or by anchoring sutures around the remaining teeth. When the two sides of the mandible become separated and unstable during surgery it is often not essential to stabilise these bone fragments.

For patients undergoing major oral surgery, **placing a feeding tube at the time of surgery should be considered,** as many patients may choose not to eat immediately following surgery.

Following surgery, patients should be provided with adequate analgesia and nutrition via the feeding tube (Figure 190). The patient should be monitored for signs of bleeding and kept calm to reduce the risk of hypertension during anaesthetic recovery as this may risk re-bleeding from the surgical site.

When fed orally, soft food should be offered, and chew toys avoided to prevent damage to intraoral sutures. Patients may initially require assistance by hand feeding to aid prehension of food.

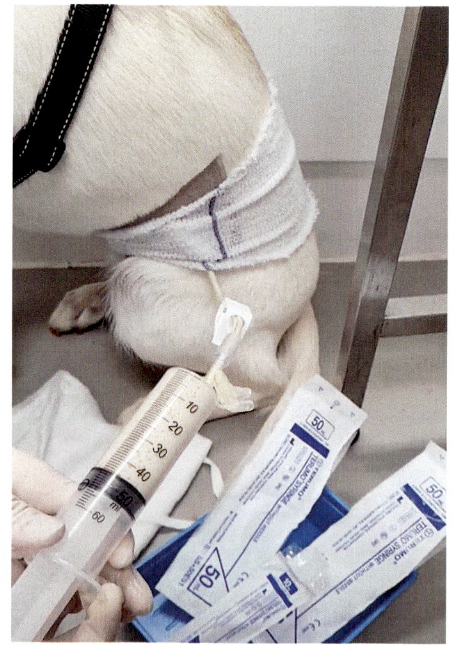

Figure 190. Gastrostomy tube feeding.

Ear Surgery

Anatomy of the Ear (Figures 191 and 192).

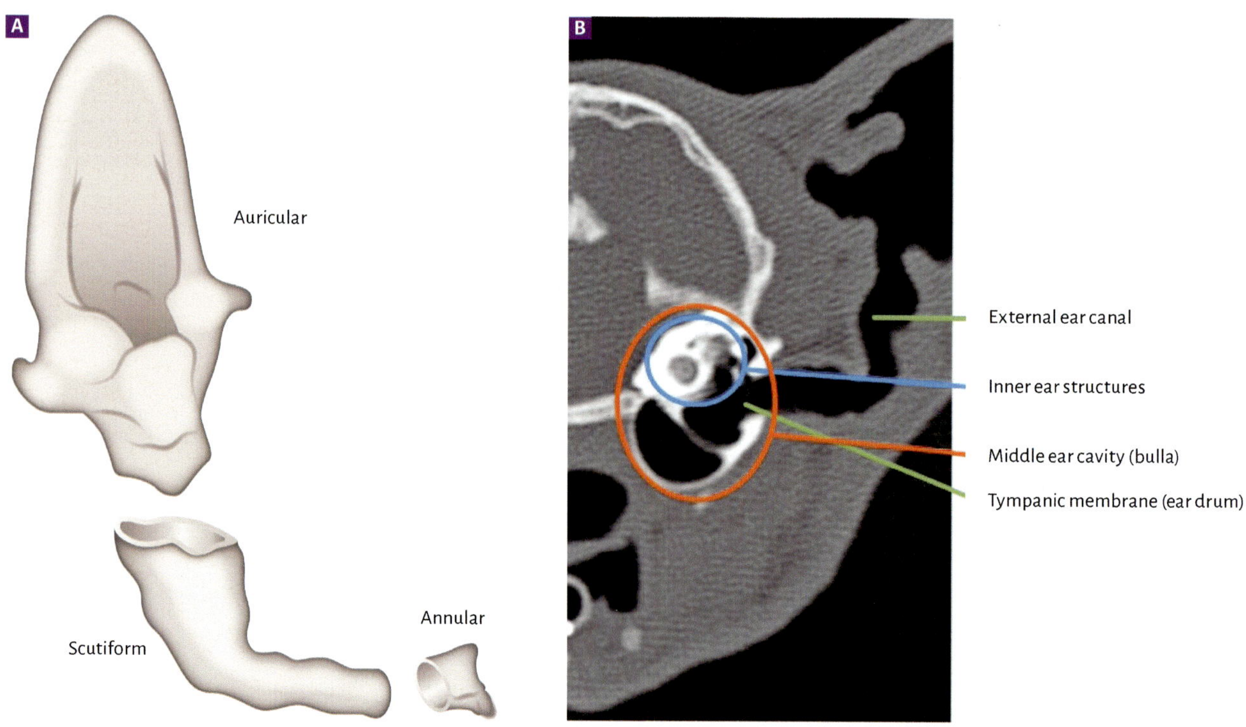

Figure 191. A. Ear cartilages; **B.** Anatomy of the ear as seen on a CT scan.

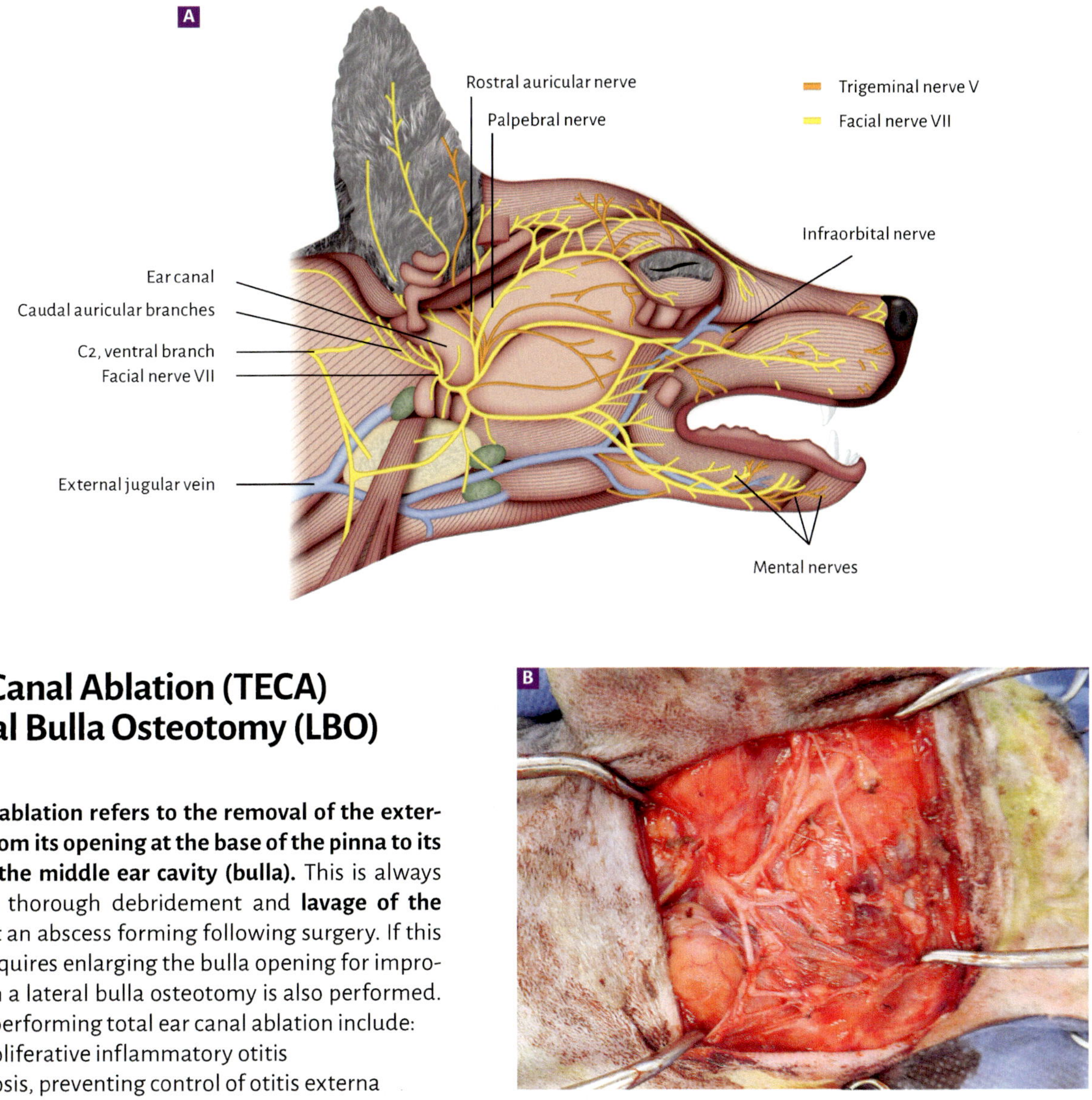

Figure 192. A. Facial nerve anatomy; **B.** Facial nerve dissection following removal of the parotid salivary gland as surgery.

Total Ear Canal Ablation (TECA) and Lateral Bulla Osteotomy (LBO)

Total ear canal ablation refers to the removal of the external ear canal, from its opening at the base of the pinna to its attachment to the middle ear cavity (bulla). This is always combined with thorough debridement and **lavage of the bulla** to prevent an abscess forming following surgery. If this debridement requires enlarging the bulla opening for improved access, then a lateral bulla osteotomy is also performed. Indications for performing total ear canal ablation include:

- chronic proliferative inflammatory otitis
- aural stenosis, preventing control of otitis externa
- otitis media
- aural tumours and cholesteatoma
- non-neoplastic epithelial proliferative disease of the middle ear.

Preoperative assessment depends on the nature of the disease. Chronic ear infections are frequently **the result of allergic skin disease,** and so full dermatological investigation is warranted. To assess the extent of infection or a mass lesion, advanced 3-D imaging with MRI (Figure 193) or CT allows thorough assessment and preoperative planning. MRI may be preferred for patients with clinical signs of otitis interna (nystagmus, head tilt), as this allows assessment of the inner ear structures, meninges, and brain.

CT is preferred for assessment of the bone, for 3-D assessment of abscesses or tumours, and for imaging the neck and thorax in patients with tumours (for staging prior to surgery). (Figure 194).

In addition to a basic surgical kit, there are several surgical instruments required for accessing and thoroughly debriding the inside of the tympanic bulla:

- **Gelpi retractors:** two or three pairs are needed to adequately retract tissue around the ear canal to maximise the surgeons view and enable identification of important structures, such as the facial nerve. An alternative is the lone-star retractor which is a frame with elasticated hooks which can retract in multiple directions simultaneously.
- **Rongeurs:** different shapes and sizes of rongeurs are useful for enlarging a bulla osteotomy opening.
- **Curettes:** are required for scooping contents from the bulla.

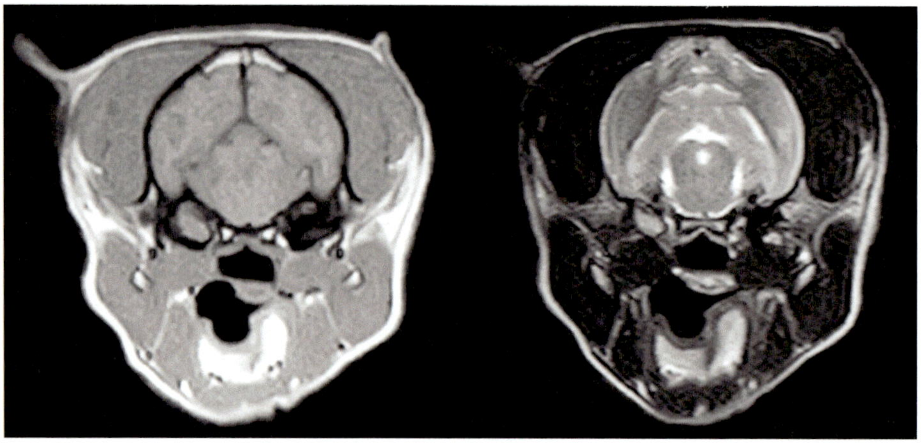

Figure 193. T1 and T2 weighted transverse MRI images through a dogs head at the level of the tympanic bullae.

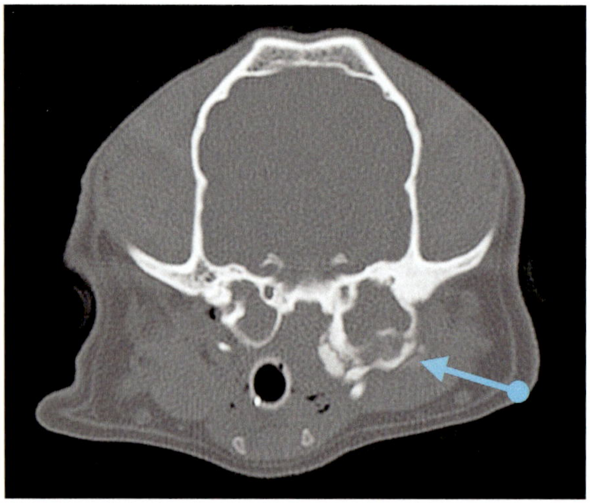

Figure 194. CT image revelling a left sided cholesteatoma.

- **Dandy nerve hook:** is useful as a blunt, bent-tipped probe for feeling around the inside of the bulla and freeing the epithelial lining.
- **Alligator forceps:** and or fine mosquito forceps are useful for reaching into the bulla to grasp and remove foreign material and loose debris.
- **Flush and suction:** needed to thoroughly lavage the bulla at the end of surgery. There is a risk of bleeding from the retroglenoid vein which exits the skull just adjacent to the bulla, and so having ice cold saline, bone wax and topical haemostatic agents on standby is also appropriate.

A total ear canal ablation requires the patient to be positioned in **lateral recumbency,** with the head supported with sandbags to stabilise as needed. The surgeon dissects the ear canal from the attached surrounding muscles, before amputating the ear canal from the bulla. Any residual tissue is removed from the entrance to the bulla, followed by thorough lavage and suction of the bulla. Care is taken not to over-traumatise the delicate vestibulocochlear structures of the inner ear whilst undertaking meticulous and thorough cleaning of the bulla. Samples from the ear canal and bulla are submitted for culture and histopathology.

Following TECA surgery, **patients are deaf in the operated ear.** Aural surgery may be painful, especially on ears which are chronically inflamed and hypersensitised prior to surgery. Multimodal analgesia during and after surgery should be considered.

Complications of surgery may result from overzealous debridement of the bulla, leading to vestibular dysfunction, with head tilt and nystagmus, which may need management with steroids and sedation until the signs abate. Insufficient debridement of the bulla and ear canal epithelium can result in para-aural abscess formation (Figure 195), which can occur at any time following surgery.

Trauma to the facial nerve may result in a lack of ability to blink the eye on the affected side, as well as drooping of the lips. Food may accumulate in the affected side of the mouth or drop from the mouth and the eye requires lubrication (at least for a few weeks after surgery) to prevent desiccation. With minor trauma or stretching the nerve may regain function over weeks to months, but with more severe trauma or inadvertent sectioning, loss of function will be permanent.

Ventral Bulla Osteotomy

Middle ear disease in cats is common as a primary condition, **due to polyp formation** (Figure 196) as a result of previous viral infections. In cats with polypoid disease, the polyp may extend into the external ear canal or along the Eustachian tube into the nasopharynx, but the disease can be managed by debriding the bulla only and removing the polyp wherever it extends. This is usually achieved by ventral bulla osteotomy.

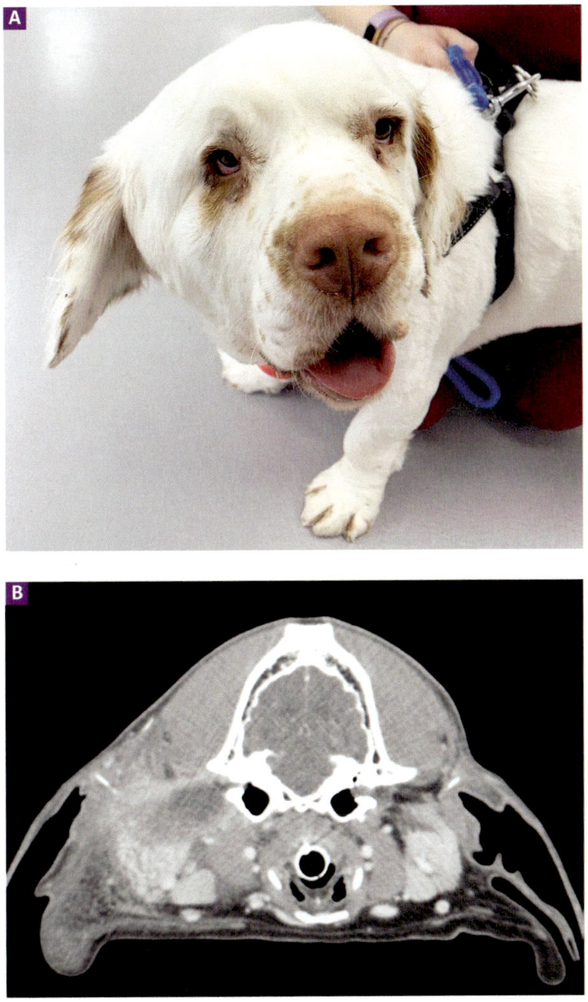

Figure 195. A. Patient with right sided facial swelling due to a para-aural abscess; **B.** The same patient's para-aural abscess seen on CT.

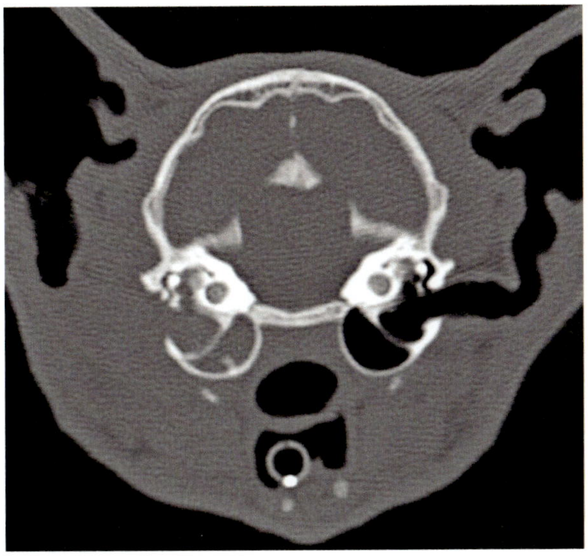

Figure 196. CT of a cat with filling of the right sided tympanic bulla and horizontal ear canal with an inflammatory polyp.

Position the cat in dorsal recumbency with the neck fully extended and supported (e.g. with a pack of surgical swabs). An incision is made directly over the bulla, which can be palpated midway between the caudal aspect of the mandible and the larynx.

The tissues overlying the bulla are bluntly dissected, the periosteum elevated with a Freer elevator and the bulla opened using either a Steinman pin or drill bit held in a Jacob's Chuck or a high-speed burr. The cat's bulla is divided into two chambers by a septum. These chambers both require exploration, debridement, and lavage.

Complications of surgery are similar to those for TECA-LBO. Additionally, in the cat the sympathetic nerves to the eye travel through the wall of the bulla and thorough debridement and lavage inevitably irritates these, leading to Horner's syndrome (third eyelid protrusion, constriction of the pupil and drooping of the upper eyelid) in all cats following surgery. These signs are more apparent when the patient is relaxed. This usually resolves within 4–6 weeks following surgery.

Ophthalmic Surgery

Ophthalmic surgery is its own speciality with a wide variety of specialist instrumentation and surgical techniques, beyond the remit of this text. This is a summary of the broad principles that apply to ophthalmic surgery.

Anatomy of the Eye

Light passes through the cornea and aqueous humour in the anterior chamber and is then focussed by the lens to project an image (through the vitreous humour) onto the retina at the back of the eye. Damage to the normally translucent structures of the eye result in a visual deficit. (Figure 197).

Eyelid Surgery

Eyelid surgery is often performed to remove mass lesions and correct congenital malformations which cause entropion (inversion) or ectropion (eversion) of the eyelids. The latter conditions are associated with damage to the ocular surface and or eyelids and loss of the windscreen-wiper function for protection of the cornea and spreading of the tear film.

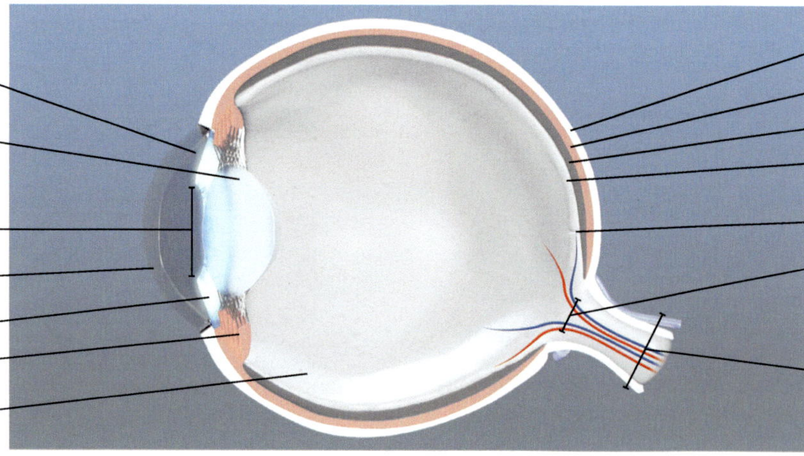

Figure 197. Eye anatomy.

When preparing for eyelid surgery, **lubricating jelly should be placed on the ocular surface** to provide protection and prevent cut hairs from entering the conjunctival sac; this is then rinsed away with the adherent hairs. The periocular area is gently scrubbed using sterile 4×4 gauze sponges soaked with povidone-iodine solution (**not scrub solution** as this contains a soaping agent which damages the ocular surface) diluted with saline (1:50, 0.2% solution), alternating with sterile saline. The conjunctival sac, including both sides of the nictitating membrane, is cleansed with the same dilute iodine solution using sterile cotton-tipped applicators to remove mucus and debris. Finally, povidone-iodine solution and saline should be used to rinse the corneal surface and the conjunctiva. The contralateral eye is lubricated with artificial tear ointment or taped closed for protection if it is not also undergoing surgery.

Eyelid surgery must be performed in such a way so as to perfectly appose the eyelid margin and **keep suture ends away from the cornea,** to prevent rubbing on the corneal surface which could cause ulceration. Many surgeons use the magnification of an operating microscope or loupes to ensure greater surgical precision.

Prolapse of the nictitating membrane gland (a.k.a. cherry eye) is another common procedure. The prolapsed gland may be removed or **preferably sutured back into a pocket** within the nictitating membrane (third eyelid).

Corneal Surgery

Common reasons for surgery of the cornea are to repair perforations due to scratches or penetrating foreign bodies, and management of deep ulcerations which are not responsive to topical medical treatment. Surgery of the cornea and lens requires a central eye position for surgery and for the eye to be stable for these delicate procedures. Hence anaesthetic techniques using **neuromuscular blocking agents** to temporarily paralyse the patient, or retrobulbar local anaesthetic bloods are useful to achieve this.

Delicate ophthalmic surgery usually requires magnification with an **operating microscope.** The surgeon sits and uses an arm rest to minimise un-necessary movements and maximise precise movement. Small, shorter, more delicate versions of the common surgical instruments are made specifically for ophthalmic surgical use (Figure 198). These often have a spring and latch mechanism rather than a ringed grip and ratchet locking mechanism.

- **Conjunctival pedicle grafting** (Figure 199) **is a technique whereby flaps of the conjunctival tissue from the margin of the eye are elevated,** maintaining their blood supply, and then sutured in place to cover corneal injuries; this provides tissue to reinforce the defect but also to provide blood supply to the normally avascular cornea. This does lead to scarring and opacification of the cornea but allows repair and maintenance of a severely damaged eye.
- **Corneoconjunctival transposition (CCT)** (Figure 200): is a technique whereby corneal tissue from the edge of the eye is advanced to the centre to repair defects in the visual axis and maintain a translucent cornea for improved vision following surgery.
- **Conjunctival grafting:** it is also possible to graft corneal tissue from deceased donors to repair conjunctival defects.

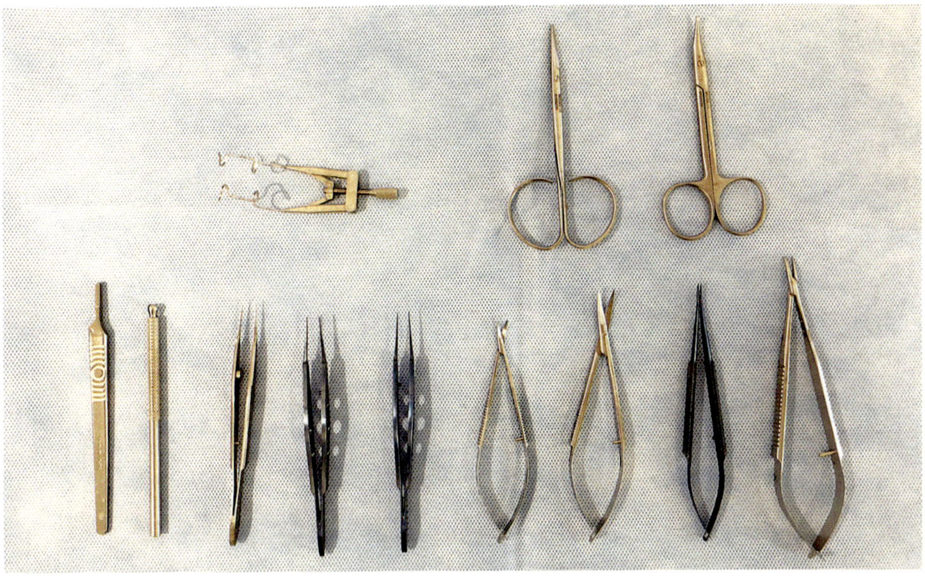

Figure 198. Ophthalmic kit.

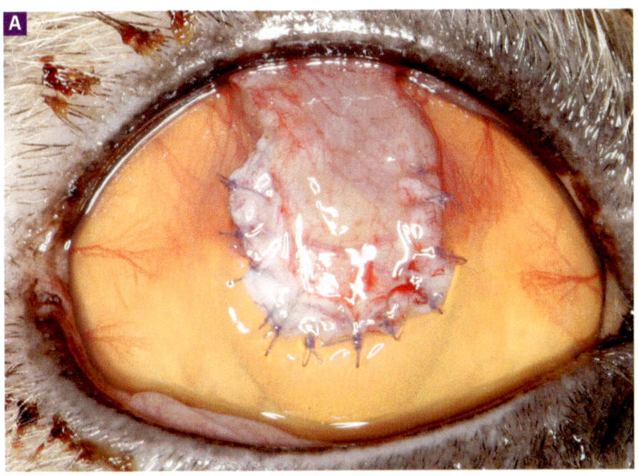

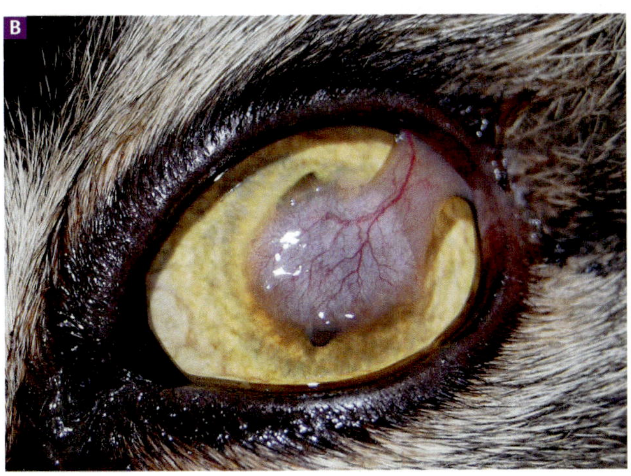

Figure 199. A. Conjunctival pedicle graft; **B.** Following healing and suture absorption. (Figures A and B courtesy of James Oliver, from "Feline Ophthalmology: The Manual" Mitchel and Oliver, ISBN 978-84-16315-11-6, May 2015).

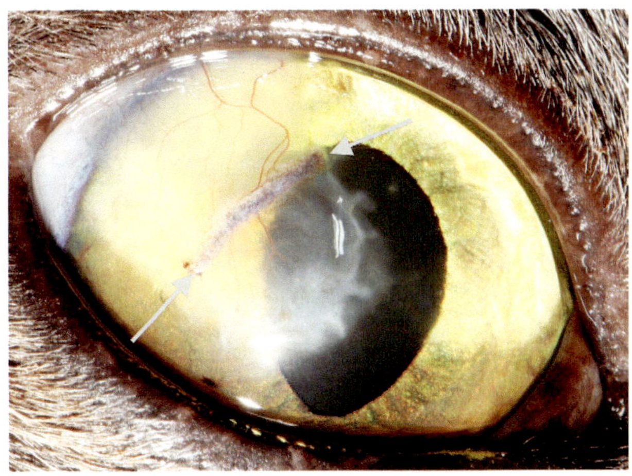

Figure 200. Corneoconjunctival transposition (Figure courtesy of James Oliver, from "Feline Ophthalmology: The Manual" Mitchel and Oliver, ISBN 978-84-16315-11-6, May 2015.

Lens Surgery

- **Lendectomy:** is the surgical removal of the lens, for patients with cataracts or lens luxation. This involves incision into the eye and release and removal of the lens as one piece.
- **Phaecoemulsification** (Figure 201): this is a procedure whereby the lens capsule is opened within the eye and a lens, which has become a mature cataract, is ultrasonically broken down into tiny fragments and aspirated, leaving most of the capsule in place; this then allows placement of an artificial lens within the remaining portion of the capsule.

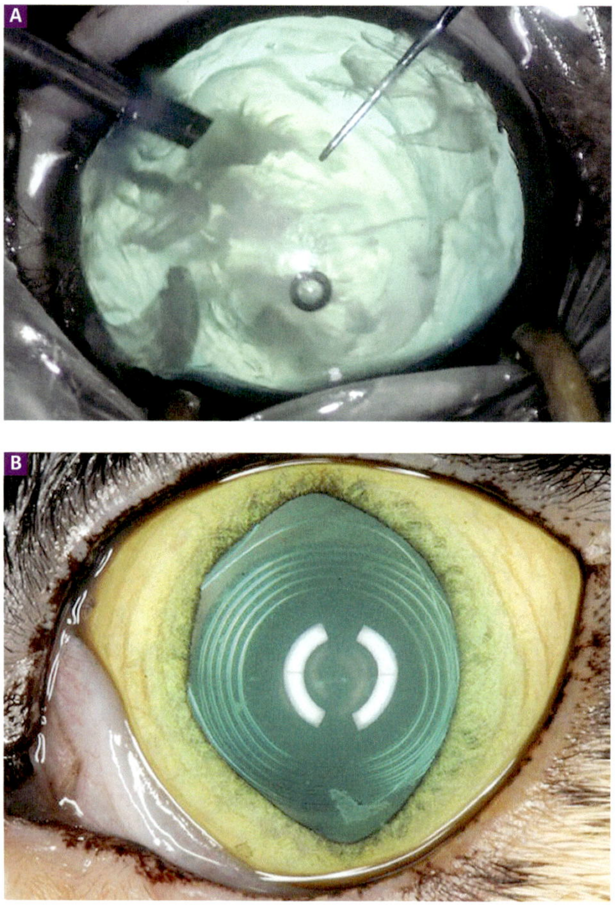

Figure 201. A. Phaecoemulsification (Figure courtesy of Ines Margarida Marino Freitas, Dick White Referrals); B. Artificial lens placed after phacoemusification (Figure courtesy of James Oliver, From "Feline Ophthalmology: The Manual" Mitchel and Oliver, ISBN 978-84-16315-11-6, May 2015.

Enucleation

The eye may be removed due to irreparable damage due to trauma, intraocular infection, neoplasia, or glaucoma (elevated intraocular pressure causing severe pain and blindness). When removing an eye, it is possible to perform different extents of removal in different circumstances:

- **Enucleation** (Figure 202): this is the term for surgical removal of the entire globe of the eye, i.e. everything contained within the sclera and the cornea. It is performed via a transconjunctival approach, and the eyelid margins removed, or by first suturing the eyelids together with a transpalpebral approach.
- **Evisceration:** this is a technique reserved for a painful, non-visual eye free from infection and neoplasia, whereby the internal contents of the globe are removed and replaced with a silicone implant to maintain cosmesis.
- **Exenteration** (Figure 203): this is a more radical surgical technique to remove not only the globe but the entire contents of the orbit, i.e. the extraocular muscles, vessels and optic nerve which sit behind the eye. This may be necessary to manage abscessation of the region or tumours invading the cone of tissues behind the eye.

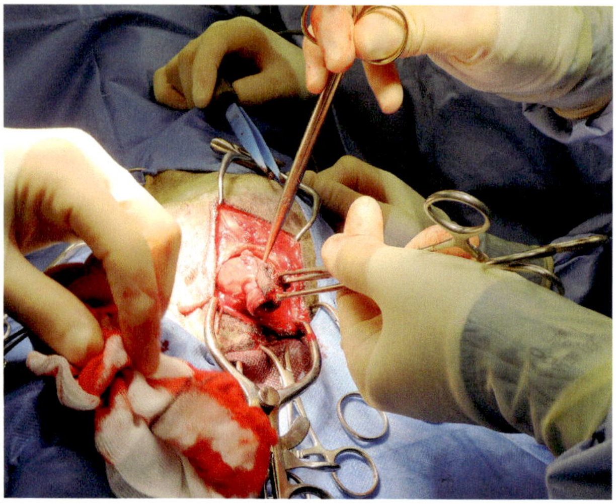

Figure 202. Intraoperative photograph of a patient undergoing transpalpebral enucleation.

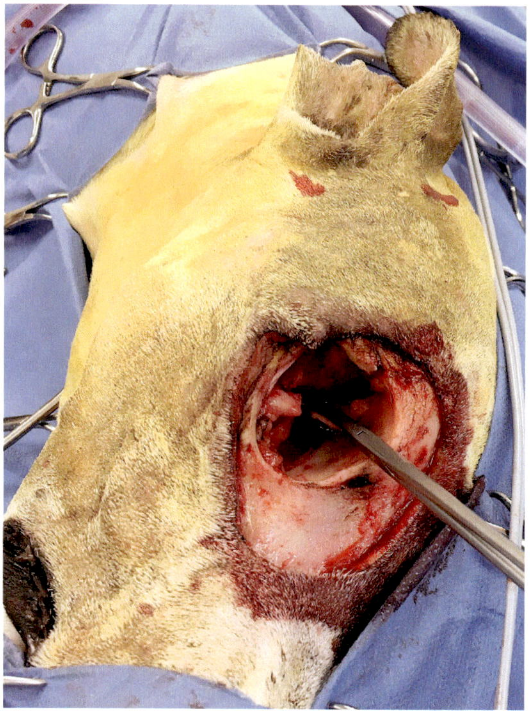

Figure 203. Intraoperative photograph of a patient undergoing exenteration to manage a periorbital sarcoma.

Bibliography

- Andrews, S.J., Thomas, T.M., Hauptman, J.G. and Stanley, B.J. (2018) Investigation of potential risk factors for mesenteric volvulus in military working dogs. *Journal of the American Veterinary Medical Association*, 253 (7), 877–885.
- Cronin, A.M., Pustelnik, S.B., Owen, L. and Hall, J.L. (2019) Evaluation of a pre tied ligature loop for canine total lung lobectomy. *Veterinary Surgery*, 48 (4), 570–577.
- Deroy, C., Hahn, H., Bismuth, C., Ragetly, G., Gomes, E. and Poncet, C. (2019) Simplified minimally invasive surgical approach for prophylactic laparoscopic gastropexy in 21 cases. *Journal of the American Animal Hospital Association*, 55 (3), 152–159.
- Frykfors von Hekkel, A.K., Pegram, C. and Halfacree, Z.J. (2020) Thoracic dog bite wounds in dogs: A retrospective study of 123 cases (2003 2016). *Veterinary Surgery*, 49 (4), 694–703.
- Glickman, L.T., Glickman, N.W., Schellenberg, D.B., Raghavan, M. and Lee, T. (2000) Non-dietary risk factors for gastric dilatation-volvulus in large and giant breed dogs. *Journal of the American Veterinary Medical Association*, 217 (10), 1492–1499.
- Glickman, L.T., Glickman, N.W., Schellenberg, D.B., Raghavan, M. and Lee, T.L. (2000) Incidence of and breed-related risk factors for gastric dilatation-volvulus in dogs. *Journal of the American Veterinary Medical Association*, 216 (1), 40–45.
- Gobello, C., Castex, G., Klima, L., Rodrı guez, R. and Corrada, Y. (2003) A study of two protocols combining aglepristone and cloprostenol to treat open cervix pyometra in the bitch. *Theriogenology*, 60 (5), 901–908.
- Greenhalgh, S.N., Reeve, J.A., Johnstone, T., Goodfellow, M.R., Dunning, M.D., O'Neill, E.J., Hall, E.J., Watson, P.J. and Jeffery, N.D. (2014) Long-term survival and quality of life in dogs with clinical signs associated with a congenital portosystemic shunt after surgical or medical treatment. *Journal of the American Veterinary Medical Association*, 245 (5), 527–533.
- Hayes, G.M., Reynolds, D., Moens, N.M., Singh, A., Oblak, M., Gibson, T.W., Brisson, B.A., Nazarali, A. and Dewey, C. (2014) Investigation of incidence and risk factors for surgical glove perforation in small animal surgery. *Veterinary Surgery*, 43 (4), 400–404.
- Hunt, G.B., Tisdall, P.L., Liptak, J.M., Beck, J.A., Swinney, G.R. and Malik, R. (2001) Skin fold advancement flaps for closing large proximal limb and trunk defects in dogs and cats. *Veterinary Surgery*, 30 (5), 440–448.
- Ladlow, J. (2018) Brachycephalic Obstructive Airway Syndrome–an update. *BSAVA Companion*, 3, pp.4-13.
- Matiasovic, M., Halfacree, Z.J., Moores, A., Nelissen, P., Woods, S., Dean, B., Chanoit, G. and Barnes, D.C. (2018) Surgical management of impalement injuries to the trunk of dogs: a multicentre retrospective study. *Journal of small animal practice*, 59 (3), 139–146.
- Meakin, L.B., Gilman, O.P., Parsons, K.J., Burton, N.J. and Langley Hobbs, S.J. (2016) Colored indicator undergloves increase the detection of glove perforations by surgeons during small animal orthopedic surgery: a randomized controlled trial. *Veterinary Surgery*, 45(6), 709–714.
- Morrice, M., Polton, G. and Beck, S. (2019) Evaluation of the histopathological extent of neoplastic infiltration in intestinal tumours in cats. *Veterinary medicine and science*, 5 (3), 307–316.
- Morrice, M., Polton, G. and Beck, S. (2019) Evaluation of the extent of neoplastic infiltration in small intestinal tumours in dogs. *Veterinary medicine and science*, 5 (2), 189–198.
- Raghavan, M., Glickman, N., McCabe, G., Lantz, G. and Glickman, L.T. (2004) Diet-related risk factors for gastric dilatation-volvulus in dogs of high-risk breeds. *Journal of the American Animal Hospital Association*, 40 (3), 192–203.
- Risselada, M., Ellison, G.W., Bacon, N.J., Polyak, M.M., Van Gilder, J., Kirkby, K. and Kim, S.E. (2010) Comparison of 5 surgical techniques for partial liver lobectomy in the dog for intraoperative blood loss and surgical time. *Veterinary Surgery*, 39 (7), 856–862.
- Rosenbaum, J.M., Coolman, B.R., Davidson, B.L., Daly, M.L., Rexing, J.F. and Eatroff, A.E. (2016) The use of disposable skin staples for intestinal resection and anastomosis in 63 dogs: 2000 to 2014. *Journal of Small Animal Practice*, 57 (11), 631–636.
- Schwartz, Z. and Coolman, B.R. (2018) Disposable skin staplers for closure of linear gastrointestinal incisions in dogs. *Veterinary Surgery*, 47 (2), 285–292.
- Schwartz, Z. and Coolman, B.R. (2018) Closure of gastrointestinal incisions using skin staples alone and in combination with suture in 29 cats. *Journal of Small Animal Practice*, 59 (5), 281–285.
- Stillion, J.R. and Letendre, J.A. (2015) A clinical review of the pathophysiology, diagnosis, and treatment of pyothorax in dogs and cats. *Journal of Veterinary Emergency and Critical Care*, 25 (1), 113–129.
- Swinbourne, F., Jeffery, N., Tivers, M.S., Artingstall, R., Bird, F., Charlesworth, T., Doran, I., Freeman, A., Hall, J., Hattersley, R. and Henken, J. (2017) The incidence of surgical site dehiscence following full thickness gastrointestinal biopsy in dogs and cats and associated risk factors. *Journal of Small Animal Practice*, 58 (9), 495–503.
- Ward, M.P., Patronek, G.J. and Glickman, L.T. (2003) Benefits of prophylactic gastropexy for dogs at risk of gastric dilatation–volvulus. *Preventive veterinary medicine*, 60 (4), 319–329.
- Wilson, D. and Monnet, E. (2016) Risk factors for the development of aspiration pneumonia after unilateral arytenoid lateralization in dogs with laryngeal paralysis: 232 cases (1987–2012). *Journal of the American Veterinary Medical Association*, 248 (2), 188–194.

Test

Answers on Page 422

1. Which of these is not one of Halstead's principles for handling soft tissues in surgery?
a. Gentle tissue handling.
b. Meticulous haemostasis.
c. Strict asepsis.
d. Creation of dead space.

2. What is the name of the retractor shown below?
a. Finochietto.
b. Balfour.
c. Gelpi.
d. Weitlander.

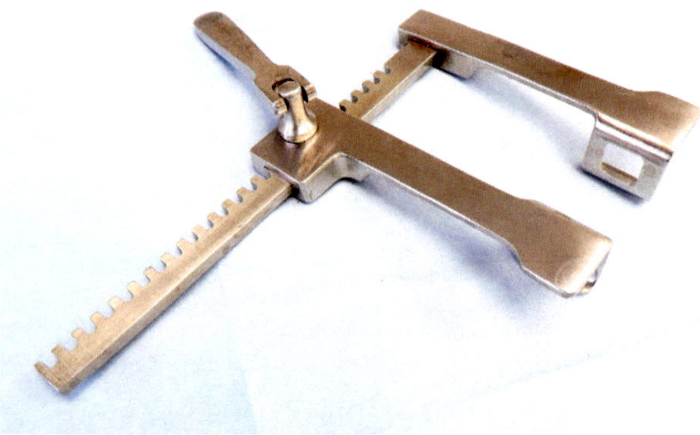

3. To which category of surgery is a gastrotomy for removal of a foreign body assigned?
a. Clean.
b. Clean-contaminated.
c. Contaminated.
d. Dirty/Infected.

4. Which breed of dog is predisposed to gallbladder mucocoele?
a. Border Terrier.
b. Labrador.
c. Coton de Tulear.
d. French Bulldog.

5. Which of these cartilages is not associated with the larynx?
a. Arytenoid.
b. Thyroid.
c. Auricular.
d. Cricoid.

6. Which of these suture materials creates the most intense tissue reaction?
a. Catgut.
b. Maxon® (polyglyconate).
c. Vicryl® (polyglactin 910).
d. Nylon® (polyamide).

7. What is the name of the retractor shown below?
a. Senn.
b. Malleable.
c. Langenbeck.
d. Army and Navy.

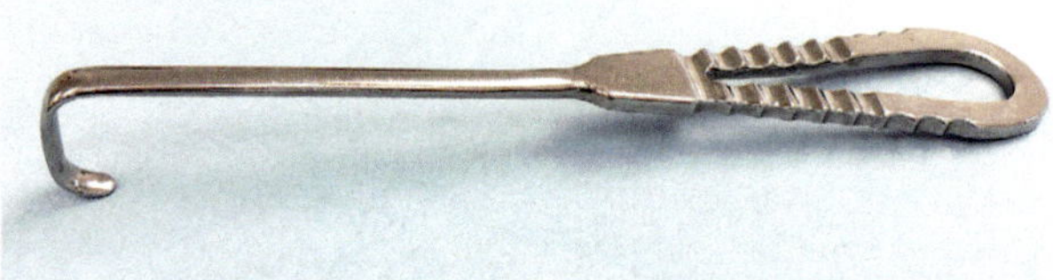

8. What is the meaning of the term "enteroplication"?
a. Anchoring the stomach to the body wall to prevent volvulus.
b. Suturing loops of bowel alongside one another to prevent intussusception.
c. Anchoring the colon to the body wall to prevent rectal prolapse.
d. Suturing a loop of bowel to another to protect an enterotomy site.

9. Which of these is not a function of the spleen?
a. Synthesis of clotting factors.
b. A reservoir of 10–20% of red blood cells.
c. Maturation of red blood cells following production in the bone marrow.
d. Immunological function in lymphoid follicles.

10. What is the Branham reflex?
a. Bradycardia noted immediately after ligation of a portosystemic shunt.
b. Tachycardia noted immediately after ligation of a portosystemic shunt.
c. Tachycardia noted immediately after ligation of a patent ductus arteriosus.
d. Bradycardia noted immediately after ligation of a patent ductus arteriosus.

Clinical Case 1

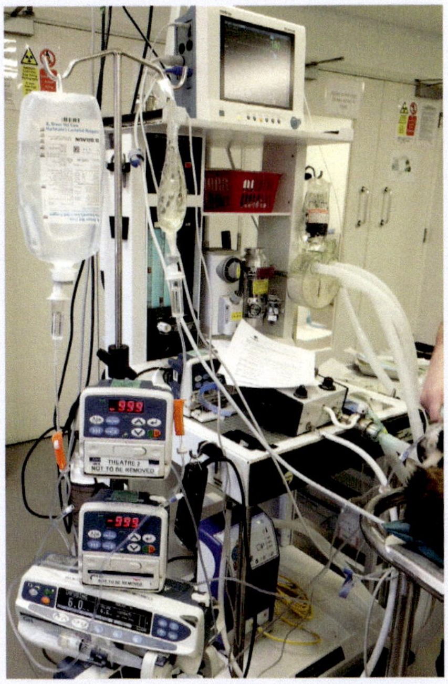

PRESENTATION

Your reception team take a call this evening from Mrs Roberts regarding her dog Geoffrey – an 8-year-old entire male, St Bernard. He has been retching non-productively for the last half an hour. He had had a quiet afternoon, had been chasing a ball in the garden before having his dinner just over an hour ago. He is now getting weaker, and Mrs Roberts will need to call on a neighbour to help lift Geoffrey into the car to come to the practice for assessment.

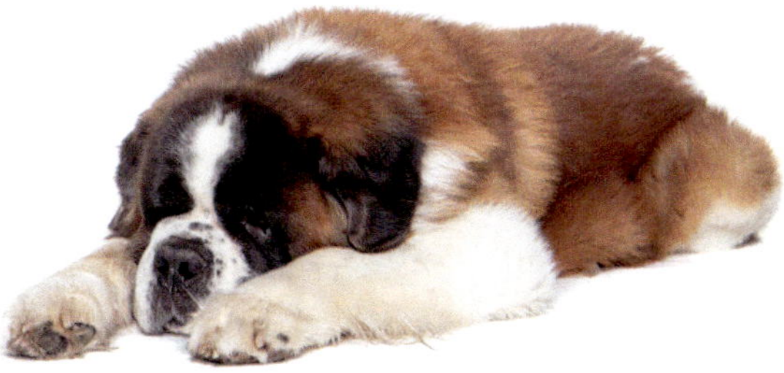

The vet suspects a gastric dilatation/volvulus and asks you to prepare for its arrival.

1. **List the equipment you prepare for helping triage and stabilise Geoffrey on his arrival.**

Geoffrey is assisted into the practice on a trolley as he is now weak. His abdomen is markedly distended and tympanic on palpation. A gastric tube is lubricated and passed into his mouth and down to the stomach. This releases a large amount of air and fluid from the stomach.

2. **How long a length of tube should be passed to reach the stomach?**

Geoffrey's peripheral pulses are weak and thready, and his heart rate is nearly 200 bpm.

3. **What might be the cause(s) of the tachycardia and hence the next steps in Geoffrey's treatment?**

INVESTIGATION

A bedside blood gas analyser reveals elevated lactate and metabolic acidosis.

4. **How do you treat Geoffrey for these findings?**

A right lateral abdominal radiograph is taken consciously whilst further intravenous fluids are being administered.

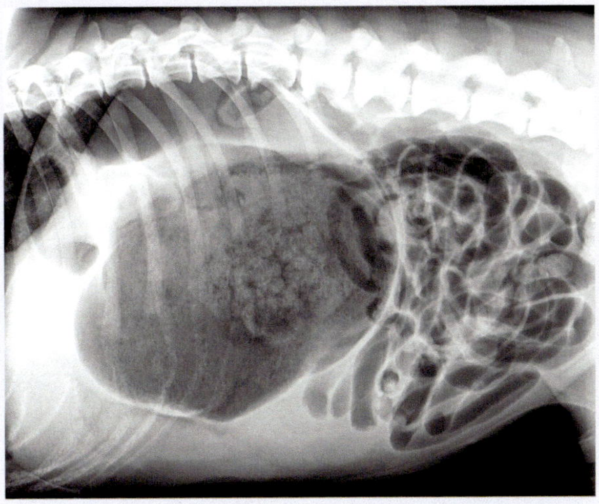

5. The following signs are all present in the radiograph, but which confirms the diagnosis of gastric volvulus?

a. Gas filling of the stomach.

b. Displacement of the intestines caudally.

c. Poor serosal detail due to free abdominal fluid.

d. Malpositioning of the gastric axis – with an invert C shape to the stomach.

SURGICAL TREATMENT

The surgeon completes a surgical request form as shown, with a basic instrument kit and some additional specialist items.

INSTRUMENT REQUESTS			
Basic kit			
Ligasure	Precise		
	5mm		Short
	10mm		Long
Harmonic Scalpel			Mono
			Bipolar
			Shears
Cautery	Mono		Bipolar
Gelpi	Mini	Med	Large
Gosset	Small		Large
Finochietto	Small		Large
Drill / Saw	Arthrex		
	Minidriver		
	Colibri		
Stapler (Size)	TA GIA Endo GIA		
	30 60 90		
Suction	Poole	Frazier	Yankauer
Scope	2.7mm Cysto		
	5mm Lap 30°		
	10mm Lap 0°		
Caesarian Drape	Laparoscopy Kit		
4 Quarter Drapes	Pin & Wire Kit		
Bowl	Ophthalmic Kit		
Lap Sponges	Biopsy Kit		
Syringes	2.3 5 10 20 50		
Saline	100 500 1000		

6. Select the additional requested instruments from the following table:

Mosquito	Kelly	Cocker
Poole	Yankauer	Frasier
Satinsky	Gossett	Langenbeck
DeBakey	Babcock	Allis

Before induction of anaesthesia the 'Sign In' part of the Surgical Safety Checklist is completed:

SIGN IN (to be read out loud)

Before induction of anaesthesia

Has the patient identity been confirmed?
□ Yes
Has a surgical request form been completed?
□ Yes
What is the procedure to be undertaken?

Do we have consent for the procedure?
□ Yes: Written / Verbal

Have the anaesthetic machine and monitor checks been completed?
□ Yes
Has a patient warming device been prepared?
□ Yes □ No, not required for this patient
Have CBC, MBC, coagulation times been checked?
□ Yes □ Not required

What is the ASA Status of the patient?
□ I □ II □ III □ IV □ V □ E
Is the patient currently receiving any medications?
□ No □ Yes:

Antibiotics to be administered after induction?
□ No □ Yes:

Does the patient have any known allergies?
□ No □ Yes:
Difficult airway/aspiration risk?
□ No □ Yes, and equipment/assistance available
Risk of >10% blood loss?
□ No □ Yes: transfusion planned?
Blood type? ___________
Previous transfusions? □ Yes □ No
Are blood products available?

Has an internal referral request form been completed?
□ Yes / Surgeon confirmed not required

PATIENT DETAILS	
Last name:	
First name:	
Breed/Age:	
Patient Number:	

7. What is the ASA Status of the patient?

a. I.

b. IIE.

c. III.

d. IVE.

8. Is the patient at risk of aspiration? Yes / No

9. What equipment should be made available?

Geoffrey is anaesthetised, intubated and an orogastric tube replaced whilst he is clipped and prepared for surgery. Epidural morphine and levobupivicaine are administered for analgesia.

Prior to the first incision, once the surgical team have draped the patient and set out the required equipment, the Time Out is performed:

TIME OUT (to be read out loud)

Before start of surgical intervention

Have all team members introduced themselves by name and role?
□ Yes

Confirm the procedure and feeding tube requirement:
□ Checked as planned / Noted changes to plan:

Are there any critical or unexpected steps you want the team to know about?

Are there any patient specific concerns?
□ No □ Yes:

Do we need to notify ICU to prepare for recovery?
□ No □ Yes

Has the sterility of the instruments been confirmed?
□ Yes
Have electrosurgical devices been connected and turned on?
□ Yes
Have Instruments and swabs been counted?
□ Yes (Tally swabs below)
Are there any equipment issues or concerns?
□ No □ Yes:

Have pre-operative antibiotics been administered?
□ Not requested □ No □ Yes:
Has pre-surgical imaging been reported?
□ Yes / not applicable
Is essential imaging displayed?
□ Yes / not applicable
Has the air conditioning been set to 21°C?
□ Yes

SWAB & SHARP TALLY					
		Counted In		Counted Out	
10x10	**20x20**				
Cotton tips					
Needles					
Blades					

10. What are the specific anaesthetic/surgical concerns for this patient?

At surgery the gastric dilatation and volvulus are confirmed. The stomach is repositioned. The stomach wall appears healthy and so a tube gastropexy is performed. The spleen is also healthy and so left in situ.

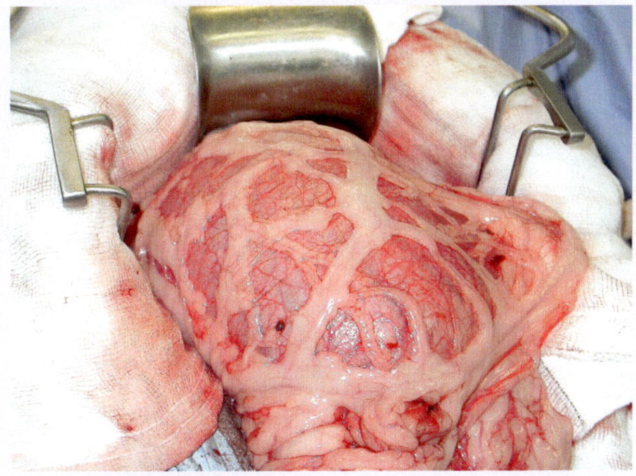

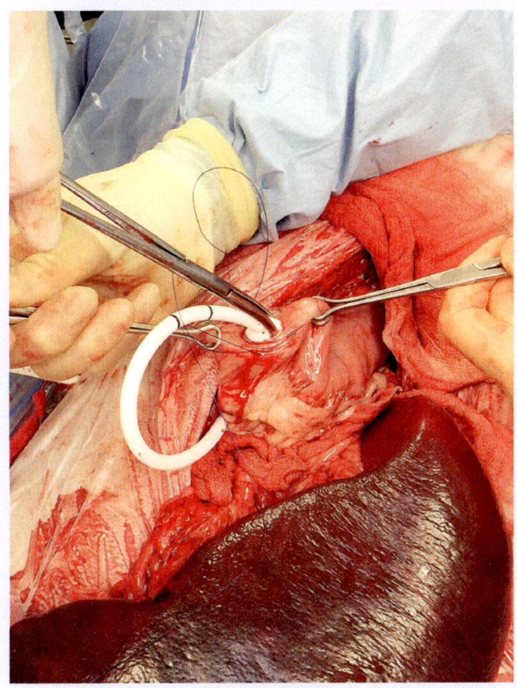

At the end of surgery, the final part of the surgical safety checklist is completed:

END OF SURGERY (to be read out loud)

Before any team member leaves theatre

Name of procedure undertaken?

What are the key concerns for recovery and management of this patient?

Post-operative requirements:
- ☐ **Medications:**
- ☐ **Checks:**
- ☐ **Feeding:**

Is a buster collar required?
☐ Hard ☐ Soft ☐ None

Is a bandage or dressing required?
☐ No ☐ Primapore ☐ Other:

Are instrument, swabs and sharp counts complete?
☐ Yes

Are throat packs, rectal swabs and purse strings removed?
☐ Yes

Have the specimens been labelled & preserved?
☐ Yes

Nominee to sign out & submit specimens?

Have any equipment problems been identified?
☐ No ☐ Yes:

SIGN OUT

Before nominee leaves the prep room

Have the laboratory request forms been completed and specimens collected?
☐ **Yes. Signed:**

ACCOUNT COMPLETION	
Before scanning records	**Y**
Post-op medications been dispensed?	
Has the procedure been priced & logged? (correct date/surgeon/cost centre)	
Internal Referral Fee / Soft Tissue Reports List	

11. What are the key concerns for recovery and management of this patient?

12. What are our postoperative requirements with regards to medication, checks and feeding to manage these concerns?

Due to the team's meticulous attention to detail and swift treatment, Geoffrey made an uneventful recovery from surgery and was discharged 2 days later.

Clinical Case 2

PRESENTATION

Toby is a 12-year-old neutered male Labrador. He arrives at your practice as an emergency in respiratory distress, with severe stridor, having been taken on a walk on the hottest day so far this year. His owner, Mrs Trimble, suggest he has had increased airway noise on exercise over the last six months and occasionally wretches after eating. He is gasping and appears moderately cyanotic in the waiting room.

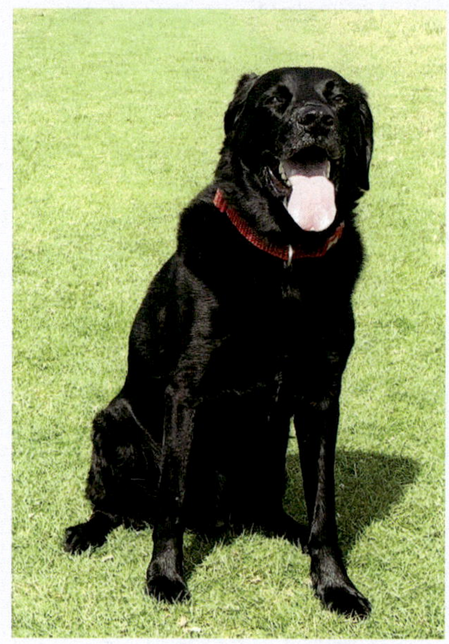

1. What are your immediate concerns with regards to stabilising Toby?

INVESTIGATION

2. Now that Toby is calm and settled, what further investigations need to be considered?

Blood results are within normal limits. Toby has no abnormalities on thorough general physical examination or neurological examination beyond the upper respiratory noise due to suspected laryngeal dysfunction.

Airway assessment is performed under a light plane of anaesthesia. Structurally the larynx appears normal – with no obvious mass lesions or swelling. Functionally, there is relatively normal movement on the right side but absent movement on the left side.

3. What is the diagnosis?

Three radiographic views of the thorax are taken with inflation and a right lateral view of the neck. No additional abnormalities are noted.

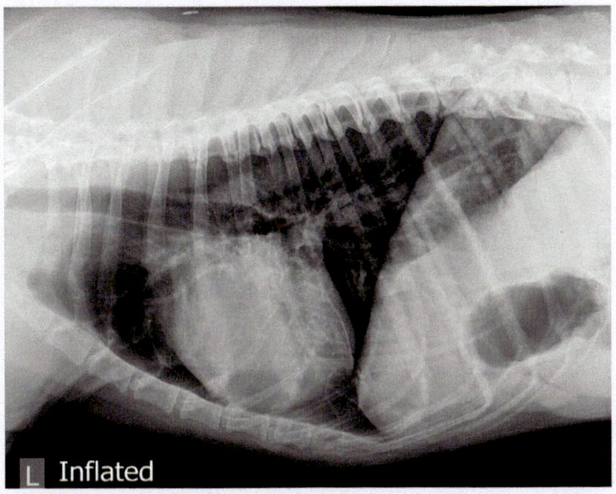

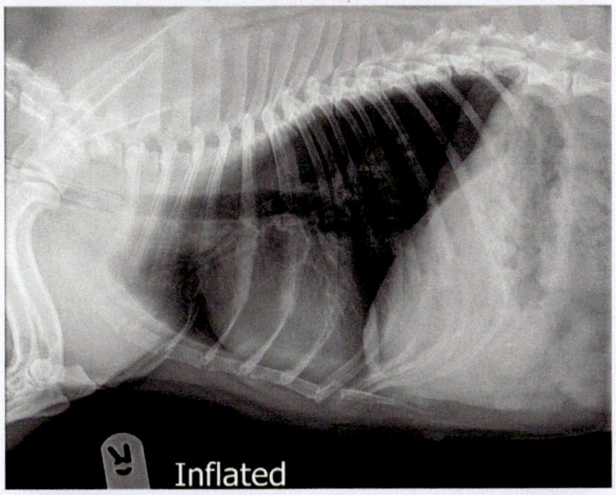

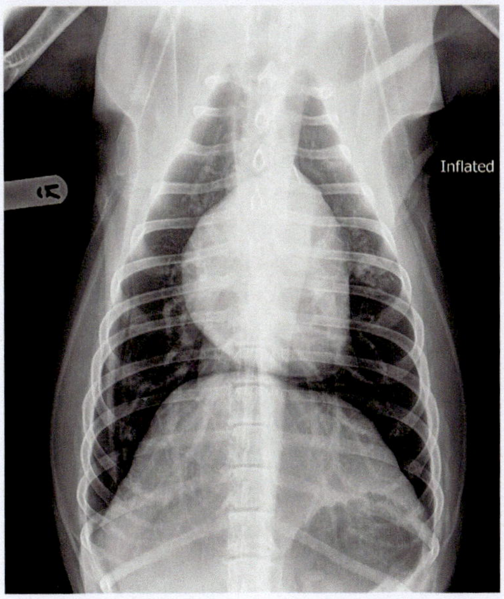

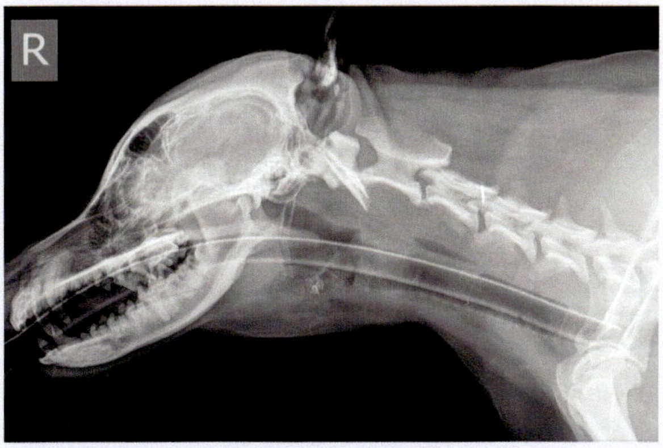

SURGICAL TREATMENT

The veterinary surgeon discusses the findings with Mrs Trimble, who agrees that Toby should undergo airway surgery.

4. What surgery is likely to be performed?

5. How should Toby be clipped and positioned for this surgery?

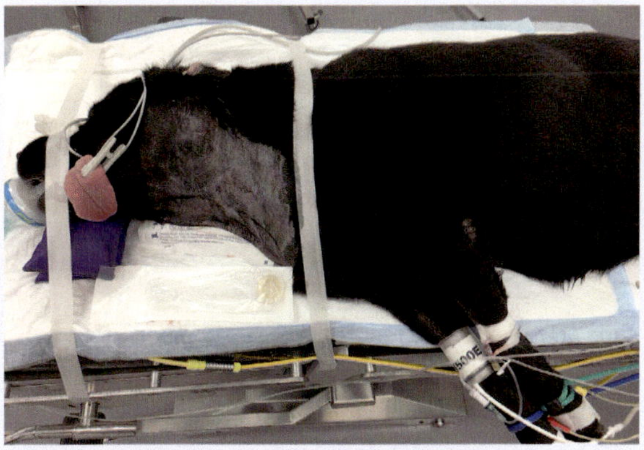

6. List the surgical instruments which have been prepared (from left to right).

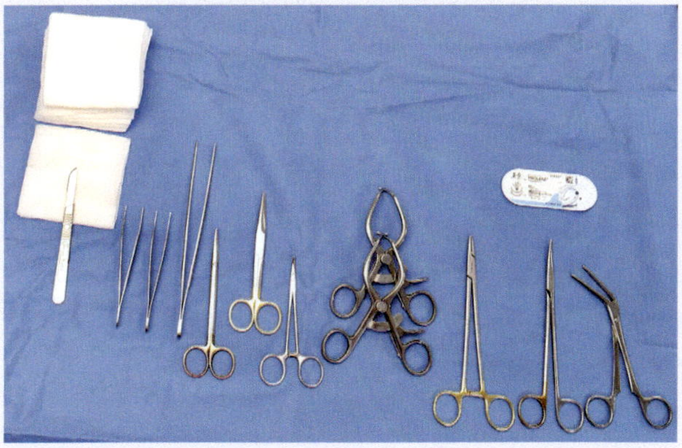

Surgery is performed to access the left side of the larynx to place sutures from the left arytenoid cartilage to the cricoid and thyroid cartilages to move the arytenoid and hence the left vocal fold to the side, into an "always open" position.

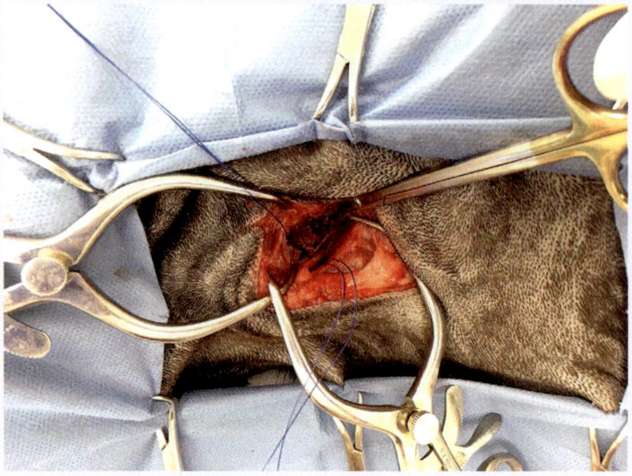

POSTOPERATIVE CARE

7. What are the postoperative concerns for Toby? Based on these concerns, help construct a nursing plan for him.

Notes

Correct Answers:

Test

1.d
2.a
3.b
4.a
5.c
6.a
7.c
8.b
9.a
10.d

Clinical Case 1

1. List the equipment you prepare for helping triage and stabilise Geoffrey on his arrival.

- Trolley/stretcher.
- Intravenous catheters (large bore).
- Intravenous fluids (isotonic crystalloids/colloids/hypertonic saline).
- Drip pumps.
- Orogastric tube, bucket, lubricant to aid passage.
- Methadone for analgesia.
- Clippers.
- Skin prep.
- ECG.
- Blood pressure monitor/cuff.
- Biochemistry analyser turned on (bedside blood gas analyser if available).

2. How long a length of tube should be passed to reach the stomach?

This can be premeasured using the distance from his nose to his elbow as a guide and marking the tube with tape.

3. What might be the cause(s) of the tachycardia and hence the next steps in Geoffrey's treatment?

- **Shock** (Hypovolaemic/distributive) – large bore intravenous catheters are placed in both forelimbs and crystalloid fluids administered as rapidly as the fluid pumps will allow.
- **Pain** – methadone is administered intravenously.

4. How do you treat Geoffrey for these findings?

High volume intravenous fluid therapy with Hartmann's solution/Lactate ringers' solution to improve perfusion and buffer the acidosis.

5. Which confirms the diagnosis of gastric volvulus?

d) Malpositioning of the gastric axis – with an invert C shape to the stomach.

6. Select the additional requested instruments.

Poole, DeBakey, Kelly, Gossett, Babcock.

7. What is the ASA Status of the patient?

d) IVE.

8. Is the patient at risk of aspiration?

Yes.

9. What equipment should be made available?

Suction machine and appropriate tip to pass down the oesophagus/endotracheal tube.

10. What are the specific anaesthetic/surgical concerns for this patient?

Anaesthetic:

- Risk of release of inflammatory mediators with derotation of the stomach.
- Risk of bleeding.
- Pain.

Surgical:

- Possible necrosis of the stomach wall which might need resection.
- Possible splenic torsion also which might require removal.

11. What are the key concerns for recovery and management of this patient?

- Hypotension.
- Regurgitation/aspiration pneumonia.
- Septic peritonitis (from leakage around the gastrostomy tube).
- Pain.
- Ileus.
- Pancreatitis.
- Incisional dehiscence.
- Surgical site infection.
- Arrhythmia (ventricular tachycardia).
- Recurrent gastric dilatation.
- Urinary retention.

12. **What are our postoperative requirements with regards to medication, checks and feeding to manage these concerns?**
    - Continue intravenous fluid therapy and monitor urine output, recheck renal parameters and lactate following anaesthetic recovery.
    - Hourly assessment of gastric distension or tympany – drain stomach via the gastrostomy tube if needed.
    - Methadone as required based on pain scoring every 2 hours.
    - Placement of an indwelling urinary catheter to allow monitoring of urine output and manage urinary retention following the epidural.
    - Continuous ECG monitoring for arrhythmia.
    - Hourly heart and respiratory rate and effort assessment initially then tapering.
    - Eight hourly temperature assessment to monitor for fever in case of peritonitis / sepsis.
    - Bland, low-fat diet (in case of pancreatitis) to be started early following anaesthetic recovery, either orally or via the gastrostomy tube – but monitoring gut sounds and residual gastric content before next feed to assess for ileus.

Clinical Case 2

1. **What are your immediate concerns with regards to stabilising Toby?**
    - Oxygen supplementation (oxygen cage/flow-by/nasal prongs).
    - Active cooling.
    - Sedation to alleviate anxiety.
    - Establish intravenous access when calm enough to do so without additional stress.

2. **What further investigations need to be considered?**
    - Thorough general physical examination, including thoracic auscultation and pulse assessment to screen for lower airway and cardiac causes of dyspnoea.
    - Neurological assessment.
    - Complete blood cell count, serum biochemistry, T4 and TSH to assess thyroid function.
    - Airway functional examination under a light plane of anaesthesia.
    - Thoracic and cervical radiography or computed tomography (CT).

3. **What is the diagnosis?**
    Left sided laryngeal hemiplegia (paralysis).

4. **What surgery is likely to be performed?**
    A left sided arytenoid lateralisation (tie-back).

5. **How should Toby be clipped and positioned for this surgery?**
    - Right lateral recumbency.
    - The neck supported with a sandbag / foam wedge / pack of swabs.
    - Forelimbs tied back.
    - The head may be secured in position with positioning aids or adhesive tape.
    - The left lateral and ventral aspects of the neck should be clipped, 15 cm cranial and caudal to the larynx.
    - It may be considered to use long anaesthetic circuit tubing so that the head of the patient can be positioned away from the anaesthetic machine to give the surgeon and anaesthetist space to work.

6. **List the surgical instruments which have been prepared.**
    - 10x10 cm Gauze swabs.
    - Scalpel handle with No10 Scalpel blade.
    - Addson Brown Thumb Forceps.
    - Addson Thumb Forceps.
    - DeBakey Thumb Forceps.
    - Metzenbaum Scissors.
    - Mayo Scissors.
    - Mosquito Haemostatic Forceps.
    - Mini Gelpi Retractors.
    - Mayo Hegar Needle Holders.
    - Suture Scissors.
    - Galliban Forceps.

7. **What are the postoperative concerns for Toby? Based on these concerns, help construct a nursing plan for him.**

    Aspiration pneumonia:
    - Food should be withheld until the surgeon has assessed that the patient has fully recovered from anaesthesia and regained a normal gag reflex. Often this may mean waiting for 24 hours following surgery.
    - When fed, patients should be hand fed soft balls of food to control the speed of eating – to ensure each mouthful is successfully swallowed before the next is offered.

- Dusty/crumbly dry foods and very liquid foods should be avoided as these will be at greater risk of being aspirated.
- Some surgeons recommend avoiding swimming, but there is no scientific evidence to support the need for this restriction.

Suture failure and hence recurrence of clinical signs:

- Interference with the surgical incision should be prevented using a soft collar.
- The patient should be kept calm and/or discharged in timely fashion when fully awake if stressed in the hospital environment and barking excessively.

Seroma:

- Dissection of the soft tissues over the larynx may predispose to fluid accumulation at the surgical site. Cold compression immediately postoperatively may be of benefit in preventing fluid accumulation and warm compression will improve blood flow to the area to aid fluid absorption in the event of seroma formation.

Pain:

- Arytenoid lateralisation is not typically noted to be a painful procedure.
- Levobupivicaine infiltration or splash block into the surgical site can aid perioperative analgesia.
- Opioid administration following arytenoid lateralisation should be carefully considered as there is evidence to suggest this may increase the risk of regurgitation and aspiration pneumonia postoperatively. NSAIDs and paracetamol should be considered when appropriate for the patient.
- (Progressive neurological dysfunction – longer term, in patients with polyneuropathies).

Notes

Orthopaedic Procedures

Alison Mann

Chapter Summary:

- **Different fracture types and options for their treatment including forelimb, hindlimb and skull.**
- **Orthopaedic equipment including basic instrumentation, plating kits, external fixation kits, joint surgery, spinal surgery and arthroscopy.**
- **Use, care and maintenance of orthopaedic equipment.**
- **Principles and mechanics for specific joint surgical procedures including joint replacement.**
- **Pathophysiology of different conditions of the spine and specific surgical procedures.**
- **Pros and cons of a variety of rehabilitation techniques. The importance of their role in the patient after specific surgical procedures.**

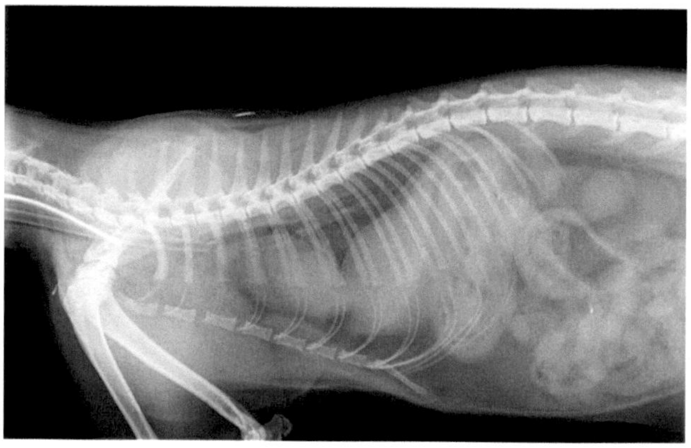

Figure 1. In this case the patient had a diaphragmatic rupture which was addressed and stabilised before any form of fracture fixation took place.

Fractures

In veterinary practice, animals with fractured bones are common and usually presented after a trauma such as a road traffic accident or fall from a height. The veterinary nurse (VN) plays many roles in the care of these patients, from triage of the newly arrived animal to assisting in theatre for fracture repair.

This chapter aims to equip the VN with the knowledge to provide optimal patient care, understand the veterinary surgeon's (VS) decisions, and be an efficient assistant at every stage of the patient's care.

Fractures occur when bone is subject to a force greater than its strength to withstand that force. Importantly, fractures often occur due to trauma and whilst fractures are rarely life-threatening, the concurrent injuries might be. Therefore, **when a patient presents post-trauma, although the fracture may be obvious, it is important to take a holistic approach and perform a full body system check.**

In some patients, the fracture might not even be repaired for a few days as the patient needs time to stabilise after the initial trauma (Figure 1). For example, in cats pelvic fractures can have a high level of morbidity and mortality due to concurrent injuries; such as thoracic trauma, internal haemorrhage, and urinary tract injury (Gant et al., 2019).

These internal injuries take precedence over fracture repair, with the cat requiring a workup including packed cell volume, radiographs (potential urethrogram to assess damage to the urinary system), and possibly a blood transfusion. Scapula or humeral fractures often have concurrent thoracic or soft tissue injury due to their location and the amount of soft tissue surrounding the structures.

If stabilisation is required and it is possible to place a **Robert Jones bandage (RJB) or a splint this may help with pain relief and prevent further injury.**

The main forces that cause fractures are bending, compression, shearing, tension and torsion (Figure 2). When the VS decides on the most appropriate method for fracture fixation, they take these forces into account because the method of fracture fixation needs to counteract them (Kapler and Dycus, 2015). Without this, the fracture may not heal and the fixation may even fail, leading to further surgery and an increased risk of infection.

The direction of fracture lines and the number of fracture lines are determined by the forces acting on them at the time of injury, as well as their velocity. High velocity forces are more likely to result not only in fracture of the bone (often comminuted) but also in damage to the surrounding soft tissue.

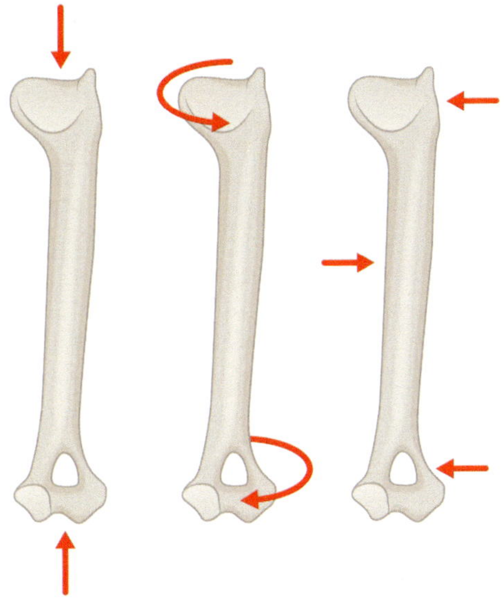

Figure 2. Main forces on the bone that can cause fractures.

Treatment for a fracture depends upon factors (Figure 3) such as the location of the fracture, the forces acting upon it, and the availability of equipment and expertise. Ultimately the treatment decision is down to the VS but the role of the VN is such that knowledge of the fracture, the method of repair, and patient considerations are important to enable appropriate, holistic care of that patient.

Once the patient is stable and any life-threatening injuries dealt with, the fracture should be assessed, and a treatment plan decided on. The considerations on how to repair a fracture can be split into three categories:

- mechanical
- biological
- clinical.

Table 1 discusses these categories and the factors that come under each category.

Table 1. Considerations for fracture repair. (Fossum, 2007).

Mechanical factors	· how many limbs are affected? · size of patient · activity levels of the patient · whether the fracture is reducible or not
Biological factors	· age/health of the patient · open/closed fracture · high energy vs low energy fracture · open reduction vs closed reduction · skill of the surgeon
Clinical factors	· compliance of the owner postoperatively · patient cooperation · limb function postoperatively

For example, there are different considerations in an elderly patient compared to a younger patient; similarly, a patient that may be difficult to manage postoperatively has different considerations to a more compliant animal (Figure 3).

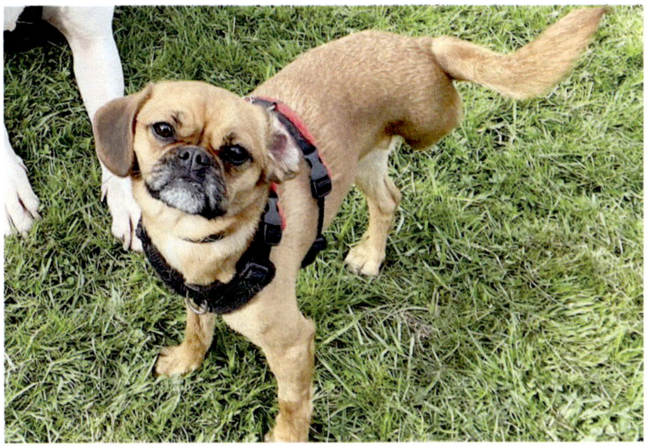

Figure 3. This patient would need very different treatment considerations for a fracture repair compared to a dog with four limbs.

Specific Fractures

Open

A communication between the fracture and the outside environment carries a higher risk of infection. The communication may be due to bone breaking through the soft tissue or something external penetrating the soft tissue to the bone. **In these cases, the use of plates and screws is discouraged, and an external fixator may be the best option,** which also facilitates wound management.

Pathological

These fractures are often due to weakness in the bone caused by a bone tumour, such as osteosarcoma. **When an osteosarcoma is diagnosed, it is important to establish if metastasis has occurred with further imaging.** Sometimes the kindest option is to euthanize the patient if this is the case. If there is no spread the affected limb is often amputated, provided this gives the animal a good quality of life afterwards.

Pathological fractures can also occur due to **nutritional hyperparathyroidism.** In this condition there are low blood calcium levels due a diet low in calcium (e.g. all meat based). To counteract this, the body reduces calcium excretion from the kidneys and absorbs calcium from the bones, which weakens them (Tomsa, 1999). Nutritional hyperparathyroidism is rarely seen due to the availability of commercially balanced diets.

Physeal

Physeal fractures affect the physis (or growth plate) of the bone in a young animal. These fractures are further classified using the Salter-Harris classification system (Table 2).

Table 2. Salter-Harris classification system. (Piermattei et al., 2006).

Salter-Harris grade	Presentation
1	Separation of epiphysis from metaphysis at the growth plate.
2	Corner of metaphyseal bone fractured with displacement of fragment at the growth plate.
3	Fracture through the epiphysis and growth plate but not including the metaphysis.
4	Fracture through the epiphysis, metaphysis and growth plate, could be same fracture line or different.

Avulsion

An avulsion fracture is one where the fragment of bone includes the insertion for a muscle, tendon, or ligament. One of the more common sites for this type of fracture is the tibial tuberosity at the insertion of the quadriceps muscle (Gower et al., 2008) (Figure 4).

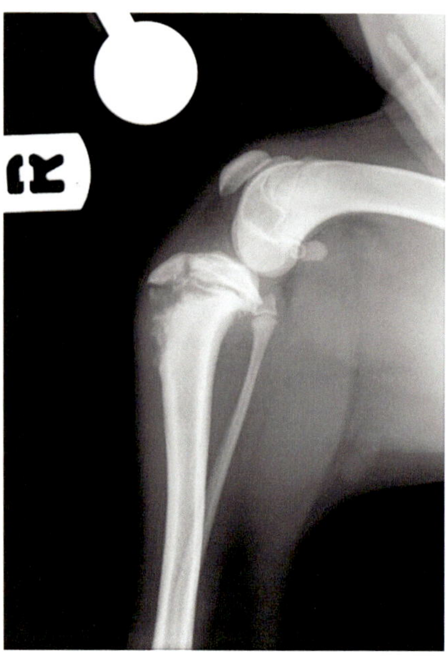

Figure 4. An avulsion fracture of the tibial tuberosity. Courtesy from Dra. Marta Soler, HCV Universidad de Murcia.

Principles of Fracture Repair

Some fractures may heal without the need for surgery. Simple fractures, where the fracture line does not run all the way through the bone or where there is no displacement of the fragments, can be treated by external coaptation such as a splint or a Robert Jones bandage (RJB).

Fractures which require surgical treatment are referred to as reducible or non-reducible.

- **Reducible.** If a fracture is reducible, this means the surgeon can bring the fragments together in alignment using specific instruments to assist, then a bone plate and screws to hold the fragments together whilst the bone heals. When this is achieved, the load the animal bears after fracture fixation is shared between the bone and the plate (Conzemius and Swainson, 1999).
- **Non-reducible.** Alternatively, a non-reducible fracture, where fragments cannot be realigned, is often treated with an external skeletal fixator or a bone plate and screws to create a bridge across the area between fragments. This means the plate and screws take on the entire load until the bone starts to heal, meaning the implants need to be strong enough to withstand all forces upon them (Conzemius and Swainson, 1999).

Surgical repair of a fracture which involves dissecting through soft tissue layers to find and reduce it is called open fracture reduction. When the fracture fragments can be aligned and placed back together with little or no gap in between the fragments this results in direct union (Houlton, 2016). The surgeon uses instruments such as bone holding forceps and fragment reducing forceps to manipulate the fragments, realign them and hold them in alignment until a plate is placed and secured with screws (Figure 5).

When anatomic reduction is not possible, the surgeon must ensure the limb is aligned and maintains the same length regardless that the fragments cannot be aligned. This is called indirect union. An example of how the VS achieves this is to use an intramedullary or Steinmann pin to engage the furthest two aspects of the fracture, and then place either an external fixator or a plate which bridges the gap and takes the load whilst the fracture heals. Indirect union involves the formation of a soft callus which mineralizes into a hard callus before the formation of cortical bone by osteoblasts (Houlton, 2016).

One type of closed reduction is to support the limb with a cast, splint, or Robert Jones bandage (RJB) whilst healing occurs. This in only appropriate for non-displaced, simple, or greenstick fractures. Also, the joints proximal and distal to the fracture site must be supported by the bandage for this method to work, therefore this choice is not appropriate for humeral or femoral fracture repair. A Velpeau sling could be used for

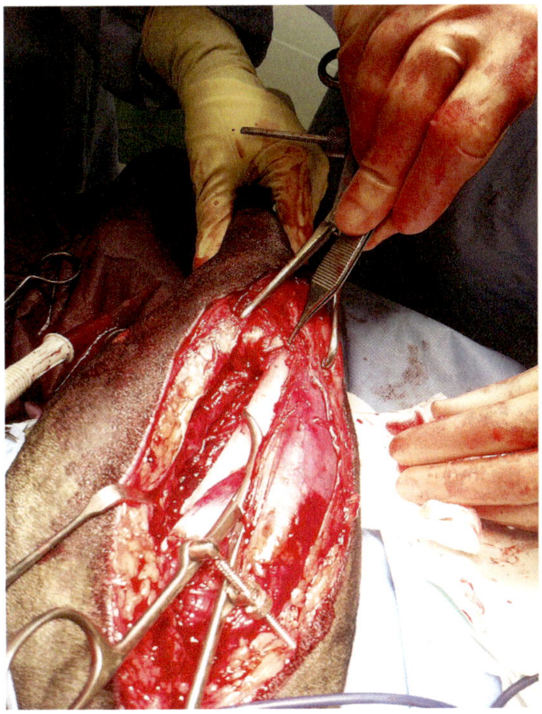

Figure 5. Open fracture repair with soft tissue retraction and manipulation of the fracture back into alignment. In this picture, the surgeon is using a pair of fragment reducing forceps to hold the fracture together whilst the plate is prepared.

non-displaced fractures of the scapula and humerus. External skeletal fixators (ESF) are also a type of closed reduction, when there is no dissection of soft tissue to access the fracture site. Intraoperative fluoroscopy may be beneficial in these cases.

Minimally invasive plate osteosynthesis involves placing a bone plate over the fracture without accessing the fracture site to manipulate the fragments into alignment. This can be used for simple, minimally displaced fractures or fractures where the plate acts as a buttress for fragments which cannot be aligned. To do this, small, incisions are made proximal and distal to the fracture site to facilitate placing the plate and screws (Perione et al., 2020). The theory behind this is preservation of soft tissue and blood supply to the fracture site with the aim of speeding up fracture repair and reducing the risk of complications associated with infection. Intraoperative fluorosocopy is required for this approach to ensure that the plate and screws are in the correct position.

Fracture Reduction Methods

Bone Plates and Screws

There are three main uses for bone plates in fracture repair:

1. **Fracture compression:** compression is only successful when the fracture fragments are fully reduced and well aligned (Kapler and Dycus, 2015). With this method the load on the bone postoperatively is shared between the bone and the plate. This method can only be used if the fragments can be fully aligned (Conzemius and Swainson, 1999).
2. **Neutralization:** this is when screws are all placed in a neutral, non-compressive way. This method can be used alone but is often used alongside lag screws or intramedullary pins and cerclage wire. By using this method the load on the bone postoperatively is shared between the bone and the implants used (Conzemius and Swainson, 1999).
3. **Buttress or bridging plate:** this is when the fracture fragments cannot be aligned (Figure 6). An intramedullary (IM) or Steinmann pin is driven through the furthest ends of the fracture to help align the fragments and then a plate is placed with screws in the proximal and distal parts of the fracture with the main part of the plate bridging the gap between the fragments. This helps to maintain alignment and length of the limb. Used alone, plates are exposed to bending which is why it is often used alongside an IM pin to counteract these forces (Kapler and Dycus, 2015). Used in this way, the plate and pin take on the load, giving the bone time to heal. Alongside this, a bone graft can help reduce the risk of implant failure (Conzemius and Swainson, 1999).

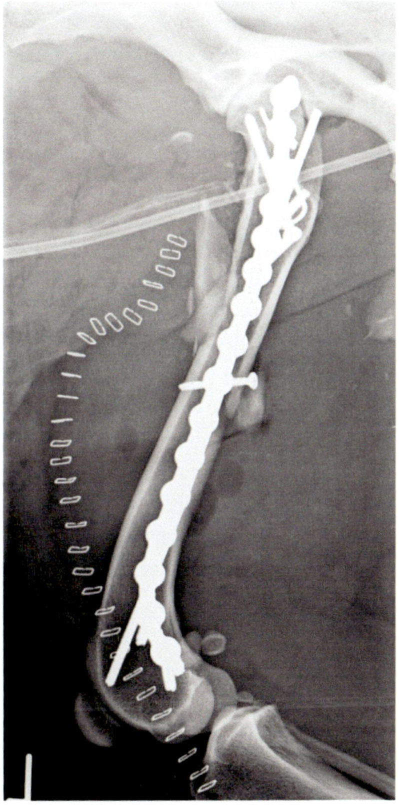

Figure 6. The plate in this radiograph has been applied in a buttress fashion.

A wide variety of plates and screws are available for veterinary use, many have the same function, but manufacturers call them different things.

There are also a variety of sizes and shapes of bone plate appropriate for different fracture sites, pictures are found in the section on instrumentation. The correct size depends on measurements taken by the VS before surgery. **Screw size should not exceed 25–30% the diameter of the bone and the plate size should be the same as the screw size** (e.g. 2.7 screws with a 2.7 plate) (Conzemius and Swainson, 1999).

Dynamic Compression Plates (DCPs)

Dynamic compression plates (DCPs) are commonly used but have been superseded by locking plates and screws. DCPs have oval gliding holes, where one side of the oval hole is sloped. They are used with a specially designed drill guide, with one side for drilling holes for compression (gold) and one side for drilling a neutral hole (green). The surgeon can use whichever end of the drill guide is appropriate. However, **this method compresses the plate and bone interface, which may reduce the blood supply to the fracture and may be undesirable.** Also, the requirement to contour the plate to the shape of the bone adds to the surgical time.

To improve blood supply, limited contact dynamic compression plates (LC-DCPs) are available, which have notches cut into the underside to aid blood supply (Roe, 2020). Both DCPs and LC-DCPs are contoured to fit the shape of the bone and there are a variety of plate benders available for this purpose. This has the disadvantage of requiring additional surgical time, especially if the plate needs contouring to a bone such as the acetabulum (Conzemius and Swainson, 1999).

Locking Plates

Locking plate technology means that (unlike the DCP where there is compression and therefore movement of the bone) **the screw** (which has a thread in the head) **engages with the thread in the hole of the plate. Because of this, the bone does not move.** This has a number of advantages such as better blood supply as there is no compression of the bone-plate interface and plate contouring is not necessary. Also, where appropriate placing a mono cortical screw works because the screw head engages with the plate which prevents loosening from occurring (which it may do with conventional plates and screws). There are some disadvantages however, such as the inability to place screws at an angle and they are more expensive than traditional plates.

Locking compression plates (LCP) have combination holes which allow the VS to choose either locking or compression when placing the screw. There are many types of locking plate available from different manufacturers, but the outcome is often the same and comes down to surgeon preference.

Lag Screws

Lag screws are screws which are placed directly into the bone without the use of a plate. They can be used on their own or to hold together two fragments of a more complex fracture alongside a bone plate. There are two methods of placing a lag screw.

1. The surgeon uses a partially threaded screw which only engages with the furthest fragment. When the screw is tightened, this brings the fragments together.
2. The surgeon drills a hole (correct for the size of screw) but can then over drill (use the next size drill bit up) the nearest fracture fragment so that when they tighten the screw the thread only engages with the furthest fracture fragment and therefore compresses the fragments together as the screw is tightened.

Both methods have the same outcome (Moores, 2016). The screw needs to be placed perpendicular to the fracture line (Conzemius and Swainson, 1999). (Figure 7)

Interlocking Nails

Interlocking nails are used for the repair of long bone fractures. They are designed to counteract the rotational forces associated with the traditional Steinmann pin, and also reduce the risk of pin migration. They contain holes in the proximal and distal parts where screws are placed, guided by an external jig to allow the surgeon to know where the holes are without fluoroscopic guidance (Wheeler et al., 2004).

The nail can serve as a buttress for comminuted fractures, or the fracture can be reduced before insertion of the nail (McLauglin, 1999).

External Skeletal Fixators (ESF)

The most commonly used type of external skeletal fixators (ESF) system for fracture repair is the linear system. This uses pins (either half or full pins) which are placed through predrilled holes in the bone (via stab incisions in the skin) and held in place with clamps, connected to linear bars (Palmer, 2012).

Indications for ESF use include comminuted fractures, open fractures, articular fractures, or those with overlying wounds where plate and screw placement would be an infection risk. Advantages to this system include that it is minimally invasive to the surrounding soft tissues and the system can be dismantled in stages, which promotes bone healing by loading when it is appropriate to do so (Johnson and DeCamp, 1999) (Figure 8).

There are **three main categories of configurations for ESFs** (Figure 9). Once the ESF is in place the fracture heals directly or indirectly, depending on whether the fragments are closely aligned or not. **Pins may be full** (going through the bone to

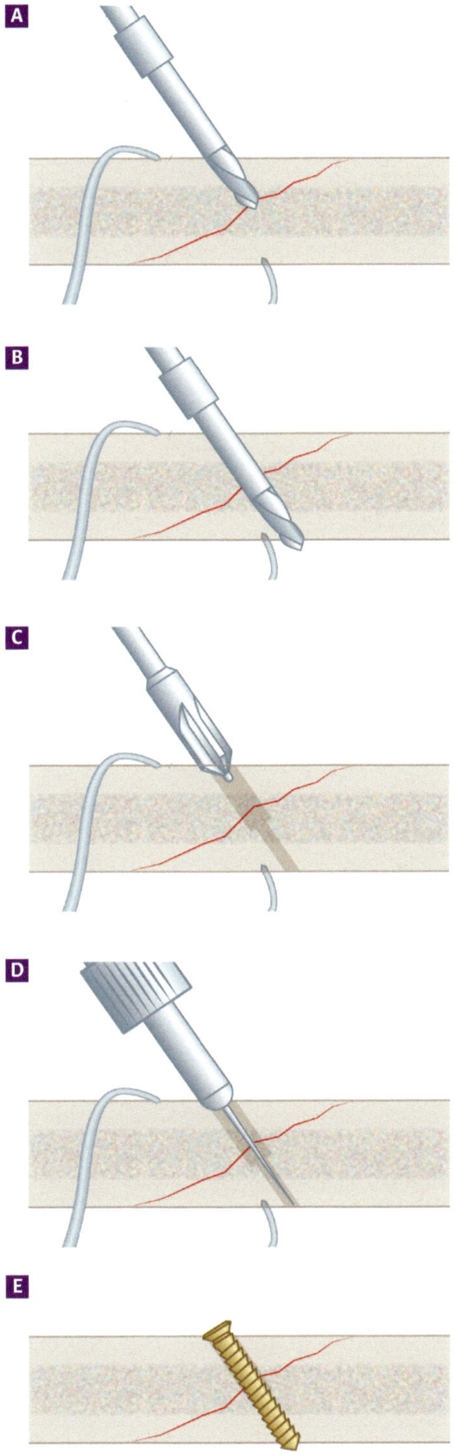

Figure 7. Lag screw placement. **A.** Firstly the nearest part is drilled using a drill bit the same width as the external diameter of the screw to be used (e.g. 4.5 mm screw then use a 4.5 mm drill bit); **B.** Secondly the furthest part of the bone is drilled according to the internal diameter of the screw (e.g. using a 4.5 screw then a 3.2 mm drill bit is used); **C.** The surgeon may use a countersink to accommodate the screw head; **D.** The length of screw is determined using a depth gauge. **E.** The screw is inserted.

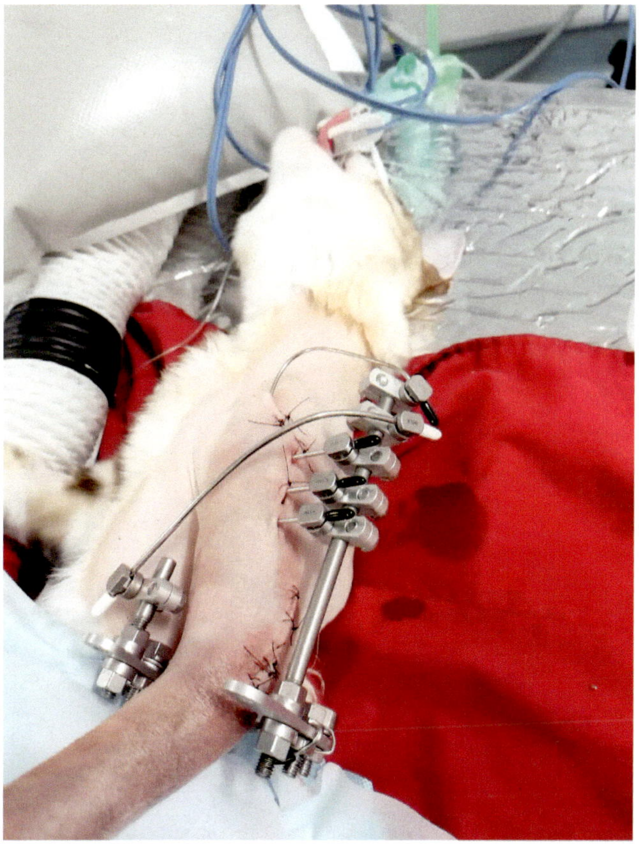

Figure 8. A cat with a hybrid ESF on its humerus.

the other side) **or half** (not penetrating all the way through) depending on the required configuration. The most proximal and distal pins tend to be full pins with others in between being half pins (Ness, 2006). Factors the surgeon takes into consideration include how long the ESF will remain in place and how stiff the configuration needs to be; in turn this depends on the age of the patient and type of facture. Some pins (such as smooth or negative threaded pins) are prone to loosening and not suitable for a long term ESF configuration (Langley-Hobbs et al., 1996).

Aspects that increase the stiffness of an ESF include pin diameter (which should never exceed 25% of the bone diameter.), threaded pins (better withstand loosening), and the number of pins in the proximal and distal fragments (up to a maximum of four per fragment, after which it makes no further difference to stiffness) (Palmer, 2012).

Postoperatively, wounds present around the ESF frame need treating accordingly using whatever method is appropriate to promote wound healing such as wet to dry dressings or non-adherent dressings. These should be tended to every two days for the first 8–10 days (Palmer, 2012). This often requires sedation or general anaesthesia (GA).

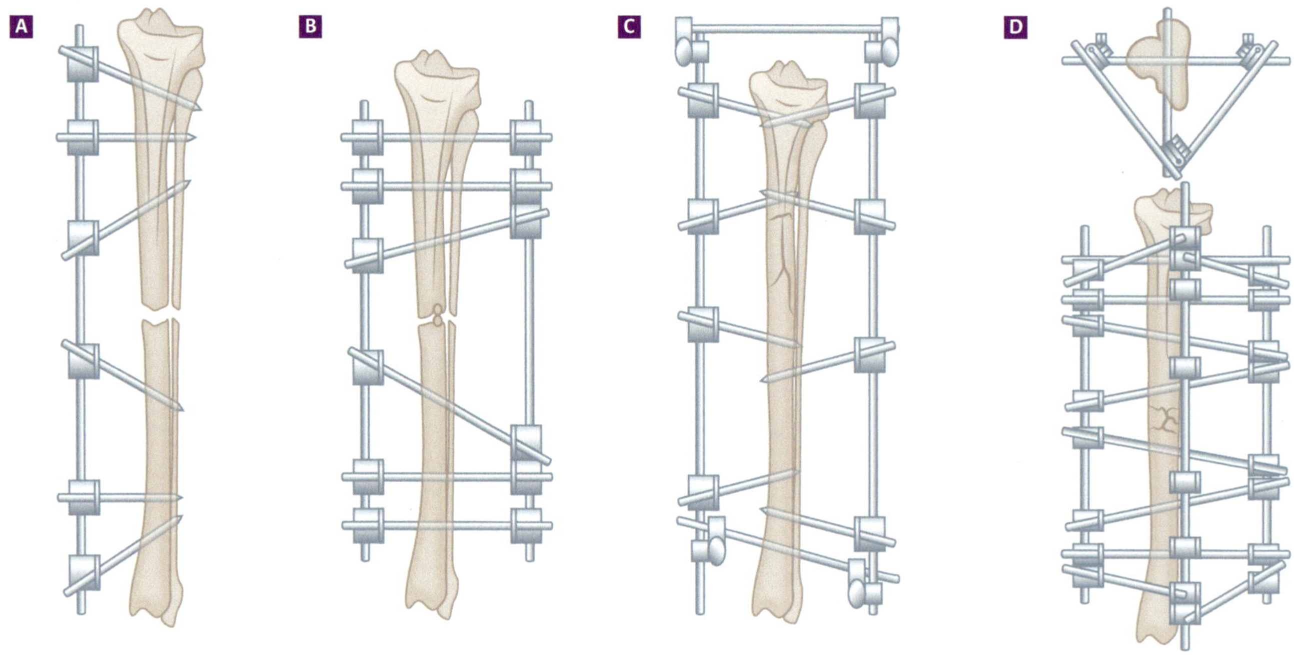

Figure 9. The different ESF configurations. **A.** Unilateral-Uniplanar; **B.** Unilateral-Biplanar; **C.** Type 2, Bilateral-Uniplanar; **D.** Type 3, Bilateral-Biplanar. (Palmer, 2012).

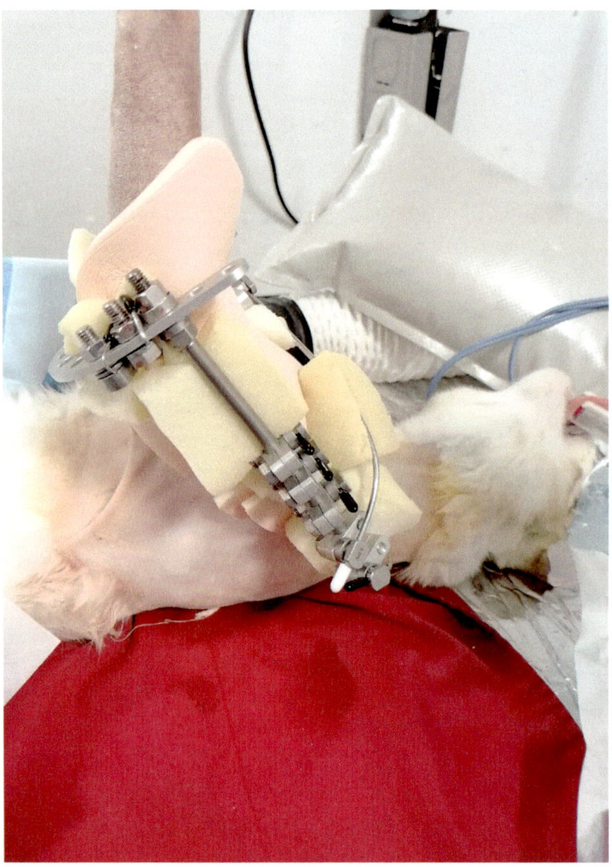

Figure 10. Sponges, holding an absorbent dressing against the pin holes, also note the bungs to protect the sharp ends of the arthrodesis wires.

The pin holes around the frame need to be treated the same as any postoperative wound and covered with a non-adherent dressing. Small incisions can be made in the dressing to fit around the pin holes. To stop the dressings from slipping, they are held in place with sponges placed between the dressings and the connecting bars (Palmer, 2012) (Figure 10). The outer frame is then covered with the usual padding, conforming, and cohesive layers. After a few days, these pin holes can be left open. This also allows for observation of any discharge or swelling. Some literature talks about cleaning the area around the pins, but in the authors experience leaving the dried scab is a good natural protection. Some argue that cleaning, however, leaves a clear tract for any drainage of discharge.

The sharp ends of the pins should be covered to avoid injury to personnel or the patient. There are commercially available rubber covers designed for this purpose.

Wounds

Traumatic fractures are often associated with wounds, which also need treating at the time of surgery. As already discussed, open fractures and those associated with a large open wound may be treated with an ESF, but the risk of infection is higher when open wounds are present.

When preparing these patients for surgery it is important to **place sterile lubricating jelly into the wound,** so that when clipping the area hair does not enter it. The jelly (and hair) is then wiped away after clipping. Before surgery, the wound should be flushed with sterile saline to flush away anything with the potential to cause contamination, and the site prepared as for any other surgery but taking care not to get prep solution into the wound.

Maxillofacial and Skull Fractures

A major consideration when repairing jaw fractures is to ensure good jaw alignment and that the dentition (including tooth roots) are not damaged in the process (Zacher and Marretta, 2013).

Many treatment options are non-surgical such as dental bonding, interdental wiring, wire around the mandible, BEARD (bignathic encircling and retaining device), or a tape muzzle. The jaw is, after all, non-weight bearing and so the theory behind fixation is slightly different.

A common injury in cats is separation of the mandibular symphysis. The main treatment option is to use cerclage wire or a thick suture to encircle the area, using a large gauge needle through which the wire or suture is threaded from the inside to outside of the jaw.

Plates, screws and pins, if used incorrectly can damage tooth roots or nerves and cause infection, however, the use of bone plates is an option for comminuted fractures.

ESF can also be used on maxillofacial fractures using positive end threaded pins to reduce pin migration, for comminuted fractures or those with a large degree of soft tissue damage (Zacher and Marretta, 2013).

For some repairs an endotracheal tube may need to be placed via a pharyngotomy to allow the surgeon full access to the oral cavity to place bone plates or an ESF (Duke, 1999).

Considerations for patients with jaw fractures include:

- The animal may not be able to eat or drink normally and a feeding tube is required. Often, due to the degree of head trauma, naso-oesophageal tubes are contraindicated and so oesophagostomy or gastrostomy tubes are preferable.
- If the fixation method means the patient cannot open their mouth properly, should they vomit or regurgitate then this risks aspiration. Ensure that there is a way of allowing the animal to fully open its mouth if it becomes distressed. A pair of rongeurs for dental bonding or scissors for nylon line or suture by the animal's kennel means that the items are easily available if needed.
- If the animal has a history of vomiting or regurgitation then many non-surgical methods may not be suitable.
- Many of the non-surgical methods such as tape muzzles and BEARD sutures may not be suitable for brachycephalic patients.
- Dogs often cannot pant normally with some of these methods and so overheating may be a risk.
- Unrepairable fractures of the mandible or maxilla may require mandibulectomy or maxillectomy.

Orthopaedic Equipment, Care, and Maintenance

To be an efficient scrub and circulating nurse, a good knowledge of different instruments and their uses is vital. It is often the role of the veterinary nurses and support staff to maintain the instruments in good working order and to clean, sterilise and store instruments and kits in optimum conditions.

This section uses pictures to identify some of the common instruments used in fracture repair including plates and screws. Having a knowledgeable theatre nurse as part of the scrub team really makes a difference to the efficiency of surgical procedures as they can preempt what the surgeon may need, clean instruments as they are handed back and also keep the trolley tidy so that instruments can be found easily.

Basic Instruments Used in Fracture Repair

- **Periosteal elevator:** to scrape soft tissue and periosteum from bone (Figure 11).
- **Fragment reducing forceps:** once a fracture is reduced these forceps hold the fragments together whilst the implants are prepared (Figure 12).
- **Bone holding forceps:** hold onto fracture fragments and help manipulate them back into position (Figure 13).
- **Hohmann:** a handheld retractor used to retract soft tissue from the surgical field, comes in a variety of sizes (Figure 14).
- **Gelpis:** a self-retaining retractor which improves access and holds soft tissue away from a surgical field, they come in small, medium, large, odd leg or deep reach (Figure 15).
- **Langenbecks:** a handheld retractor used to retract soft tissue from the surgical field (Figure 16).
- **Drill bits:** used to drill holes in bone. The size of drill bit used depends on the size of screw/plates required (Table 3). These need changing after a few uses as they become blunt.
- **Drill guides:** help guide the drill bit and protect

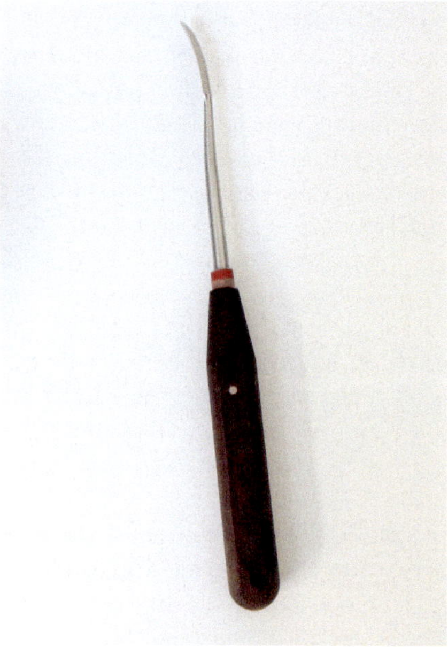

Figure 11. Periosteal elevator.

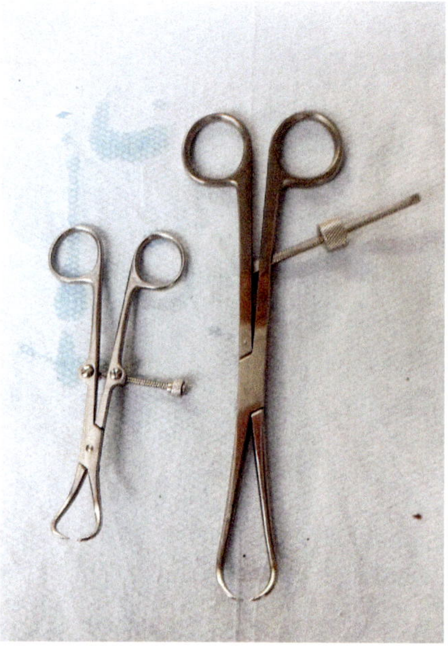

Figure 12. Fragment reducing forceps or pointed reduction forceps.

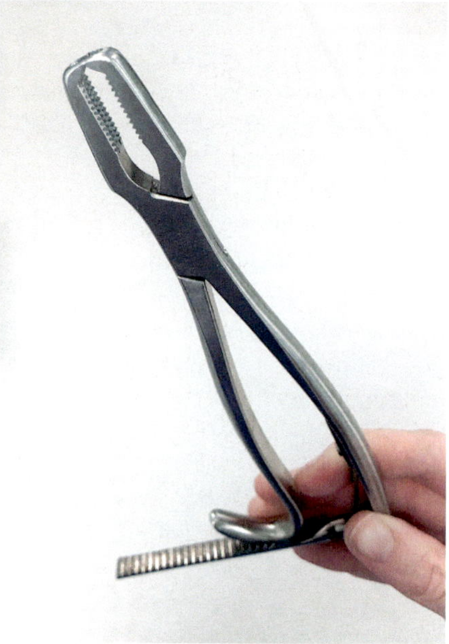

Figure 13. Bone holding forceps.

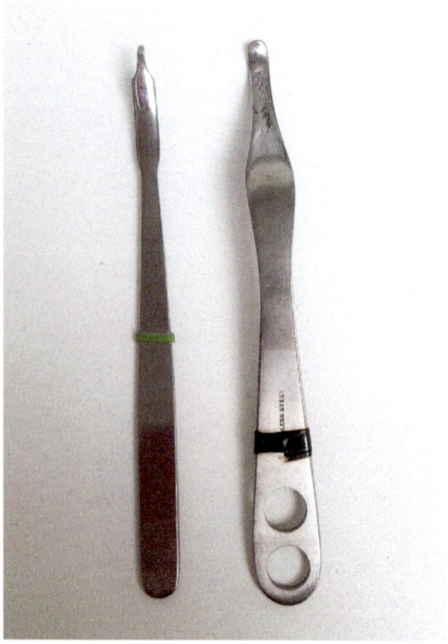

Figure 14. Hohmann retractor.

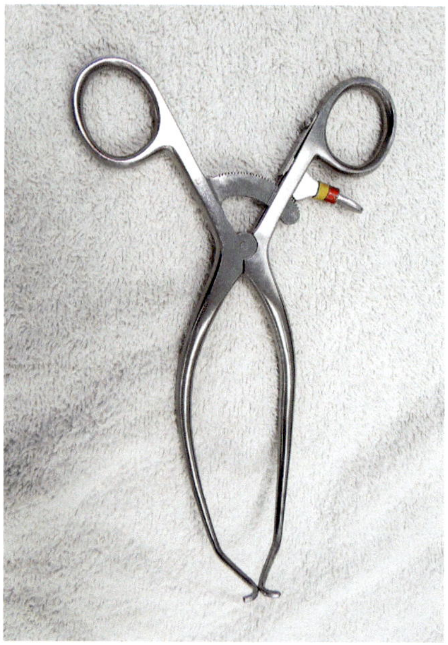

Figure 15. Gelpi retractor.

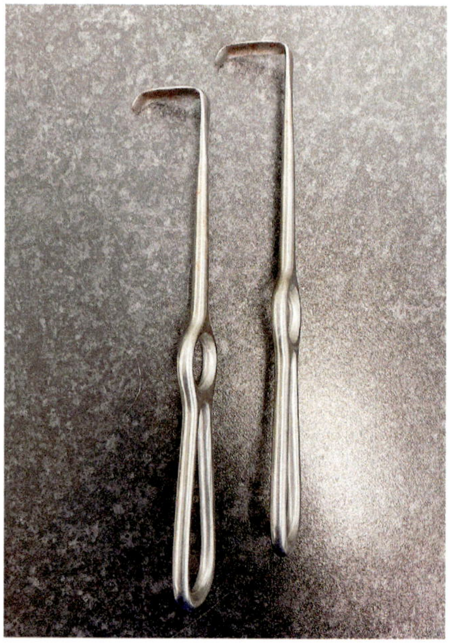

Figure 16. Langenbeck retractor.

Table 3. A guide to drill bit sizes.

Screw size	Drill bit required
1.5	1.1
2.0	1.5
2.7	2.0
3.5	2.5
4.5	3.2
5.5	4.0

surrounding soft tissue from getting caught in the drill bit (Figure 17).

- **DCP drill guide** (Figure 18).
- **Locking drill guide:** allows greater control when drilling a hole and also protects surrounding soft tissue. Locking drill guides have a thread which allows them to engage with the plate to ensure the hole is drilled perpendicular to the bone to ensure the threads engage as required (Figure 19).
- **Depth gauge:** once the hole has been drilled the surgeon

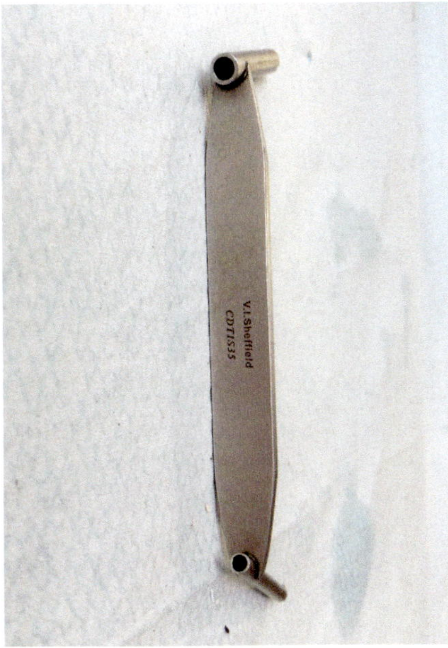

Figure 17. Drill guide.

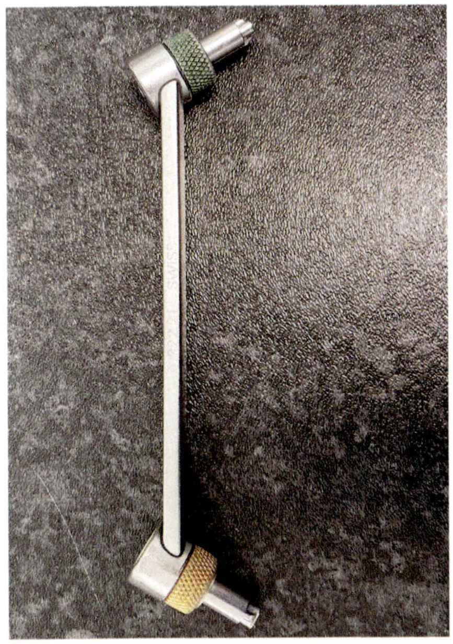

Figure 18. DCP drill guide.

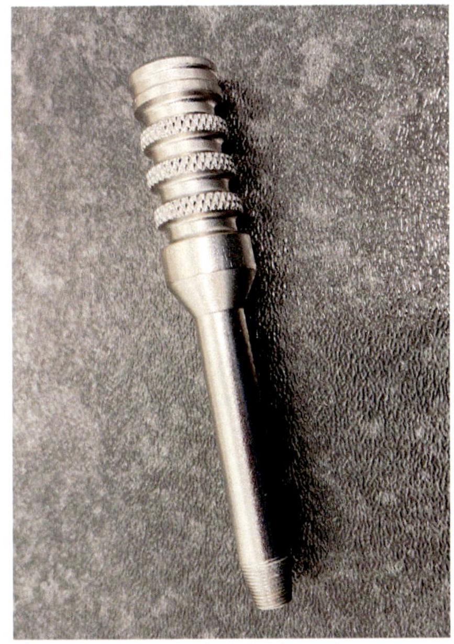

Figure 19. Locking drill guide, for use when placing locking screws, the end screws into the plate hole whilst the hole is drilled.

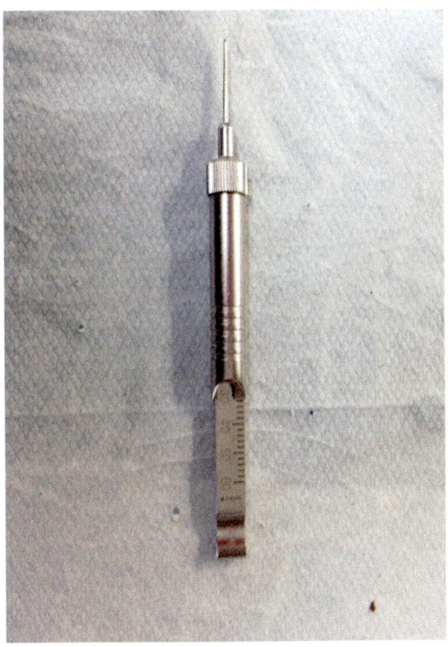

Figure 20. Depth gauge.

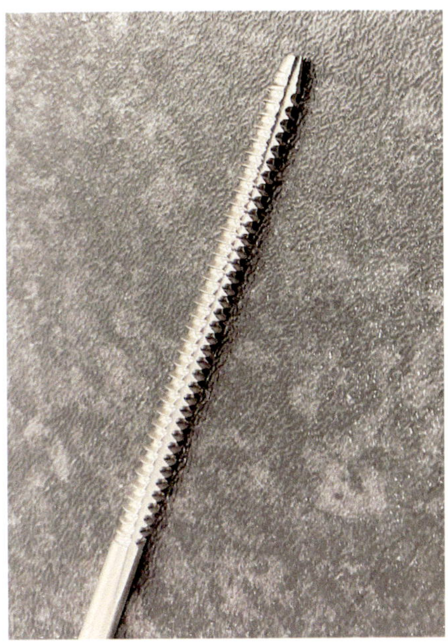

Figure 21. Tap.

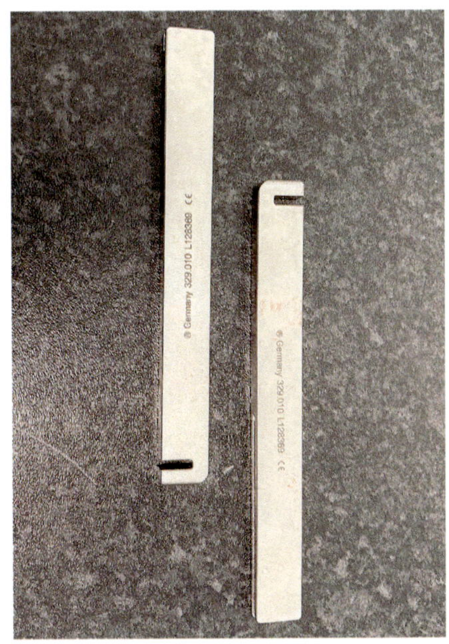

Figure 22. Plate benders.

needs to know what length of screw to place, and the depth gauge is used to calculate this (Figure 20).

- **Tap:** if using a non-self-tapping screw, the surgeon needs to make the thread in the bone for the screw to engage with the bone. The tap is used for this as it cuts a thread in the bone. If using self-tapping screws this is not needed (Figure 21).
- **Screwdrivers:** used to place screws in the bone. These come in a variety of sizes and also head shapes depending on the shape of the screwhead.
- **Plate benders:** help to contour plates to the shape of the bone to which it is applied (Figure 22).

Plates

Dynamic Compression Plate (DCP)

When drilling for compression, the gold end of the drill guide is used and this drills a hole off centre, furthest away from the fracture line, towards the end of the oval hole with the sloping shoulder. When the screw is placed, the screw travels down the slope and therefore, the fracture is compressed as the screw tightens and is forced towards the centre of the hole down the sloping edge (Figure 23).

Limited Contact DCP (LC-DCP)

A variation on the DCP, the plate has grooves on the underside which improves blood supply to the periosteum. There is no gap in the middle of these plates meaning that holes are spaced evenly and designed so compression can be achieved in either direction (Figure 24).

Reconstruction Plates

These plates can be contoured in all directions due to their design. This does, however, make them less strong and they should only be used for fractures when forces are low. Holes are oval but not gliding, as with the DCP. This means the plate can only be used to provide neutralisation or buttress support, not compression (Conzemius and Swainson, 1999).

Veterinary Cuttable Plates (VCP)

These are bought in long lengths and then cut to size as needed, they can also be stacked when needed. The holes are round which limits any angulation of the screws and also means the plate can only provide neutralisation or buttress support, similar to reconstruction plates (Conzemius and Swainson, 1999) (Figure 25).

Acetabular Plates

Specifically contoured to fit the acetabulum (Figure 26).

Supracondylar

Shaped like a hockey stick, these plates are specifically designed to fit the lateral edge of the distal femur (Figure 27).

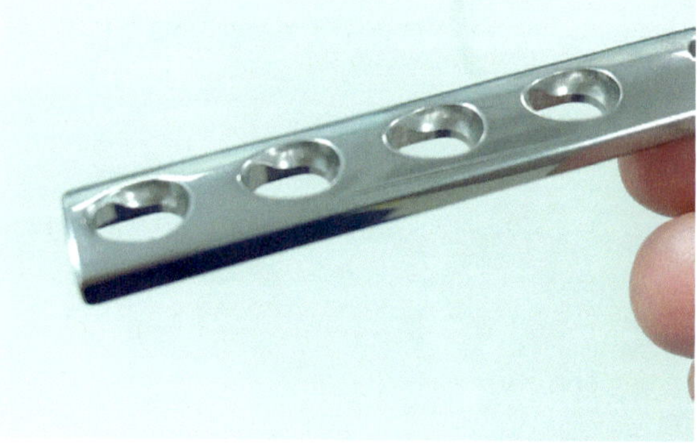

Figure 23. DCP plate: note the sloping edge at one side of the oval hole for compression of the fracture.

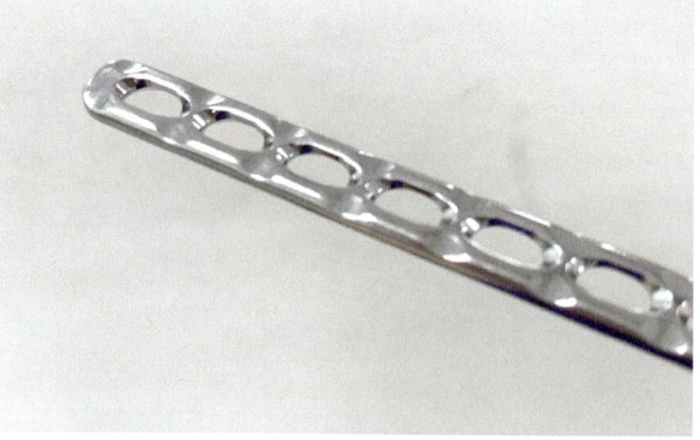

Figure 24. The underside of an LC-DCP plate with the notches cut out in order to help with blood supply to the fracture site.

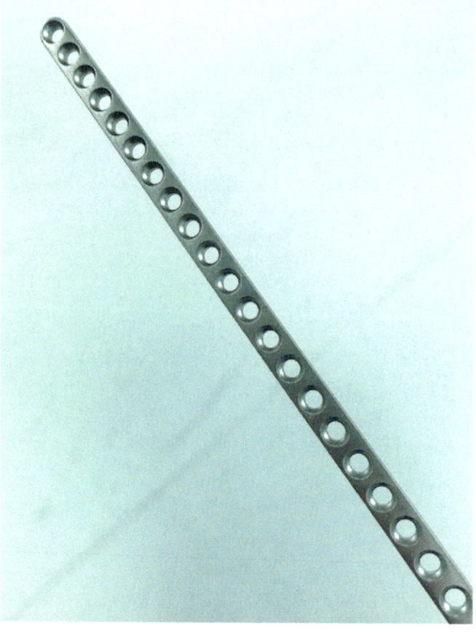

Figure 25. Veterinary cuttable plate (VCP).

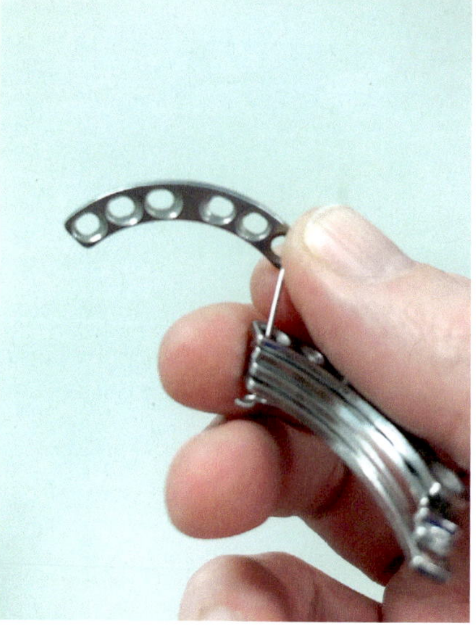

Figure 26. Acetabular plate.

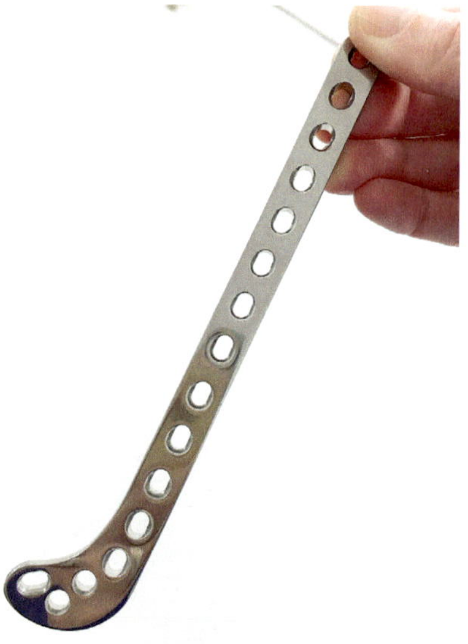

Figure 27. Supracondylar plate.

Locking Plates

Locking plate technology means that unlike the DCP where there is compression and therefore movement of the bone, the screw (which has a thread in the head) engages with the thread in the hole of the plate. Because of this, the bone does not move. This has a number of advantages such as better blood supply as there is no compression and contouring of the plate is not necessary which saves time. Also, if the surgeon wants to place a mono cortical screw this will work because the screw head is engaged with the plate and therefore loosening will not occur (which can occur with conventional plates and screws). There are some disadvantages however, such as the inability to place screws at an angle and they are more expensive than traditional plates.

There are a variety of locking plates available from different manufacturers.

Locking Compression Plates (LCP)

Locking compression plates (LCP) have combination holes which allow the VS to choose either locking or compression when placing the screw.This can be used as a combination of locking and compression plate as one end of the hole (the end furthest from the middle) has a thread and one end has a sloping edge for compression (Figure 28).

Pancarpal Arthrodesis/ Pantarsal Arthrodesis Plates (PCA/PTA)

These plates accept two different screw sizes with the screws on the proximal half being bigger than the screws on the distal end (i.e. 3.5 then 2.7). The plates are tapered at the bottom in order to help with soft tissue cover due to the lack of available soft tissue in this location (Figure 29).

Screws

Cortical

These can be identified by their narrower thread. These screws engage with either one or both bone cortices.

Cancellous

These are identifiable by having a wider/deeper thread compared to cortical screws. These screws are superseded by cortical screws for most things, and the narrow inner body of the cancellous screw can sometimes lead to screw breakage. A partially threaded cancellous screw can be used as a lag screw (Figure 30).

Self-tapping

These screws cut their own thread in bone as they are screwed into place, which means that tapping beforehand is not required.

Non-self-tapping

If using these screws, the surgeon must cut a thread first.

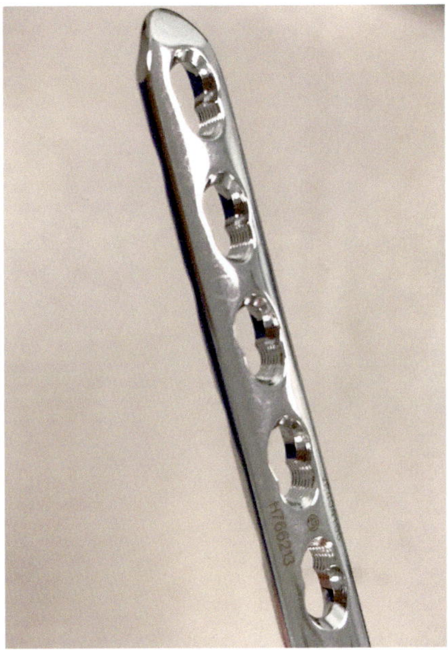

Figure 28. Locking compression plate.

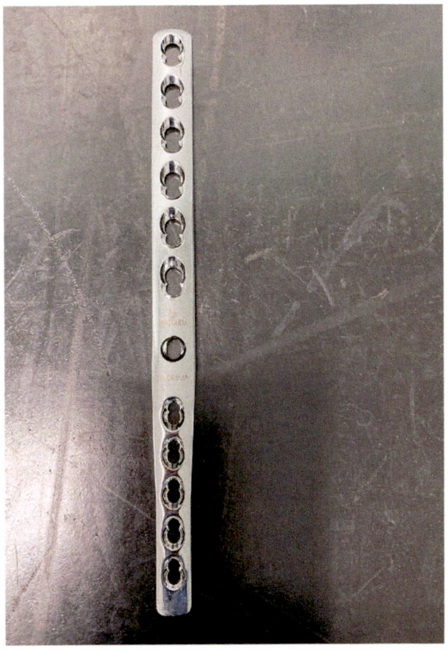

Figure 29. Pancarpal arthrodesis plate, note how it is narrower at the distal end to allow for closure of soft tissue around the plate without too much tension.

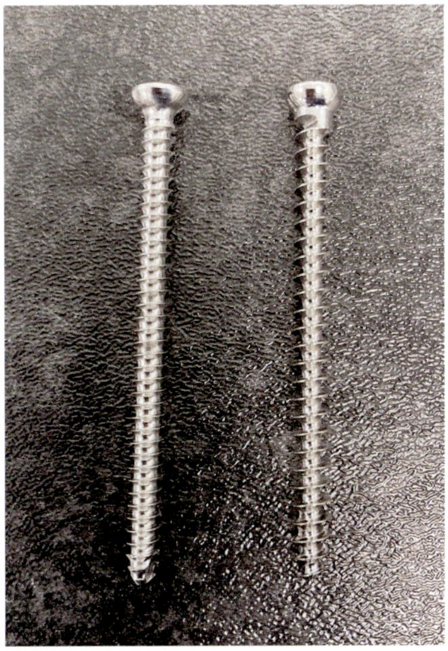

Figure 30. Cortical and cancellous screws.

External Fixation Instrumentation

Half Pins

Threaded at the end, these go through both cortices of the bone but do not go through the skin surface furthest from insertion. The thread may be long enough to engage with both cortices or short enough to only engage with the furthest cortex (Figure 31).

Full Pins

Threaded in the centre, these pins go all the way through both cortices and out through the skin at the other side (Figure 32).

Negative vs Positive Pins

Negative threaded pins have the pin thread cut into the shaft diameter (Figure 33). This can create a weakness at the point where the thread starts, making it susceptible to bending forces. Positive profile pins have the thread added onto the shaft diameter making them stronger (Figure 31).

External Connecting Bars

The connecting clamps thread onto these in order to hold the pins in place. They can be made of stainless steel, carbon fibre, or titanium (Figure 34).

Linkage-SK Clamps

These can be taken apart to place on the connecting bars and are available as double or single clamps (Figure 35).

Kirschner Clamps

These are available as single or double clamps. They cannot

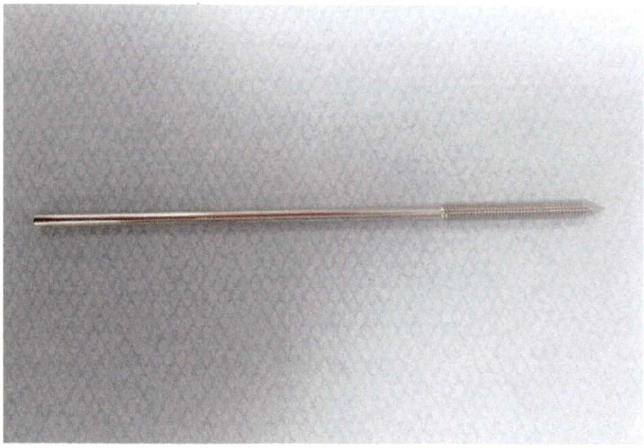

Figure 31. Half pin (positive thread).

Figure 32. Full pin.

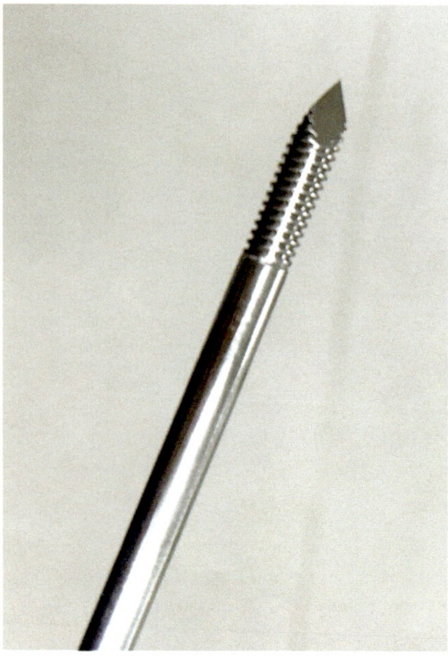

Figure 33. Negative thread, for comparison with the pin in Figure 31.

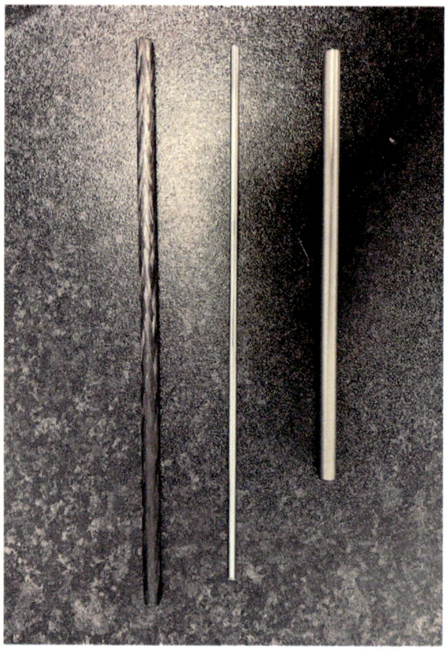

Figure 34. A selection of connecting bars.

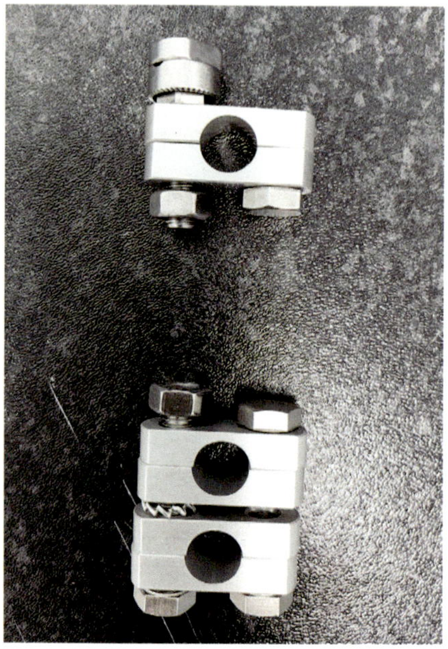

Figure 35. Single and double SK clamps.

be taken apart and so once the frame is in place the surgeon cannot add or take any clamps away. Also they cannot accept positive threaded pins unless the pins are preplaced and the clamp is attached onto the end.

As a result, SK clamps are used more frequently.

Circular ESF

Used for fracture fixation, they have the ability to distract or compress fractures and are **used for the correction of limb deformities.** The external rings are connected to wires which are drilled through bone. The wires used can have a trocar or bayonet point (Kirschner) or have a bead positioned halfway along (called olive wires).

The wires can be tightened with a wire tensioner both at the time of placing or weeks after if required. The bead on the olive wire helps with fracture reduction when tightened. The wires are fixed to the rings with cannulated fixation bolts and these bolts are tightened when needed using spanners. The rings are connected externally by threaded rods. Rings can be full circle, five eighths, or stretch ring.

Hinges can be used in the circular ESF setup to account for natural bends at joints.

Powered Equipment

Orthopaedics and neurology often requires the use of drills and burrs. Burrs are often air powered from a medical air outlet. Drills can be air powered, battery, or mains powered. **Some of the drills used are similar to household DIY drills. These cannot be sterilised and are therefore covered with a sterile covering to allow use during surgery.** These drills are being replaced by drills which can be sterilised and are battery powered, making them more portable and easier to use.

As with all powered items these need a degree of maintenance, such as oiling at regular intervals (depending on make) and care must be taken when cleaning as many cannot be submerged in water.

Drills often come with different attachments depending on what the surgeon requires such as saws, Jacobs chuck, quick release drills, and wire drivers.

Maintenance of Orthopaedic Instruments

Orthopaedic surgery requires a huge variety of kit, depending on the surgical procedure. This equipment needs regular maintenance to prevent any perioperative issues which could potentially mean extra surgical time.

Drill bits can become blunt and cause iatrogenic trauma to the bone as it heats up. Therefore, these should be changed regularly. If a hospital carries out a lot of orthopaedic surgery, it is useful to have a stock of drill bits to replace blunt ones when needed. Indeed, cannulated drill bits should only be single use as they are difficult to clean and because the way they are used means arthrodesis wires may be retained inside. Again a stock of these is useful.

Any instrumentation which can be taken apart for cleaning should be dismantled, for example many drill guides can be disassembled. Blood and tissue can get inside these items and so a thorough clean cannot be carried out unless they are dismantled.

Powered equipment requires servicing and so it is helpful to have at least two of each item with one available for use when the other is being repaired or serviced. Saw blades should be replaced when blunt and it is important any problems with kit, such as blunt drill bits and blunt saw blades, are communicated to the sterilising team so that these items are dealt with appropriately.

Storage of Kits

It is useful to have specific kit bundles for surgeries, for example a stifle kit for arthrotomies, containing everything the surgeon might need all in one box. This can be more efficient than opening lots of individual instruments. Many instrumentation manufacturers have fracture kits available which come in different sizes according to the size of plate being placed. For example, a fracture kit for placing 3.5 mm screws and a plate contains everything needed to do this, such as the correct size drill bits, drill guides, and screwdrivers (Figure 36). These are often provided in metal boxes which can be wrapped in paper before sterilising.

To help with sustainability, metal boxes are now available which have inner metal baskets which holds the kits. The circulating member of staff removes the lid of the metal box at the time of surgery and the sterile assistant then removes the inner basket. This negates the need to wrap the boxes in paper. These are specifically designed for steam autoclaving and have filters in the lid and holes for steam to escape (Figure 37).

In larger hospitals it is useful to have a team of people whose sole responsibility is sterilising. This person or team can be in charge of maintenance and repairs as well as regular inspection of kits, ordering, and stock control. For example, if there are a lot of fracture repairs or TPLOs carried out in a practice or

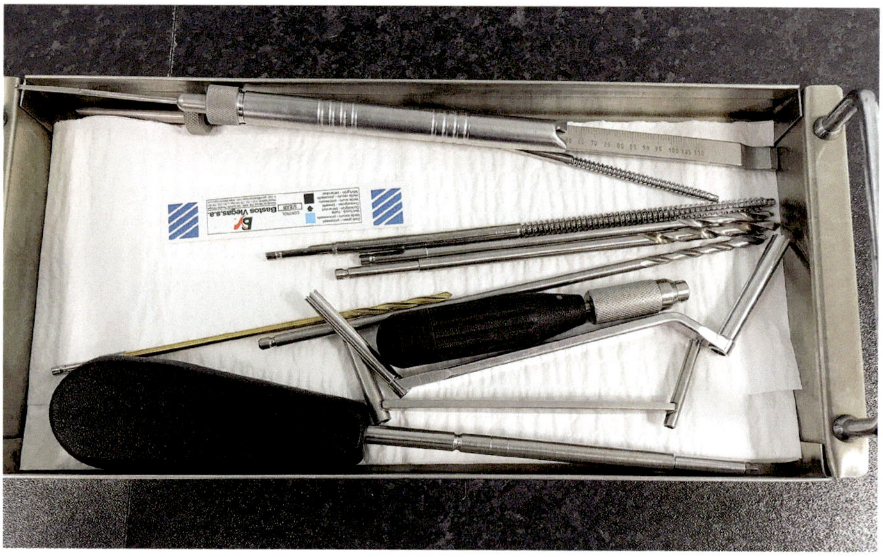

Figure 36. A 4.5 fragment kit, containing all the instruments needed to place 4.5 screws.

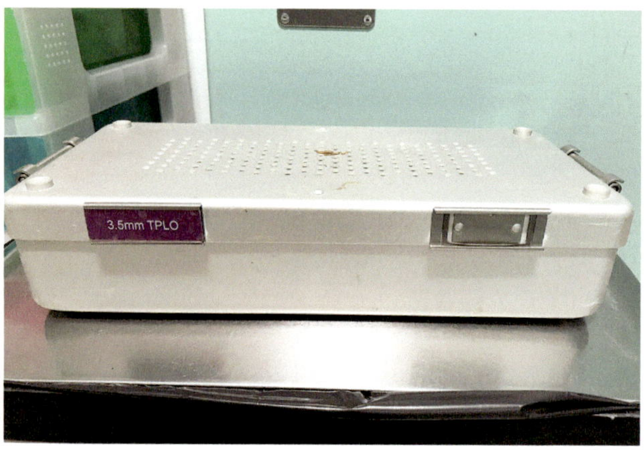

Figure 37. A metal box containing a basket of sterile kit for the scrubbed assistant to remove at the time of surgery.

hospital, plates and screws need to be ordered regularly. It is a good idea to have minimum amounts of stock, perhaps with someone from the sterilising team responsible for ordering these items weekly.

Having a room or space designated for storing kit is very useful, especially in larger hospitals. Kits in the kit room need the dates of sterilization checking monthly and anything which is out of date (three months for steam autoclaving) should be resterilised. Using a system similar to pharmacy stock control for sterilised instruments means the oldest sterilised kit is used first to reduce the need to keep resterilising time-expired kits.

When using paper wrapping, make sure the integrity of the paper is checked before opening to ensure it has not been damaged, this should be checked when placing the item on the shelf after sterilising but also by the person who puts a kit together. The paper wrapping can become prone to ripping, especially after steam autoclaving. This is another advantage of the metal boxes for kits.

Conditions of the Joints and Surgical Treatment Options

The aim of this section is to give the veterinary nurse the knowledge to understand the common joint diseases that may present. This knowledge is used when helping owners understand conditions and decide on the best course of treatment for their pet. Although the VN cannot diagnose or suggest treatment, they can provide owners with advice to aid them in the decision-making process.

Being knowledgeable about the joint surgeries helps the VN to understand why a particular surgery is undertaken and help with the efficiency of circulating and scrub staff in theatre as it enables them to thoroughly prepare for surgeries.

Elbows

Luxations

Elbow luxations are typically the result of trauma. The radius and ulna tend to luxate laterally, as the medial condyle of the humerus prevents medial luxation (Tomsa et al., 1999). The same trauma often results in avulsion or rupture of the ligaments which hold the elbow joint together. In this scenario, or with chronic luxations, then surgery is required. However, if the luxation is acute with no damage to the supporting soft tissue then a closed approach to repair is indicated first. For the most severe cases, elbow arthrodesis is an option, but this reduces the mobility of the joint.

Subluxations of the elbow joint often occur due to elbow incongruity (see elbow dysplasia). This may happen due to early growth plate closure from a trauma that went undetected at the time, which in turn leads to shortening of the radius or ulna. To realign these bones the ulna may need to undergo osteotomy (to lengthen it) or osteotomy (to shorten it). The ulna is usually the bone that undergoes surgery since the radius bears more of the patient's weight and if it is cut then a plate is required to stabilize it (Piermattei et al., 2006).

Elbow Dysplasia

There are a few conditions discussed below, which come under the umbrella of elbow dysplasia. The causes can be multifactorial, including genetic and environmental. **Elbow dysplasia is often diagnosed in young, growing dogs and mainly affects larger breeds** such as Labradors, Golden Retrievers, German Shepherds, and Bernese Mountain Dogs (Vezzoni and Benjamino, 2021).

Ununited Anconeal Process (UAP)

The anconeal process is a bony prominence on the end of the ulna, which is attached to a growth plate which is a primary centre of ossification in the growing dog. Normally, by 20 weeks of age, the anconeal process attaches itself to the proximal ulna. In the case of UAP this does not happen and the anconeal process remains detached (Vezzoni and Benjamino, 2021). Surgical intervention includes the removal of this process, preferably by arthroscopy. The use of lag screws could also be considered but implant failure can occur and the outcome is no more successful than removal of the piece of bone, which is less invasive when done arthroscopically. There are also reports of this being treated by a combination of a lag screw and proximal ulna osteotomy (Krotscheck et al., 2000).

Osteocondrosis Dessicans (OCD) of the Medial Humeral Condyle

In young dogs the joint surfaces are covered in cartilage, which eventually turns to bone with a small amount of cartilage remaining. In some animals the cartilage remains and becomes thickened. As a result of this thickening nutrients cannot get to it and so the cartilage dies to form a flap in the elbow joint. The flap of cartilage can be removed by arthroscopy or via an open approach to the elbow joint, but the former method is less invasive (Vezzoni and Benjamino, 2021).

Ununited or Fragmented Coronoid Process

The coronoid process is a bony prominence on the ulna. In some animals this develops a crack or fissure, and in some cases completely separates from the ulna. This often occurs with the coronoid process on the medial or inner side of the ulna, in young dogs that are still growing. Surgery is carried out arthroscopically to remove the piece of bone. As with the above disorder, an open approach can be considered but arthroscopy is less invasive (Temwichitr et al., 2010).

Surgical Options

Arthroscopy

For many of the above disorders of the elbow, arthroscopy can be used for diagnosis (alongside radiographs/CT) and treatment if appropriate.

For arthroscopy a camera, light source, and a variety of scope sizes (with the correct size cannula) are required as well as a kit of fine, long instruments which can fit down an arthroscopy cannula (Figure 38).

Useful instruments to include are a selection of meniscus knives, grasping forceps, probes, milling drill, and curettes.

Arthrotomy

The other approach to a joint is called an arthrotomy; this

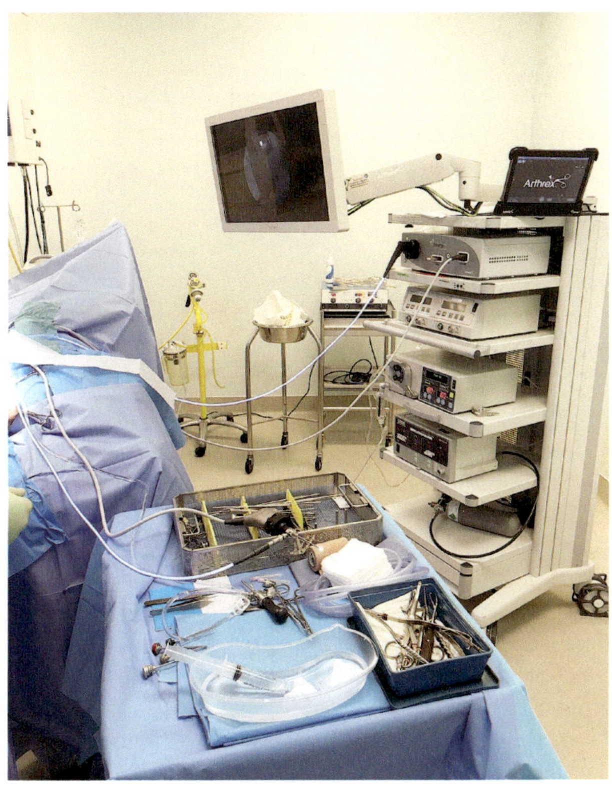

Figure 38. An arthroscopy tower.

involves surgically opening the joint space to have a look inside. This carries a higher risk of joint infection and is more painful that minimally invasive arthroscopy. However, the instrumentation and equipment required to perform an arthrotomy is less expensive.

Incomplete Ossification of the Humeral Condyle (IOHC)

At birth, the lateral and medial condyles of the humerus are separated by cartilage, which normally starts to ossify by 10–12 weeks with full ossification by 32 weeks of age. In the case of IOHC this ossification has not occurred, which results in elbow pain and lameness in skeletally immature dogs and if left untreated can predispose to humeral condylar fractures (Moores, 2012).

Spaniels are overrepresented with this condition; they often present with a condylar fracture in one forelimb and when the contralateral limb is radiographed, there is also an incidental finding of a fissure in that limb (Butterworth and Innes, 2001).

IOHC is normally treated surgically as conservative treatment is not normally sufficient and can end in fracture of one or both humeral condyles. Fractures of both humeral condyles (often referred to as a Y fracture) is technically challenging and requires surgical approaches to both sides of the distal humerus with plates on either side.

Treatment for IOHC involves placing a screw across the humeral condyle. This is termed a positional screw, but a lag screw method is an alternative with a partially threaded screw to achieve compression (Butterworth and Innes, 2001).

Hips

Luxations

Hip luxation is mainly caused by some kind of trauma, such as a road traffic accident (RTA). The hip is well supported by muscle and soft tissue, and so a large force is required to produce luxation, therefore there are often other significant injuries, such as chest trauma (Fossum, 2007). Some hip luxations can be treated by closed reduction, depending on injury to the joint capsule. The number of days after injury has an influence on whether or not closed reduction is effective due to muscle contracture. After successful closed reduction, an Ehmer sling should be applied (Fossum, 2007). The amount of time this should be left on depends on how stable the hip joint feels after reduction. Hips that reluxate need surgical stabilisation (Figure 39).

Open reduction aims to place the femoral head back into the acetabulum and secure it to prevent reluxation. The method used depends on the severity of damage to the joint capsule. In some cases opening the joint capsule, placing the femoral head back in the acetabulum and closing the joint capsule is sufficient. If there is too much damage to the joint capsule to achieve reduction then sutures and toggle pins are used to anchor the hip joint and hold it in place until the joint capsule is healed (Fossum, 2007).

A toggle pin technique is where a toggle is placed in the acetabulum with suture attached to the toggle and then threaded through tunnels in the femur. This creates a prosthetic ligament to hold the hip joint in place (Gemmill and Oxley, 2018).

An ilieofemoral suture is similar to the toggle pin technique, with the aim of holding the joint in place. Bone tunnels are drilled through the greater trochanter and the ventral aspect of the ilium and suture placed through them, which are held in place with suture anchors. The femur is internally rotated whilst the suture is tightened. This method again, creates a prosthetic ligament whilst the joint capsule heals (Gemmill and Oxley, 2018).

Another technique is the placement of a temporary transarticular pin which stays in place for approximately four weeks whilst the joint heals. A hole is drilled through the femoral

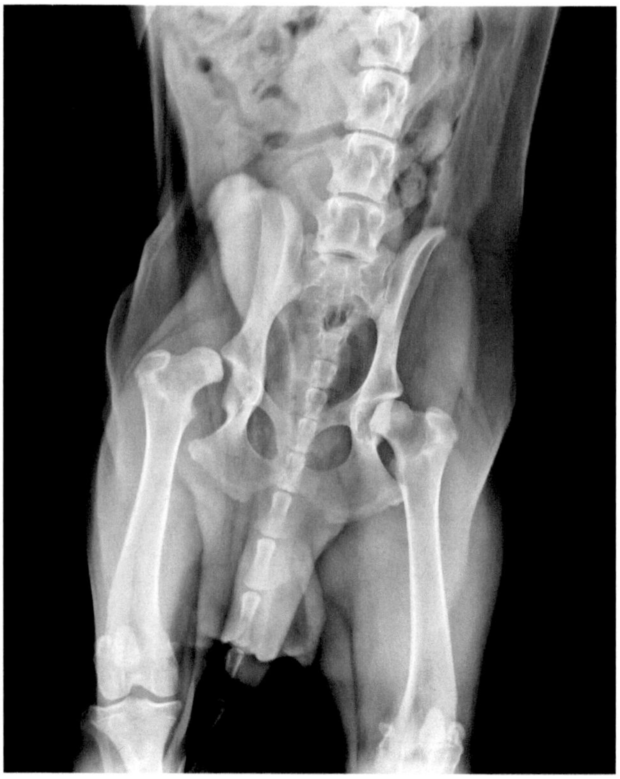

Figure 39. A traumatic hip luxation of the right hip.

neck and head through to the other side of the pelvis. A Steinman pin is driven through the hole and the pin bent over at the end to prevent migration (Gemmill and Oxley, 2018).

Femoral head and neck ostectomy and total hip replacement are also treatment options for severe or chronic hip luxation, these are discussed in the next section on hip dysplasia.

Hip Dysplasia

Hip dysplasia is relatively common in dogs and consists of hip laxity, remodelling of the joint due to the structures not sitting as a ball and socket joint, which leads to osteoarthritis later in life.

The clinical findings of hip dysplasia differ according to the age of the animal. Dogs younger than 12 months of age often present with acute signs of the disease, whilst dogs over 15 months of age present with more chronic disease leading to osteoarthritis (Piermattei et al., 2006).

Young dogs often show unwillingness to exercise and pain in the hindlimbs with a short hindlimb gait. On examination the vet may find a positive Ortolani test, which is produced when the femoral head clicks as it subluxates in and out of the acetabulum. Radiographs may also show microfractures in the acetabulum from where the hip subluxates and bears extra weight through a particular point of the acetabulum (Piermatti et al., 2006).

In older dogs, the pain of hip dysplasia is associated with osteoarthritis and the degeneration of cartilage due to the normal aging process or secondary to abnormal development of the hip.

Surgical Treatment Options for Hip Dysplasia

Pubic Symphysoidesis

Performed at 12 to 16 weeks of age, this procedure involves using diathermy electrocautery to induce the closure of the growth plates at the pubic symphysis. This then means the acetabulum rotates to cover more of the femoral head (Fossum, 2007).

Due to the age at which this needs to be carried out to be effective, the procedure is rarely utilized as owners often do not see the signs of hip dysplasia so young (Barthelemy and Parsons, 2020).

Pelvic Osteotomy

This procedure is carried out in young dogs, normally younger than 6 months of age, before some of the changes associated with hip subluxation become apparent, such as bone formation in the acetabulum or damage to the femoral head. The idea is that the acetabulum is rotated to allow the femoral head to become more stable in the acetabulum. The surgeon may choose to carry out a triple pelvic osteotomy (TPO), which involves cuts to the ischium, pubis and ilium or double pelvic osteotomy (DPO) which omits the cut to the ischium. Some evidence suggests there are fewer complications associated with a DPO approach. The rotation is held by a TPO/ DPO plate set at a certain angle of rotation depending on preoperative planning (Piermatti et al., 2006) (Figure 40).

Femoral Head and Neck Excision

This is considered a salvage procedure for the elimination

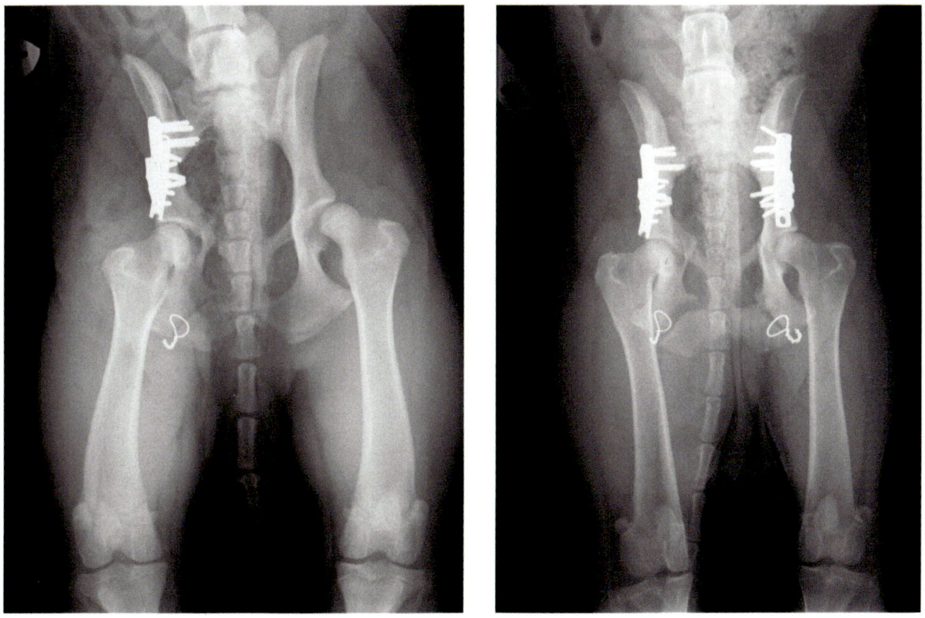

Figure 40. Postoperative view of a triple pelvic osteotomy. Courtesy from Dr. Marta Soler, HCV Universidad de Murcia.

of pain associated with hip dysplasia and degenerative joint disease. Abnormalities of the gait persist with some limb shortening, so it is not recommended for animals requiring a degree of athletic ability afterwards. It is often the treatment of choice when there are financial constraints. This procedure is also appropriate for femoral head and neck fractures, and chronic hip luxation (Piermatti et al., 2006).

Total Hip Replacement

This surgery involves remodelling of the acetabulum with an acetabular cup and inserting a femoral stem component followed by femoral head prosthesis. There are two main systems used for this: cemented (acetabular cup and femoral stem) or **cementless** (biological fixation). Implants are available in a range of sizes, including for cats (Figure 41).

The surgery is technically challenging and the decision to carry out the surgery not taken lightly. All treatment options should be thoroughly discussed with the owners. Surgeons are required to have carried out a relevant course. There is also the need for a scrub team, including a nurse, to keep surgery time as efficient as possible and reduce the risk of infection (Figure 42).

Avascular Necrosis of the Femoral Head

A disease of small breed dogs, thought to have a genetic component, caused by aseptic necrosis of the femoral head. On radiographs the femoral head appears flattened or has a moth eaten appearance. The condition can be uni or bilateral and is normally diagnosed in the first year after birth. Treatment is normally femoral head ostectomy or total hip replacement (Figure 43).

Stifles

Patella Luxation

This is when the patella displaces from the trochlear groove where it should sit normally. This condition is thought to have a genetic component but can also be caused by trauma or after surgery on the hindlimb. Luxation is normally medial, generally affects small dog breeds, and varies in severity which is identified by different grades (Table 4).

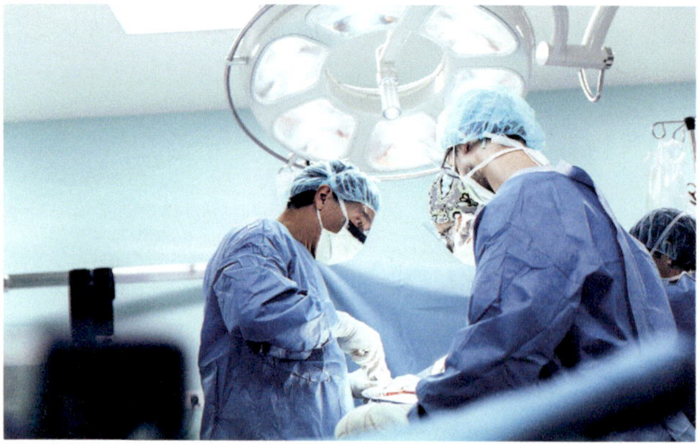

Figure 42. The scrub team at work during a total hip replacement.

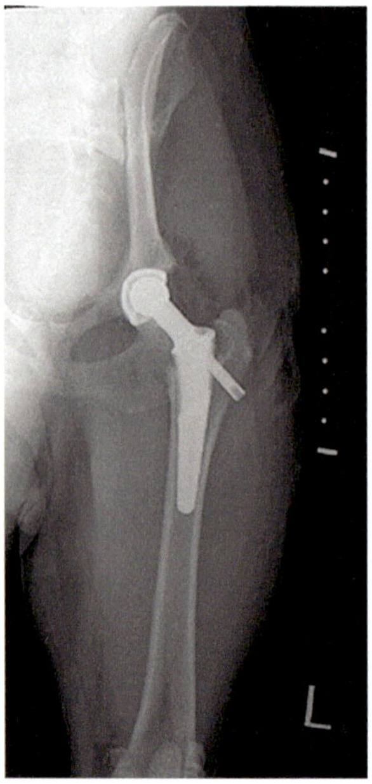

Figure 41. A postoperative view of a total hip replacement.

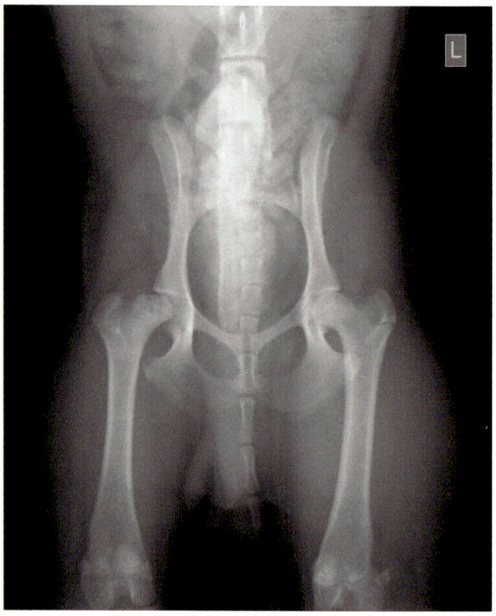

Figure 43. A hip joint with avascular necrosis of the femoral head. Courtesy from Dr. Marta Soler, HCV Universidad de Murcia.

Table 4. Grades of patella luxation. (Piermattei et al, 2006).

Grade	Signs
Grade 1	Patella can be luxated but returns to normal when released.
Grade 2	Patella luxates on stifle flexion or manual luxation but returns to position on extension or if manual replacement occurs.
Grade 3	Patella continuously luxates unless manually replaced (normally reluxates when hand removed).
Grade 4	Patella continuously luxates and cannot be manually replaced.

The mechanism that holds the patella in position is called the extensor apparatus. This includes the distal quadriceps muscle, patella, and the patella ligament. When in normal alignment the patella sits in the trochlear groove. If the mechanism is not aligned during development, the patella can luxate. The absence of the patella in the trochlear groove means the groove does not deepen enough to house the patella, making it prone to luxation (Maddox, 2017).

Owners normally report their dog has a skipping gait of the hindlimbs when exercising.

Surgical treatment options aim to deepen the trochlear groove (sulcoplasty) or better align the extensor apparatus. Sulcoplasty is the deepening of the trochlear groove in the distal femur. There are a number of methods for achieving this:

- **Trochlear block recession.** A rectangular piece of bone is removed using a hand held saw. The trochlear bed is then deepened with a modular osteotome and the rectangular wedge replaced.
- **Wedge recession sulcoplasty.** A V-shaped wedge segment is removed using a handheld saw. A second cut is made to make the V-shape slightly wider (cut only on one side, normally the side away from the patella). The original wedge of bone is then replaced (Fossum, 2007). See Figure 44 for comparison between this recession and the trochlear block.
- **Transposition of the tibial tuberosity** aims to realign the extensor apparatus, which enables the patella to sit within the trochlear groove. To do this, the tibial tuberosity, (which is the insertion for the patella tendon) is cut, reallocated, and held in place with arthrodesis wires. Bone heals quicker than tendons and this is why the bone is cut rather than any other soft tissue (Kowaleski, 2014).

Cranial Cruciate Ligament (CCL) Rupture

The cranial cruciate ligament prevents internal rotation and cranial displacement of the tibia against the femur. Injury is normally chronic and occurs over time, often due to conformational abnormalities. Acute injury, although not common, can still occur due to hyperextension or sharp internal rotation of the stifle joint (Farrell, 2018).

There is research showing links with breed, size, and neuter status when it comes to cruciate disease with large and giant

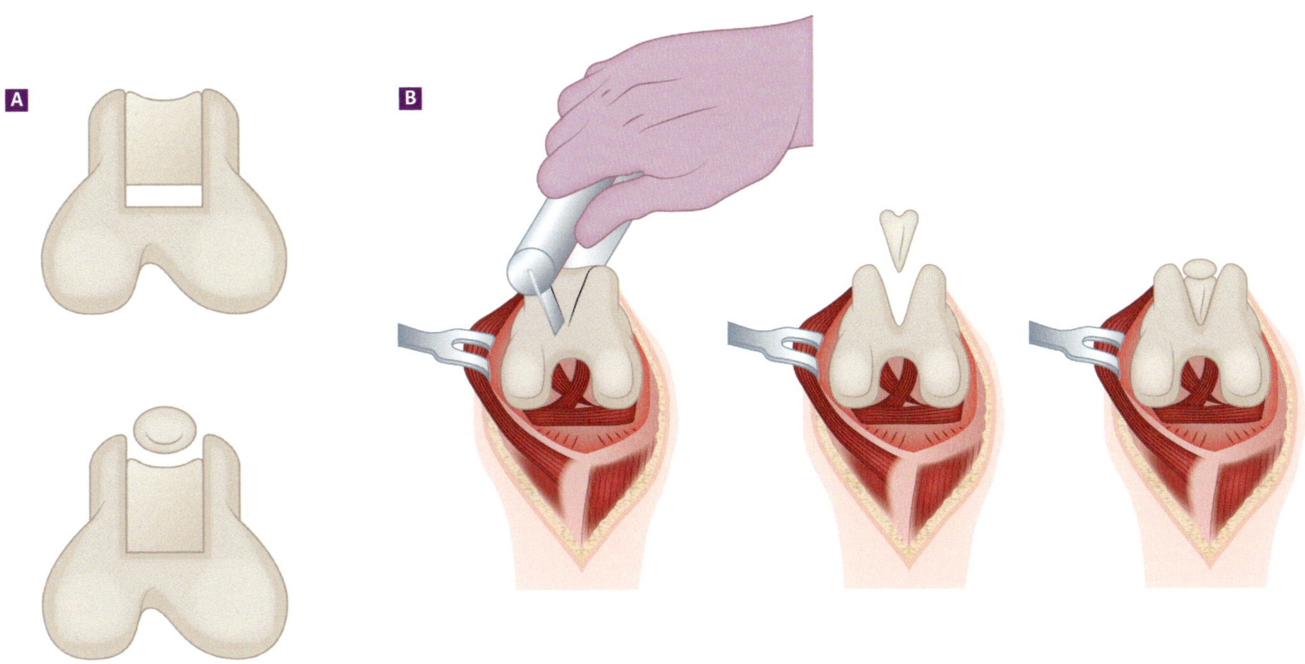

Figure 44. A comparison of the trochlear block sulcoplasty (**A**) and a wedge recession (**B**).

breed dogs overrepresented, as well as neutered male and female dogs (Witsberger, 2008).

Treatment Options for CCL Rupture

As with most orthopaedic disease there is always the conservative treatment option. A combination of controlled exercise, weight control, and NSAIDs can all contribute to improvements but there is a lot of research to suggest that surgery brings the most favourable outcome. There are also other considerations such as owner finances, owner compliance and expertise/equipment available.

Regardless of the surgery chosen to correct the disease, the surgeon normally examines the stifle joint itself. This is to examine the meniscus as this can become damaged following rupture of the cruciate ligament. Any damaged meniscus is normally removed and the joint capsule is closed before moving onto the next stage of the surgery. This can be done either as an arthrotomy or an arthroscopy.

Extracapsular Repair

Extracapsular simply means the repair is done outside of the joint capsule. A thick piece of monofilament Nylon® suture passes round the back of the stifle from the lateral fabella to the proximal tibia. The suture is then passed through bone tunnels drilled in the tibial tuberosity and the suture is held in place with metal crimps (Farrell, 2018).

Although this method still exists and is considerably cheaper than other methods there are other options which have superseded this such as a tibial plateau levelling osteotomy and tibial tuberosity advancement.

Tibial Plateau Levelling Osteotomy (TPLO)

There is evidence to suggest the angle of the tibial plateau has a direct effect on cruciate ligament injury. When there is injury to the cruciate ligament the angle of the tibial plateau has an effect on the movement of the femur relative to the tibia. **The aim of a TPLO surgery is to reduce the tibial plateau angle (TPA) to stabilise the risk of cranial tibial thrust** (Farrell, 2018).

A degree of preoperative planning is required for this procedure. The surgeon must calculate the current tibial plateau angle and calculate what they would like it to be. This allows them to calculate the amount of rotation needed once the osteotomy of the proximal tibia is carried out. The surgeon also uses preoperative radiographs to work out what size TPLO plate and screws to use and what size saw blade is needed to make the crescent shaped cut in the tibia. The plate and screws are applied once the bone has been cut and rotated in order to hold the bone in its new position.

Tibial Tuberosity Advancement

This surgery aims to keep the patella tendon angle at less than 90 degrees to counteract the cranial tibial thrust, which occurs when the cruciate ligament is deficient.

As with a TPLO, there is some preoperative planning which needs to take place for a TTA. The tibial crest is cut with a saw, moved forward, and held in place with a cage or plate that fill the gap and fixes to the bone with screws (Farrell, 2018).

There are a number of modifications to this technique with regards to how the tibial crest is held in its position.

The outcomes of both TPLO and TTA are similar and so the choice is often surgeon and hospital dependant, however, there is evidence to suggest that long term there may be a better return to function (analysed with force plates) with a TPLO. The body of evidence is not strong, however, with some studies saying there is no difference in outcome certainly with TPLO and TTA (Boudrieau, 2009).

Conditions of the Spine and Surgical Treatment

As with many disorders, neurological conditions (Table 5) can be acute or chronic. Acute presentations include RTAs, seizures, and paraplegia. Chronic presentations are more subtle and may be described by the owner as being intermittent.

With many acute injuries it can be obvious what has contributed, however, a full workup is still needed to localise the injury. Nonetheless, in the case of RTA a full neurological examination may be contraindicated.

Table 5. Some common definitions used to describe neurological conditions.

Plegia	Total loss of function.
Hemiplegia	Limbs on one side affected.
Paraplegia	Pelvic limbs affected.
Monoplegic	One limb affected.
Paresis	Weakness.
Ataxia	Lack of coordination.

Chronic presentations require a full neurological work up by the vet, as well as a full history (including any travel), and vaccination status.

The Spinal Column

The spinal column is made up of vertebrae through which the spinal cord runs and also the nerves which originate there. In between each vertebra lie the vertebral discs. Within the vertebral disc there is the outer layer, known as the annular ligament, and the inner nucleus pulposus (Gillam, 2017). (Figure 45).

Conditions of the Cervical Spine

Fractures of the Cervical Spine

Fractures of the cervical spine affecting the vertebrae may result in compression of the spinal cord and nerve roots. Fractures may occur as a result of RTA, running head first into a solid object, hanging, or tumours (pathological).

Treatment depends on the severity of the spinal cord compression and the instability present. Correction aims to realign the vertebrae and remove compression of the spinal cord. This is achieved by external splinting or internal fracture fixation.

Surgical fixation is often associated with a quicker recovery and hence shorter hospitalisation times, however, surgery in the cervical region of the spine is associated with potential perioperative mortality. Although the exact cause for such a high complication rate is unknown, one research paper talks about damage to the central nervous system associated with surgical manipulation. This could cause problems with respiration leading to cardiac arrest. The same study also talks about postoperative tracheal necrosis and pneumonia due to retraction of the trachea during surgery (Thomas et al., 1991).

Non-surgical treatment remains an option, provided it is started as early as possible with immediate immobilisation increasing the likelihood of a good outcome (Hawthorne et al., 1999).

Surgical repair aims to relieve any compression of nerves in the spinal cord and stabilise the vertebrae. Vertebral body fractures, disc extrusions, and atlantoaxial subluxation due to trauma are often repaired by a ventral approach whereas fractures of the dorsal lamina of C1 and C2 may be repaired by a dorsal approach (Fossum, 2007).

Surgical repair may involve the careful placement of Steinmann pins or screws. Polymethylmacralate (PMMA) cement is often used alongside these to prevent loosening (Fossum, 2007).

Atlantoaxial Subluxation

Although this condition can be trauma related, it is more often associated with breeding and genetics and affects small breed dogs such as Yorkshire Terriers and Toy Poodles.

It occurs due to fracture, hypoplasia, or malformation of the dens, which normally stabilises the atlas and axis (the first two vertebrae in the spinal column). Alternatively, or in addition, there can be failure of the ligamentous attachments or fracture/malformation of the other ligamentous attachments between the atlas and axis. Failure of the ligaments or the dens gives rise to laxity between the two bones. This predisposes to spinal cord and nerve root compression. Clinical signs can vary in severity from mild neck pain, tetraparesis, and even respiratory arrest (Olby, 2014).

Treatment with an external splint may be sufficient whilst the ligaments heal but if neurological deficits are already present, surgery is indicated although there can be a high perioperative risk associated with this procedure, as discussed in the section about cervical fractures.

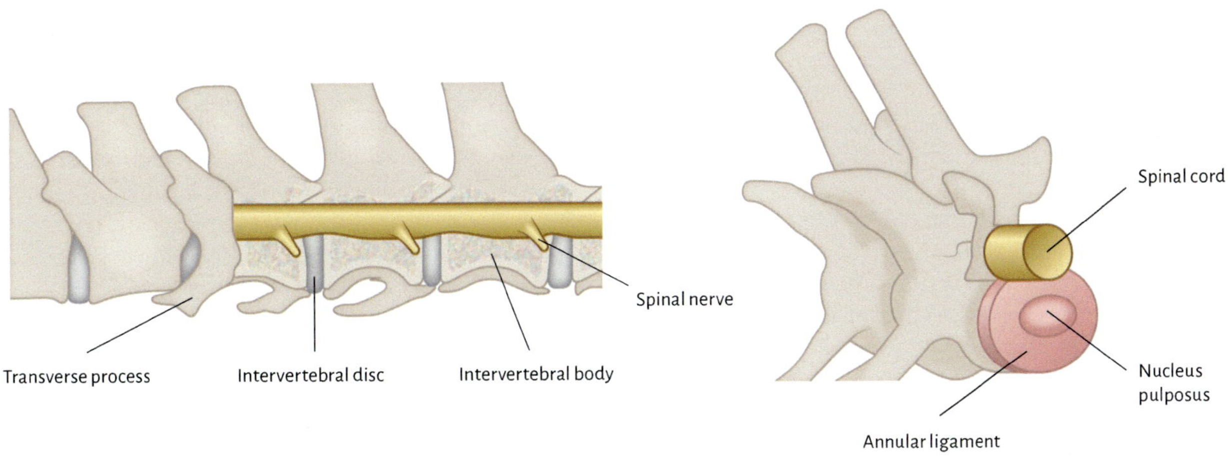

Figure 45. The normal anatomy of the vertebrae and intervertebral discs.

Depending on the surgical technique, the surgeon may perform a dorsal or a ventral approach. Screws or pins are placed ventrally to hold the bones in place once the subluxation or luxation is repaired and these can be stabilised with PMMA cement to prevent loosening. However, due to the size of some of these patients, the placement of screws can be very challenging.

An implant known as a Kishigami hook may be used, which is similar to tension banding (as with some avulsion fractures) and these are placed dorsally. The benefit is there is no risk of damage to the spinal column by incorrectly placed screws or wires (Pujol, 2010).

As with other surgery of the cervical spine, if the dog survives the first 48 hours postoperatively, the prognosis is generally good.

Caudal Cervical Spondylomyelopathy

This disease is common in **Dobermann Pinschers** and other large breed dogs. The cause is unknown but could be a combination of nutritional, traumatic, hereditary, or acquired factors (Fossum, 2007). There are a number of conditions within this disease, of which a dog may have one or many of those individual conditions (Box 1).

Box 1. Conditions which Can Contribute to Caudal Cervical Spondylomyelopathy.
(Fossum, 2007).

- **Chronic disc disease.**
- **Congenital malformations.**
- **Vertebral tipping.**
- **Hypertrophied ligaments.**
- **Spinal canal stenosis.**

Conservative treatment generally has a good outcome, and this is often desirable due to financial reasons. Also, as this disease is so prevalent in Dobermanns a conservative approach may be preferable to surgery due to the potential for the dog to also suffer from dilated cardiomyopathy (daCosta, 2010).

The decision to opt for surgery is based on clinical signs, neurological deficits, pain, and what the owners would like as a long-term outcome for their dog (daCosta, 2010). Because the disease has so many contributing factors there remain many surgical options depending on the prevailing aspect of the disease.

In essence, surgery aims to decompress the spinal cord, but this may be through removal of disc material (via dorsal laminectomy, hemilaminectomy, or ventral slot), distraction, and stabilisation of vertebrae (daCosta, 2010).

Fracture of the Thoracic or Lumbar Spine

Fractures of this region of the spinal column are more common than cervical fractures, with **RTA the most frequent cause.** Studies report that the most common area of the spinal column to fracture is the lumbar region followed by sacrococcygeal, thoracic, and cervical (Bruce et al., 2008).

Treatment can be conservative (with the use of splints) or surgical. Conservative treatment has a good success rate, but **should the patient show pain after 72 hours, spinal cord compression, or worsening neurological signs then surgery is indicated** (Bruce et al., 2008). This should be weighed up against outcomes which show surgery has a quicker return to function. Other benefits include shorter hospitalisation times (including less chance of decubitus ulcers and urine scalding), starting rehabilitation sooner, and decreasing the amount of nursing care required, especially if the dog is a large breed (McKee, 2016).

For fractures of the **cervical spine, repair commonly involves pins, screws and PMMA cement.** Bone plates can also be applied to the vertebral body, but care must be taken with locking plates as the direction and angle of the screw is determined by the engagement of the plate hole and the thread, and so the surgeon does not have as much control (McKee, 2016).

Plastic plates are available with the advantage of not requiring full surgical exposure as they sit on the dorsal lamina on either side of the dorsal spinous processes. They are flexible and secured in between the spinal processes (Fossum, 2007).

Intervertebral Disc Disease

Intervertebral disc disease results in compression of the spinal cord either by disc extrusion or disc protrusion. As discussed previously, the intervertebral discs are composed as **an annulus ligament which surrounds an inner nucleus pulposus.** The nucleus pulposus is normally a well hydrated gelatinous structure which naturally becomes slightly more dehydrated over time hence losing some of its hydroelastic function. This occurs more quickly in chondrodystrophic breeds such as Dachshunds and Basset hounds (Brisson, 2010). This gives rise to extrusion of the inner nucleus pulposus from the annulus and causing compression of the spinal cord. This is known as a **disc extrusion or Hansen type 1 disc.**

Similarly, there is a **Hansen type 2 disc** or a disc protrusion whereby the annulus ligament may weaken and cause the nucleus pulposus to bulge. This is a more chronic disease presentation in older dogs and is more prevalent in larger breeds such as German Shepherds, Labradors, Rottweilers, and Dalmatians (Brisson, 2010).

Diagnosis and Treatment

If disc extrusion occurs in the cervical region, the dog presents with neck pain, with or without tetraparesis or tetraplegia, depending on the severity of spinal cord compression (Olby, 2014). If it occurs in the thoracolumbar spine, the hindlimbs are more commonly affected leading to hemiparesis or hemiplegia.

Diagnosis of disc disease is based on history, clinical signs, neurological exam to localise the region of the extruded disc, and diagnostic imaging such as radiography, myelography, computed tomography (CT), or magnetic resonance imaging (MRI). Practices that do not have access to these modalities may choose to refer the patient at this stage for diagnostic imaging with surgery if indicated (Figure 46).

Conservative management can be attempted for dogs that only show very mild symptoms of spinal cord compression, but often disc extrusion requires surgical correction especially when causing tetra or paraplegia. Conservative management consists of strict cage rest with non-steroidal anti-inflammatory medication. Surgery should be considered however, if neurological signs worsen (Olby, 2014).

There is also supporting evidence to suggest if a dog presents without pain perception then surgery should be done as soon as practically possible. By delaying surgery, this may worsen the outcome, however, this may need to be considered against the risk of carrying out surgery at unsociable hours when there are fewer people around to provide patient care (Martin et al., 2020).

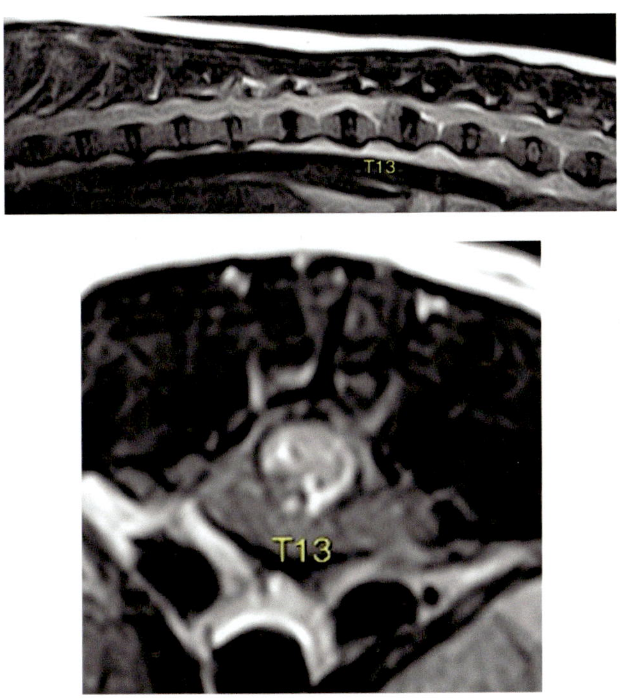

Figure 46. An MRI scan showing a disc extrusion. Courtesy from Dr. Marta Soler, HCV Universidad de Murcia.

A disc extrusion in the cervical region is best approached via a ventral slot procedure. This approach is used to get access to the ventral vertebral spinal canal in the cervical region with the aim of decompressing the spinal cord. By using this approach, less soft tissue and bony dissection is needed (Sturges and Dickinson, 2014). However, there are vital structures which require retraction such as the oesophagus, laryngeal nerves, and large vessels.

Patient positioning tip

If a long enough anaesthetic circuit is available, having the head away from the anaesthetic machine is helpful to avoid personnel having to work in small spaces. Sandbags or a cradle help hold the patient in dorsal recumbency, with an additional sandbag placed under the neck to help open the disc spaces. The forelimbs should be tied caudally.

Haemorrhage is a risk with many approaches to the spine due to nearby venous sinuses, it is therefore useful to have suction available and some form of haemostatic product to hand.

Due to the retraction of the laryngeal nerve there may be respiratory compromise postoperatively. This is uncommon but all patients should be monitored closely in the immediate postoperative period.

Disc material that has extruded into the thoracolumbar area of the spine can be approached by a hemilaminectomy procedure, provided the disc material is lateralised to one side or the other.

The disc material is accessed by the surgeon making a window in the lamina of the vertebrae, depending on which side the disc material is located. For this approach, the patient is positioned in sternal recumbency.

This approach carries the risk of haemorrhage due to the proximity of the venous sinuses but also pneumothorax as there is a risk of accidentally creating a hole into. the thoracic cavity.

A dorsal laminectomy approach is used when the area to be accessed is in the dorsal aspect of the spinal column. It can be used along any aspect of the vertebrae from cervical to lumbar spine. If the part of the spinal column has a dorsal spinous process then this may be removed to allow access also.

This approach is also good for tumour removal, spinal stenosis and cervical spondylomyelopathy (Sturges and Dickinson, 2014).

Disc Protrusion

Hansen type 2 discs are treated conservatively with cage rest and anti-inflammatories provided the symptoms are only mild. Worsening symptoms may lead to the need for surgery. Hemilaminectomy is often used as the approach for type 2 discs but due to the protrusion often being ventral to the spinal cord there is the need for manipulation of the spinal cord, potentially leading to worsening of neurological signs. A corpectomy procedure may therefore be carried out instead which involves a more ventral approach thus avoiding too much manipulation of the spinal cord (Salger et al., 2014).

Instrumentation (Figure 47):

- **Tissue forceps** (Adsons and dissecting forceps) used to help tissue manipulation on approach and closure of the surgical wound.
- **Mayo scissors** (curved and straight) used for blunt dissection and cutting sutures.
- **Needle holders** for holding suture needles when closing the layers.
- **Metzenbaum scissors** used for fine dissection.
- **Periosteal elevator** for manipulating soft tissue off bone.
- **Scalers** used to help with drilling to gauge the depth (they are the same as a dental scaler and have indentations at certain points).
- **Curette** which helps to remove disc material or collect bone grafts.
- **Freer elevator** for more delicate removal of soft tissue from bone.
- **Artery forceps** (mosquito) useful for helping to remove disc material.
- **Rongeurs** in a variety of sizes including a number of microspinal rongeurs. Used to remove bone when drilling the bony window to visualise the spinal canal.
- **Gelpi** (medium) for self-retaining retraction of soft tissues when making a surgical approach and to maintain visualisation.
- **Nerve hooks** for the retraction of delicate tissue.
- **Allis tissue forceps** for atraumatic manipulation on soft tissue.
- **Scalpel handle.**
- **Osteotome.**

Postoperative Nursing Care of Neurological Patients

Surgical Wound Care

In the immediate postoperative period whilst still in the operating theatre, **an adhesive dressing should be placed over the wound;** gloves should be worn to apply the dressing and for any further dressing changes. Normally it is enough for the dressing to be in place for 24–48 hours, until the patient has formed a natural fibrin seal to protect the wound from infection.

At this stage, the patient may also benefit from **cold packs placed around the surgical site,** which have an analgesic effect and also prevent postoperative swelling and bruising.

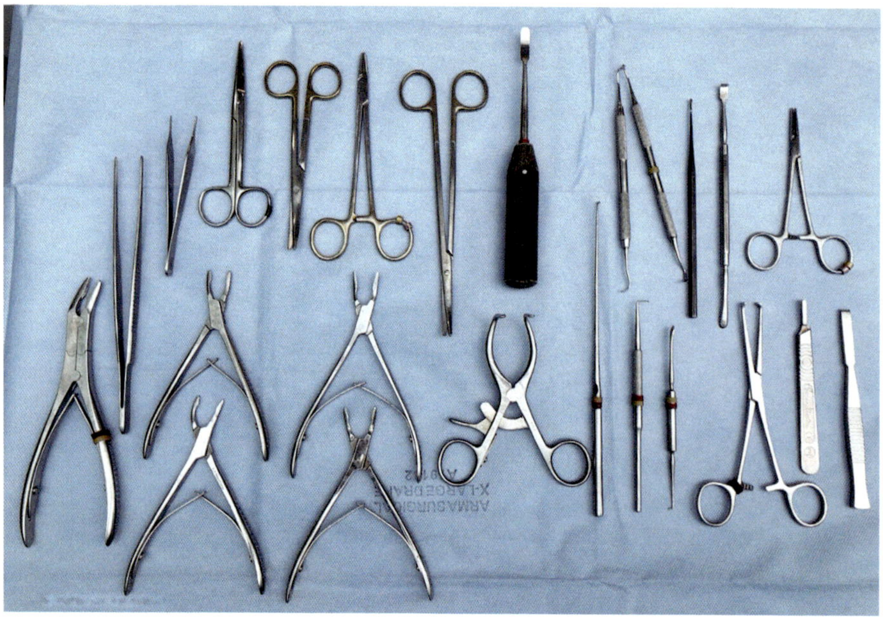

Figure 47. An example of a spinal kit.

The surgical wound should be monitored for haemorrhage, excessive swelling, and seroma formation. It should be ensured that the patient cannot interfere with the wound by using appropriate aids to stop this, such as an Elizabethan collar.

Nutrition and Fluid Therapy

Any surgical patient requires adequate nutrition in order to reduce recovery and hospitalisation times, as well as reduce healing times of wounds and surgical sites. It is therefore imperative that patients are allowed to eat as soon as possible after surgery, once it is safe to do so. Neurological patients, however, tend to be stressed and anxious about their condition due to the effects on the body and the inability in some cases, to mobilise. As a result they may be less inclined to eat.

Owner questionnaires at admit are useful in allowing the patient care team to devise their holistic nursing strategy for their patients and are especially important for neurological patients as they could be hospitalised for longer than other surgical patients. Knowing what the patient normally eats allows the VN to provide something similar and also take into consideration any allergies. If this was not done at patient admit (which may happen if the owner was distressed) then the VN could call the owner postoperatively to ask some questions about what food their pets like to eat.

Cooked chicken and fish are tempting for many patients, and something else which may help is spending some time bonding with the patient through hand feeding. Getting the owner to visit and spend some time with their pets is also a good way to tempt them to eat. Daily requirements for nutrition should be calculated for the patient once eating and split into 3–4 meals a day.

If a patient is still reluctant to eat it is important their hydration is maintained using fluid therapy, if the VN is concerned that a patient is not eating then this should be communicated to the VS.

If a patient cannot mobilise well, it can be dangerous to leave water bowls in their kennels in case they fall in and cannot move away. It may be safer to offer water at timely intervals, adding this onto the orders on the hospitalisation sheet so it is not forgotten.

Bladder Management

Bladder dysfunction may be a side effect of intervertebral disc disease and may give rise to urinary tract infections (UTIs). There are several methods available for emptying the bladder of these patients but the **longer this is required, the higher the risk of UTI.** It is therefore advantageous to allow the patient to void urine themselves once this ability has returned (Bubenik and Hosgood, 2008). It is difficult to know when a patient can voluntarily void urine when the patient has an indwelling catheter and this option should be used only when unavoidable, especially as research indicates the risk of UTI increases with patient age, each additional day of catheterisation, and the use of antibiotics. (Bubenik et al., 2007).

Compared to other methods, **manual expression may be preferable** in the postoperative period as long as it is well-tolerated by the patient. The patient, however, should still be taken out onto a suitable substrate so they can attempt to void urine by themselves first.

The use of an ultrasound scanner to measure bladder size is useful (Figure 48). This can be used to check how much urine is still in a bladder after voluntary urination by the patient (the urination may just be bladder overflow) or measure bladder size to determine when manual expression is next needed. The VS may indicate at what size the bladder needs to be before manual expression is undertaken.

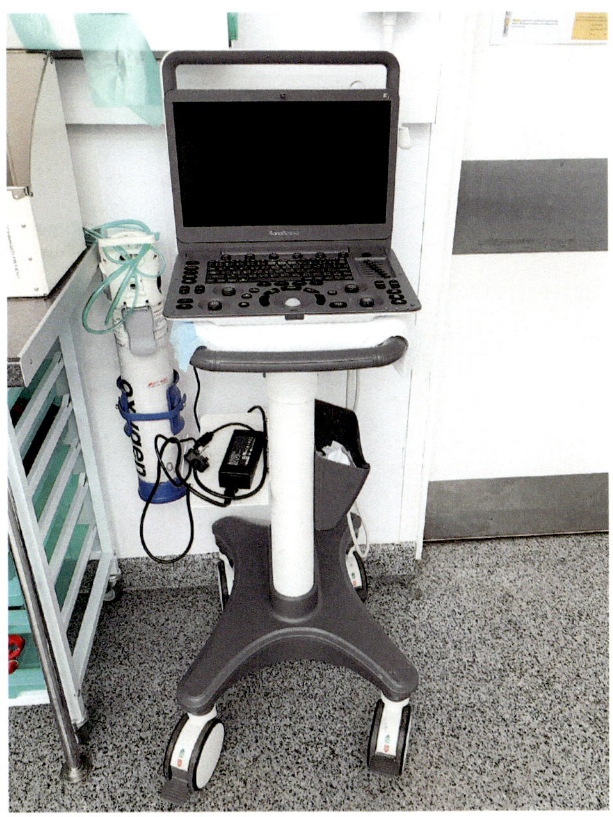

Figure 48. An ultrasound scanner for use in a neurological ward.

There are some patients where indwelling catheterisation is the best option. It may be more advantageous to place an indwelling catheter in large, fearful, and potentially aggressive patients where manual expression or regular movement is difficult.

Male Dog: Technique for Placing an Indwelling Urinary Catheter

- Hands should be washed and sterile gloves worn.
- An assistant restrains patient/prepares patient.
- Penis exposed from prepuce and wiped over with dilute iodine (Figure 49 A).
- Catheter inserted into urethra and fed in until urine is seen in the catheter. It should not be forced if there is a lot of resistance (Figure 49 B).
- The bladder should be emptied and catheter removed.
- OR if an indwelling catheter: the bulb should be inflated to the desired amount and attached to a collection bag/bung (Figure 49 C).

Bitch: Technique for Placing an Indwelling Urinary Catheter

- Chemical restraint likely to be necessary.
- Placing the catheter may be easier in dorsal recumbency.
- The area around the vulva should be cleaned and clipped.
- Speculum (if using) should be inserted until urethral orifice can be seen.
- If no speculum available, a finger should be inserted with catheter alongside and it should feed into the urethral orifice.
- The rest of the technique is as for male dogs.

Skincare

Neurological deficits may mean the patient cannot lift their limbs properly and para or tetraplegic patients cannot lift their feet from the ground. This can give rise to the patient **scuffing hair and skin off their feet.** This may have already happened before the patient arrives at the practice and avoiding further damage is important. To do this **paw coverings** such as cohesive bandages, drip bags (although this may affect placement of feet in a patient trying to establish voluntary movements) or commercially available foot covers should be used. The skin on the patient's feet should be examined daily as part of routine checks.

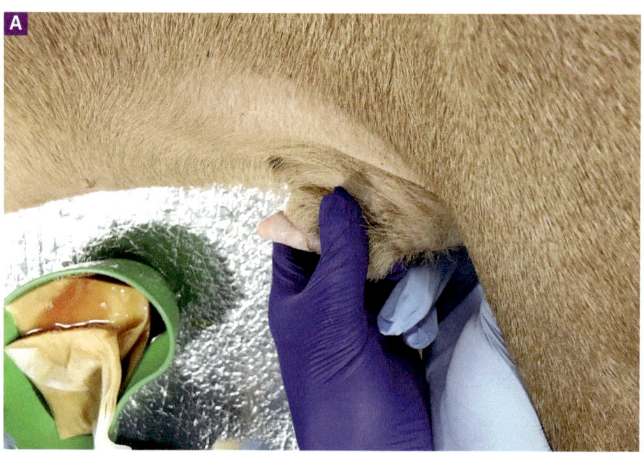

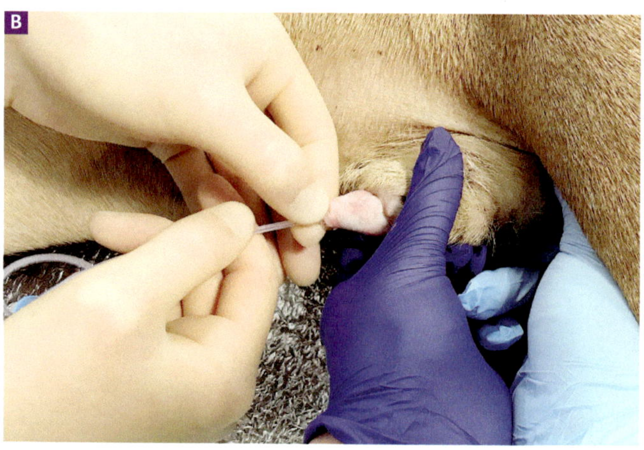

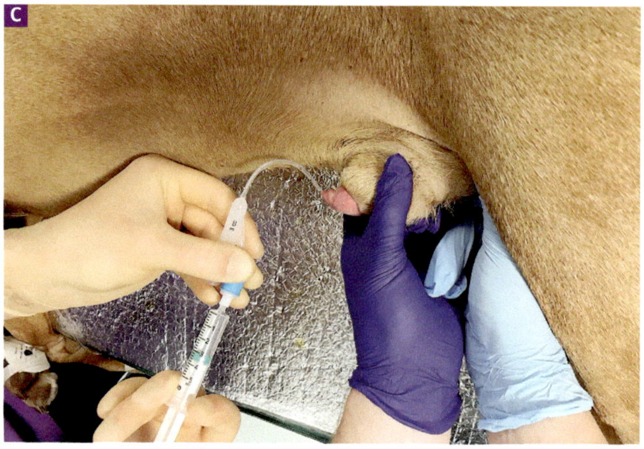

Figure 49. A. An assistant should extrude the penis and clean it with diluted iodine antiseptic solution; **B.** Whilst wearing sterile gloves, the lubricated end of the catheter should be gently inserted into the urethral orifice; **C.** Once in the bladder, sterile water should be injected to inflate the bulb to keep the catheter in place (the catheter will have a volume where the water is injected).

It is useful to pass a sling under the abdomen of a patient that cannot walk properly, and similarly a sling can lift a smaller patient's paws off the ground when walking over rough surfaces.

Neurological patients are particularly at risk of **decubital ulcers and bed sores.** It is imperative these patients have plenty of bedding, especially if recumbent postoperatively. Special mattresses are commercially available, but duvets, blankets, and Vetbed® are also useful. Bony prominences such as elbows and the greater trochanter are high risk for pressure sores so it should be ensured that these areas are routinely checked twice a day for any signs of soreness.

Recumbent patients should be turned every 2–4 hours (including positioning in sternal recumbency).

Urine scalding may occur and, as with sores, the patient may present with urine scalding. Adequate and regular bladder management help prevent this, which includes ensuring the bladder is fully emptied after the patient voids urine or after manual bladder expression.

Vetbed® is excellent at wicking away fluid from the patient, paired up with incontinence sheets underneath them, to soak up any urine should the patient urinate in their bed. Bedding should always be checked and changed as necessary when the patient is out of their kennel.

The skin around the perineum and caudal abdomen should be checked as part of routine checks. **If the skin is sore then the area should not be clipped** as this may further exacerbate the irritation and also take away one of the body's natural protective barriers, the hair. Barrier creams stop air getting to the skin, which is counterproductive, instead the VS should be consulted who may be able to prescribe some cream.

Respiration

Respiration should be routinely monitored as part of regular TPR checks but for patients that have had a ventral surgical approach; particular attention should be paid to their respiratory rate and effort. The trachea and larynx are often retracted during a ventral approach, which can cause iatrogenic damage to these structure and the recurrent laryngeal nerves. This can potentially cause **respiratory difficulties or increase the risk of aspiration pneumonia.** A rise in respiratory rate or breathing difficulties should be reported to the VS.

Patients with brachycephalic obstructive airway syndrome (BOAS) also need their respiration monitored closely as they are at higher risk of regurgitation which could potentially lead to aspiration pneumonia. Unfortunately, French Bulldogs commonly suffer from IVDD in the cervical region and often suffer from BOAS. In the worst cases, patients may require ventilatory support, but this is uncommon.

Patients with atlanto axial subluxation can have respiratory failure due to location of the compression of the spinal cord. They can present with this as part of their disease but again, could suffer respiratory failure peri or postoperatively.

Introduction to Rehabilitation

When muscle, cartilage and bone are not used they undergo atrophy; examples of these circumstances include cruciate ligament disease or hip dysplasia, where normal weight bearing does not occur. Rehabilitation, such as the use of hydrotherapy, can also benefit healthy dogs as an adjunct to a normal exercise routine or to help with weight loss.

The benefits of rehabilitation include:

- decreased oedema
- improved muscle tone and reduced muscle wastage
- improved quality of movement
- bonding with owner/care provider
- change to usual exercise routine (e.g. dog having hydrotherapy instead of usual walks).

The evidence base for veterinary rehabilitation is minimal, **with the majority of evidence for the benefits coming from human medicine.** However, this is changing and the ability to quantify the effects of rehabilitation is helping to increase the evidence base in veterinary patients. Use of tape measures to measure muscle mass, goniometers, force plates and treadmills can all help quantify the effects of rehabilitation.

As with all aspects of patient care, rehabilitation should be holistic and suited to each individual patient and their needs, temperament, surgical condition, and the required outcome.

When limbs are not used there is a degree of muscle wastage and stiffness within the joints. At the very least, the aims of rehab are to prevent this happening. Other benefits of rehab include patient stimulation, bonding, and quicker recovery and therefore discharge from the clinic.

Any rehabilitation techniques must be **under the direction of a VS** and only carried out by trained personnel.

This section discusses some of the common rehabilitation techniques available to veterinary patients. The various techniques may not be suitable for all patients and contraindications are listed at the end of each section.

Massage Therapy

Techniques

Stroking

This technique is good way of introducing a physiotherapy session, especially if the patient is anxious. It involves a gliding movement of the hands over the entire body from head to tail (Figure 50).

Effleurage

Effleurage is when the hands stroke from proximal to distal, for example in the limbs, the hand is placed gently around the limb and an even pressured stroking movement is used up the limb in the direction of lymphatic and venous return (Figure 51).

Petrissage

This is the use of rhythmic pressure and release to improve circulation and flow of lymph (Figure 52).

Tapotement

This includes striking the body with the hands whilst the wrists remain relaxed, so the touch is springy. There are a number of techniques for this, such as using the sides of the hands, the fists, knuckles, and hands in a cupping motion (Figure 53).

Contraindications

- pyrexia
- shock
- unstable fractures
- neoplasia
- open wounds.

Passive Range of Motion (PROM)

This is when the person giving the physiotherapy (rather than the patient) moves the limb through the full range of normal motion. It is useful for non-ambulatory patients, chronic degenerative conditions, and those recovering from spinal surgery. Passive movements include flexion and extension of all the joints in either a specific limb or in all limbs, as instructed by the VS. It is important to ensure the joints are supported at all times and if a patient shows signs of pain, anxiety or stiffness, movements should never be forced.

Another option is to make a bicycling motion with the limbs, which simulates how the limb normally goes through the motion of walking. This is, again, useful for patients with neurological disorders that may be non-ambulatory (Figure 54).

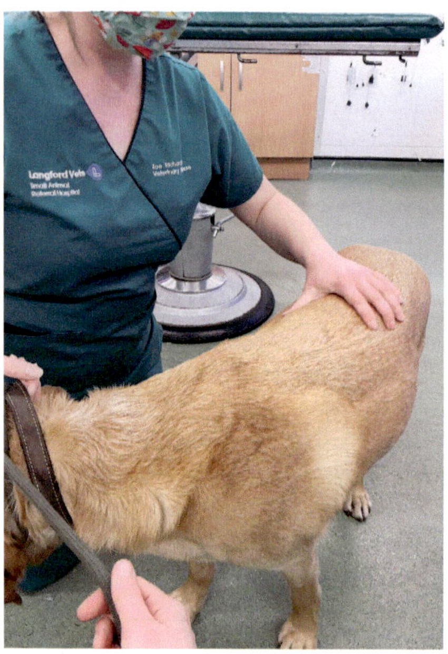

Figure 50. Stroking.

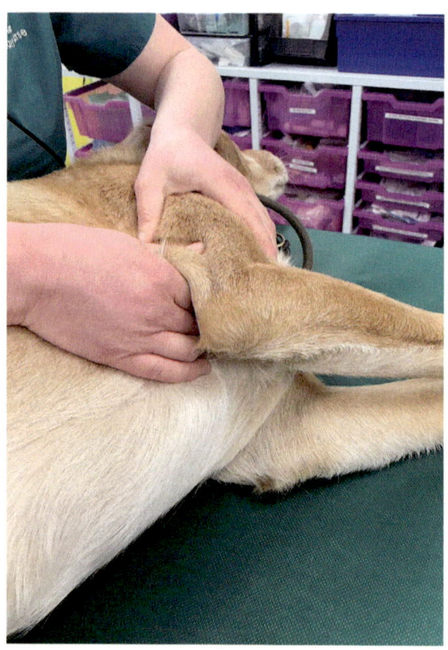

Figure 51. Effleurage.

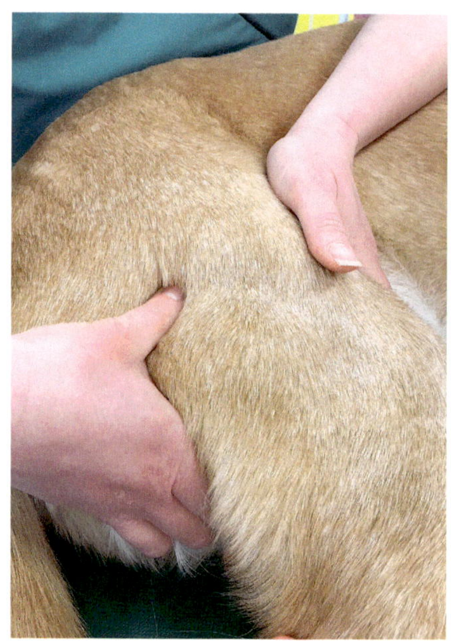

Figure 52. Pettrisage.

Contraindications

- acute injury to tendons/ligaments/muscle/bone
- unstable fractures.

Heat and Cold Therapy

Cryotherapy

Cryotherapy (cold) is useful in the immediate postoperative period to reduce tissue inflammation and pain. However, evidence shows that to get a temperature change in deeper tissues, the cold must be present for 20 minutes (Wright et al., 2020). The simplest way of applying cold is to wrap an ice-pack in a towel and hold it over the area, but cold compression units are also available. **Care should be taken when applying cold over a superficial metal implant as the latter conducts the cold and the effects last longer.** It is advisable to avoid placing cold directly over metallic implants but instead placing the cold in the surrounding area.

Thermotherapy

Thermotherapy (heat) increases blood flow (and therefore oxygenation) to the tissues and provide analgesia, again making this useful in the postoperative period. Cryotherapy is the preferred treatment of choice for the first 72 hours, with heat applied after this stage (Burnett and Wardlaw, 2012). There appears to be less evidence for thermotherapy than cryotherapy but studies have found that heat for 10 minutes has an effect on the temperature of the deep tissues, which does not further increase with longer application times.

Warm packs wrapped in a towel and placed over the area to be treated is an easy way to provide superficial heat. Deeper heat can be provided by therapeutic ultrasound by trained personnel.

Contraindications

- inflammation
- neoplasia
- decreased circulation
- open wounds
- pyrexia.

Remember, neither heat or cold should be applied directly to the skin.

Electrotherapy

Techniques

Laser

Photobiomodulation (or laser) emits a light which stimulates a response and change in cells. Laser therapy is thought

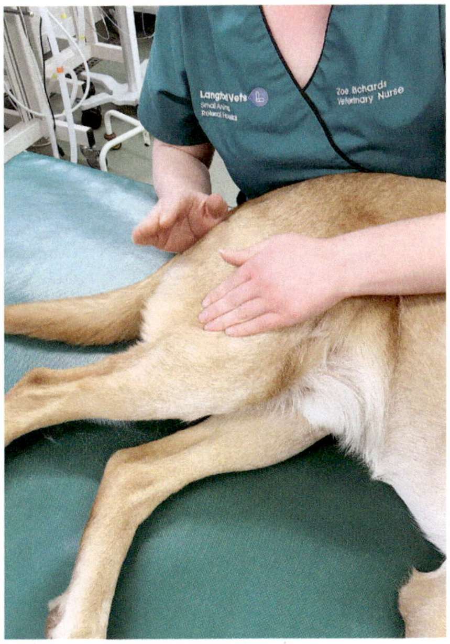

Figure 53. Tapotement.

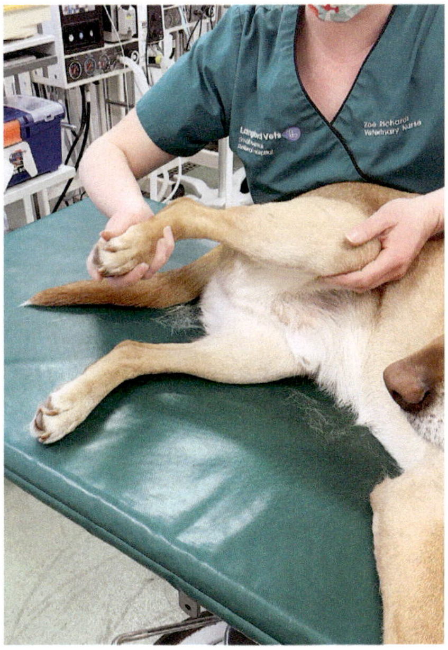

Figure 54. An example of PROM: bicycling the hind limbs.

to have many uses including pain relief, reduction of inflammation. and the promotion of healing. The therapeutic laser discussed here is different to the laser used in some minimally invasive surgeries, such as laser ablation of ectopic ureters (Pryor and Millis, 2015).

Evidence this method has a significant effect on tissue healing is questionable, with the majority of research done on rats. There does seem to be an increase in practices adapting the use of low-level lasers to help with wound healing and so hopefully more evidence will emerge in the future.

Ultrasound

Ultrasound can be absorbed by tissues such as tendons, ligaments, and scar tissue to help enhance the repair of these tissues. It can also reduce the amount of scar tissue by enhancing the tensile strength of the collagen fibres (Sharp, 2010).

Electrical Nerve Stimulation

This is either the use of neuromuscular electrical stimulators (NMES) which stimulate peripheral nerves in order to bring about a response from the patient, or transcutaneous electrical nerve stimulators (TENS), which can be used for pain relief. NMES are useful in patients who cannot contract their own muscles, for example, those with paraplegia. The unit can produce either twitching with lower frequencies or visible muscle contractions with higher frequencies (Sharp, 2010).

Contraindications

- epileptic patients
- patients with pacemakers
- compromised circulation/ischaemic tissues
- tumours.

Therapeutic Exercises

This involves a number of different exercises to get the patient to move in certain ways which aim to enhance function, promote wellness, and optimize overall health (Table 6).

Table 6. The four main types of therapeutic exercise. (Sharp, 2010).

Strength	Running, hill walking, dancing, swimming.
Endurance	Swimming, trotting, treadmill.
Flexibility	Crawling under objects, stepping over objects, stair climbing, weaving.
Balance and proprioception	Wobble boards, trampolines, walking on a variety of surfaces.

It is rare that this is carried out in the veterinary practice as the patient is likely be fully recovered by the time these exercises became an option. These are usually carried out either by the owner or at specific appointments with a veterinary physiotherapist or similar.

The exercises are carried out to enhance recovery from injury but also as a way to strengthen muscles and improve proprioception.

Hydrotherapy

This is the use of water, normally in the form of a swimming pool or an underwater treadmill. Not only is it useful for rehabilitation but also as a complementary training method or alternative exercise for healthy dogs (Figure 55).

Buoyancy in the water means the animal can move its limbs through the full range of motion without any strain through the limbs (Tomlinson, 2012). Similarly, on underwater treadmills, the deeper the water, the less weight is loaded through the limbs, hence increasing the flexion and extension of joints (Levine et al., 2002).

Contraindications

- fear of water
- recent surgery or open wounds
- cardiovascular issues
- pain.

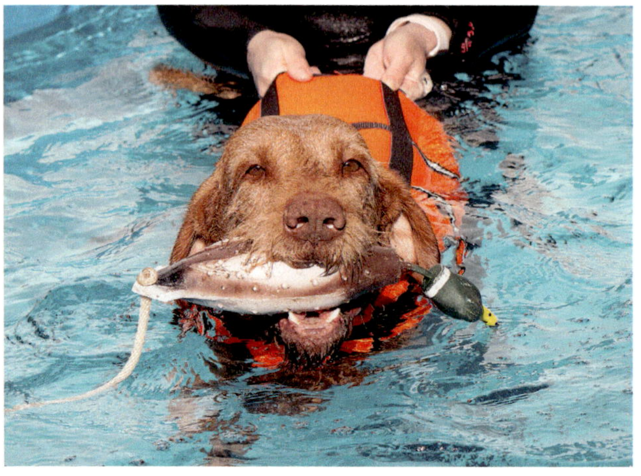

Figure 55. A dog having hydrotherapy.

References

■ Barthelemy, N. and Parsons, K. (2020) When should we consider total hip replacement for dysplastic dogs. Accessed online: https://veterinary-practice.com/article/when-should-we-consider-total-hip-replacement-for-dysplastic-dogs

■ Boudrieau, R.J. (2009) Tibial plateau levelling osteotomy or tibial tuberosity advancement? *Veterinary Surgery*, 38(1), 1–22.

■ Brisson, B.A. (2010) Intervertebral disc disease in dogs. *Veterinary Clinics: Small Animal Practice*, 40(5), 829–858.

■ Bruce, C.W., Brisson, B.A. and Gyselinck, K. (2008) Spinal fracture and luxation in dogs and cats. *Veterinary and Comparative Orthopaedics and Traumatology*, 21(03), 280–284.

■ Bubenik, L.J., Hosgood, G.L., Waldron, D.R. and Snow, L.A. (2007) Frequency of urinary tract infection in catheterized dogs and comparison of bacterial culture and susceptibility testing results for catheterized and noncatheterized dogs with urinary tract infections. *Journal of the American Veterinary Medical Association*, 231(6), pp. 893–899.

■ Bubenik, L. and Hosgood, G. (2008) Urinary tract infection in dogs with thoracolumbar intervertebral disc herniation and urinary bladder dysfunction managed by manual expression, indwelling catheterization or intermittent catheterization. *Veterinary Surgery*, 37(8), 791–800.

■ Burnett, J.M. and Wardlaw, J.L. (2012) Physical rehabilitation for veterinary practices. *Today's Vet. Pract*, 2, 14–20. Accessed online https://todaysveterinarypractice.com/physical-rehabilitation-for-veterinary-practices/

■ Butterworth, S.J. and Innes, J.F. (2001) Incomplete humeral condylar fractures in the dog. *Journal of Small Animal Practice*, 42(8), 394–398.

■ Conzemius, M. and Swainson, S. (1999) Fracture fixation with screws and bone plates. *Veterinary clinics: Small Animal Practice*, 29(5), 1117–1133.

■ da Costa, R.C. (2010) Cervical spondylomyelopathy (wobbler syndrome) in dogs. *Veterinary Clinics: Small Animal Practice*, 40(5), 881–913.

■ Duke, T. (1999) Dental and maxillofacial surgery. In Seymour, C. and Gleed, R. (eds) *BSAVA Manual of Small Animal Anaesthesia*. Gloucester: BSAVA.

■ Farrell, M. (2018) The stifle. In Arthurs, Brown and Petit (eds) *BSAVA manual of canine and feline musculoskeletal disorders. 2nd edition*. Gloucester: BSAVA.

■ Fossum, T. (2007) *Small animal surgery*. Missouri: Elsevier.

■ Gant, P., Asztalos, I., Kulendra, E., Lee, K. and Humm, K. (2019) Retrospective evaluation of factors influencing transfusion requirements and outcome in cats with pelvic injury (2009–2014): 122 cases. *Journal of Veterinary Emergency and Critical Care*, 29(4), 407-412.

■ Gemmill, T. and Clements, D. (2016) *BSAVA Manual of Canine and Feline Fracture Repair and Management*. Gloucester, BSAVA.

■ Gemmill, T and Oxley, B. (2018) The hip. In Arthurs, Brown and Petit (eds) *BSAVA manual of canine and feline musculoskeletal disorders. 2nd edition*. Gloucester: BSAVA.

■ Gillam, S. (2017) Intervertebral disc herniation. Accessed online https://todaysveterinarynurse.com/articles/intervertebral-disc-herniation/

■ Gower, J.A., Bound, N.J. and Moores, A.P. (2008) Tibial tuberosity avulsion fracture in dogs: a review of 59 dogs. *Journal of Small Animal Practice*, 49(7), 340–343.

■ Hawthorne, J.C., Blevins, W.E., Wallace, L.J., Glickman, N. and Waters, D.J. (1999) Cervical vertebral fractures in 56 dogs: a retrospective study. *Journal of the American Animal Hospital Association*, 35(2), 135–146.

■ Johnson, A.L. and DeCamp, C.E. (1999) External skeletal fixation: linear fixators. *Veterinary Clinics of North America: Small Animal Practice*, 29(5), 1135–1152.

■ Kapler, M and Dycus, D. (2015) A Practitioner's Guide to Fracture Management. *Todays Veterinary Practice*. Accessed online: https://todaysveterinarypractice.com/selection-of-fixation-technique-and-external-coaptation/

■ Kowaleski, M. (2014) Tibial tuberosity transposition: Step by step'. Accessed online https://www.vetfolio.com/learn/article/tibial-tuberosity-transposition-step-by-step

■ Krotscheck, U., Hulse, D.A., Bahr, A. and Jerram, R.M. (2000) Ununited anconeal process: lag-screw fixation with proximal ulnar osteotomy. *Veterinary and Comparative Orthopaedics and Traumatology*, 13(04), 212–216.

■ Langley Hobbs, S.J., Carmichael, S. and McCartney, W. (1996) Use of external skeletal fixators in the repair of femoral fractures in cats. *Journal of small animal practice*, 37(3), 95–101.

■ Levine, D., Tragauer, V. and Millis, D. L. (2002) Percentage of Normal Weight-Bearing During Partial Immersion at Various Depths in Dogs. *Proceedings of the 2nd International Symposium on Rehabilitation and Physical Therapy in Veterinary Medicine*. Knoxville, Tennessee.

■ Maddox, M. (2017) Luxating patellas: Pathology and treatment options. Accessed online https://todaysveterinarynurse.com/articles/luxating-patellas-pathology-and-treatment-options/

■ Martin, S., Liebel, F.X., Fadda, A., Lazzerini, K. and Harcourt Brown, T. (2020) Same day surgery may reduce the risk of losing pain perception in dogs with thoracolumbar disc extrusion. *Journal of Small Animal Practice*, 61(7), 442–448.

■ McKee, M. (2016) The spine. In Gemmil, T and Clements, D.(eds) *BSAVA manual of canine and feline fracture repair*. Gloucester: BSAVA.

■ McLaughlin, R. (1999) Internal fixation: intramedullary pins, cerclage wires, and interlocking nails. *Veterinary clinics of North America: Small Animal Practice*, 29(5), 1097–1116.

■ Moores, A.P., Agthe, P. and Schaafsma, I.A. (2012) Prevalence of incomplete ossification of the humeral condyle and other abnormalities of the elbow in English Springer Spaniels. *Veterinary and Comparative Orthopaedics and Traumatology*, 25(03), 211–216.

■ Moores, A.P. (2016) Biomechanical basis of bone fracture and fracture repair. In *BSAVA manual of canine and feline fracture repair and management*. Gloucester, BSAVA, pp. 20–31.

- Ness, M.G. (2006) Treatment of inherently unstable open or infected fractures by open wound management and external skeletal fixation. *Journal of small animal practice*, 47(2), 83–88.
- Olby, N. (2014) Tetraparesis. In Platt and Olby (eds) *BSAVA manual of canine and feline neurology*. Gloucester, BSAVA.
- Palmer, R.H. (2012) External fixators and minimally invasive osteosynthesis in small animal veterinary medicine. *Veterinary Clinics: Small Animal Practice*, 42(5), 913–934.
- Peirone, B., Rovesti, G.L., Baroncelli, A.B. and Piras, L.A. (2020) Minimally invasive plate osteosynthesis fracture reduction techniques in small animals. *Veterinary Clinics: Small Animal Practice*, 50(1), 23–47.
- Piermattei, D. L., Flo, G. L. and DeCamp, C. E. (2006) *Handbook of small animal orthopaedics and fracture repair*. Missouri, Elsevier.
- Pryor, B. and Millis, D.L. (2015) Therapeutic laser in veterinary medicine. *Veterinary Clinics: Small Animal Practice*, 45(1), 45–56.
- Pujol, E., Bouvy, B., Omana, M., Fortuny, M., Riera, L. and Pujol, P. (2010) Use of the Kishigami atlantoaxial tension band in eight toy breed dogs with atlantoaxial subluxation. *Veterinary Surgery*, 39(1), 35–42.
- Roe, S. (2020) Biomechanics of fracture fixation. *Veterinary clinics of North America Small Animal Practice*. Vol 50, no 1, 23–47.
- Salger, F., Ziegler, L., Böttcher, I.C., Oechtering, G., Böttcher, P. and Flegel, T. (2014) Neurologic outcome after thoracolumbar partial lateral corpectomy for intervertebral disc disease in 72 dogs. *Veterinary Surgery*, 43(5), 581–588.
- Sharp, B. (2010) Physiotherapy and physical rehabilitation. In *BSAVA manual of canine and feline rehabilitation, supportive and palliative care*. Gloucester, BSAVA, pp. 90–113.
- Sturges, B. K and Dickinson, P. J. (2014) Principles of neurosurgery. In Platt and Olby (eds) *BSAVA manual of canine and feline neurology*. Gloucester, BSAVA.
- Temwichitr, J., Leegwater, P.A. and Hazewinkel, H.A. (2010) Fragmented coronoid process in the dog: a heritable disease. *The Veterinary Journal*, 185(2), 123–129.
- Thomas, W. B., Sorjonen, D. C. and Simpson, S. T. (1991) Surgical management of atlanto axial subluxation in 23 dogs. *Veterinary Surgery*. 20(6), 409–412.
- Tomlinson, R. (2012) Use of canine hydrotherapy as part of a rehabilitation programme. *The Veterinary Nurse*, 3(10), 624–629.
- Tomsa, K., Glaus, T., Hauser, B., Flückiger, M., Arnold, P., Wess, G. and Reusch, C. (1999) Nutritional secondary hyperparathyroidism in six cats. *Journal of small animal practice*, 40(11), 533–539.
- Vezzoni, A. and Benjamino, K. (2021) Canine Elbow Dysplasia: Ununited Anconeal Process, Osteochondritis Dissecans, and Medial Coronoid Process Disease. *Veterinary Clinics: Small Animal Practice*, 51(2), 439–474.
- Witsberger, T.H., Villamil, J.A., Schultz, L.G., Hahn, A.W. and Cook, J.L. (2008) Prevalence of and risk factors for hip dysplasia and cranial cruciate ligament deficiency in dogs. *Journal of the American Veterinary Medical Association*, 232(12), 1818–1824.
- Wheeler, J.L., Cross, R.A., Stubbs, W.P., Guerin, R.S. and Lewis, D.D. (2004) Intramedullary interlocking nail fixation in dogs and cats: biomechanics and instrumentation. *Compendium*. Accessed online: http://vetfolio-vetstreet.s3.amazonaws.com/mmah/b1/819a8eeec843b4b47fd6da070ec882/filePV_26_07_519.pdf
- Wright, B., Kronen, P.W., Lascelles, D., Monteiro, B., Murrell, J.C., Robertson, S., Steagall, P.V.M. and Yamashita, K. (2020) Ice therapy: cool, current and complicated. *Journal of Small Animal Practice*, 61(5), 267–271.
- Zacher, A.M. and Marretta, S.M. (2013) Oral and maxillofacial surgery in dogs and cats. *Veterinary Clinics: Small Animal Practice*, 43(3), 609–649.

TEST

ANSWERS ON PAGE 462

1. **A bone tumour can be responsible for a pathological fracture, what can be another cause of pathological fractures?**
   a. Hyperthyroidism.
   b. Pregnancy.
   c. Hyperparathyroidism.
   d. Cushings disease.

2. **In a double pelvic osteotomy, the osteotomies are carried out on the ilium and the pubis. In a triple pelvic osteotomy, which extra part of the pelvis has an osteotomy carried out?**
   a. Acetabulum.
   b. Femur.
   c. Ischium.
   d. Greater trochanter.

3. **Why is a pancarpal arthrodesis plate thinner at the distal end than the proximal end?**
   a. To help with soft tissue coverage where soft tissue is minimal.
   b. Because the bone is thinner.
   c. To preserve blood supply.
   d. So that less screws are required.

4. **What is the preferred surgical approach to a disc extrusion in the cervical spine?**
   a. Hemilaminectomy.
   b. Corpectomy.
   c. Ventral slot.
   d. Fenestration.

5. **When is neuromuscular electrical stimulation the most effective?**
   a. In paraplegic patients.
   b. Postoperative fracture repair.
   c. Osteoarthritis.
   d. Postoperative THR.

6. **When referring to instrument categories, what is a Gelpi?**
   a. A handheld retractor.
   b. A self-retaining retractor.
   c. An abdominal retractor.
   d. A plate used for fracture repair.

7. **What orthopaedic disease is a Tibial Plateau Levelling Osteotomy carried out for?**
   a. Patella luxation.
   b. Fracture of the tibia.
   c. Hip dysplasia.
   d. Cruciate disease.

8. **When referring to bone plates, what does DCP stand for?**
   a. Dynamic compression plate.
   b. Direct compression plate.
   c. Dynamic core plate.
   d. Direct core plate.

9. **What is cryotherapy?**
   a. The use of heat to promote healing.
   b. A type of massage therapy.
   c. The use of cold to promote healing and provide analgesia.
   d. A type of electrical stimulation therapy.

10. **What is the jelly-like material called inside the annulus ligament within intervertebral discs?**
   a. Nucleus pulposus.
   b. Cerebral spinal fluid.
   c. Annular fluid.
   d. Collagen.

CLINICAL CASE 1

Ben is a 4-year-old Miniature Dachshund. He was admitted the previous day after going acutely off his hind limbs with a complete loss of sensation.

1. **What is it called when there is total loss of sensation in the hindlimbs?**

The Veterinary Surgeon (VS) diagnosed paraplegia and after a CT scan, Ben was diagnosed with a disc extrusion at T13–L1. Due to the loss of sensation, the VS opted for surgery straight away.

2. **What surgical approach would the VS have carried out to access the extruded disc material from T13–L1 on the right-hand side?**

Ben returned from surgery late in the evening, his surgery was successful, and he recovered well from his general anaesthetic.

The next day at rounds you would like to discuss nursing considerations with the surgeon.

3. **What considerations would you like to discuss?**

For each of the above considerations:

4. **What would be your recommendations? (NB: These will need to be "prescribed" by the VS before beginning).**

Considerations would already be in the table, please write in their suggestions.

Consideration	Nursing care suggestions
Nutrition and fluid therapy	
Bladder management	
Physiotherapy/ Rehabilitation	
Pain relief	

5. **What else could help with Ben's holistic care whilst he is hospitalised?**

Clinical Case 2

A couple has just come out from a vet consult to discuss their Labrador who has been diagnosed with hip dysplasia. They have been given treatment options but feel quite overwhelmed and would like to discuss in more detail what the different options entail.

1. **Their dog is 9 months old, so which two options are not applicable as a form of treatment?**
2. **What are the non-surgical options available to them?**
3. **What are the pros and cons of the remaining surgery options?**

Notes

Correct Answers:

Test

1. c
2. c
3. a
4. c
5. a
6. b
7. d
8. a
9. c
10. a

Clinical Case 1

1. **What is it called when there is total loss of sensation in the hindlimbs?** Paraplegia.

2. **What surgical approach would the VS have carried out to access the extruded disc material from T13–L1 on the right-hand side?** Hemilaminectomy.

3. **What considerations would you like to discuss?**
   - **Pain relief.** What is the plan for Ben's pain relief? Should he be pain scored?
   - **Nutrition and fluid therapy.** What are the plans for fluids whilst Ben is not eating?
   - **Bladder management.** Ben may need help to empty his bladder. What will be his bladder management plan?
   - **Physiotherapy/Rehabilitation.** Should Ben be started on some rehabilitation to help keep the muscles in his hind limbs from starting to atrophy?

4. **What would be your recommendations?**

Consideration	Nursing care suggestions
Nutrition and fluid therapy	· Find out from the owner what Ben likes to eat and offer this. · Suggest the owners could visit and bring some food if Ben is still reluctant. · Keep on maintenance fluid requirements until eating (as long as there are no other losses such as vomiting or diarrhoea).
Bladder management	· Use an ultrasound scanner to check the bladder size. · When it gets to a certain size express the bladder. · Do not express before then as you need to give Ben the chance to urinate for himself. · Check once you have expressed the bladder that it is empty.
Physiotherapy/ Rehabilitation	· Start some passive range of motion exercises. · Consider the use of a Neuromuscular Electrical Stimulation.
Pain relief	· Should Ben be pain scored? What score would indicate action is needed? · Could the surgical wound be cold compressed to help with swelling and pain?

5. **What else could help with Bens holistic care whilst he is hospitalised?** The use of a questionnaire or asking the owners questions during a telephone conversation or visit.

Clinical Case 2

1. **Their dog is 9 months old, so which two options are not applicable as a form of treatment?**
   - Pubic symphysiodesis.
   - Triple pelvic osteotomy.

2. **What are the non-surgical options available to them?**
   - Hydrotherapy.
   - Pain relief. Likely in the form of NSAIDs.
   - Weight management.

   These would help with symptoms but not the progression of the disease.

3. **What are the pros and cons of the remaining surgery options?**
   - FHNE (femoral head and neck excision)
     - Pros: not too technically demanding, could be done at the practice and not need referral, therefore the cheaper option. Not too invasive or long a procedure, dog may be home the next day. Although there is a risk of infection, it is not as great as with a THR as there are no implants being placed.
     - Cons: limb shortening, physiotherapy required afterwards for optimum limb function although unlikely will regain 100% function. If there is a degree of muscle wastage already then may take a little longer and physio before the procedure may help. Is a surgical procedure so there is an infection risk and also risk from the GA.
   - THR (total hip replacement)
     - Pros: good return to function and a very high portion of dogs will be pain free.
     - Cons: more expensive, risk of infection and this would be worse than FHNE due to implants. There is also the risk of luxation and fracture, but all efforts would made to reduce this in the immediate postoperative period.

Notes

Surgical Sampling, Surgical Complications, and Wound Management

Darren Barnes

Chapter Summary:

- **Collection, analysis and handling of surgical samples to maximise the chance of a diagnosis.**
- **Early identification of surgical complications and how to minimise them.**
- **Managing surgical complications.**
- **Wound management. Handling challenging cases.**
- **Postoperative management after discharge and how to communicate this to the client.**
- **The importance of clinical governance in a veterinary practice.**

Surgical Sampling

Surgical sampling is the process of collecting tissue or fluid to aid diagnostics and optimise patient treatment. There are numerous ways to sample tissues, with the most appropriate means depending on the clinical condition, the tissue affected, and the impact of the findings on patient treatment thereafter. For example, a slow growing lump on the skin may warrant a diagnosis for surgical planning to determine the margins required to achieve a surgical cure, whereas a ruptured splenic tumour resulting in an emergency admission requires emergency surgical treatment in spite of the diagnosis and preemptive sampling is not appropriate.

Methods of Biopsy

Fine Needle Aspirate (FNA)

Fine needle aspirates (Figure 1) are the **least invasive and least traumatic** means of tissue sampling. This achieves a **small sample of cells,** which are smeared on a slide and hence does not reflect the tissue's architecture. However, cytological analysis often gives a helpful insight into tissue pathology.

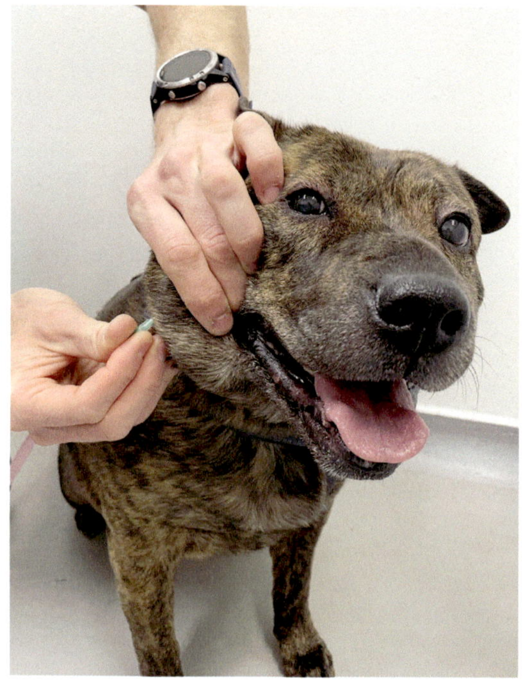

Figure 1. Fine needle aspirate (FNA).

FNAs are helpful in assessing:

- the cell types in a lump or swelling
- staging of tumours by sampling draining lymph nodes, liver, and spleen.

FNAs do not provide information on tumour grades since this depends on the architecture of the tissue and the interaction/invasiveness of the tumour within the surrounding tissue.

The advantage of FNAs is they can be obtained without surgery for superficial lesions in the conscious patient, or with the guidance of ultrasound under sedation for deeper lesions. Sometimes a lesion found during surgery warrants FNA sampling for urgent cytological analysis to guide the procedure itself.

Fine needle samples are obtained **by inserting a hypodermic needle into the abnormal tissue in multiple directions,** with or without the application of gentle suction on the attached syringe. The sample is sprayed onto a slide, using the syringe, then smeared smoothly across the centre of the slide to create a monolayer of cells, labelled, and submitted.

Core Needle Biopsy

Core needle biopsies provide the smallest samples for **histopathological assessment of tissue architecture.** The principle is similar to a FNA, but uses a purpose designed, larger bore needle sampling device. Due to their larger, more traumatic nature, **heavy sedation or general anaesthesia are generally warranted.** Samples may be obtained percutaneously with or without the guidance of ultrasound. These techniques are also used in some circumstances for intraoperative abdominal organ biopsy as discussed later.

Tru-Cut® Biopsies

Tru-Cut® needles (Figure 2) are spring loaded, large gauge needles (typically 14–18 gauge; the gauge size is the number of needles of that type that fit side by side within one inch; **the larger gauge, the smaller the needle**). These have an inner needle/stylet, with a cut out notch in the side. The stylet is advanced into the tissue, the outer needle advanced over the stylet (cutting the tissue free), leaving a core sample within the cut out section of the stylet. The needle is then withdrawn, the outer needle retracted, and the sample collected from the inner stylet by teasing out with a fine hypodermic needle to minimise handling of the sample.

Usually, a few samples are taken by redirecting the biopsy needle in different directions, via the same stab incision through the skin, in order to maximise the chances of an accurate diagnosis.

Jamshidi™ Needle Biopsies

The Jamshidi™ needle (Figure 3) is a trephine needle suitable for **bone and bone marrow biopsy,** to obtain a cylindrical sample of tissue, a core biopsy specimen. It is a cylindrical needle with a tapered cutting tip. These needles have stylets, used to advance them through soft tissue overlying the bone and through the cortical bone if only a medullary/marrow sample is required. With the stylet removed, a syringe should be attached to aspirate the bone marrow or advance the outer sheath of the needle to harvest a core bone sample.

Punch Biopsy

Biopsy punches are disposable instruments with a sharp cylindrical blade which is advanced perpendicularly into the surface of the tissue. They are **used for superficial lesions** (e.g. of the skin) (Figure 4) or to sample deeper tissues using a surgical approach to expose the tissue.

Biopsy punches are available as **cylinders of varying diameters, from 1 mm to 8 mm.** The depth of the sample obtained is limited by the length of the cutting blade. Following application of the punch, the tissue sample should be gently lifted to prevent squash artefact, and the base cut free with Metzenbaum scissors or a scalpel blade, (as the punch only cuts along the sides of the sample).

These biopsies leave a cylindrical tissue defect, which is **sutured closed** (e.g. in the skin) or filled with a haemostatic sponge (e.g. in the liver).

Incisional Biopsy

An incisional biopsy (Figure 5) is a surgical procedure to harvest a larger sample. This technique is used to sample skin masses, lymph nodes, and the intestine affected by diffuse changes. A **V-shaped wedge of tissue** is cut out of the lesion to facilitate suturing to close the defect. A sample is taken from

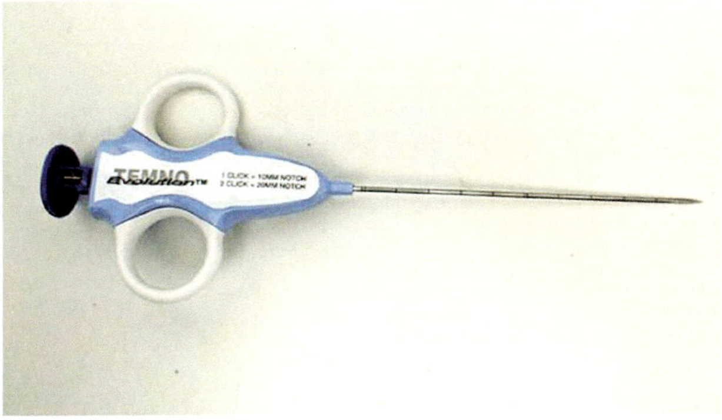

Figure 2. Tru-Cut® needle.

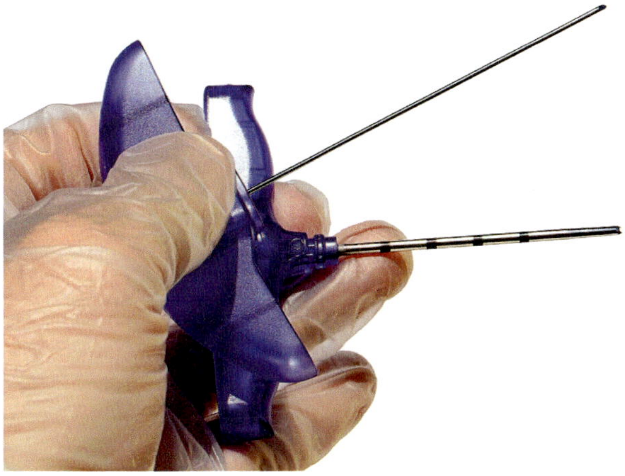

Figure 3. Jamshidi™ needle.

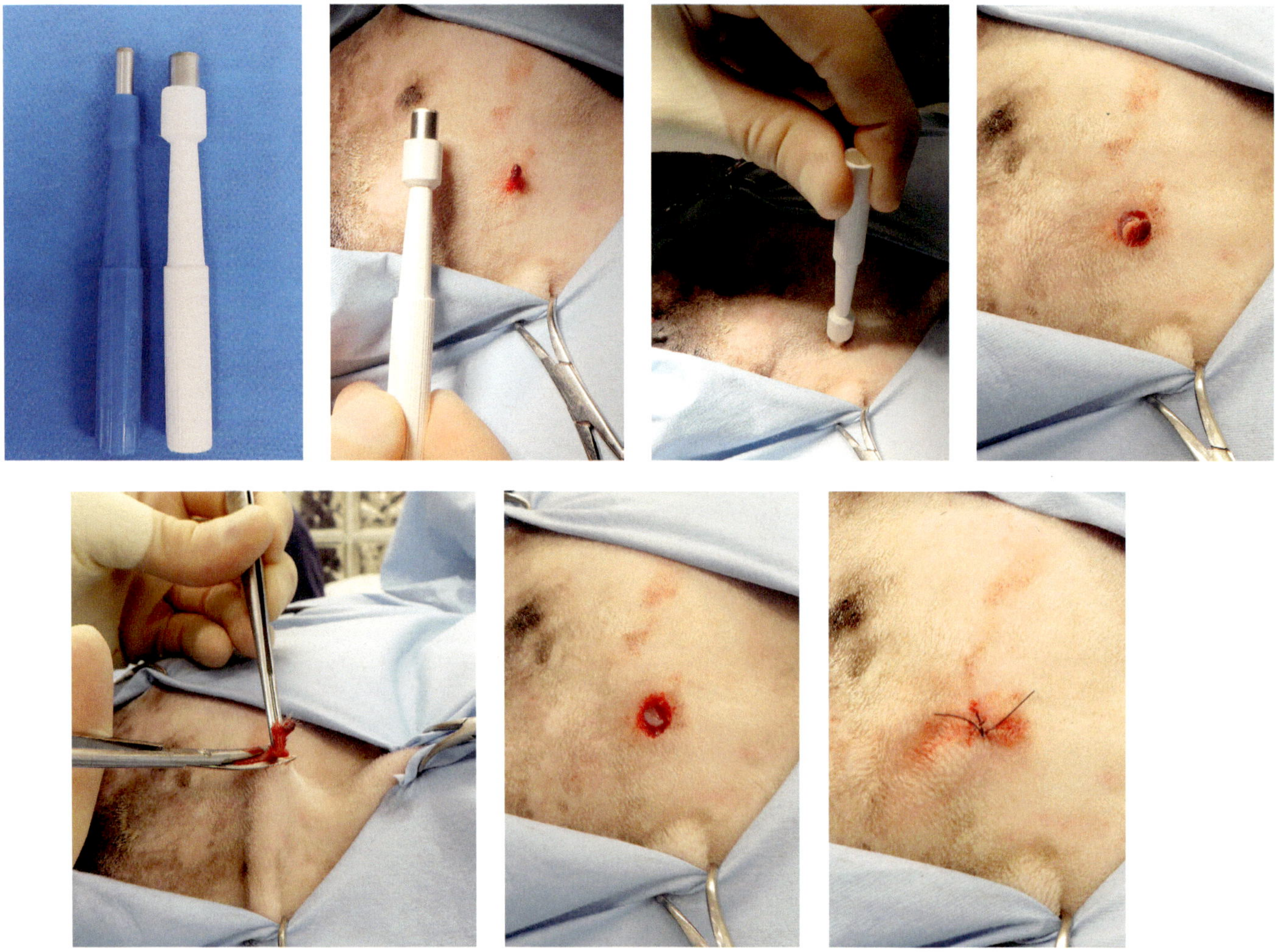

Figure 4. Punch biopsy of a skin lesion. The punch makes a circular incision and when removed the island of skin is lifted and the base cut with a blade or Metzenbaum scissors. The defect can often be closed with a single interrupted suture as shown.

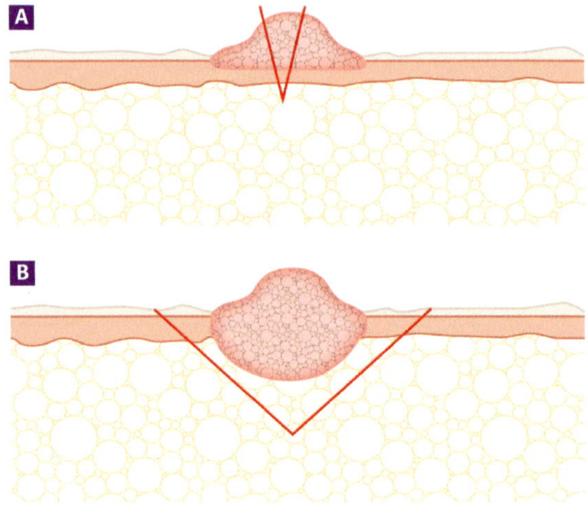

Figure 5. Incisional biopsy (**A**); excisional biopsy (**B**).

the edge of the lesion to **include some of the normal surrounding tissue,** so the pathologist can assess the interaction or invasion of the abnormal tissue with the surrounding tissue.

This technique is used to sample a tissue, such as a tumour, prior to a more definitive treatment. Hence, the biopsy should be planned so the biopsy site can be removed along with the main lesion, to prevent seeding of cancer cells along the biopsy tract.

Excisional Biopsy

Excisional biopsy (Figures 5B and 6) **is the complete surgical removal of a lesion** prior to a definitive histopathological diagnosis. This technique is used when complete removal of the mass is achievable. Excisional biopsies may be **marginal** (when only the lesion itself is shelled out within its capsule) or **wide** (removed in bloc with a perimeter or normal appearing tissue).

A risk of marginal excision is leaving disease behind, in the event of a locally invasive process such as a mast cell tumour or a soft tissue sarcoma. Hence this technique is only appropriate when wide excision is not achievable (and adjunctive chemotherapy and or radiotherapy should be considered), or in a location where a second procedure to achieve a clean margin is possible.

Wide excisional biopsy may be unnecessarily aggressive for larger lesions but might be appropriate for some smaller lesions with copious loose surrounding tissue, which are not amenable to sampling prior to surgery.

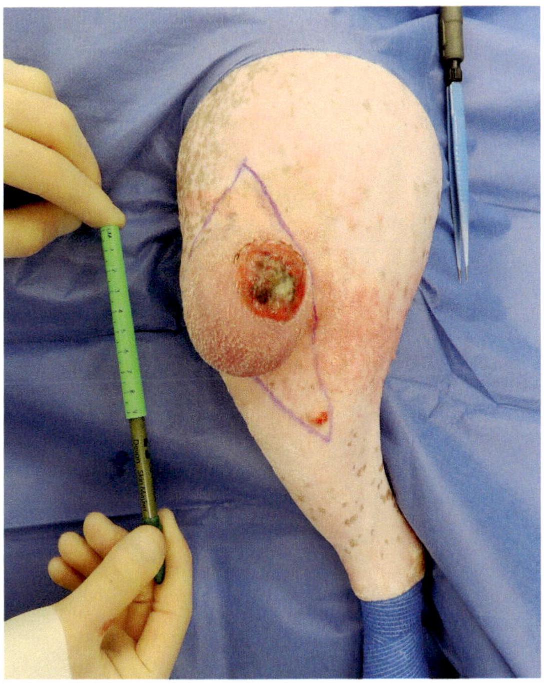

Figure 6. Excisional biopsy of an ulcerated and necrotic skin mass.

Endoscopic Biopsy

Endoscopic biopsy requires specialised endoscopic biopsy instruments such as cup biopsy forceps, punch biopsy forceps, or self-tying suture loops which lasso the periphery of a lobe of tissue e.g. liver or lung. (Figure 7).

Tissue Biopsy

Skin and Subcutaneous Tissues

Skin lesions may be biopsied by various means: **incisional, excision, or punch biopsies** for more superficial skin changes; with **Tru-Cut® needle biopsies or larger incisional biopsies** for deeper lesions such as large skin tumours. (Figure 8).

Larger tumours may have areas of necrosis or abscessation at their centre, (due to outgrowing their blood supply) and **biopsy of the mass margin is indicated** or an **ultrasound guided**

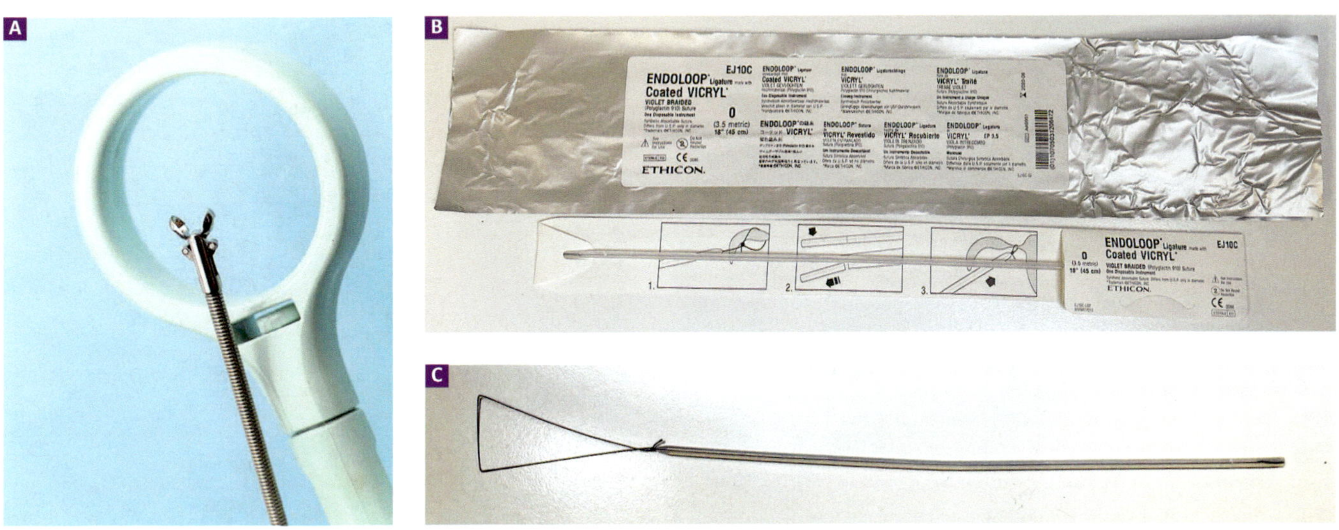

Figure 7. A. Endoscopic biopsy cup forceps; **B** and **C.** Endoloop – pretied loop of suture.

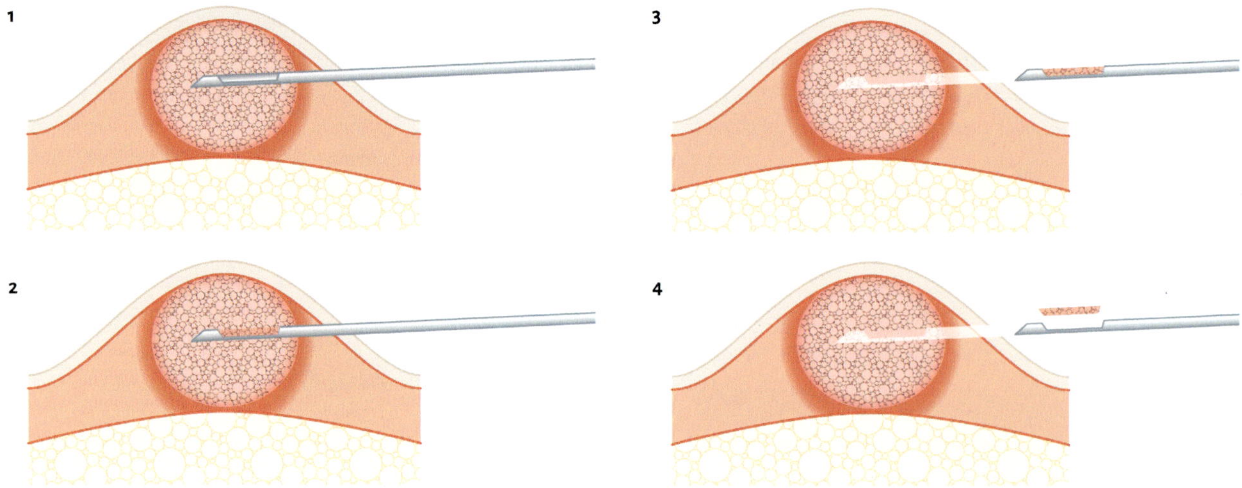

Figure 8. Tru-Cut® biopsy of mass. The needle outer sheath is drawn back prior to insertion into the tissue to be sampled. Then when in position the trigger is fired which advances the outer sheath, isolating a tissue sample within the core of the needle which is then withdrawn. The sheath is drawn back again outside of the patient to allow extraction of the sample. Needles may be used multiple times within the same lesion for the same patient to collect multiple samples.

Tru-Cut® biopsy to ensure sampling of vascularised tissue. In the case of sarcomas it is essential to obtain a deep tissue sample to ensure sampling of the mass itself rather than the pseudocapsule of surrounding inflammatory tissue.

Larger samples or multiple small samples from different areas of a lesion, maximise the chances of an accurate diagnosis as some lesions contain areas of inflammation, necrosis, or cavitation, and occasionally, areas which appear more or less aggressive (in the case of carcinomas).

Lymph Node

Lymph nodes are commonly biopsied to stage tumours, often at the time of tumour removal. When possible, **the entire draining lymph node is removed,** but an incisional biopsy is appropriate if removing the lymph node interferes with the vascular supply to an organ, e.g. within the mesentery in the abdomen.

Liver

For accessible lesions, fine needle aspirates or ultrasound guided Tru-Cut® core needle biopsies help avoid major vessels in the liver and surrounding tissues.

Open surgical biopsies from the lobe surfaces are usually performed using the punch biopsy technique, with the void filled with a haemostatic sponge. Peripheral samples from the caudal edges of the lobes are taken using **the guillotine method;** tying a loop of suture around the tissue to control bleeding. With smaller samples, clamping the periphery of the liver tissue with a haemostat for a few seconds is sufficient to control bleeding, with a small tissue sample cut from beyond the haemostat.

When laparoscopy is performed (Figure 9), **5 mm cup biopsy forceps** are used to grasp small bites of tissue from the edge of the liver, with haemorrhage limited by the crushing of the forceps for 30 seconds, and then twisting of the sample to separate it from the liver lobe. Following sampling, biopsy sites should be visually inspected to check for bleeding, before completing the procedure.

With all liver biopsy techniques, care should be taken not to bite too deeply into the liver tissue where large vessels might cause significant bleeding.

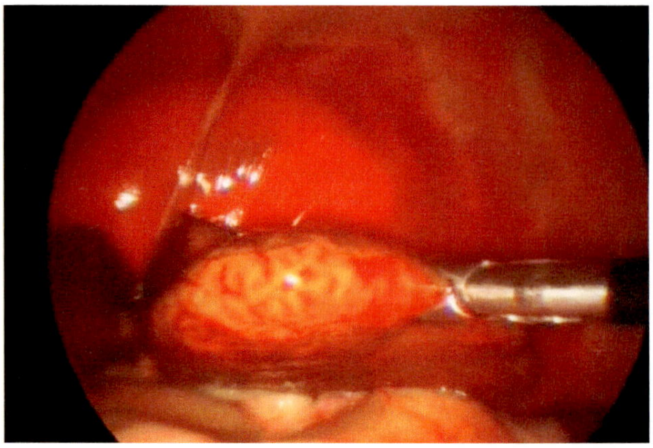

Figure 9. Laparoscopic liver biopsy being harvested using cupped biopsy forceps.

Bleeding is the most serious complication of liver biopsy and coagulation tests are advocated prior to biopsy, and after the procedure the patient should be monitored overnight for signs of internal bleeding; this includes regular assessment of vital parameters and ultrasound examination to check for free abdominal fluid.

Kidney

Kidney biopsy (Figure 10) **is rare, due to a significant risk of bleeding,** plus the damage to the renal tissue causes additional insult to renal function. In rare circumstances which do require renal biopsy, only the renal cortex is sampled, since sampling the medulla carries a significant risk of life threatening haemorrhage. Hence, the kidney should be physically stabilised and the Tru-Cut® technique used (guided by ultrasound or at laparoscopy), or a small wedge biopsy taken during open surgery. After wedge biopsy, the renal capsule should be sutured with mattress sutures or sealed with cyanoacrylate glue.

Again, **prebiopsy coagulation testing** should be performed due to a significant risk of haemorrhage.

Intestine

Flexible endoscopy facilitates minimally invasive biopsy of the stomach, duodenum, and colon. Biopsies are obtained by grasping the internal lining of the bowel with cup biopsy forceps, but sample size is limited by the size of the biopsy channel through which the instrument passes, and also **limited to the superficial, internal mucosal layer of the bowel wall.** This is often sufficient to diagnose inflammatory conditions or superficial growths, but deeply penetrating infiltrative disease or full thickness masses require surgical biopsy. The latter is necessary to sample the jejunum and ileum, which are beyond the reach of flexible endoscopy.

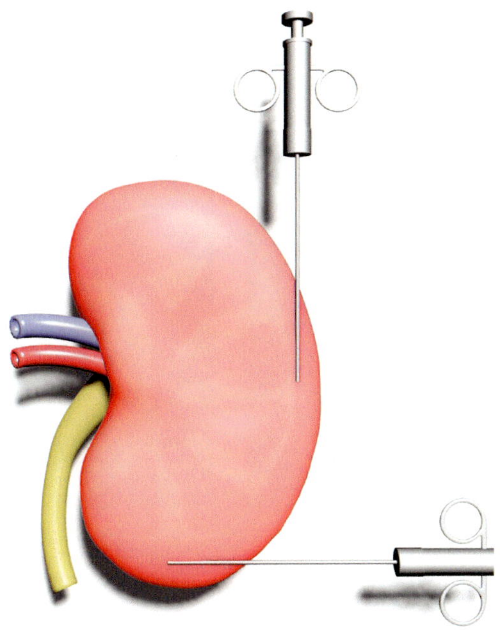

Figure 10. Tru-Cut® biopsy of the renal cortex.

Full thickness biopsy of the intestinal tract is obtained during **coeliotomy, or a miniature laparotomy** which uses an Alexis® wound retractor to create a portal to expose a loop of bowel. An externalised bowel loop minimises the risk of abdominal contamination, with the lumen compressed orad and aborad to the biopsy site by surgical assistant's fingers or Doyen clamps to contain the bowel contents.

The punch biopsy technique can harvest a full thickness biopsy (4 mm punch for cats, 4–6 mm for dogs depending on the dog's size) or alternatively an incisional biopsy technique can be used. The bowel wall defect should be sutured closed, and leak tested by insufflation with saline injected into the bowel lumen. The loop should then be lavaged and replaced into the abdominal cavity. (Figure 11).

Pancreas

Biopsy of the pancreas (Figure 12) is usually with the **suture guillotine method** (as described above for the liver) but care should be taken not to disrupt the blood supply to the duodenum: hence biopsies are harvested from the **tip of the right limb of the pancreas** (if representative of the tissue pathology). **Pancreatic biopsy is performed only if essential** as handling the pancreas instigates an inflammatory response which may result in pancreatitis following surgery.

Lung

Lung biopsies are rarely performed, and an airtight seal of the lung is essential to prevent pneumothorax postoperatively. **A thoracic drain** should be placed to remove the air introduced into the thorax at surgery and allow for monitoring thereafter.

Lung biopsy includes an endoscopic, suture guillotine, technique, e.g. using a pretied surgical loop to lasso the periphery of the lung lobe. Alternatively, the lung margin can be biopsied by sealing it with a bipolar vessel sealing device or surgical staples.

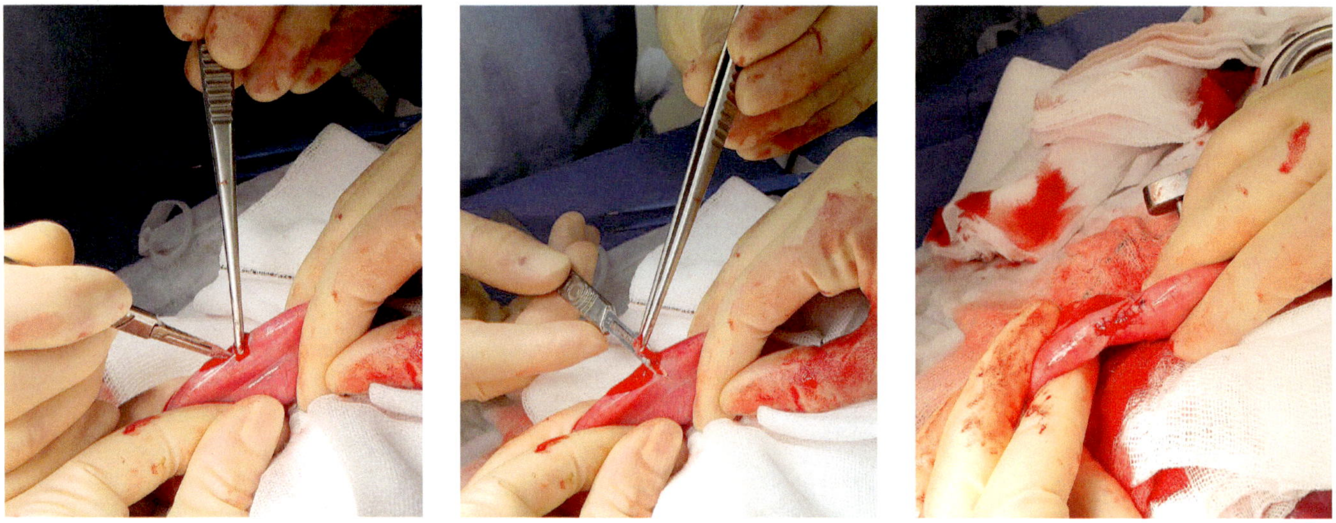

Figure 11. Small intestinal incisional biopsy. Figures courtesy of Jackie Demetriou.

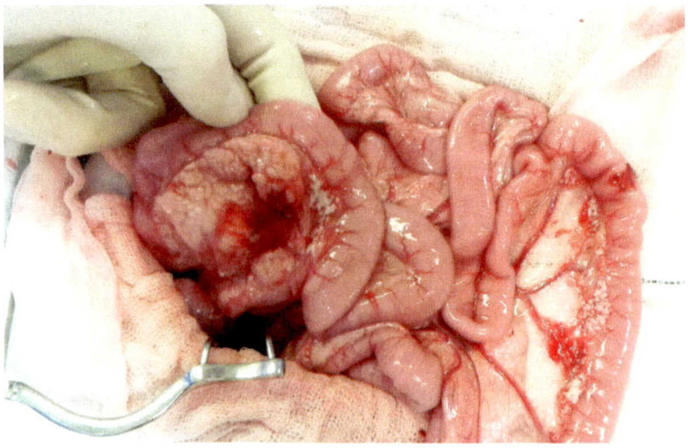

Figure 12. Photograph of the small intestine and pancreas of a cat.

Bone

Clip and aseptically prepare the skin overlying the bone (based on X-ray or CT findings, see Figure 13) should be clipped and prepared aseptically, and a stab incision made over the biopsy site. Unlike soft tissue biopsies, a bone biopsy should be harvested **from the centre of the lesion,** to avoid only sampling reactive changes surrounding the lesion.

A Jamshidi™ needle with the stylet in place, should be advanced through the skin to the level of the bone. The stylet should then be removed, and the outer core needle advanced whilst rotating it on its axis like a corkscrew, back and forth through the tissue. Once the needle has advanced across the lesion, the needle should be rocked back and forth to disrupt the base of the core to allow extraction within the needle. As the needle has a slight bevel, a probe should be passed from the tip of the needle to extract the sample from the base of the needle.

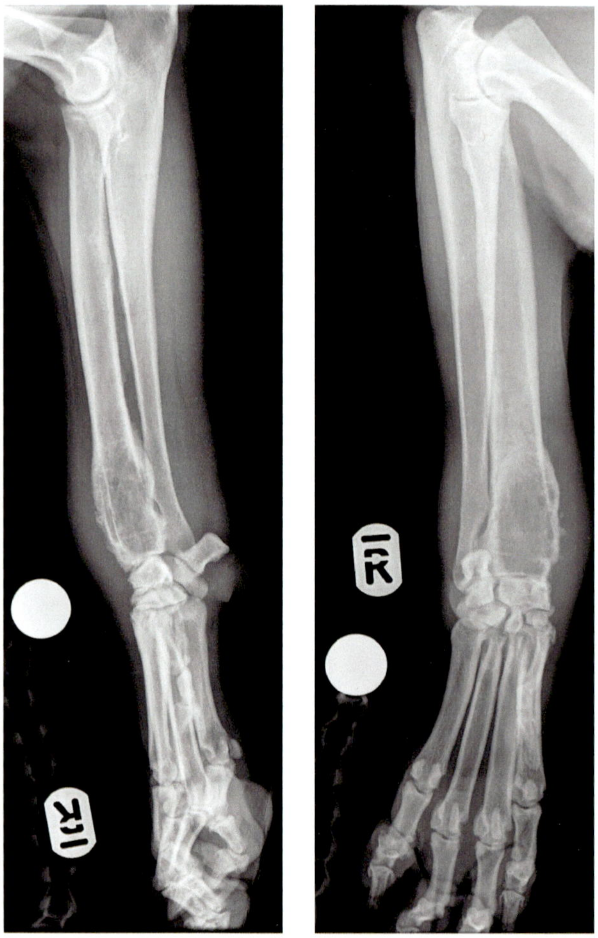

Figure 13. Mediolateral and dorsopalmar views of the antebrachium, carpus and digits of a large breed dog with an osteosarcoma affecting the distal radius. Note the lysis of the bone, with surrounding expansion of the cortices and significant soft tissue swelling.

Multiple samples should be taken through the same entry point, by redirecting the needle in at different angles.

Biopsy Handling and Processing

Appropriate handling, processing, and submission of the biopsy sample are as important as how the sample was obtained, to maximise the benefit and optimise patient outcome. No biopsy procedure is benign and so as much information as possible should be extracted from the sample to fully benefit the patient.

Postbiopsy Tissue Handling

All tissue removed from a patient (with the exception of gonads following routine elective neutering) should be considered for pathology assessment, as an opportunity to achieve an accurate diagnosis.

For the maximum benefit to the patient, the tissue sample must be handled and processed appropriately to ensure meaningful pathological assessment. All samples should be handled as atraumatically as possible since crush artefacts may limit pathological interpretation. Also, samples should be processed in a timely fashion, since undue delay results in tissue degradation.

When multiple small tissue samples are collected, such as with endoscopic biopsy techniques, the samples should be placed directly into a sterile cassette to aid processing and minimise the risk of loss (Figure 14). Alternatively, the samples should be collected on the paper insert from a suture material packet, for transfer into a submission pot, minimizing handling.

Marking

Following collection of an excisional biopsy or complete tissue resection, the surgeon needs to know if the procedure completely removed the diseased tissue and affected a surgical cure, (especially for oncology surgery). Therefore, it is important that tissue is submitted in a way that preserves its structure, integrity, and orientation so the pathologist's view of the tissue is not impaired. It is also helpful to take surgical photos, before surgery and after surgery, to illustrate the appearance of the mass.

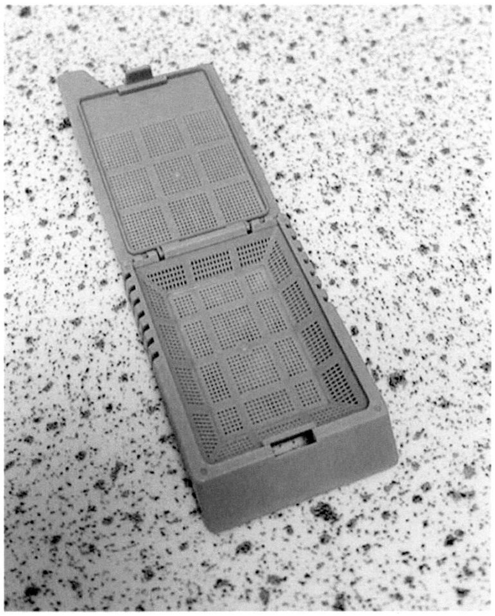

Figure 14. Pathology sample cassette.

Some tissues (such as the skin, subcutaneous tissue, underlying fascia, and muscle) glide over each other causing disruption of the tissue planes after removal, which hinders assessment by the pathologist. For this reason, the periphery of the tissue planes should be suture tagged to maintain the alignment during fixation and processing. To do this simple interrupted sutures should be placed through all tissue layers at the corners or 12, 3, 6, and 9 o'clock positions around the perimeter. Alternatively, a continuous suture can be placed around the entire perimeter of the tissue to stabilise the margins.

Another aid for the pathologist is to **mark the cut surface of the tissue with ink** to highlight the surgical margin (Figure 15). Red and purple inks should be avoided as these are similar to the colour of commonly used histology stains.

In addition, specific ink colours or additional suture tags should be used to identify areas of special interest, for example an area where the surgical margin is at its narrowest due to anatomical considerations.

Fixation

Incisions should be made into larger samples (such as entire spleens) to allow adequate fixation. This is done at **intervals of 2–3 cm in systematic parallel incisions,** which do not extend all the way through the tissue, to allow infiltration of the formalin without completely disrupting tissue architecture. (Figure 16).

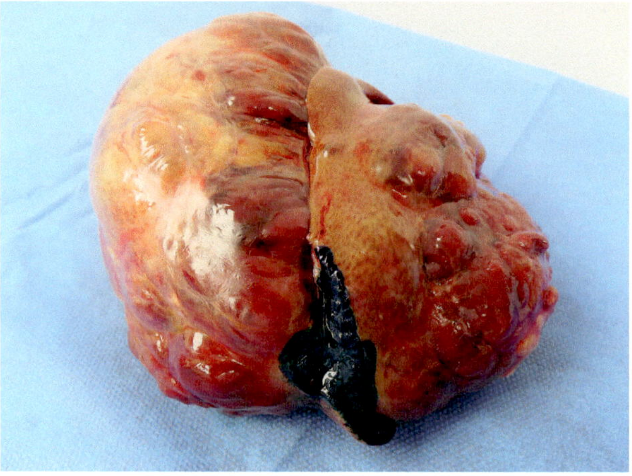

Figure 15. Ink staining of the surgical margin following removal of a large liver tumour.

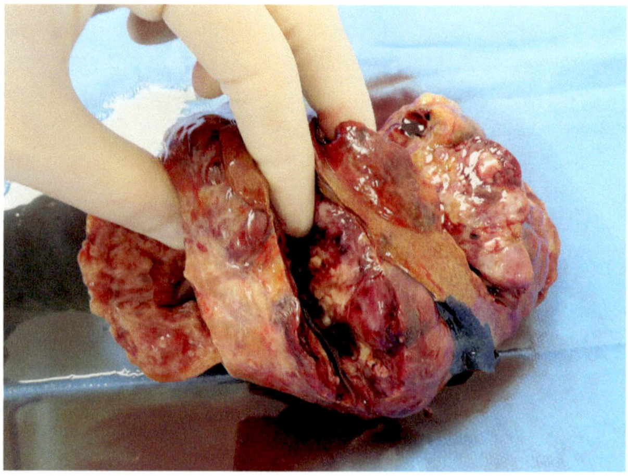

Figure 16. Tissue slicing of the same sample as in figure 15, to allow the penetration of the formalin to fix the tissue adequately. Previous staining of the surgical margin allows the pathologist to be confident in assessing the completeness of tumour removal, as the slicing has penetrated the tumour tissue directly.

If a lesion affects bone meaning amputation is required, only the lesion and surrounding tissue should be submitted. This means unwanted tissue should be removed after the surgery, to limit the amount of material sent for testing.

Following marking, suture tagging, and trimming, biopsy samples should be placed as soon as possible in 10% neutral buffered formalin (formal saline), although ink marked samples should be allowed to dry prior to fixation to prevent the ink washing out. In order to allow adequate fixation, the samples should be submerged in a volume of formalin that is **at least ten times their own volume.**

Pathology Request Forms

It is essential all submissions are **adequately labelled** with each individual sample detailed on the pathology submission form. Sample interpretation requires the pathologist to be as fully informed as possible about the case, the tissue sampled, and the orientation of that tissue. No matter how good the sample and how well a surgery is performed, if the pathologist is not fully informed they cannot provide the best possible, essential diagnostic information for optimal treatment of the patient.

The patient signalment and summary of the clinical presentation are essential. As are the location and suspected identity of the tissue. Ideally, surgical photos should be sent to orientate the pathologist, as well as diagnostic imaging if appropriate.

Whilst not every practice has their own in house pathologist, it is worth bearing in mind that the pathologist is usually available on the phone to discuss how they would prefer samples submitted, to maximise interpretation of that sample.

Surgical Complications

Surgical Site Infection

Since the first surgeons started operating, postoperative infections have always been a concern. This risk has been mitigated **by the development of surgical asepsis and appropriate use of prophylactic antibiotics;** however, infection continues to be a concern and a frustrating complication of surgery, especially with the advancement of surgical procedures and particularly associated with surgical implants.

Surgical site infections affect patient morbidity and mortality, treatment cost, hospitalisation time, owner and veterinary staff frustration, and also pose a risk to other patients and public health.

Infection is defined as the invasion and growth of microorganisms within body tissues. Most surgeries are associated with a degree of inflammation (redness, swelling, heat, pain) but it is critical to understand when this is normal or excessive, in order to treat infection promptly. In the era of widespread antimicrobial resistance, it is also essential to encourage appropriate and justifiable **antibiotic stewardship.**

The risk of development of infection varies between patients and surgical procedure, and is associated with several factors, including:

- **Microbial concentration** at the incision site and within the operated tissues. This is reduced by appropriate surgical site preparation and preparation of the operating room environment and surgical team.

- Microbial virulence.
- Appropriate use of perioperative **antimicrobial prophylaxis.**
- Antimicrobial resistance.
- **Systemic and local tissue immunity:** this may be affected by systemic disease, obesity, and immunosuppressive therapy.
- **Tissue injury:** arising from presurgical trauma, the procedure, surgical environment, and postoperative tissue insult due to postoperative management. It is shown that increased time between clipping the surgical site and first incision leads to an increase in infection rate, suspected due to microtrauma to the skin which allows bacterial proliferation.
- **Surgical and anaesthetic duration:** in particular intraoperative hypotension is associated with increased infection risk.
- The presence of **foreign material and implants.**

Surgical site contamination at the time of surgery is classified as follows:

- **Clean:** minimally traumatic, elective surgery, performed on uninfected tissue, with no break in aseptic surgical technique, closed primarily.
- **Clean contaminated:** controlled entering of a hollow muscular viscus, or a minor break in aseptic surgical technique.
- **Contaminated:** a fresh, open, traumatic wound, or incision into a site with acute nonpurulent inflammation, or surgery with a major break in aseptic technique.
- **Dirty/infected surgery:** associated with pus, a perforated viscus, or a traumatic wound with devitalised tissue, foreign material, or faecal contamination of more than four hours duration (outside the golden period hence allowing time for bacterial invasion and/or proliferation within the wound).

It is important to understand that identifying the presence of bacteria within a surgical site is not necessarily associated with infection and, conversely, failure to culture a microbial growth from a tissue or fluid sample does not exclude surgical site infection. Thus classification is based on **wound appearance, identification of pathogens, and clinical judgement** based on patient assessment, imaging findings and pathology sample analysis.

Classification of Surgical Site Infections (SSIs)

A standard classification system for SSIs in human surgery was developed by the US Centers for Disease Control and Prevention (CDC), also widely used in veterinary surgery, based on three tiers (Figure 17):

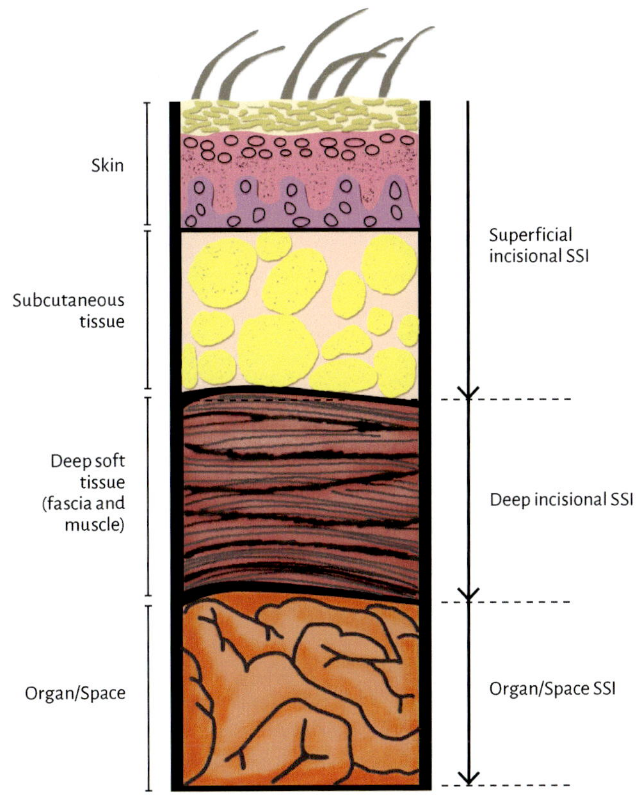

Figure 17. An illustration of the typical tissue planes which may be affected by a surgical site infection.

Superficial Incisional SSI

- occurs within 30 days of surgery
- affects only the skin and/or subcutaneous tissue
- clinically superficial incisional SSIs must demonstrate at least one of the following:
  - purulent discharge
  - organisms isolated from an aseptically collected fluid or tissue sample
  - pain/tenderness, local swelling, redness **or** heat, **and** the incision is reopened by the surgeon **unless** culture is negative.

Deep Incisional SSI

- occurs within 30 days of surgery or one year if an implant is placed
- affects the deep soft tissues (muscle and fascia) of the surgical site
- clinically deep incisional SSIs must demonstrate at least one of the following:
  - purulent drainage coming from the deep soft tissue layer

- spontaneous dehiscence of the deep soft tissue layers **or** deliberate surgical opening of this layer to allow drainage in a patient with fever, local pain **or** tenderness, **unless** culture is negative
- abscessation or demonstration of infection by histopathology or diagnostic imaging of the deep soft tissues.

Organ/Space SSI

- occurs within 30 days of surgery or one year if an implant is placed
- affects any area of an incision other than the superficial and deep incisional layers (e.g. a bone, body cavity or visceral organ)
- clinically organ/space SSIs must demonstrate at least one of the following:
  - purulent drainage from a drain placed within the affected organ/space
  - organisms isolated from an aseptically collected sample from the affected organ/space
  - abscess or other evidence of infection on direct examination, during reoperation or by histopathology or radiology
  - diagnosis of an organ/space SSI by the attending clinician.

Incidence of a Surgical Site Infection

Surgical site infection rates for clean surgical procedures affect around **2–3% of surgical patients.** Rates are slightly higher (around 5%) for clean elective orthopaedic procedures and are likely to be higher for contaminated and dirty procedures, in spite of the routine and appropriate use of antibiotics. **Every practice should survey and monitor their infection rates,** which are then reviewed as part of clinical governance to highlight peaks in infection rates and allow identification of possible causes and resolutions. Active surveillance of infections is essential as without this more than a quarter of surgical site infections may not be reported back to the surgeon.

Infection Prevention and Control

Infection prevention is best achieved by controlling the known risk factors for surgical site infection by means of:

- **Aseptic preparation of the patient, surgical team and operating room environment:**
  - use of well-maintained clippers and atraumatic clipping to minimize skin trauma;
  - skin preparation should be thorough but not harsh, using products for the recommended contact time;
  - prevention of recontamination after preparation; and
  - appropriate patient draping, along with surgical team gowning and gloving.
- **Perioperative antimicrobial prophylaxis:**
  - with appropriate aseptic preparation, clean surgical procedures should not require the routine use of prophylactic antibiotics;
  - prophylactic perioperative antibiotics are appropriate for use with clean contaminated procedures;
  - delivery of perioperative antibiotics to reach an appropriate tissue concentration at the time of the first surgical incision; and
  - perioperative antibiotics with a postoperative antibiotic course based on surgical sampling are appropriate for contaminated and infected/dirty surgical procedures, with the duration of antibiosis judged on a case by case basis with respect to the tissue affected, the nature of the contaminants, and both local and systemic patient factors which might affect immunity and resolution of infection.
- **Minimising surgical trauma (including surgical duration):**
  - attention to Halsted's principles helps to preserve tissue integrity and minimise the immunological response to surgery and the associated risk of infection;
  - many veterinary studies show that an increasing duration of surgery is associated with an increased infection risk; and
  - prolonged surgery allows increased exposure of the surgical site to environmental contaminants and may also be associated with greater tissue dissection and trauma, and perhaps a less precise surgery in the hands of less experienced surgeon.
- **Minimum anaesthetic duration:**
  - studies also highlight a correlation between anaesthesia duration and infection risk, which is partly afforded by the surgical duration, but also the effects of anaesthesia, including hypotension and hypothermia impacting on immunity and so ensuring efficient use of time whilst anaesthetised is imperative, ensuring swift transitions between induction, diagnostics, skin preparation and surgery etc. whilst minimising hypotension and hypothermia.
- **Postoperative wound care:**
  - a fibrin seal forms to protect a surgical incision within 6–10 hours following surgery provided this process is not disrupted by excessive movement, interference with the incision or incisional discharge. From this stage the wound has a weak but protective seal to external contamination;

- prior to this it is essential the surgical incision is protected with an appropriate dressing and/or sealant spray or glue; and
- thereafter the incision must be protected from mutilation by the patient with use of appropriate exercise restriction, collars/dressings/body suits as needed until complete healing of the incision.

– **Treatment of comorbidities:**
  - any disease or medication that compromises a patient's immunity potentially increases the risk of surgical site infection. Endocrinopathies (e.g. Cushing's, hypothyroidism, diabetes) and obesity are demonstrated to increase the risk of surgical site infection in dogs; and
  - medical control of these disease states may reduce risk for these patients.

Specific Surgical Site Infections

Sepsis

Sepsis (or septic shock) is defined as the systemic inflammatory response to an infectious cause. Criteria for defining systemic inflammatory response syndrome differ between the dog and cat (Table 1).

Tabla 1. Criteria for defining systemic inflammatory response syndrome. (Silverstein and Otto, 2012).

SIRS Criteria	Cats	Dogs
Temperature	<37.8 °C or >40 °C	<37.2 °C or >39.2 °C
Heart rate	<140 bpm or >225 bpm	>140 bpm
Respiratory rate	>40/min	>30/min
White blood cell count	<5 x 10^9/l or >19 x 10^9/l	<4 x 10^9/l or >12 x 10^9/l

Dogs initially show an increase in cardiac output due to a range of compensatory mechanisms, with tachycardia, tachypnoea, hyperaemia, bounding pulses, accelerated capillary refill times and hyperthermia.

As these **compensatory mechanisms are exhausted,** cardiac output drops due to a combination of systemic vascular dilation and impaired myocardial function, resulting in hypotension, pale mucous membranes, weak pulses, hypothermia and increased capillary refill time. This reduction in perfusion leads to multiple organ dysfunction.

In cats, the situation is less clearly defined, with patients often presenting with hypothermia, bradycardia, pallor, and nonspecific pain.

Treatment of sepsis is based on **early recognition and aggressive circulatory resuscitation** both by restoring circulating volume and vascular tone, combined with source control and antibiotic therapy of the specific septic focus.

Septic Peritonitis

Septic peritonitis (Figure 18) **is defined as inflammation and infection within the peritoneal cavity.** Septic peritonitis most frequently results from bacterial contamination due to leakage from the gastrointestinal tract after incisional breakdown, perforation by an intestinal foreign body, external bite

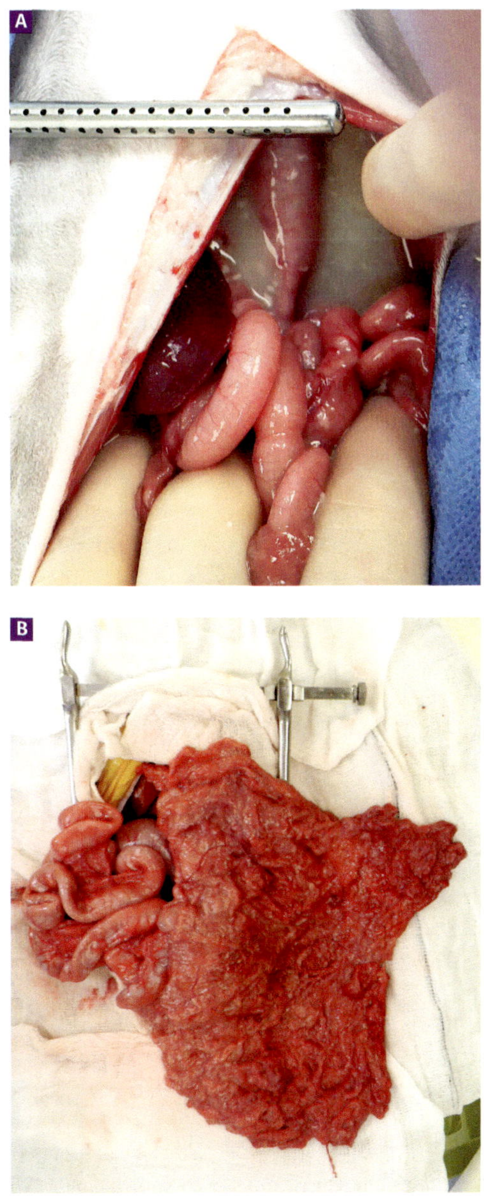

Figure 18. Photographs taken of the abdominal contents in patients with septic peritonitis. **A.** In a cat; **B.** In a dog.

wound, erosion due to ulceration, neoplastic disease, or avascular necrosis due to torsion/strangulation or intussusception. Septic peritonitis may also result from leakage from the urogenital tract, biliary system, rupture of a visceral abscess or body wall puncture.

Clinical Signs

The clinical signs associated with septic peritonitis are highly variable but include varying degrees of **abdominal distension with free fluid accumulation, abdominal pain, pyrexia, and nonspecific signs of illness** such as anorexia, vomiting, depression, and lethargy. Cats with septic peritonitis are commonly hypothermic. As discussed with generalised sepsis, the cardiovascular system often progresses from a state of compensation for hypovolaemia to decompensation. Septic peritonitis should be considered as a cause for sepsis in any patient having undergone recent gastrointestinal surgery, suffering blunt trauma or penetrating injury to the abdominal wall.

The **praying posture** is a typical stance taken by dogs with abdominal pain: standing on the hind limbs but stretched out and recumbent on the thoracic limbs.

Auscultation of the intestines reveals reduced intestinal sounds due to **ileus.** If unfamiliar with the normal sounds of the intestinal tract, listening to clinically well patients is useful. When assessing patients with abdominal disease or following abdominal surgery it is helpful to **serially assess intestinal sounds** and score as either: absent, reduced, normal or increased.

Diagnosis

Diagnosis of septic peritonitis is suspected on the basis of clinical history and examination findings, and **confirmed by observation and analysis of free abdominal fluid.** Free gas within the abdomen may be present following recent abdominal surgery (for a few weeks after surgery), but otherwise should not be present and if identified suggests peritoneal perforation.

Free gas or fluid may be observed on abdominal radiography, but **smaller volumes are detected by ultrasonography** of the abdomen, paying specific attention to areas where fluid commonly pools: between the caudal margins of the liver lobes, at the apex of the bladder, and adjacent to the kidneys on each side. Ultrasound may be used to guide aspiration of small pockets of fluid for analysis. In experienced hands ultrasound may also aid in the confirmation of the source of abdominal contamination. In the absence of ultrasound availability, blind abdominocentesis or **diagnostic peritoneal lavage** (infusing 20 ml/kg of saline into the abdomen through a catheter placed just caudal to the umbilicus and then draining for analysis) may be performed.

Abdominal fluid from patients with septic peritonitis (Figure 19) appears **varyingly turbid** (cloudy), dependent on the cellularity. Analysis reveals a high cellularity >5 x 10^9/l with a predominance of **toxic and degenerative neutrophils** and the presence of **intracellular bacteria** confirms the diagnosis. In the absence of intracellular bacteria, their presence in the fluid may be detected indirectly, by means of their metabolic function, which **reduces the fluid glucose and produces increased lactate** in comparison to those in the circulation of the patient.

Treatment

Treatment of septic peritonitis has the following goals:

- **Reestablish circulating fluid volume and electrolyte balance:** by the provision of intravenous fluid therapy and vasopressor support. Hypoalbuminaemia and associated reduction in colloid oncotic pressure are common due to protein rich fluid loss. Hence administration of fresh frozen plasma or human serum albumin may be necessary in severely affected patients.
- **Surgical abdominal drainage, debridement, repair of leakage, lavage** (Figure 20): as soon as the patient is adequately stabilised to undergo anaesthesia, exploratory coeliotomy should be performed to identify and manage the source of contamination and clean the peritoneal cavity. Lavage with 200–300 ml/kg of isotonic warm crystalloid solution is recommended. Following debridement and lavage the surgeon will consider if closing the abdominal cavity is appropriate, or if closed suction drain placement or open peritoneal drainage are required.
- **Antibiosis:** broad spectrum antibiotics are instituted pending cultures of samples taken at the time of diagnosis or surgery.

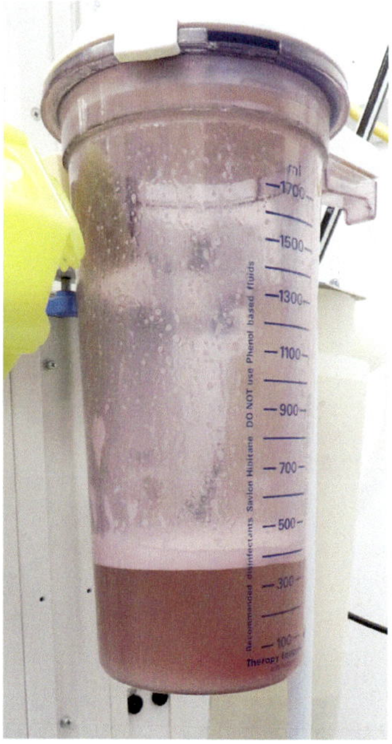

Figure 19. Suction jar containing effluent from the abdomen in a patient with septic peritonitis. This is foul smelling and turbid (cloudy).

- **Nutritional support:** placement of a feeding tube at the time of surgery.
- **Analgesia:** a multimodal approach should be considered. NSAIDs are contraindicated in hypotensive, hypovolaemic patients.

Prognosis

The prognosis for septic peritonitis is guarded, despite aggressive treatment from multidisciplinary specialist teams, with roughly 50% of cases surviving. Early diagnosis and intervention are essential.

Pyothorax

Pyothorax (Figure 21) **is the accumulation of septic exudate within the thoracic cavity.** Infection in the thoracic cavity is most commonly the result of thoracic puncture wounds or due to inhaled, migrating foreign bodies, but may also result as a complication of intrathoracic surgery for other indications. Pyothorax leads to inflammation of the pleural lining of the thoracic cavity and the mediastinal tissues and mediastinal lymph nodes.

Clinical Signs

The clinical signs associated with pyothorax include **dyspnoea, tachypnoea, pyrexia, and lethargy.**

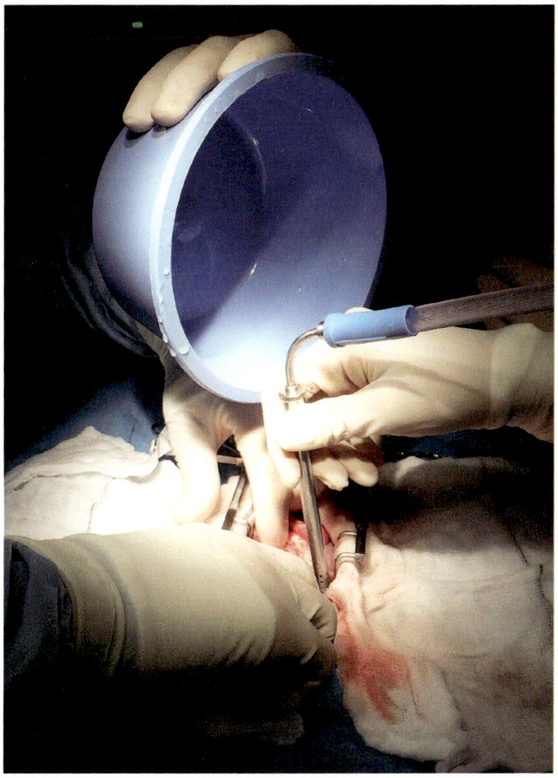

Figure 20. Abdominal lavage.

Diagnosis

Diagnosis of pyothorax is based on clinical signs and thoracocentesis, following thoracic imaging, by either radiography (X-ray or CT) or thoracic ultrasonography. **The fluid is protein rich, and the predominant cell type is degenerate neutrophils** similar to that noted with septic peritonitis. With larger volumes of effusion, pulmonary auscultation may reveal dull lung sounds or crackles.

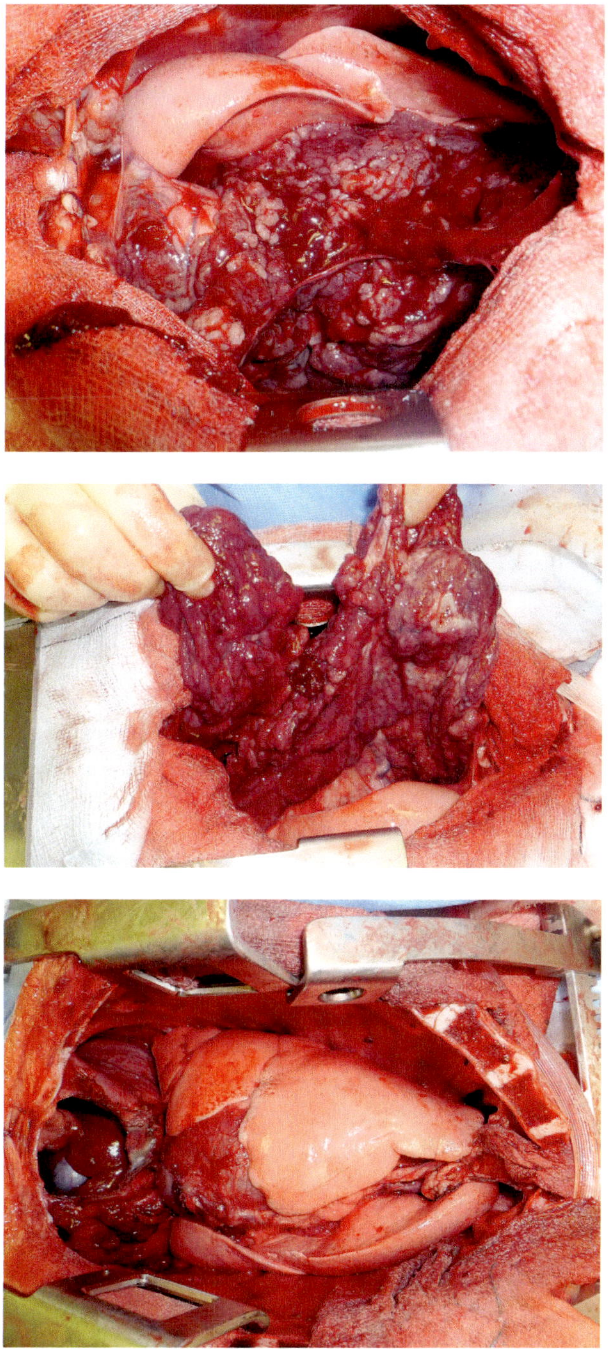

Figure 21. Photographs of the thorax of a dog with pyothorax before and after removal of the thickened and inflamed mediastinal tissues. Figures courtesy of Daniela Murgia.

Treatment

Treatment of pyothorax is similar to that of infection at other sites, with the following goals:

- **Reestablish circulating fluid volume and electrolyte balance:** by the provision of intravenous fluid therapy and vasopressor support. Hypoalbuminaemia and the associated reduction in colloid oncotic pressure are common due to the loss of protein rich fluids. Hence administration of fresh frozen plasma or human serum albumin should be considered in severely affected patients.
- **Drainage, debridement, lavage:** depending on the nature of the pyothorax, conservative management or surgical debridement are indicated, and placement of a thoracic drain essential. If the mediastinum is intact (it often is not following thoracic surgery) bilateral thoracic drains are placed to achieve adequate drainage. Open surgical debridement is usually reserved for cases with compartmentalised abscesses or retained foreign bodies which are removed to resolve the infection. Lavage is performed at surgery following debridement, and/or via the thoracic drains in conservatively managed cases.
- **Antibiosis:** broad spectrum antibiotics are instituted pending cultures of samples taken at the time of diagnosis or surgery.
- **Analgesia:** a multimodal approach is ideal. Local analgesic techniques should be considered, including administration of levobupivicaine via the thoracic drain following fluid aspiration.

Septic Arthritis

Septic arthritis (Figure 22) **is a microbial infection within a synovial joint.** As a complication of orthopaedic surgery, septic arthritis is most commonly bacterial in nature, most frequently resulting from *Staphylococcus* or *Streptococcus species* from the skin flora.

There are a number of risk factors associated with increased risk for septic arthritic following joint surgery:

- **Procedural factors:**
  - placement of an implant
  - open surgery compared to arthroscopic surgery
  - prolonged surgical time
  - presence of periarticular infection (e.g. dermatitis at the surgical incision site).
- **Patient factors:**
  - previous surgery at the same site (e.g. revision surgery)
  - reduced blood supply to the joint
  - immunosuppression (e.g. steroid administration, Cushing's disease).

Clinical signs

Clinical signs associated with septic arthritis include:

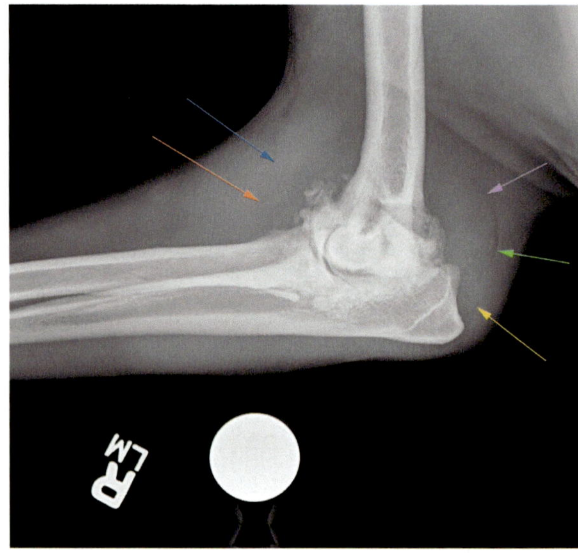

Figure 22. Radiograph of the right elbow of a Labrador with a septic arthritis with cellulitis and swelling of the limb and severe lameness. The arrows indicate the severe swelling of the joint capsule. Note the severe arthritic change which is a risk factor for septic arthritis.

- pain on joint manipulation/lameness (often peracute in onset: owners may not report lameness at all, then the patient gets up from rest and develops a non-weight bearing lameness without obvious explanation)
- joint swelling (surrounding cellulitis with severe cases)
- redness around the joint
- heat on palpation of the joint
- discharging sinus
- lymphadenomegaly of the draining lymph node
- pyrexia (uncommon)
- systemic depression (uncommon).

Diagnosis

Diagnosis of septic arthritis is by **arthrocentesis** (Figure 23) **and joint fluid analysis.** The skin should be clipped over the joint and prepared aseptically. Arthrocentesis should be performed and the fluid assessed with cytological evaluation and submission for culture and sensitivity testing. Fluid samples should be submitted in blood culture medium when despatched out of hours or to an external laboratory, to improve the chance of a positive culture in affected cases.

Grossly, joint fluid from affected joints is more profuse than usual, turbid (cloudy), and have reduced viscosity (more watery and less stringy). As with other septic fluid analyses, neutrophils predominate. Although identification of intracellular bacteria is confirmatory for diagnosis of septic arthritis, this is only seen in a small minority of cases. Culture of joint fluid in enrichment medium increases the sensitivity of diagnosis. Synovial biopsy should be considered in cases where septic arthritis is suspected but cannot otherwise be confirmed clinically.

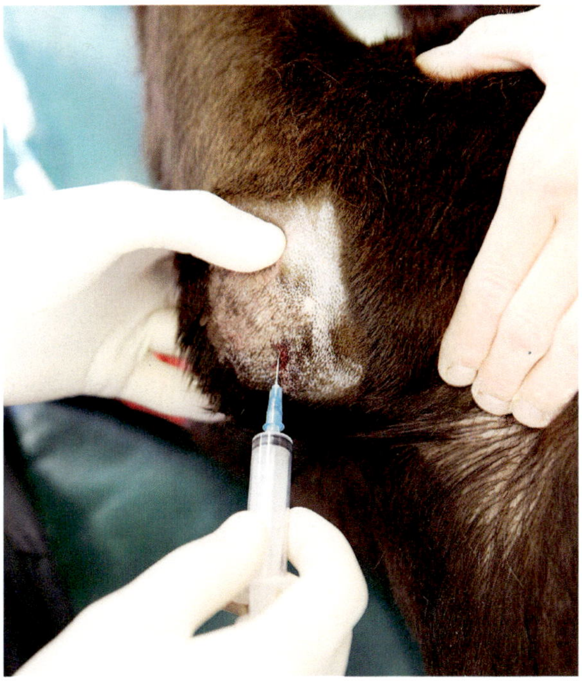

Figure 23. Arthrocentesis.

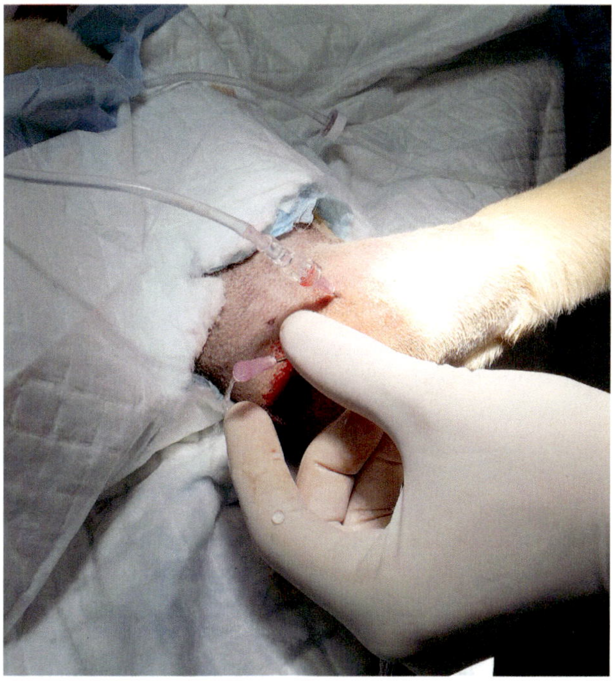

Figure 24. Joint lavage.

Treatment

Treatment of septic arthritis involves a combination of the following approaches:

- **Antibiotic administration:** broad spectrum intravenous antibiotic administration for at least 24 hours is indicated pending cytological analysis, and culture and sensitivity results where infection is suspected based on clinical signs and gross joint fluid appearance. Thereafter antibiotics are selected on the basis of culture and sensitivity testing results. Antibiotics are continued for 4–6 weeks, with repeat arthrocentesis advocated prior to discontinuation of therapy. In some circumstances intra-articular antibiotics may be considered, possibly in cases when joint penetration is limited or systemic treatment options are limited or have undesirable risks due to systemic side effects with some resistance infections.
- **Joint aspiration and irrigation:** following sampling of the joint fluid, remaining fluid in the joint should be drained as completely as possible. Placement of a second needle into the joint and connecting to a pressurised fluid bag or fluid pump allows copious lavage through the joint (Figure 24). The importance of this step is not completely known and often does not seem to be required for successful treatment of septic arthritis.
- **Multimodal analgesia.**

Prognosis

Clinical improvement is expected with appropriate antibiotic therapy within 24–48 hours. Once improvement is noted antibiotics are switched from parenteral to oral administration.

Multidrug-resistant (MDR) Infections

As the name would suggest, multidrug-resistant infections are bacterial infections of surgical sites or wounds, where the bacteria show in vitro resistance to at least one drug in each of three different classes of antimicrobial.

Culture and sensitivity testing of a swab, aspirate, or tissue sample is required for diagnosis. There may be a clinical suspicion of MDR infection with failure to respond to first line antimicrobial administration, but culture and sensitivity testing should be performed to guide antibiotic selection rather than empirical selection of a second line treatment.

Risk Factors

Risk factors for development of MDR infections are similar to those for other surgical site infections, including:

- duration of anaesthesia
- duration of surgery
- placement of surgical implants
- immunocompromise
- surgical contamination.

Factors which specifically increase the risk of a surgical site infection being associated with a MDR organism:

- previous antibiotic exposure/administration
- preoperative patient colonisation with MDR organisms,

e.g. methicillin resistant *Staphylococcus aureus* (MRSA) or methicillin resistant *Staphylococcus pseudointermedius* (MRSP).

Treatment

Once culture sensitivity results are returned, the appropriate antibiotics available should be considered. Often the veterinary surgeon needs to consider if any antibiotics which are suggested to be effective against the MDR infection (if any are identified) are appropriate to use in the patient due to the risk of **adverse reactions,** drug interactions with other medications, predicted penetration of the site of infection, and social responsibility in use of the treatment, which may often require the off licence use of antibiotics used for treatment of life-threatening infections in humans.

Treatment very frequently requires **removal of infected implants** or prolonged courses of antibiotics alongside agents which might aid in the decontamination of implants by disruption of the biofilm layer which may have developed over their surface, where bacteria can lie dormant and evade the immune system of the patient. For example **disinfectant solutions** (including polyhexanide) used to lavage open wounds and tris-EDTA or tetra-EDTA to lavage contaminated cystostomy tubes or subcutaneous ureteral bypass (SUB) devices.

Open wounds or incisions which have dehisced due to MDR infections, are usually **managed as open wounds.** This allows surface decontamination with disinfectants and debridement. Wounds often heal uneventfully in spite of MDR infections, but if the wound is closed, this contains the infection and may lead to dehiscence of the closed wound.

Prevention

Prevention of MDR infections includes reducing factors which increase the risk of surgical site infection. The judicious use of antibiotics is only for appropriate cases and for the optimised duration of treatment in order to limit the development of resistant strains of bacteria.

Within the hospital environment, **prevention of cross-contamination of patients** is imperative, and hence adherence to infection control measures discussed previously, as well as appropriate isolation of patients who may potentially harbour infection and those at increased risk of infection. For example a patient with an open wound should not be housed in proximity to an immunocompromised patient undergoing surgery or a patient undergoing elective orthopaedic surgery e.g. for total hip replacement.

General Complications

Unfortunately occasional complications occur after surgery performed by even the most experienced hands. Certain measures can help to minimise the risk of complications at the time a surgery. Others are important from a postoperative management perspective to prevent complications occurring during the early phases of wound healing, both in the hospital environment and when discharged to the care of the patient's owners. **Ensuring adequate client education is imperative** at this stage. The key to management of complications is often **early recognition** to minimise the impact of the complication and take measures to address and overcome that complication.

Dehiscence

Dehiscence is the term used to describe **the undesirable opening up of a surgical incision following suture closure.** Dehiscence may occur as the result of:

- infection
- mechanical disruption due to:
    - rubbing
    - scratching
    - licking
    - tension on the wound edges
- necrosis (Figures 25, 26 and 27) of the wound edges secondary to:
    - infection
    - disruption of the blood supply by:
        - surgical damage
        - presurgical trauma (e.g. due to a crushing injury)
        - ischaemia due to overtight bandaging/suturing
- malnutrition/endocrine disease.

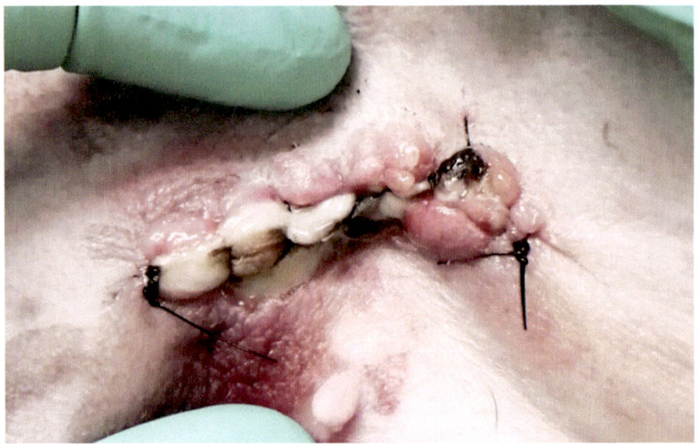

Figure 25. An abdominal incision which shows necrosis of the skin margins, with surrounding inflammation and bruising.

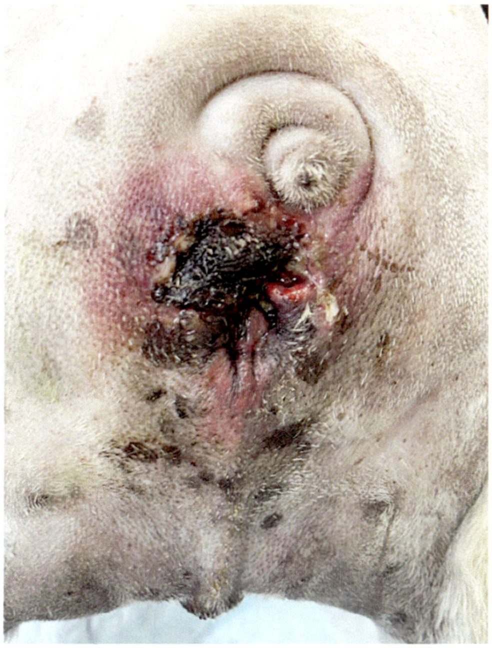

Figure 26. Necrosis of the perianal skin following a perianal tumour removal with partial dehiscence.

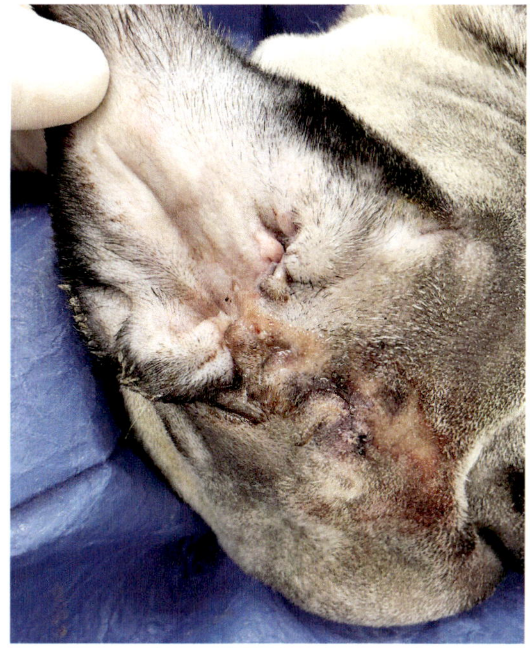

Figure 28. Incisional discharge from a total ear canal ablation surgical site.

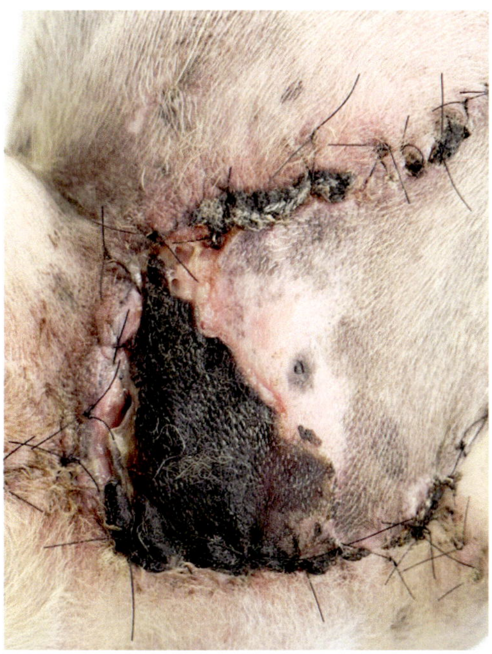

Figure 27. Necrosis and partial dehiscence of the tip of a skin flap seven days after surgery.

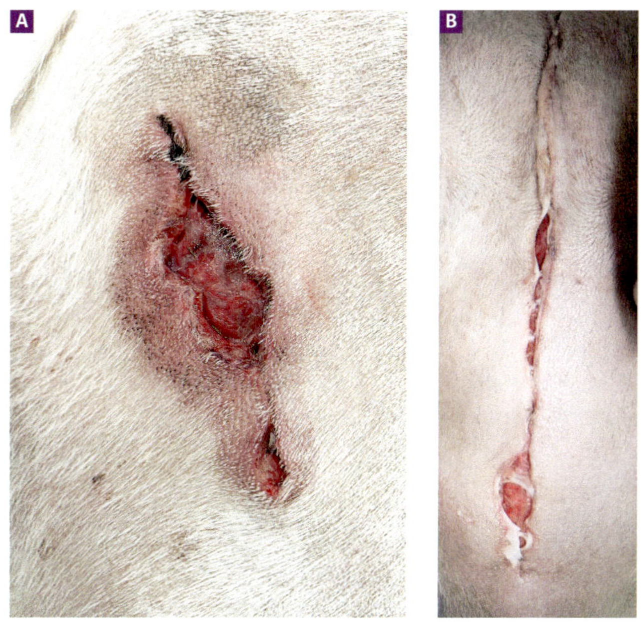

Figure 29. A. Partial dehiscence of a surgical incision with surrounding inflammation; **B.** Incomplete dehiscence of an extensive abdominal incision with partial necrosis of the incision and a minimal rim of surrounding inflammation.

Incisions should be monitored closely for discharge and gap formation (Figures 28 and 29). Should this occur, then swabs should be taken from around the wound for culture and sensitivity testing, and it should be cleaned with saline or topical wound disinfectants such as polyhexanide solution. If there is an opening of part of a long incision which has been closed with continuous sutures which run the length of the incision, placing interrupted skin sutures or staples should be considered to prevent further progression of the dehiscence. Necrotic tissue should be debrided from the wound edges. Broad spectrum antibiotic therapy should be considered to prevent contamination of the now open wound, pending the results of culture and sensitivity testing. The wound should be appropriately covered with a sterile dressing, which is capable of absorbing discharge from the wound

Following assessment for infection, the wound should be managed as an open wound or (if infection is managed or found not to be a causal factor in the dehiscence of the wound and other factors are adequately assessed), repeat wound closure may be considered.

Deeper tissue planes, rather than the skin, may dehisce, for example an incisional hernia associated with the abdominal wall. Dehiscence of appendicular muscle/fascial layer closures may lead to loss of function or more commonly seroma formation (discussed further below). The consequences of deep incisional dehiscence are specific to the surgery undertaken and hence influence the specific signs of dehiscence and monitoring strategies employed to assess for these. Generally, any swelling or pain associated with an incision should be assessed, as should a deterioration or loss of limb function.

Suture Reaction

Suture material is a foreign body and as such elicits an immune response. The degree of response varies with the suture material. Modern synthetic materials elicit less immune response than historically used natural materials, such as cat gut. Multifilament or braided sutures are more prone to wicking bacteria and hence associated with greater incisional infection rates, and therefore should not be routinely used in the skin.

Intradermal skin closure is also associated with a greater degree of inflammation (not infection) within the skin than simple interrupted skin sutures, likely due to the increased quantity of suture material placed within the dermal layer.

Use of polymerised caprolactam (e.g. Supramid®, Vetafil®) for skin suturing is associated with a greater degree of suture reaction and suture tract formation compared to monofilament Nylon®, as these materials are nonsterile and their multifilament nature means that bacteria is wicked within their substance. Such tissue reactions usually rapidly resolve following suture removal.

Haemorrhage

Postoperative haemorrhage is a common complication which can occur after any surgical procedure.

Haemorrhage in the surgical patient can be classified into three main categories:

1. **Primary bleeding:** bleeding that occurs during surgery. This should be managed during the procedure. Quantitative assessment of blood loss is made by measurement of fluid collected in suction jars (Figure 19) and weighing blood soaked swabs.
2. **Reactive bleeding:** occurs within 24 hours of surgery, usually as the result of ligature slippage or a missed vessel. These vessels are often missed intraoperatively due to hypotension and vasoconstriction, meaning that bleeding only occurs once the blood pressure normalises postoperatively. The surgeon should assess the risk and consequences of postoperative haemorrhage and institute appropriate monitoring during the postoperative period.
3. **Secondary bleeding:** occurs 7–10 days postoperatively, often due to erosion of a vessel from a spreading infection or abrasion by a surgical drain or surgical.

Clinical Features and Assessment of Reactive Bleeding

Bleeding from the surgical incision may be seen, or an accumulation of swelling under the skin at the surgical site. (Figure 30).

– Major cavitary bleeding presents as **haemorrhagic shock,** with signs including tachycardia, dizziness, agitation, and decreased urine output. One of the most sensitive signs is a raised respiratory rate.

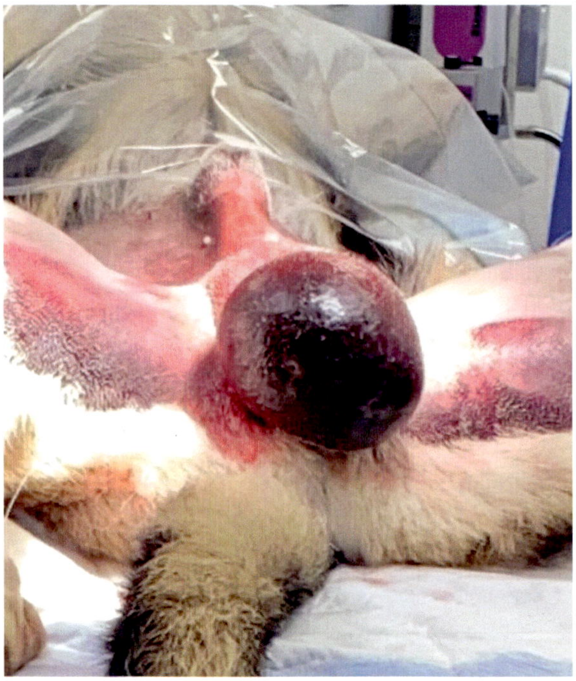

Figure 30. A scrotal haematoma due to persistent bleeding following a castration surgery.

- **Hypotension** is often a late sign as initially compensatory mechanisms adapt to maintain blood pressure, and only when this reserve capacity is exceeded by changes in vascular resistance and heart rate, does blood pressure begin to drop.
- **Examination of the patient** includes a thorough exposure looking for bleeding, systematic palpation of the surgical area looking for swelling, discolouration, and undue pain.
- **Vital parameters** include heart rate, pulse quality, mucous membrane colour and respiratory rate and effort which should be monitored intensively following surgery that carries a risk of postoperative haemorrhage, tracking trends and gradually reducing sensitivity of monitoring as long as parameters remain stable.

If there is a clinical suspicion of postoperative bleeding, fast and efficient management reduces overall morbidity and mortality.

In a patient with suspected haemorrhage:
- intravenous access should be established/maintained;
- direct, cold compression should be applied to the bleeding site (if visible);
- the patient should be reviewed urgently by the veterinary surgeon;
- imaging, initially by point of care ultrasound (POCUS) may be appropriate to assess for fluid accumulation and sampling to confirm haemorrhagic effusion; and
- blood transfusion/aspiration and autotransfusion in the case of moderate to severe postoperative haemorrhage may be performed.

Haemorrhage at specific sites:
- postoperative haemorrhage in the cervical region can have catastrophic consequences on breathing due to swelling resulting in airway obstruction; and
- intra-abdominal bleeding may be apparent due to the observation of the Cullen sign; bruising around the umbilicus.

Seroma

A seroma is the accumulation of serous or serosanguinous fluid under the skin at a surgical site. Seromas result from effusion from a wound bed within an area of dead space under the skin. Seromas commonly occur at sites where there is excessive space under the skin, such as in the ventral cervical region, axilla, or inguinal regions.

Seroma is also a common consequence of deep incisional dehiscence, i.e. of muscle layer disruption or tearing. Excessive movement encourages seroma formation.

Prevention

Seroma formation is reduced by minimising the undermining of tissues during surgery, managing dead space by adequate tissue reapposition at the time of surgical closure, including the placement of walking sutures, or by placing surgical drains or compressive bandages. **Exercise restriction** is also key in the postoperative period both to prevent deep suture layer disruption but also to minimise movement between tissue planes which may promote seroma formation.

Treatment

When seromas occur, management is aimed at **reducing the factors that contributed to fluid accumulation** e.g. by exercise restriction and compression; as well as **increasing the rate of fluid reabsorption,** which includes warming the area to increase local blood flow and aid fluid reabsorption.

Needle drainage may be considered but risks the introduction of infection as well as not eliminating the cause of the seroma, and so recurrence is common. Rarely, surgical opening of the incision to allow drainage or placement of a closed suction drain is considered where other measures are insufficient to adequately reduce the fluid accumulation, e.g. for a ventral neck seroma causing respiratory compromise due to airway obstruction.

Bandage Complications

Bandages play many useful roles in the management of surgical patients, but there are risks linked with their application and maintenance. An inappropriate or slipped bandage may cause:
- **Tourniquet:** reduced perfusion to tissue within or distal to the bandage, in the worst instance leading to loss of the extremity.
- **Pressure sores:** open wounds propagated by rubbing over bony prominences (Figures 31 and 32).
- **Harbour infection:** wet/soiled dressings wick bacteria to the wound surface and allow surgical site contamination.

Endocrine/Metabolic Complications

Hypocalcemia

Hypocalcemia may result following **parathyroidectomy** for removal of a functional parathyroid tumour, or inadvertent parathyroidectomy or parathyroid tissue devascularisation following a thyroidectomy procedure.

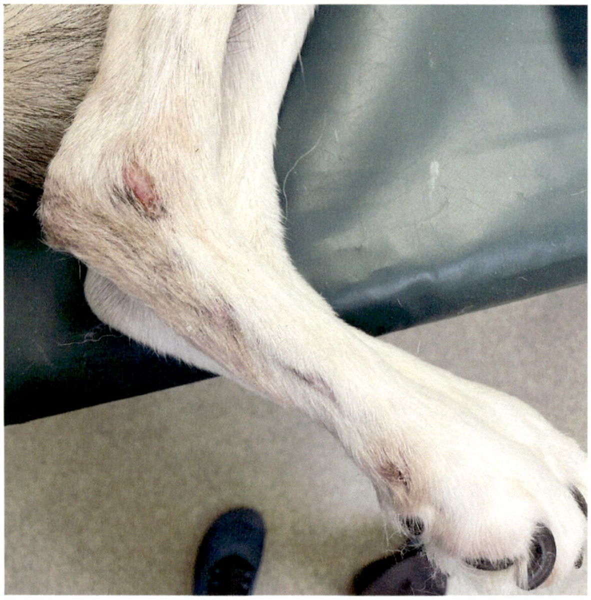

Figure 31. Early pressure sores over the lateral malleolus of the fibula and the 5th metatarsophalangeal joint.

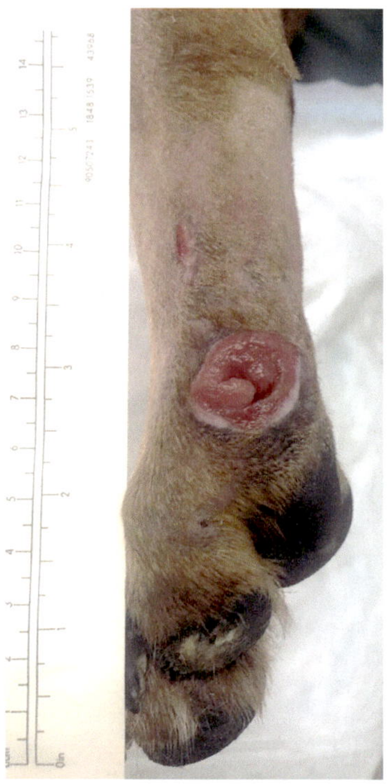

Figure 32. Deep pressure sore over the 5th metatarsophalangeal joint.

Clinical Signs

Clinical signs of hypocalcemia include **muscle twitching, facial pruritus (rubbing), loss of appetite, weakness, lethargy, and in severe cases, seizures.**

Hypocalcemia most commonly becomes apparent **two to six days following surgery,** although can occur up to three weeks after surgery. For this reason it is common to keep patients **hospitalised for serial ionised calcium level checks** following surgery. Ionised calcium is the active form of the total calcium within the blood stream. The non-ionised portion of calcium in the blood is bound to albumin and is not active.

In patients with acute signs of hypocalcemia, 10% calcium gluconate is administered by slow intravenous injection (over 10 to 20 minutes) to effect. Ideally, the patient is **monitored by ECG for** bradycardia and arrhythmias during intravenous calcium administration. The patient is then treated with a continuous rate infusion of calcium.

When the patient is stable enough to accept oral medication, **calcium and oral vitamin D** (to increase calcium absorption from the intestine) should be administered.

Hyperglycaemia/Hypoglycaemia

Hyperglycaemia may occur in diabetic patients or in surgery to remove an insulinoma (insulin secreting pancreatic tumour). Initially it causes polydipsia and polyuria, but if untreated may result in urinary tract infection due to glycosuria and eventually diabetic ketoacidosis. Insulin administration is necessary to treat protracted hyperglycaemia.

Hypoglycaemia may occur in very young patients, and those with impaired or reduced hepatic function, such as those with porto-systemic shunts and with sepsis. Hypoglycaemia causes weakness, lethargy, and in severe cases seizures. Hypoglycaemia is initially managed by feeding/oral glucose administration if the patient is able to accept oral feeding, and intravenous dextrose administration in the acute setting.

Porto-systemic Shunt Attenuation Surgery

- **Hypoglycaemia** (as discussed above) is common in patients undergoing treatment of porto-systemic shunts, due to their small size and reduced hepatic function.
- **Portal hypertension** is more common in patients undergoing complete suture ligation than in patients undergoing gradual shunt occlusion.
    - Clinical signs include evidence of hypovolaemic shock, abdominal pain and distention, and diarrhoea or vomiting.
    - In the acute setting, patients are managed with analgesics and sedatives, if needed, to keep them comfortable and relaxed. Supportive care includes oxygen, warmth, intravenous crystalloids, colloids, gastrointestinal protectants (e.g. omeprazole and sucralfate) and systemic antibiotics.

- **Post-attenuation neurological syndrome (PANS):** postoperative seizures develop in roughly 5% of dogs and cats after shunt attenuation and are most common in cats and in small-breed dogs with extra-hepatic shunts. Seizures may occur up to three days after surgery and are not associated with hypoglycaemia (although this should be checked for), hyperammonia, or surgical technique.
    - Clinical signs include lethargy, facial twitching, ataxia, muscle fasciculation, blindness, and abnormal vocalisation which are often apparent before generalised seizure activity. The cause of postoperative seizures is unknown and unpredictable.
    - **Initial treatment** includes intravenous boluses of diazepam. Additional antiepileptic medications including levatiracetam, phenobarbital, and bromide are then loaded to effect. In severe cases, propofol CRI may be required initially whilst other medications are loaded.

The prognosis is poor for animals with postoperative seizures, with only 50% of patients surviving and those that do are often left with long term neurological dysfunction.

Airway Complications

Airway Obstruction

Following any surgical intervention within (e.g. surgery for BOAS or laryngeal mass removal) or around the airway (e.g. arytenoid lateralisation, ventral neck exploration for management of stick injuries or thyroid tumours), there is a risk that inflammation and swelling may lead to obstruction or external compression of the airway and compromise breathing (Figures 33 and 34). This is especially true of patients undergoing treatment for BOAS, whereby the swelling, compounded by tachypnoea due to stress (from hospitalisation and surgical treatment) and potentially regurgitation may lead to decompensation of a patient who was on the verge of respiratory disaster prior to treatment.

Airway obstruction may be acute or progressive in onset, and usually evident as **increased respiratory noise and effort.**

Management is through sedation to alleviate stress (which compounds the respiratory dysfunction), oxygen therapy, and then airway assessment and securing an airway if necessary. Securing an airway may be challenging in these patients with a tracheostomy (temporary or permanent) or further laryngeal surgery may be required to alleviate the obstruction. (Figure 35).

The key to management of airway obstruction patients, is awareness of the risk, being prepared, and adequate monitoring of the patient, whilst having sufficient staff available to intervene if needed.

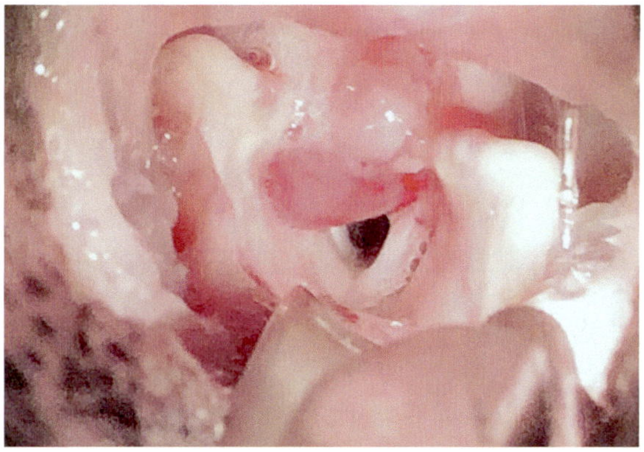

Figure 33. Laryngeal tumour seen on intubation compromising the airway from dorsally to the left of midline.

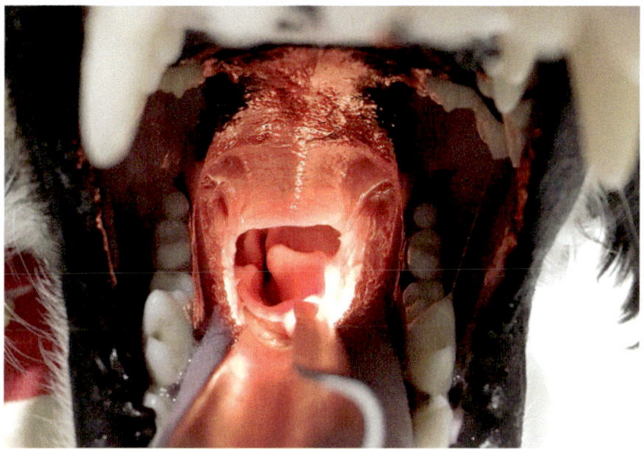

Figure 34. Displacement of the larynx to the right due to left sided swelling resulting from a cervical abscess due to a penetrating stick injury.

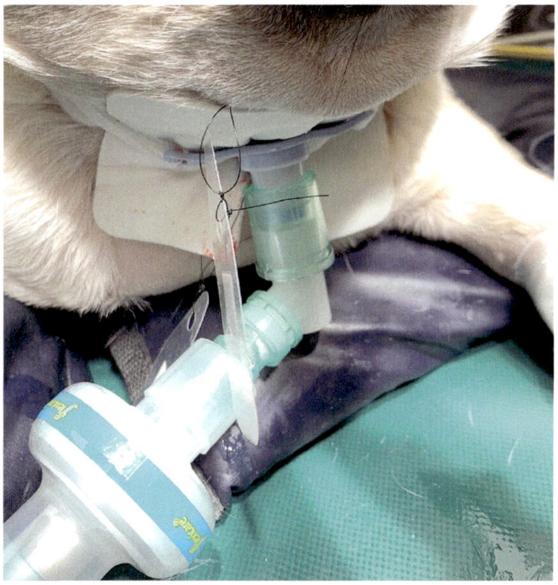

Figure 35. Surgical placement of a temporary tracheostomy tube with tagged sutures placed in tracheal rings either side of the incision to facilitate tube replacement. Figure courtesy of Rachel Hattersley.

Aspiration Pneumonia

Aspiration pneumonia is not uncommon following airway surgery or in **patients at risk of regurgitation,** particularly during anaesthesia and the immediate postoperative recovery. During surgery the airway is secured with a cuffed endotracheal tube, but during anaesthetic recovery, when the endotracheal tube is no longer tolerated the patient is still at increased risk of regurgitation and the effects of sedation mean they are unable to consciously protect their own airway.

Patients most at risk include those experiencing:
- lengthy anaesthetics
- multiple repositioning, e.g. orthopaedic procedures with pre and postoperative imaging
- manipulation of the upper gastrointestinal tract
- brachycephalic patients, which typically have oesophageal hiatal dysfunction
- arytenoid lateralisation as this surgery reduces airway protection against aspiration.

Patients with aspiration pneumonia are typically tachypnoiec to dyspnoeic with varying degrees of hypoxia as a result of the degree of pulmonary dysfunction. Their oxygen saturation should be assessed with **pulse-oximetry** and **blood gas analysis** to guide and monitor response to oxygen therapy. Oxygen is administered as flow by, either by nasal prongs, intranasal catheter, high-flow intranasal administration, or positive pressure ventilation under sedation on a slide scale of disease severity. Acute aspiration events are managed by suction of the upper airway to clear obstruction and help prevent further fluid aspiration. Patients may also present with milder signs of coughing and pyrexia.

Antibiotic therapy should be administered intravenously. Initial antibiotic choice is broad spectrum. If feasible and safe to do so, bronchoalveolar lavage or tracheal wash should be performed to directly sample bacteria from the airway for culture and sensitivity testing.

Thoracic imaging should be considered to confirm the diagnosis. Radiographic changes can lag behind clinical signs by around 48 hours and their utility is limited by the need for sedation or anaesthesia to obtain good quality images. POCUS as discussed in the diagnostic imaging chapter may be more helpful in unstable patients, with B-lines observed in affected areas of the lung field.

Pleural Effusion/Pneumothorax

Following intrathoracic surgery, initially fluid or accumulation is most frequently the result of:
- **haemothorax:** intrathoracic haemorrhage
- **pneumothorax:** air leakage from the lower airways.

In the longer term, pleural fluid or air is likely due to:
- **haemothorax:** indicative of lower grade haemorrhage
- **pneumothorax:** slow air leakage or progressive erosion of sutures or a tumour through the airway
- **pyothorax:** due to surgical site infection
- **chylothorax:** with damage to the thoracic duct
- **neoplastic effusion:** due to carcinomatosis (spread of carcinoma tumours to the thoracic wall).

Whatever the cause, the accumulation of fluid within the thorax causes **progressive loss of reserve respiratory function** causing tachypnoea and increased respiratory effort. Hence these signs should be investigated by performing thoracic radiography or TFAST. If an effusion or pneumothorax is identified this should be drained. If the volume is low and slow to accumulate, initial **one-off needle drainage** may suffice, but if fluid is rapidly accumulating or there is a large volume with a concern for ongoing production then **a drain should be placed** to allow ongoing monitoring and quantification of the fluid production.

Any liquid aspirated from the pleural space should be analysed; starting with a visual assessment:
- **Bloody fluid:** the PCV of the fluid should be compared to that of the patient's circulation; if these numbers are similar this indicates intrathoracic haemorrhage.
- **Pyothorax:** the fluid may appear brown, cloudy and foul smelling. However milder infections are only apparent on cytological analysis with the identification of a predominance of neutrophils, with phagoctyosed bacteria.
- **Chylothorax:** the fluid appears like strawberry milkshake, and is confirmed by assessing triglycerides and cholesterol for comparison with the values from the blood.

If the pneumothorax or pleural effusion fails to resolve with drainage and appropriate medical therapy (if available) then further surgical intervention may be required.

Orthopaedic Complications

Implant Failure

Orthopaedic surgery frequently involves **the placement of metal implants.** In most cases the implants are temporary, i.e. for the duration of bone healing, however implants are seldom removed unless they cause interference with normal function or become infected. Some implants are required permanently for example those placed during joint replacement surgeries. In either event the implant selected should be strong enough to tolerate the strain of load bearing and gentle activity, although might not be sufficient to tolerate higher strains or more extreme activity. **Overload of the implant**

before bone healing occurs may result in implant failure (Figure 36). Implant failure may be acute with a single episode of heavy overload, or cyclic loading may progressively lead to weakening and failure.

Depending on the nature of the implant and the mechanism of overload, failure may occur in a number of ways:

- failure of the bone-to-implant interface by pulling out of the implants or fracture of bone around the implants
- implant breakage
- implant bending causing malalignment.

Bone Healing Complications

Bone takes longer to heal than most soft tissues and following bone injury and orthopaedic surgery **prolonged rest and recovery are needed.** Bone healing is faster in younger patients, in areas of good blood supply, in healthy, well-nourished patients and given adequate rest and stability in the form of splinting or orthopaedic implants. In general a long bone fracture in a young puppy will heal in two to four weeks, whereas in an adult this may take six to eight weeks or longer in a geriatric patient.

- A **delayed union** is defined as a fracture that has not healed in the timeframe expected for that fracture to have healed in that patient. A delayed union may go on to heal given time, if the conditions are optimised to allow healing to continue.
- A **non-union** is defined as a fracture where healing has not taken place and the body's attempts to heal the fracture have stopped. Non-union fractures do not heal without further surgical intervention.
- A **malunion** is a fracture which has completely healed, but in an undesirable position, e.g. with a torsional (twist), valgus (bent outwards), or varus (bent inwards) deformity.

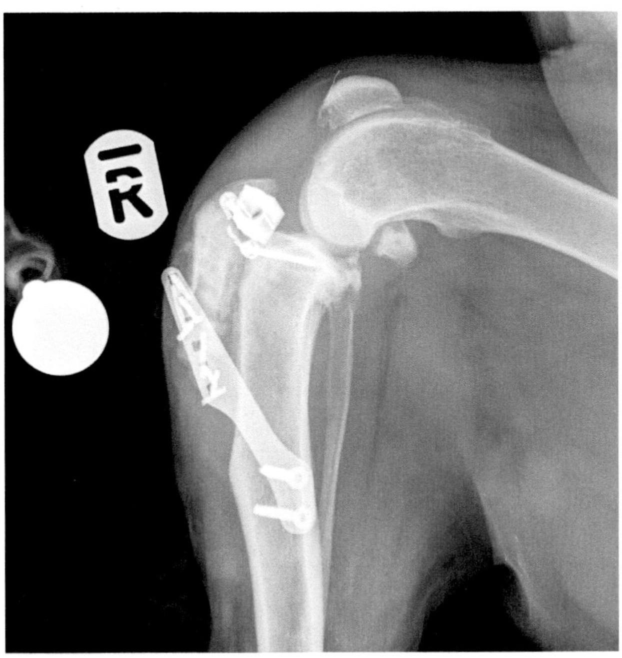

Figure 36. Implant failure: this image shows both implant breakage and failure of the bone-to-implant interface following a TTA (tibia tuberosity advancement) surgery.

Causes of delayed/non-union are similar to those noted as causes of dehiscence for soft issue wounds, and include:

- inadequate immobilisation of the fracture site
- inadequate reduction of the fracture ends (too big a gap)
- loss of blood supply (due to the original trauma +/- the surgical technique)
- infection
- loss of bone (due to the trauma leaving a gap)
- general health factors which affect healing: e.g. immunosuppression, old age, endocrine diseases.

Orthopaedic reassessment is usually performed by **repeating radiographs after an appropriate interval (usually four to six weeks)** after surgery to assess implant positioning, limb alignment, and bone healing. Radiographs may be taken sooner in very young, growing patients or if there is a change in limb usage which might suggest a problem with the surgical site.

If bone healing is not proceeding as expected, treatment may require prolonged rest, or in the worst case further surgery to realign or stabilise the bones, and possibly to consider the placement of a **cancellous bone graft** to help stimulate the healing process.

Osteoarthritis

Osteoarthritis (Figure 37) is the name given to degenerative disease of the joints, which in dogs and cats occurs **secondary to joint injury or instability.** Osteoarthritis is a progressive disease, whereby radiographically, spurs of **new bone** form around the periphery of the joint, where the joint capsule attaches to the bone. There may be an **increase in synovial fluid,** which shows evidence of mild, chronic inflammation with **increased numbers of monocytes** on cytology.

Osteoarthritis will always result and progress following any joint injury, but surgical stabilisation of an unstable joint or debridement of a pathological process helps to slow the rate of progression. Chronic instability or infection as a complication of orthopaedic surgery or additional trauma due to a less precisely performed orthopaedic surgery, result in a more rapid rate of progression of osteoarthritis and worse long term outcome for the joint.

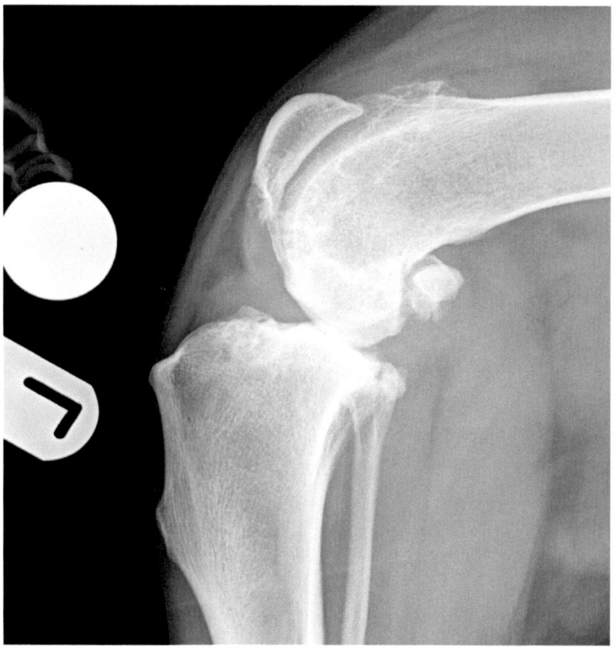

Figure 37. Osteoarthritis: this image shows a severely osteoarthritic stifle. Note the irregular bone formation on the proximal trochlear groove, on both proximal and distal poles of the patella (which should be smooth and rounded) and on the tibial plateau.

Osteoarthritis is best prevented. Treatment for osteoarthritis is limited to joint replacement or excision surgeries (e.g. femoral head and neck excision) or management strategies which aim to slow the rate of osteoarthritis progression:

- **weight control**
- **regular, controlled exercise** including physiotherapy and hydrotherapy to maintain muscle strength to support weak joints
- **analgesia** (including non-steroidal anti-inflammatory medications when appropriate)
- **nutraceuticals/joint supplements** which help to reduce joint inflammation and may aid the development of fibrocartilage (scar tissue formation) within the joint.

Contracture

Muscle contracture and fibrosis resulting in irreversible stiffness and loss of movement is uncommon with orthopaedic injuries in dogs and cats, but is most frequently noted in the **quadriceps muscles following femoral fracture** repair in immature patients. The key to prevention of this irreversible change is in rapid return to mobilisation and stretching of the quadriceps muscles following fracture repair. The condition is thought to result from a form of **compartment syndrome,** with swelling of the muscles with a tight fascial sheath which limits swelling and hence swelling restricts blood flow to the affected muscles.

Wound Classification

Wounds are defined as any surface disruption to the body or an internal surface of an organ. There are a wide variety of aetiologies and resultant patterns of injury from wounds. **There is no one system for wound classification,** but it is helpful to assess wounds based on the surface defect, the extent of deep and surrounding tissue trauma, and the level of contamination.

Classification of Cutaneous Wounds Based on Aetiology/Appearance

Incision

A **surgical incision** (Figure 38) is a unique term used to describe the precise and deliberate, sharp, minimally traumatic separation of tissue with a scalpel in the hands of a surgeon, in order to achieve a purposeful treatment of an underlying pathology or to perform an elective diagnostic or therapeutic procedure.

There is a clear distinction between surgical incisions and wounds. Although a surgical incision is a form of wound, it is referred to as an incision, **reserving the term wound for injuries of traumatic origin.**

Laceration

Laceration is the term used for a wound created by **a sharp object moving parallel to the skin surface.** (An incision is a special type of deliberately created laceration). Lacerations generally create minimally contaminated, or clean, regular, linear wounds, which gape open as a result of the elasticity and tension in the surrounding skin.

- Lacerations are frequently associated with broken glass, the edges of tin cans, or barbed/razor wire.
- Lacerations tend to bleed freely, which aids in wound lavage but are associated with significant external blood loss if wounds are extensive or deep. This type of wound is however usually **amenable to lavage and primary closure** at an early stage due to the minimal contamination and surrounding tissue trauma/contusion. It is essential however **the wound is fully explored** to the full depth of penetration so as not to misidentify injury to deeper tissues, e.g. tendon or ligament disruption with superficial trauma to the distal limbs.

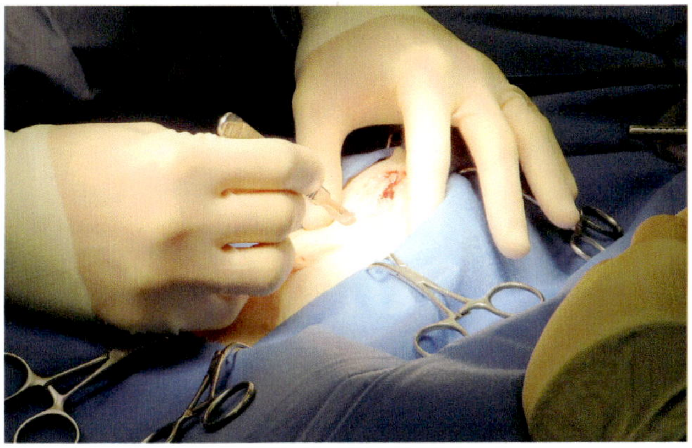

Figure 38. Surgical incision.

Abrasion

An abrasion is the superficial injury caused to the epidermis and dermis of the skin due to **frictional contact parallel to the surface of the tissue.** In practice, this term describes wounds of similar aetiology with deeper trauma to the underlying tissue, with the more specific term shearing injury used for deeper injuries to the limbs.

- Abrasions are commonly encountered in small animal veterinary practice, most frequently resultant from road traffic trauma, when the patient is trapped between a moving vehicle and the road.
- Abrasions are usually **heavily contaminated** with microorganisms and debris from the abrading surface, with contamination deeply embedded within the wound, such that thorough wound cleaning and debridement is required in the initial stages of wound management.

Puncture

A puncture is caused by a sharp object moving perpendicular to the skin surface, perforating the surface, creating an entry wound, a path of deeper tissue trauma and then potentially an exit wound. Needle sticks are the simplest form of puncture wound, but rarely associated with surrounding tissue trauma or a significant cutaneous injury. More common are puncture wounds associated with more significant trauma, such as **impalement injuries and bite wounds.** Less common are insect and snakebite wounds and firearms injuries.

Bite Wounds

Bite wounds (Figure 39) **are puncture wounds caused by teeth,** usually the canine teeth, and frequently complicated by **crushing injury** to the deeper tissue, contusion, tearing, and laceration of the local tissue due to lateral movement during injury; as well as **inoculation of contaminants** including hair and bacteria under the skin surface. The combination of a closed wound, with poor drainage, contused muscle, damaged blood supply, and seroma or haematoma formation create an ideal medium for bacterial proliferation within the wound.

A relatively small cutaneous wound may be of little significance, however **thorough assessment of the unseen injury to the deeper tissues** should be made, either by diagnostic

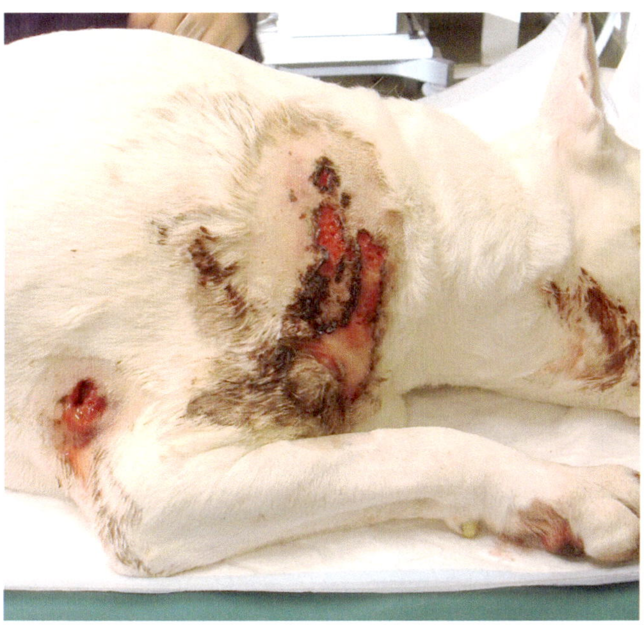

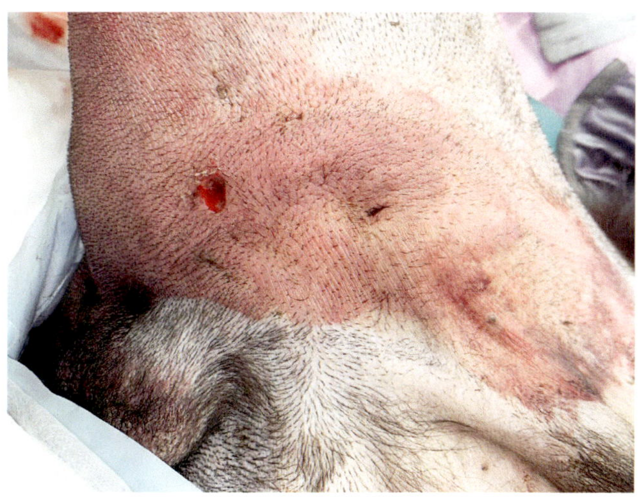

Figures 39. Bite wounds from a dog fight show small punctures to the skin but extensive surrounding bruising and, more importantly, there will be extensive tissue damage under the skin's surface.

imaging investigation or surgical exploration depending on the degree of trauma and the region of the body traumatised i.e. thoracic CT or radiography may be preferred for assessment of bite wounds over the thorax to evaluate for thoracic cavity penetration, thoracic wall disruption and intrathoracic pathology, e.g. pneumothorax, whereas abdominal ultrasonography may be preferred for injury to the abdominal wall, to assess for intraabdominal effusion and tissue trauma.

Impalement Injury

Impalement injuries are generated by the patient's own momentum, usually from chasing and retrieving sticks. Injuries are most commonly to the oropharynx but may also include injury to the trunk. Stick injuries (Figures 40, 41 and 42) cause trauma and bleeding from the initial puncture, but fragmentation of the stick results in persistent contamination and a septic focus for abscess formation, and hence, require urgent thorough exploration either by open surgery, or by endoscopic examination, lavage and debridement of the tract created by the injury.

As with other penetrating injuries, the exterior wound may only be the tip of the iceberg with respect to deeper tissue trauma.

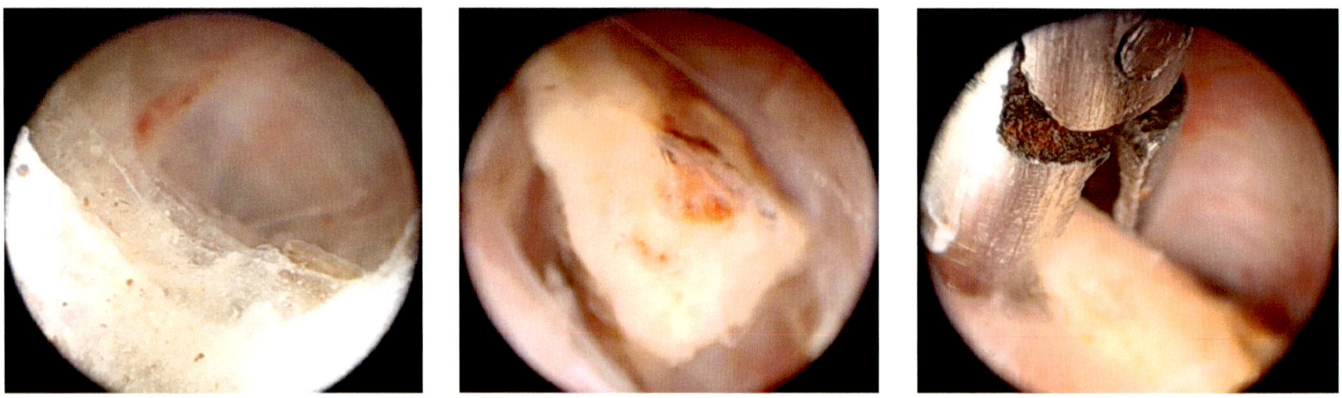

Figure 40. Rigid endoscopic images of the tract created by an oral stick injury reveal small fragments of the stick, which are retrieved with endoscopic forceps under visualisation.

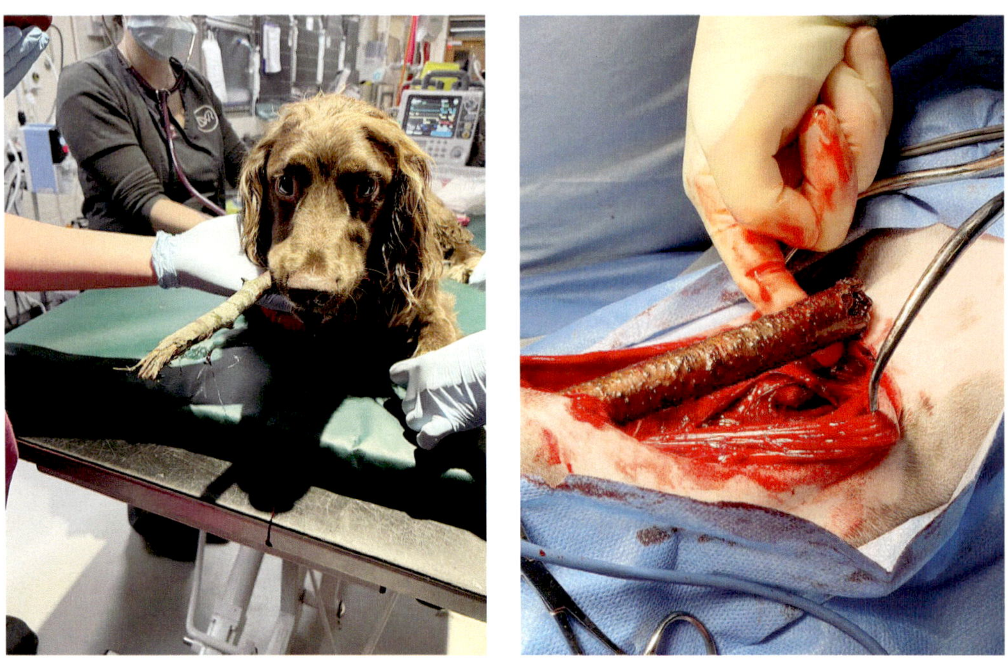

Figure 41. Photographs of a patient suffering a penetrating stick injury, which was then removed under surgical guidance by ventral neck exploration. Figures courtesy of Daniela Murgia.

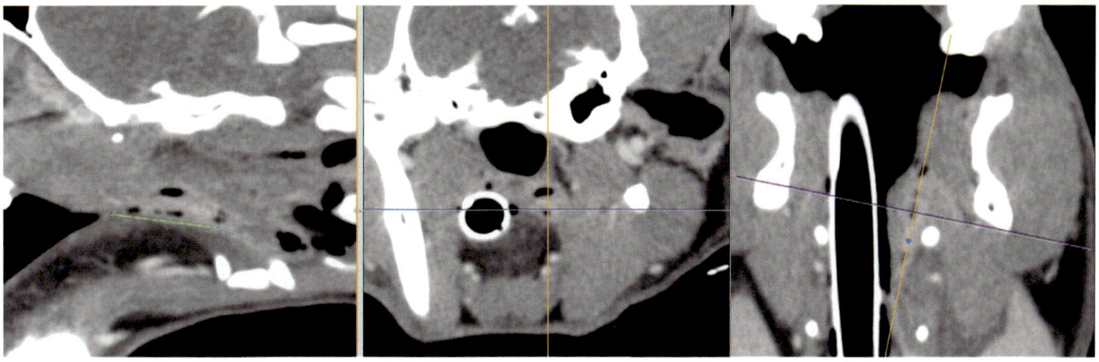

Figure 42. Stick injury CT – note the line of black gas bubbles through the tissue along the path of penetration.

Firearms Injury

Gunshot wounds are complex and varied. The type of injury created depends on the impact velocity and the type of firearm. The kinetic energy of the missile is transferred to the patient's tissues:

- **Low velocity shotguns** typically create small diameter entry and exit wounds and lacerate and compress a tract of tissue along their path, dragging skin, hair and debris in from the entry site.
- **High velocity rifle bullets** create a compressive wave as energy is transferred to tissue and tend to tumble through the tissue following entry, causing extensive internal trauma and creating large exit wounds.

Insect, Arachnid, and Snakebites

These are specific puncture wounds, **complicated by the consequences of toxic substances** inoculated into the tissues. The severity of these tissue effects is highly variable based on the species of creature involved, which varies with geographical location. These effects may be local with tissue inflammation, ischaemia, and necrosis, or more widespread systemic disease and anaphylaxis.

Avulsion

Avulsion refers to the forcible tearing of tissue from its underling attachments. These injuries can result from catching the skin on a perpendicular penetrating projection, such as barbed wire, whilst running. (Figure 43). Avulsions may also occur with bite wounds from fights with other dogs, badgers or foxes, and not infrequently can affect the tissue covering the mandible. (Figure 44).

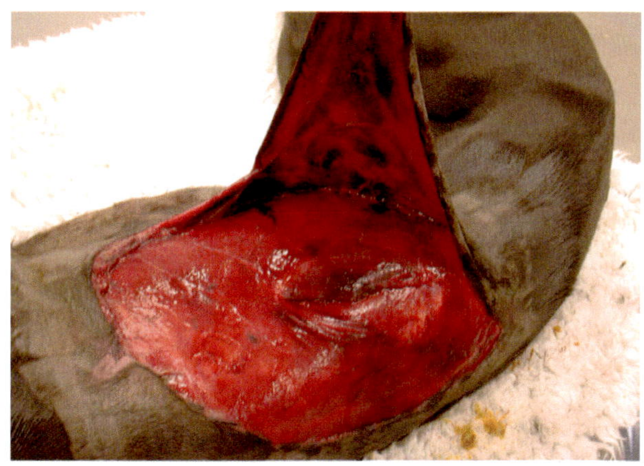

Figure 43. Avulsion of the skin of the flank of a Greyhound.

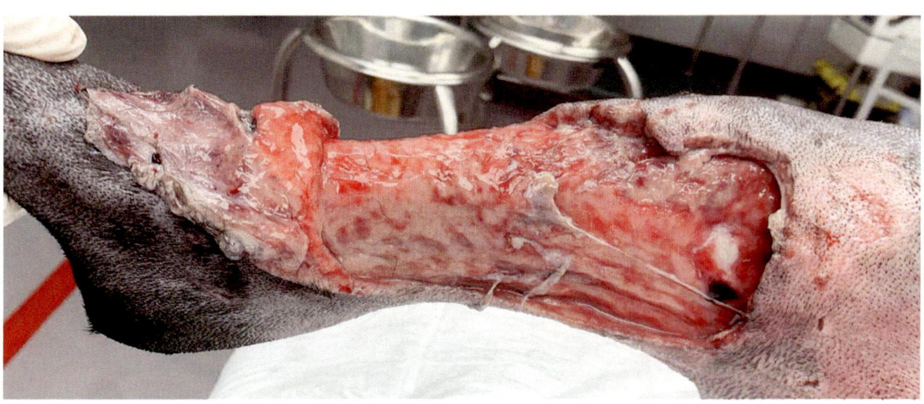

Figure 44. Avulsive bite wound over the tibia of a Labrador.

Avulsions may lead to extensive tissue loss and frequently concurrent injuries to deeper tissue, including orthopaedic injuries.

Degloving

Degloving injury is an avulsion with the loss of skin from an extremity, usually a limb, whereby the layer of tissue removal is equivalent to taking off a glove. Commonly the aetiology of degloving is mechanical due to trauma, with tearing off of the skin from the underlying tissue, through the plane of loose subcutaneous tissue which attached the layers. This is often seen with road traffic injury to the distal limb (or tail) where the extremity becomes trapped between the tyres and the road. (Figures 45 and 46). These injures may be combined with abrasive wounds and the accompanying contamination.

Degloving injuries result from physiological causes as a consequence of loss of blood supply to the extremity with trauma, leading to a delayed devitalisation and sloughing of the compromised skin over a number of days following the original injury.

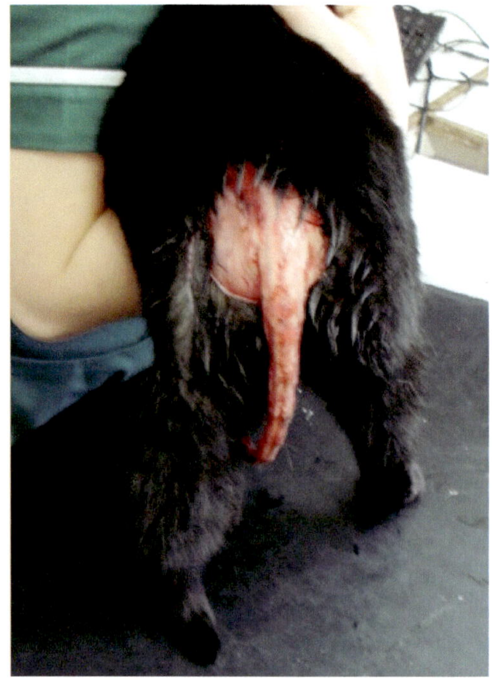

Figure 45. Degloving of a cat's tail likely due to a road traffic accident.

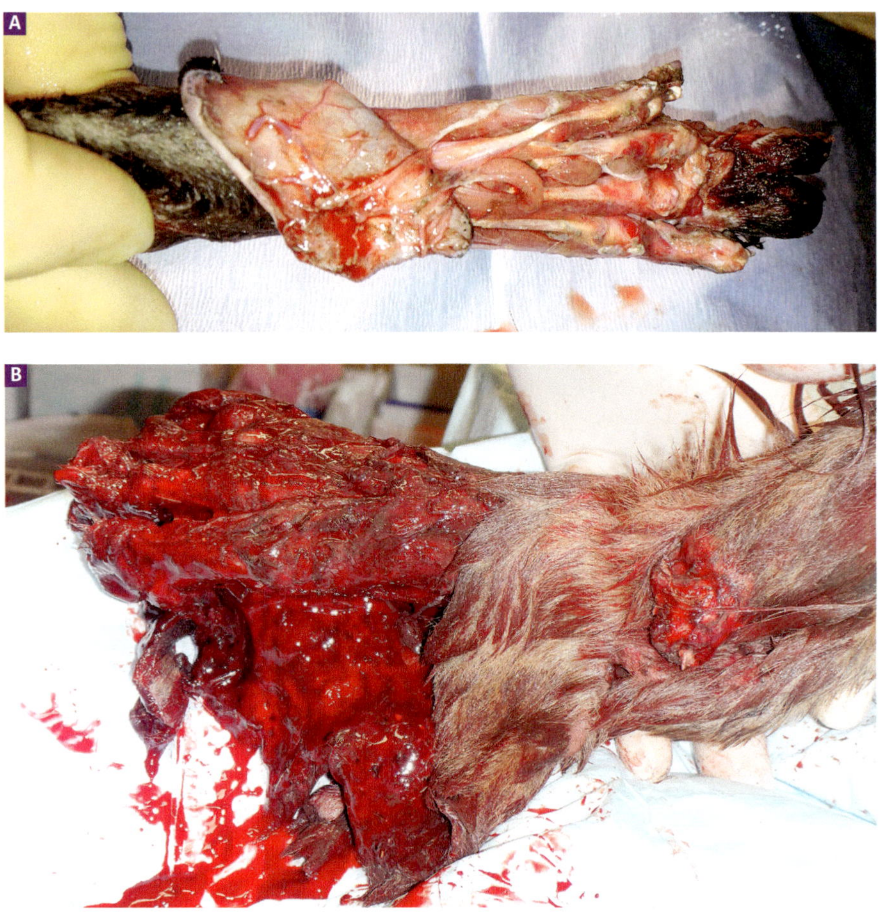

Figure 46. Extensive degloving injuries to the pes of a cat (**A**), dog with extensive haemorrhage and contamination (**B**).

Shearing Injury

Shearing injuries are a specific type of **combined avulsion and abrasive wounds,** which usually result from road traffic trauma, but affect one side (usually medial) of the distal limb of (usually young) animals. They involve complete loss of skin and underlying soft tissues and frequently loss of ligaments and bone from the affected carpus or tarsus with contamination with debris and joint exposure. These wounds are hence prone to infection. They are also challenging to manage due to inability to close extensive defects as a result of a lack of locally available tissue, as well as also frequently result in joint instability. They may require ligament reconstruction and long term support with splinting or external skeletal fixation. (Figure 47).

Burns

Burns are injuries which can be caused by extremes of temperature, but also by electricity, radiation or caustic chemicals.

- **Hyperthermic burns** result from scalding with hot water, car exhausts, or iatrogenic heat pad injuries. The distribution of these wounds is characteristic of the cause of the injury, with heat pad induced injuries seen following anaesthesia, affecting the dorsum or flanks, and scalding injuries depending on if the scald results from jumping into the hot fluid or spillage from above.
- **Hypothermic burns,** such as frostbite usually affect extremities as a result of reduced peripheral perfusion.
- **Chemical burns** caused by caustic chemicals such as battery acid, may affect the pads of the feet, or the oral cavity and oesophagus if ingested.
- **Electrical burns** result from puppies chewing through unearthed electrical cables.
- **Radiation burns** are a frequent sequelae of radiotherapy in referral oncological practice.

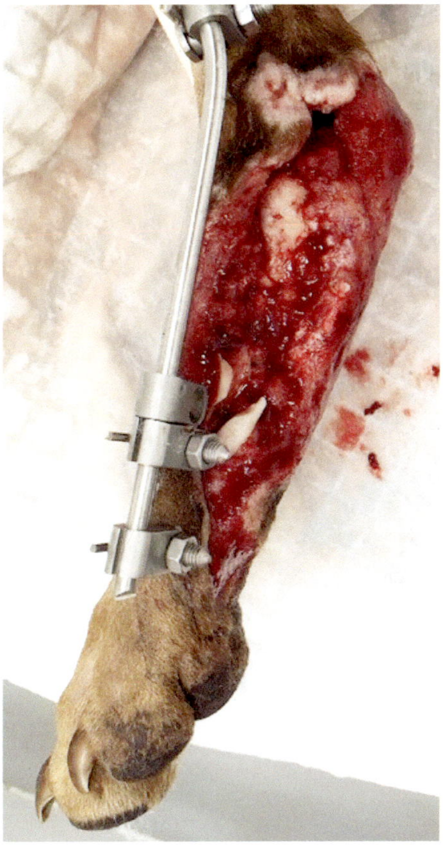

Figure 47. Shearing injury to the tarsus and metatarsus stabilised with a transarticular external skeletal fixator due to ligament loss and subsequent joint instability.

Burns are classically classified by the depth of tissue penetration:

- **First degree** (1st): affect only the epidermis of the skin. These heal without major cosmetic impact, by regeneration of the epidermis.
- **Second degree** (2nd): affect the epidermis and the dermis of the skin. Damage of the dermis and associated adnexal structures results in scarring.
- **Third degree** (3rd): affect the full thickness of the skin and variable amounts of the underlying tissue, and often require reconstructive surgery.

Burns may also be classified based on the surface area of the patient's surface affected. One method is called the rule of nines. Whereby the head accounts for 9% of the body surface area, as do each of the forelimbs, the hind limbs each account for two lots of 9%, and the trunk the remaining four lots of 9%.

The Veterinary Burn Card is based on the size of a standard credit card, which is 8.5 cm x 5.3 cm or 45 cm^2. The extent of the burn is assessed in terms of **the number of credit cards it takes to cover the wound.** The patient's body surface area can by estimated from their body weight using standard conversion charts and hence the total percentage of the body surface area of the patient affected by the burn calculated. (Figure 48).

The pathophysiology of burn wounds is poorly understood but results in severe fluid loss from the wound surface, electrolyte derangements, acidosis, azotaemia, and anaemia.

Cast Associated Soft Tissue Injury (CASTI)

Casts and bandages are frequently the cause of wounds over pressure points (e.g. the olecranon of the elbow, calcaneus of the tarsus, and metacarpophalangeal/metatarsophalangeal joints on either side of the manus/pes. These occur in roughly two thirds of patients with long standing casts or bandages. (Figure 49).

Veterinary Burn Card

To calculate the burn percentage of the total body surface area (% TBSA):

1. Measure the burn with this burn card. How many burn cards are needed to cover the burn completely?
2. Weigh the patient. Convert the weight to surface area in m² using the conversion tables on the back of this burn card.
3. Apply theses numbers to the following formula:

% TBSA burn = (number of cards x 0.45)/m²

EXAMPLE: 21 kg dog; burn size = 15.5 burn cards
Burn area = (15.5 x 0.45)/0.76 = 9.2% TBSA

Weight to surface area
CONVERSION TABLES

Dogs						Cats			
kg	**m²**	**kg**	**m²**	**kg**	**m²**	**kg**	**m²**	**kg**	**m²**
1	0,10	20	0,74	46	1,28	1,0	0,100	6,0	0,330
2	0,15	21	0,76	48	1,32	1,5	0,131	6,5	0,348
3	0,20	22	0,78	50	1,36	2,0	0,159	7,0	0,366
4	0,25	23	0,81	52	1,41	2,5	0,184	7,5	0,383
5	0,29	24	0 83	54	1,44	3,0	0,208	8,0	0,400
6	0,33	25	0,85	56	1,48	3,5	0,231	8,5	0,416
7	0,36	26	0,88	58	1,51	4,0	0,252	9,0	0,432
8	0,40	27	0,90	60	1,55	4,5	0,273	9,5	0,449
9	0,43	28	0,92	62	1,58	5,0	0,292	10,0	0,464
10	0,46	29	0,94	64	1,62	5,5	0,311		
11	0,49	30	0,96	66	1,65				
12	0,52	32	1,01	68	1,68				
13	0,55	34	1,05	70	1,72				
14	0,58	36	1,09	72	1,75				
15	0,60	38	1,13	74	1,78				
16	0,63	40	1,17	76	1,81				
17	0,66	42	1,21	78	1,84				
18	0,69	44	1,25	80	1,88				
19	0,71								

Figure 48. Actual size (8.5 cm x 5.3 cm) burn card.

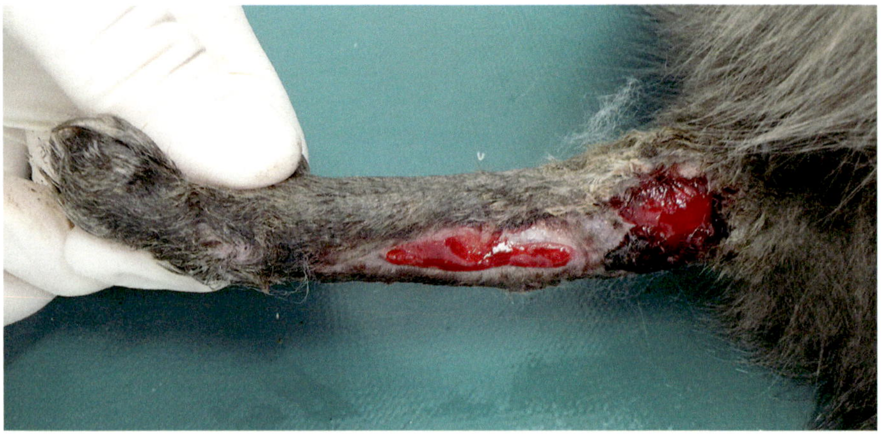

Figure 49. Cast associated soft tissue injury (CASTI).

Classification of Wound Contamination

Classification of wound contamination is similar to that for surgical site contamination:

- **Clean:** the only truly clean wound is a surgical incision following a strict aseptic surgical technique. All other types of wounds are considered contaminated, to varying degrees.
- **Contaminated:** a traumatic wound is contaminated. The ideal opportunity to manage a traumatic wound is within the golden period six hours following trauma, prior to significant bacterial proliferation. During this window of opportunity, debridement and lavage of the wound may prevent contamination become an established infection. Appropriate early management of these cases may allow primary wound closure.
- **Infected:** a figure of 10^5 bacteria per gram of tissue or millilitre of fluid has been suggested to indicate wound infection, however this varies with the extent and type of tissue trauma, host immunity, and vascular supply to the wound bed. Bite wounds for example have a high propensity for infection due to tissue crushing and trauma, with delayed necrosis even with low initial bacterial loads.

Classification of Open Fractures

Fractures associated with open wounds are at risk of contamination, infection and as a result impaired healing. The effects of infection on bone healing are potentially disastrous for limb function. Such fractures are referred to as open fractures. (Figure 50).

These are classified based on severity using the **Gustilo-Anderson Classification System:**

- **Type I:** an open fracture, with a wound of less than 1 cm. The surrounding soft tissues are mildly to moderately contused. These skin wounds are frequently created by penetration by a shard of bone from the inside out. The fracture ends frequently then retracts back within the wound.
- **Type II:** an open fracture, with a wound larger than 1 cm without extensive soft tissue damage.
- **Type III:** an open fracture with extensive soft tissue injury, e.g. avulsive or degloving injuries.
  - **Type IIIa:** an open fracture with adequate soft tissue coverage of the fractured bone despite extensive wounds.

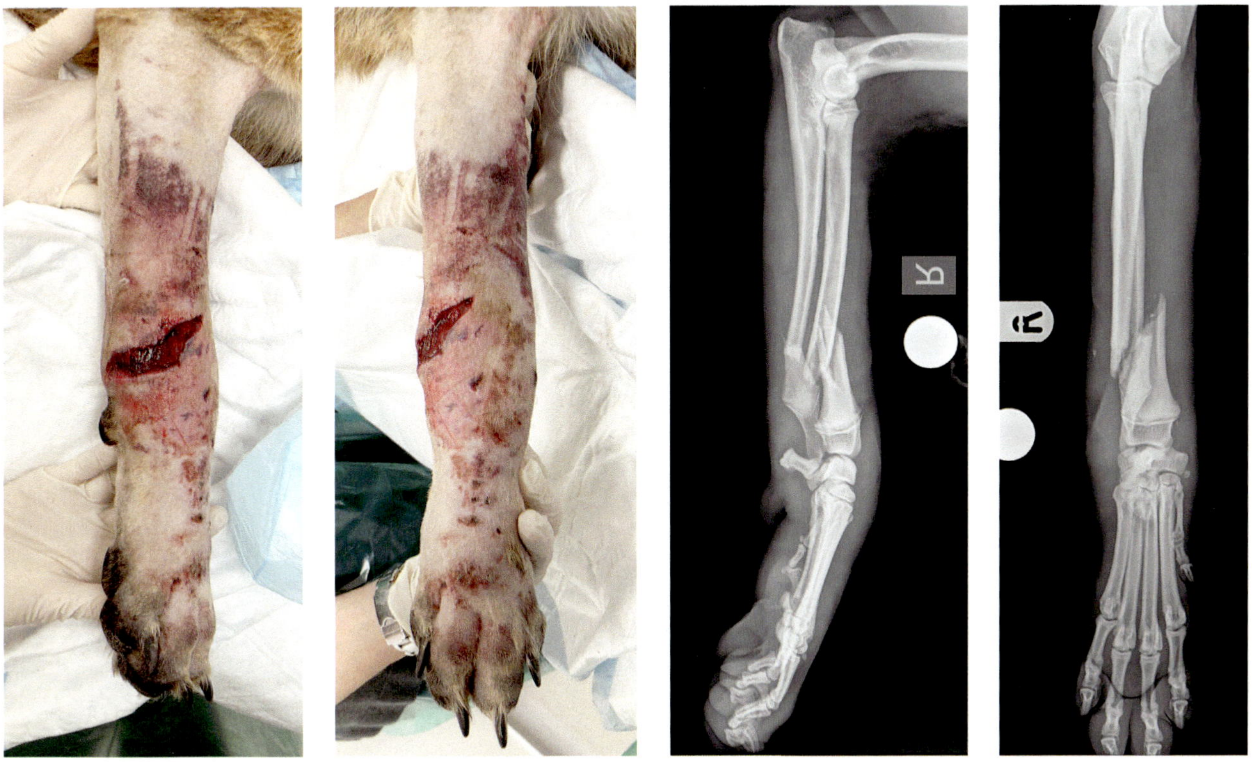

Figure 50. Mediolateral and dorsopalmar photographs and radiographs of the antebrachium of a large breed dog with a type II open fracture of the distal diaphyseal radius and ulna.

- **Type IIIb:** an open fracture with extensive soft tissue loss, periosteal stripping and bone exposure. These fractures are usually heavily contaminated.
- **Type IIIc:** an open fracture associated with an arterial injury requiring repair.

Classification of Muscle, Tendon, and Ligament Injuries

The term **sprain is used to describe ligament injuries.** The term **strain describes injuries to muscles and tendons** (Figure 51).

They are classified as follows:
- Grade 1: fibres of the affected ligament are stretched but not torn.
- Grade 2: fibres of the affected ligament are partially torn.
- Grade 3: the ligament is completely ruptured.

Differentiation of the grade of injury to a muscle, tendon, or ligament is **based on the degree of instability of a joint:**
- **Grade 1** injuries result in pain, but minimal to no residual instability.

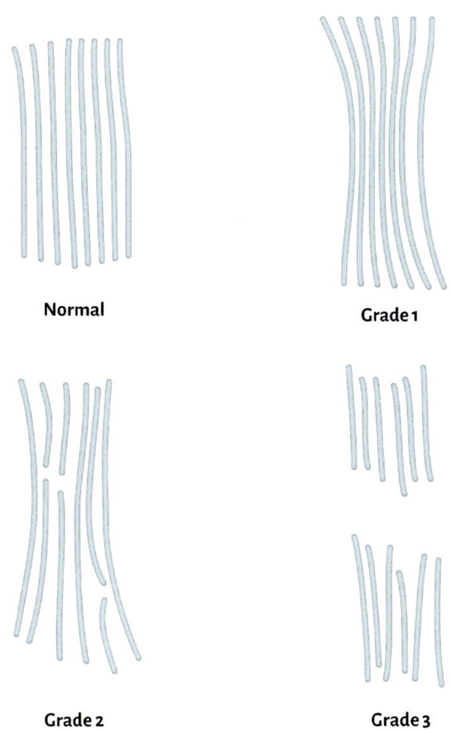

Figure 51. Classification of sprains and strains.

- **Grade 2** injuries allow varying degrees of increased range of motion, but usually an abrupt end point to the movement.
- **Complete tears** are associated with unrestricted movement of the joint in the direction normally prevented by the damaged structure.

With regards to management:
- Grade 1 injuries usually heal with adequate r**est and analgesia.** Support may be required, to aid analgesia.
- Less severe grade 2 injuries may heal if **adequately supported** with bandages/splints/orthotics to prevent loading and progression of the injury.
- More severe grade 2 and grade 3 injuries require **surgical management** to repair or replace the damaged structure, or prevent the requirement for the damaged structure, e.g. by performing a TPLO operation for a rupture cranial cruciate ligament or arthrodesis to fuse an unstable carpus. (Figures 52 and 53).

Open Wound Management and Dressings

Wound management is commonplace in veterinary practice. Wounds vary in aetiology from clean surgical incisions to contaminated, traumatic wounds. All wounds undergo the same basic natural process to try to heal. **Healing is prevented when the balance of constructive factors is outweighed by negative influences on the wound healing process.**

The role of the veterinary surgical team is to tip the balance of influences in the direction of promoting wound healing and doing this in such a way as to minimise morbidity for the patient and cost for the client, as protracted wound management can prove expensive. (Figure 54).

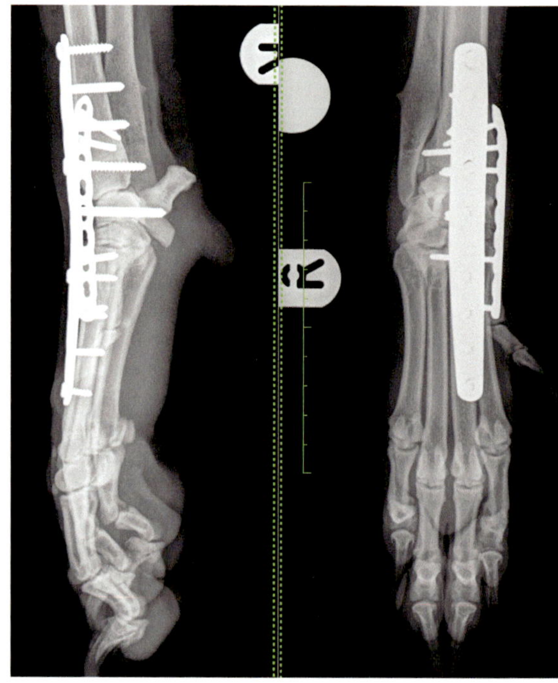

Figure 53. Pancarpal arthrodesis is a surgical fusion of the carpus by removal of the joint cartilage, filling the defects with bone graft and then rigidly immobilising the joint with orthopaedic implants.

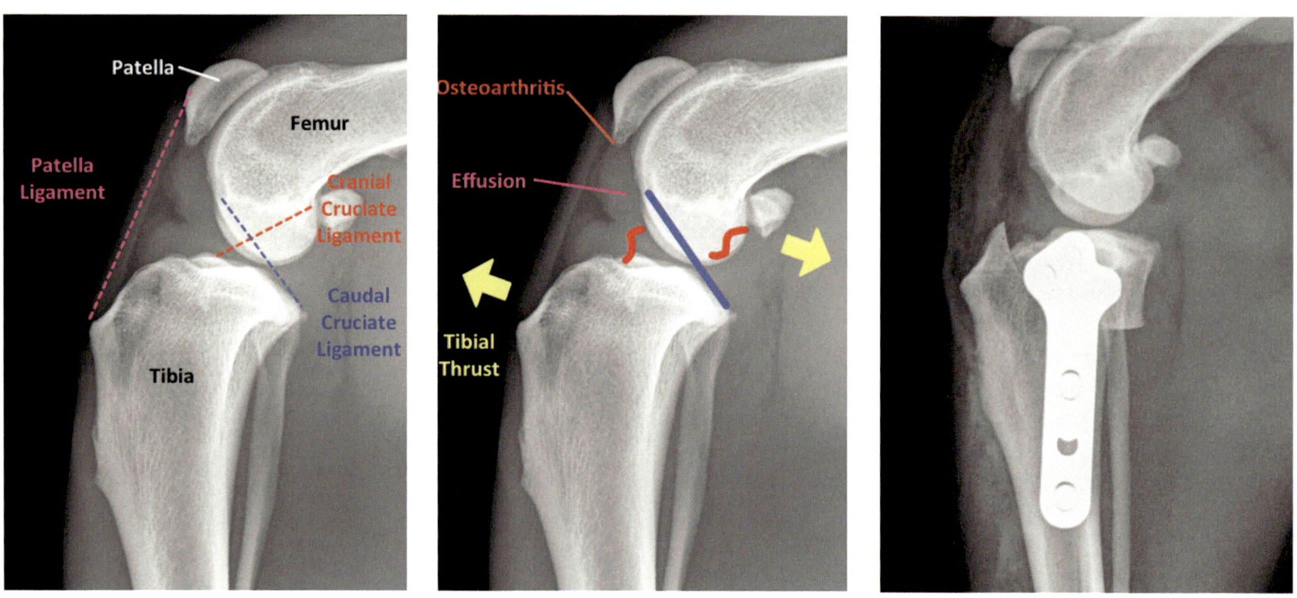

Figure 52. TPLO surgery aims to provide dynamic stability to the stifle in a patient following loss of integrity of the cranial cruciate ligament by altering the load bearing through the top of the tibia.

WOUND HEALING
Negative influences

- **Local:**
  - Contamination
  - Infection
  - Self-trauma
  - Necrotic tissue
  - Seroma
  - Foreign material
  - Neoplasia
  - Poor blood supply
  - Mechanical disruption
- **Systemic:**
  - Anaemia
  - Hypoproteimaemia
  - Malnutrition
  - Obesity
  - Endocrine disease

Figure 54. Negative influences on wound healing.

Open Wound Management

When presented with a patient with an open wound, it is essential not to focus solely on the wound (unless there is profuse bleeding or an open body cavity which requires immediate life-saving intervention), but ensure **a full clinical history is taken** including appreciating the aetiology of the wound, as well as thorough, **complete physical examination** so that additional clinical findings are not overlooked.

For example, puncture wounds to the chest may appear relatively minor at first glance, but knowing the patient was attacked by a larger dog, picked up and shaken raises concerns for crush injury to the body wall, pneumothorax, broken ribs, whiplash and head injury, all of which are of greater concern than the skin defects which might be initially observed.

Goals of Open Wound Management

The aim of wound management is to **optimise the conditions for body's natural wound healing process.** (Figure 80 Chapter 6).

Important considerations include:
- **prevention of further contamination** of the wound (skin preparation)
- wound **decontamination**
- **promotion of granulation tissue** formation, epithelialization, and contraction.

Skin Preparation

Wounds should be filled with sterile gel lubricant (Figure 55) to keep them moist and to prevent adhesion of further skin and hair debris during clipping and preparation of the surrounding skin. The wound may be temporarily closed with towel clips or skin staples where the edges can be opposed.

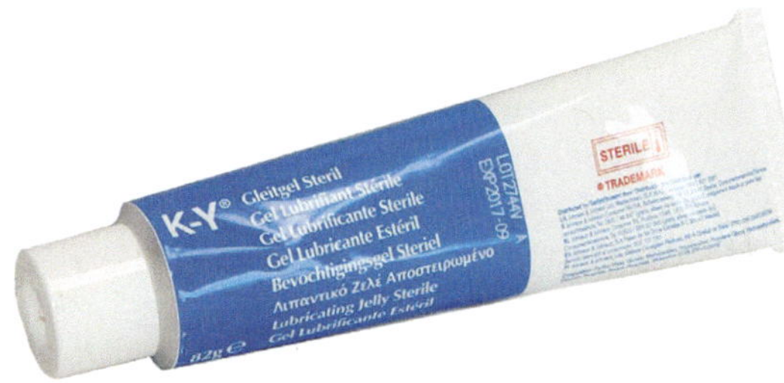

Figure 55. Sterile gel lubricant.

Hair at the wound edges should be removed with scissors dipped in mineral oil so the hair sticks to the blades rather than falling into the wound. The affected body region should be extensively clipped and prepared, as if for surgery, even if surgery is to be delayed, in order to achieve adequate decontamination of the wound and prevent recontamination from the surrounding area once the wound is dressed.

Wound Decontamination

Following adequate preparation of the surrounding tissue, the wound itself (Figure 56) must be decontaminated by a combination **of lavage, debridement, and administration of antibiotic therapy.** These steps may be taken in parallel, with initial lavage prior to debridement and a subsequent final lavage before wound dressing or closure.

Lavage: the principle of lavage of a wound is to dilute the bacterial contamination and to mechanically remove debris from the wound.

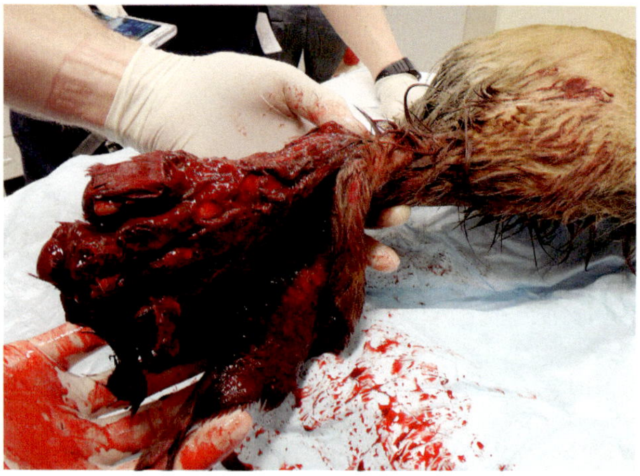

Figure 56. A heavily contaminated degloving wound following a road traffic accident.

Once the periphery of the wound has been clipped and prepared, temporary skin staples or towel clips should be removed.

Gross contamination and necrotic tissue may simply be rinsed away with tap water, using a jug, under the tap, or using a shower head. Tap water is hypotonic and nonsterile but is cheap and easily available for the initial flush of the wound. (Figure 57).

Thereafter, **the wound should be managed aseptically** to reduce contamination further. **The ideal lavage solution is sterile and isotonic;** either 0.9% sodium chloride, lactated Ringers or Hartmann's solution may be used. They should be used in large volumes to dilute any residual contamination. Pressures of 7–8 psi are recommended for displacement of debris from wounds. **This can be generated using a 35 ml syringe and an 18–19G needle.** Others use a fluid bag with three way tap, syringe, and needle attached for refilling.

A quick, simple, and effective method is to use an 18G needle (pink) inserted into the port of a fluid bag, firmly squeezing the bag. (Figure 58).

Sterile saline is also available in pressurised spray canisters, ready for ease of use.

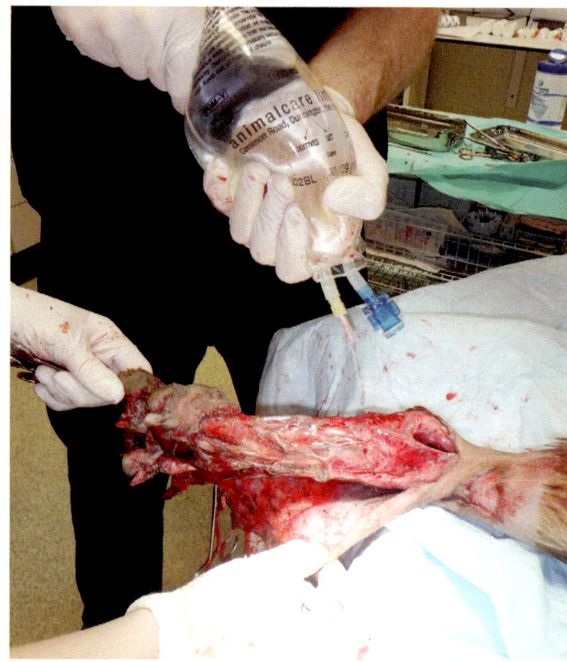

Figure 58. Lavage of the wound with sterile isotonic saline.

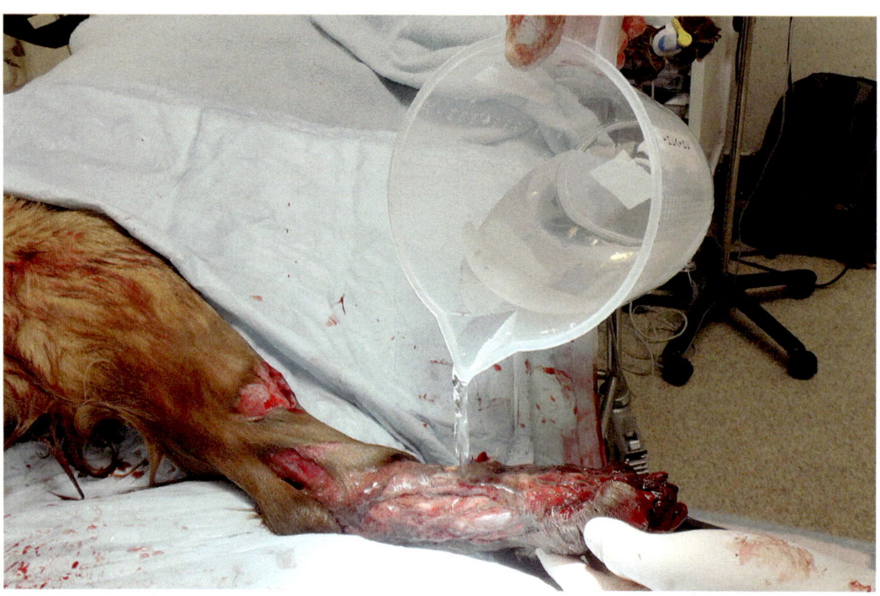

Figure 57. Tap water lavage.

Debridement

Debridement is the removal of necrotic or devitalised tissue and foreign debris from the wound. This reduces the burden for debridement by macrophages within the wound bed, and helps limit infection. Good debridement of a wound often converts a contaminated wound into one which may be surgically closed. This process may require a staged approach (**layered debridement**) in order to reassess tissue viability on a daily basis in order to limit initial overzealous removal of tissue. Whilst loose skin and subcutaneous fat may be removed relatively ruthlessly, the surgeon needs to be sparing of bone, tendons, and ligaments, and in areas around large blood vessels.

- **Sharp debridement:** refers to the use of surgical instruments to cut away an area of compromised tissue. (Figure 59).
- **En bloc debridement:** is the complete surgical excision of a wound in a region with no vital structures and sufficient skin to close the wound following removal of the compromised tissue.
- **Non-surgical debridement:** may be performed using debridement dressings, enzymatic agents or maggots.

Antibiotic Therapy

Following lavage and debridement wound swabs or tissue samples should be taken for culture and sensitivity testing. **Broad spectrum intravenous antibiotic therapy** should be initiated to help slow the invasion of bacteria within the wound bed. Antibiotic penetration to the wound site may be limited if vascular supply to the region is compromised. Penicillins (e.g. amoxycillin) or first generation cephalosporins (e.g. cephalosporins) are appropriate first line antibiotic choices. With suspicion of anaerobic bacterial involvement, potentiated amoxycillin or clindamycin are appropriate. **Fluoroquinolones should not be used as first line antibiotics** but instead reserved for use following culture and sensitivity testing.

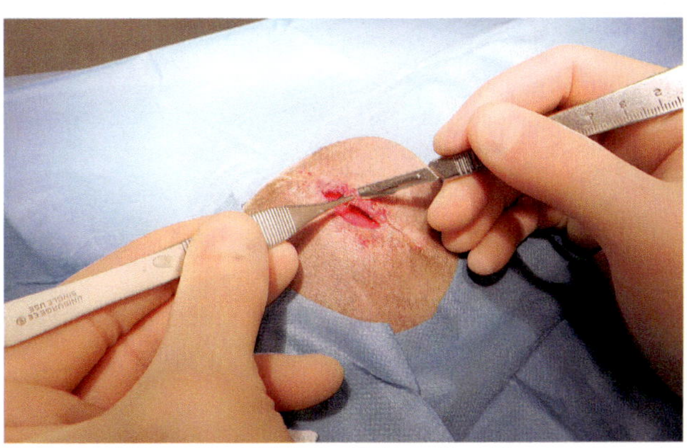

Figure 59. Sharp debridement.

Topical antibiotics should not be used on wounds as they are rapidly diluted and washed out of the wound and are associated with higher rates of multidrug-resistant infections and contact sensitivity in the surrounding skin. **Hence antibiotics should be administered systemically.**

The use of **topical disinfectant agents** has historically been controversial. Chlorhexidine may be used as a 0.05% solution, but **at stronger concentrations is toxic** not only to contaminants but also to host cells including fibroblast and epithelial cells.

499

Newer antibacterial wound products have been developed, such as polyhexanide (Prontosan® wound irrigation solution) (Figure 60) which have been shown to be nontoxic to host cells and to speed the rate of granulation tissue formation when used to manage open wounds in humans. These wound solutions are expensive but are an appropriate choice for the final rinse of the wound following high volume lavage and decontamination with isotonic crystalloid solutions. They also have some residual antibacterial action within the wound.

Following these steps to prepare the skin surrounding the wound, and then decontaminating the wound as thoroughly as is reasonably possible in the first instance, the veterinary surgeon may consider open wound management when the wound:

- is too large to allow closure
- is still too contaminated, but in bloc excision of the wound would result in loss of delicate or structural tissues

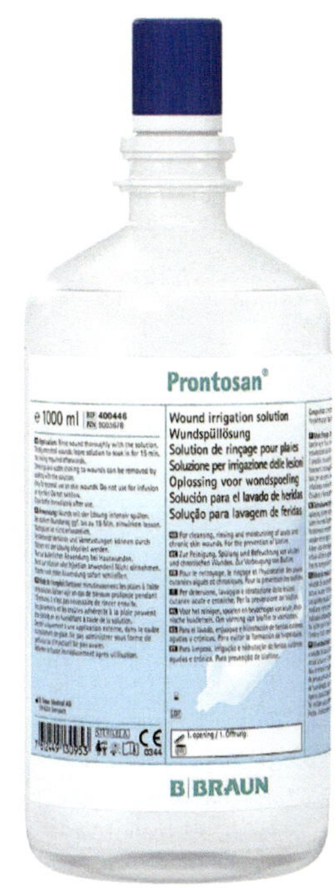

Figure 60. Prontosan (polyhexanide) solution®.

which must be maintained, such as ligaments, tendons and nerves
– has regions of tissue where viability is questionable, and the surgeon chooses to wait and see if this tissue survives rather than debriding overzealously in the first instance.

At this stage the wound must be dressed until the time of reassessment.

Once the wound is converted to a clean wound the surgeon faces the decision to close the wound or continue to manage the wound as an open wound and allow healing by second intention.

The wound should only be closed if:

– there is sufficient tissue to allow tension free closure
– there is no devitalised tissue or foreign material within the wound
– there are no signs of contamination or infection
– the adjacent available skin is healthy.

Wound Dressings

Functions of Dressings and Topical Wound Products

Dressings provide a physical covering of a wound and have a number of functions with respect to the management of a wound:

– aid haemostasis
– debridement
– promote wound healing
– protect the wound from the environment and the patient
– absorb exudate
– eliminate dead space
– apply or relieve pressure
– administer topical medications
– modulate pain.

The ideal dressing provides an optimal combination of these benefits for each individual patient's wound, whilst also being:

– nontoxic
– nonirritant
– nonallergenic
– absorbent
– sterile
– cost effective
– vapour permeable.

Other topical wound products may be used in combination with a dressing to augment their function. These may be liquid or gel formulations, which are applied directly to the wound.

Many veterinarians use the same dressing for management of all wounds without considering the phase of wound healing and dressing properties required to facilitate wound healing. Choosing an inappropriate dressing is not necessarily harmful but might not promote healing as rapidly as possible.

Following the progression of wound healing, initially, open wounds frequently produce a large volume of exudate and contain necrotic debris which requires removal and so **dressings which aid debridement, with high absorbency are indicated.**

As healing progresses, the requirement for debridement and absorbance of exudate reduces and **encouragement of granulation tissue formation** is important.

Occlusive dressings are then indicated once there is no infection present and the wound is fully granulated, to provide a moist, warm healing environment to promote epithelialisation and to protect the surface of the wound (note, it is an old wives' tale that wounds need to be left open to the air; instead a moist, warm, protected environment is preferred).

Dressing Classification

There are a number of criteria under which wound dressings are classified:

– active (interactive or bioactive)/passive
– absorbent/nonabsorbent
– adherent/nonadherent
– permeable/occlusive.

Examples of each category are discussed in the next section. (This list is not exhaustive).

Commonly Used Dressings and Topical Wound Products

These commonly used types of dressing and topical wound products are categorised with respect to their function in the sequence of wound healing. However many of the dressings have more than one function/utility but are listed only once although they may fit into more than one category.

Haemostatic Products

Alginates (e.g. Algosteril®, Algisite M®, Tegagen®, Kaltostat®)

Alginates are derived from seaweed and must be moistened before application. When moist they release calcium into the

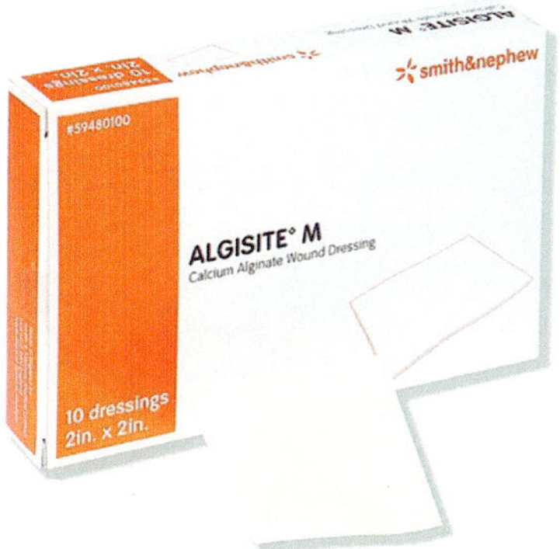

Figure 61. Algisite®.

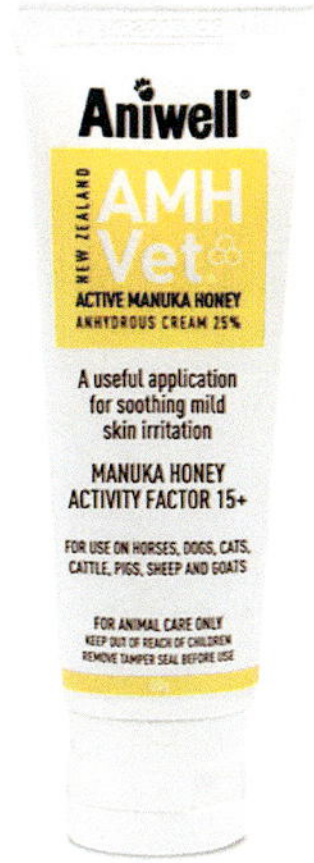

Figure 62. Medical grade Manuka honey.

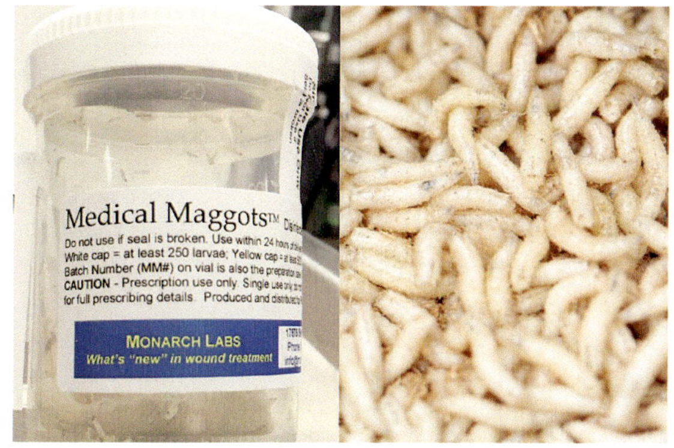

Figure 63. Medical grade maggots.

wound, which aids coagulation and stimulates the formation of granulation tissue. They are also able to absorb wound exudate to form a gel, which can be lavaged from the wound. They do however require a second dressing layer to keep them in place. The fibres can be irritant to surrounding tissue and so should be trimmed to fit within the wound bed. (Figure 61).

Debridement Products

Honey

Manuka honey (Figure 62) is a relatively inexpensive topical wound product which is natural and nontoxic. **The high sugar content draws fluid from the wound, reducing tissue oedema, and aiding wound debridement.** Honey also lowers the pH of the wound to around pH 5, plus has natural antibacterial properties, which help decontaminate the wound bed. Honey for use on wounds needs to be **medical grade** to be specific pathogen free (spf), due to the risk of clostridial spores in regular honey.

Some experts dislike the sticky brown consistency, which resembles a purulent discharge, and instead prefer to use other antibacterial topical products that are more efficient.

Gauze Swabs (wet to dry, dry to dry)

Lint free, woven, sterile, gauze swabs, such as those used for surgery, make cheap and efficient, adherent, absorbent dressings, which rapidly aid debridement of the wound. They are applied dry to highly effusive wounds (**dry to dry**), or wet to less effusive wounds (**wet to dry**), and then allowed to dry out over 12–24 hours before removal, which helps to strip away debris from the wound.

Wet to dry dressings are commonly moistened with saline; however antibacterial solutions may also be considered (e.g. polyhexanide solution).

Removal is painful and requires sedation or general anaesthesia, which needs to be repeated for frequent changes. These dressings also risk damaging healthy tissue and so must be accurately placed and only used where appropriate.

When placing a gauze dressing, in order to maximise debridement, the surface contact must be maximised with the gauze unfolded and packed into every crevice within the wound.

Maggots (Figure 63)

Stage 1 larval maggots digest liquid protein and hence produce accurate and efficient debridement of the wound. They must however be medical grade.

When they develop into stage 2 larvae, their mouthparts are then capable of damaging intact skin but feed on wound exudate and necrotic tissue preferentially. They should be left on superficial wounds for a maximum of three days before being removed and replaced with a new batch.

These are not a simple option to keep on the shelf ready for use but might be useful if ordered in for specific cases, for those that can stomach applying them and removing them afterwards.

Hydrocolloids (e.g. Tegasorb®, Granuflex®, Cutinova®, Compeed®) (Figure 64)

These are adhesive dressings capable of absorbing a moderate volume of fluid, leading to a change in texture. They gently debride the wound and provide a moist environment, encouraging granulation and epithelialisation. They are also waterproof, and commonly used for management of decubital ulcers and blisters in humans, however due to their expense and lack of adherence to small animal skin, they are seldom used in the veterinary field.

Hydrogels (Figure 65)

Hydrogels are gel consistency, topical wound agents, which

interact with the wound, conform to the uneven surface, hydrate debris to aid removal, but also provide a moist wound environment for encouragement of granulation tissue formation. They require a second dressing to keep them in place and provide a barrier function. They also have a cool, soothing effect providing a degree of analgesia.

Basic hydrogels, such as Intrasite® allow anaerobic bacterial growth **and are contraindicated for infected wounds.** Prontosan® wound gel contains polyhexanide (a disinfectant) which helps to maintain a sterile wound environment. Nu-Gel® also contains alginates, which help to promote granulation tissue formation.

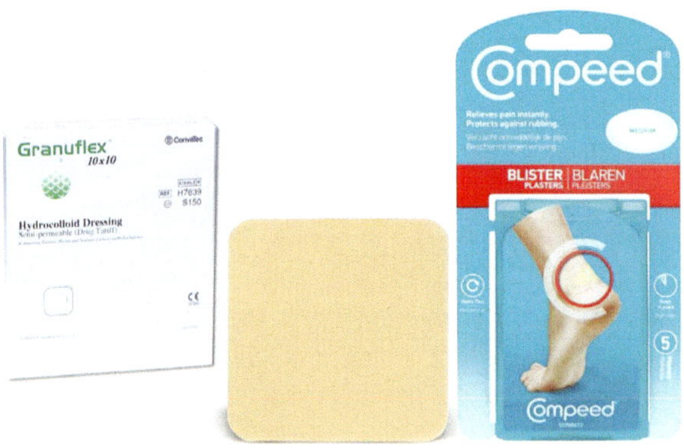

Figure 64. Hydrocolloids.

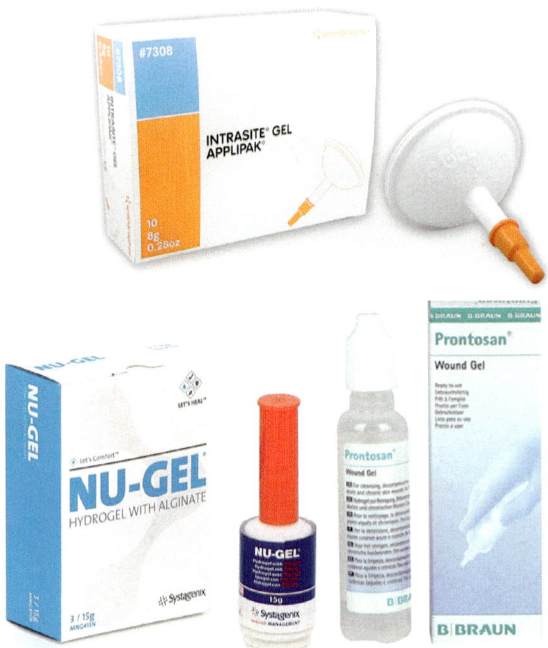

Figure 65. Hydrogels.

Debriding Ointment (e.g. Dermisol®) (Figure 66)

Mixtures of weak acids and propylene glycol in a cream debride wounds by causing differential swelling of healthy and necrotic tissue. They may be used early in the management of contaminated wounds but are toxic to healthy granulation tissue due to their acidity and so should be discontinued as this begins to form.

Absorbent Dressings

Hydrophilic Polyurethane Foams

These foams act primarily to absorb fluid from the wound. They come in a variety of shapes and sizes for use in cavities and on the surface of wounds. They maintain a moist wound environment which allows granulation tissue formation and epithelialisation. They may absorb up to ten times their own weight in fluid from the wound. (Figure 67).

These dressings usually have a semipermeable outer coating and so must be used the right way up. They have a pink outer surface which is intended to mimic the skin of the human patients for whom they are designed.

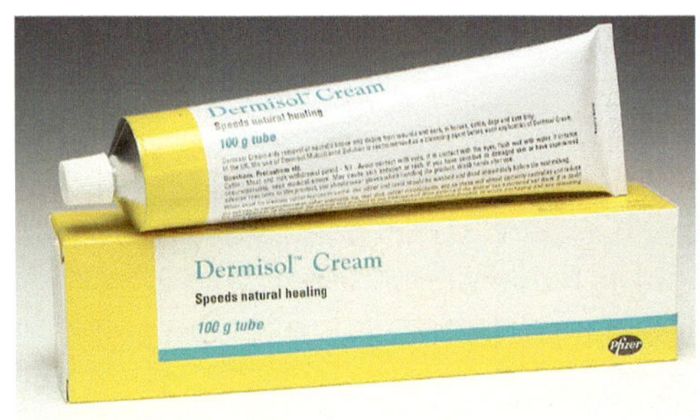

Figure 66. Dermisol®.

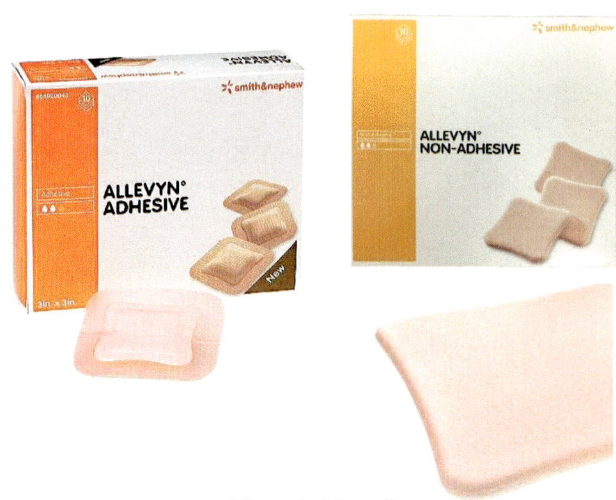

Figure 67. Allevyn®.

Nappies

Nappies are designed to be the ultimate in fluid absorbers and are useful in the management of some highly effusive wounds (Figure 68). They may be weighed prior to placement and following removal to allow calculation of fluid losses via the wound. They are not produced to be sterile but may be individually packed and sterilised in ethylene oxide prior to use. The main risk with nappies is that they may be toxic and caustic and so it is essential the patient cannot interfere with them.

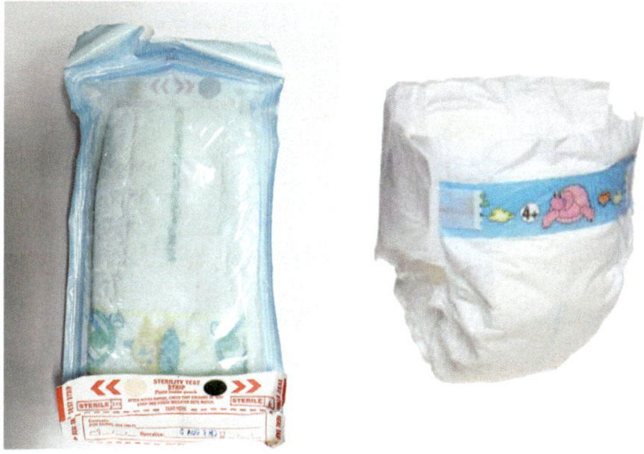

Figure 68. Nappies.

Negative Pressure Wound Therapy (NPWT)

Negative pressure wound therapy (Figure 69) **is the application of suction to a wound through a gauze or foam dressing using a specialised suction device.** An airtight seal is created around the gauze or foam using vapour permeable film dressing material. This is covered with a padded bandage to prevent traumatisation and puncture of the dressing which would result in leakage and trigger an alarm from the suction device.

Negative pressure wound therapy is shown to reduce tissue oedema, improve tissue perfusion, promote granulation tissue formation, with greater vascular development and remove wound exudate.

Negative pressure wound therapy is indicated following the debridement phase, in order to promote granulation tissue formation, but also used to help achieve drainage, tissue immobilization, and promote vascularisation with free skin grafts. Another advantage of negative pressure wound therapy dressings, is that for effusive wounds, the effusion is removed from the wound bed and into the storage cannister, meaning dressings can remain in place for up to three to four days at a time between changes, meaning the patient might require less frequent intervention and sedation.

Patients remain connected to the suction pump continuously whilst the dressing is in place, requiring it to be carried (or placed in a harness pack on larger dogs) when walking.

Antibacterial Dressings

Silver

Silver sheet dressings (e.g. Acticoat®) contain nanocrystals of silver (Figure 70). These release silver ions into the wound, which **in vitro inhibit the growth of virtually all bacteria and fungi.**

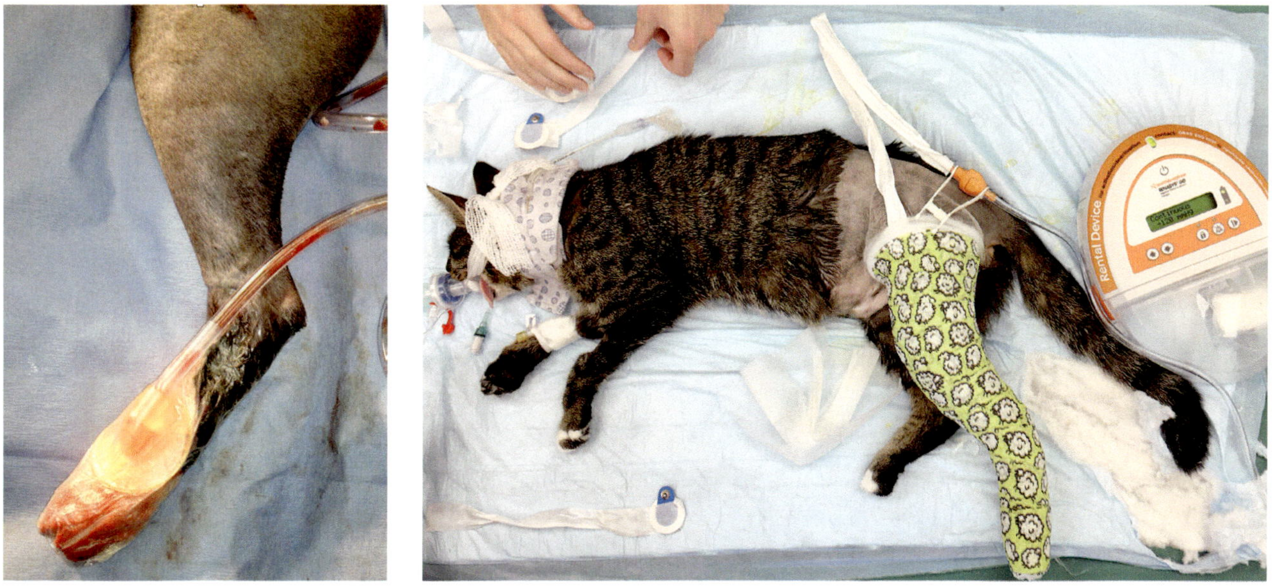

Figure 69. Negative pressure wound therapy (NPWT).

Silver sulphadiazine cream (Flamazine®) may be applied to the surface of the wound, or to fill a wound cavity. This treatment is often used for **Gram-negative sepsis** in human burn patients, with action demonstrated against *MRSA*, *Pseudomonas* and *Enterococcus spp.* Silver dressings are also available as sheets which may be applied to the surface of the wound.

Promotors of Granulation/Epithelialisation

Aloe Vera

Acemannan is a chemical found in aloe vera, which activates macrophages and fibroblasts and hence accelerates the rate of granulation tissue formation. For use on open wounds, purified, sterile versions of the product should be used.

Collagens (e.g. Collamend®, Biosist®, Emovet®)

In human and veterinary wounds, these dressings reduce wound contraction and promote early epithelialisation over the incorporated collagen. They have however not been shown to lead to an overall improvement in the rate of wound healing. **They should not be used in infected wounds.** Evidence to support their use is limited at present.

Moisture Retention Dressings

Perforated Polyurethane Membranes (PPM) (Figure 71)

These are gas permeable, thin (hence a low absorbance capacity) dressings with a low adherence. Over open wounds, when left in place too long then capillary loops may grow into the holes in the dressing, causing adherence and bleeding/pain on removal.

These are most frequently used as a short term covering for a closed surgical incision but are often also used to provide a light covering for wounds in the latter stages of healing. They are manufactured as isolated sheets (e.g. Melolin®, Zorbpad®) or with an adhesive perimeter strip to adhere around the wound or surgical site (e.g. Primapore®).

Vapour Permeable Films (Figure 72)

Minimal Adherence Dressings

These dressings have the specific purpose of reducing adherence to the wound bed. They provide no absorbency themselves and wick fluid through to their outer surface and hence require a secondary absorbent layer. They are most commonly used over free skin grafts to minimise disruption of graft take when dressings are changed in the first week after surgery.

Paraffin Gauze

Paraffin gauze (Figure 73) provides a low adherence protecting layer over the wound, which wicks fluid through to the secondary layer. The paraffin component leaves a sticky residue on the wound, and may itself inhibit epithelialisation, but these dressings are relatively inexpensive and so frequently used to cover skin grafts with a minimally adherent layer.

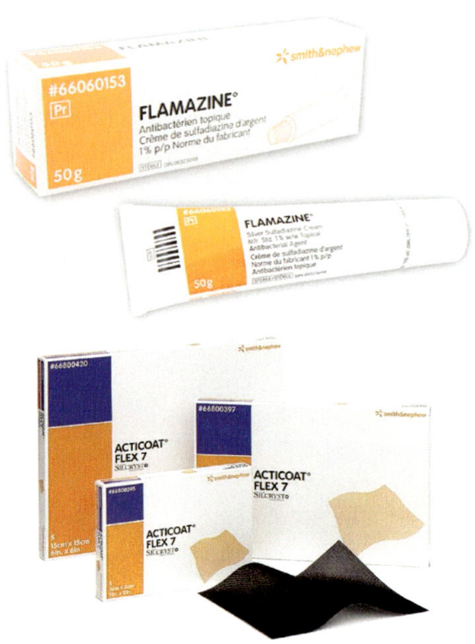

Figure 70. Silver sulfadiazine wound ointment and Nanocrystalline wound dressings.

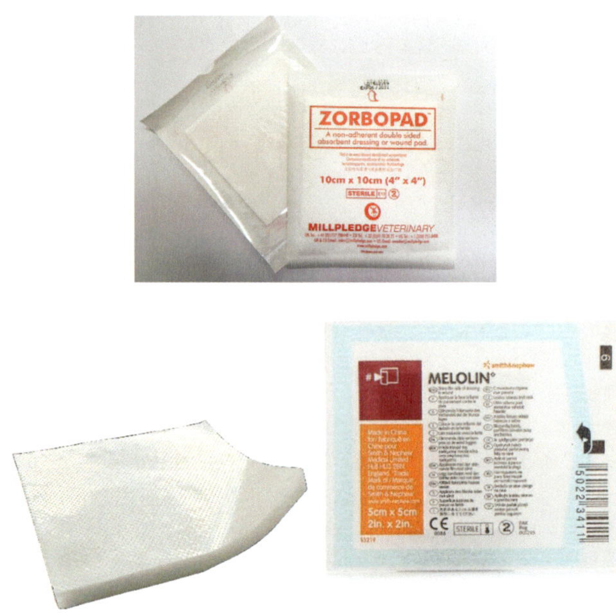

Figure 71. Perforated polyurethane membrane dressings.

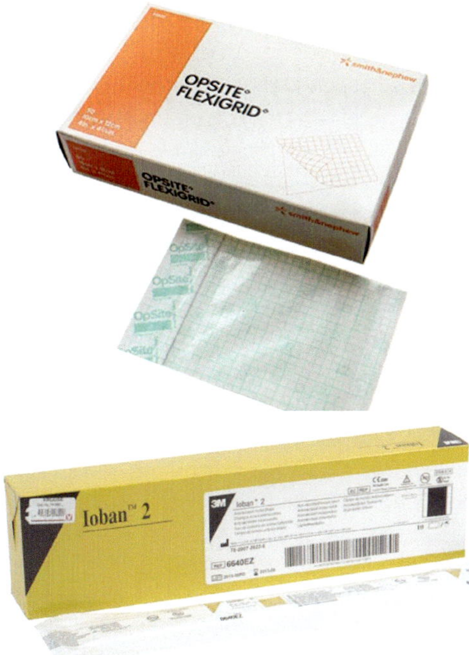

Figure 72. Vapour permeable films.

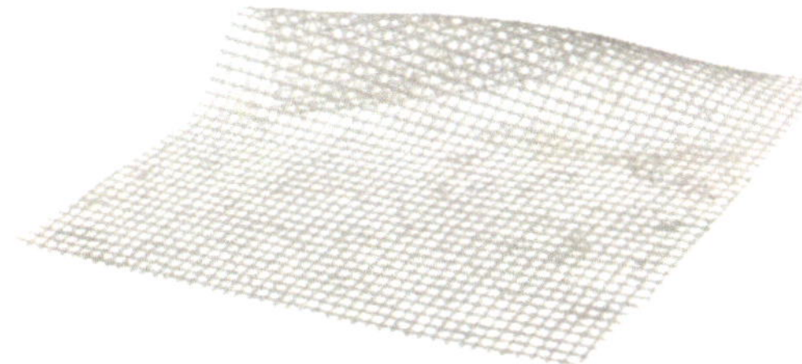

Figure 73. Paraffin gauze.

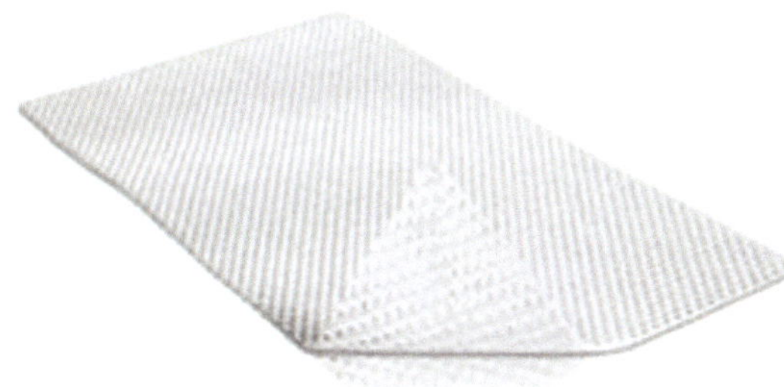

Figure 74. Silicone mesh.

Silicone Mesh (e.g. Mepitel®)

This is a medical grade silicone dressing, which is soft and easy to apply (Figure 74). The mesh allows fluid to pass through the dressing to a secondary layer, but unlike paraffin gauze is not coated with paraffin to achieve this low adherence, and so has no harmful effect on the wound.

However, these are expensive, but can be washed and sterilised in an autoclave for a second use on the same patient.

Barrier Films (e.g. Opsite Spray™, Cavilon™)

These spray on dressings provide a **waterproof film** when dried on, which helps to protect the skin surrounding an effusive wound or bodily orifice, e.g. from urine scalding. They may help with adherence of other dressings.

Bandaging and Supports

Functions of Bandages

Bandages (Figure 75 and 84) are placed for a variety of reasons in different circumstances, from a first aid temporary covering to provide pressure to a bleeding wound, to a supportive

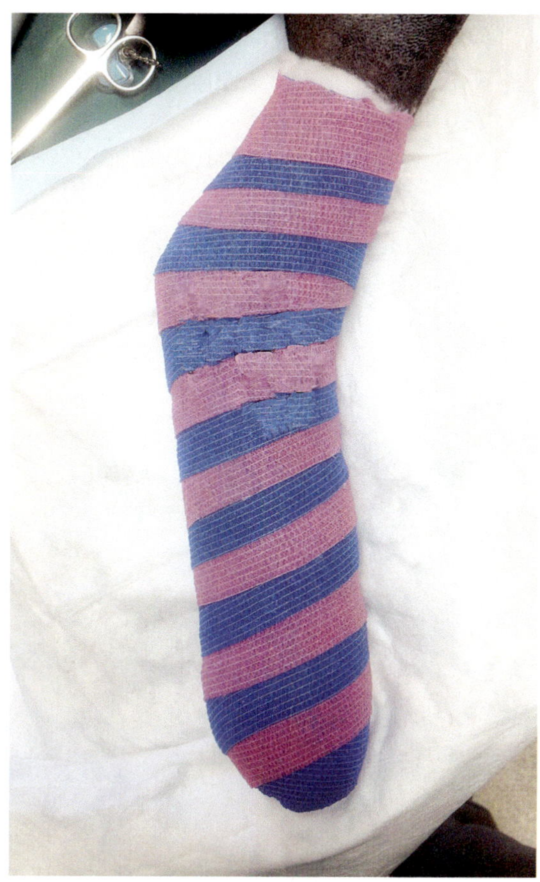

Figure 75. Bandaged limb.

stabilising bandage used to immobilise a fractured bone, and to allow healing and alleviate pain associated with movement at the fracture site. Ultimately, the functions of bandages include:

- aid haemostasis
- promote healing
- protect wounds from the environment and the patient
- absorb exudate
- eliminate dead space
- apply or relieve pressure
- modulate pain
- improve aesthetics
- restrict or allow safe movement
- immobilise, stabilise, and/or support underlying structures.

The ideal bandage provides an optimal combination of these benefits for the patient, depending on the nature of their injuries. Hence each bandage is tailored to the individual patient's needs and risks, rather than repeating a standard formula used for all bandaging.

Bandaging Layers

(See Figure 76).

Primary Contact Layer

The primary contact layer is the dressing that is in direct contact with the wound bed. The type of dressing is selected on a case by case basis, dependent on the stage of wound healing and degree of exudation from the wound.

Intermediate (secondary) Layer

The primary contact layer is held in place by the outer layers of the bandage. The outer layers are typically applied circumferentially to the limbs, tail, head and trunk. (Figure 77).

The intermediate layers function is to hold the primary layer in position and provide additional support, absorbence capacity, padding and protection. Cotton wool was historically used, but a variety of synthetic and natural similar products are now available. They have different densities which provide different levels of absorbency, and stiffness and support, and may be selected appropriately for an individual bandage. For example, a Robert-Jones type bandage to support a broken limb requires a denser and thicker, more supportive bandage than a light padded covering to protect a healing superficial wound.

When applying a bandage to a limb, it is common to **leave the toenails of the third and fourth digits accessible through the open end of the bandage** to allow assessment every few hours for evidence of swelling/divergence, pain, hypothermia, hyperthermia, and changes in sensation. It is essential that only the nails are exposed as any vascularised tissue which is not adequately supported by the bandage is at risk of swelling and biological tourniquet from above (Figures 78 and 79). When the pes requires dressing due to wounds or incisions at this level, the toes are completely wrapped within the bandage. Padding is placed between the digits to prevent pressure sores, especially if the paw has been clipped and in thin skinned breeds.

The secondary layer material typically generates minimal tension as they have no elasticity. They should be applied smoothly and evenly but cannot be used to create any compression.

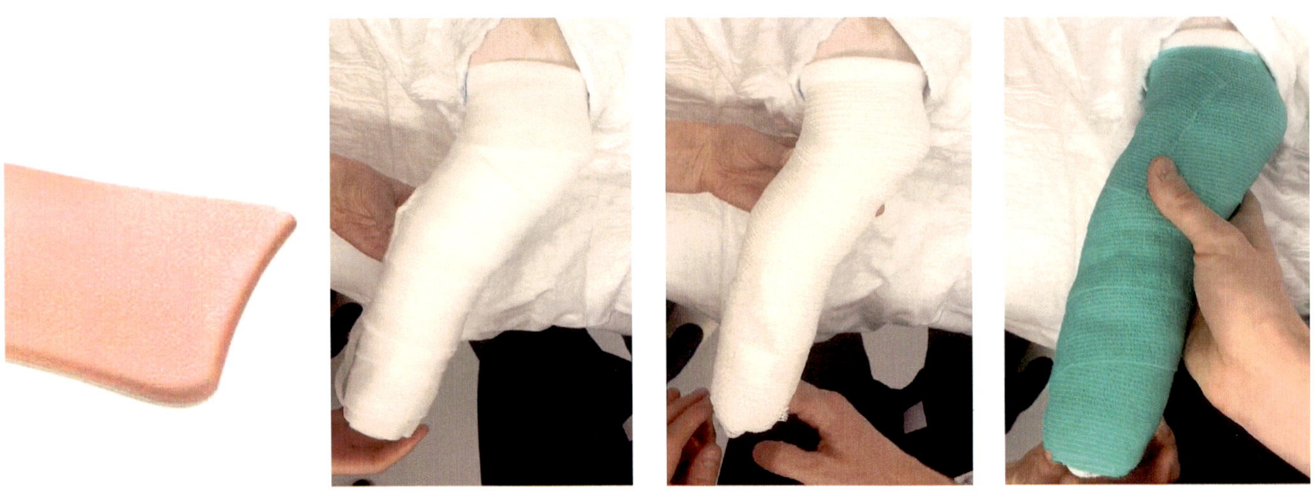

Figure 76. Bandage layers.

Outer (tertiary) Layer

The function of the outer layer is to generate the required level of pressure and support under the bandage (Figure 80). The pressure may be required to control haemorrhage, prevent swelling, support and stabilise underlying tissue and hold other bandage layers in position.

Materials used may be elastic or inelastic, adhesive, or cohesive (selfadhesive), porous, or waterproof and come in a variety

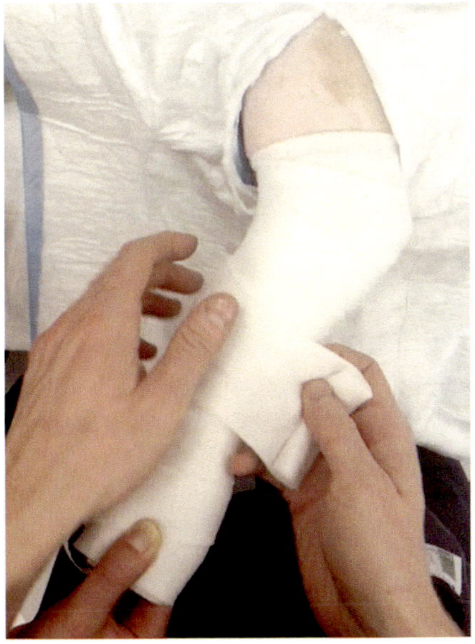

Figure 77. Intermediate layer.

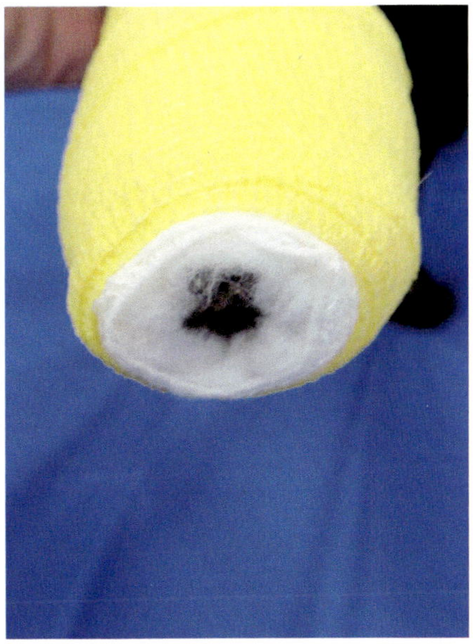

Figure 78. View of the end of the limb demonstrating that the toe nails are still visible.

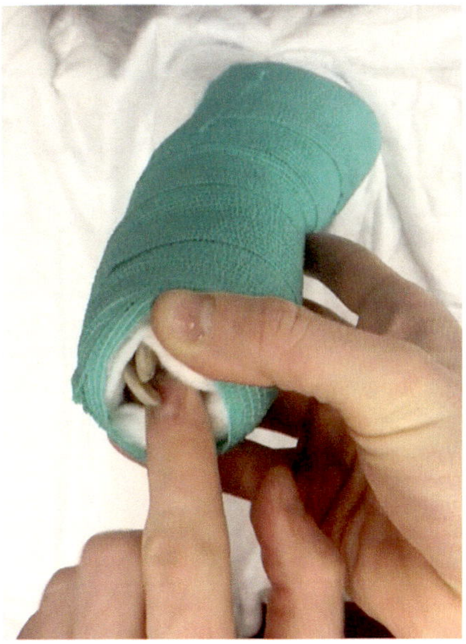

Figure 79. Toes being palpated to checked for excessive swelling, coldness or warmth and discomfort.

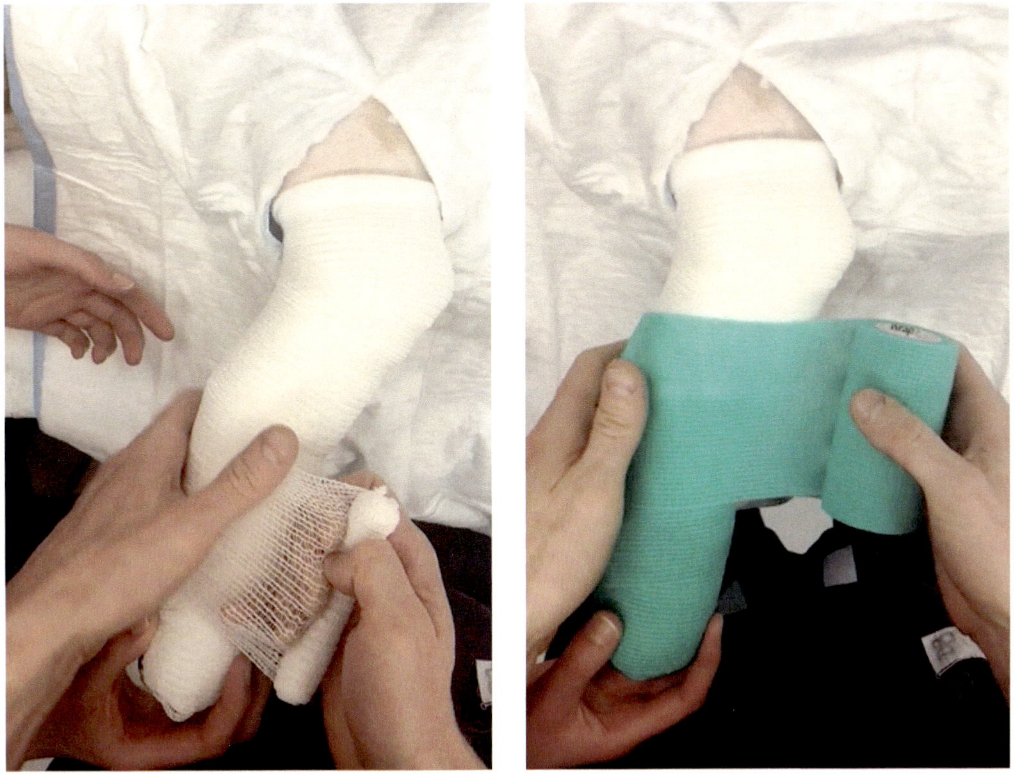

Figure 80. Application of tertiary conforming and protective layers of a bandage, ensuring even tension along the limb during application.

of widths. Often more than one tertiary layer is used to make the best compromise of these properties, using an inelastic, porous, nonadhesive layer to conform the secondary layer and apply the required pressure and support, then covered with a cohesive, water repellent layer applied loosely over the top to maintain and protect the underlying layers.

Anchoring a Bandage to Prevent Slipping

Stirrups

Limb bandages tend to slip distally due to the tapering shape of canine and feline limbs. **Stirrups** (Figure 81) **are strips of adhesive tape placed lengthways along the limb,** beyond the toes, which are then reflected and adhered to the tertiary layer of the bandage, to provide friction and prevent the bandage slipping.

Tape Overlay Strips

Similarly bandages on the torso tend to slip caudally, and so placing **a strip of adhesive tape on the skin/fur at the cranial extent of a body bandage,** before then placing a bandage with a 50% overlap with this strip, then allows a second layer of adhesive tape to be placed to secure the cranial end of the tertiary bandage layer to the original tape strip.

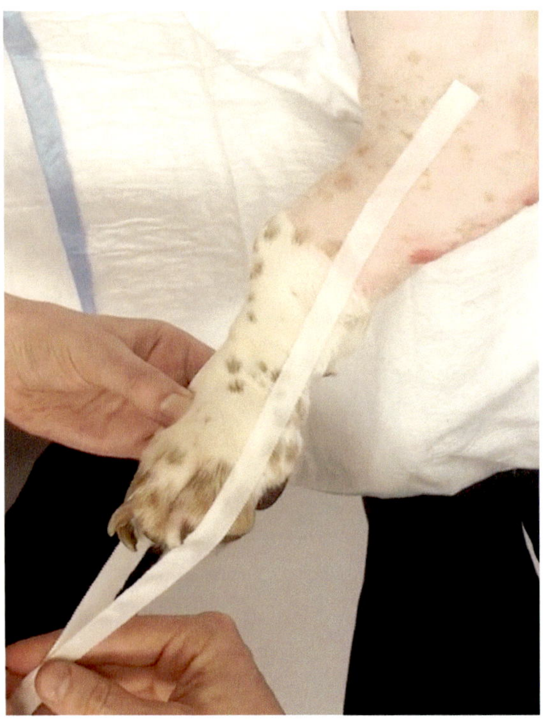

Figure 81. Stirrups being anchored to the limb before bandage placement.

- **Elasticated adhesive tape should never be placed circumferentially around the body or a limb, as it will tighten, especially if it becomes wet, creating a biological tourniquet.**
- **Hence strips should be placed three quarters of the way around the body.**

Tie-over/Bolus Dressings

Some regions of the body are not amenable to circumferential bandaging, and so a primary contact layer may be secured in position by **lacing umbilical (Nylon®) tape between loosely placed skin sutures.** (Figure 82).

Alleviation of Pressure Points

Pressure relief can be achieved by creating an empty space under a bandage to off load the pressure from the outer layers over a bony prominence. This is achieved by the use of **a ring doughnut of padding placed with the central opening over the bony prominence** which requires protecting (Figure 83). Care must be taken not to displace the doughnut as additional bandage layers are circumferentially applied over the top.

Doughnuts can be made (Video 1) by cutting slices of foam pipe insulation.

In some situations, pressure relief over a bony prominence is achievable by **reducing the prominence of the bone,** i.e. by

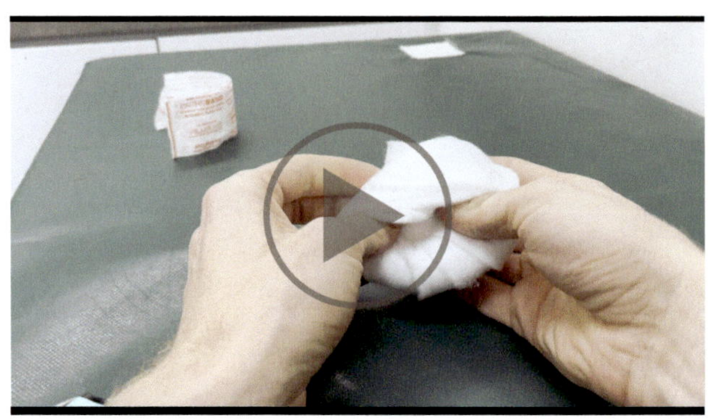

Video 1. A video called "Making a doughnut" can be found in this site: https://publicationen.improveinternational.com.

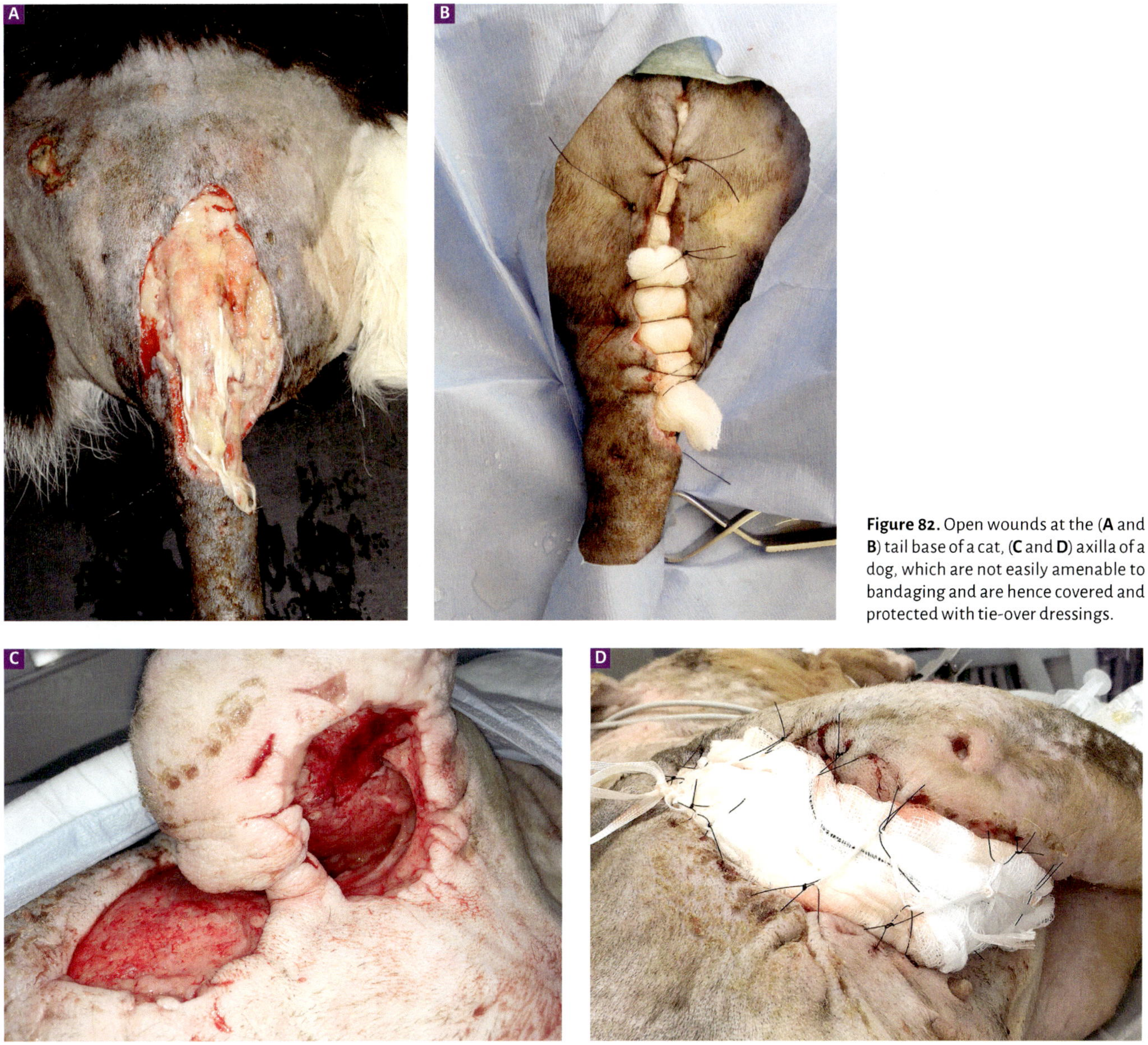

Figure 82. Open wounds at the (**A** and **B**) tail base of a cat, (**C** and **D**) axilla of a dog, which are not easily amenable to bandaging and are hence covered and protected with tie-over dressings.

splinting the elbow in full extension to reduce the prominence of the olecranon, or the tarsus to achieve something similar for the calcaneus.

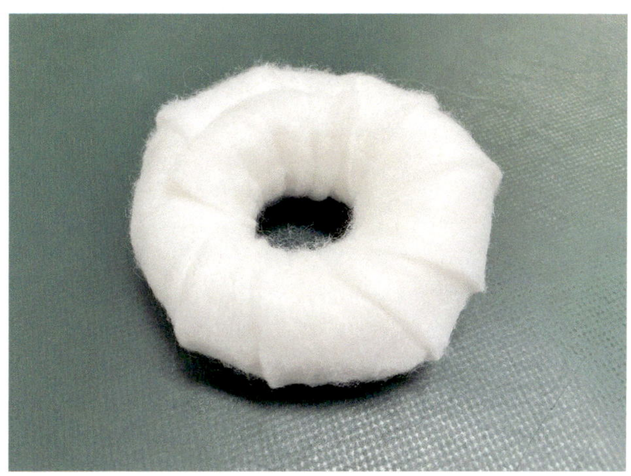

Figure 83. Doughnut.

Application and Changing a Bandage

Applying the Bandage

Circumferential bandage layers should be applied with a 50% overlap with the previous layer. The layers should be applied with even tension and without folds or wrinkles to prevent ridges forming, which might result in areas of increased pressure when the outer conforming layers are placed.

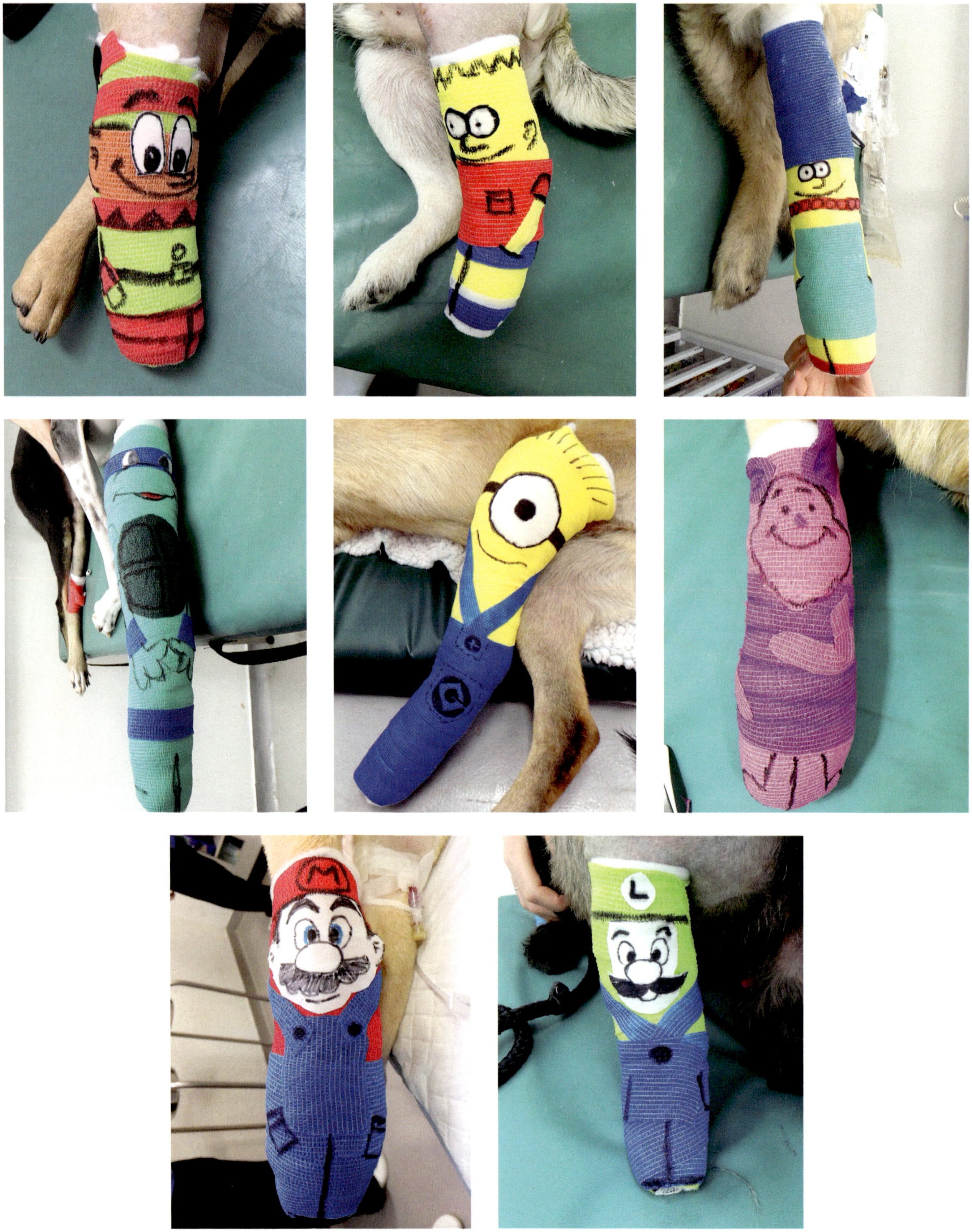

Figure 84. Bandage art.

Laplace's law applies to the application of bandages. **In general, limbs become narrower more distally, the pressure gradient of a bandage applied evenly increases from proximal to distal.**

$$P = (N \times T) / (R \times W)$$

Pressure = (**N**umber of layers x **T**ension) / (**R**adius of the limb x **W**idth of bandage)

The exception to this rule is proximal to the carpus and tarsus as in most patients the limb here becomes narrower, hence, an even thickness bandage results in higher pressure above the carpus or tarsus, which risks creating a biological tourniquet. For this reason, it is essential that additional padding (intermediate layer) is placed at this level to fill the void, such that when the outer, conforming layers are placed, they form an even or widening column as they are placed up the leg. This is achieved by overlapping by more than 50% for an appropriate number of turns at this level.

It is the tertiary layer which is critical in generating the required (and not excessive) pressure under the bandage and for which knowledge of this equation is essential.

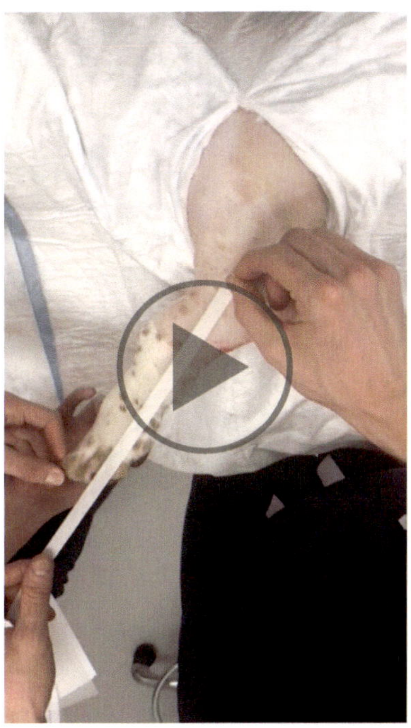

Video 2. A video called "Bandaging" can be found in this site: https://publicationen.improveinternational.com.

Changing the Bandage

The primary layer (dressing) should be changed when it has become saturated (strike through), or when its properties are no longer appropriate for the stage of wound healing and/or the amount of exudate. If moisture from the wound reaches the outer layers of a dressing or bandage, there is potential for bacteria and contaminants to wick in from the outside to the wound surface resulting in infection.

Fluid production from a wound typically reduces over time, and so can the interval between dressing changes. Infected wounds are usually more exudative and hence require more frequent interventions. Initially a highly effusive and contaminated wound needs **dressing changes every 12–24 hours.** A wound sealed with healthy granulation tissue, which produces minimal discharge, might only require changes every three to four days.

- **If a dressing becomes adherent to the wound bed, it should be moistened with sterile saline or 2% lidocaine for a few minutes to minimize trauma to the wound bed and discomfort for the patient.**
- **This does not apply to wet to dry dressings which are intended to adhere to the wound bed in order to help strip away contamination on removal, hence patients require analgesia and usually sedation or anaesthesia for removal of wet to dry dressings.**

Bandages which are placed to prevent swelling or limit movement in the absence of a wound are left in place for longer, although require close monitoring for evidence of complications.

Protection of Bandages

Protection from the Environment

It is essential bandages are kept clean and dry to prevent wicking inwards of bacteria and maceration of the skin if damp and so **waterproof boots** must be used when the patient is walked outside. It is also essential the boot is removed when inside to allow the bandage to breathe. An inexpensive, but durable boot can be crafted from a dry empty, used drip fluid bag. (Figures 85 and 86).

Protection from the Patient

The patient must be prevented from traumatizing or displacing the bandage, and from urinating or defaecating on the bandage. This is achieved with the use of Elizabethan collars or muzzles. For recumbent patients without indwelling urinary catheters, the bandage can be wrapped in a protective layer of an incontinence sheet. Patients require adequate analgesia to prevent the desire to traumatise the dressing due to pain, and some patients may also require sedation.

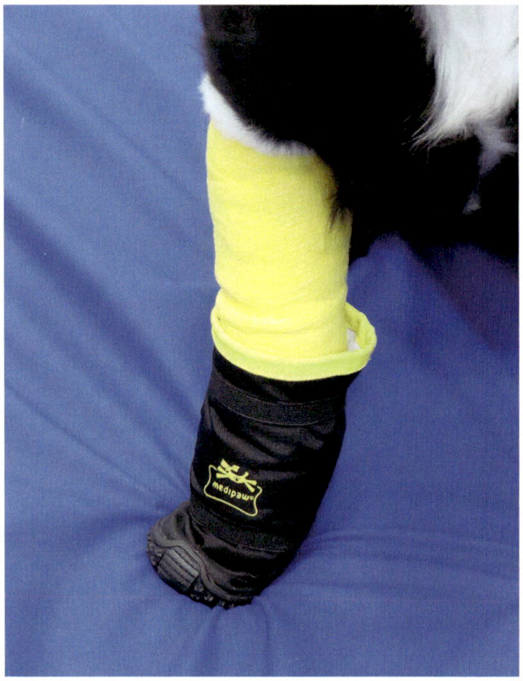

Figure 85. Boot cover.

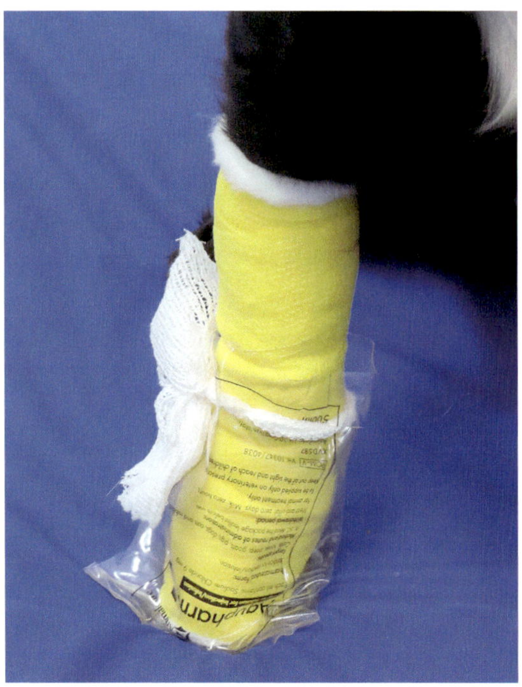

Figure 86. Drip bag boot.

Bandage Related Complications

Bandaging is as much an art form as a science:
- bandaging **too tightly** reduces perfusion of the tissue under the bandage;
- bandaging **too loosely** results in slippage, which might expose a wound, reduce support to the limb, or lead to gathering of the bandage at a distal joint, which might impair blood flow below that level;
- **too lightweight** a bandage may provide insufficient support and allow rapid striking through of fluid from a wound under the bandage which might then secondarily allow wicking of microorganisms from the outside, into the wound; and
- **too heavy and bulky** a bandage impairs a patient's limb function and ability to groom and express normal behaviour more than is necessary.

Hence bandage application must be suited to the specific requirements of the patient and the condition requiring the bandage. Bandages also require regular monitoring.

Bandages require close monitoring for:
- **Getting wet:** this may result in contamination of the wound and maceration of the underlying skin.
- **Slippage down the leg:** this may lead to uncovering of the wound, loss of support and risk of tourniquet if it results in a tightening at the level of a joint.
- **Damage from the environment/patient:** leading to loss of support or wound protection.
- **Swollen toes:** may indicate a tourniquet effect higher up the leg.
- **Excessively warm or cold toes:** may indicate a tourniquet effect, with reduced egress or inflow of blood to the distal limb.
- **Any unusual smell:** indicating necrotic tissue or wound discharge.
- **Any discharge/fluid striking through the bandage:** indicating the need for a dressing change.
- **Worsening limb use** or the patient paying increased attention to the bandage or attempting to chew at the bandage: which might suggest pain due to a loss of support, infection, pressure sore, or loss of blood supply.
- **Swelling of the head and neck** and restricted ability to breathe if the bandage wraps around the patient's body; which might require emergency removal of the bandage.

Splints, Slings, Casts, and Orthotics

In patients where immobilisation of a joint or joints is required, soft dressings may not be sufficient and so incorporation of more rigid components is required.

Splints and Slings

When temporary restriction of joint movement is required, a rigid strut or splint between the outer bandage layers on one side may suffice. This is often in the form of a prefabricated plastic splint which is cut to size and incorporated into the bandage. (Figure 87).

Alternatively, **fiberglass casting material** can be used for a custom-made splint of a specific shape and size for a particular patient. The casting material is applied lengthways up and down the limb, in layers until of sufficient thickness and moulded to the shape of the patient's limb. When custom making a splint, it is important to bear in mind that fibreglass casting material has some inherent elasticity and **shortens following placement but before it sets.**

Custom made fibreglass splints can be reapplied following a bandage change on the same patient, provided a similar bandage is applied below the splint to ensure a good fit.

Splints are useful for partly restricting movement and may be enough to support a fractured limb prior to repair in combination with a supportive bandage, or to limit a joint's movement following management of a luxation. However, they should not be relied upon to manage a fracture in their own right.

A **spica splint** (Figure 88) is a specific name for a laterally applied forelimb splint usually applied to **support and immobilise a shoulder joint.** The splint extends up over the trunk and requires a body bandage as well as a bandage along the length of the limb.

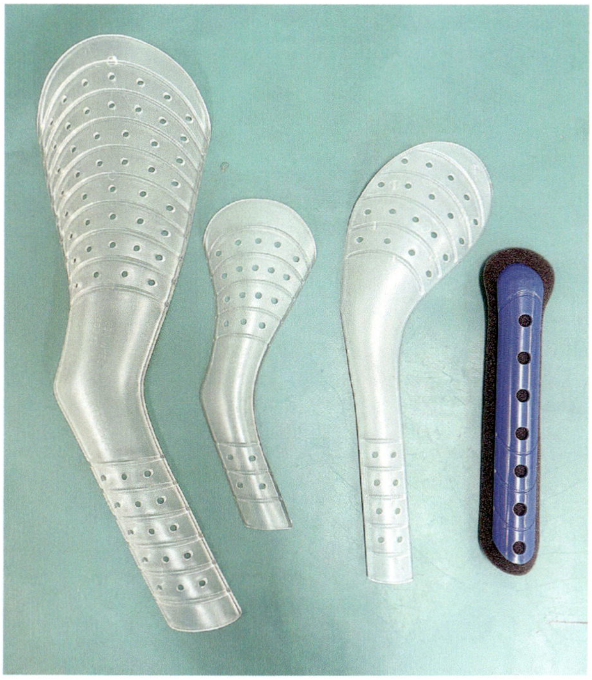

Figure 87. Prefabricated splints.

Slings are soft supports which immobilise and rest joints in a flexed position, often anchored around the body. Examples include the **Velpeau sling,** which offloads the forelimb and **Ehmer sling,** which has traditionally been used following hip luxation, although recently its utility has been questioned. (Figure 89).

Casts

Casts are circumferential splints, traditionally made from plaster of Paris, but nowadays more commonly made from purpose made fibreglass casting material. This is kept in

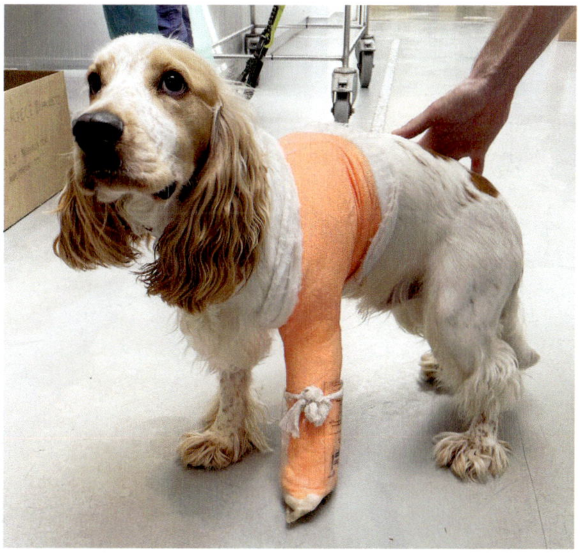

Figure 88. Spica splint.

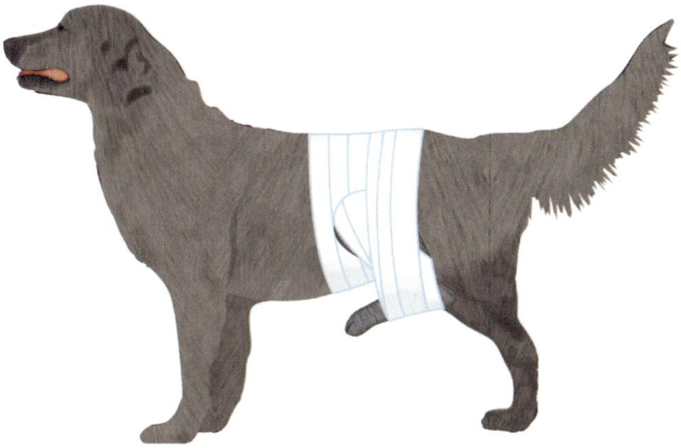

Figure 89. Ehmer sling.

airtight packages and dowsed in water to activate the chemical reaction, which is associated with heat production (an exothermic reaction) and leads to hardening of the fibreglass.

Casts are used to immobilise certain fractures of long bones and usually only considered in young patients with **incomplete, minimally, or non-displaced fractures.** Adequate immobilisation requires **complete immobilisation of the joint above and below the fracture site, which is only possible for a fracture distal to the elbow or stifle joint.**

Cast materials should be placed over the top of sufficient soft padding to protect the soft tissues, but not an excessive amount, which might allow movement within the cast. Usually 3–4 layers of soft padding will suffice but this varies with patient size. The soft padding should extend sufficiently proximal to the cast to prevent rubbing.

Cast material is placed following the conforming tertiary layer of the bandage and **wrapped with a 50% overlap** usually aiming for a total thickness of four layers of cast material to create sufficient thickness and stiffness for an average sized patient. (Figure 90).

At the time of application splitting the cast along two opposite edges should be considered, to create a **bivalve cast** (Figure 91) **to facilitate its removal and replacement** without the need for general anaesthesia, (due to the noise and patient stimulation associated with the use of a cast saw). The cast saw can also cut windows over possible pressure points to prevent sores if appropriate, e.g. over the calcaneus.

Cast saws have **oscillating saw blades,** rather than rotating blades, which minimise the risk of trauma to soft tissue, as the latter usually move with the blade unless tightly tethered. Nevertheless, care should be taken to avoid soft tissue trauma when splitting a cast with a saw.

Adherence of the cast material to the conforming layer below can also hamper removal, and so placement of a layer of stockinet between these layers facilitates removal.

Orthotics

Orthotics or orthoses are used as a solution for long term immobilization. They are often manufactured to the specific requirements of the patient, based on their size and the joint(s) requiring support and the degree of restriction needed. (Figure 92).

Orthotics are designed for long term use for the **management of more severe strains or sprains,** which can take many months to heal; or to off load surgical repair of ruptured tendons or ligaments. They may also be used as non-surgical solutions for unstable joints in patients with comorbidities at high risk for surgical intervention. (Figure 93).

One classification system grade (Figure 94) as:

- **Grade 1 support:** a soft, flexible neoprene (wetsuit material) joint support.
- **Grade 2 support:** a similar soft support, but with restrictive straps limiting movement in specific directions.

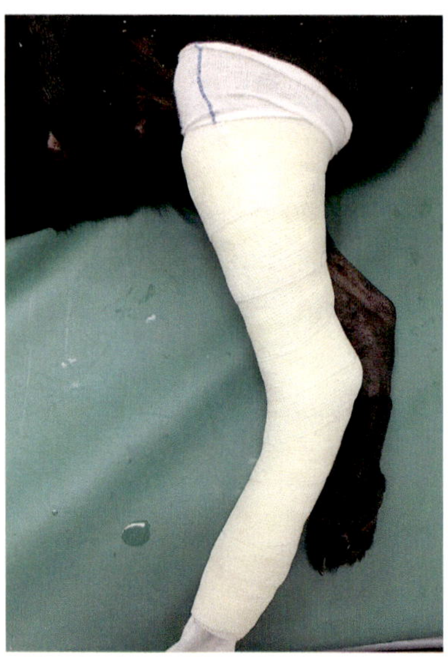

Figure 90. A cast is applied over a stockinette to facilitate removal with separation from the bandage materials underneath.

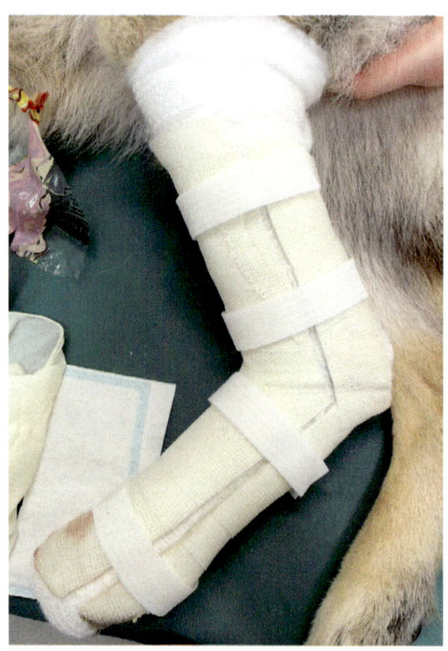

Figure 91. Bivalve cast: following cast placement and setting of the cast material, the cast is split on opposing sides and then taped back together to facilitate removal and replacement in a conscious or sedated patient.

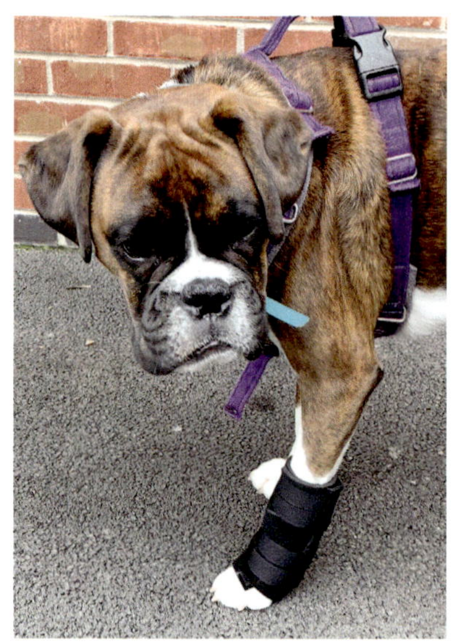

Figure 92. Carpal orthotic.

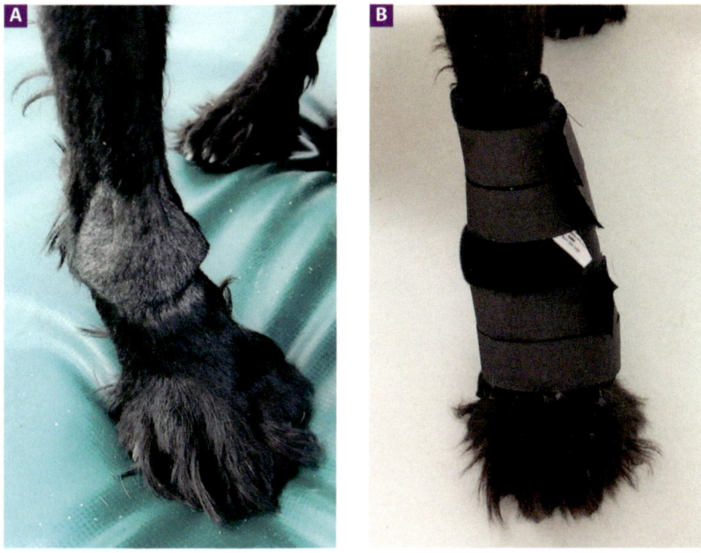

Figure 93. A. Carpal swelling and varus deformity due to joint collapse subsequent to severe polyarthritis; **B.** The same carpus supported with an orthotic.

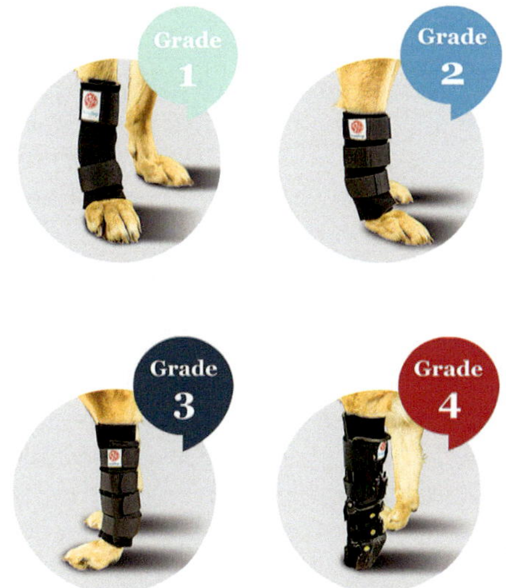

Figure 94. Orthotic grades (with acknowledgement to Scandi Orthopedic for this image).

- **Grade 3 support:** incorporate a custom moulded thermoplastic sheet, which acts as a splint.
- **Grade 4 support:** are custom made, rigid carbon fibre boots (like ski boots) which either completely restrict or only allow certain amounts of movement in specific directions.

Orthotics are designed to be easily removed and replaced by the patient's owners and secured in place with Velcro straps. This allows parts of the device to be replaced and/or washed.

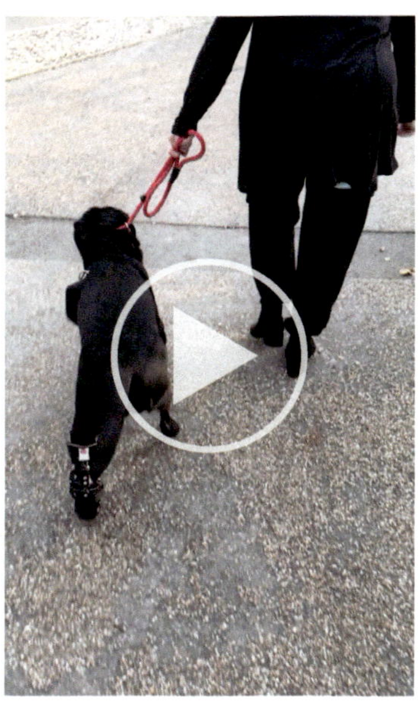

Video 3. A video called "Grade 4 tarsal orthotic" can be found in this site: https://publicationen.improveinternational.com.

Patients may initially be introduced to the orthotic for short periods at a time, e.g. just for exercise, although they are usually well tolerated. Video 3 shows a patient with a grade 4 orthosis placed to protect a tarsal collateral ligament injury; the patient is walking out of hospital immediately following the initial fitting.

Postoperative Management

Postoperative management of patients is equally as important as the surgery performed. It is essential to ensure the patient has the safest and best possible recovery from surgery and minimise the risk of postoperative complications. Surgical nurses play a vital role during patient recovery including monitoring recovery and discussing concerns with the overseeing veterinary surgeon. The surgical nurse is responsible for ensuring adequate nutrition and analgesia and is often instrumental in relaying important information regarding ongoing care to clients, such that care is continued successfully at home.

Monitoring the Surgical Site

Immediately following surgery, surgical incisions require a **protective covering** until the fibrin seal has formed, which usually takes between **6 and 12 hours.** Thereafter the incision is usually left uncovered (unless specifically indicated otherwise e.g. bandaging to provide support or limit swelling) to allow for visual monitoring and assessment.

The covering is often a **sterile adhesive dressing,** but in areas of high movement or contamination cyanoacrylate adhesive layers or spray on dressing materials such as Cavalon™ or Op-site Spray™ may be appropriate, e.g. for perianal incisions.

Surgical incisions should be monitored for **redness, swelling, pain, and heat** (the four signs of inflammation), as well as for **bruising, discharge, dehiscence, and necrosis.** If the initial dressing becomes saturated, the dressing should be changed to prevent wicking of bacteria from the external surface to the wound surface. Depending on the rate of saturation, it might be appropriate to upgrade the dressing to one with a greater absorptive capacity. Assessing and documenting the volume and nature of discharge and informing the veterinary surgeon in case further action is required to manage, treat, or sample the discharge is imperative.

Infection may be suspected based on the presence of incisional discharge, dehiscence, or the presence of any of the signs of inflammation. The clinical suspicion of infection should prompt appropriate isolation of the patient and protection of other hospitalised patients, plus continued monitoring, and sampling of the wound to confirm and categorise the infection and facilitate appropriate treatment.

Postoperative Haemorrhage

Postoperative haemorrhage (reactive or secondary bleeding) should be monitored by documenting visible bleeding from the surgical incision or any accumulation of swelling under the skin at the surgical site as a haematoma (and associated with undue pain at the surgical site).

Vital parameters (including heart rate, pulse quality, mucous membrane colour and respiratory rate and effort) should be monitored intensively in patients with postoperative haemorrhage. Trends should be tracked and intensity of monitoring should be gradually reduced as long as parameters remain stable. The veterinary surgeon should define thresholds for intervention should vital parameters stray beyond certain acceptable levels of variation or blood loss.

In cases of suspected haemorrhage:

- intravenous access should be established/maintained
- direct, cold compression should be applied to the bleeding site (if visible)
- urgent review by the veterinary surgeon should be sought
- imaging, initially by point of care ultrasound (POCUS) should be performed, to assess for fluid accumulation and sampling to confirm haemorrhagic effusion
- blood transfusion/aspiration and autotransfusion should be considered in the case of moderate to severe postoperative haemorrhage.

Warmth, Cooling, and Compression

Warmth

Application of warmth to a surgical site aims to promote blood flow by causing vasodilation, the natural response to dissipate heat from the tissue. Hence warmth is applied to skin of compromised blood supply, to encourage vasodilation and blood flow within the tissue, e.g. following a skin graft of a skin flap transfer procedure, or to a distal limb following trauma and fracture repair which have resulted in reduced blood flow to the foot and a cold extremity.

Warmth also provides comfort and analgesia to some patients, in particular helping to relax injured muscles allowing improved range of motion and flexibility and reducing pain and stiffness in joints affected by osteoarthritis.

Warmth and improved vascular supply may be beneficial to improve drainage and hence reabsorption of seromas.

Warmth is applied by using a hot water bottle, warm wheat bag, or heat pad, wrapped in a clean covering to prevent contamination of the surgical site and to minimise cross contamination between patients. (Figure 95).

Application of warmth is not advised for areas of acute inflammation, including open wounds, areas of active bleeding, and tumours and care should be taken when applying heat to areas of reduced sensation.

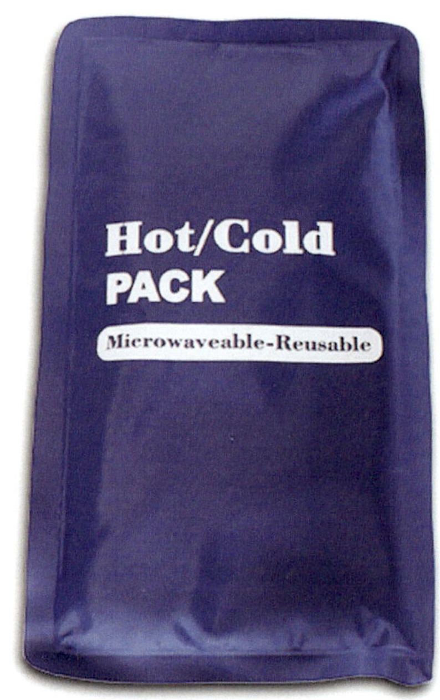

Figure 95. Hot/cold pack.

Cooling

Cooling a surgical site aims to reduce:

- inflammation
- pain
- blood flow: which may aid haemostasis with mild to moderate surgical site bleeding
- oedema
- muscle spasm
- metabolic demand.

Cooling is applied by using an ice pack, frozen peas, or cold pack wrapped in a clean covering (such as a laparotomy swab and cling film) to prevent contamination of the surgical site and to minimise cross contamination between patients.

Cooling is associated with the **Hunting reaction, whereby there is a reactive hyperaemia,** with vasodilation and increase in temperature, which occurs 20–40 min following application of a cold pack.

Cooling therapy should be used with caution in patients with reduced sensation or circulatory problems.

Compression

Compression of a surgical site helps provide **support, reduce oedema/bleeding and soft tissue swelling.**

Compression, in combination with cooling, helps compound the potential benefits and there are specialised devices specifically designed to apply compression and cooling to patient limbs following appendicular surgery. Alternatively, bandaging helps provide ongoing support and compression.

Bandages and Slings

The functions of bandages are mentioned in pages 505 and 506. Splints may be added to bandages to further restrict movement if required. Slings are supportive straps which take the weight of a limb and prevent load bearing. The most commonly used slings are the **Velpeau and Ehmer slings.**

A Velpeau sling supports the forelimb in a flexed position, e.g. following a scapula fracture managed conservatively. The Ehmer sling supports the hind limb in flexion, e.g. following reduction of a craniodorsal hip luxation. **Hobbles** may also be placed between the tarsi to prevent limb abduction, whilst not limiting weight bearing, e.g. to limit recurrence of ventral hip luxation. (Figure 96). Both bandages and slings require careful follow-up monitoring (see **Bandage related complications section**) to ensure correct usage and maximum benefit to the patient's recovery.

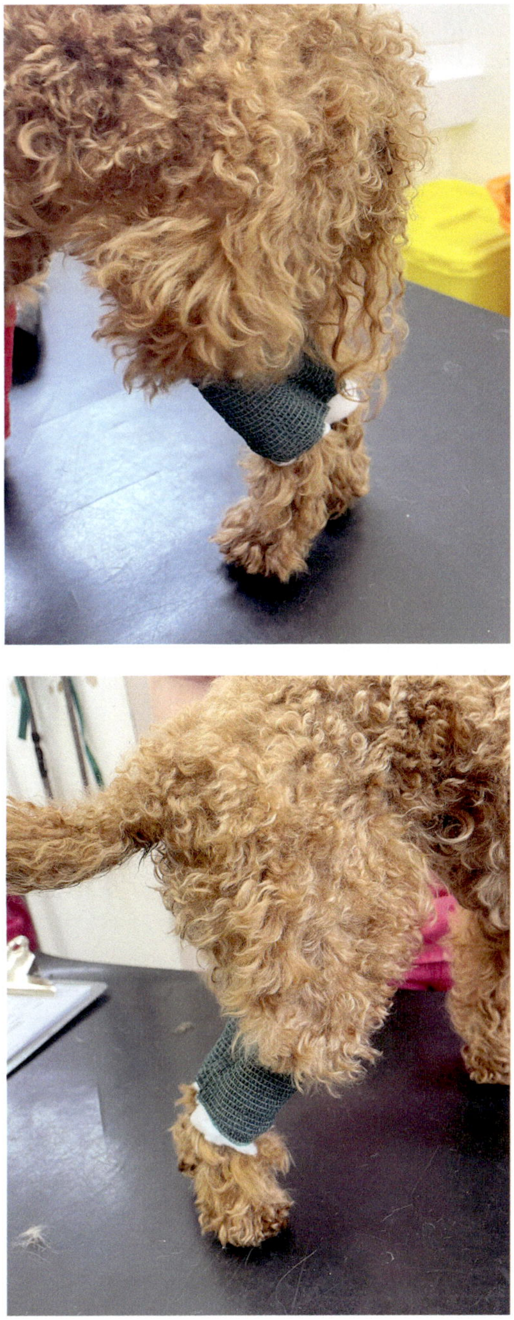

Figure 96. Hobbles. Images provided by Joy Fenner.

Pain Assessment

Multimodal Analgesia

Multimodal analgesia is key to control pain via a variety of methods to prevent wind up. This includes a range of medicinal options, stabilisation and heating/cooling strategies, as well as physiotherapy and massage techniques.

Local Anaesthetics

Local anaesthetic drugs directly impede sensory nerve conduction, blocking pain signals. **Preemptive local anaesthetic blocks** may reduce postoperative pain sensation. These may be administered locally to the area undergoing surgery by infiltration or administration around nerves proximal to the surgical site, or indeed into the epidural space.

Postoperatively, **local anaesthetic dosing via wound diffusion catheters,** epidural catheters, or thoracic drains helps to reduce the requirement for systemic medications and the associated side effects.

NSAIDs

Non-steroidal anti-inflammatories (NSAIDs) are the most common analgesics for systemic use to manage inflammatory pain associated with surgery. **NSAIDs are contraindicated in hypovolaemic patients,** those with preexisting renal or hepatic disease, or those who suffer vomiting or gastroduodenal disease. **Most NSAIDs should be administered with food,** due to risk of adverse reactions, which can be problematic in inappetant patients following surgery, (due to stress, pain associated with the surgery, or nausea due to the effect of other analgesic medications).

Opioids

Opioids (including methadone, morphine, buprenorphine) are frequently used perioperative analgesics due to their relatively low risk of adverse responses at therapeutic doses in small animal species. They may however commonly **affect gut motility and cause nausea,** sometimes requiring coadministration of antiemetic medication to counteract this effect. Dosing is commonly based on pain scoring assessment postoperatively.

Others

There are many other additional analgesics which can be considered in parallel to the options discussed above depending on the nature of the painful stimulus and hence the type of pain, as well as contraindications for the use of other analgesic options. These include paracetamol, gabapentin, amantadine, ketamine, and lidocaine; often administered as constant rate infusions.

Pain Scoring

Pain scoring assessments should be repeated at regular intervals. These intervals are gradually extended as time passes following surgery and the level of analgesia required becomes more predictable and hopefully reduces. Ideally pain scoring assessment is performed as repeatably as possible, by the same team caring for the patient, and using a standardised and validated scale for assessment of degree of pain, for example the short form of the Glasgow composite pain scoring system. http://www.isvra.org/PDF/SF-GCPS%20eng%20owner.pdf

This scoring system is validated for use following soft tissue surgery but may be less applicable to orthopaedic procedures or to some specific cases. **The scores are interpreted in the light of the specific patient and other parameters.** Elevations in heart rate, temperature, blood pressure, or respiratory rate/effort are nonspecific but may be indicators of pain in nonresponsive patients, although can also be altered by many other systemic conditions.

Monitoring Vital Parameters

Vital parameters vary for a multitude of reasons between patients and even within an individual patient. Only by regular monitoring, in parallel with medical interventions, can the veterinary team interpret changes which may indicate a clinical deterioration or demonstrate the effect of medical interventions. The veterinary surgeon will often request regular assessment of a patient's vital parameters but should also **give values for those parameters which represent a cause for concern in that individual patient and require their immediate attention for further intervention.** Review of the recent therapeutic interventions, and knowledge of the known/anticipated disease affecting the patient aids interpretation and therefore how to treat the altered parameters.

Heart Rate

In dogs, tachycardia is caused by many factors, from being a normal response to exercise, excitement, fear, or acute pain under the influence of adrenaline (the fight or flight response), or due to reduction in cardiac output due to shock, (e.g. hypovolaemic, distributive or cardiogenic), anaemia, hypoxia or the effect of some medications (e.g. adrenaline, thyroxine, etc).

Bradycardia is less common but occurs due to the effects of sedative medications, (particularly α-2 agonists), hypothermia, pericarditis, hyperkalaemia, (e.g. due to urinary tract rupture or obstruction), hypocalcemia, hypomagnesaemia, and with severe neurological, respiratory and gastrointestinal disease.

Respiratory Rate/Effort

Tachypnoea or dyspnoea; an increase in respiratory rate or effort is caused by:

- panting due to stress, anxiety, pain or hyperthermia/pyrexia
- upper respiratory obstruction due to conformation, airway collapse, foreign bodies, inflammation, or tumours
- pulmonary disease e.g. pneumonia, oedema, contusions, tumours, bronchitis, bronchospasm due to allergy

- pleural disease e.g. pleural effusion, pneumothorax
- chest wall/diaphragmatic disease/injury e.g. rib fractures, phrenic nerve injury, congenital malformations (e.g. PPDH/ pectus excavatum)
- abdominal distension pressing on the diaphragm
- metabolic acidosis.

Blood Pressure

Hypertension is caused by pain, anxiety, stress, chronic kidney disease, Cushing's disease (hyperadrenocorticism), phaeochromocytoma (an adrenal gland tumour), or vasopressor medications.

Hypotension may occur due to shock (e.g. hypovolaemic, distributive, cardiogenic or anaphylactic), or the effects of many sedative and anaesthetic medications.

Temperature

Hypothermia may result from anaesthesia/sedation causing homeostatic dysfunction, active cooling, or shock.

Hyperthermia/pyrexia may result from overheating, muscle activity, (including seizures), pain, drug reactions (e.g. opioid administration in cats), infection or systemic inflammation.

Mentation

Patient mentation should be monitored for changes in strength, awareness and interaction with surroundings and for other neurological signs including head tilting, head pressing, twitching and seizures.

Mentation is quantitatively assessed using the modified **Glasgow Coma Scale** (Table 2), which helps to guide prognosis for patients with neurological signs. Scoring is based on assessment of motor activity, brainstem reflexes and level of consciousness and combining these 3 scores to produce an overall MCGS Score.

Whilst each of these parameters is interpreted individually, it is often the combination of changes which guide the clinician as to the cause and therefore the necessary therapeutic intervention.

Drain and Catheter Care

Thoracic Drains

An essential part of most thoracic surgery is provision for the **removal of fluid** (air, blood, inflammatory fluid, chyle) which may accumulate within the thorax following surgery. Usually,

Table 2. Modified Glasgow Coma Scale.

Modified Glasgow Coma Scale	Score
Motor activity	
· Normal gait, normal spinal reflexes.	6
· Hemiparesis, tetraparesis or decerebrate rigidity.	5
· Recumbent, intermitent extensor rigidity.	4
· Recumbent, constant extensor rigidity.	3
· Recumbent, constant extensor rigidity with opisthotonos.	2
· Recumbent, hypotonia of muscles, depressed or absent spinal reflexes.	1
Brainstem reflexes	
· Normal PLR and oculocephalic reflexes.	6
· Slow PLR and normal to reduced oculocephalic reflexes.	5
· Bilateral unresponsive miosis with normal to reduced oculocephalic reflexes.	4
· Pinpoint pupils with reduced to absent oculocephalic reflexes.	3
· Unilateral, unresponsive mydriasis with reduced to absent oculocephalic reflexes.	2
· Bilateral, unresponsive mydriasis with reduced to absent oculocephalic reflexes.	1
Level of consciousness	
· Occasional periods of alertness and responsive to environment.	6
· Depression or delirium, capable of responding, but response may be inappropriate.	5
· Semicomatose, responsive to visual stimuli.	4
· Semicomatose, responsive to auditory stimuli.	3
· Semicomatose, responsive only to repeated noxious stimuli.	2
· Comatose, unresponsive to repeated noxious stimuli.	1

MCGS Score	Prognosis
3–8	Grace
9–14	Guarded
15–18	Good

these fluids are not overly viscous and so narrow gauge drains are commonly used to reduce postoperative morbidity.

Maintenance

The drain is anchored to the skin at the point of entry, by sutures through eyelets on the drain or by a finger trap suture. **This point of the entry should be treated aseptically** as a surgical incision and is a potential entry point for nosocomial infection and should therefore be covered and regularly cleaned, inspected, and recovered. (Figure 97).

Whilst essential for removing fluids from the thorax, if not kept well closed and sealed drains are a risk for allowing air entry into the thorax. Hence **at least two methods should be used for closing off the drain,** i.e. a clamp on the drain itself, a turned off three way tap, and bungs on the outlets of the drain/three way tap. Junior members of staff should be trained and monitored for their use of three way taps for this purpose as their misuse is a common cause of problems associated with thoracic drainage.

It is also paramount that the drain is adequately **protected from patient interference,** by the use of a hard, Elizabethan collar, and often also a body suit to prevent removal by the rear paws in cats.

Ongoing Drainage

Drainage of the thorax may be intermittent or continuous. Intermittent drainage is usually performed by a trained nurse or veterinarian, using a syringe, with an aseptic technique and ensuring the chest drain remains sealed closed at all times to prevent air entry. Continuous drainage is less frequently used and requires connection to a dedicated pump or suction device but may be considered for cases where high volumes of air are leaking inside the thorax (in order to prevent a tension pneumothorax). (Figure 98).

The frequency of thoracic drainage will be advised by the surgeon. The initial frequency depends on the rate of fluid accumulation and risk associated with that fluid accumulation. Generally, the frequency of drainage is reduced over time as the productivity of the drain diminishes, until it is removed. The presence of a drain itself in the thorax causes production of a small volume of inflammatory fluid (often suggested to be up to 2 ml/kg/day).

To harvest fluid, **the patient may need to be repositioned in different recumbencies;** this is to allow the fluid or air within the thorax to be in contact with the drain. Air rises within the thorax, whereas fluid falls under gravity; so the position of the drain (from knowledge of its placement at surgery or postoperative radiographs) should be considered and the predicted location of the fluid.

Drainage Records

The volume and nature of fluid removed should be clearly recorded to allow the veterinary surgeon to adjust the frequency of drainage and consider drain removal.

Of particular concern is the removal of substantial volumes of blood from the thorax. The PCV of the fluid removed is compared to that in the patient's circulation to assess the active intrathoracic haemorrhage. If a large volume of frank blood is drained, it may be advisable to aseptically collect the blood into syringes or a blood collection bag preloaded with citrate anticoagulant, so **the blood is available for autotransfusion** if required.

Turbid, cloudy liquid drained from the chest, especially if it progressively increases in volume, may indicate surgical site infection and fluid analysis by cytology and white blood cell counts are advocated for comparison with previous samples.

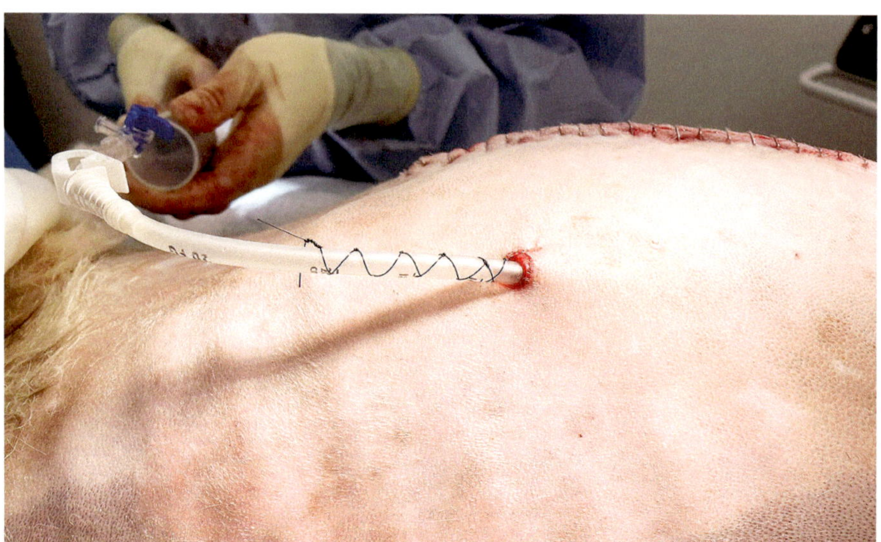

Figure 97. A chest drain secured to the thoracic wall with a friction suture and undergoing drainage using a three way tape and a gate clamp to prevent leakage. Figure courtesy of Joy Fenner.

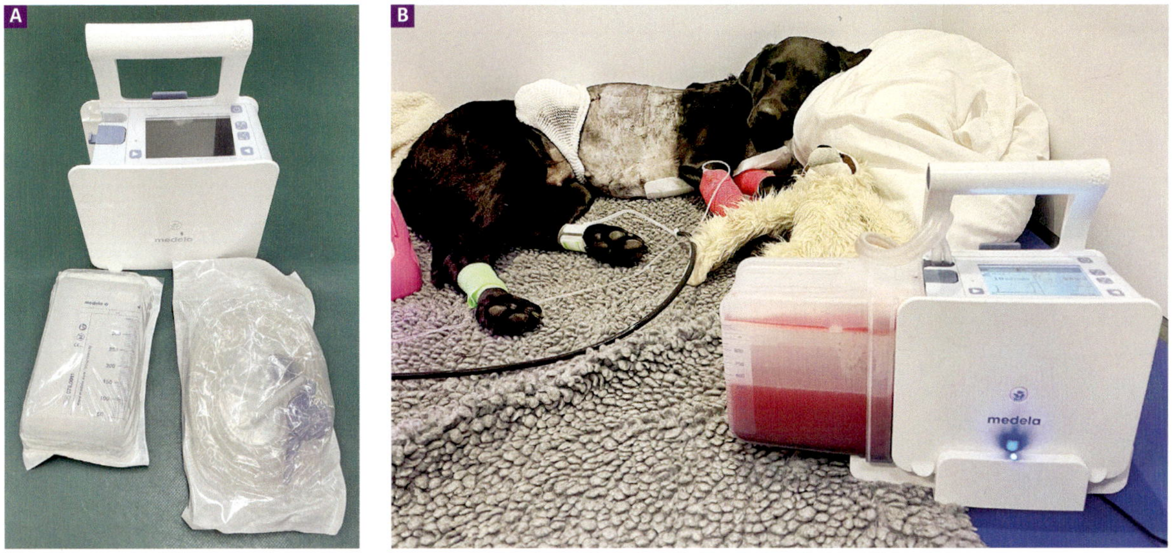

Figure 98. A. Components of the continuous thoracic drainage system (pump, fluid collection canister and connection tubing); **B.** Assembled system attached to a patient following surgical management of pyothorax.

Drain Removal

Thoracic drains should be removed aseptically. The sutures anchoring the drain should be cut, which should allow the drain to be gently withdrawn without resistance in the unsedated patient. The tip of the drain should be saved and submitted to the laboratory for bacteriology testing (if desired) for hospital infection monitoring or as indicated by the patient's status.

Closed Suction Drains

Closed suction drains are tubes with variable numbers and types of fenestrations which are placed into surgical sites and exit via a stab incision which is separate from the main surgical incision. They attach to containers which apply negative pressure to drain fluid which accumulates at the surgical site, out into a collection chamber. (Figure 99).

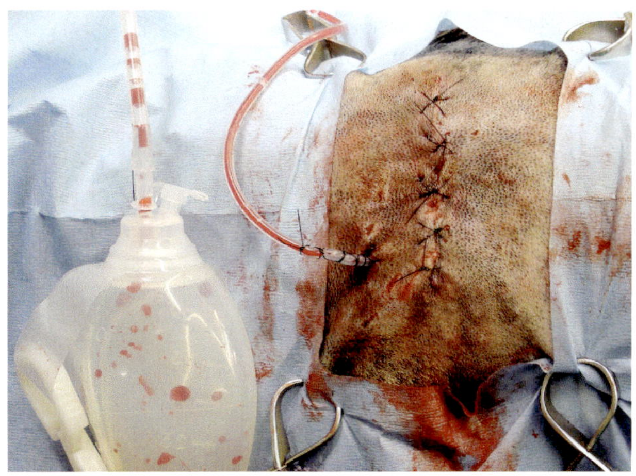

Figure 99. Active suction drain placed into a wound cavity at surgery. Note the drain exits via a small stab incision, separated from the main incision. The drain is secured to the skin at the exit point with a friction suture.

As with thoracic drains, closed suction drains are potential portals of entry for surgical site infections and should be kept covered to prevent contamination. Drains should be handled wearing gloves and the tubing occluded with atraumatic (to prevent puncture of the tubing) forceps during drainage to prevent back flow into the surgical site. Drainage canisters should be emptied and the quantity and nature of the fluid drained recorded, before the drain is reactivated, (usually by squeezing to empty before reattaching) and the tube is unclamped.

How often the canister is emptied depends on the productivity of the drain. It should be checked regularly, but **only emptied when more than 50% full,** to minimise handling and risk of contamination.

Drains requires **an airtight seal** to be effective, and so when placed superficially initial **activation is delayed for 6–12 hours** until the fibrin seal has formed to seal the wound and prevent air being sucked into and contaminating the surgical site. For deeper surgical sites, where an airtight seal is formed immediately, the drain is activated during surgery. To maintain the integrity of the system, the drain and collection device must be adequately protected from patient interference, by the use of a hard Elizabethan collar and securing the drain and collection device to a harness or collar, contained within a body stocking as shown in Figure 100.

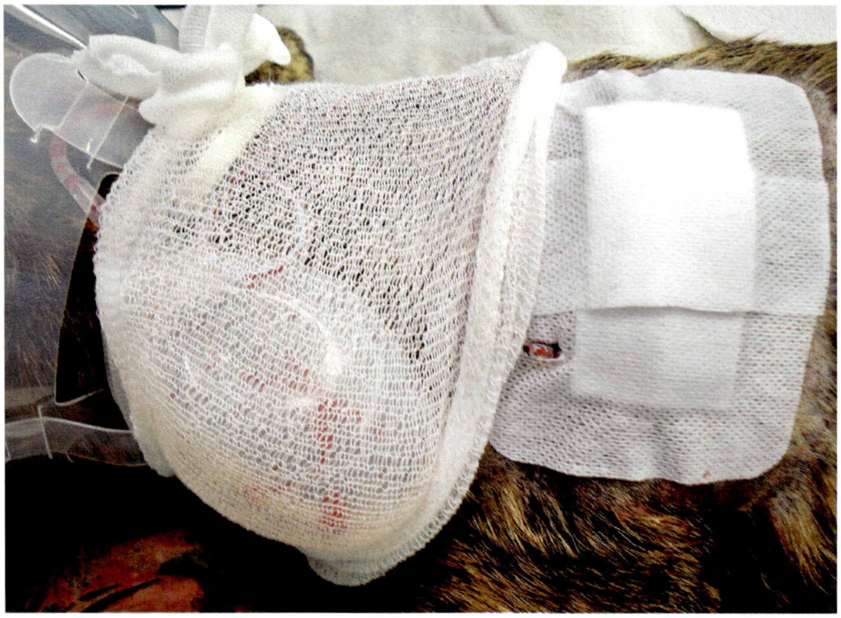

Figure 100. A closed suction drainage canister secured to the patient's Elizabethan collar as well as being retained within a light circumferential neck bandage. Note the drain entry through the skin is covered with an adhesive dressing.

As with thoracic drains, the fluid volume should be monitored and the drain removed when the quantity of discharge has reduced to a level anticipated due to the presence of the drain itself.

Abdominal Drains

Abdominal drains are structurally the same as the closed suction drains placed within the dead space of other wounds but refer to their use within the abdominal cavity. Abdominal drains are placed to aid the management of uroabdomen, or postoperatively in cases of septic peritonitis, to allow ongoing drainage and monitoring of abdominal effusion following surgical treatment.

They are placed and managed similarly to closed suction drains at other sites, however they are often highly productive, especially following initial placement and therefore require more frequent monitoring and emptying. The consequences of ascending surgical site infection are catastrophic and so the previously noted instructions regarding aseptic management and prevention of back flow are imperative.

Vascular Catheters

Vascular access catheters should be inspected regularly for **security of fixation, evidence of inflammation or infection, and flushed to check and maintain patency.** Assessment requires periodic redressing which is performed aseptically.

Arterial and venous lines should be clearly differentiated by appropriate labelling to ensure proper use. Arterial lines are used postoperatively for repeat blood gas analysis and/or for invasive blood pressure monitoring but should not be used for medical administration.

Central venous catheters and long stay catheters should be managed similarly to shorter, peripheral lines, although asepsis and security against dislodgement are even more critical as replacement is more challenging and requires general anaesthesia.

Urinary Catheters

Following surgery urinary catheters are placed for a number of reasons:

- for accurate measurement of urine output
- prevention of urine scalding in a recumbent patient
- draining the bladder in a patient who has received epidural anaesthesia
- keeping a bladder empty following urinary tract repair/trauma to prevent urine leakage/urethral stenosis.

Urinary catheters are a risk for nosocomial infection as discussed previously in this chapter. Hence placement should be performed aseptically and the catheter handled and drained aseptically. **The catheter should be maintained in place for the minimum time necessary** as duration of placement is associated with the risk of development of urinary tract infection.

Urinary catheters may be drained intermittently (commonly every three to four hours) or attached to a closed collection system for continuous drainage. The latter is more appropriate in cases which have suffered trauma to the urinary tract, whereby keeping the lower urinary tract decompressed to minimise leakage is recommended but comes with the risk of twisting and patient interference with the connecting tubing. **Hence closed collection systems should be monitored regularly, and urine output assessed every few hours to ensure they remain patent.** Urinary catheters should not be maintained as an open system without a collection bag or bung to seal the catheter as this represents an unnecessarily high risk of ascending infection and prevents quantification of urine output assessment.

In a normotensive, well perfused and hydrated patient, urine output is in the range of 2–4 ml/kg/hr. In the event of reduced or absent urine production, the urinary catheter and bedding should be checked for leaks. If no leaks are identified, then the bladder should be palpated or inspected using point of care ultrasound (POCUS) to check for filling which is not being adequately drained. The latter may occur due to malpositioning, obstruction, or too high a pressure being applied to the catheter causing luminal collapse during draining.

If obstruction is suspected, then aseptic injection of a small volume of sterile water for injection or saline infusion into the bladder via the catheter may alleviate the obstruction or be used to check patency; this is confirmed using POCUS in Doppler mode to visualise the flow within the bladder. **Anuria (the absence of urine pooling within the bladder) is as an emergency,** which should be managed in consultation with the overseeing veterinary surgeon.

Cystostomy tubes (Figure 101) **are a special case of urinary drainage catheter, placed directly into the bladder via the inguinal body wall.** They are placed to allow urinary diversion in cases of urethral trauma, stenosis/stricture, tumours obstructing urinary drainage from the bladder neck, and in cases of reflex dyssynergia whereby the bladder loses tone and the ability to contract to an empty state. In these cases, either a long Foley catheter, mushroom-tipped catheter, or a low profile tube are placed.

Urinary catheters are secured and protected from the patient similarly to drains used at other locations, although Foley catheters are usually prevented from dislodgement by sufficient inflation of the balloon within the bladder.

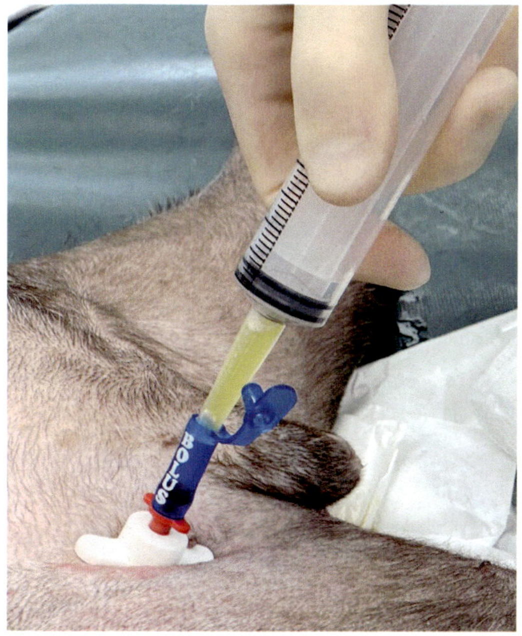

Figure 101. A low-profile cystostomy tube undergoing drainage.

Nutrition

A full review of the nutritional requirements of the surgical patient is beyond the scope of this chapter.

In brief, healthy patients undergoing surgery only require their current diet at the same quantity and frequency. Patients are generally not fed 8–12 hours before anaesthesia to allow for gastric emptying and minimal risk of regurgitation preoperatively but can **resume normal feeding as soon as adequately recovered from surgery.** Preoperative starvation times are reduced in immature patients at risk of hypoglycaemia with prolonged starvation. It may be necessary to tempt with a different diet to stimulate appetite in the postoperative period, or use bland or low fat diets in patients undergoing gastrointestinal surgery or who have undergone manipulation of the pancreas (hence at greater risk of postoperative pancreatitis). Energy requirements during hospitalization, where activity is restricted, **are estimated as the resting energy requirement (RER).**

$$\text{RER (kcal/day)} = (30 \times \text{BW}) + 70$$

or

$$\text{RER (kcal/day)} = 70 \times \text{BW}^{(0.75)}$$

(where BW is body weight in kilograms)

Severely traumatised patients typically have energy requirements exceeding or up to twice resting energy requirements because of the extent of the injuries.

Convalescent diets are formulated to be more calorific, with higher levels of protein and fat, to be more palatable, and have a homogeneous texture suitable for syringe administration via feeding tubes in patients not capable of taking adequate oral nutrition.

Feeding requirements should be clearly documented, to ensure surgical patients receive adequate nutrition.

A more thorough discussion of nutritional support of critical patients can be found in Wernerman J., 2005.

Type of Nutrition

Enteral feeding is the provision of nutrients to the patient using at least a portion of the gastrointestinal tract; this may be oral or via a feeding tube. Enteral nutrition is the preferred option for provision of nutrients whenever there is adequate function of the digestive tract. Indeed, the enterocytes which line the gastrointestinal tract receive their own nutrition solely from the intestinal contents, hence a minimum trickle feeding with carbohydrates (e.g. baby rice) and vitamin B12 should be attempted.

Parenteral nutrition is the provision of nutrients intravenously. This provision aims to provide the partial or total nutritional requirements of the patient, known as partial parenteral nutrition (PPN) or total parenteral nutrition (TPN). Parenteral nutrition is significantly more expensive to administer and risks complications including thromboembolism and infection, and metabolic complications such as hyperglycaemia, electrolyte and acid base disturbances, and refeeding syndrome.

Timing of Nutrition

Many studies confirm the survival and recovery benefits of patients who receive early nutrition following surgery. For healthy patients which can be fed orally, this means resuming normal feeding as soon as the patient has adequately recovered from anaesthesia to feed and not risk regurgitation or aspiration of the food. For more systemically unwell patients or those undergoing more invasive surgeries, the patient's ability should be considered and the likelihood of taking oral feeding postoperatively.

Factors to consider include:

- extent of surgery
- level of discomfort following surgery
- analgesic requirement following surgery and adverse effects of those medications: e.g high doses of opioids cause sedation and nausea, lidocaine CRIs frequently result in profound nausea, ketamine CRIs may be highly sedative
- patients anxiety and propensity for eating in the hospital environment
- prior history of, or expectation of pancreatitis, particularly for abdominal procedures involving manipulation of the pancreas
- surgical interference with bowel function, e.g. with major bowel resection, or if a portion of the bowel requires postoperative rest, e.g. the oesophagus following oesophageal foreign body removal resulting in ulceration and oesophagitis.

If the surgical team anticipate the patient may not receive adequate oral nutrition postoperatively, then **placing a feeding tube at the time of surgery** to help to manage the nutritional requirement should be considered.

If patients have suffered a prolonged period of inappetence or starvation prior to surgery then feeding should be reintroduced progressively to **prevent refeeding syndrome,** which may cause electrolyte disturbances. Typically feeding begins at 33% RER in the 24 hours following surgery and is then increased to 66% and 100% RER over the following 48 hours if feeding is well tolerated.

Feeding Tubes

Naso-oesophageal (NO) Tubes

Naso-oesophageal (NO) tubes (Figure 102) are considered in patients too unstable to undergo general anaesthesia for placement of other tube types, and where **only short term nutrition** is required. These tubes have narrow lumens, limiting what can be fed, and are the least well tolerated of the feeding tube options. NO tubes are contraindicated for patients with oesophageal dysfunction, with an abnormal gag reflex, or those at increased risk of regurgitation and aspiration pneumonia.

Other complications of NO tube placement include epistaxis, rhinitis, sneezing, and premature tube removal by the patient.

Pharyngostomy (P) Tubes

Pharyngostomy (P) tubes are placed from the left side of the neck, into the oropharynx at the back of the oral cavity, and then passed into the oesophagus. They are contraindicated in patients with oesophageal disease and dysfunction and those at risk of regurgitation or aspiration as with NO tubes. The tube diameter is generally larger allowing administration of blended foods of thicker consistency than is possible via an NO tube. These tubes may cause inappetency in some patients, including most cats, and have therefore been superseded by oesophagostomy tubes.

Oesophagostomy (O) Tubes

Oesophagostomy (O) tubes (Figure 103) are similar to pharyngostomy tubes, but **placed more caudally in the neck, directly into the oesophagus** from a cut down through the skin. Contraindications are as for P and NO tubes, with the advantages of a larger tube diameter shared with P tubes, but less irritation to the pharynx has a less significant effect on patient appetite.

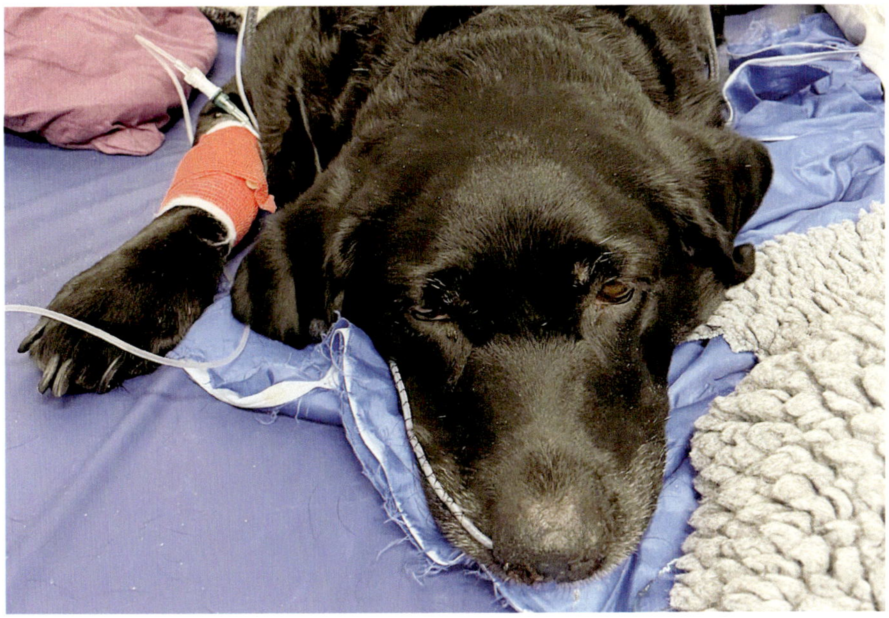

Figure 102. Naso-oesophageal tube.

Placement requires general anaesthesia. Tubes are generally placed on the left side as the oesophagus sits to the left of the midline. A square of skin over the side of the neck should be clipped and prepared aseptically. Attention should be paid to the location of the jugular vein. A pair of large, curved artery forceps or a specialised O tube introducer is passed into the oesophagus, which is then elevated towards the skin, stretching and tenting the skin over the tip of the instrument, midway along the length of the neck. A number 11 blade is then used to cut down onto the instrument and the tube passed from the outside into the oesophagus. In the case of curved artery forceps the tube is grasped and withdrawn its full length through the mouth up to the syringe connector valve and then advanced back down into the oesophagus. The bend of the tube exiting the mouth is then pushed into the oropharynx as the syringe connector is gently withdrawn, until a pop is noted as the tube straightens from the skin incision to be directed caudally along the oesophagus. **A radiograph should be taken to confirm correct placement,** with the end located in the distal oesophagus, caudal to the heart base and the exit point secured to the skin with either a friction suture or purpose designed butterfly clip.

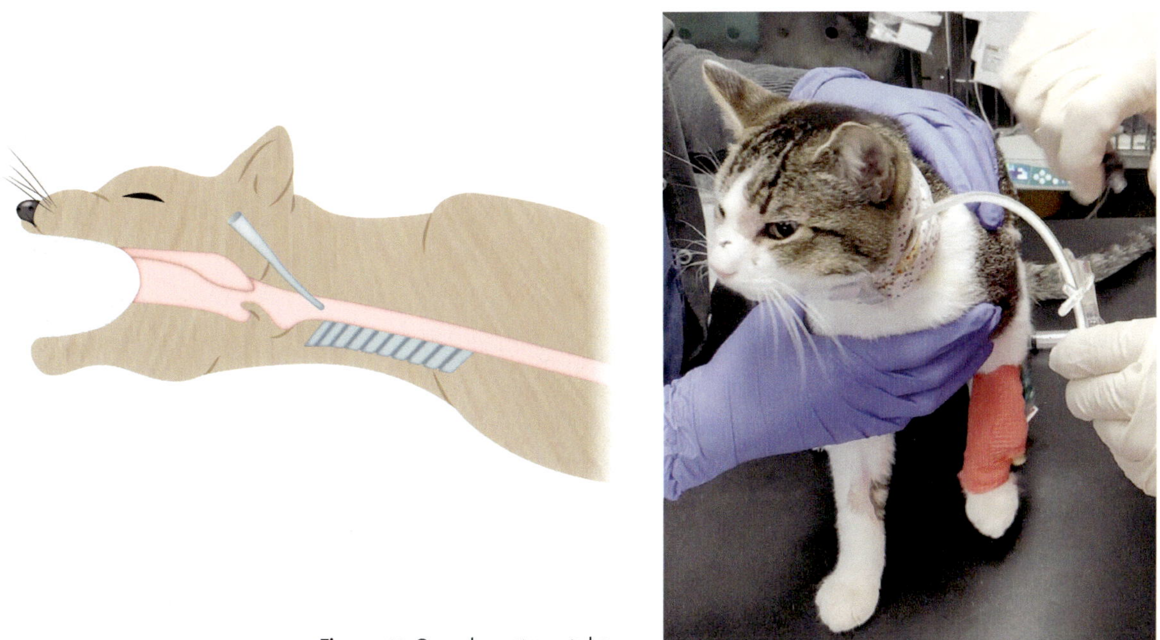

Figure 103. Oesophagostomy tube.

The major risks of placement are haemorrhage and nerve injury, both of which are minimised by awareness of the location of the jugular vein before placement and adequate tenting of the tissue over the intraoesophageal instrument to minimise dissection and maximise displacement of the vital neuromuscular structures. The other common complication is discharge associated with the entry site, which requires regular cleaning and care to protect the surrounding skin.

Method for Tube Feeding (Video 4)

Before each feed, the tube's entry point should be checked, ensuring that it is securely attached to the skin and the tube is correctly placed. Aspiration of the tube should show negative pressure if the tube is correctly placed within the lumen of an empty oesophagus. If either air or fluid is aspirated the veterinary surgeon should be contacted immediately as the tube may be displaced. If the tube placement appears correct, a test dose of water should be administered slowly to check this does not result in coughing or gagging and to check tube patency. Thereafter, the patient should be gently restrained, with head elevated, and the feed slowly administered (at a rate similar to the patient swallowing when feeding naturally). After the feed, the tube should be flushed with water once again before clamping, sealing, and securing to the patient. **The daily food allowance is typically spread over six smaller feeds to limit the volume administered per feed.** In severely debilitated patients, trickle feeding may be administered as a constant rate infusion via a pump at 10% of RER. O tubes may be removed at any time as soon as they are no longer needed. The affixing suture is released, and the tube withdrawn. The stoma usually seals within 24–48 hours.

Gastrostomy (G) Tubes

Gastrostomy (G) tubes (Figure 104) are large bore tubes placed during surgery within the abdominal cavity, which **pass directly through the body wall and into the lumen of the stomach.** The tube is placed caudal to the last rib on the left side, lateral to the rectus abdominal muscles and mammary tissue. The tube then passes through a purse-string suture into the fundus of the stomach. The stomach is then secured to the body wall within the abdomen to minimise the risk of tube displacement or leakage. Externally the tube is secured in place with a friction suture.

Gastrostomy tubes bypass the upper gastrointestinal tract and are used in patients with oesophageal disease, dysfunction, or injury and those at risk of regurgitation or aspiration. They are simple and quick to place in patients undergoing other abdominal procedures but are an invasive procedure for patients not undergoing abdominal surgery and so their placement is weighed up in light of other patient factors.

The main risks of placement are of **leakage around the stoma,** which can cause skin incisional inflammation, or of greater

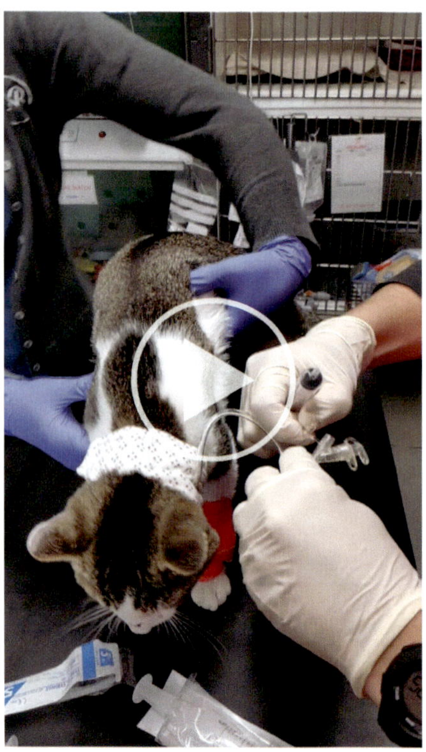

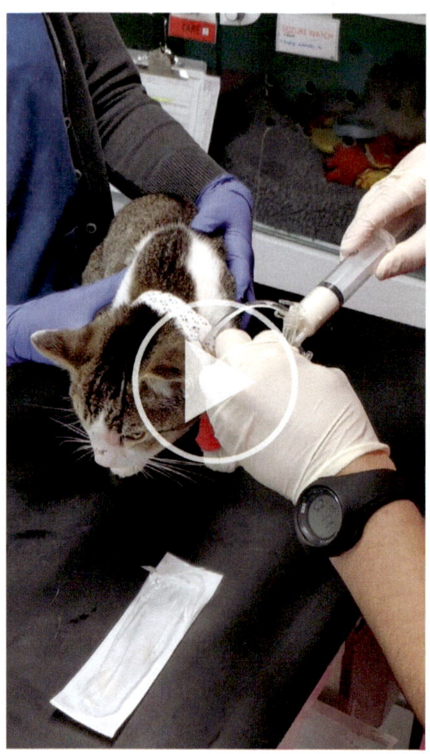

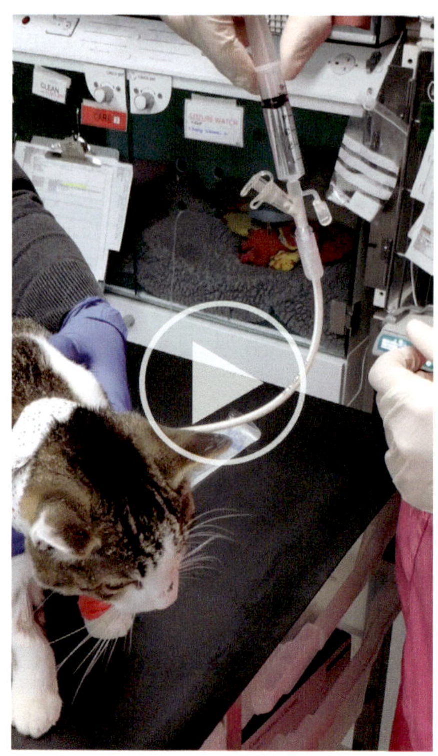

Video 4. Three videos called "O tube feed 1", "O tube feed 2" and "O tube feed 3" can be found in this site: https://publicationen.improveinternational.com.

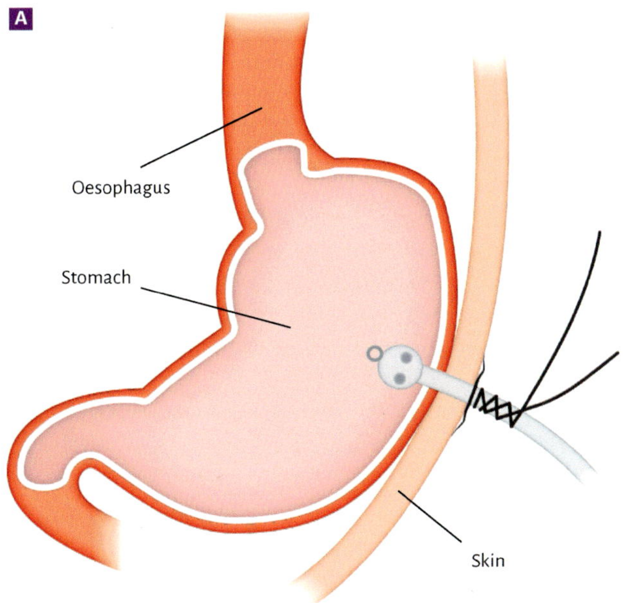

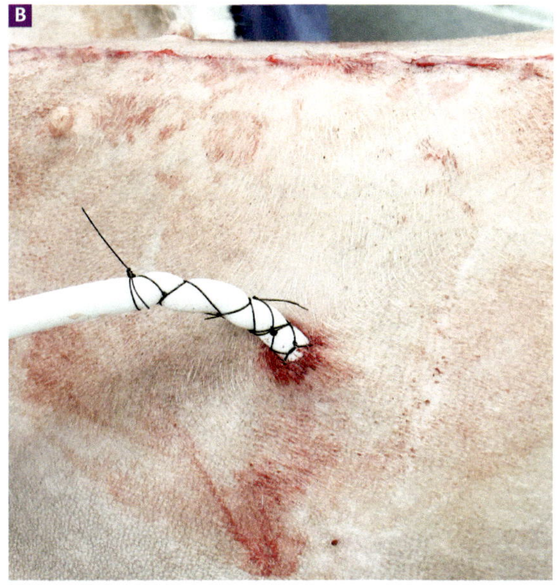

Figure 104. A. Gastrostomy tube placement; **B.** Gastrostomy tube exit.

significance but lower risk with correct placement, **septic peritonitis.** Mushroom tipped catheters are preferred over Foley catheters, as the balloon of a Foley catheter may rapidly degrade and burst in the acidic stomach lining and cause tube displacement.

Most surgeons advise leaving a gastrostomy tube in place for at least 10 days, even if not required, to allow a mature stoma and internal adhesions to form and minimise the risk of disruption due to tube removal.

G Tube Removal (Video 5)

The tube is unhitched from the body bandage or harness and shortened to allow passage of a probe which deforms the mushroom tip into a more linear tube, which is then firmly pulled through the stoma, whilst bracing the body wall either side of the stoma. The stoma usually seals within 24–48 hours.

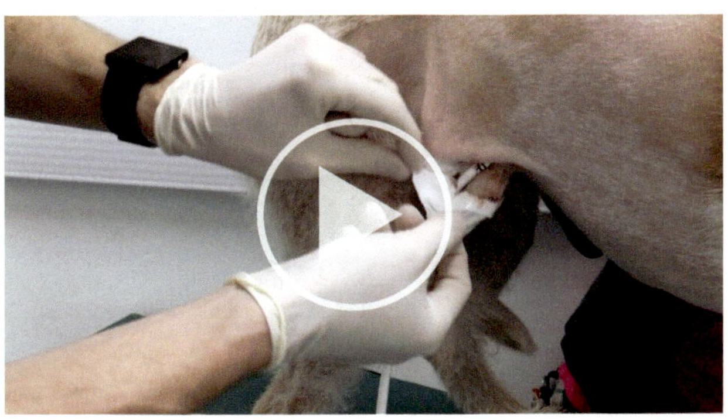

Video 5. A video called "G tube removal" can be found in this site: https://publicationen.improveinternational.com.

If tubes are required for long term use, once a mature stoma has formed, they may be exchanged for a low-profile tube. The low-profile tube sits flush with the skin surface and is less likely to be caught or inadvertently pulled out by the patient.

Administration of food via a gastrostomy tube is similar to that via an oesophagostomy tube, although as the tube resides within the stomach, aspiration prior to feeding does not produce negative pressure, but instead aspirates air or residual gastric content or bile.

Percutaneous Endoscopic Gastrostomy (PEG) Tubes

Percutaneous endoscopic gastrostomy (PEG) tubes (Figure 105) are functionally identical to gastrostomy tubes but are placed minimally invasively under endoscopic guidance from the stomach, with the patient in right lateral recumbency.

The major difference is the tube is anchored in place only by the mushroom tip and the external suture or tube clamp which sits against the body wall. Failure of either of these anchoring points results in tube displacement and septic peritonitis. For this reason, it really is essential the tube is kept in place for at least 10–14 days to allow mature internal adhesions to form at the level of the stoma.

Feeding via a PEG tube is similar to feeding via a gastrostomy tube.

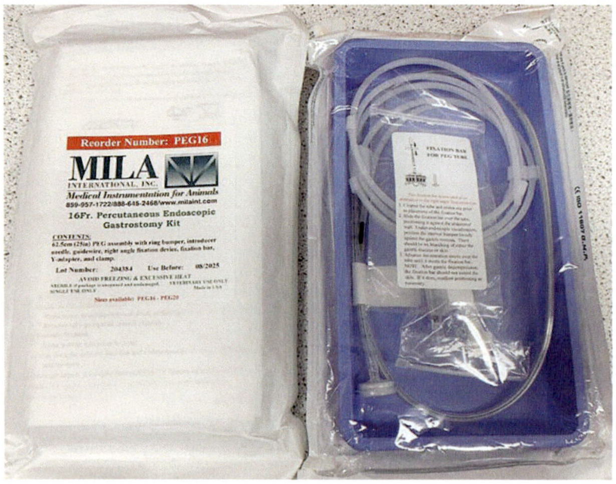

Figure 105. Percutaneous endoscopic gastrostomy tube.

Jejunostomy (J) Tubes

Jejunostomy (J) tubes are surgically placed tubes which enter the jejunum directly via the abdominal wall, via a suture secured stoma. These tubes also risk major complications with septic peritonitis, in the event of dislodgement, and cannot be secured with a mushroom tip due to the limited diameter of the bowel lumen, and therefore are the least commonly placed feeding tubes. Their advantage is in **bypassing the stomach and pancreas** in patients with gastric outflow disorders or diseases affecting gastric motility. The other downside to this is that food must be of an appropriate composition for jejunal digestion and must be trickle fed via a syringe driver as a constant rate infusion.

The risk of tube displacement is reduced by placing a jejunostomy tube via a gastrostomy tube and various systems are designed for J through G placement, which also allows administration to or drainage from the stomach plus food delivery directly into the jejunum with a tube continuing through the pylorus from the stomach.

Assessment of Intestinal Motility

Ileus is the term used to describe atony, lack of motility in the intestine. Ileus results in fluid accumulation in the stomach, with distension, discomfort, and impaired nutrition.

Gut motility is assessed using diagnostic ultrasound to observe waves of peristalsis or sequential assessment of gastric distention. Serial radiography of the abdomen following barium swallow also allows tracking of intestinal transit.

Cage side, some assessment may be made by **auscultating the bowel for sounds of movement.** This requires some practice auscultating the gut of normal fit and healthy patients. It is typical to hear intermittent gurgling and dripping sounds in all quadrants of the abdomen. When recording and documenting intestinal sounds, they may be difficult to quantify, but can be qualitatively described as absent, reduced, normal or increased (hypermotile).

In patients with gastric feeding tubes (G or PEG tubes) it is possible to monitor gastric residual contents from the previous feed, at the time of feeding, by completely draining the gastric contents. If the gastric content is low volume, this is replaced along with the feed to be administered.

In patients with ileus, **prokinetic medications** (e.g. metoclopramide, cisaprid) may help improve intestinal transit.

Controlled Exercise and Physiotherapy

Controlled Exercise

Following surgery, generally exercise is restricted, but requirements may differ depending on the nature of the surgery performed.

After any surgery, minimising interference with the wound and the sutures is necessary and so restraining the patient to exercise on a lead permits a degree of control to allow restraint from selfmutilation and from damage to the surgical site from abrasion of the area in undergrowth, for example when out for toilet breaks.

For surgeries of the major body cavities, exercise should be restricted to prevent increases in intracavitary pressures which might exceed the bursting strength of the sutures. Wound healing begins with inflammation and debridement before the proliferative phase and maturation, which then results in a return to preinjury tissue strength. Hence there is a lag phase where wound strength reduces after surgery before becoming stronger. (Figure 106).

In the early phase, wound strength relies on the sutures and fibrin seal. The strength of different tissues returns at different rates. Skin heals quicker than muscle and fascia, which in turn heal faster than bone. Hence the nature of the surgery determines the duration of restraint from exercise, which might overcome the strength of the healing wound.

On this basis, a surgery to remove a small skin mass, under no tension, require only 10 days of rest. An extensive abdominal

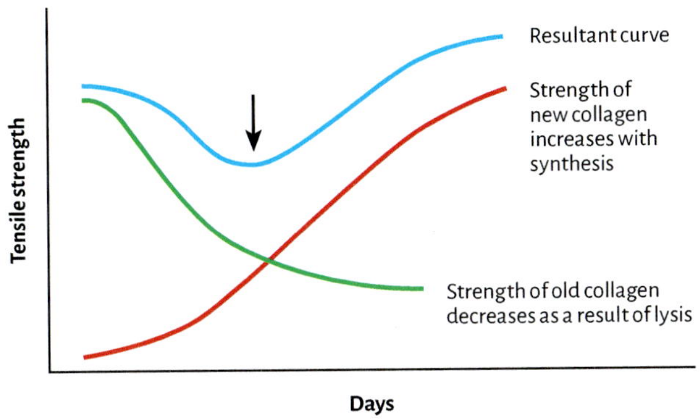

Figure 106. Wound healing strength.

exploration reliant on healing of the abdominal wall fascia for strength requires a month before return to full uncontrolled activity (e.g. chasing balls and jumping ditches). An orthopaedic osteotomy procedure or fracture repair takes two months for adequate uncomplicated recovery in a healthy young adult patient. Note that increasing age, metabolic or endocrine disease, malnutrition, infection, and other factors increase the times for normal tissue healing and this should be **taken into consideration on a case by case basis.**

Particularly important are specific exercises aimed at maintaining muscular strength and joint support. **For bone healing, a degree of loading encourages remodelling** and strengthening of the bone appropriately (Wolfe's Law) during the maturation and remodelling phase, so gentle, controlled activity and some specific exercises may be advocated by the veterinary surgeon and/or physiotherapist.

Physiotherapy and Hydrotherapy

Low Level Laser and Therapeutic Laser Therapy

Low level laser therapy is suggested to have a photochemical effect to enhance wound healing. This works by increasing leukocyte infiltration, growth factors and hence neovascularisation and fibroblast proliferation to repair the tissue damaged by the surgical trauma.

Massage Therapy

Massage produces beneficial effects for the patient by a number of mechanisms:

- **Vascular:**
  - improved venous and lymphatic return
  - removal of waste products
  - improved arterial blood flow
  - supply of oxygen and nutrients
  - improved tissue elasticity
  - warmth.
- **Mechanical:**
  - releasing adhesions
  - passive stretching and increased range of motion.
- **Endorphins:**
  - relaxation and endorphin release aid analgesia.
- **Neurological:**
  - improve sensory function
  - improve muscle tone in weak muscles.

Massage therapy is contraindicated in patients with:

- infection (local or systemic)
- hypotension/shock
- open wounds
- thromboembolic disease
- coagulopathies
- malignancies affecting the area of treatment.

Massage techniques should be selected under direction of a physiotherapist. There are many different massage techniques:

- effleurage (stroking)
- petrissage (kneading)
- rubbing (friction)
- shaking/vibration
- percussion/tapotement (clapping).

Passive Range of Motion Exercises

Passive range of motion exercises aim to:

- maintain joint range of motion
- increase joint fluid production and circulation and hence joint nutrition
- improve muscle and tendon flexibility
- improve neuromuscular stimulation
- improve vascular and lymphatic drainage in immobile patients.

Patients should be comfortable and tolerate manipulation. Passive range of motion exercises may be beneficial immediately following a joint surgery, or in paralysed patients to help to maintain their joint function. Range of motion exercises may be isolated to a single joint, or applied to the limb as a whole e.g. by performing cycling movements ensuring flexion and extension of each of the joints.

Stretching

Stretching is the forced elongation of a contracted muscle or tendon. There are different ways to perform stretching, which are beyond the scope of this chapter, but stretching aims to:

- increase joint range of motion
- decrease muscle pain associated with tension.

Passive stretching is applied by external force by the surgical nurse or physiotherapist, and performed after warming the muscles/tendons to be stretched. The patient either stands or lies in lateral recumbency but is ideally as relaxed as possible. The structures are stretched and held for 30 seconds to the point of causing mild discomfort and this is repeated four to five times. Ideally stretching is repeated two to four times per day. Goniometry helps monitor gains in joint range of motion as the result of improved flexibility.

Hydrotherapy

The indications for hydrotherapy are wide and variable, but include:

- rehabilitation after orthopaedic surgery for joint stabilisation or fracture repair
- rehabilitation of patients after spinal injuries and surgery
- muscle building and improvement of joint function in patients with hip or elbow dysplasia.

Exercising in water provides a number of benefits:

- buoyancy reduces loading of joints by the weight of the patient with increasing water depth in a pool or underwater treadmill;
- the density and viscosity of the water increases the resistance to movement and hence the work of the muscles; and
- if not completely submerged the patient may pick their limbs up and step over the surface of the water and hence actively increase their range of motion of the joints of the limbs.

Other forms of physiotherapy include therapeutic ultrasound, electrical stimulation, extracorporeal shock wave therapy, nuclear magnetic resonance therapy, magnetic therapy, and joint support with orthotics (which are beyond the scope of this chapter).

Client Communication

Client Education

Postoperative patient management does not stop or suddenly change in nature when a patient leaves the hospital environment. However, at some point during recovery, the risk of catastrophic complication reduces, as does the patient's reliance on continuous monitoring and injectable analgesia.

At this stage the veterinary surgeon discusses the relative risks of being away from the specialist attention within the hospital environment, balanced with the benefits of a reduction in stress and anxiety by being at home and returning to a normal environment, even if initially restricted within that environment.

At the right time, patient care is handed over to the owner. This might also be dependent to some degree on client availability and ability to administer specific postoperative care at home. At that time, it is essential that the client is given clear instruction on how to care for their pet at home, with guidelines of what should be considered normal and what should be considered of concern, and the recommended course of action in the event of noting any of these concerns. There is always potential for unexpected or unforeseen complications and the **default position should always be to seek the attention of the veterinary surgeon** in this eventuality.

Discharge Instructions

It is essential to **provide succinct, clear written instructions** covering the pertinent points for clients to take away from the discharge consultation. Often there is a large amount of information to take onboard and the client might be emotional to see their pet again and/or be overwhelmed by the description of the surgical treatment undertaken. It is essential the client is clear about their responsibilities for the patient in the postoperative period. Having these clearly documented as a discharge checklist help ensure clients are adequately prepared and that information can be shared with others in the household assisting with care over the coming days.

The discharge checklist acts as a succinct way of reviewing the client has what they need. The list may include confirmation the client has been given information regarding:

- wound management instructions, e.g. inspection, cleaning, hot/cold packing
- activity restriction instructions
- collars, bandages and protective coverings and the need for these to be monitored and changed appropriately
- correct medications, dosages, and timing of next due dose
- specific instructions for managing a feeding tube/drain/catheter
- information on when and how to report back on the patient's progress.

This checklist is **signed off by the veterinary surgeon or nurse responsible for discharging the patient, and by the client,** with a copy stored in the patient file. With complex instructions, it is best to ask the client to reiterate the instructions to demonstrate they have taken it onboard and understand the instructions.

With regards to use of feeding tubes and draining catheters, providing hands on demonstrations with the patient or a stuffed toy with similar tubes attached is helpful for client training. Video recordings of how treatments are administered in the hospital environment are helpful for demonstration purposes to clients and provide a resource for clients to refer to when at home.

Review and Reporting Back

Clients should be counselled on the importance of patient review to assess if the patient is progressing as anticipated. Early detection of clinical concerns allows for early intervention which may prevent complications escalating. Clients are usually asked to return for reassessment at a suitable interval following hospital discharge, to allow a review in the level of the patient's restriction depending on an adequate recovery. This varies with the surgery type, as orthopaedic injuries frequently have a more protracted recovery than most soft tissue surgeries. Patients with open wounds require the most frequent and intensive ongoing reassessment. In the long term, as wound healing progresses, dressing changes become less frequent and indeed wound management is taken on by the client, who can track ongoing progress of the wound photographically, providing periodic updates remotely to the veterinary team.

In some cases, it is beneficial for **the client to keep records** of their animal's recovery for review, including drain volumes (when drains are kept in place long term), to allow for intervention if drain volumes are increasing or drain removal when volumes are adequately reduced.

Clinical Governance

Clinical governance is a continuing process of reflection, analysis, and improvement in professional practice for the benefit of the patient and the client owner. (Figure 107).

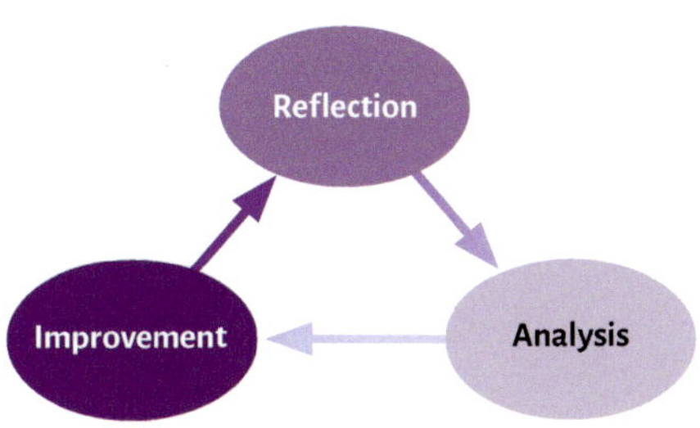

Figure 107. Diagram showing the cyclical process of clinical governance.

The Royal College of Veterinary Surgeons guidance for veterinary surgeons and veterinary nurses advises that clinical governance includes:

- **keeping up to date** with continuing professional development (CPD) and new developments relevant to the area of work
- **reflecting upon performance,** preferably in the form of a learning diary, and making appropriate changes to practice
- **reflecting upon any unexpected critical events** and learning from the outcome and making appropriate changes to practice
- **critically analysing** the evidence base for procedures used and making appropriate changes to practice
- **reflecting upon communication** with other members of the work team and making appropriate changes to practice
- reflecting upon **communication with clients** and making appropriate changes to practice
- **assessing professional competence** in consultation with more experienced or better qualified colleagues and limiting your practice appropriately.

https://www.rcvs.org.uk/setting-standards/advice-and-guidance/code-of-professional-conduct-for-veterinary-surgeons/supporting-guidance/clinical-governance/

Clinical Governance: Animal Safety

Patient welfare should always be first and foremost in the minds of veterinarians and veterinary nurses and as such patient safety is paramount to prevent unnecessary morbidity or mortality.

Standard Operating Procedures (SOPs)

Veterinary staff should be adequately trained for the specific tasks they are undertaking, and veterinary practices should have clear protocols in the form of standard operating procedures (SOPs) in place to ensure all staff are familiar with procedures for ensuring patient safety. If following review and analysis of a protocol, an improvement is decided upon and implemented, this should be clearly communicated to the whole veterinary team.

SOPs should include the implementation of checklists including anaesthetic checklists, surgical safety checklists and case handover checklists.

Critical Incidents

In the event of any critical incident, such as unexpected medical or surgical complications or serious complaint, all staff involved should conduct a **no blame meeting and record all the details** as soon as possible after the incident, with an opportunity for reflection of training and protocols in attempt to prevent similar occurrences in the future.

A record should be created for the incident, which documents:

- What has happened?
- Why did it happen?
    - systemic factors
    - human factors
    - patient factors
    - owner factors
    - communication factors
    - other
- What has been learned?
- What changes have been implemented?
    - CPD/training required
    - new or updated protocols/checklists/guidelines
- Is further audit required?
- Other.

Asking for Help

It is important to accept that no one member of the veterinary team is best placed to provide the optimal treatment for every patient with any medical or surgical complaint. Staff should be aware that **referral to a more appropriate veterinary surgeon** either within the practice or referral to another practice at any time is an option to the client and might be in the best interests of the patient.

No one should be above accepting their own limitations and hence with respect to patient safety and optimising clinical outcome, **assistance should be sought when appropriate.** This also applies to nursing colleagues, who should voice when they have concerns and not be afraid to ask for help from other members of the nursing team or veterinary surgeons.

Clinical Effectiveness

Veterinary practices should review and analyse their own performance, on a team and an individual level, in order to constructively analyse outcomes of procedures and training in such a way to ensure best possible patient outcomes.

Team Coordination

There may be more than one way to perform a specific task in the veterinary practice, and so a **common understanding among the team** on the specific methods chosen and implemented in the practice is key to the cohesion and understanding within the team.

Regular clinical meetings should take place for the veterinary and nursing team, with participation of all clinical staff encouraged. These meetings are an opportunity for all team members to share ideas and experiences, with the goal of improving clinical effectiveness, by improving patient safety, outcomes of procedures and treatments, as well as the well-being of the team members. Points of discussion should be documented and recorded and then an action plan created to **make any resultant changes arising** from the meeting, with **a period of review and reflection** and future discussion of the efficacy of the changes.

The practice should, over time, build up a manual used as clinical guidance available to all staff members. Team meetings are an opportunity to review SOPs and ensure they are in line with best practice guidelines, supported by the evidence base and revised as a result if this is not the case. The practice manual can hence be continually reviewed and updated.

Clinical Audit

Clinical audit is a review of the practice outcomes for commonly performed protocols and procedures, to ensure that those outcomes are in line with expectations, based on previous experience within the practice, but also compared to standard benchmark reference values (www.vetaudit.co.uk).

Audit data can be used to monitor the outcome of changes implemented following review and reflection of previous audit findings.

Continuing Professional Development (CPD)

Continuing professional development is an essential part of keeping up to date in the ever changing world of veterinary medicine and surgery. There are constant developments with regards to new treatment options, both medical and surgical, and publications of data of comparisons of outcomes from different treatments in the form of abstract publications, presentations, and journal articles. Information should be critically appraised based on the strength of that evidence, as demonstrated in the pyramid of evidence (Figure 108), which shows the hierarchy of the strength of evidence, relative to the frequency of availability of the data.

Continuing professional development should be encouraged and supported by the veterinary practice with respect to making time available and providing funding for training. This may be in the form of organising clinical clubs or journal clubs, training in the use of newly available equipment or medication, and in attending externally provided training courses. This development should be monitored with individual performance review to assess staff development.

Whilst it may not be possible for every team member to attend every training event, the feedback from individuals regarding interesting information from CPD courses to the rest of the practice team should be encouraged to help share and expand the common wealth of knowledge within the team. This information can then be considered for inclusion into practice protocols, where appropriate.

Within the practice, staff should have access to suitable up to date reference material to help them research and develop their knowledge and provide a resource to refer to for support in clinical decision making.

Patient and Client Experience

Key to the patient and client experience is both having the appropriate treatment options for the patient and management of the patient, but also communication, both within the veterinary team to ensure that the planned treatment protocol is implemented as scheduled but then also between the veterinary team and the client. Communication in both directions is essential to transfer the required treatment information but then also to receive and report feedback, which can then be reviewed and analysed to help improve protocols in the future.

Communication within the Veterinary Team

Patient treatment records should be clearly documented, clearly legible, and available to read for all those caring for the patient. These are legal documents which should be checked and countersigned by the overseeing veterinary surgeon. Treatment records include adequate provision of analgesia and regular assessment with a defined pain scoring protocol as deemed appropriate for the individual patient's needs.

Continuity of care for patients must be established between clinical staff by having protocols and checklists for case handovers, such as conducting patient rounds.

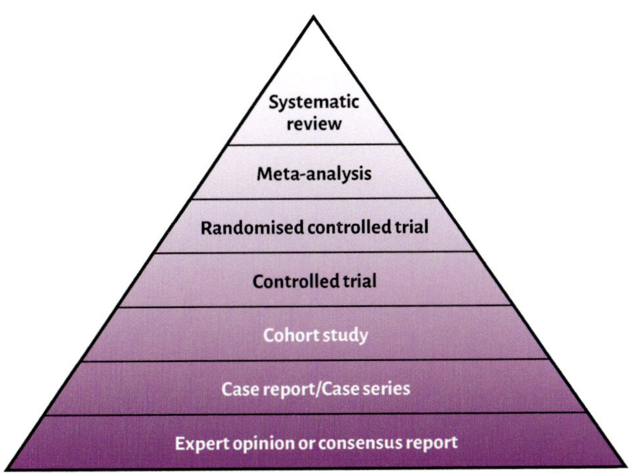

Figure 108. The evidence-based medicine pyramid which shows the highest quality, strongest evidence, which is available in the smallest quantities at the top of the pyramid, with increasing quantities of less rigorous evidence descending the pyramid.

Communication to the Client

The veterinary team should have a clear and effective means of communicating with clients. Nonspecific practice information including names of staff may be shared on uniforms, name badges, posters and display boards and use of websites. The practice should have defined protocols and staff training for dealing with members of the public.

Any electronic marketing communications presented or sent to the client must comply with local legal restrictions on use of personal data.

Specific patient care instructions should be provided to the client in writing where appropriate, in the form of discharge notes and legally compliant labelling of medications.

Receiving Communication from the Client

The practice should have a means to receive and monitor feedback from clients in place, including having a transparent procedure for complaints.

All complaints received and the responses made should be recorded and documented. Complaints should be audited and reviewed by the relevant members of the veterinary team and management in order to analyse the cause of the complaint, whether this be based on clinical grounds or communication thereof. Complaints are considered personal data and this information should be handled in accordance with local laws.

Bibliography

- Adams R.J., Doyle, R.S., Bray, J.P., Burton, C.A. (2014) Closed Suction Drainage for Treatment of Septic Peritonitis of Confirmed Gastrointestinal Origin in 20 Dogs. *Veterinary Surgery.* 43(7), 843–51.
- Burgess, B.A. (2018) Prevention and surveillance of surgical infections: A review. *Veterinary Surgery.* 48(3), 284–90.
- Garcia Stickney, D.N., Thieman Mankin, K.M. (2017) The impact of post-discharge surveillance on surgical site infection diagnosis. *Veterinary Surgery.* 3rd ed. 44(1), 2–8.
- Kieves, N.R., Bergh, M.S., Zellner, E., Wang, C. (2016) Pilot study measuring the effects of bandaging and cold compression therapy following tibial plateau levelling osteotomy. *Journal of Small Animal Practice.* 57(10), 543–7.
- Matiasovic, M., Halfacree, Z.J., Moores, A., Nelissen, P., Woods, S., Dean, B., Chanoit, G., Barnes, D.C. (2017) Surgical management of impalement injuries to the trunk of dogs: a multicentre retrospective study. *Journal of Small Animal Practice.* 59(3), 139–46.
- Meeson, R.L, Davidson, C., Arthurs, G.I. (2011) Soft-tissue injuries associated with cast application for distal limb orthopaedic conditions. *Veterinary and Comparative Orthopaedics and Traumatology.* 24(2), 126–31.
- Silverstein, D.S., Otto, C.M. (2012) Sepsis. In Greene, C.E. (ed.) *Infectious diseases of the dog and cat,* 4th ed, St Louis, Elsevier.
- Wernerman, J. (2005) Guidelines for nutritional support in intensive care unit patients: a critical analysis. *Curr Opin Clin Nutr Metab Care.* 8(2), 171–5.

Test

Answers on Page 540

1. **Which of the following is not an appropriate method for taking intestinal biopsies?**
    a. Incisional biopsy.
    b. Endoscopic grab biopsy.
    c. Punch biopsy.
    d. Ultrasound-guided Tru-Cut® biopsy.

2. **What is the name of the following biopsy needle?**

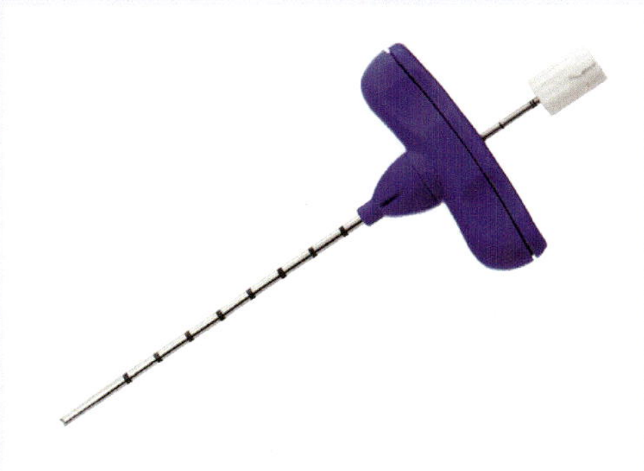

    a. Tru-Cut®.
    b. Jamshidi™.
    c. Veress.
    d. Ni-Ting.

3. **Which of the following dressing types aid haemostats in an open wound?**
    a. Alginate.
    b. Hydrogel.
    c. Hydrophilic polyurethane foam.
    d. Paraffin gauze.

4. **Which of the following is the name for a specific bandage used to immobilise the elbow following closed reduction of a luxated elbow?**
    a. Ehmer sling.
    b. Velpeau sling.
    c. Spica splint.
    d. Robert Jones.

5. **Which of the following is the strongest form of scientific evidence?**
    a. Systematic review.
    b. Controlled trial.
    c. Case series.
    d. Expert opinion.

6. **What should be done with very large histopathology samples to speed their fixation in formalin?**
    a. Only submit a small sample to the pathologist.
    b. Use a stronger concentration of formalin.
    c. Make deep slices into the tissue to allow penetration of the formalin.
    d. Inject formalin into the tissue.

7. **Which of these terms refers to a fracture which has healed at an inappropriate angle?**
    a. Non-union.
    b. Malunion.
    c. Delayed union.
    d. Retrograde union.

8. **Which of these properties of dressings best applies to paraffin gauze dressings (e.g. Jelonet™)?**
    a. Absorbent.
    b. Adhesive.
    c. Active.
    d. Permeable.

9. **Which feeding tube type would be most appropriate for a patient with a history of pancreatitis, undergoing removal of a large stomach tumour?**
    a. NO tube.
    b. O tube.
    c. NG tube.
    d. J tube or J through G tube.

10. **Which level of evidence should be considered to have the least weight when comparing treatment options for a patient?**
    a. The opinion of an expert.
    b. Systematic review/meta-analysis.
    c. Controlled trial.
    d. Case report.

Clinical Case 1

Bruno, a 7-year-old Parsons terrier underwent a cranial closing wedge osteotomy to surgically manage a right cranial cruciate ligament injury. His owner neglected to use the buster collar and Bruno chewed open the surgical site. Hence the appearance of the open wound when presented to you ten days after surgery. Bruno is reported to otherwise be in excellent general health. He was toe touching on the operated leg.

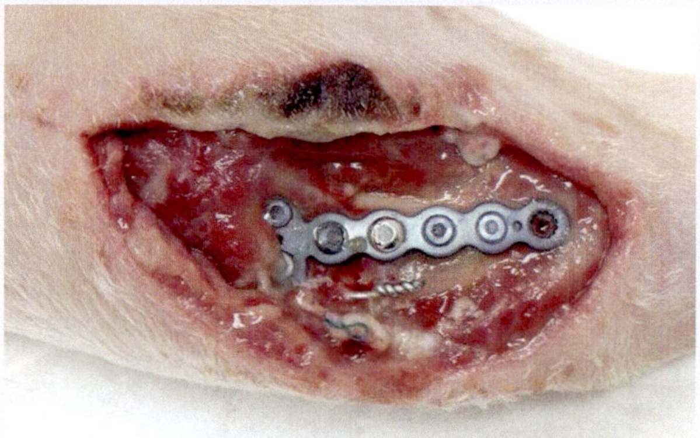

You prepare for the vet whilst they are gaining consent from the client for management of this wound.

1. What equipment do you prepare in anticipation of management of this wound?

Under sedation, radiographs are taken to assess the bone and implant integrity. The wound is swabbed with a bacteriology swab, then packed with water based lubricating gel and clipped, then cleaned around with dilute chlorhexidine solution. The wound itself is then surgically debrided, lavaged with sterile saline and then polyhexanide solution, before being packed with a wet to dry dressing, held in place by a tie-over dressing, anchored through sutures placed around the periphery.

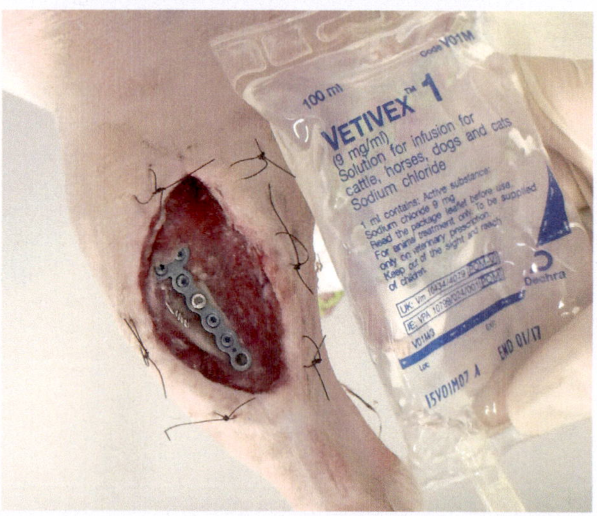

2. Other than the wet-to-dry dressing, which alternative debridement dressings could be placed into this wound initially to achieve further debridement?

3. Should this patient be treated with antibiotics at this stage? Explain your reasoning.

Culture of the wound yields a profuse growth of *Staphylococcus pseudointermedius* with sensitivity pattern as follows:

Amoxicillin	Resistant
Potentiated amoxicillin	Resistant
Cephalexin	Resistant
Doxycycline	Resistant
Tetracycline	Resistant
Enrofloxacin	Resistant
Marbofloxacin	Intermediate
Amikacin	Sensitive
Gentamicin	Sensitive
Chloramphenicol	Sensitive
Fucidic acid	Resistant

4. How might this infection be described?

The vet decides to prescribe marbofloxacin at a high dose due to the significant risk of acute kidney injury associated with the use of aminoglycosides (amikacin/gentamicin).

5. How does this infection affect your management of Bruno in the hospital?

Bruno was treated with intravenous antibiotics for three days and underwent daily dressing changes. When the wound discharge was then minimal, he returned to surgery (at the end of the day in a dirty procedures room) to undergo wound closure. He was discharged on a six-week course of antibiotics with a buster collar in place and made a full recovery. Bone healing was however delayed, and implant removal was required after five months, due to recurrent infection (likely as the result of biofilm formation on the surgical implants).

Reflective exercise: prophylactic use of antibiotics in your practice

- Make a list of the surgical procedures undertaken in your clinic this week or the last 10 surgical procedures you have been involved with.
- For each case, categorise the surgery as clean/clean-contaminated/contaminated/infected.
- On the basis of your classification, should the patient receive antibiotics at all/perioperatively/perioperatively and postoperatively?
- Was this the case for the cases you have been involved with? If not, consider what was the justification for their use in your specific case?

Clinical Case 2

Coco, a 5-year-old, neutered, male, domestic shorthaired cat was found hiding in a garden shed by his owner, Mrs Lambert, 4 days after going missing. The cat is severely dehydrated, pyretic (40.5 °C) and lethargic and has an open wound over the left scapula. When encouraged to move the cat is not bearing weight on its left forelimb.

An initial clipping of Coco's wound is performed but paused when the extent of the wound is appreciated.

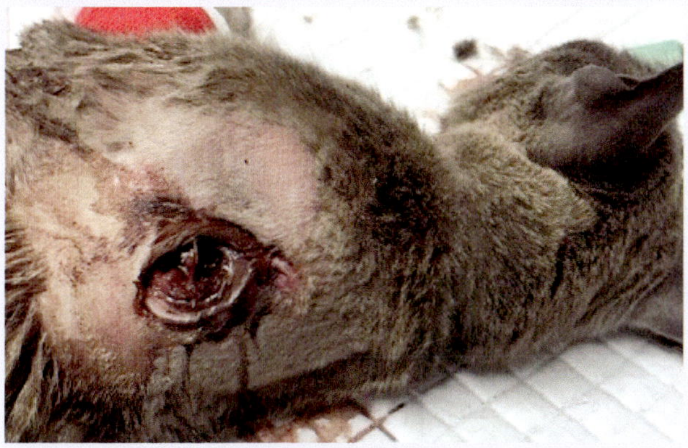

Following baseline blood tests, analgesia and starting fluid therapy the cat is anaesthetised for assessment of the wound. An X-ray is taken.

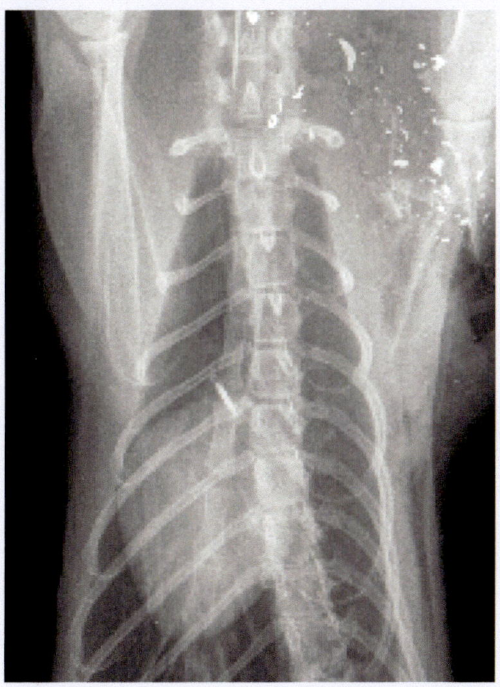

1. What can you see on the X-ray?

Closer inspection of the wound reveals that it is infested with maggots!

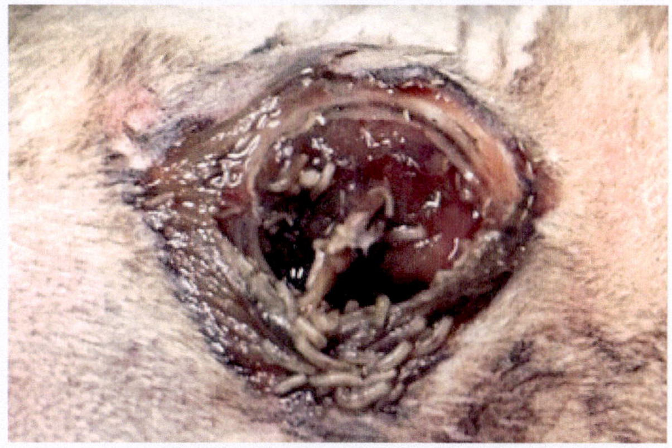

Coco then undergoes surgical preparation of the wound and surrounding skin.

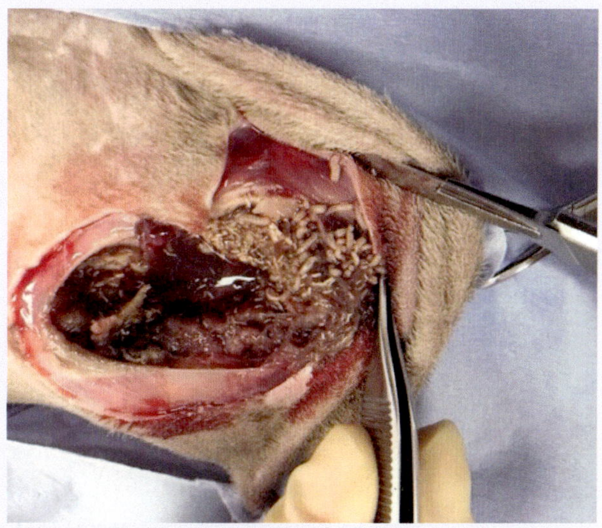

Surgical sharp debridement of the wound is performed, removing the devitalised and necrotic tissue and thoroughly lavaging the wound bed.

2. What solutions may be used to lavage the wound before debridement?

Tissue samples are also taken for bacteriology testing.

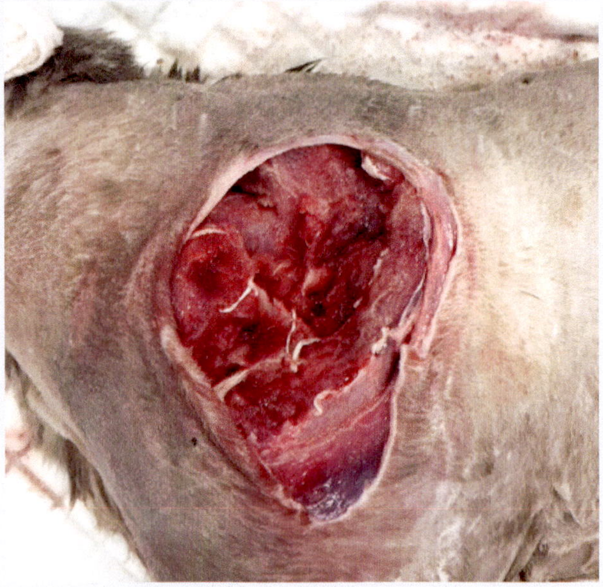

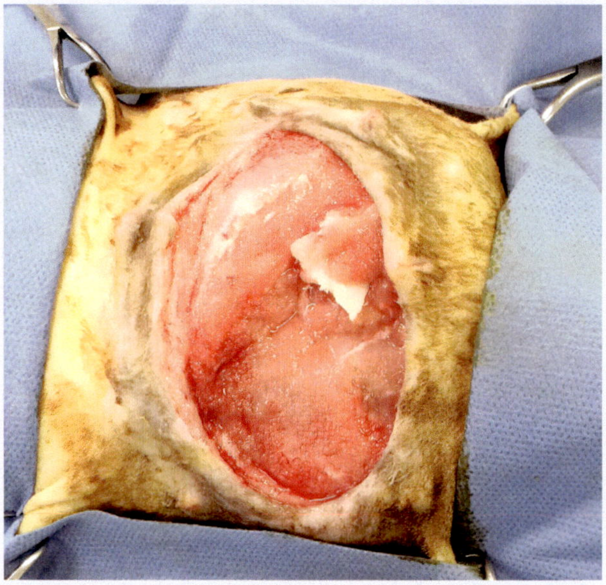

3. **What solutions may be used to lavage the wound after debridement?**

Following debridement, a negative pressure wound therapy dressing is placed over the wound.

4. **What are the potential benefits of negative pressure wound therapy?**

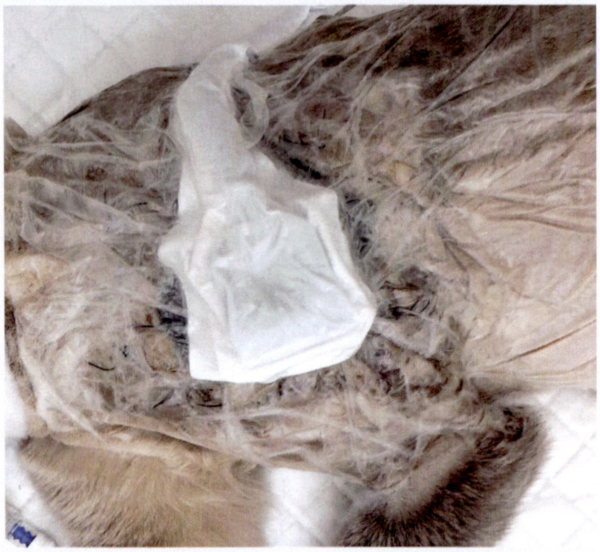

Four days later Coco's negative pressure dressing is removed, and the wound appears clean and has started to granulate.

Coco is now receiving appropriate antibiotics based on the culture results taken previously. The cat is also clinically in a better condition to undergo a surgery to now excise and close the wound, with a closed suction drain in place.

5. **What is the term used to describe wound closure after a period of open wound management?**

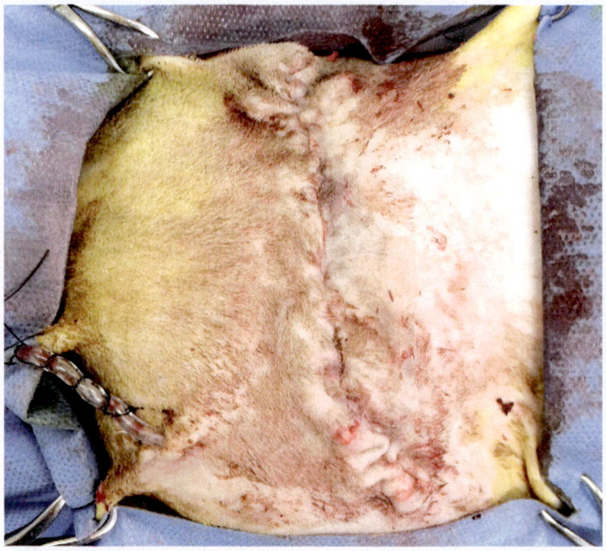

6. **What is the function of the closed suction drain?**

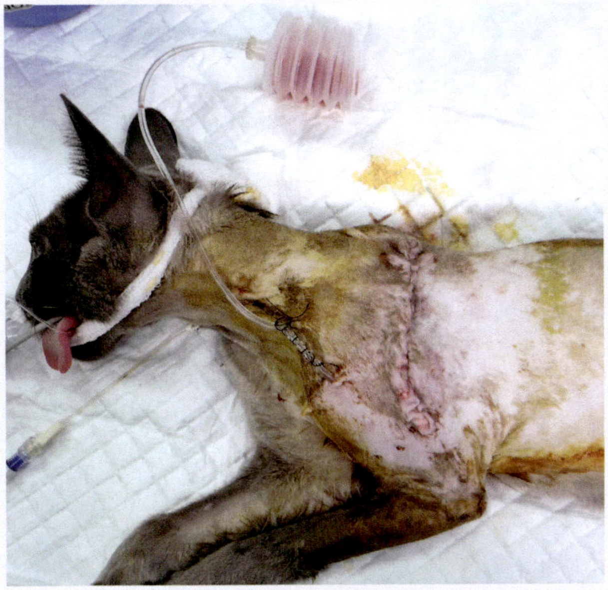

7. If Coco weighs 4 kg, at what stage would you consider removing the drain?

8. What other management measures might we consider in order to minimise fluid production within the wound following closure?

Coco was hospitalised for 3 days for analgesia and drain management. He was then discharged with 2 weeks of meloxicam and antibiotics and was cage rested for 6 weeks to allow his scapula fracture to heal. He made a full recovery.

Correct Answers:

Test

1. d
2. b
3. a
4. c
5. a
6. c
7. b
8. d
9. d
10. a

Clinical Case 1

1. **What equipment do you prepare in anticipation of management of this wound?**
    - Intravenous catheter.
    - Analgesia.
    - Sedation.
    - X-ray machine.
    - Water based lubricating gel to pack the wound.
    - Clean clippers.
    - Dilute chlorhexidine/povidone iodine /polyhexanide solution.
    - Bacteriology swab.
    - Basis surgical instrument pack.
    - Suture material.
    - Surgical gloves/gown/hats/face masks.
    - Bandage materials.

2. **Other than the wet-to-dry dressing, which alternative debridement dressings could be placed into this wound initially to achieve further debridement?**
    - Manuka honey.
    - Maggots.
    - Hydrogels.
    - Hydrocolloids.
    - Dermisol (debridement ointment).

3. **Should this patient be treated with antibiotics at this stage? Explain your reasoning.**
   Yes, broad spectrum first line antibiotics e.g. amoxicillin clavulanate.

   The open wound is likely infected, but if not is at risk of infection as it is not sealed with granulation tissue. The presence of exposed bone and an orthopaedic implant also increased the risk and the consequence of infection in this patient.

4. **How might this infection be described?**
   Multidrug-resistant (MDR) or Multidrug-resistant *Staphylococcus pseudointermedius* (MRSP).

5. **How does this infection affect your management of Bruno in the hospital?**
   Bruno requires isolation and barrier nursing wearing full PPE to prevent transmission of the superbug to other hospitalised patients. He will require bandage changes which should be performed at the end of the working day and in a dedicated area, which can be thoroughly deep cleaned afterwards.

Clinical Case 2

1. **What can you see on the X-ray?**
    - An open fracture of the left scapula.
    - Metallic debris from a gunshot injury in the surrounding tissue.
    - Subcutaneous gas accumulation over the left thoracic wall.

2. **What solutions may be used to lavage the wound before debridement?**
   Initially, the wound is so contaminated that any clean lavage solution may be used. Initially high volume of tap water may even be used, then rinsing with isotonic sterile saline or better Hartmann's/Lactate ringers solution. It would be wasteful to use antiseptic solutions on a highly contaminated wound at this stage.

3. **What solutions may be used to lavage the wound after debridement?**
   Further isotonic sterile saline or Hartmann's/Lactated ringers or even an antiseptic solution such as polyhexanide.

4. **What are the potential benefits of negative pressure wound therapy?**
    - To promote granulation tissue formation.
    - To provide ongoing drainage.
    - To allow further stabilisation of the patient, whilst minimising further anaesthetic episodes over the next few days.

5. **What is the term used to describe wound closure after a period of open wound management?**
   Delayed primary closure.

6. What is the function of the closed suction drain?

To remove fluid which forms within the wound, to prevent seroma formation and to minimise dead space.

7. If Coco weighs 4 kg, at what stage would you consider removing the drain?

Ideally the drain production would be down to less than 2 ml/kg/day, so 8 ml/day, although we might consider keeping the drain in for 48–72 hours minimum if drain production is initially low to promote adhesion of the skin to the underlying tissue if there is a large dead space; this will depend on the method of suture the wound closed.

8. What other management measures might we consider in order to minimise fluid production within the wound following closure?

- Warm compression of the wound for 10 minutes 3–4 times daily for 10 days following surgery.
- Minimise activity of the patient, by enforcing cage rest.

Notes

Notes